CURRENT
SURGICAL THERAPY - 2

Current Therapy Series

Bayless:
Current Therapy in Gastroenterology and
Liver Disease
Bayless, Brain, Cherniack:
Current Therapy in Internal Medicine
Brain, Carbone:
Current Therapy in Hematology–Oncology
Callaham:
Current Therapy in Emergency Medicine
Cameron:
Current Surgical Therapy
Cherniack:
Current Therapy of Respiratory Disease
Dubovsky, Shore:
Current Therapy in Psychiatry
Ernst, Stanley:
Current Therapy in Vascular Surgery
Foley, Payne:
Current Therapy of Pain
Fortuin:
Current Therapy in Cardiovascular Disease
Garcia:
Current Contraceptive Management
Garcia, Mastroianni, Amelar, Dubin:
Current Therapy of Infertility
Garcia, Mikuta, Rosenblum:
Current Therapy in Surgical Gynecology
Gates:
Current Therapy in Otolaryngology—
Head and Neck Surgery
Glassock:
Current Therapy in Nephrology and Hypertension
Grillo, Austen, Wilkins, Mathisen, Vlahakes:
Current Therapy in Cardiothoracic Surgery
Jeejeebhoy:
Current Therapy in Nutrition
Johnson:
Current Therapy in Neurologic Disease
Kass, Platt:
Current Therapy in Infectious Disease
Krieger, Bardin:
Current Therapy in Endocrinology and Metabolism
Lichtenstein, Fauci:
Current Therapy in Allergy, Immunology
and Rheumatology
Long:
Current Therapy in Neurologic Surgery
McGinty, Jackson:
Current Therapy in Orthopaedic Surgery
Nelson:
Current Therapy in Neonatal-Perinatal Medicine
Nelson:
Current Therapy in Pediatric Infectious Disease
Parrillo:
Current Therapy in Critical Care Medicine
Provost, Farmer:
Current Therapy in Dermatology
Resnick, Kursh:
Current Therapy in Genitourinary Surgery
Rogers:
Current Practice of Anesthesiology
Trunkey, Lewis:
Current Therapy of Trauma
Welsh, Shephard:
Current Therapy in Sports Medicine

CURRENT
SURGICAL THERAPY – 2

JOHN L. CAMERON, M.D., F.A.C.S.

Warfield M. Firor Professor and Chairman
Department of Surgery
The Johns Hopkins University
School of Medicine

Chief of Surgery
The Johns Hopkins Hospital
Baltimore, Maryland

1986

B.C. DECKER INC • Toronto • Philadelphia
The C.V. MOSBY COMPANY • Saint Louis • Toronto • London

Publisher   **B.C. Decker Inc.**
3228 South Service Road
Burlington, Ontario   L7N 3H8

B.C. Decker Inc.
P.O. Box 30246
Phildelphia, Pennsylvania   19103

Sales and Distribution

United States
and Possessions   **The C.V. Mosby Company**
11830 Westline Industrial Drive
Saint Louis, Missouri   63146

Canada   **The C.V. Mosby Company, Ltd.**
5240 Finch Avenue East, Unit No. 1
Scarborough, Ontario   M1S 4P2

United Kingdom, Europe   **Blackwell Scientific Publications, Ltd.**
and the Middle East   Osney Mead, Oxford OX2 OEL, England

Australia   **Holt-Saunders Pty. Limited**
9 Waltham Street
Artarmon, N.S.W. 2064
Australia

Japan   **Igaku-Shoin Ltd.**
Tokyo International P.O. Box 5063
1-28-36 Hongo, Bunkyo-ku, Tokyo 113, Japan

Asia   **Holt-Saunders Asia Limited**
10/F, Inter-Continental Plaza
Tsim Sha Tsui East
Kowloon, Hong Kong

Current Surgical Therapy   ISBN 0–941158–70–5

Library of Congress catalog card number: 85-072316

10   9   8   7   6   5   4   3   2   1

CONTRIBUTORS

HERAND ABCARIAN, M.D., F.A.C.S.

Professor of Surgery, University of Illinois College of Medicine; Chairman, Section of Colon and Rectal Surgery, Cook County Hospital, Chicago, Illinois

Anal Stricture (Stenosis)

MARTIN D. ABELOFF, M.D.

Associate Professor of Oncology and Medicine, The Johns Hopkins University School of Medicine; Chief of Medical Oncology, The Johns Hopkins Hospital Oncology Center, Baltimore, Maryland

Disseminated Breast Cancer

MARTIN A. ADSON, M.D.

Professor of Surgery, Mayo Medical School; Consultant, Department of Surgery, Mayo Clinic, Rochester, Minnesota

Colorectal Cancer Metastatic to the Liver: Resection

JOHN ALEXANDER-WILLIAMS, Ch.M., M.D., F.R.C.S., F.A.C.S.

Honorary Clinical Senior Lecturer, University of Birmingham; Consultant Surgeon and Chairman, Gastroenterology Group, The General Hospital, Birmingham, England

Remedial Operation for Postgastrectomy and Postvagotomy Syndromes

MARIA ALLO, M.D.

Assistant Professor of Surgery, The Johns Hopkins University School of Medicine; Surgeon-in-Chief (Acting), Division of Surgical Endocrinology and Oncology, Medical Director, Surgical Intensive Care Unit, The Johns Hopkins Hospital, Baltimore, Maryland

Nontoxic Goiter

RUDOLPH ALMARAZ, M.D., Ph.D.

Assistant Professor of Surgery and Oncology, The Johns Hopkins University School of Medicine; Surgeon-in-Charge, Surgical Oncology and Endocrinology, The Johns Hopkins Hospital, Baltimore, Maryland

Breast Cancer: Stage I and II

JOHN R. ANDERSON, M.B., Ch.B., B.Sc., F.R.C.S.

Senior Lecturer, Department of Surgery, University of Glasgow Faculty of Medicine; Consultant Surgeon, The Royal Infirmary, Glasgow, Scotland

Volvulus of the Colon

ARTHUR H. AUFSES, Jr., M.D.

Franz W. Sichel Professor of Surgery and Chairman, Department of Surgery, Mount Sinai School of Medicine of the City University of New York; Director, Department of Surgery and Surgeon-in-Chief, The Mount Sinai Hospital, New York, New York

Granulomatous Colitis

J. BRADLEY AUST, M.D., Ph.D.

Professor of Surgery and Chairman, Department of Surgery, University of Texas Medical School at San Antonio; Chief of Surgery, Medical Center Hospital, San Antonio, Texas

Skin Tumor

R. ROBINSON BAKER, M.D.

Professor of Surgery and Oncology, The Johns Hopkins University School of Medicine; Director, Thoracic Surgical Service and Director, Breast Clinic, The Johns Hopkins Hospital, Baltimore, Maryland

Thyroid Cancer

CHARLES M. BALCH, M.D., F.A.C.S.

Professor and Head, Division of Surgery, University of Texas Medical School at Houston; Head, Division of Surgery and Chairman, Department of General Surgery, M. D. Anderson Hospital and Tumor Institute, Houston, Texas

Melanoma

ROBERT W. BARNES, M.D.

Professor and Chairman, Department of Surgery, University of Arkansas College of Medicine; Attending Surgeon, McClellan Veterans Administration Hospital, Little Rock, Arkansas

Venous Thrombosis

ARTHUR E. BAUE, M.D.

Associate Dean for Clinical Affairs and Professor of Surgery, Saint Louis University School of Medicine, Saint Louis, Missouri

Shock

ROBERT W. BEART, Jr., M.D.

Associate Professor of Surgery, Mayo Medical School; Head, Section of Colon and Rectal Surgery, Mayo Clinic and Mayo Foundation, Rochester, Minnesota

Radiation Enteritis and Proctitis

WILLIAM R. BELL, M.D.

Professor of Medicine and Radiology, Department of Medicine, The Johns Hopkins University School of Medicine, Baltimore, Maryland

Abnormal Bleeding

JOHN J. BERGAN, M.D.

Magerstadt Professor of Surgery and Chief, Division of Vascular Surgery, Northwestern University Medical School; Attending Surgeon, Northwestern Memorial Hospital, Chicago, Illinois

Femoropopliteal Occlusive Disease

GAIL E. BESNER, M.D.

Clinical Fellow in Surgery, Harvard Medical School; Senior Resident in Surgery, Brigham and Women's Hospital, Boston, Massachusetts

Peripheral Arterial Embolus

HENRI BISMUTH, M.D.

Professor of Surgery, Université de Paris Sud, Orsay, France; Surgeon and Chairman, Department of Surgery, Hôpital Paul Brousse, (Villejuif) Paris, France
Bile Duct Tumor

GEORGE E. BLOCK, M.D., F.A.C.S.

Thomas D. Jones Professor of Surgery, University of Chicago Pritzker School of Medicine; Attending Surgeon and Section Head, General Surgery, University of Chicago Medical Center, Chicago, Illinois
Obstruction of the Large Bowel

LESLIE H. BLUMGART, B.D.S., M.D., F.R.C.S.

Professor of Surgery, Royal Postgraduate Medical School; Director, Department of Surgery, Hammersmith Hospital, London, England
Postcholecystectomy Syndrome

SCOTT J. BOLEY, M.D.

Professor of Surgery and Pediatrics, Albert Einstein College of Medicine of Yeshiva University; Chief of Pediatric Services, Hospital of the Albert Einstein College of Medicine (a division of Montefiore Medical Center), Bronx, New York
Mesenteric Ischemia

JOHN S. BOLTON, M.D.

Clinical Assistant Professor, Department of Surgery, Louisiana State University School of Medicine in New Orleans; Attending Surgeon, Ochsner Clinic and Alton Ochsner Medical Foundation, New Orleans, Louisiana
Colorectal Cancer Metastatic to the Liver: Infusion Chemotherapy

DAVID L. BOUWMAN, M.D., F.A.C.S.

Associate Professor, Department of Surgery, Wayne State University School of Medicine; Attending Surgeon, Harper-Grace Hospital and Detroit Receiving Hospital, Detroit, Michigan
Pancreatic Pseudocyst

JOHN C. BOWEN, M.D., F.A.C.S.

Associate Chairman and Director of Surgical Education, Ochsner Clinic and Alton Ochsner Medical Foundation, New Orleans, Louisiana
Colorectal Cancer Metastatic to the Liver: Infusion Chemotherapy

EDWARD L. BRADLEY III, M.D.

Piedmont Professor of Surgery, Emory University School of Medicine; Attending Surgeon, Emory University Hospital, Atlanta Veterans Administration Hospital, and Piedmont Hospital, Atlanta, Georgia
Pancreatic Abscess

CARL E. BREDENBERG, M.D.

Professor of Surgery and Vice Chairman, Department of Surgery, State University of New York Upstate Medical Center at Syracuse, Syracuse, New York
Adult Respiratory Distress Syndrome

GREGORY B. BULKLEY, M.D., F.A.C.S.

Associate Professor of Surgery; Director of Surgical Research, Active Staff, The Johns Hopkins University School of Medicine, Baltimore, Maryland
Small Bowel Obstruction
Mesenteric Vascular Occlusive Disease

JAMES F. BURDICK, M.D.

Associate Professor, Department of Surgery, The Johns Hopkins University School of Medicine; Surgeon and Director of the Transplant Service, The Johns Hopkins Hospital, Baltimore, Maryland
Abdominal Aortic Aneurysm

JOHN F. BURKE, M.D.

Helen Andrus Benedict Professor of Surgery, Harvard Medical School; Chief of Trauma Services, Massachusetts General Hospital, Boston, Massachusetts
Fluid and Nutritional Management of the Burn Patient

JOHN L. CAMERON, M.D., F.A.C.S.

Professor and Chairman, Department of Surgery, The Johns Hopkins University School of Medicine; Chief of Surgery, The Johns Hopkins Hospital, Baltimore, Maryland
Budd-Chiari Syndrome
Acute Cholangitis

C. JAMES CARRICO, M.D.

Chairman, Department of Surgery, University of Washington School of Medicine, Seattle, Washington
Abdominal Trauma

FRANK B. CERRA, M.D.

Professor of Surgery and Director of Critical Care, Nutrition, and Clinical Metabolism, University of Minnesota Medical School — Minneapolis; Staff Surgeon, University of Minnesota Hospitals and Clinics of the University of Minnesota Health Sciences Center and Saint Paul-Ramsey Hospital and Medical Center, Minneapolis, Minnesota
Clostridial Gas Gangrene of the Extremity

TZU-MING CHANG, M.D.

Assistant Professor of Surgery and Attending Surgeon, Tri-Service General Hospital, Taipei, Taiwan
Peptic Ulcer

LAURENCE Y. CHEUNG, M.D.

Professor of Surgery, Washington University School of Medicine, Saint Louis, Missouri
Benign Gastric Ulcer

GAYLORD L. CLARK, M.D.

Assistant Professor, The Johns Hopkins University School of Medicine; Attending Hand Surgeon, Union Memorial Hospital and Orthopaedic Attending Staff, The Johns Hopkins Hospital, Baltimore, Maryland
Infection of the Hand

ORLO H. CLARK, M.D.

Professor of Surgery, University of California, San Francisco, School of Medicine; Surgical Service, Veterans Administration Medical Center, San Francisco, California
Hyperparathyroidism

ISIDORE COHN, Jr., M.D., M.Sc.(Med), D.Sc.(Med)

Professor and Chairman, Department of Surgery, Louisiana State University School of Medicine in New Orleans; Surgeon-in-Chief, Louisiana State University Service at

Charity Hospital, New Orleans, Louisiana
Preoperative Bowel Preparation

MARVIN L. CORMAN, M.D.
Department of Colon and Rectal Surgery, Sansum Medical Clinic, Inc., Santa Barbara, California
Anal Incontinence

NATHAN P. COUCH, M.D.
Associate Professor of Surgery, Harvard Medical School; Surgeon, Department of Surgery, Brigham and Women's Hospital, Boston, Massachusetts
Extracranial Occlusive Cerebral Vascular Disease

E. STANLEY CRAWFORD, M.D.
Professor of Surgery, Baylor College of Medicine; Senior Attending Surgeon, The Methodist Hospital, Houston, Texas
Ruptured Abdominal Aortic Aneurysm

ROBERT D. CROOM III, M.D.
Associate Professor of Surgery, University of North Carolina at Chapel Hill School of Medicine, Chapel Hill, North Carolina
Primary Common Duct Stones

JOHN M. DALY, M.D., F.A.C.S.
Jonathan E. Rhoads Professor of Surgical Science and Chief, Division of Surgical Oncology, University of Pennsylvania School of Medicine, Philadelphia, Pennsylvania
Preoperative Nutritional Assessment

CHI V. DANG, M.D., Ph.D.
Fellow in Medicine, Department of Medicine, The Johns Hopkins University School of Medicine, Baltimore, Maryland
Abnormal Bleeding

RICHARD H. DEAN, M.D.
Professor of Surgery and Head, Division of Vascular Surgery, Department of Surgery, Vanderbilt University School of Medicine, Nashville, Tennessee
Renovascular Hypertension

THOMAS L. DENT, M.D.
Professor of Surgery, Temple University School of Medicine, Philadelphia, Pennsylvania; Chairman, Department of Surgery, Abington Memorial Hospital, Abington, Pennsylvania
Colorectal Polyposis

CLIFFORD W. DEVENEY, M.D.
Associate Professor, University of Pennsylvania School of Medicine, Visiting Professor, Medical College of Pennsylvania; Chief, Surgical Service, Philadelphia Veterans Administration Medical Center, Philadelphia, Pennsylvania
Zollinger-Ellison Syndrome

ALAN R. DIMICK, M.D.
Associate Professor of Surgery, University of Alabama School of Medicine; Director of the Burn Center, University of Alabama Hospitals, Birmingham, Alabama
Cold Injury

BROWN M. DOBYNS, M.D., Ph.D.
Emeritus Professor of Surgery, Case Western Reserve University School of Medicine; Associate Director, Department of Surgery, Cleveland Metropolitan General Hospital, Assistant Surgeon, University Hospitals, Associate Surgeon, Lutheran Hospital, and Visiting Surgeon, St. Lukes Hospital, Cleveland, Ohio
Hyperthyroidism

ARTHUR J. DONOVAN, M.D.
Professor and Chairman, Department of Surgery, University of Southern California School of Medicine; Director of Surgery, Los Angeles County–USC Medical Center, Los Angeles, California
Unusual Forms of Breast Cancer

WILLIAM R. DRUCKER, M.D., F.A.C.S, F.R.C.S.(C)
Professor and Chairman, Department of Surgery, University of Rochester School of Medicine and Dentistry; Surgeon-in-Chief, The Strong Memorial Hospital, Rochester, New York
Fluid and Electrolyte Therapy

DAVID L. DUDGEON, M.D.
Associate Professor, Departments of Surgery and Pediatrics, The Johns Hopkins University School of Medicine; Attending Surgeon and Deputy Director, Department of Pediatric Surgery, The Johns Hopkins Hospital, Baltimore, Maryland
Acute Appendicitis

FREDERIC E. ECKHAUSER, M.D.
Associate Professor of Surgery, University of Michigan Medical School; Chief, Division of Gastrointestinal Surgery, Section of General Surgery, University Hospitals, Ann Arbor, Michigan
Periampullary Cancer
Unusual Pancreatic Tumors

FREDERICK R. EILBER, M.D.
Professory of Surgery, Division of Surgical Oncology, University of California, Los Angeles, UCLA School of Medicine, Los Angeles, California
Soft Tissue Sarcoma of the Extremity

JEAN EMOND, M.D.
Research Fellow, Hepatobiliary Unit, Hôpital Paul Brousse, (Villejuif) Paris and Université de Paris Sud, Orsay, France; Recipient of Eleanor B. Pillsbury Fellowship, Department of Surgery, University of Illinois College of Medicine, Chicago, Illinois
Bile Duct Tumor

RAYMOND ENGLUND, M.D.
Fellow, Division of Vascular Surgery, Department of Surgery, Vanderbilt University School of Medicine, Nashville, Tennessee
Renovascular Hypertension

H. PAT EWING, M.D.
Cardiothoracic Surgeon, Surgery Clinic of Tupelo and Staff Thoracic Surgeon, North Mississippi Medical Center, Tupelo, Mississippi
Pneumothorax

VICTOR W. FAZIO, M.B., B.S., F.R.A.C.S., F.A.C.S.
  Chairman, Department of Colon and Rectal Surgery, The Cleveland Clinic Foundation, Cleveland, Ohio
Anal Cancer: Squamous Cell Cancer and Melanoma

MARK K. FERGUSON, M.D.
  Assistant Professor, Department of Surgery, University of Chicago Pritzker School of Medicine; Staff Physician, Section of Thoracic Surgery, University of Chicago Hospitals, Chicago, Illinois
Esophageal Tumor

CHARLES O. FINNE III, M.D.
  Clinical Instructor, Division of Colon and Rectal Surgery, University of Minnesota Medical School — Minneapolis, Minneapolis, Minnesota
Presacral Tumor and Cysts

JOSEF E. FISCHER, M.D., F.A.C.S.
  Christian R. Holmes Professor and Chairman, Department of Surgery, University of Cincinnati College of Medicine, Cincinnati, Ohio
Enterocutaneous Fistulas

RONALD H. FISHBEIN, M.D.
  Associate Professor of Surgery, The Johns Hopkins University School of Medicine, Baltimore, Maryland
Anal Fissure, Anorectal Abscess, and Fistula-in-Ano

DONALD E. FRY, M.D., F.A.C.S.
  Professor of Surgery, Case Western Reserve University School of Medicine; Chief, Surgical Service, Cleveland Veterans Administration Hospital, Cleveland, Ohio
Tumor, Cysts, and Abscesses of the Spleen

HAROLD V. GASKILL III, M.D.
  Assistant Professor of Surgery, University of Texas Medical School at San Antonio; Attending Physician, Medical Center Hospital, San Antonio, Texas
Skin Tumor

HUGH GATELY, M.D.
  Cardiovascular Fellow, Baylor College of Medicine and The Methodist Hospital, Houston, Texas
Ruptured Abdominal Aortic Aneurysm

WILLIAM A. GAY, Jr., M.D.
  Professor and Chairman, Department of Surgery, University of Utah School of Medicine, Salt Lake City, Utah
Tumor of the Chest Wall

ALFRED S. GERVIN, M.D., F.A.C.S.
  Associate Professor of Surgery, Director of Emergency Medical Services, and Director of Trauma Service, Virginia Commonwealth University Medical College of Virginia School of Medicine, Richmond, Virginia
Retroperitoneal Injury

ARMANDO E. GIULIANO, M.D.
  Associate Professor of Surgery, Division of Surgical Oncology, University of California, Los Angeles, UCLA School of Medicine, Los Angeles, California
Fibrocystic Disease of the Breast
Soft Tissue Sarcoma of the Extremity

HERBERT E. GLADEN, M.D.
  Assistant Professor of Surgery, The Johns Hopkins University School of Medicine; Assistant Chief, Surgical Service, Veterans Administration Hospital, Baltimore, Maryland
Short Bowel Syndrome

STANLEY M. GOLDBERG, M.D., F.A.C.S.
  Clinical Professor of Surgery and Director, Division of Colon and Rectal Surgery, Department of Surgery, University of Minnesota Medical School — Minneapolis, Minneapolis, Minnesota
Hemorrhoids

JERRY GOLDSTONE, M.D.
  Professor of Surgery, University of California, San Francisco, School of Medicine, San Francisco, California
Occlusive Disease of the Upper Extremity

RICHARD D. GOODENOUGH, M.D.
  Instructor in Surgery and Fellow in Vascular Surgery, University of Rochester School of Medicine and Dentistry, Rochester, New York
Postoperative Intra-abdominal Infection

HERBERT B. GREENLEE, M.D.
  Professor and Vice Chairman, Department of Surgery, Loyola University of Chicago Stritch School of Medicine, Maywood, Illinois; Chief, Surgical Service, Veterans Administration Hospital, Hines, Illinois
Ascites

WARD O. GRIFFEN, Jr., M.D., Ph.D.
  Professor, Temple University School of Medicine; Executive Director/Secretary-Treasurer, American Board of Surgery, Philadelphia, Pennsylvania
Lumbar, Obturator, and Spigelian Hernias

JACOB C. HANDELSMAN, M.D.
  Associate Professor of Surgery, The Johns Hopkins University School of Medicine, Baltimore, Maryland
Chronic Ulcerative Colitis

JAMES D. HARDY, M.D.
  Professor and Chairman, Department of Surgery, University of Mississippi School of Medicine; Surgeon-in-Chief, University Hospital — University of Mississippi Medical Center, Jackson, Mississippi
Adrenal Cortex

STEVEN G. HARPER, M.D.
  Resident in Surgery, Abington, Memorial Hospital, Abington, Pennsylvania
Colorectal Polyposis

J. MICHAEL HENDERSON, M.B., Ch.B., F.R.C.S., F.A.C.S.
  Associate Professor of Surgery and Assistant Director of Clinical Research Facility, Emory University School of Medicine, Atlanta, Georgia
Portal Hypertension

ROBERT E. HERMANN, M.D.
  Clinical Professor of Surgery, Case Western Reserve University School of Medicine; Chairman, Department of General Surgery, The Cleveland Clinic Foundation,

Cleveland, Ohio
Acute and Chronic Cholecystitis

VIRGINIA M. HERRMANN, M.D.

Assistant Professor, Department of Surgery, Saint Louis University School of Medicine, Saint Louis, Missouri
Ischemic Colitis

ROBERT W. HOBSON II, M.D.

Professor and Vice Chairman, Department of Surgery, and Chief, Section of Vascular Surgery, University of Medicine and Dentistry of New Jersey, New Jersey Medical School, Newark, New Jersey
Intra-arterial Injections and Infusions

W. JOHN B. HODGSON, M.D., M.S., F.R.C.S., F.A.C.S.

Associate Professor, Department of Surgery, New York Medical College; Chief, Gastrointestinal Surgery, Westchester County Medical Center, Valhalla, New York, and Consultant, Veterans Administration Medical Center, Bronx, New York
Pilonidal Sinus and Cyst

JAMES W. HOLCROFT, M.D.

Professor, Department of Surgery, University of California, Davis, School of Medicine, Davis, California
Small and Large Bowel Injury

HERBERT C. HOOVER, Jr., M.D.

Associate Professor of Surgery and Chief, Division of Surgical Oncology, State University of New York at Stony Brook, Stony Brook, New York
Rectal Prolapse

LOREN J. HUMPHREY, M.D., Ph.D.

Clinical Professor of Surgery, University of Missouri — Kansas City School of Medicine; Chief, Surgical Oncology, Truman Medical Center–West, Kansas City, Missouri
Lobular Carcinoma In Situ

ANTHONY L. IMBEMBO, M.D.

Professor and Vice Chairman, Department of Surgery, Case Western Reserve University School of Medicine; Director, Department of Surgery, Cleveland Metropolitan General Hospital, Cleveland, Ohio
Gastric Restrictive Procedure for Morbid Obesity

SHUNZABURO IWATSUKI, M.D.

Associate Professor of Surgery, University of Pittsburgh School of Medicine; Attending Surgeon, Veterans Administration Hospitals, Presbyterian-University Hospital, and Children's Hospital of Pittsburgh, Pittsburgh, Pennsylvania
Liver Tumor

MARTIN D. JENDRISAK, M.D.

Instructor in Surgery, Department of Surgery, Washington University School of Medicine; Instructor, Department of Surgery, Division of General Surgery, Barnes Hospital, Saint Louis, Missouri
Recurrent and Persistent Primary Hyperparathyroidism

STEPHEN N. JOFFE, M.B., B.Ch., M.D., F.R.C.S., F.A.C.S.

Professor of Surgery, University of Cincinnati College of Medicine, Cincinnati, Ohio
Pancreatic Islet Cell Tumor

CRAIG A. JOHANSON, M.D.

Associate Clinical Professor of Medicine, University of California, San Francisco, School of Medicine, San Francisco, California
Endoscopic Sclerotherapy for Esophageal Varices

RENNER M. JOHNSTON, M.D.

Clinical Associate Professor, Department of Orthopaedics, University of Minnesota Medical School — Minneapolis; Chairman, Department of Orthopaedics, Park Nicollet Medical Center, Minneapolis, Minnesota
Open Treatment of Pelvic Fractures

IAN T. JONES, M.B., B.S., F.R.A.C.S., F.R.C.S.

Clinical Associate, Department of Colon and Rectal Surgery, The Cleveland Clinic Foundation, Cleveland, Ohio
Anal Cancer: Squamous Cell Cancer and Melanoma

R. SCOTT JONES, M.D.

Stephen H. Watts Professor and Chairman, Department of Surgery, University of Virginia School of Medicine; Surgeon-in-Chief, University of Virginia Medical Center, Charlottesville, Virginia
Liver Cysts

GEORGE L. JORDAN, Jr., M.D., M.S.(Surg)

Distinguished Service Professor of Surgery, Baylor College of Medicine; Chief of Staff, Harris County Hospital District Neighborhood Clinics, Attending in Surgery, The Methodist Hospital, and Consultant in Surgery, The Veterans Administration Medical Center, St. Lukes Episcopal Hospital, and Texas Children's Hospital, Houston, Texas
Pancreatic and Duodenal Injury

DONALD L. KAMINSKI, M.D.

Professor of Surgery, Saint Louis University School of Medicine, Saint Louis, Missouri
Ischemic Colitis

ROGER G. KEITH, M.D., F.R.C.S.(C), F.R.C.S., F.A.C.S.

Associate Professor of Surgery, University of Toronto Faculty of Medicine; Department of Surgery, St. Michael's Hospital, Toronto, Ontario, Canada
Chronic Pancreatitis

JOHN M. KELLUM, M.D.

Professor, Department of Surgery, Virginia Commonwealth University Medical College of Virginia School of Medicine; Surgeon, Department of Surgery, Medical College of Virginia Hospitals, Richmond, Virginia
Small Bowel Diverticular Disease

MARVIN M. KIRSH, M.D.

Professor of Surgery, Section of Thoracic Surgery, University of Michigan Medical School, Ann Arbor, Michigan
Acute Caustic Burn of the Esophagus

WALTER LAWRENCE, Jr., M.D.

Professor and Chairman, Division of Surgical Oncology and Director, Massey Cancer Center, Virginia Commonwealth University Medical College of Virginia School of Medicine, Richmond, Virginia
Gastric Tumor

HAROLD H. LINDNER, A.B., M.D., F.A.C.S.
Clinical Professor of Surgery and Topographic Anatomy, University of California, San Francisco, School of Medicine, San Francisco, California
Epigastric, Umbilical, and Ventral Hernias

ALEX G. LITTLE, M.D.
Associate Professor, University of Chicago Pritzker School of Medicine; Chief, Section of Thoracic Surgery, University of Chicago Medical Center, Chicago, Illinois
Esophageal Motility Disorder

PAUL LoGERFO, M.D.
Professor of Surgery, Columbia University College of Physicians and Surgeons, New York, New York
Thyroiditis

CHARLES E. LUCAS, M.D.
Professor of Surgery, Wayne State University School of Medicine, Detroit, Michigan
Liver Injury

GREGORY LUNA, M.D.
Instructor, Department of Surgery, University of Washington School of Medicine, Seattle, Washington
Abdominal Trauma

JOHN A. MANNICK, M.D.
Moseley Professor of Surgery, Harvard Medical School; Surgeon-in-Chief, Department of Surgery, Brigham and Women's Hospital, Boston, Massachusetts
Extracranial Occlusive Cerebral Vascular Disease

ARLIE R. MANSBERGER, Jr., M.D.
Professor and Chairman, Department of Surgery, Medical College of Georgia School of Medicine; Chief of Surgery, Medical College of Georgia Hospital and Clinics, and Chief Surgical Consultant, Veterans Administration Medical Center, Augusta, Georgia
Acute Renal Failure

VITO MANTESE, M.D.
Resident in Surgery, Saint Louis University Medical Center, Saint Louis, Missouri
Pulmonary Thromboembolism

JACQUELINE McCLARAN, B.S., M.D., C.C.F.P.
Assistant Professor of Family Medicine, McGill University Faculty of Medicine; Acting Director, McGill Centre for Studies in Age and Aging, Montreal, Quebec, Canada
Preoperative Assessment of the Elderly Patient

AMANDA M. METCALF, M.D.
Fellow, Gastroenterology Unit, Mayo Clinic and Mayo Foundation, Rochester, Minnesota
Radiation Enteritis and Proctitis

FABRIZIO MICHELASSI, M.D.
Assistant Professor of Surgery, University of Chicago Pritzker School of Medicine; Attending Surgeon, University of Chicago Medical Center, Chicago, Illinois
Obstruction of the Large Bowel

DAVID O. MOORE, M.D.
Assistant Instructor, Department of Surgery, University of Mississippi School of Medicine; Chief Resident, General Surgery, Department of Surgery, University of Mississippi Medical Center, Jackson, Mississippi
Adrenal Cortex

JON F. MORAN, M.D.
Associate Professor and Chairman, Department of Thoracic and Cardiovascular Surgery, University of Kansas Medical Center School of Medicine, Kansas City, Kansas
Paraesophageal Hernia

ANDREW M. MUNSTER, M.D., F.R.C.S, F.A.C.S.
Associate Professor of Surgery and Plastic Surgery, The Johns Hopkins University School of Medicine; Director, Baltimore Regional Burn Center, Baltimore, Maryland
Burn Wound

GORDON F. MURRAY, M.D.
Professor and Chief, Division of Cardiothoracic Surgery, West Virginia University School of Medicine, Morgantown, West Virginia
Tracheal Stenosis

GEORGE L. NARDI, M.D.
Professor of Surgery, Harvard Medical School; Visiting Surgeon, Massachusetts General Hospital, Boston, Massachusetts
Gallstone Ileus

MOREYE NUSBAUM, M.D.
Professor of Surgery, University of Pennsylvania School of Medicine; Chief, Division of Gastrointestinal Surgery, The Graduate Hospital, Philadelphia, Pennsylvania
Tumor of the Small Bowel

LLOYD M. NYHUS, M.D., F.A.C.S.
Warren H. Cole Professor and Head, Department of Surgery, University of Illinois College of Medicine; Surgeon-in-Chief, University of Illinois Hospital, Chicago, Illinois
Groin Hernia

CHARLES S. O'MARA, M.D.
Clinical Instructor in Surgery, University of Mississippi School of Medicine, Jackson, Mississippi
Dead Foot

STANLEY E. ORDER, M.D., Sc.D.
Willard and Lillian Professor and Director, Radiation Oncology, The Johns Hopkins Hospital and Oncology Center, Baltimore, Maryland
Breast Cancer: Surgical Staging and Radiation Therapy

MARK B. ORRINGER, M.D.
Professor of Surgery and Head, Section of Thoracic Surgery, University of Michigan Medical School, Ann Arbor, Michigan
Esophageal Reflux

BRUCE J. PARDY, B.Med.Sc., Ch.M., F.R.C.S., F.R.A.C.S.
Consultant Surgeon, Department of Surgery, Newham General Hospital, London, England
Raynaud's Syndrome

EDWARD PASSARO, Jr., M.D.

    Professor of Surgery, University of California, Los Angeles, UCLA School of Medicine; Chief, Surgical Service, Veterans Administration Medical Center, Los Angeles, California

Peptic Ulcer

CARLOS A. PELLEGRINI, M.D.

    Associate Professor, University of California, San Francisco, School of Medicine; Attending Surgeon, Veterans Administration Medical Center, San Francisco, California

Postoperative Wound Infection

BRUCE A. PERLER, M.D.

    Assistant Professor of Surgery, The Johns Hopkins University School of Medicine; Director of the Vascular Laboratory and Clinics, Attending Vascular Surgeon, The Johns Hopkins Hospital, and Consultant in Vascular Surgery, Francis Scott Key Medical Center, Baltimore, Maryland

Buerger's Disease
Diabetic Foot

HENRY A. PITT, M.D.

    Associate Professor of Surgery, The Johns Hopkins University School of Medicine, Baltimore, Maryland

Liver Abscess

RAYMOND POLLAK, M.B., F.R.C.S.

    Assistant Professor, Department of Surgery, University of Illinois College of Medicine; Attending Surgeon, University of Illinois Hospitals and Clinics, Chicago, Illinois

Groin Hernia

RICHARD A. POMERANTZ, M.D.

    Senior Resident in General Surgery, University of Michigan Medical School, Ann Arbor, Michigan

Periampullary Cancer

JULIAN W. PROCTOR, M.D.

    Assistant Professor, Radiation Oncology, The Johns Hopkins University School of Medicine, Baltimore, Maryland

Breast Cancer: Surgical Staging and Radiation Therapy

TERENCE QUIGLEY, M.D.

    Clinical Instructor of Surgery, University of California, San Francisco, School of Medicine, San Francisco, California

Occlusive Disease of the Upper Extremity

SESHADRI RAJU, M.D.

    Professor of Surgery, University of Mississippi School of Medicine; Staff Surgeon, University Hospital and Director, Doppler Laboratory, University Medical Center, Jackson, Mississippi

Lower Extremity Varicosities

JOHN J. RICOTTA, M.D.

    Associate Professor of Surgery, University of Rochester School of Medicine and Dentistry; Associate Surgeon, Strong Memorial Hospital, Rochester, New York

Tibioperoneal Arterial Occlusive Disease

LAYTON F. RIKKERS, M.D.

    Professor and Chairman, Department of Surgery, University of Nebraska College of Medicine, Omaha, Nebraska

Hepatic Encephalopathy

DAVID B. ROOS, M.D.

    Clinical Professor of Surgery, University of Colorado School of Medicine; Presbyterian Denver Hospital, Denver, Colorado

Thoracic Outlet Syndrome

JOEL ROSLYN, M.D.

    Assistant Professor, Division of General Surgery, University of California, Los Angeles, UCLA School of Medicine; Attending Surgeon, UCLA Medical Center, Los Angeles, California, and Staff Surgeon, Sepulveda Veterans Administration Medical Center, Sepulveda, California

Asymptomatic Cholecystitis

FRED W. RUSHTON, M.D., F.A.C.S.

    Clinical Assistant Professor, Department of Surgery, University of Mississippi School of Medicine, Jackson, Mississippi

Recurrent Inguinal Hernia

ROBB H. RUTLEDGE, M.D.

    Clinical Associate Professor of Surgery, University of Texas Southwestern Medical School at Dallas, Dallas, Texas; Staff Surgeon, Harris Hospital, Fort Worth, Texas

Antibiotic Selection in Biliary Tract Surgery

CHARLES R. SACHATELO, M.D.

    Professor of Surgery, University of Kentucky College of Medicine; Attending Physician, Department of Surgery, University of Kentucky Medical Center, Lexington, Kentucky

Penetrating Injury to the Neck

MICHAEL G. SARR, M.D.

    Assistant Professor, Department of Surgery, Mayo Medical School, Rochester, Minnesota

Barrett's Esophagus

ROBERT C. SAVAGE, M.D.

    Clinical Instructor in Surgery, Division of Plastic Surgery, Harvard Medical School, Boston, Massachusetts

Lymphedema of the Extremity

JOHN L. SAWYERS, M.D.

    John Clinton Foshee Distinguished Professor of Surgery and Chairman, Department of Surgery, Vanderbilt University School of Medicine, Nashville, Tennessee

Esophageal Perforation

SEYMOUR I. SCHWARTZ, M.D., F.A.C.S.

    Professor of Surgery, Department of Surgery, University of Rochester School of Medicine and Dentistry; Senior Surgeon, The Strong Memorial Hospital, Rochester, New York

Splenectomy for Hematologic Disorders

ROGER SHERMAN, M.D., F.A.C.S.

    Professor of Surgery, Emory University School of Medicine; Chief of Surgery, Grady Memorial Hospital, Atlanta, Georgia

Splenic Injury

MARIO SIMI, M.D.

    Associate Professor of Surgery, University of Rome, La Sapienza Medical School; Assistant Chief of Surgery, VIth Surgical Clinic, Umberto I Polyclinic, Rome, Italy

Crohn's Disease of the Small Bowel

JAMES V. SITZMANN, M.D., F.A.C.S.
Assistant Professor of Surgery, The Johns Hopkins University School of Medicine, Baltimore, Maryland
Intravenous Hyperalimentation in the Surgical Patient

DAVID B. SKINNER, M.D.
Professor and Chairman, Department of Surgery, University of Chicago Pritzker School of Medicine, Chicago, Illinois
Esophageal Tumor

KENNETH W. SMITH, M.D., F.A.C.S.
Clinical Instructor, Department of Surgery, University of Texas Medical School at Houston; Clinical Instructor, Department of Surgery, Baylor College of Medicine, Houston, Texas
Solitary Rectal Ulcer Syndrome

DAVID I. SOYBEL, M.D.
Research Fellow, Department of Surgery, Washington University School of Medicine, Saint Louis, Missouri
Benign Gastric Ulcer

VINCENZO SPERANZA, M.D., F.A.C.S.
Professor of Surgery, University of Rome, La Sapienza Medical School; Chief of Surgery, VIth Surgical Clinic, Umberto I Polyclinic, Rome, Italy
Crohn's Disease of the Small Bowel

BRUCE E. STABILE, M.D.
Associate Professor of Surgery, University of California, Los Angeles, UCLA School of Medicine; Assistant Chief, Surgical Service, Veterans Administration Medical Center, Los Angeles, California
Peptic Ulcer

THOMAS E. STARZL, M.D., Ph.D.
Professor of Surgery, University of Pittsburgh School of Medicine; Attending Surgeon, Veterans Administration Hospital, Presbyterian-University Hospital, and Children's Hospital of Pittsburgh, Pittsburgh, Pennsylvania
Liver Tumor

WILLIAM E. STRODEL, M.D.
Associate Professor of Surgery, University of Michigan Medical School; Director of Surgical Endoscopy, Division of Gastrointestinal Surgery, Section of General Surgery, University Hospital, Ann Arbor, Michigan
Unusual Pancreatic Tumors

PAUL H. SUGARBAKER, M.D.
Assistant Professor, Uniformed Services School of the Health Sciences; Head, Section of Colorectal Cancer Surgery Branch, National Cancer Institute, National Institute of Health, Bethesda, Maryland
Colorectal Tumor

CHOICHI SUGAWA, M.D.
Associate Professor, Department of Surgery, and Chief of Surgical Endoscopy Unit, Wayne State University School of Medicine, Detroit, Michigan
Mallory-Weiss Syndrome

PANAGIOTIS N. SYMBAS, M.D.
Professor of Surgery, Emory University School of Medicine, Atlanta, Georgia
Diverticulum of the Esophagus

COLIN G. THOMAS, Jr., M.D.
Professor of Surgery, Department of Surgery, University of North Carolina at Chapel Hill School of Medicine, Chapel Hill, North Carolina
Primary Common Duct Stones

JEREMY NOWELL THOMPSON, M.A., F.R.C.S.
Research Fellow, Royal Postgraduate Medical School; Honorary Senior Registrar, Hammersmith Hospital, London, England
Postcholecystectomy Syndrome

NICHOLAS L. TILNEY, M.D., F.A.C.S., F.R.C.S.
Professor of Surgery, Harvard Medical School; Surgeon, Brigham and Women's Hospital, Boston, Massachusetts
Peripheral Arterial Embolus

RONALD G. TOMPKINS, M.D., Sc.D.
Instructor in Surgery, Harvard Medical School; Assistant in Surgery, Massachusetts General Hospital, Boston, Massachusetts
Fluid and Nutritional Management of the Burn Patient

RONALD K. TOMPKINS, M.D., M.Sc., F.A.C.S.
Professor and Chief, Division of General Surgery, University of California, Los Angeles, UCLA School of Medicine; Attending Surgeon, UCLA Medical Center, Wadsworth Veterans Administration Medical Center, Los Angeles, California, and Sepulveda Veterans Administration Medical Center, Sepulveda, California; Honorary Staff, Cedars-Sinai Medical Center, Los Angeles, California
Asymptomatic Cholecystitis

L. WILLIAM TRAVERSO, M.D., F.A.C.S.
Assistant Clinical Professor of Surgery, Uniformed Services University of the Health Sciences, Bethesda, Maryland; Staff Surgeon, Departments of General, Vascular, and Thoracic Surgery, The Mason Clinic, Seattle, Washington
Biliary Cysts: Choledochal Cyst and Caroli's Disease

DONALD D. TRUNKEY, M.D.
Professor of Surgery, University of California, San Francisco, School of Medicine; Chief of Surgery, San Francisco General Hospital, San Francisco, California
Vascular Injury

JEREMIAH G. TURCOTTE, M.D.
Frederick A. Coller Professor of Surgery and Chairman, Department of Surgery, University of Michigan Medical School, Ann Arbor, Michigan
Periampullary Cancer
Unusual Pancreatic Tumors

KEVIN TURLEY, M.D.
Associate Professor, University of California, San Francisco, School of Medicine; Attending Surgeon, H. C. Moffitt Hospital, San Francisco, California
Hemothorax

MARSHALL M. URIST, M.D., F.A.C.S.
Associate Professor of Surgery and Chief, Division of Sur-

gical Oncology, University of Alabama School of Medicine at Birmingham, Birmingham, Alabama
Solitary Neck Mass

JON A. van Heerden, M.B., Ch.B., M.S.(Surg.), F.R.C.S.(C), F.A.C.S.
Professor of Surgery, Department of Surgery, Mayo Graduate School of Medicine, Rochester, Minnesota
Pheochromocytoma

MALCOLM C. VEIDENHEIMER, M.D., C.M., F.R.C.S.(C), F.A.C.S.
Lecturer on Surgery, Harvard Medical School; Chairman, Department of General Surgery and Chief, Section of Colon and Rectal Surgery, Lahey Clinic Foundation, Boston, Massachusetts
Diverticular Disease of the Colon

FRANK J. VEITH, M.D.
Professor of Surgery, Albert Einstein College of Medicine of Yeshiva University; Chief, Division of Vascular Surgery, Hospital of the Albert Einstein College of Medicine (a division of Montefiore Medical Center), Bronx, New York
Mesenteric Ischemia

FREDERICK W. WALKER, M.D.
Assistant Professor of Surgery, The Johns Hopkins University School of Medicine; Associate Surgeon-in-Chief, Sinai Hospital of Baltimore, Baltimore, Maryland
Thoracic Wall Trauma

WILLIAM A. WALKER, M.D.
Medical Fellow, Division of Colon and Rectal Surgery, Department of Surgery, University of Minnesota Medical School — Minneapolis, Minneapolis, Minnesota
Hemorrhoids

ALEXANDER J. WALT, M.B., Ch.B., F.R.C.S., F.R.C.S.(C), F.A.C.S.
Professor and Chairman, Department of Surgery, Wayne State University School of Medicine; Chief of Surgery, Harper-Grace Hospital, Detroit, Michigan
Pancreatic Ascites and Pancreatic Pleural Effusions

KENNETH W. WARREN, M.D., F.A.C.S.
Lecturer in Surgery Emeritus, Harvard Medical School; Surgeon, New England Baptist Hospital, Boston, Massachusetts
Common Duct Exploration
Sclerosing Cholangitis

W. DEAN WARREN, M.D., F.A.C.S.
Joseph B. Whitehead Professor of Surgery and Chairman, Department of Surgery, Emory University School of Medicine, Atlanta, Georgia
Portal Hypertension

ANDREW L. WARSHAW, M.D.
Associate Professor of Surgery, Harvard Medical School; Associate Visiting Surgeon, Massachusetts General Hospital, Boston, Massachusetts
Acute Pancreatitis

JOSEPH T. WATLINGTON, M.D.
Senior Fellow in Nephrology, Department of Medicine, Medical College of Georgia School of Medicine, Augusta, Georgia
Acute Renal Failure

LAWRENCE W. WAY, M.D.
Professor of Surgery, University of California, San Francisco, School of Medicine; Chief of Surgical Service, San Francisco Veterans Administration Medical Center, San Francisco, California
Biliary Stricture

DONALD W. WEAVER, M.D., F.A.C.S.
Associate Professor of Surgery, Wayne State University School of Medicine, Detroit, Michigan
Retained Common Duct Stones

SAMUEL A. WELLS, Jr., M.D.
Bixby Professor and Chairman, Department of Surgery, Washington University School of Medicine; Surgeon-in-Chief, Barnes Hospital, Saint Louis, Missouri
Recurrent and Persistent Primary Hyperparathyroidism

ANTHONY D. WHITTEMORE, M.D.
Assistant Professor of Surgery, Harvard Medical School; Surgeon, Department of Surgery, Brigham and Women's Hospital, Boston, Massachusetts
Extracranial Occlusive Cerebral Vascular Disease

G. MELVILLE WILLIAMS, M.D.
Professor of Surgery and Chief, Division of Transplantation and Vascular Surgery, The Johns Hopkins University School of Medicine, Baltimore, Maryland
Aortoiliac Occlusive Disease

WALTER G. WOLFE, M.D.
Professor of Surgery, Duke University School of Medicine, Durham, North Carolina
Pulmonary Thromboembolism

CREIGHTON B. WRIGHT, M.D.
Professor of Clinical Surgery, Department of Surgery, University of Cincinnati College of Medicine, Cincinnati, Ohio
Intra-arterial Injections and Infusions

JAMES S. T. YAO, M.D., Ph.D.
Professor of Surgery, Division of Vascular Surgery, Northwestern University Medical School; Attending Surgeon and Director, Blood Flow Laboratory, Northwestern Memorial Hospital, Chicago, Illinois
Femoral and Popliteal Aneurysms

ALBERT E. YELLIN, M.D., F.A.C.S.
Professor of Surgery, University of Southern California School of Medicine; Senior Attending Surgeon and Chief, Vascular Surgery, Los Angeles County — USC Medical Center, and Attending Surgeon, Hospital of the Good Samaritan and Kenneth Norris Cancer Center, Los Angeles, California
False Aneurysm and Arteriovenous Fistula

PREFACE

The first edition of *Current Surgical Therapy* received very favorable critical review. This, plus the warm response I have received personally from medical students, residents, and practicing surgeons concerning the value of the book, encouraged me to prepare a second edition. It could be argued that a two-year interval between editions is too short, that advances in surgical management do not occur with the rapidity to justify a revision of the book so soon. However, the present work is in truth a new volume and not a new edition; each of the 135 chapters included in the first edition is written by a different author. Thus, the combination of the two editions will provide the surgeon with a broader perspective for each disease or disorder.

The chapters are written in a personalized manner; each author deals with his or her topic, outlining a personal therapeutic regimen and operative technique. Generally, the reader will find one technique of management as practiced by a recognized expert, even though we acknowledge that controversy may exist and that more than one approach to treatment is acceptable.

This edition has expanded to include 181 authors and 148 chapters. New to this edition are solitary rectal ulcer syndrome, infusion chemotherapy of metastases to the liver, endoscopic sclerotherapy for esophageal varices, Budd-Chiari syndrome, biliary cysts, surgical staging and irradiation in breast cancer, pelvic fracture, presacral tumor and cyst, preoperative assessment of the elderly patient, acute renal failure, abnormal bleeding.

If detailed information concerning clinical presentation, diagnosis, and pathophysiology of surgical diseases is what you require, you should consult one of the several excellent textbooks of surgery. On the other hand, if you seek the most up-to-date, complete, and practical coverage of treatment of commonly encountered surgical diseases, then *Current Surgical Therapy - 2* should satisfy your need.

John L. Cameron
December, 1985

PREFACE TO THE FIRST EDITION

There are several excellent textbooks of surgery. Every surgeon has at least one and usually more. Often they are one, two, or even more editions old, and are only infrequently opened. They remain useful because of sections on clinical presentation, diagnosis, and pathophysiology. Many, however, devote only limited attention to treatment, and these sections rapidly become dated. In no surgical text that I know is surgical therapy the main thrust. Thus, for most practicing surgeons standard texts have limited usefulness. Staying current with surgical therapy has been difficult, requiring reading the current litearture, attending local, regional, and national surgical meetings, and participating in a variety of continuing medical education projects. These means of staying abreast of current surgical therapy can be inefficient, may be costly, and certainly are haphazard.

Current Surgical Therapy was conceived and has been designed to provide the general surgeon with a text focusing entirely on surgical management. Each of the 135 chapters covers a surgical disease seen with predictable frequency by general surgeons, and presents helpful, practical, up-to-date information on surgical management. Each author has been chosen not only for his or her national prominence in a field, but more importantly because he or she is actively involved in patient care. I believe the general surgeon now has a means to update his surgical treatment every two years with successive editions of *Current Surgical Therapy*, and can be assured that in no area has he fallen behind or missed an important new development. When an unfamiliar problem is referred to a surgeon, it is time consuming to search the current literature for new developments. This text will alleviate this burden by providing the current treatment regimen outlined by a prominent clinician. I believe this text will function as effectively for the surgeon as its medical counterpart has for the internist.

Initially, I was somewhat concerned that without illustrations it would be difficult to discuss surgical therapy. However, early in the project I found that operative procedures and technical tips could be described easily by experienced surgeons without figures and with no difficulty. Considerations of patient selection, timing of therapy, pre– and postoperative care, choice of suture material and instruments, adjuvant therapy, follow-up, and so on account for the success and skill of the experts who have written for us. I am very pleased with this book and am indebted to the many contributors for their outstanding efforts. My family, as always, paid a price for my efforts, and I am appreciative of their understanding. I also would like to thank the publisher, Brian Decker, for his ideas, encouragement, optimism, and endless patience. However, the greatest burden of this book fell, as everyone knows who has ever written or edited a word for publication, to my secretary, Cindy Tucciarella. To her I would like to offer my most special thanks.

John L. Cameron, M.D.
January, 1984

CONTENTS

THE ESOPHAGUS

Esophageal Perforation 1
John L. Sawyers

Esophageal Motility Disorder 3
Alex G. Little

Diverticulum of the Esophagus 6
Panagiotis N. Symbas

Esophageal Reflux 9
Mark B. Orringer

Barrett's Esophagus 14
Michael G. Sarr

Paraesophageal Hernia 16
Jon F. Moran

Acute Caustic Burn of the Esophagus . . . 19
Marvin M. Kirsh

Esophageal Tumor 22
Mark K. Ferguson
David B. Skinner

THE STOMACH

Benign Gastric Ulcer 27
Laurence Y. Cheung
David I. Soybel

Mallory-Weiss Syndrome 31
Choichi Sugawa

Gastric Tumor 34
Walter Lawrence, Jr.

Gastric Restrictive Procedure for
Morbid Obesity 39
Anthony L. Imbembo

Peptic Ulcer 43
Tzu-Ming Chang
Bruce E. Stabile
Edward Passaro, Jr.

Zollinger-Ellison Syndrome 46
Clifford W. Deveney

Remedial Operation for Postgastrectomy
and Postvagotomy Syndromes 49
John Alexander-Williams

SMALL BOWEL

Small Bowel Obstruction 57
Gregory B. Bulkley

Crohn's Disease of the Small Bowel 63
Vincenzo Speranza
Mario Simi

Tumor of the Small Bowel 69
Moreye Nusbaum

Small Bowel Diverticular Disease 72
John M. Kellum

Mesenteric Vascular Occlusive Disease . . 74
Gregory B. Bulkley

Enterocutaneous Fistula 81
Josef E. Fischer

Short Bowel Syndrome 84
Herbert E. Gladen

LARGE BOWEL

Diverticular Disease of the Colon 90
Malcolm C. Veidenheimer

Chronic Ulcerative Colitis 92
Jacob C. Handelsman

Granulomatous Colitis 95
Arthur H. Aufses, Jr.

Obstruction of the Large Bowel 97
Fabrizio Michelassi
George E. Block

Volvulus of the Colon 100
John R. Anderson

Rectal Prolapse 103
Herbert C. Hoover, Jr.

Solitary Rectal Ulcer Syndrome 105
Kenneth W. Smith

Radiation Enteritis and Proctitis 109
Amanda M. Metcalf
Robert W. Beart, Jr.

Ischemic Colitis 110
Donald L. Kaminski
Virginia M. Herrmann

Colorectal Polyposis 114
Thomas L. Dent
Steven G. Harper

Colorectal Tumor 118
Paul H. Sugarbaker

Anal Cancer: Squamous Cell Cancer
and Melanoma 124
Victor W. Fazio
Ian T. Jones

Preoperative Bowel Preparation 126
Isidore Cohn, Jr.

Acute Appendicitis 129
David L. Dudgeon

Hemorrhoids 132
William A. Walker
Stanley M. Goldberg

Anal Fissure, Anorectal Abscess,
and Fistula-in-Ano 137
Ronald H. Fishbein

Anal Stricture (Stenosis) 139
Herand Abcarian

Anal Incontinence 144
Marvin L. Corman

Pilonidal Sinus and Cyst 150
W. John B. Hodgson

THE LIVER

Liver Abscess 153
Henry A. Pitt

Liver Cysts 157
R. Scott Jones

Liver Tumor 160
Shunzaburo Iwatsuki
Thomas E. Starzl

Colorectal Cancer Metastatic to the
Liver: Resection 164
Martin A. Adson

Colorectal Cancer Metastatic to the
Liver: Infusion Chemotherapy 169
John C. Bowen
John S. Bolton

PORTAL HYPERTENSION

Portal Hypertension 176
W. Dean Warren
J. Michael Henderson

Endoscopic Sclerotherapy for
Esophageal Varices 180
Craig A. Johanson

Ascites 183
Herbert B. Greenlee

Hepatic Encephalopathy 187
Layton F. Rikkers

Budd-Chiari Syndrome 189
John L. Cameron

GALLBLADDER AND BILIARY TREE

Asymptomatic Cholecystitis 193
Joel Roslyn
Ronald K. Tompkins

Acute and Chronic Cholecystitis 195
Robert E. Hermann

Common Duct Exploration 198
Kenneth W. Warren

Retained Common Duct Stones 201
Donald W. Weaver

Primary Common Duct Stones 204
Colin G. Thomas, Jr.
Robert D. Croom III

Acute Cholangitis 208
John L. Cameron

Biliary Stricture 211
Lawrence W. Way

Postcholecystectomy Syndrome 212
Jeremy N. Thompson
Leslie H. Blumgart

Biliary Cysts: Choledochal Cyst
and Caroli's Disease 216
L. William Traverso

Gallstone Ileus 219
George L. Nardi

Sclerosing Cholangitis 220
Kenneth W. Warren

Bile Duct Tumor 223
Henri Bismuth
Jean Emond

Antibiotic Selection in Biliary Tract
Surgery 226
Robb H. Rutledge

THE PANCREAS

Acute Pancreatitis 232
Andrew L. Warshaw

Pancreatic Abscess 235
Edward L. Bradley III

Pancreatic Pseudocyst 238
David L. Bouwman

Pancreatic Ascites and Pancreatic
Pleural Effusions 241
Alexander J. Walt

Chronic Pancreatitis 245
Roger G. Keith

Periampullary Cancer 249
Frederic E. Eckhauser
Richard A. Pomerantz
Jeremiah G. Turcotte

Unusual Pancreatic Tumors 256
Jeremiah G. Turcotte
Frederic E. Eckhauser
William E. Strodel

Pancreatic Islet Cell Tumor 258
Stephen N. Joffe

THE SPLEEN

Splenectomy for Hematologic
Disorders 263
Seymour I. Schwartz

Tumors, Cysts, and Abscesses
of the Spleen 265
Donald E. Fry

Hernia

Groin Hernia 268
Raymond Pollak
Lloyd M. Nyhus

Recurrent Inguinal Hernia 271
Fred W. Rushton

Epigastric, Umbilical, and
Ventral Hernias 274
Harold H. Lindner

Lumbar, Obturator, and
Spigelian Hernias 278
Ward O. Griffen, Jr.

Endocrine Glands

Adrenal Cortex 281
David O. Moore
James D. Hardy

Pheochromocytoma 288
Jon A. van Heerden

Nontoxic Goiter 291
Maria Allo

Thyroid Cancer 295
R. Robinson Baker

Hyperthyroidism 298
Brown M. Dobyns

Thyroiditis 303
Paul LoGerfo

Hyperparathyroidism 306
Orlo H. Clark

Recurrent and Persistent Primary
Hyperparathyroidism 310
Martin D. Jendrisak
Samuel A. Wells, Jr.

The Breast

Fibrocystic Disease of the Breast 315
Armando E. Giuliano

Breast Cancer: Stage I and II 317
Rudolph Almaraz

Breast Cancer: Surgical Staging and
Radiation Therapy 321
Julian W. Proctor
Stanley E. Order

Unusual Forms of Breast Cancer 324
Arthur J. Donovan

Lobular Carcinoma in Situ 326
Loren J. Humphrey

Disseminated Breast Cancer 329
Martin D. Abeloff

Chest Wall

Thoracic Wall Trauma 333
Frederick W. Walker

Tumor of the Chest Wall 336
William A. Gay, Jr.

Pneumothorax 339
H. Pat Ewing

Hemothorax 343
Kevin Turley

The Trachea

Tracheal Stenosis 345
Gordon F. Murray

Vascular System

Abdominal Aortic Aneurysm 349
James F. Burdick

Ruptured Abdominal Aortic Aneurysm .. 352
E. Stanely Crawford
Hugh Gately

Femoral and Popliteal Aneurysms 355
James S. T. Yao

False Aneurysm and Arteriovenous
Fistula 357
Albert E. Yellin

Extracranial Occlusive Cerebral
Vascular Disease 360
John A. Mannick
Anthony D. Whittemore
Nathan P. Couch

Aortoiliac Occlusive Disease 364
G. Melville Williams

Femoropopliteal Occlusive Disease 366
John J. Bergan

Tibioperoneal Arterial Occlusive
Disease 369
John J. Ricotta

Occlusive Disease of the Upper
Extremity 373
Terence Quigley
Jerry Goldstone

Dead Foot 376
Charles S. O'Mara

Peripheral Arterial Embolus 381
Gail E. Besner
Nicholas L. Tilney

Buerger's Disease 385
Bruce A. Perler

Intra-arterial Injections and Infusions 388
Robert W. Hobson II
Creighton B. Wright

Renovascular Hypertension 390
Raymond Englund
Richard H. Dean

Raynaud's Syndrome 392
Bruce J. Pardy

Thoracic Outlet Syndrome 395
David B. Roos

Mesenteric Ischemia 399
Frank J. Veith
Scott J. Boley

Diabetic Foot 405
Bruce A. Perler

Lower Extremity Varicosities 409
Seshadri Raju

Venous Thrombosis 412
Robert W. Barnes

Pulmonary Thromboembolism 421
Walter G. Wolfe
Vito Mantese

Lymphedema of the Extremity 423
Robert C. Savage

TRAUMA AND EMERGENCY CARE

Abdominal Trauma 427
Gregory Luna
C. James Carrico

Shock 433
Arthur E. Baue

Adult Respiratory Distress Syndrome 438
Carl E. Bredenberg

Liver Injury 442
Charles E. Lucas

Pancreatic and Duodenal Injury 444
George L. Jordan, Jr.

Small and Large Bowel Injury 448
James W. Holcroft

Splenic Injury 451
Roger Sherman

Retroperitoneal Injury 454
Alfred S. Gervin

Vascular Injury 458
Donald D. Trunkey

Burn Wound 460
Andrew M. Munster

Fluid and Nutritional Management
of the Burn Patient 466
Ronald G. Tompkins
John F. Burke

Penetrating Injury to the Neck 470
Charles R. Sachatello

Cold Injury 474
Alan R. Dimick

Pelvic Fracture 476
Renner M. Johnston

SKIN AND SOFT TISSUE

Skin Tumor 479
Harold V. Gaskill III
J. Bradley Aust

Presacral Tumor and Cysts 482
Charles O. Finne III

Melanoma 487
Charles M. Balch

Soft Tissue Sarcoma of the Extremity 492
Armando E. Giuliano
Frederick R. Eilber

Solitary Neck Mass 495
Marshall M. Urist

Infection of the Hand 498
Gaylord L. Clark

Clostridial Gas Gangrene
of the Extremity 501
Frank B. Cerra

PRE- AND POSTOPERATIVE CARE

Fluid and Electrolyte Therapy 504
William R. Drucker

Intravenous Hyperalimentation
in the Surgical Patient 512
James V. Sitzmann

Postoperative Wound Infection 518
Carlos A. Pellegrini

Preoperative Nutritional Assessment 522
John M. Daly

Preoperative Assessment of the
Elderly Patient 525
Jacqueline McClaran

Postoperative Intra-abdominal
Infection 532
Richard D. Goodenough

Acute Renal Failure 535
Arlie R. Mansberger, Jr.
Joseph T. Watlington

Abnormal Bleeding 543
Chi V. Dang
William R. Bell

THE ESOPHAGUS

ESOPHAGEAL PERFORATION

JOHN L. SAWYERS, M.D.

Esophageal perforation is an acute surgical emergency. It is considered the most serious and frequently the most rapidly lethal perforation of the intestinal tract. Contamination of the mediastinum with corrosive fluids, food matter, and bacteria may lead to cardio-respiratory embarrassment, shock, major fluid losses, and fulminating infection. However, with prompt, aggressive surgical treatment, survival should be expected in most patients.

ETIOLOGY

Iatrogenic injuries are the most common cause of esophageal perforation and are frequently due to endoscopy and bougienage. With the use of the fiberoptic endoscope, the incidence of endoscopy perforations has decreased. In 1976, Silvis reviewed 211,410 fiberoptic esophagogastroscopic procedures and found a perforation rate of 0.03 percent, the mortality rate following perforation being 4.3 percent. The cricopharyngeal region of the esophagus is the site most commonly perforated by endoscopy. The abdominal segment of the esophagus is the other area at highest risk. Hydrostatic or pneumatic dilators for achalasia have been a frequent cause of iatrogenic esophageal perforation.

External trauma from penetrating gunshot or knife wounds may injure the esophagus. The incidence of esophageal perforations from external trauma has been increasing in recent years, especially in hospitals with busy trauma services. A Gastrografin swallow examination usually demonstrates the site of the perforation. Blunt trauma to the neck more often injures the airway, but may avulse the esophagus from the pharynx.

Intraoperative injury to the esophagus may occur during operations around the esophagus. Such injuries have been reported during vagotomy operations, hiatal hernia repairs, and antireflux procedures (Nissen fundoplication). Immediate recognition of the injury, good exposure of the point of the perforation and primary suture repair should result in little morbidity. Unfortunately, many of these injuries are not recognized until late in the postoperative period or at postmortem examination.

Foreign bodies ingested by children and mentally disturbed patients may result in esophageal perforation. Straight pins or open safety pins, chicken bones, toothpicks, and artificial dentures have been the foreign bodies most commonly involved in esophageal perforations in our institution. Removal of the foreign body with operative repair of the esophageal perforation is the preferred method of management.

Ingestion of corrosive agents may result in a necrotizing esophagitis with perforation. Alkalis are the most common cause of this type of esophageal injury. Acids may pass through the esophagus so rapidly that severe necrosis and erosion occur in the stomach rather than the esophagus. Primary repair of esophageal perforations from caustic injuries is usually impossible. Esophageal exclusion procedures are more appropriate to handle these complicated problems, with later esophageal reconstruction using a colon bypass.

CLINICAL PRESENTATION

In a review of 110 patients sustaining esophageal perforation at the Vanderbilt University Medical Center, 27 patients had a cervical esophageal perforation, 63 had thoracic esophageal perforations, and 20 had abdominal esophageal perforations.

The signs and symptoms vary in relation to the location of esophageal perforation and are shown in Table 1. The triad of chest pain, fever, and crepitus, when present, should establish the diagnosis of thoracic

TABLE 1 Signs and Symptoms of Esophageal Perforation (% of Cases)

	Area of Perforation		
	Cervical (27)*	Thoracic (63)*	Abdominal (20)*
Neck pain	80	0	0
Chest pain	10	75	13
Abdominal pain	0	25	60
Dyspnea	10	33	6
Temperature elevation	30	69	47
Crepitus	90	20	0

* Number of patients

esophageal perforation. Contrast roentgenographic studies with a water-soluble medium demonstrated the perforation in all but one of our patients who had this diagnostic examination.

TREATMENT

The treatment of esophageal perforation, regardless of the site, should be operative intervention with an attempt at primary closure of the perforation. The primary repair should be buttressed, if possible, to prevent subsequent leak at the suture line. A pleural flap is generally used for repair of thoracic esophageal perforations.

The time between perforation and operative repair greatly influences the prognosis. The mortality rate in our series increased from 6 to 54 percent when treatment was delayed more than 24 hours.

The surgeon's judgment becomes important in managing esophageal perforations of long standing. There is little advantage to placing sutures in an esophageal wall that obviously will not hold them. Adequate drainage is essential for these patients. Multiple procedures have been described. It is our feeling that resection or diversion should be used when primary closure of the esophagus cannot be achieved. Reconstruction of the esophagus, usually by colon interposition, can be done later.

Selective nonoperative management for thoracic esophageal perforations has been advocated by Cameron and associates. Eight patients with intrathoracic esophageal disruptions were treated successfully without operation. The criteria, however, are rigid. The esophageal disruption must be contained in the mediastinum, or between the mediastinum and visceral lung pleura; the cavity must drain back into the esophagus; and the patient must have minimal symptoms with minimal signs of clinical sepsis. Patients are given broad-spectrum antibiotics and maintained on parenteral hyperalimentation until the esophagus heals.

BOERHAAVE'S SYNDROME (SPONTANEOUS PERFORATION)

Boerhaave's syndrome, or spontaneous rupture of the esophagus, is associated with forceful vomiting. Boerhaave described the syndrome in 1724 when he performed an autopsy on Baron Wasserauer, who was an admiral of the Dutch fleet. The baron had induced vomiting by taking emetics at the end of a very large dinner. He died 18½ hours later. The autopsy performed by Boerhaave showed a linear tear present on the left side of the esophagus just above the diaphragm. This is the characteristic site of spontaneous perforation of the esophagus. An anatomic weakness exists in the left lateral wall of the distal esophagus. Vomiting causes rapid distention of the esophagus in the segment immediately above the diaphragm, leading to spontaneous rupture. Laceration of the esophagus in Boerhaave's syndrome varies from 2 to 20 cm in length. The mucosal tear usually

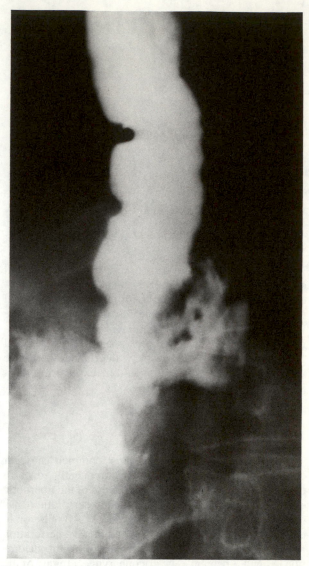

Figure 1 Gastrografin swallow demonstrates extravasation of the radiopaque dye outside the lower esophagus in a patient with spontaneous esophageal perforation (Boerhaave's syndrome).

extends further than that of the muscle layers. The edges of the esophageal tear become irritated by regurgitated gastric secretions with rapid development of inflammation. The resulting edema and friability make suture closure difficult if perforation is not treated within 24 hours of injury.

Patients who sustain esophageal rupture following emesis have a characteristic presentation of forceful vomiting followed by acute severe pain, which may be localized initially to the upper abdominal and retrosternal area. Later, the pain may be referred to the patient's back. Patients have difficulty staying in a recumbent position. As the condition progresses, dyspnea may develop followed by vascular collapse. Physical examination may reveal epigastric tenderness and abdominal wall resistance, but to a lesser degree than is seen in patients with a perforated duodenal ulcer. Mediastinal emphysema may be found on the chest film along with a left pleural effusion.

Because spontaneous esophageal rupture occurs infrequently, physicians tend not to think of the disorder. Many patients are diagnosed as having acute pancreatitis, myocardial infarction, perforated ulcer, dissecting abdominal aneurysm, or spontaneous pneumothorax. If the condition is thought of, the diagnosis can be made by a Gastrografin swallow examination (Fig. 1). If the Gastrografin esophagogram fails to show a leak, a barium esophagogram is done. Barium gives better contrast and may demonstrate a small leak. A prior Gastrografin study rules out large perforations, permitting a barium esophagogram to be used.

Treatment of spontaneous perforation of the esophagus in patients diagnosed within 24 hours of perforation is immediate thoracotomy to close the site of the perforation and wide drainage of the mediastinum. The only delay in operation should be for emergency resuscitative measures. Antibiotics to cover both gram-positive and gram-negative organisms are started prior to operation. In the last decade, no patient with spontaneous perforation of the esophagus has died in our institution when treatment was initiated within 24 hours of perforation. The mortality rate in patients in whom treatment was delayed longer than 24 hours is 25 percent.

COEXISTING ESOPHAGEAL DISORDERS

Definitive treatment of coexisting esophageal disorders is usually mandatory in treating esophageal perforations. Patients who have sustained perforation from pneumatic dilation for achalasia should have closure of the perforation and esophagocardiomyotomy carried out at the same time. Perforations secondary to carcinoma of the esophagus generally demand resection of the esophageal malignant tumor. As so eloquently stated by Skinner, "simple repair of a perforation above an obstructing esophageal lesion or in the presence of free acid-peptic reflux cannot be expected to succeed."

ESOPHAGEAL MOTILITY DISORDER

ALEX G. LITTLE, M.D.

The physiologic functions of the esophagus are to transport ingested food into the stomach and to return gastric contents to the stomach following gastroesophageal reflux episodes. Although gravity plays a role in esophageal transport, the most important component is peristalsis. Peristaltic or sequential esophageal contractions follow swallows (primary peristalsis) and reflux of gastric contents into the esophagus (secondary peristalsis). Disruptions in these normal peristaltic patterns are termed esophageal motility disorders. Normal aging processes are reflected in an increasing incidence of simultaneous, spontaneous, and repetitive esophageal contractions, and so the occurrence of these mild abnormalities is not necessarily pathologic. In addition, many disorders of esophageal motility are nonspecific, cause only minimal symptoms, and are secondary to other primary disorders such as gastroesophageal reflux. I will discuss only those primary, pathologic esophageal motility disorders that the surgeon may be called upon to treat. The focus will be on selection of patients, techniques, and results of surgical intervention. The approaches to be described are summarized briefly in Table 1. Surgery for esophageal motility disorders is palliative surgery and functional surgery. The diseased organ is left in place, and it is unrealistic to expect its function to improve or change in any way. For this reason, it is important for surgeons and patients to understand that, although significant improvement will result, the patient may continue to be aware of mild symptoms and sensations following a "successful" operation.

ACHALASIA

Patients with achalasia are characterized as having dysphagia to solids and liquids, regurgitation, and sequelae of pulmonary aspiration. The age of onset is variable. X-ray examination demonstrates an enlarged esophagus and a distal and tapered narrowing when barium contrast studies are performed. The extent of dilatation depends on the duration of the disease. The diagnosis is established by esophageal manometry which documents the absence of peristalsis. Only simultaneous, not sequential, esophageal contractions are present. In addition, manometry shows distal esophageal sphincter (DES) relaxation with swallowing to be either absent or incomplete. These two manometric features are the diagnostic hallmarks of this disorder. They are functionally significant in that the esophagus, functioning without benefit of esophageal peristalsis, empties only when the hydrostatic pressure caused by the column of retained food

TABLE 1 Esophageal Motility Disorders

Motility Disorder	Symptoms		Diagnosis	Treatment
Achalasia	Dysphagia, regurgitation/ aspiration	Manometry:	Nonrelaxing or incompletely relaxing DES, aperistalsis	Pneumatic dilation for most patients; esophagomyotomy and modified Belsey for failure or complications of dilations
Zenker's diverticulum	Dysphagia, regurgitation/ aspiration	X-ray study:	Pharyngoesophageal diverticulum	Cricopharyngeal myotomy and diverticulopexy
		Manometry:	Cricopharyngeal dysfunction	
Thoracic esophageal diverticulum	Dysphagia regurgitation/ aspiration	X-ray study:	Midesophageal or epiphrenic diverticulum	Distal esophageal myotomy, diverticulectomy, and modified Belsey
		Manometry:	Distal esophageal dysfunction	
Scleroderma	Reflux symptoms, dysphagia if stricture	Manometry: pH Monitoring:	No distal motor activity Acid reflux	Transthoracic Belsey Mark IV
Diffuse spasm	Chest pain, dysphagia	Manometry:	Simultaneous, repetitive and prolonged contractions, occasional peristalsis	Usually medical; myotomy and modified Belsey for selected patients

is high enough to overcome the DES pressure.

Treatment is aimed at correction of the functional distal obstruction produced by the partially relaxing or nonrelaxing DES. Pneumatic dilation, rather than hydrostatic dilation or simple bougienage, has proved to be a safe and effective means of initial treatment in most patients. The dilator consists of a cylindrical, distensible bag fastened about the end of a flexible rod. The bag is positioned across the gastroesophageal junction and rapidly inflated with air. The goal is to distend and actually disrupt the muscle fibers constituting the DES while the more redundant mucosa remains intact. Reported complications include a less than 5 percent incidence of esophageal perforation and an acceptably low incidence of subsequent gastroesophageal reflux caused by the decrease in DES pressure. Variable results are reported, but at least 75 percent of patients obtain satisfactory relief of dysphagia with no more than two pneumatic dilation sessions, requiring no additional therapy. Accordingly, for most patients surgical intervention should follow two attempts at pneumatic dilation. As results of pneumatic dilation decrease after two sessions and complications increase, two sessions are a sufficient trial. Surgery is therefore indicated for patients with continued symptoms following two pneumatic dilations and may be considered earlier in select cases such as the very young, in whom long-term results of dilation can be expected to deteriorate.

Surgical treatment for achalasia was initiated by Heller, who described a double myotomy on both sides of the esophagus. This has evolved to current surgical treatment, which consists of a single surgical esophagomyotomy of the distal esophagus. Again, treatment is aimed at correcting the functional obstruction produced by the nonrelaxing DES. The procedure is performed through a left thoracotomy through the sixth intercostal space. The esophagus is mobilized from the inferior pulmonary vein to the hiatus, which is dissected and freed from its attachments. This hiatal mobilization allows the myotomy to be carried on to the gastric wall under direct vision so that there is no question of complete division of the muscular fibers at the cardia, which are responsible for the manometric DES. If all these fibers are not divided, dysphagia will persist. The myotomy is begun at the level of the inferior pulmonary vein on the anterior esophagus, between the vagal nerves, and carried down onto the stomach so that all the distal esophageal musculature is divided. A blunt tip scissor, such as the Mayo type, is the safest instrument to use. The myotomy is begun by cutting at right angles in a longitudinal orientation between two forceps lifting the esophageal muscle. The mucosa is pushed away by the scissor's tip, and the plane between the mucosa and circular muscle is easily recognized. It is important that the myotomy be widened by mobilization of the muscular layers from the mucosa for a sufficient distance to ensure that rehealing between the muscle edges will not occur and produce recurrent dysphagia. The height or proximal extent of the myotomy that is required has not been established. Most surgeons perform a short myotomy to address only the DES. I have recently produced evidence that the disordered peristalsis of the esophageal body may contribute to dysphagia, and accordingly, I now extend the proximal myotomy upward near the aortic arch. This has not produced any increase in morbidity or complications. Air insufflation into the esophagus through a nasal tube, following the myotomy, provides a check for mucosal injuries, which are localized by air leaking from the esophagus.

With the cardia fully mobilized, gastroesophageal reflux will result unless an antireflux procedure is added. A Nissen procedure produces a DES pressure of a magnitude that the aperistaltic esophageal body cannot overcome and dysphagia will result. The procedure of choice is a Belsey Mark IV fundoplication. Because of the myotomy, only four horizontal mattress stitches—two on each side of the myotomy—are used in this fundoplication, rather than the standard six, but otherwise it is performed in the same way as for primary gastroesophageal reflux. Hiatal stitches are placed posteriorly to the cardia and tied so that a finger can easily pass through the hiatus alongside the esophagus. Some surgeons feel that this operation should be done without mobilizing the hiatus, thus eliminating the need for an antireflux procedure. I believe that this increases the risk both of reflux, if incompetence of the cardia is inadvertently produced and an antireflux procedure is not added, and of insufficient distal extension of the myotomy by obscuring the anatomy of the gastroesophageal junction. This is suggested by the failure rate of this technique, as high as 20 percent, the recurrent dysphagia being attributable to an insufficient myotomy, or complications of reflux, or both.

Surgical mortality for the myotomy and modified Belsey should be no more than 1 to 2 percent, and that is the experience at The University of Chicago Medical Center. Complications are usually pulmonary in nature, secondary to the effects of thoracotomy on a patient who may have been chronically regurgitating and aspirating material from the esophagus. It is important to place a nasoesophageal tube prior to operation to prevent aspiration during induction of anesthesia. Long-term surgical results are good, with 85 to 90 percent of patients having excellent results. Failures are due to incomplete distal myotomy or development of gastroesophageal reflux leading to stricture formation. With the approach I have described, both these causes of failure should be uncommon.

ZENKER'S DIVERTICULUM

Although traditional focus in patients with Zenker's or pharyngoesophageal diverticula has been on the diverticulum itself, this is inappropriate. All these patients have a motility disorder involving the cricopharyngeus muscle or upper esophageal sphincter (UES). This functional abnormality of the UES, characterized manometrically by either a high UES pressure or lack of coordination between pharyngeal contraction and cricopharyngeal (UES) relaxation, produces high pressures in the posterior pharynx, which lead to development of this mucosal diverticulum and cause dysphagia and regurgitation. That this is true is shown by the presence of symptoms in patients with small diverticula and by the prompt recurrence of both symptoms and the diverticulum in patients who are treated by diverticulectomy alone.

Accordingly, just as achalasia is treated by relieving functional obstruction of the DES, surgical treatment of Zenker's diverticulum must include a cricopharyngeal myotomy to relieve the functional obstruction at the UES. The operation can be performed from either side, but is more frequently done through the left neck because the diverticulum tends to protrude in that direction. The prevertebral space is entered by dissecting between the strap muscles medially and the carotid sheath laterally. In the prevertebral space the diverticulum is found and dissected sufficiently to permit identification of its neck. The myotomy is performed from the neck of the diverticulum

downward or distally for a distance of 3 to 4 cm. Further extension is unnecessary as the manometric extent of the UES is no greater than this. A short, less than 1 cm, proximal extension is advisable to ensure complete division of all fibers of the cricopharyngeus, but further extension is meddlesome as it may interfere with pharyngeal function. The myotomized muscle is mobilized sufficiently to prevent primary rehealing and, following completion, air is instilled via a nasal tube to check for the presence of a mucosal disruption.

Following myotomy, surgical opinion differs as to care of the diverticulum itself. I perform diverticulopexy, suspending the diverticulum from the prevertebral fascia behind the pharynx by means of Prolene sutures. Gravity drainage is promoted, and the sac is partially obliterated by the through-and-through sutures. This approach leaves no esophageal suture line, and the patient begins oral intake the first day following surgery and is discharged within another few days. Other surgeons prefer resection of the diverticulum with either staple or manual closure of the posterior mucosa. When resection is chosen, too aggressive mucosal traction and resection can produce an iatrogenic stricture. Long-term results are comparable for both techniques, but I prefer diverticulopexy over diverticulectomy for the stated reasons.

When diverticulopexy is performed in conjunction with a cricopharyngeal myotomy, the complication rate is low. In my last 17 patients, the only complication was in a patient requiring simultaneous pulmonary lobectomy for an aspiration-caused lung abscess. I have seen no important complications in patients undergoing only myotomy and diverticulopexy. Long-term results are good as patients are permanently relieved of dysphagia. Many patients experience minimal but recognizable aspiration episodes while eating for the first few weeks following surgery. This is probably a result of disruption of pharyngeal function secondary to pharyngeal mobilization, and resolves quickly.

DIVERTICULUM OF THE THORACIC ESOPHAGUS

Symptomatic diverticula of the thoracic esophagus can all be shown to have an associated motility disorder of either the distal esophagus or, particularly with epiphrenic diverticula, of the DES. Although traction diverticula due to inflamed mediastinal lymph nodes can occur, symptomatic diverticula are related to these nonspecific esophageal motility disorders. Most frequently encountered in my experience are a high pressure or nonrelaxing DES or spastic activity within the distal or middle esophagus. Patients are not relieved of their symptoms of regurgitation or dysphagia if diverticulectomy alone is performed. Additionally, experience with diverticulectomy shows a high complication rate owing to suture line leakage, not surprising when one considers the presence of a functional distal obstruction.

Accordingly, when symptoms necessitate treatment, surgical myotomy is imperative. Regardless of the location of the diverticulum, midesophageal or epiphrenic, I perform the myotomy from the level of the diverticulum through the DES following mobilization of the cardia. It is not clear whether this distal myotomy is critical in all cases, but I hesitate to perform an operation that is less than definitive. With reconstruction by means of a modified Belsey Mark IV operation, as described for achalasia, results are good, and neither dysphagia nor gastroesophageal reflux results. When myotomy is adequate, treatment of the diverticulum itself is optional. Usually diverticulectomy is performed to eliminate the risk of retention esophagitis or even carcinoma within the diverticular mucosa. It is important to close the neck of the diverticulum in two layers, mucosal and muscular. It is also important to minimize traction on the diverticulum at the time of excision as this will draw esophageal mucosa into the neck, and excision and transection may result in an iatrogenic stenosis.

When the operation is performed with a concomitant myotomy, mortality and morbidity rates are low. Our experience with 10 such patients shows no mortality and only one complication, a vascular event not directly related to the surgical procedure. Long-term results are good, with complete elimination of regurgitation and significant improvement in dysphagia.

COLLAGEN VASCULAR DISORDERS

Scleroderma is the most common of these entities that produce esophageal disease. Involvement of smooth muscle leads to loss of motor function in the distal esophagus and a low-pressure DES. Incompetence of the cardia with gastroesophageal reflux and the inability of the esophageal body to clear refluxed materials are combined, increasing the probability of complications such as stricture. Although as a group these patients are a higher surgical risk than the routine patient, surgery for control of reflux should not be deferred until serious complications such as fibrous stricture develop. This complication may necessitate resection and organ interposition, which is to be avoided when possible in these patients.

Surgery is therefore indicated when, despite adequate medical management, important esophagitis such as mucosal ulceration is documented. At this stage, an antireflux procedure of the standard type is usually sufficient. Because of the esophageal muscular involvement and resulting ineffective motor function, A Belsey Mark IV antireflux repair is preferable because it results in a lower DES pressure than, for example, a Nissen fundoplication. The operation is performed through the left chest. This approach allows extensive esophageal mobilization so that the repair can be placed below the diaphragm without tension.

DIFFUSE ESOPHAGEAL SPASM

This is a rare disorder when rigorously defined. There are reports in the surgical literature describing experience with what is called diffuse esophageal spasm, but described only as "disordered esophageal motility." At present, this diagnosis is made on the basis of specific manometric findings, which include the presence of occasional true peristalsis and frequent repetitive, simultaneous, and prolonged contractions. High-pressure contractions are not required for the diagnosis. These patients may have chest pain or dysphagia or a combination, but chest pain is probably more common. Interestingly, the pain rarely can be documented to correlate with the abnormal manometric examination. It is therefore not surprising that surgical intervention for relief of chest pain provides unsatisfactory and unreliable results. When dysphagia is a prominent symptom, a long myotomy from beneath the arch of the aorta through the DES is more likely to provide good results. Because most or all of the esophageal body is involved in this disorder, a long myotomy is indicated.

DIVERTICULUM OF THE ESOPHAGUS

PANAGIOTIS N. SYMBAS, M.D.

Esophageal diverticula occur at the upper, middle, and lower ends of the esophagus. The diverticula of the upper esophageal end, the so-called pharyngoesophageal or Zenker's diverticula, and those of the lower end, labeled epiphrenic diverticula, are pulsion type with the esophageal mucosa protruding through the muscular layer of the esophagus. The middle esophageal diverticula are traction type and result from paratracheal and parabronchial node infection and scarring.

The diagnosis of the diverticula of the esophagus is made by esophagography. Esophagoscopy is an unnecessary and potentially dangerous diagnostic test, and if done, it should be performed for the diagnosis of other suspected coexisting esophageal diseases. Esophagoscopy should be done carefully to avoid possible perforation of the diverticulum.

PHARYNGOESOPHAGEAL OR ZENKER'S DIVERTICULUM

Zenker's diverticulum occurs at the inlet of the esophagus in the triangular space between the oblique fibers of the inferior pharyngeal constrictor muscle and the transverse fibers of the cricopharyngeal muscle. The development of the pharyngoesophageal diverticulum is usually due to failure of relaxation of the cricopharyngeus muscle during contraction of the pharyngeal constrictor muscle, resulting in the increase of the cephaled intraluminal pressure and protrusion of esophageal mucosa through this triangular space. Therefore the diverticulum is a pulsion type, its wall is composed of esophageal mucosa that protrudes through the triangular space first posteriorly and then commonly projects to the left side of the esophagus.

The majority of Zenker's diverticula, 70 to 80 percent, occur during adulthood and after the age of 60. Their symptoms are dependent on the size of the diverticulum and usually consist of dysphagia, sonorous swallowing, regurgitation, and aspiration of food and mucus.

The treatment of pharyngoesophageal diverticula is surgical; medical therapy is not effective. Although treatment is not urgent, it should be initiated within a reasonable period after the diagnosis has been made. The progressive diverticula enlargement and the accompanying complications, which include aspiration, pneumonitis, pulmonary abscess, and ultimately, inanition secondary to esophageal obstruction in the advanced stages of the disease, can be avoided by early treatment.

The operation is done under general anesthesia with a cuffed endotracheal tube in place, which provides protection against intraoperative aspiration of diverticular contents and permits safe control of ventilation and oxygenation.

Either a transverse or vertically oriented left cervical incision bordering the sternocleidomastoid muscle is used. After the platysma and the omohyoid muscles are incised, the retropharyngeal space and the diverticulum are exposed by laterally retracting the sternocleidomastoid muscle and the underlying carotid artery, and jugular vein, while the thyroid gland and larynx are retracted medially. If necessary, the inferior thyroid artery and the middle thyroid vein may be divided to facilitate exposure of the diverticulum. The diverticulum is grasped with forceps and elevated into the wound to permit its thorough mobilization. Surrounding tissues are carefully separated from the diverticulum by sharp dissection so that the neck of the mucosal sac and the surrounding ring of the muscular defect are clearly defined. Care must be taken to limit the mucosal dissection to the diverticulum to avoid encroachment on the true esophageal lumen.

After the diverticulum has been freed to its neck, a small right-angle clamp is passed under the transverse fibers of the cricopharyngeus muscle, which forms a sling bordering the inferior margin of the neck of the diverticulum. This permits accurate and careful division of the cricopharyngeus muscle. Since the length of the upper esophageal sphincter is somewhat longer than the width of this band of muscle, the myotomy is continued into the upper part of the cervical esophagus for a total length of 3 to 5 cm. The underlying mucosa is then freed from the surrounding muscular tissue to allow slight mucosal protrusion which prevents healing of the myotomy. The

diverticulum is then resected and the esophageal mucosa is sutured or preferably stapled. In either instance care must be taken to avoid excision of too much mucosa, which would limit the esophageal lumen. To avoid this complication, an indwelling esophageal stent of suitable size, a Maloney No. 50 dilator, is positioned before diverticulectomy.

A stapling device is then placed at right angle to the long axis of the esophagus, across the mucosa of the diverticulum at its neck, activated, and the diverticulum is excised.

If a stapling device is not available, after the diverticulum is removed, the esophageal mucosal defect is closed at a right angle to the long esophageal axis with interrupted 3–0 absorbable sutures, with the knots tied in such a manner as to lie within the lumen of the esophagus.

After the mucosa is satisfactorily closed, either with sutures or, preferably, with staples, the muscular and fascial layers of the hypopharynx and upper esophagus are approximated in a transverse direction over most of the mucosal suture line for protection.

A Penrose drain is then positioned away from the suture line and brought out through the incision, and the platysma muscle and skin are closed with interrupted sutures. Oral alimentation is begun 2 or 3 days after operation, and patients are usually ready for dismissal from the hospital within a few days.

The risk of surgery is low, the hospital mortality being less than 2 percent. Complications include esophagocutaneous fistula, vocal cord paralysis, and recurrence of the diverticulum. The incidence of the first two complications is low, and with the addition of cricopharyngeal myotomy to the diverticulectomy, the postoperative recurrence rate is far lower than it was in the past.

MIDESOPHAGEAL DIVERTICULUM

Midesophageal diverticula occur in the midesophagus opposite the trachea or left main bronchus and are due to granulomatous infection, tuberculosis, or, more frequently, histoplasmosis of the paratracheal or parabronchial nodes. This can lead to traction of the neighboring esophageal wall segment and the development of the traction diverticulum. They commonly develop from the anterior or right lateral esophageal wall. Their apex is usually higher than their stoma, which is wide, allowing free filling and emptying of the diverticula without stagnation. As a result, symptoms produced by them, which is the requirement for surgical treatment, are extraordinarily rare. When in the extremely rare case symptoms due to the diverticulum develop diverticulectomy may be required. The resection of the diverticulum is done through a thoracotomy at the fifth intercostal space. After the right lung is collapsed, the mediastinal pleura is opened at the level of the diverticulum, and the esophagus just proximal and distal to the diverticulum is dissected free and encircled with tape. The diverticulum then is carefully dissected from the adjacent structures to which it is usually adherent with dense adhesions. The base of the diverticulum is then stapled with a stapling device longitudinally, parallel to the esophageal axis. A parietal pleural flap is then developed and wrapped around the esophagus to cover the esophageal suture line, enhance healing, and add protection from subsequent leakage from the suture line.

EPIPHRENIC DIVERTICULUM

Epiphrenic diverticula, like those occurring in the upper end of the esophagus, are pulsion type, their wall being composed of esophageal mucosa protruding through the muscular esophageal layer. The epiphrenic diverticulum most often occurs in middle age, usually on the right side and in conjunction with other diseases of the esophagus, diffuse spasm, achalasia, or hiatal hernia. They are commonly due to neuromuscular esophageal dysfunction with incoordinated opening of the distal esophageal sphincter and an increase of the intraluminal esophageal pressure proximal to it. Usually their clinical manifestations are those of the esophageal diseases coexisting with the diverticula (dysphagia, odynophagia, or regurgitant esophagitis). When the diverticula become large, they may produce symptoms of their own. The diagnosis of epiphrenic diverticulum is made, as in diverticula at other esophageal sites, by esophagography.

However, before surgical therapy is instituted, the previously mentioned esophageal diseases that coexist with the epiphrenic diverticula should be excluded. Diverticulectomy without concomitant correction of such esophageal abnormalities results in failure to ameliorate the patients complaints and may lead to disruption of the esophageal suture line with its consequences. Therefore esophageal motility and pH studies in addition to esophagography should be done preoperatively in all patients, and the subsequent operative procedure should be tailored according to the results of these studies.

In general, the need for therapy of an epiphrenic diverticulum is determined by the presence or absence of symptoms. A patient with an asymptomatic epiphrenic diverticulum requires no therapy. However, operation is clearly indicated when symptoms are progressive or have become severe. Progressive enlargement of the diverticulum, progressive dysphagia, and regurgitation with or without symptoms of aspiration are indications for surgical therapy irrespective of the duration of symptoms.

The operative procedure is done through a left thoracotomy since the lesion is typically located within several centimeters of the esophagogastric junction, and there is almost universal need for an associated esophageal myotomy. This incision gives excellent access to the lesion and provides ample exposure for the performance of the myotomy, regardless of the side on which the diverticulum present. Even from a left-sided approach, an epiphrenic diverticulum presenting to the right can be managed easily by simple rotation of the esophagus after its mobilization.

A double-lumen endotracheal tube is used for the administration of anesthesia and ventilation; this facilitates the esophageal exposure by collapsing the left lung while providing adequate ventilation for the patient through the right lung. The thoracotomy is done through the left seventh intercostal space. The mediastinal pleura is opened, and the distal esophagus is mobilized and encircled by two Penrose drains, one above and one below the diverticulum.

The diverticulum is carefully dissected from the peridiverticular tissue up to its neck, so that only the mucosal layer is present at the anticipated level of transection. As in the pharyngoesophageal diverticulum, care must be taken to avoid overgenerous excision of mucosa with subsequent narrowing of the esophagus. Again a No. 50 Maloney dilator is inserted into the esophagus under direct guidance to avoid perforation of the diverticulum, which is subsequently transected at its base. The defect of the esophageal mucosa is either sutured or, preferably, stapled in the same manner as in Zenker's diverticulectomy. However, the stapler device is positioned parallel to the long axis of the esophagus, which is then activated and the diverticulum excised.

After completion of the diverticulectomy, an esophagomyotomy is then performed. The type and extent of myotomy depends on the nature of the motility disorder. Achalasia and diffuse spasm of the esophagus are the most commonly encountered motility disorders associated with epiphrenic diverticula. In the case of a patient with achalasia, a modified Heller myotomy is carried out. The myotomy is usually made on the left anterolateral surface of the esophagus, but its location can be altered, depending on the site of the diverticulectomy suture or staple line. The muscular incision extends for 6 to 7 cm and is restricted almost entirely to the distal esophageal musculature and crosses the esophagogastric junction only far enough to complete transection of the circular muscles of the sphincter zone. If diffuse spasm is present, however, the myotomy is appropriately extended to encompass the entire area of abnormal motility. The muscle is then dissected from the underlying mucosa to allow it to protrude through the incision and prevent subsequent healing of the myotomy.

An antireflux procedure is also done if regurgitant esophagitis is demonstrated in the preoperative studies. The thoracotomy is then closed in a conventional manner with intercostal tube drainage. Oral feedings are permitted within a few days of operation after an esophagography has verified the integrity of the esophageal suture line, and the patient is usually ready for dismissal within a week after the operation.

The results of epiphrenic diverticulotomy with an associated esophagomyotomy are good, and postoperative complications and recurrence of either symptoms or the diverticulum are rare.

ESOPHAGEAL REFLUX

MARK B. ORRINGER, M.D.

Gastroesophageal reflux results from incompetence of the lower esophageal sphincter mechanism and may occur whether or not a hiatal hernia is present. Symptoms from gastroesophageal reflux correlate poorly with the degree of esophagitis present. Thus the patient with severe pyrosis and heartburn may have little, if any, endoscopic esophagitis, while others may present with dysphagia from a stricture and advanced esophagitis without having experienced significant reflux symptoms in the past. It is therefore critical that patients with documented abnormal gastroesophageal reflux on barium esophagogram or pH monitoring of the distal esophagus undergo esophagoscopy so that esophagitis can be detected in its earlier and more easily treatable stages. *Prevention*, then, is the most important factor in the treatment of a peptic esophageal stricture, i.e., controlling gastroesophageal reflux *before* mural fibrosis occurs. The early diagnosis of reflux esophagitis is hampered both by the poor correlation between symptoms and severity of esophagitis and by the notorious inability of the barium esophagogram to detect reflux esophagitis reliably and consistently. The endoscopic grading system for esophagitis proposed by Belsey provides a more objective and meaningful description of the gross pathologic changes seen than the traditional designation of "mild," "moderate," or "severe" esophagitis, which have inherent wide variations and meaning between observers.

ENDOSCOPIC GRADES OF ESOPHAGITIS

Esophagitis has been graded endoscopically by Skinner and Belsey (1967) as follows:

Grade I   Distal esophageal mucosal erythema (which may obscure the esophagogastric squamocolumnar epithelial junction).

Grade II Mucosal erythema with superficial ulceration, typically linear and vertical and with an overlying fibrinous membranous exudate that is easily wiped away, leaving a bleeding surface (often misinterpreted as "scope trauma" by the inexperienced endoscopist).

Grade III Mucosal erythema with superficial ulceration and associated mural fibrosis—a dilatable "early" stricture.

Grade IV Extensive ulceration and fibrous luminal stenosis; may represent irreversible panmural fibrosis.

It is clear from an understanding of the pathophysiology of reflux esophagitis and the foregoing grading system that the roentgenographic designation of a "mild" esophageal stricture in fact indicates an *advanced* stage of esophagitis. It is usually wrong to infer that a "mild" stricture as noted on roentgenogram represents a process that has been detected early enough to require only conservative therapy.

INDICATIONS FOR ANTIREFLUX SURGERY

Failure of Medical Management

Perhaps 80 to 85 percent of patients with abnormal gastroesophageal reflux respond to a medical antireflux regimen, including elevation of the head of the bed on blocks (4- to 6-inch), antacids after meals and at bedtime, refraining from eating for several hours before bedtime, smaller more frequent meals, and weight reduction. Although the H_2 inhibitors (e.g., cimetidine) should not be used for a prolonged period or on a daily basis, a single dose at bedtime may control the majority of nocturnal acid reflux symptoms. Only when such a regimen has failed to relieve reflux symptoms after a conscientious 3- to 6-month trial should a patient with incapacitating symptoms be regarded as a candidate for antireflux surgery. The impact of reflux on daily living should not be underestimated. Patients may be virtually exhausted from having to sleep upright at night to prevent acid regurgitation. Conversely, the construction worker who can sleep comfortably at night with the head of his bed elevated and the use of antacids finds little solace when he must bend over at work to lift a heavy load of bricks and promptly regurgitates his lunch. Thus, "failure of medical management," that "gray zone" of indications for antireflux surgery, is open to wide interpretation and requires an honest assessment of the impact of gastroesophageal reflux on the individual patient's life style. Thus patients with symptomatic reflux and no esophagitis or grade I endoscopic esophagitis require an antireflux operation in only a small percentage of cases, primarily when their symptoms are clearly refractory to medical therapy or adversely affect a comfortable life style.

Ulcerative Esophagitis

The presence of ulcerative (grade II) esophagitis at esophagoscopy is generally an indication for an antireflux procedure. The majority of patients with this degree of inflammation may respond to intensive medical therapy with healing of the ulceration, only to relapse once again the moment the stringent antireflux program is relaxed.

Stricture

Early in my training I was taught that the presence of an esophageal stricture represented advanced esophagitis in a patient in whom an antireflux operation was long overdue. However, I have subsequently learned that this dictum is not absolute. Perhaps 25 percent of patients with reflux strictures complain only of dysphagia, not pyrosis, heartburn, or regurgitation of gastric contents. They simply do not have an acid-sensitive esophagus that responds to acid with pain. When their stricture is dilated and their dysphagia relieved, they are grateful, satisfied patients. In such individuals, institution of an aggressive antireflux medical regimen and periodic outpatient esophageal dilations, perhaps once or twice a year, provide excellent therapy. It should be remembered that antireflux surgery has a definite incidence of morbid complications which must be heavily weighed in a patient who is totally asymptomatic after dilation of a stricture. However, in the majority of patients with grade III or IV esophagitis, dilation and a medical program for reflux control fail to provide adequate relief of symptoms of esophagitis, and an antireflux operation is indicated.

Recurrent Aspiration

Respiratory symptoms are elicited in perhaps 25 percent of patients with gastroesophageal reflux and range from frank aspiration of gastric contents into the tracheobronchial tree to a subjective complaint of shortness of breath in the supine position. Relatively few patients give a classic history of awakening at night choking on regurgitated stomach acid that has been inhaled into their lungs, causing wheezing and a burning feeling over both lung fields. Such patients are definite candidates for antireflux surgery to prevent ongoing damage to their lungs from chemical pneumonitis. On the other hand, not all respiratory symptoms in patients with reflux are due to aspiration, as acid in the esophagus may trigger vague retrosternal discomfort and subjective dyspnea, perhaps related to reflux-induced esophageal spasm. The surgeon must therefore exercise caution in attributing all respiratory symptoms to aspiration, which may easily become an overrated indication for antireflux surgery.

Bleeding

Bleeding from reflux esophagitis is seldom massive and is usually intermittent, presenting clinically as occult blood loss anemia. When bleeding is documented endoscopically, the presence of concomitant grade II or more ulcerative esophagitis constitutes an indication for antireflux surgery.

Barrett's Esophagus

The presence of a Barrett's esophagus (columnar epithelium-lined lower esophagus) is a more controversial indication for antireflux surgery. Once believed to be of congenital origin, the columnar epithelium-lined lower esophagus is now almost universally accepted as an acquired condition resulting from reflux esophagitis. As the normal esophageal squamous epithelium is denuded by chronic acid regurgitation, the lower esophagus may be reepithelialized by the upgrowth of gastric epithelium, which grows five times faster than squamous epithelium. Thus the esophagus comes to be lined by columnar epithelium of gastric origin, which may become dysplastic and ultimately develop into carcinoma. The potential for malignant degeneration in Barrett's esophagus has, in my opinion, been overestimated at approximately 15 percent. This figure has usually been based on series of patients who already have adenocarcinoma of the distal esophagus associated with a Barrett's esophagus. The true incidence of carcinoma developing in a Barrett's esophagus is not actually known, and may be as low as 1 to 2 percent. Thus if there is esophageal ulceration in the Barrett's esophagus when it is diagnosed on esophageal biopsy, an antireflux operation is usually indicated. If there is no ulceration, however, medical therapy may suffice. The columnar epithelial lining does not revert back to squamous epithelium after antireflux surgery, even though the associated reflux esophagitis may heal. Thus the decision to do an antireflux operation for a Barrett's esophagus is not clear-cut. However, if biopsies demonstrate the presence of severe dysplasia or carcinoma in situ in the columnar epithelium, a strong argument can be made for esophagectomy before frank carcinoma develops.

Paraesophageal or Combined Sliding and Paraesophageal Hiatal Hernia

The final indication for an antireflux operation is the presence of a large paraesophageal or combined sliding and paraesophageal hiatal hernia. A pure paraesophageal hiatal hernia is unusual, most patients with paraesophageal hernias having some component of a sliding hernia as well. Furthermore, in the process of mobilizing the herniated stomach out to the chest and away from the diaphragmatic hiatus so that complete reduction into the abdomen is possible, disruption of the esophagogastric junction and supporting structures is inevitable. Therefore reconstruction of the esophagogastric junction with an antireflux operation is part of the operative repair of large paraesophageal or combined sliding and paraesophageal hiatal hernias.

CHOOSING AN ANTIREFLUX OPERATION

The virtues of one standard antireflux operation over another have been exaggerated; although the three leading antireflux procedures in this country—the Hill posterior gastropexy, the Belsey Mark IV, and the Nissen fundoplication—differ from one another in technique, all share a number of common features and a similar mechanism of action. Each requires the placement of sutures either into esophageal or periesophageal tissues to maintain a 3- to 5-cm segment of distal esophagus below the diaghragm, where the influence of positive intraabdominal pressures provides a compressive force that prevent reflux. The hiatus is narrowed behind the esophagus in all repairs. Thus, regardless of whether the operation is done transabdominally (the Hill or Nissen repairs) or transthoracically (the Belsey or Nissen repairs), the end result is the same—a short segment of distal esophagus under the influence of positive intra-abdominal pressure. Competent well-trained surgeons who are comfortable with any of these procedures can achieve excellent results in terms of *initial* reflux control. Except when coexisting intra-abdominal disease, for example, cholelithiasis or peptic ulcer disease, requires a trans-abdominal approach, there is really no difference in the immediate end result among the standard antireflux operations. The incidence of intraoperative splenic injury is higher in transabdominal operations; that of vagal nerve injury is greater with transthoracic repairs. Fortunately, both are low. An antireflux operation can be performed through a limited thoracotomy without the potential for an incisional hernia or subsequent bowel obstruction from adhesions. Thus, the idea that a transthoracic hiatal hernia repair is a much bigger operation than a transabdominal repair is not really valid.

There is a prevailing notion in North America that a 360-degree fundoplication is contraindicated in the presence of esophageal motor dysfunction such as achalasia or scleroderma, the rationale being that a hypo-tensive, poorly emptying esophagus may be functionally obstructed by the wrap. This is simply not the case. In Europe, a Nissen fundoplication has been performed following an esophagomyotomy for achalasia in hundreds of patients and long-term results have been excellent. The key is a loose, short wrap performed over a large intra-esophageal bougie. A partial (Belsey) fundoplication can obstruct an atonic esophagus just as assuredly as a total Nissen wrap if it is performed incorrectly. In my own experience, therefore, a hypomotility disorder of the esophagus is not a contraindication to total fundoplication in the patient requiring reflux control.

If the standard antireflux operations differ little in mechanism of action, morbidity, or initial reflux control, what factors should indicate a need to use any approach other than one of these three? A discussion of these follows.

RECURRENCE RISK FACTORS

It has been known for years that a reflux stricture or severe periesophagitis, if present at the time of a Belsey hiatal hernia repair, greatly increases the incidence of recurrent reflux or hernia in long-term follow-up of these patients. Two groups of factors emerge as being responsible for this increased recurrence rate: (1) those that result in tension on the repair, and (2) those that inter-fere with the healing of sutures placed into either esophageal or periesophageal tissues. Thus, the presence of severe reflux esophagitis with secondary esophageal shortening not only interferes with the performance of a tension-free reduction of the distal esophagus into the abdomen, but the associated intramural inflammation jeopardizes healing of the esophageal sutures used in the fundoplication. And if these considerations apply to patients undergoing a Belsey repair, they must also be

applicable in patients having either a Hill or Nissen repair, since all of these operations require either esophageal or periesophageal sutures and the fixation of a 3- to 5-cm segment of distal esophagus below the diaphragm.

It is thus possible to assess each patient coming to operation for control of gastroesophageal reflux in terms of existing conditions that might predispose him to recur-rent reflux or hernia after any of the standard repairs (Table 1). In addition to reflux esophagitis, periesophagitis associated with either reflux esophagitis or a prior lower esophageal operation interferes with the placement and subsequent healing of the esophageal sutures of the standard repairs. Relative esophageal shortening may be found in patients with longstanding large combined sliding and paraesophageal hiatal hernias. And just as obesity and chronic obstructive pulmonary disease with repeated coughing increases intra-abdominal pressure and therefore the incidence of abdominal incisional hernias, these factors must also result in more tension at the diaphragmatic hiatus and therefore an increased incidence of recurrent herniation and disruption of the hernia repair. Patients demonstrating any of these ''recurrence risk factors'' are, in my opinion, candidates for the transthoracic esophagus-lengthening Collis gastroplasty followed by a 360-degree Nissen fundoplication, the so-called Collis-Nissen procedure. The rationale for this approach is simple. The gastroplasty tube provides not only additional ''esophageal'' length, thereby eliminating tension on the repair, but also a resilient gastric tube around which to perform the fundoplication without the need for the tenuous esophageal sutures of the standard hernia repairs.

TECHNIQUE OF THE COLLIS-NISSEN OPERATION

If the patient has a benign peptic stricture, dilation to a 40 French (F) Hurst-Maloney bougie is performed after the induction of general anesthesia. Strictures that can be dilated per os to a 40 F dilator can inevitably be dilated intraoperatively to the 56 F or larger range. If the patient has no stricture, but rather another indication for the Collis esophageal lengthening procedure, a 54 F or 56 F Hurst-Maloney bougie is positioned in the esophagus prior to turning the patient to his right side. Through a posterolateral thoracotomy in the seventh intercostal

TABLE 1 Recurrence Risk Factors

I. Factors affecting the reliability and healing of esophageal or periesophageal sutures
  A. Reflux esophagitis
  B. Periesophagitis
    1. Reflux esophagitis
    2. Previous operation
II. Factors resulting in increased tension on the repair
  A. Esophageal shortening
    1. Reflux esophagitis
    2. Large combined sliding and paraesophageal hernia
  B. Chronic pulmonary disease
  C. Obesity

---

space, the distal esophagus is mobilized and encircled with a Penrose drain. In the presence of extensive mediastinal inflammation or periesophagitis, no attempt is made to mobilize the esophagus higher than the inferior pulmonary vein, since additional length will be gained distally by the gastroplasty procedure. The gastric fundus is mobilized into the chest through the diaphragmatic hiatus as for a standard Belsey or transthoracic Nissen repair, dividing four to six high short gastric vessels between clamps. Care is taken to avoid injury to the vagus nerves or the spleen.

If indicated, intraoperative dilation of a peptic stricture is performed, supporting the area of stenosis from without as progressive Hurst-Maloney bougies are passed from above, occasionally forcefully, up to the size of a 56 F to 60 F dilator. The gastroplasty tube is constructed with a 54 F or 56 F dilator across the esophagogastric junction, displaced against the lesser curvature of the stomach. The gastrointestinal anastomosis (GIA) surgical stapler is applied to the stomach against the dilator, usually once, and the result is a 5-cm extension of the functional distal esophagus. The staple suture line is oversewn with a 4–0 polypropylene Lembert stitch. Silver slip markers are placed at the new esophagogastric junction. A 3- to 4-cm Nissen fundoplication is then performed around the gastroplasty tube with the large esophageal dilator still in place. Each 2–0 silk suture used in the repair passes first through gastric fundus, then through the gastroplasty tube, and then through the gastric fundus again. The silk suture line is oversewn with a 4–0 polypropylene Lembert stitch. The dilator is removed, the fundoplication is reduced below the diaphragm, and the previously placed No. 1 silk crural sutures are tied to narrow the hiatus until it admits the surgeon's index finger comfortably alongside the distal esophagus. A nasogastric tube is inserted. Silver clips are placed at the edge of the diaphragmatic hiatus. The repair results in a 3- to 5-cm tension-free intra-abdominal segment of functional "esophagus," encircled completely by the gastric wrap.

CLINICAL EXPERIENCE WITH THE COMBINED COLLIS-NISSEN OPERATION FOR GASTROESOPHAGEAL REFLUX AND ITS COMPLICATIONS

In our department, the Collis-Nissen operation has been performed in 209 patients ranging in age from 18 to 86 years. The indications for the combined Collis-Nissen approach included factors I believe predispose to recurrent reflux after the standard hiatal hernia operations as I have already defined. It was initially postulated that the need for an esophagomyotomy for esophageal spasm might diminish the ability of the distal esophageal muscle to hold the sutures used in the subsequent fundoplication. Of our 112 patients with reflux esophagitis, peptic strictures were present in 41 (20%). Among this group were 22 patients with scleroderma reflux esophagitis. Twenty-six percent of our patients had undergone prior operations at the esophagogastric junction, including 21 transthoracic and 22 abdominal hiatal hernia repairs. Preoperative evaluation in all patients included barium swallow

examination and esophagoscopy. Esophageal manometry and acid reflux testing were performed in 92 percent of these patients.

There have been two postoperative deaths in the series for an operative mortality of 0.9 percent, and neither was the direct result of the technique of the antireflux procedure. Two patients with extensive periesophageal adhesions from prior antireflux operations developed gastroplasty tube leaks postoperatively. One required an esophagectomy and later colonic interposition. The other leak closed spontaneously after drainage. In one patient undergoing intraoperative dilation, the stricture was perforated. Another patient was operated on within 7 hours of sustaining a perforation of the stricture during attempted dilation elsewhere. In both of these latter patients, a transient leak occurred at the site of closure of the injury, but responded well to drainage, and the patients continued to undergo stricture dilation until there was spontaneous closure. Two patients bled from the edge of hypertrophied muscle following an esophagomyotomy for spasm, and one patient required abdominal exploration for bleeding from a divided short gastric vessel.

Of our 209 patients, 48 have either died of causes unrelated to their esophageal disease or have not been followed for a minimum of 6 months. Postoperative personal interviews and repeat esophageal function tests have been performed 6 months or more after surgery in 161 (77%) of the patients. Seventy-three percent have been restudied at 6 months; 78 percent at one year; 53 percent at 2 years; 35 percent at 3 years; and 20 percent at 4 years. The average follow-up in this group is now 31 months.

Subjectively, based on the patient's response to standard postoperative questioning during personal interviews, 93 percent have no symptoms of reflux; 3 percent have mild intermittent heartburn for which they take an occasional antacid, but are still able to sleep horizontally without reflux symptoms; and 4 percent (six patients) have developed severe recurrent reflux symptoms which have necessitated institution of a vigorous antireflux regimen and eventually reoperation. The overall *subjective* recurrence rate has therefore been 7 percent (11 of 161 patients). Eighteen patients (11%) have acknowledged experiencing some degree of early satiety or "gas bloats" after operation. However, in only three has this been associated with marked abdominal distress. In fact, a number of extremely obese patients have regarded their postoperative early satiety as an asset, for it has forced them to eat in smaller amounts and allowed them to lose weight whereas standard weight reduction diets had failed for years. We have obtained a history of postoperative dysphagia, no matter how slight, in 62 patients (39%). Among this group, however, 22 patients have had such mild transient slow emptying of the esophagus that no treatment has been required; six of these patients had esophageal spasm preoperatively, and nine had peptic strictures. Forty patients, or 25 percent of the entire group, have required postoperative dilations, 12 of these having had preoperative spasm and 22 strictures. Because 38 percent of patients with esophageal spasm preoperatively have required some esophageal dilations postoperatively, we no longer use the Collis-Nissen reconstruction of the esophagogastric junction in patients undergoing an esophagomyotomy and believe that either a modified Belsey or a loose Nissen fundoplication is preferable.

Objective assessment of the results of the Collis-Nissen procedure has been obtained with manometry and acid reflux testing. Esophageal function tests were repeated in our first 107 consecutive Collis-Nissen patients within 3 months of operation to be certain that initial reflux control was in fact being achieved. *No* patient in this group was found to have abnormal reflux. Over the period of follow-up to 60 months, average high pressure zone pressures and length have been relatively constant at approximately 11 mm Hg and 4 cm respectively. A total of 22 patients have been found to have abnormal reflux with the pH electrode for an overall *objective* recurrence rate of 14 percent. However, ten of these patients have no reflux symptoms.

Among 36 patients with peptic strictures treated with intraoperative dilation and the combined Collis-Nissen operation, the average follow-up is now 41 months. Ninety-four percent of these patients have no reflux symptoms. However, 61 percent have required further bougienage after the initial intraoperative dilation. It should be emphasized, however, that despite the need for postoperative dilations, between 60 and 70 percent of these patients with strictures have required no more than 1 or 2 outpatient dilations a year after their antireflux procedures. All patients with strictures had markedly abnormal reflux as determined by the pH electrode preoperatively. Postoperatively, 17 percent of these patients have demonstrated abnormal reflux, and 83 percent have had good reflux control.

These data showing gratifying subjective and objective evidence of reflux control after the combined Collis-Nissen procedure justify its use in patients who have a predisposition to recurrent reflux after a standard hiatal hernia repair. Long-term follow-up for at least 5 years will be required before this approach can be said to have proved its value in controlling gastroesophageal reflux and its complications.

MANAGEMENT OF THE UNDILATABLE PEPTIC ESOPHAGEAL STRICTURE

The vast majority of strictures secondary to reflux esophagitis are dilatable either per os or forcefully at the time of the antireflux repair. In patients with dense panmural fibrosis that results in fracturing of the esophagus during attempted dilation, the criterion of a

"nondilatable" stricture has been met, and resection is indicated. Thus, in patients in whom dilation of a stricture per os to a 40 F bougie is not possible, the colon is prepared preoperatively in the event that intraoperative dilation is not possible and resection with a short segment colonic interposition is necessary. As an alternative, particularly in elderly patients, a transhiatal total esophagectomy with a cervical esophagogastric anastomosis provides excellent relief of reflux symptoms. An intrathoracic esophagogastric anastomosis should *never* be performed for benign esophageal disease, since the inevitable development of gastroesophageal reflux and secondary esophagitis results in recurrent dysphagia in a major percentage of these patients.

I strongly oppose the practice of performing an intrathoracic fundoplication in patients in whom esophageal shortening prevents a tension-free intra-abdominal wrap. This operation creates a man-made paraesophageal hiatal hernia with all of its potential for mechanical complications. For the same reason, the Thal-Woodward procedure is not optimal, since this approach not only relies on the healing of the open diseased esophagus to which the gastric fundus is sutured, but it also requires a intrathoracic fundoplication to control reflux and therefore accepts the inherent potential complications of this intentionally constructed paraesophageal hernia.

ANGELCHIK PROSTHESIS

During the past ten years, the Angelchik silicone gel prosthesis has been popularized as an effective antireflux operation. The concept of slipping a collar around the esophagogastric junction through an abdominal incision is appealing because of its simplicity. Unfortunately, there appears to be *at least* a 10 percent incidence of major complications associated with this operation, including migration of the ring into the chest through the diaphragmatic hiatus, slippage of the ring onto the body of the stomach, erosion through the esophagus, and dysphagia. As occurs in other parts of the body where silicone has been implanted, a fibrous capsule develops around the prosthesis, further contributing to the potential for dysphagia from stricture formation. The concept of placing a semirigid prosthesis around a portion of the intestinal tract that is constantly exposed to motion of the adjacent diaphragm is extremely worrisome. In my opinion, there is little justification for placing a ring of foreign body around the distal esophagus when a fundoplication using autogenous tissue achieves the same goal of reflux control with proven safety and far less potential for complications.

BARRETT'S ESOPHAGUS

MICHAEL G. SARR, M.D.

Barrett's esophagus is a condition in which the squamous lining of the lower esophagus has been replaced by a columnar epithelium, the so-called columnar-lined lower esophagus. This columnar lining involves a variable mosaic of three types of columnar epithelium—a specialized intestinal type with goblet cells, a junctional type resembling the epithelium of the gastric cardia, and a fundic type containing both parietal cells and chief cells. Barrett's esophagus has recently become a topic of heightened interest to gastroenterologists and surgeons alike because of its increasingly recognized incidence and because of its association with adenocarcinoma of the esophagus.

PATHOGENESIS

Although Barrett's esophagus was originally thought to result from a congenitally short esophagus with resultant intrathoracic stomach, current evidence overwhelmingly suggests that Barrett's esophagus is an acquired columnar metaplasia occurring in response to chronic acid-peptic reflux. Evidence supporting the acquired nature of this entity is multifactorial and includes the clinical observation of the orad progression of this columnar epithelium over time, the demonstration of objective evidence of gastroesophageal reflux in virtually all these patients, and the development of several animal models in which chronic gastroesophageal reflux eventuates in a columnar metaplasia of the injured squamous epithelium of the lower esophagus.

CLINICAL PRESENTATION

The majority of patients recognized as having Barrett's esophagus present with symptoms or complications related to gastroesophageal reflux. Dysphagia associated with an esophageal stricture is a not uncommon initial presentation. Review of our experience at The Johns Hopkins Medical Institutions from 1975 to 1981 yielded 90 patients with Barrett's esophagus. Symptoms of heartburn, regurgitation, dyspepsia, or dysphagia were present in over 90 percent (84/90). However, 7 percent (6/90) presented without symptoms of gastroesophageal reflux, but with evidence of chronic blood loss or with nonspecific abdominal complaints and were recognized only serendipitously as having Barrett's esophagus. Some investigators have suggested that development of Barrett's epithelium in certain patients with the most severe and persistent gastroesophageal reflux may ''protect'' the patient from the usual symptom complex of heartburn and dyspepsia; these patients present later only after dysphagia ensues secondary to stricture formation. A history of exposure to alcohol and tobacco is the rule.

PREVALENCE

The exact prevalence of Barrett's esophagus is unknown because an undefined percentage of patients are asymptomatic. However, in patients who can be identified clinically to be at risk for developing Barrett's esophagus, i.e., those patients with symptoms of gastroesophageal reflux, the prevalence of Barrett's esophagus is about 8 percent. This condition is not limited to adults; children with symptomatic gastroesophageal reflux severe enough to warrant esophagoscopic evaluation have a prevalence of Barrett's epithelium that approaches 13 percent. Thus, Barrett's esophagus is not an uncommon entity.

DIAGNOSIS

The diagnosis of Barrett's esophagus requires an esophageal biopsy from an area proximal to the manometrically defined lower esophageal sphincter or from an esophageal segment confidently visualized to be above an associated hiatal hernia. Barrett's esophagus may be suspected if endoscopic examination reveals a red, friable, velvety esophageal mucosa. However, routine esophageal biopsy is strongly advised in all patients with symptoms of gastroesophageal reflux severe enough to warrant esophagoscopy; only 34 percent of patients in our experience, who were eventually demonstrated to have a Barrett's esophagus, were recognized visually by the endoscopist as harboring Barrett's esophagus at the time of esophagoscopy. Another clue to the diagnosis of Barrett's esophagus is the presence of a benign, midesophageal stricture, which is virtually diagnostic of Barrett's esophagus and warrants further investigation.

BARRETT'S ESOPHAGUS AND ADENOCARCINOMA

In recent years, adenocarcinoma of the esophagus arising from a segment of Barrett's esophagus has been recognized with increasing frequency. In one center, 20 percent of esophageal carcinomas encountered in the last 2 years were adenocarcinomas associated with Barrett's esophagus. What in the past were often considered to be adenocarcinoma of the gastric cardia extending up the distal esophagus were most probably adenocarcinomas arising from a Barrett's esophagus and extending down into the proximal stomach.

In our recent experience at The Johns Hopkins Medical Institutions (1975 to 1981), 14 percent of patients (13/90) with Barrett's esophagus presented with a concomitant adenocarcinoma of the esophagus. Moreover, in the last 3 years (1981 to 1984), we have managed 14 patients with Barrett's esophagus and adenocarcinoma. This association has raised the question of whether Barrett's esophagus represents a premalignant condition. Support for this association comes from detailed histopathologic studies of resected specimens in patients with adenocarcinoma arising in Barrett's epithelium. Areas of dysplasia and carcinoma in situ within the columnar epithelium, both adjacent to and remote from the tumor mass, were found, suggesting the progression from columnar metaplasia (Barrett's epithelium) to dysplasia, carcinoma in situ, and eventually invasive malignancy.

This is an especially interesting entity because, unlike squamous carcinoma of the esophagus which is more prevalent in blacks, adenocarcinoma arising from Barrett's esophagus is predominantly a disease of white males. Excessive smoking and alcohol intake appear to be associated as well. Patients present with symptoms of mechanical obstruction of the esophagus, many of whom (up to 40%) deny any previous symptoms of gastroesophageal reflux. One wonders whether these patients may represent a subgroup with the most severe gastroesophageal reflux who lack the usual symptoms of gastroesophageal reflux because of replacement of the squamous lining with the insensitive columnar metaplasia. Unfortunately, in these patients the reflux of acid-peptic juices continues and may serve as the irritant in the development of dysplasia.

CONTROVERSIES IN MANAGEMENT OF BARRETT'S ESOPHAGUS

Treatment of uncomplicated Barrett's esophagus should be directed at symptomatic relief, but the prevention of the complications related to gastroesophageal reflux and Barrett's esophagus, such as the development of esophageal stricture, bleeding, and adenocarcinoma, must now also be addressed. Unfortunately, good long-term studies of the natural history of Barrett's esophagus and its response to the various treatment modalities are lacking. Thus, appropriate treatment of the patient with Barrett's esophagus remains controversial.

Does Treatment Halt the Progression or Lead to the Regression of Barrett's Esophagus? No one knows. With prevention of acid-peptic reflux or with prolonged neutralization of the acid content of the stomach, one might imagine interruption of the stimulus for further columnar metaplasia and possibly the subsequent healing of the injured mucosa. Several groups have claimed that a small percentage of patients treated by successful antireflux procedures have had partial regression of their Barrett's esophagus. However, other groups have failed to see similar regression and argue that this "regression" is a sampling error of biopsy technique. Another study treated a group of patients with an intense regimen of cimetidine and oral antacids; although most patients were rendered asymptomatic, the Barrett's esophagus failed to regress in any patient.

Does Treatment Prevent the Development of Adenocarcinoma? This also is unknown. With prevention of gastroesophageal reflux, the progression of dysplasia, carcinoma in situ, and invasive neoplasia might be interrupted. However, there have been no such studies. Of interest is a patient of ours with an unresponsive esophageal stricture (and Barrett's esophagus) who had undergone a distal esophagectomy with short-segment colon interposition, a proven, highly effective antireflux procedure. Eight years later, he presented with adeno-

carcinoma of the proximal esophagus arising from a segment of residual Barrett's epithelium. This suggests that, in some patients, effective prevention of gastroesophageal reflux may not completely protect against the eventual development of malignant degeneration of the columnar metaplasia.

SUGGESTIONS IN MANAGEMENT

Barrett's esophagus by itself probably is an indication for an antireflux procedure despite the lack of conclusive evidence that prevention of gastroesophageal reflux causes stabilization or regression of the Barrett's epithelium. Although intense medical therapy may relieve bothersome symptoms, the reflux continues. The Nissen fundoplication has provided the best results in most surgeons' experience in relieving symptoms and in preventing objective gastroesophageal reflux when tested by measurements such as pH monitoring of the distal esophagus. The Hill and Belsy repairs are somewhat less reliable in preventing the reflux.

Occasionally these patients may have a shortened esophagus from the chronic scarring of persistent gastroesophageal reflux, and a transabdominal approach would be inappropriate. Under these circumstances, a transthoracic Collis-Nissen procedure is a better choice. Concomitant benign esophageal strictures in patients with Barrett's esophagus usually occur at the squamocolumnar junction and are not the woody, fibrous contractures related to chronic peptic esophagitis. Thus, they are usually easily managed by intraoperative bougienage and transient postoperative esophageal dilation if necessary. With the known association with adenocarcinoma in Barrett's esophagus, one must be certain that the stricture is not malignant.

Management of the patient with Barrett's esophagus also necessitates long-term surveillance for the development of adenocarcinoma. The risk of malignant degeneration is unknown. Several groups have suggested that, in patients recognized to have Barrett's esophagus because of symptomatic gastroesophageal reflux, the future development of adenocarcinoma is as infrequent as one cancer developing in every 125 to 425 patient years. However, a prevalence of adenocarcinoma of about 10 to 15 percent in patients presenting with Barrett's esophagus has been noted. Whether the majority of patients who develop carcinoma have no symptoms of gastroesophageal reflux and only present after the tumor mass causes dysphagia is unknown. Nevertheless, all authorities agree that the presence of Barrett's esophagus requires at least yearly esophagoscopy, routine biopsy, and probably also esophageal cytology. In addition, all exposure to alcohol and tobacco should cease.

The presence of dysplasia within the Barrett's epithelium is a much more controversial topic. With our present state of knowledge, dysplasia alone can be used as an indication for aggressive management, possibly with esophageal resection. However, dysplasia can be used as an even stronger indication for an antireflux procedure, and it does warrant an even more frequent surveillance schedule.

The presence of carcinoma in situ justifies esophageal resection. Because gastroesophageal reflux continues after a routine segmental esophagectomy with intrathoracic esophagogastrostomy, consideration should be given to removal of all the Barrett's epithelium by total thoracic esophagectomy and reconstruction with a cervical gastric pull-up or, in the younger patient with a longer life expec-

tancy, with a long-segment colon interposition. These patients would be ideal candidates for an extrathoracic, transhiatal, "blunt" esophagectomy.

When invasive adenocarcinoma develops in Barrett's esophagus, resection is indicated whenever possible. Although 5-year survival was only 15 percent in our recent series of 32 patients, palliation was excellent with a mean survival after standard esophagogastric resection of about 26 months.

PARAESOPHAGEAL HERNIA

JON F. MORAN, M.D.

Paraesophageal hernia represents a relatively uncommon but quite distinct subgroup of hiatal hernias. Less than 5 percent of patients coming to operation for hiatal hernia have a paraesophageal hernia. The less frequent occurrence of paraesophageal hernia is responsible for the confusion that often exists about the definition, natural history, and management of this disorder. Gradually over the past twenty years a number of clinics seing large numbers of patients with hiatal hernias have collected sizable series of patients with paraesophageal hernias, and from these series a better understanding of this condition and its treatment has evolved.

Definitions of paraesophageal hernia in the past focused purely on strict anatomic criteria, ignoring important pathophysiologic elements. Both paraesophageal (rolling) hernias and the much more common sliding hiatal hernias involve herniation of the stomach through the esophageal hiatus into the mediastinum. Anatomically, paraesophageal hernia implies that the gastroesophageal (GE) junction remains more nearly in its original anatomic position while the body of the stomach rolls up through the anterior portion of the dilated hiatus until a major portion of the stomach lies above the GE junction. This anatomy leads to the term "upside-down stomach" often used in describing paraesophageal hernias. In the usual sliding hiatal hernia, the GE junction remains above the herniated portion of the stomach. As a result, the angle at the GE junction (the angle of His) becomes more acute in a paraesophageal hernia and less acute in a sliding hiatal hernia.

Management of hiatal hernias is dictated not by strict anatomic definitions, but rather by a clear understanding of the pathophysiology and natural history of each condition. The pathophysiologic consequences of a sliding hiatal hernia are related to the displacement of the GE junction and the resulting incompetence of the lower esophageal sphincter. Treatment of sliding hiatal hernias focuses on elimination of GE reflux to avoid the symptoms and complications related to reflux esophagitis. The pathophysiology of paraesophageal hernia is quite distinct from

that of sliding hiatal hernia. Pure paraesophageal hernia has previously been defined as a paraesophageal herniation of the stomach into the mediastinum while the GE junction remained in an absolutely normal position below the diaphragm. In a pure paraesophageal hernia there would be no GE reflux, no esophagitis, and no secondary shortening of the esophagus. Pure paraesophageal hernias represent a minority of cases of paraesophageal hernia. Much more commonly, although the GE junction is tethered posteriorly in the esophageal hiatus, the dilated esophageal hiatus and the increased intra-abdominal pressure that encourage the stomach to herniate into a paraesophageal position also predispose to displacement of the GE junction slightly upward above the diaphragm. As a result, many paraesophageal hernias have some incompetence of the lower esophageal sphincter and coexistent reflux esophagitis.

Regardless of the precise position of the GE junction, the pathophysiology and possible complications of a hiatal hernia are quite different if there is a significant paraesophageal component compared to the usual sliding hiatal hernia. Paraesophageal hernias are quite distinct from sliding hiatal hernias in their sequelae and therefore in their management. Paraesophageal hernias are usually massive hernias as the majority of the stomach has herniated into the mediastinum. As the stomach rolls up through the anterior and lateral aspects of the esophageal hiatus, it remains covered by a parietal peritoneal hernia sac. The greater curvature of the stomach is less fixed anatomically and therefore usually forms the leading edge of the herniation. The attached omentum and transverse colon, as well as other intra-abdominal organs, may herniate through the enlarged esophageal hiatus. The distensible stomach stretches the dilated hiatus even more. Once the entire stomach has herniated with the greater curvature most cephalad, the GE junction and pylorus come together, predisposing the stomach to rotate and thus cause a volvulus. The most serious complications of paraesophageal related to the hernia itself and not to reflux or other secondary physiologic derangements. Unlike sliding hiatal hernias, paraesophageal hernias often present with complications such as gastric volvulus; incarceration of the stomach; partial or complete obstruction of the stomach, small intestine, or colon; or bleeding from an erosion or ulcer in the herniated stomach. A distended stomach in a massive paraesophageal hernia occasionally leads to severe respiratory distress from simple displacement of functioning lung. The types of complications encountered secondary to paraesophageal hernias make prompt recognition and treatment of this condition mandatory. For the most part the complications of sliding hiatal hernias progress gradually as a result of chronic reflux esophagitis. Acute, catastrophic complications are rare in sliding hiatal hernias, but relatively common in paraesophageal hernias.

PRESENTATION

Paraesophageal hernias present predominantly in patients over the age of 40. Most patients have a body habitus consistent with chronically increased intra-abdominal pressure. Paraesophageal hernia is found more often in women than in men. The very large esophageal hiatus that is invariably found in patients with paraesophageal hernias is probably the result of gradual dilatation of a congenitally widened or weakened hiatus. Often even large paraesophageal hernias are minimally symptomatic. In the absence of catastrophic complications, the usual symptoms are postprandial distress and substernal fullness attributed to dilatation of the herniated, intermittently obstructed stomach. Most patients admit to episodic heartburn, occasional regurgitation or vomiting, and intermittent dysphagia. Respiratory distress associated with eating is another common symptom in these patients. Blood loss from an ulcer or erosion in the herniated stomach may lead to melena or anemia as a presenting sign in 30 to 40 percent of patients.

Though most paraesophageal hernias present with insidious, gradually worsening symptoms, any of several acute, life-threatening complications can occur at any time without warning. Bleeding from the mucosal surface of the herniated stomach is seldom massive, but can present acutely. This bleeding usually results from a combination of overdistention of the partially obstructed herniated stomach, direct trauma to the stomach, and vascular compromise (venous or arterial) of the stomach wall. Because the damage to the stomach wall is the result of mechanical problems related to the hernia, the bleeding seldom responds to conservative treatment. Such mechanical problems require mechanical, operative treatment. Paraesophageal hernia may also present acutely as respiratory failure. In such cases the massively dilated herniated stomach compresses the adjacent lung sufficiently to cause ventilatory failure with carbon dioxide retention. This is also a mechanical problem and requires operative reduction of the hernia to allow full reexpansion of the lungs. Though the ventilatory insufficiency caused by the paraesophageal hernia is completely reversible after the stomach is decompressed and the hernia is reduced, an element of aspiration pneumonia may be superimposed at the time of acute decompensation and may continue to interfere with respiratory function postoperatively.

The most ominous presenting symptoms of paraesophageal hernias are those related to obstruction secondary to organoaxial volvulus of the stomach or incarceration of the herniated stomach. These complications present with acute substernal pain that is often mistakenly diagnosed as angina pectoris. Once the correct diagnosis is suspected, careful passage of a nasogastric tube both confirms the diagnosis and decompresses the compromised stomach. If another portion of the gastrointestinal tract is incarcerated (colon or small bowel) or if passage of a nasogastric tube is not possible, emergency operation is indicated to avoid the dire complications of volvulus or incarceration. Either volvulus or incarceration with resulting obstruction may progress to gangrene of the stomach (or other incarcerated portion of the gastrointestinal tract). The distended, obstructed viscus becomes gangrenous and then may perforate into either the abdominal cavity or the mediastinum. Once gangrene or perforation occurs, the operative mortality approaches 50 percent.

DIAGNOSIS

Roentgenographic examinations are useful to confirm the diagnosis of paraesophageal hernia whenever the history suggests this diagnosis as a possiblity. Frequently, upright posteroanterior and lateral chest radiographs reveal one or two air-fluid levels in the posterior mediastinum just behind the lower portion of the cardiac silhouette. If a nasogastric tube can be passed into the stomach without difficulty, the position of the tube in relation to the left hemidiaphragm and the esophagus may confirm the presence of a paraesophageal hernia. A definitive diagnosis may be established with an upper gastrointestinal series to delineate the position of the GE junction and the relative positions of anatomic portions of the stomach itself. An elevated, paralyzed hemidiaphragm or a chronic eventration of the left hemidiaphragm may present a similar roentgenographic appearance, with the stomach lateral and superior to the distal esophagus. However, careful contrast studies will show that the stomach is completely subdiaphragmatic. Rarely, a barium enema may be helpful in demonstrating herniation of the transverse colon through the dilated esophageal hiatus.

Esophagoscopy, either flexible or rigid, should be performed in all cases of paraesophageal hernia prior to operative repair. Esophagoscopy is useful to determine the position of the GE junction relative to the diaphragm, to assess the presence of reflux esophagitis, and to be certain that there is no esophageal stricture. All of this information is important in the planning of the operative repair of a paraesophageal hernia. If time permits, esophageal manometry and pH reflux testing can be employed as well to evaluate the competence of the lower esophageal sphincter and the need for an antireflux procedure at the time of hernia repair.

TREATMENT

The most important principle of treatment of a paraesophageal hiatal hernia is that the mere presence of a paraesophageal hernia, pure or mixed, is an indication for repair, even in a totally asymptomatic patient. This principle derives from the high incidence of serious complications secondary to volvulus or incarceration, the increased morbidity and mortality of emergent operative repair once such complications occur, the low morbidity of elective repair, and the low recurrence rate following operative repair. Obviously, the development of any of the aforementioned symptoms or complications is further indication for prompt operative treatment.

Paraesophageal hernias may be repaired transabdominally or transthoracically. The abdominal approach is usually through an upper midline incision, though a left paramedian or left subcostal incision may be used. The thoracic approach is usually through the left sixth or seventh intercostal space or the resected bed of the sixth or seventh rib. Both approaches have their advantages and their ardent advocates. In general, one should approach a paraesophageal hernia through the incision one uses most frequently to approach the esophageal hiatus. It is important that one be comfortable working through the incision chosen since the anatomy of the dilated hiatus is often distorted. However, particular aspects of an individual case may indicate the use of a specific incision. Coexistent problems in the abdomen or chest, for example, symptomatic cholelithiasis or a suspicious nodule in the left lung, may dictate the choice of incision in an elective repair of a paraesophageal hernia. It is generally easier to resect gangrenous stomach or transverse colon through the abdomen in cases with severe incarceration. In particularly complex cases, with gangrenous stomach or colon that has perforated into the mediastinum or pleural space, separate abdominal and thoracic incisions are probably indicated. The pleural space and mediastinum can be debrided and optimal drainage of the pleural space established through the usual left thoracotomy incision. Reconstruction of the gastrointestinal tract and lavage of the peritoneal cavity should be carried out through a separate abdominal incision. Other potential advantages and disadvantages of the abdominal and thoracic approaches to the repair of paraesophageal hernia will be discussed later.

Regardless of the approach chosen, the basic principles of the operative repair are the same. First, the hernia itself must be reduced below the diaphragm. Usually traction on the stomach or colon from below (transabdominally) or manual compression from the mediastinum (transthoracically) accomplishes reduction of the hernia relatively easily. When the stomach is incarcerated in the dilated hiatus, division of the anterolateral rim of the defect may be necessary to facilitate reduction. In the presence of a volvulus or incarceration, excessive pressure on the distended stomach can perforate the compromised stomach wall. Rarely, a gastrotomy is necessary initially to decompress a distended, incarcerated stomach that completely obscures the hiatal rim, preventing any division of the hiatus.

The true hernia sac of peritoneum that is present in a paraesophageal hernia must be mobilized from the posterior mediastinum and reduced below the diaphragm.

From the thoracic approach the sac is mobilized by blunt and sharp dissection from pericardium, diaphragm, and lung without necessarily opening the sac. Once the sac is mobilized the entire hernia with the sac can be reduced by pulsion back below the diaphragmatic hiatus. From the abdomen the sac is removed separately after reduction of its contents. Working from the abdomen the mobilization of an adherent hernia sac is often tedious. Complete removal of this sac is essential to avoid recurrent herniation or formation of a fluid-filled cyst in the lower posterior mediastinum.

Chronic bleeding from the herniated stomach does not require gastrotomy since it is most frequently from superficial mucosal erosions that will rapidly heal once the hernia is reduced and the stomach is no longer obstructed. A history of brisk bleeding mandates a gastrotomy with oversewing of any actively bleeding ulcer. Portions of stomach or colon that remain gangrenous following reduction and areas of frank perforation are resected by means of routine reconstructive techniques. If a decompressing gastrotomy is necessary, it is reasonable to convert this to a standard Stamm gastrostomy after the hernia is reduced. A gastrostomy allows comfortable chronic decompression of the stomach and simultaneously anchors the stomach to the abdominal wall. Although a gastrostomy is not an essential part of the repair of paraesphageal hernia, once the stomach has been opened, the potential benefits of a gastrostomy outweigh any disadvantages.

Once the contents of the hernia sac have been reduced back beneath the diaphragm, attention is turned to repair of the hernia defect. Whether an antireflux operation should be performed as well as a simple repair of the dilated hiatus remains controversial. In cases of "pure" paraesophageal hernia with no symptoms of reflux esophagitis and no evidence of esophagitis at the time of esophagoscopy, the esophagus is fixed posteriorly in the hiatus with the gastroesophageal junction tethered firmly in its normal position. In such cases, closure of the dilated hiatus with a series of interrupted nonabsorbable sutures without any antireflux procedure is sufficient. The hiatus should be narrowed so that two fingers passed through the hiatus next to the esophagus are a snug fit. In simple cases of paraesophageal hernia, repair of the hiatal defect alone results in relief of symptoms and a low recurrence rate (less than 2%). Subsequent reflux symptoms are also rare.

There is a relatively high incidence of concomitant reflux symptoms or evidence of reflux by esophagoscopy, pH monitoring, or esophageal manometry in patients with large paraesophageal hernias. Patients with "mixed" hiatal hernias naturally require an effective antireflux procedure at the time of the reduction and repair of their paraesophageal hernias. Despite preoperative manometric and roentgenographic studies and endoscopic examination at the time of repair, most surgeons have found it difficult to confidently distinguish "pure" paraesophageal hernias from "mixed" paresophageal hernias. The routine addition of an antireflux procedure to the reduction of the paraesophageal hernia and the narrowing of the dilated hiatus seems the most reasonable strategy to avoid postoperative reflux symptoms.

Through an abdominal incision, either a Nissen fundoplication or a Hill posterior gastropexy can be performed easily after reduction of the paraesophageal hernia. The Nissen fundoplication is the most consistently effective of the various antireflux procedures. After the stomach and the hernia sac have been pulled beneath the diaphragm and the diaphragmatic hiatus narrowed, as already described, with a series of interrupted sutures, the uppermost portion of the greater curvature is wrapped (360 degrees) around the intra-abdominal portion of the esophagus (2 to 4 cm). The wrap should be performed over a 48 F Maloney dilator. Only two to four nonabsorbable sutures are used to secure the wrap, being certain to anchor the wrap to the underlying esophagus to avoid upward displacement of the stomach through the wrap. The wrap must be loose enough to admit one finger easily to avoid the gas-bloat syndrome.

When operating through a thoracic incision, either a Nissen fundoplication or a Belsey partial fundoplication is the logical choice for an antireflux procedure. In patients with severe reflux esophagitis, especially if there is shortening of the esophagus, the thoracic approach is safer. Severe esophagitis causes a paraesophageal inflammation that makes mobilization of the esophagus from below hazardous, especially if the esophagus has been shortened significantly. Mobilization of the inflamed distal esophagus can be performed safely under direct vision through the usual thoracic incision. In these cases a Collis gastroplasty prior to performance of the Nissen or Belsey fundoplication allows the replacement of the fundoplication intra-abdominally without any tension on the esophagus or the diaphragmatic repair.

Through the usual thoracic incision the paraesophageal hernia sac is mobilized and the hernia sac reduced. The GE junction is mobilized and a 48 F Maloney dilator passed into the stomach from the mouth., A line of staples (5 to 6 cm) is applied along the dilator to separate a tube of the lesser curvature from the fundus of the stomach. This uncut, stapled gastroplasty effectively lengthens the esophagus. Either the Nissen fundoplication just described or a Belsey (240 degrees) fundoplication is then performed around the newly created distal esophagus. The fundoplicated stomach and distal esophagus are replaced below the diaphragm and the hiatus closed with interrupted sutures.

Regardless of the specific operative techniques employed, the stomach should be kept decompressed postoperatively with a nasogastric tube (or gastrostomy) until the distended stomach regains its normal motility. Prolonged periods of relative gastric atony are seen commonly in these patients. Oral diet is resumed and gradually advanced once gastrointestinal motility returns. With the exception of cases of preoperative perforation, repair of paraesophageal hernia carries a low morbidity even in elderly patients. The recurrence rate is low and the relief of symptoms approaches 100 percent, especially if a simultaneous antireflux procedure is performed.

ACUTE CAUSTIC BURN OF THE ESOPHAGUS

MARVIN M. KIRSH, M.D.

The nature and extent of corrosive esophageal injuries has changed drastically since 1967 with the introduction of concentrated liquid lye solutions for use as drain cleaners. Prior to this time, most of the caustics ingested were flakes or solid pellets of sodium hydroxide. Alkali swallowed in this form adhered on contact to the mucous membrane, especially those of the esophagus and the oropharynx. The burning produced in the mouth by this type of caustic caused the patient to expectorate as much as possible or drink water. The latter would tend to neutralize the burned tissues, dilute the remaining caustic, and wash it into the stomach where neutralization occurred. Consequently, the caustic resulted in burns primarily of the oropharyngeal and upper digestive tract, and segmental stricture of the esophagus was a common sequela. Injury of the stomach was a rare occurrence. Animal investigations revealed that if antibiotics and steroids were given early following ingestion of these caustics, the likelihood of stricture formation was reduced. Thus for years, therapy consisted of steroids and antibiotics during the acute stage and chronic dilation for strictures that developed later.

The ingestion of these newer concentrated lye substances results in tissue damage of unprecedented proportions and has created catastrophic situations. The high viscosity of these substances contributes to its tissue destructive effect by prolonging the duration of contact when it is applied to mucous membranes and the esophagus. The high viscosity also contributes to a rapid passage to the stomach. The pathologic sequence of events that occurs following liquid caustic ingestion is similar to that described following ingestion of the older granular lye, but with a greater frequency and severity of serious sequelae. Following granular lye ingestion, only 10 to 25 percent of the patients developed an esophageal stricture. However, most patients with a history of liquid caustic ingestion are found to have a serious (near-circumferential) esophageal burn, and almost all progress to extensive stricture formation.

Early in our experience, these patients were treated in the conventional manner (steroids, antibiotics, early dilation) with disastrous results, namely perforation and aortoesophageal fistula. Consequently, we have modified our approach to patients who have ingested these caustics.

SOLID CAUSTICS

Alkali swallowed in the solid state adheres on contact to the mucous membranes, especially those of the oropharynx and esophagus. Severe damage is more apt to occur in these areas, while the stomach is usually spared because the solids fail to reach it in sufficient quantity. If particles of alkali should enter the gastric lumen, they are diluted or neutralized by gastric acid.

The patient who ingests a solid caustic usually burns the lips, tip of the tongue, and fauces. Initial drooling may cause the caustic to drain over the chin so that circumoral burns develop. These patients do not drool chronically and are usually able to manage their saliva. Since there is rarely deep burning of the esophagus, perforation of the esophagus and resultant shock do not occur.

Examination of the oropharynx within 24 hours of the burn usually demonstrates a white-to-yellow leukocytic membrane covering the ulcers produced by the caustic. The lesions bleed easily and are painful.

Diagnosis

Although oral cavity burns can be assessed by visual examination, the question whether the esophagus has been burned and to what degree can be answered only by esophagoscopy. This should be performed within 24 hours.

Management

As a rule, the ingestion of caustic crystals almost immediately produces severe pain that causes the patient to stop further ingestion. The crystals tend to adhere to the mucous membranes of the tissues with which they first come into contact, namely, the mouth, pharynx, and the esophagus. Perforation of the esophagus can occur and should be constantly searched for, but is an infrequent occurrence following ingestion of caustic crystals. Emergency measures include early esophagoscopy and contrast roentgenographic visualization. The process of healing is observed by esophagoscopy and barium swallow repeated at 10- to 14-day intervals. The majority of patients who have ingested crystals do not suffer severe esophageal burns; however, patients who sustain severe (second- or third-degree) burns often develop an esophageal stricture. Those patients should swallow a string as soon as a liquid diet can be tolerated. Since early bougienage is associated with an increased risk of perforation, dilation is not started until healing is complete and an epithelialization mucosa is seen as far as the esophagoscope can be advanced; this may take 4 to 5 weeks. Dilation is then started and can be carried out with the mercury-filled, tapered, Hurst-Maloney bougie or the

Tucker bougie, using the previously swallowed string as a guide. Even if dilation is delayed until healing has occurred, there is still an increased risk of perforation, hemorrhage, or both when it is instituted. Therefore dilation should be carried out as carefully as possible.

LIQUID CAUSTICS

The clinical picture varies, depending on the concentration and amount of the liquid caustic agent ingested as well as the presence or absence of food in the stomach. The liquid caustic is often rapidly swallowed, causing extensive injury to the esophagus and stomach, but with less tissue injury within the mouth and pharynx. Therefore, caustic burns of the esophagus cannot necessarily be predicted from the presence and appearance or even the absence of external burns. In many cases, if the patient vomits after ingesting the caustic, he drools continuously. Substantial pain, back and abdominal pain, and rigidity are usually indicative of mediastinitis, peritonitis, or both. Hoarseness, stridor, aphonia, and dyspnea suggest either associated laryngeal edema or actual epiglottic and laryngeal destruction. With burns of the esophagus, stomach, or both, the patient is febrile and tachypneic and has a rapid pulse. Hypotension secondary to hypovolemia may be an additional complicating factor.

Examination of the lips, mouth, and oropharynx may reveal signs of tissue injury ranging from a few scattered areas of superficial mucosal erosions of the lips and tongue to deep and extensive destruction of the lingual, buccal, and pharyngeal mucosa.

Diagnosis

Since it is not possible to correlate the findings in the mouth and pharynx with esophageal changes, the only means of establishing the extent and severity of esophageal injury is by esophagoscopy, preferably within the first 24 hours of injury. The risk of esophageal perforation is low if the procedure is performed under general anesthesia and the flexible pediatric endoscope is used. Only if the endoscopist has considerable experience in performing esophagoscopy should the esophagus beyond the first burned area be visualized. Early esophagoscopy permits patients without esophageal burns to avoid prolonged hospitalization. There are several limitations to esophagoscopy, however:

1. At times it may be difficult to evaluate the depth of any burn with absolute certainty by observing superficial epithelial necrosis.
2. When a severe burn is encountered in the upper third of the esophagus, the esophagoscope is not passed beyond this area, and the involvement of the middle and lower thirds cannot be ascertained.

Despite these limitations, the advantages of early esophagoscopy are great enough that it should be carried out in all patients with suspected caustic injury to the esophagus when the hypopharynx and larynx are free from burns. Hyperemia of the esophageal mucosa with superficial desquamation of epithelium occurs with a first-degree burn. Superficial blisters, ulcers, hyperemia, and patchy membranous exudate of the mucosa are characteristic of second-degree burns. Areas with deep loss of esophageal epithelium that are hyperemic and show evidence of granulation tissue are classified as third-degree burns.

Radiologic Features

Contrast visualization of the esophagus and stomach is the best means of assessing the severity of the stomach injury. A radiocontrast esophagogram provides additional evidence of liquid caustic injury. Water-soluble agents are preferable to barium for contrast examinations in view of the increased risk of perforation. The prominent radiocontrast features include: (1) diffusely blurred esophageal margins, reflecting mucosal ulceration, sloughing, and pseudomembrane formation; (2) linear streak and plaque-like collections of contrast material due to deep necrotic ulcers with intramural dissection; (3) scalloped or straightened esophagogastric margins, probably reflecting submucosal edema and hemorrhage; (4) intraluminal and intramural retention of contrast material for prolonged periods because of esophageal atony due to intramural dissection; and (5) persistent esophageal dilation with intraluminal retention of gas secondary to diffuse muscular necrosis and possibly indicative of impending perforation.

Treatment

For many years the treatment of caustic injuries has included systemic corticosteroid therapy. Steroid therapy was based on the observation by Spain that early administration of cortisone in mice inhibited fibroplasia and formation of granulation tissue. Since 1963, 14 clinical series have appeared in the literature evaluating the role of steroids in the treatment of caustic injuries. Of the 374 patients who received steroids and in whom there were adequate esophagoscopic findings, stricture or death occurred in 16.8 percent. By contrast, there were 144 patients who did not receive steroids. The incidence of stricture or death was 20 percent, little different from that calculated for steroid-treated individuals. Steroids have been found to impair wound healing, depress the body's immune defense mechanism, and mask the signs and symptoms of infection and visceral perforation. In view of these dangers, the lack of proved efficacy, and my own personal experience, it is my conviction that steroids should not be used in the treatment of esophageal injuries caused by liquid caustics.

All individuals with physical findings indicative of caustic ingestion should be admitted to the hospital; in fact, anyone in whom there is the least suspicion of caustic ingestion should be admitted and undergo evaluation. An attempt should be made to find the container that held the ingested caustic or some of the material itself for proper identification. Hypovolemia should be treated with either whole blood or colloid-containing fluids. The patient should be carefully observed for airway obstruction. Laryngeal edema is frequently seen in the first 24 hours in association with severe caustic burns of the esophagus, and endotracheal intubation may be needed. In view of the instantaneous nature of the injury produced by liquid caustics, water or other juices to "dilute the caustic" are of little value. In fact, they may produce additional vomiting or retching that may aggravate the situation. For the same reason, emetics and gastric lavage are contraindicated. Because antibiotics have been shown to decrease both the risk of pulmonary infection and bacterial invasion through the injured esophagus into the mediastinum, they should be administered as soon as the diagnosis of esophageal injury is established. Our preference is for ampicillin (40 mg per kilogram per day in divided doses) or, in penicillin-allergic patients, clindamycin (8 to 10 mg per kilogram per day in divided doses). It should be administered intravenously until oral feedings are begun. The antibiotics are discontinued after 7 days if the patient is afebrile or continued until the fever disappears. Contrast visualization of the esophagus and stomach should be carried out shortly after admission.

Esophagoscopy is done on admission or not later than 24 hours after the ingestion. Patients in whom there are no oropharyngeal or esophageal burns and in whom the barium swallow is normal can be discharged after 24 hours of observation. A repeat barium swallow should be obtained at 1 and 2 months so that an unrecognized esophageal stricture will not be overlooked. A nasogastric tube is inserted cautiously and the stomach is aspirated. If the aspirate is basic and the alkalinity does not cease with gentle and limited irrigation, it is presumed that the stomach and esophagus are burned. Contrast visualization of the esophagus and stomach is also obtained. If there are clinical signs of perforation, peritoneal findings of peritonitis, or, on contrast examination, evidence of impending perforation, a celiotomy is performed, and if the gastric wall is ecchymotic or black, indicating a necrotic stomach, a gastrectomy is performed. At times a burn extends through the stomach wall to involve the adjacent viscera such as colon, pancreas, spleen, or small bowel. If damaged, these structures are also removed. It has now been amply demonstrated that when the stomach is necrotic following caustic ingestion, the esophagus is also necrotic or is so severely burned that a nondilatable stricture will develop within several months. Therefore, a transhiatal esophagectomy and left cervical esophagostomy should be carried out. Colon interposition is performed 4 to 6 weeks later.

If the stomach is not necrotic at celiotomy, only a gastrostomy need be performed. If the distal intraabdominal segment of esophagus is necrotic or if contrast examination shows dilation of the esophagus with retention of either swallowed air or contrast material (which implies diffuse muscular necrosis and impending perforation), transhiatal esophagectomy is performed. If neither of these abnormalities is present, the extent and severity of the esophageal injuries are assessed by careful esophagoscopy and managed with antibiotics and later dilations.

If the gastric aspirate is acidic and peritoneal signs are present, a celiotomy should be performed and gastrectomy, esophagectomy, or both carried out if indicated. When the gastric aspirate is acid (as is apt to occur when ingestion occurs on a full stomach) and there are no peritoneal signs, there is little likelihood that the stomach is seriously burned, and a celiotomy should not be performed. The extent and severity of the esophageal injuries are assessed by careful esophagoscopy and managed with antibiotics, hyperalimentation, and later dilation.

Protocol for the treatment of caustic burns of the esophagus:

Attempt to identify the caustic agent.
Place the patient on "nothing by mouth."
Correct hypovolemia.
Obtain chest roentgenogram.
Begin on intravenous antibiotics.
Perform contrast visualization of esophagus.

Perform esophagoscopy within 24 hours.
Aspirate gastric contents for pH.

A. Alkaline aspirate
1. Celiotomy—only when there are peritoneal findings of peritonitis or impending perforation on contrast examination
2. Necrotic stomach—esophagogastrectomy
3. Non-necrotic stomach—esophagoscopy
   a. Esophagus necrotic—esophagectomy
   b. Esophagus not necrotic
      (1) Antibiotics
      (2) Late dilations
      (3) No steroids

B. Acid aspirate
1. Peritoneal signs—celiotomy; esophagogastrectomy if indicated
2. No peritoneal signs
   a. Esophagoscopy
   b. Antibiotics
   c. Hyperalimentation
   d. Late dilation

ESOPHAGEAL TUMOR

MARK K. FERGUSON, M.D.
DAVID B. SKINNER, M.D.

Tumors of the esophagus are among the most challenging surgical problems. Because of the difficulty of early detection of esophageal cancer, two-thirds of patients have locally advanced or metastatic disease at the time of diagnosis. This historically results in an overall 5-year survival rate of less than 10 percent, and has spurred efforts toward earlier detection and a more radical approach in surgical and adjuvant treatment in the hope of improving survival.

The standard preoperative staging work-up includes a barium swallow, esophagoscopy and biopsy, gallium scan, bone scan, and computerized tomography of the chest and upper abdomen. Following completion of these tests, over one-third of cases are inoperable owing to contiguous involvement of other mediastinal structures by the tumor or owing to distant metastatic disease. Over one-half of patients undergo surgical exploration, and nearly all have a potentially curative or palliative resection. We do not advocate preoperative radiation therapy or chemotherapy for potentially curable cases, as there is no evidence that preoperative adjuvant therapy increases survival or is more effective than postoperative therapy. For patients found to have stage I carcinoma (T1N0M0 or T2N0M0) by pathologic staging after resection, long-term survival rates are in the range of 80 percent; therefore

preoperative adjuvant therapy is only likely to be harmful. Patients whose disease is unresectable are offered other forms of treatment to alleviate symptoms or to eliminate potential complications (Table 1).

SURGICAL TREATMENT

The choice of operation is based on the location, extent, and cell type of the tumor (Table 2). For potentially curable tumors we advocate en bloc removal of the esophagus and surrounding mediastinal structures to include the mesoesophagus and lymphatic drainage pathways. Contraindications to radical resection include involvement of lymph nodes beyond the limits of en bloc resection, an inability to obtain clear deep margins at the limits of mediastinal dissection, or distant metastases. In

TABLE 1 Treatment Modalities for Esophageal Carcinoma, All Stages Considered

Treatment	% of Cases
Resection	52%
Bypass	8%
Radiation and/or chemotherapy only	28%
Intubation	4%
None	8%

TABLE 2 Distribution of Carcinoma of the Esophagus and Cardia According to Site and Histology. All numbers are percentages

	Cardia and Lower Third	Middle Third	Cervical	Total
Squamous cell	9	25	15	49
Adenocarcinoma	30	0	1	31
Adenocarcinoma (Barrett's)	9	6	0	15
Carcinosarcoma	2	2	1	5
Total	50	33	17	100

such cases palliative (or standard) esophagectomy is done whenever possible to prevent complications such as obstruction, hemorrhage, fistula, or abscess during subsequent adjuvant treatment.

Lesions of the Cardia and Lower Third

For patients in whom the proximal extent of tumor is 10 cm or more below the aortic arch at esophagoscopy, resection is performed through a left thoracotomy. This provides optimal exposure for thorough dissection of the lower mediastinum and stomach and allows for reconstruction with an anastomosis below the level of the arch or in the neck. The incision is made through the sixth intercostal space, and thoracic exploration is performed to exclude metastases. The diaphragm is incised peripherally from the border of the sternum to the spleen to expose the upper abdomen. Abdominal exploration is performed, including the gastric nodal drainage basin and liver. If intraoperative staging confirms the preoperative clinical impression that the tumor does not extend outside the limits for resection, en bloc resection is indicated. For adenocarcinoma of the cardia extending onto the stomach, a total gastrectomy with esophagectomy extending 10 cm above the proximal extent of the lesion is performed. For adenocarcinoma or squamous carcinoma of the distal third of the esophagus, esophagectomy and partial gastrectomy is performed to include 10 cm of tissue on either side of the lesion. The omentum is separated from the transverse colon and mesocolon. The spleen is mobilized, and the splenic artery and vein are divided, leaving the spleen attached to the stomach by the short gastric vessels. Retracting the stomach superiorly, the celiac axis is exposed. The origin of the left gastric artery is divided, as is the coronary vein. The left gastric artery should be occluded with a vascular clamp prior to ligation, and the hepatic artery palpated to ascertain a normal origin of this latter vessel. Retroperitoneal lymph nodes and tissues cephalad to the pancreas are dissected upward toward the hiatus. If total gastrectomy is to be done, the right gastric and gastroepiploic arteries are divided and the gastrohepatic omentum is cleared from the liver. If only a partial gastrectomy is required, the right gastric and gastroepiploic arteries are retained and a Kocher maneuver is performed. We routinely perform a pyloroplasty or

pyloromyotomy in conjunction with esophagectomy to avoid problems with gastric emptying. The left inferior phrenic artery is ligated as it passes toward the diaphragmatic hiatus. A cuff of diaphragm surrounding the esophagus is taken with electrocautery.

The operation is continued in the chest. The parietal pleura overlying the aorta is incised from the diaphragm to the arch. The mediastinum is mobilized from the surface of the aorta, and esophageal arteries are divided as they are encountered. The dissection is carried on to the vertebral bodies, ligating and dividing the medial extent of the right intercostal vessels to free the azygos vein, which, with the thoracic duct, is left in continuity with the mediastinal specimen enveloping the esophagus. The thoracic duct and azygos vein are ligated at the hiatus and again 10 cm proximal to the superior tumor margin. The pulmonary ligament is taken to the level of the inferior pulmonary vein. The pericardium is entered and incised anterior to the pleuropericardial junction and distally as far as the diaphragm. The pericardium is divided across the back of the heart to the level of the right inferior pulmonary vein. Dissection should include all the subcarinal lymph nodes at this point. Following incision into the right pleura and dissection of the right pulmonary ligament, the lateral side of the right intercostal vessels are divided and ligated as they come off the vertebral bodies to complete the mediastinal dissection.

If a total gastrectomy is performed, the duodenum is divided distal to the pylorus, the esophagus is divided 10 cm superior to the proximal tumor margin, and the specimen is removed. Reconstruction is generally performed with colon following total gastrectomy. For tumors of the distal third of the esophagus, points for division of the stomach are selected 10 cm distal to the inferior extent of tumor on both the lesser and greater curvature. The stomach is divided and oversewn at this point. For adenocarcinoma of the lower third, after the esophagus is divided 10 cm proximal to the superior extent of tumor, an esophagogastrostomy is usually performed intrathoracically. For squamous carcinoma, subtotal esophagectomy is done because of the high incidence of multiple primary tumors. Following the en bloc resection extending 10 cm proximal to the superior extent of tumor, dissection is carried on the wall of the esophagus to the cervical region, where the esophagus is divided and later reconstructed with a colon interposition.

Lesions of the Middle Third

Middle third neoplasms of the esophagus are approached through the right fifth intercostal space. Mobilization of abdominal organs may be performed either through the diaphragmatic hiatus or through a separate midline laparotomy incision. The parietal pleura is divided on the right side of the vertebral bodies from the diaphragm to the level of the clavicles. Intercostal vessels are divided and the vertebral bodies cleared across the midline by elevating the azygos vein and thoracic duct along with the esophagus. When the aorta is reached the intercostal arteries and esophageal arteries are divided. The azygos vein is divided and oversewn at its junction with the vena cava, and the thoracic duct is divided. The esophagus is carefully mobilized from the membranous portion of the trachea, and the subcarinal lymph nodes are dissected free. A window of posterior pericardium is excised from the level of the pulmonary veins to the diaphragm. The left pleura is entered and the left pulmonary ligament is resected. The en bloc dissection is brought inferiorly to the level of the hiatus where the thoracic duct and azygos vein are again ligated and divided. When a margin 10 cm proximal to the superior extent of tumor is reached, the dissection is brought onto the wall of the esophagus and continued into the cervical region. The vagus nerves are divided distal to the recurrent nerves.

In the absence of obesity, previous intra-abdominal surgery, or inflammatory disease, the stomach may be mobilized through the esophageal hiatus. The short gastric vessels are divided and the left gastric artery divided near its origin from the celiac axis. The omentum is detached from the gastroepiploic arcade and the left gastroepiploic vessels are divided. In the event that the stomach cannot be mobilized through the hiatus, this part of the operation is performed through a separate laparotomy incision, which can be done synchronously with the intrathoracic dissection in the interest of saving time.

We generally perform reconstructive anastomoses in the neck to avoid the difficulties of a high intrathoracic anastomosis. This approach also allows simple percutaneous drainage and avoids empyema in case of a leak. The organ used for reconstruction (stomach or colon) is attached to the closed proximal stump of the esophagus. The ends of the sutures are left uncut and are pushed into the cervical prevertebral space for later retrieval through a neck incision. The specimen is removed and the chest closed.

Lesions of the Cervical Esophagus

Squamous carcinoma of the cervical esophagus is treated by total esophagectomy, bilateral modified radical neck dissections, and laryngectomy in conjunction with our head and neck surgical colleagues. In some cases it is necessary to perform a right thoracotomy to obtain adequate radical margins of resection, followed by removal of the remainder of the esophagus along its wall. In other instances an esophagectomy without thoracotomy is performed through a combined cervical and abdominal approach (to be discussed), followed by standard reconstruction.

Radical Versus Standard Esophagectomy

For cases in which radical resection is contraindicated because of widespread disease or when operative risk is prohibitive owing to poor physiologic status, a standard esophagectomy can be performed. This can eliminate symptoms of dysphagia and pain and prevents the onset of acute morbid complications, including hemorrhage, obstruction, perforation, and aspiration. The operation is approached in a manner similar to that described above, primarily based on tumor location. We excise the esophagus with a generous envelope of surrounding mediastinal tissue, but in contrast to the en bloc resection, we do not take pericardium, contralateral pleura, azygos vein, or thoracic duct. When lesions of the cardia are involved, splenectomy and total gastrectomy are not indicated for palliation.

An alternative technique for some patients is esophagectomy via a combined abdominal and cervical approach. Although we do not advocate this routinely, it is useful in patients who have carcinoma of the cardia, distal esophagus, or upper esophagus, and in whom thoracotomy presents undue risk or a strictly palliative esophagectomy is indicated. The cervical esophagus is exposed through a left supraclavicular incision extending from the midline. The sternocleidomastoid muscle and carotid sheath are retracted laterally, and the strap muscles, thyroid, and trachea are retracted medially. The middle thyroid vein is divided. It is useful to divide the muscle attachments to the clavicular head and manubrium to obtain adequate exposure and a tunnel for later reconstruction, but we do not practice routine resection of the clavicular head. Under direct vision, dissection and mobilization of the esophagus can be obtained almost to the level of the aortic arch. An upper midline laparotomy gives exposure to the hiatus. This is facilitated by an "upper hand" retractor. With retraction on the stomach the esophagus is separated from the crura and, again with blunt dissection, is mobilized to the level of the arch. Usually the lowest one and sometimes two esophageal arteries can be divided and ligated under direct vision. The specimen is then removed and reconstruction performed in a standard fashion following careful inspection for bleeding.

Reconstruction Following Resection

Reconstruction is done with either the stomach or colon following esophageal resection. Jejunum may be employed in instances in which great length is not needed or in which adequate stomach or colon is not available, although microvascular anatomoses are usually necessary for long jejunal segments. The stomach may be used for intrathoracic esophagogastrostomy following partial gastrectomy for lower third adenocarcinoma. Following total esophagectomy for squamous cell carcinomas, a cervical esophagogastrostomy may be performed if no stomach has been resected. In other cases, particularly following total gastrectomy for lesions of the cardia, colon interposition is required. We use a segment of transverse and descending colon based on the ascending branch of the left colic artery, placed in an isoperistaltic fashion. Although a larger procedure, colon interposition is preferred in patients who appear at operation to have highly favorable pathologic findings. This reduces the risk of esophagitis,

TABLE 3 Prevalence of Early Nonfatal Postoperative Complications Following Esophagectomy

Complication	% of Cases
Persistent pleural drainage or chylothorax	8
Pneumonia	6
Cardiac failure or arrhythmia	6
Bowel perforation or anastomotic leak	9
Wound infection	5

which occurs to a serious degree in about one-third of long-term survivors after esophagogastrostomy.

The colon is freed from the omentum. The estimated length of colon necessary to reach from the duodenum or gastric remnant to the cervical esophagus is measured and marked with sutures placed in the antimesenteric taenia for reference. The ascending branch of the left colic artery is identified and the wall of the colon dissected free just distal to this in preparation for division. The marginal artery is carefully preserved along the splenic flexure and transverse colon while the mesocolon is divided at its base. Often the middle colic vessels must be left with the interposition segment and care should be taken in dividing them close to their origin so as not to disrupt their connections with the marginal artery. When the dissection is complete save for division of the middle colic and marginal vessels, vascular clamps are applied to isolate the interposition segment from all blood supply except the ascending branch of the left colic artery, and the status of the circulation of the interposition segment is assessed. If the circulation is adequate, the middle colic and marginal vessels are divided, and the segment is left in place without dividing the bowel until the reconstruction route is prepared. Following division of the colon, the colocolostomy is performed first followed by the cologastrostomy or coloduodenostomy; the cervical esophagocolostomy is performed last. We bring the colon segment posterior to the stomach and perform the cologastrostomy in the body of the stomach. Tacking the remaining fundus loosely around the hiatus in a horseshoe shape helps to eliminate gastrocolic reflux and prevents herniation of abdominal organs into the chest. Whether or not a partial gastrectomy has been performed, we attempt to fashion the stomach into a tube when using it for an esophageal substitute to limit the capacity of its intrathoracic portion, avoiding some of the potential problems of reflux and aspiration. A portion of the lesser curvature is resected from the fundus to the angularis, which does not limit the length of the stomach to any extent, but does decrease its capacity by about 30 percent. Esophageal anastomoses are performed in a single layer using either a running or interrupted technique. We prefer a nonabsorbable monofilament suture, usually 5–0 stainless steel wire.

POSTOPERATIVE CARE

Radical dissection of posterior mediastinal lymphatic tissue makes careful respiratory management essential immediately following operation. All patients are maintained on positive pressure ventilation for at least 48 hours following surgery until significant diuresis indicates mobilization of sequestered fluid. Chest tubes are left in place until the drainage from each hemithorax is under 200 ml daily. Prophylactic antibiotics are given perioperatively and for 48 hours postoperatively. Generally the nasogastric tube can be removed 5 or 6 days postoperatively, and clear liquids are begun at this time. A barium swallow is obtained before the diet is advanced.

Early postoperative complications may occur in up to 50 percent of patients (Table 3). Operative mortality is about 10 percent and is usually due to myocardial infarction, technical complications, or pneumonia.

SURVIVAL

With radical en bloc resection, overall 5-year survival is approximately 20 percent. Metastases to lymph nodes and the extent of esophageal muscle penetration are independent variables affecting survival. In the absence of lymph node metastases and the absence of full-thickness wall penetration, 2-year survival is 80 percent. If one, but not both, of these factors is unfavorable, 2-year survival free of disease is about 50 percent. It is hoped that these results may be favorably modified through the use of adjuvant radiation therapy and/or chemotherapy.

SPECIAL PROBLEMS

Occasionally even palliative esophagectomy is not possible because of contiguous involvement of other mediastinal structures by the primary tumor, particularly the respiratory tree or the aorta. In selected situations we advocate bypass of these tumors, particularly when obstruction is imminent, or following the development of a respiratory esophageal fistula. In such cases esophageal exclusion, performed by dividing both the esophagogastric junction and the cervical esophagus and then bypassing this segment with substernal stomach or colon, can provide significant palliation with only moderate operative morbidity. In such instances it is valuable to drain the mediastinal esophagus with an intraluminal catheter brought out through a stab incision in the neck. This prevents perforation of the mediastinal esophagus in the case of obstruction and allows decompression of the esophagus if ventilator therapy is required following bypass for malignant respiratory esophageal fistula.

TABLE 4 Benign Tumors of the Esophagus

Leiomyoma
Hemangioma
Lipoma
Hamartoma
Adenoma
Mucocele
Chondroma
Papilloma

BENIGN TUMORS

There are a variety of rare benign tumors of the esophagus, the most common of which is the leiomyoma (Table 4). Benign lesions often are asymptomatic, but may present at an advanced size with dysphagia. The diagnosis is normally suspected on barium swallow and confirmed at esophagoscopy. When a benign tumor or cyst is suspected, it is important to avoid subjecting this mass to biopsy because fixation of the mucosa to the tumor at the biopsy site may compromise the ability to perform a simple operative excision. These tumors are removed via a thoracotomy and can be shelled out from the wall of the esophagus after overlying esophageal muscular layers are divided; thus the underlying mucosa is left intact. The divided muscle layers are reapproximated with interrupted simple sutures, and the patient can resume a normal diet within 2 to 3 days. Other benign tumors may require esophagotomy for excision. Closure of the esophagus should be performed over a large Maloney dilator to avoid narrowing the esophageal lumen.

THE STOMACH

BENIGN GASTRIC ULCER

LAURENCE Y. CHEUNG, M.D.
DAVID I. SOYBEL, M.D.

The incidence of gastric ulcer in the United States has remained relatively unchanged during the last decade. This is in contrast to the rapid decline in duodenal ulcer disease over the same period of time. Although the introduction of newer antisecretory and cytoprotective drugs in recent years has perhaps reduced the need for surgery in some patients with gastric ulcer, the propensity of gastric ulcers to bleed, perforate, and recur, as well as the difficulty of recognizing cancer in apparently benign lesions, eventually brings 35 percent of patients to surgery for this disease.

This review first briefly examines some of the current understanding of the pathophysiology of gastric ulceration which provides the rationale for medical and surgical treatment. We will then discuss the indications for, and results of, the medical and surgical therapies in use at present, with some attention to the problem of malignancy in benign-appearing lesions. Finally, we will discuss some of the problems encountered in elderly patients, since the majority of patients with benign gastric ulcer are elderly and often in poor general health.

Before we proceed, a word of caution in interpretation of clinical studies is necessary. Gasric ulceration is not a single disease, but rather a number of diseases. Much of the available clinical data are retrospective and have been collected sometimes without discrimination between type I ulcers (ulcers on the lesser curve and more proximal stomach) and type II (prepyloric ulcers) or type III ulcers (gastric ulcers associated with duodenal ulcers). It should be questioned whether different proportions of the three types of ulcer in different clinical studies of gastric ulcer biases the results of therapy. In some newer series, results of therapy in different groups of ulcer patients are separated, but patient numbers are small and follow-up is often limited to 2 or 3 years. This review focuses on an assessment of therapy for the type I gastric ulcer. The discussion of the pathophysiology and treatment of types II and II gastric ulcers is brief since their behavior and response to treatment are more like those of duodenal ulcers, which are discussed in another chapter of this text.

TYPE I OR LESSER CURVATURE ULCERS

Pathophysiology and Rationale of Therapy

The etiology of this type of gastric ulcer is probably related to a number of factors. Several potential sources of mucosal insult or weakening have been identified. Certain groups of patients taking aspirin regularly have an increased incidence of chronic gastric ulcer. Some of these ulcers have developed even in the absence of surrounding gastritis. Reflux of bile contents has also been observed in patients with chronic gastric ulcer and is commonly associated with diminished tone in the pyloric sphincter. Current hypotheses suggest that agents such as aspirin, bile salts, or alcohol compromise mucosal defenses against acid injury, but may not necessarily cause significant ulceration by themselves.

The concept of the gastric mucosal barrier refers to the mechanism by which the gastric mucosa maintains a hydrogen ion gradient between the lumen and the blood of $10^6:1$. The presence of damaging agents disrupts this barrier with subsequent back diffusion of acid from the lumen into the tissue, leading to mucosal acidification and ulceration. The increased amount of back diffusion of acid in these patients may in part explain the finding that these patients are rarely hypersecretors of acid and often hyposecretors as measured by gastric analysis. Despite the observation that the amount of acid secretion in these patients may be normal or even low, the presence of luminal acid still plays a central role in its pathogenesis. A number of studies have shown that virtually all patients with gastric ulcer secrete enough acid to provide a luminal pH of 3.5 or less. In addition, many conventional medical and surgical therapies rely on inhibition of acid secretion or on prevention of acid contact with the ulcer and do in fact facilitate ulcer healing. Therefore, it appears that acid may not be primary in the etiology of gastric ulcer, but its presence is essential in the development of gastric ulcer. The continued presence of luminal acid may be responsible for the complications of ulcer disease such as bleeding, perforation, or obstruction.

It has been suggested that in certain areas of the stomach the mucosal layer may be relatively susceptible to damage. Oi et al reported 170 cases of type I gastric ulcer, all of which appeared within 2 cm of the border zone containing antral and fundic tissue. When multiple ulcers were present, all were in proximity to the zone. The hypothesis that the zone represents a locus of decreased resistance is supported by observations that with increasing age this zone migrates cephalad along the lesser curvature and that the majority of ulcerations in older patients also tend to be located on a more proximal part of the stomach. This hypothesis is also consistent with some older clinical observations that benign gastric ulcers that healed spontaneously or were only locally excised often recurred in the same location. Thus, it suggests why hemigastrectomy, which includes the excision of both the ulcer and the border zone, offers the lowest incidence of recurrences.

Medical Treatment

The medical management of gastric ulcers involves certain considerations. First, up to 10 percent of all gastric ulcers and perhaps 3 percent with benign roentgeno-graphic appearance prove to be malignant. In general, if medical therapy is planned, we believe that all gastric ulcers should be examined endoscopically and six to ten biopsies of each lesion should be obtained. If the ulcer recurs or fails to heal by 8 to 12 weeks, we repeat endoscopy for additional biopsies to again exclude malignancy. A second consideration is that although 60 percent of type I gastric ulcers may heal without specific therapy, approximately 70 percent of these ulcers recur within 1 to 2 years. Even if the ulcers heal with specific therapy, recent studies suggest a high rate of recurrence unless patients are maintained on at least prophylactic doses of medication. The long-term rates of recurrence (over 5 years) with prophylaxis have not been well documented, and the long-term side effects of maintenance doses of the various medications are also unknown.

Table 1 summarizes the results of medical management of benign gastric ulcers with placebo, antacid, cimetidine, or sucralfate. The numbers are pooled from a variety of studies in the United States, United Kingdom, and Europe. As already mentioned, spontaneous healing

with placebo alone is 44 percent by 6 weeks and 68 percent by 12 weeks. Antacids improve the rate of healing, but it has not been well documented whether they prevent recurrences. Histamine H_2 antagonists accelerate healing to 90 percent by 12 weeks and, with maintenance doses, appear to reduce the incidence of recurrence. Nevertheless, some 10 to 25 percent of patients treated wtih cimetidine or ranitidine suffer recurrence in 1- to 2-year follow-up. The proportion of these patients returning with emergency complications such as bleeding and perforation has not been well defined, but several case reports have indicated that sudden discontinuation of these medications can precipitate these serious complications.

Sucralfate is a basic aluminum salt of sulfated sucrose and is viscous at acid pH. It adheres to the ulcer base, protecting it from further erosion by acid-pepsin and bile contents. It improves the healing rate of gastric ulcer, although perhaps not as well as in duodenal ulcers. Since its activity depends, in a sense, on the presence of the ulcer, there is no clear rationale for its use to prevent recurrence. Accordingly, the recurrence rate during prophylactic use of sucralfate appears to be higher than with H_2 blockers. Other agents including carbenoxolone, colloidal bismuth, and prostaglandins have been used with success in some patients, but these agents are not available at present for general use in the United States.

On the basis of these figures, the current recommendations for conservative management of a clearly benign type I gastric ulcer might include an initial trial of sucralfate, particularly if a source of injury such as aspirin or alcohol could be identified and removed. A first recurrence would be treated by an H_2 antagonist, which could be continued prophylactically after healing. Several studies have shown that a first recurrence heals as readily as the initial lesion. A second recurrence is, at the present time, an indication for surgery.

Surgical Treatment

Elective surgery should be considered for patients with more than one recurrence, those with lesions in which

TABLE 1 Gastric Ulcer Healing with Conventional Medical Therapies

	6 Weeks % Healed	12 Weeks % Healed	1 Year With Prophylaxis % Recurred	Major Side Effects
Placebo	44	68	70–80	--
Antacid	61	84	--	Changes in bowel habits Mineral imbalances
H_2 Antagonists cimetidine/ranitidine	75	90	15–25	Gynecomastia Thrombocytopenia Leukopenia Mental disturbances
Sucralfate	70	85	35–50	Constipation Phosphate binding

Data derived largely from two review articles:
  1. Brogden RN et al. Drugs 1984; 27:194–209.
  2. Lewis JH. Arch Int Med 1983; 143:264–274.

malignancy cannot be exluded, and those who are stabilized following admission for complications such as occult or mild bleeding, or obstruction. Long-term results (5 years or more follow-up) with surgical therapy for benign gastric ulcer are shown in Table 2. In low-risk patients the operative mortality is less than 1 percent for most vagotomy procedures and slightly higher for gastric resections. Gastric resection is attended by a greater number of postoperative complications, but is associated with fewer recurrences and fewer reoperations. "Quality of life," as recorded using the Visick grading system, thus appears to be no different, overall, between patients undergoing vagotomy procedures and those undergoing resection. From these considerations, hemigastrectomy including the excison of gastric ulcer is the procedure of choice. Vagotomy is not necessary for most patients undergoing hemigastrectomy for benign gastric ulcer of type I. Vagotomy may be performed in addition to hemigastrectomy in selected patients with gastric ulcer such as those under 35 years of age with hypersecretion of acid, in patients taking steroids or nonsteroidal inflammatory agents, and in uremic or alcoholic patients.

The reconstruction of the gastrointestinal tract following hemigastrectomy depends on the location of the ulcer and on the presence or absence or inflammation or scarring of the first portion of duodenum. Since most type I gastric ulcers do not involve the pylorus or first portion of duodenum, Billroth I reconstruction can usually be performed without technical difficulty or the fear of a compromised anastomosis. Reports in the literature suggest that a Billroth I reconstruction may be "more physiologic" with respect to postgastrectomy syndromes, but this is far from a universal opinion.

The highly selective vagotomy with ulcer excision merits special attention. This operation is said to preserve antral motility and storage function, and to prevent alkaline reflux into the stomach. It has had impressive 2- to 3-year cure rates in the hands of a few surgeons. However, with longer periods of follow-up and in the hands of other surgeons, the recurrence rates are similar to those obtained with nonselective vagotomy and drainage procedures. In addition, it has not been established whether patients with biliary reflux in fact benefit from the preservation of pyloric function. Finally, if Oi's hypothesis is correct, this operation does not address the problem of the locus of decreased resistance. Although this operation may be beneficial for patients who will not tolerate a major gastric resection, it has not yet been proved to be the procedure of choice for all patients with type I gastric ulcer.

Benign-appearing lesions can harbor malignancy and, if detected in the ulcer stage, may be curable in half the cases. Ulcers should be excised whenever possible and sent for frozen section. If multiple ulcers are present, biopsies should be taken from all gross ulcers for sectioning. Giant ulcers and ulcers near the esophagogastric junction have a higher incidence of complications such as bleeding and possibly a higher incidence of malignancy. If a hemigastrectomy including the ulcer can be done by carefully placing clamps along the lesser curvature without narrowing the esophagogastric junction, this is the preferred procedure. If this cannot be accomplished technically, ulcer excision with distal gastric resection or with vagotomy and pyloroplasty is recommended. Interest has been revived recently in Pauchet's operation, which is a distal resection in continuity with a "tongue" of lesser curve tissue including the ulcer. This tongue can be fashioned to include posterior or anterior ulcers. In elderly patients with severe atherosclerosis, dissection of the esophagogastric junction and ligation of the short gastric vessels may compromise blood supply to an anastomosis in this area. Overall, however, this operation merits further appraisal.

Emergency surgery is indicated for perforation and for uncontrolled hemorrhage. Unlike prepyloric or channel ulcers, type I gastric ulcer rarely causes gastric outlet obstruction. Rebleeding within the same hospitalization or endoscopic visualization of a vessel within the ulcer crater ought to be indications for urgent surgical intervention. Emergency surgery carries a much worse prognosis with 10 to 40 percent mortality, depending on risk factors. These factors include age over 65 years, poor general health, and specific liver, cardiac, or pulmonary ailments such as cirrhosis, active hepatitis, chronic

TABLE 2   Elective Operation for Benign Gastric Ulcer

Procedure	Operative Mortality	Operative* Morbidity	% Recurrence (5 Years)	% Reoperation For Ulcer	% of Patients Visick I and II At 5 Years
Highly selective vagotomy (with ulcer excision)	0–2%	0–5%	8–25% (5 yr)	5–10%	70–80%
Vagotomy and drainage (with ulcer excision)	0–5%	1–10%	10–25% (5 yr)	5–10%	70–85%
Hemigastrectomy (with BI or BII reconstruction)	1–5%	5–15%	2–10% (5 yr)	1–2%	75–85%

Data compiled from a variety of studies reported in the United States, United Kingdom, and Scandinavian countries.
* Includes pulmonary, renal, hepatic complications of surgery as well as wound infection, dehiscence, bleeding, or anastomotic breakdown.

obstructive lung disease, aspiration, congestive heart failure, or arrhythmia. Complications of emergency conditions such as hypotension, electrolyte imbalance, or sepsis with or without abscess formation are often the primary causes of death. Significant improvements in the survival of patients presenting with emergency complications are now being achieved with early admission to an intensive care unit for correction of electrolyte imbalances and for aggressive repletion of blood and blood volume.

The decision concerning the type of operative procedures for gastric ulcer with complications such as perforation and bleeding depends on the general condition of the patient and the degree of peritoneal soiling in the case of perforation. If possible, the treatment of choice is hemigastrectomy including excision of the ulcer. In younger patients, especially those with prior history of ulcer disease, such definitive therapy prevents the higher recurrence rates associated with simple closure or excision of the ulcer with or without vagotomy.

For patients who are unstable or in poor general health, there is a place for vagotomy and drainage when used in conjunction with excision of the ulcer or closure of the perforation. This is the expedient alternative to gastric resection in poor risk patients, but the recurrence rates are high. Ten percent of patients treated this way for bleeding gastric ulcer will rebleed. In some studies, 20 to 30 percent of patients with perforated type I gastric ulcers treated with vagotomy, drainage, and closure eventually required gastrectomy, and 85 percent of these patients continued to experience ulcer-related symptoms.

One final point worth mentioning is that the incidence of malignancy in bleeding, perforated, or obstructing gastric ulcers has been reported as high as 2, 8, and 10 to 15 percent, respectively. Therefore, the ulcer should be excised whenever possible during an emergency operation. If the ulcer is not excised during this initial surgery, endoscopy and biopsy should be performed when the patient has recuperated from the operation.

Gastric Ulcer in the Elderly Patient

Age alone is not a contraindication to surgical treatment. However, elderly patients have a higher incidence of systemic diseases. They present more frequently with complications and often delay in seeking medical attention. Lower operative mortality and early recognition of complications can be achieved by an aggressive approach to diagnosis with endoscopy, early surgery for complications, observation in the intensive care unit with Swan-Ganz catheterization for hemodynamic monitoring, and attention to blood volume, coagulation parameters, and electrolytes.

In some of these elderly patients with chronic pulmonary disease, we place a gastrostomy tube to avoid a nasogastric tube. This allows more aggressive pulmonary toilet. In occasional patients with poor nutritional status, we may consider the placement of a jejunostomy tube for postoperative feeding. The pH of the gastric aspirate should be monitored, and antacids are administered when the pH is less than 4. Antacids with a high content of sodium should be avoided. Because of possible interference with absorption of drugs such as digoxin or quinidine, the serum levels of these drugs should be measured. Following recovery from gastrectomy, the elderly patient is more prone to develop iron or vitamin B_{12} deficiency anemias and metabolic bone diseases due to fat malabsorption. Hemoglobin, hematocrit, blood smears, and serum alkaline phosphatase levels are followed more frequently in these patients following gastrectomy.

TYPES II AND III GASTRIC ULCERS

Gastric ulceration does occur in some patients with chronic duodenal ulcer disease. Dragstedt proposed that this is a result of altered antral pyloric motor function secondary to the presence of duodenal ulcer. This altered pyloric function or gastric outlet obstruction would then lead to antral stasis and would subsequently result in release of increased amounts of gastrin. The high level of circulating gastrin would cause hypersecretion of acid, leading to development of the gastric ulcer (type III). Prepyloric ulcers or pyloric channel ulcers (type II) can also be considered Dragstedt ulcers or ulcers similar in characteristics to duodenal ulcers. Therefore, both type II and type III gastric ulcers can be treated medically and surgically as in patients with duodenal ulcer disease, as discussed in another chapter of this text. The preferred surgical procedure for these ulcers would include resection of the ulcer and a procedure that will decrease the amount of acid secretion. The recommended procedure is vagotomy and antrectomy to include the ulcer. The reconstruction, Billroth I or Billroth II, depends on the inflammatory status of the duodenum. Because these are essentially hypersecretory ulcers, it is important to perform vagotomy in addition to hemigastrectomy in this group. Vagotomy and drainage procedure alone is an acceptable alternative, but is clearly a second choice.

MALLORY-WEISS SYNDROME

CHOICHI SUGAWA, M.D.

The Mallory-Weiss syndrome consists of upper gastrointestinal bleeding caused by a linear nonperforating laceration of the proximal gastric mucosa associated with sudden increases in intra-abdominal pressure. This injury usually results from vomiting, retching, or violent coughing.

In 1929, Mallory and Weiss, pathologists at the Boston City Hospital, detailed the case histories of 15 patients who developed massive hematemesis following prolonged bouts of retching and vomiting during an alcoholic debauch. Four of them succumbed and at autopsy demonstrated a linear "fissure-like" ulceration of the mucosa of the gastric cardia, one of which extended across the gastroesophgeal junction. They attributed these lacerations to increased intragastric pressure produced as a consequence of vomiting and were able to reproduce the lesions in two cadavers by applying pressure to the stomach while simultaneously occluding the pylorus and proximal esophagus. For several decades thereafter, the Mallory-Weiss "syndrome" was considered to be a rare but often lethal entity, invariably associated with massive blood loss. With the advent of the widespread use of fiberoptic endoscopy, however, it has become apparent that the Mallory-Weiss tear is far more common than previously supposed, that blood loss is usually minimal, and that the condition is almost always self-limiting and innocuous.

A wide variety of events may initiate the Mallory-Weiss tear including vomiting, retching, coughing, straining, hiccupping, gastroscopy, seizure, childbirth, lifting, and cardiopulmonary resuscitation.

Mallory-Weiss lacerations occur most often in middle-aged male adults and are rare in children. The typical tear is short (1 to 2 cm), is invariably solitary, and is confined to the gastric mucosa in more than 75 percent of instances. The majority of Mallory-Weiss tears are located just below the gastroesophageal junction on the lesser curvature of the stomach (52% to 78%), 8 to 23 percent are located on the greater curvature of the stomach, 10 to 18 percent are on the posterior surface, and 4 to 7 percent are on the anterior surface.

The Mallory-Weiss syndrome seems to occur more frequently in patients with an established hiatal hernia. In addition, a significant number of patients have a transient hiatal hernia observed only during retching or at the beginning of the endoscopic examination. The Mallory-Weiss syndrome is generally accepted to be the result of a large transient transmural pressure gradient between the intra-abdominal and intrathoracic compartments at the gastroesophageal junction. When the gastroesophageal junction is vigorously elevated above the diaphragm during violent retching or vomiting, the gradient results in dilatation of the gastroesophgeal junction and mucosal tearing. The location and direction of the mucosal tear relate to the geometric configuration of the stomach and esophagus. A tear will occur where the tension is greatest. The stomach may be considered as a cylinder, and therefore the tension required to tear the mucosa in the longitudinal direction is one-half that required to produce a tear in the transverse direction.

In about 10 percent of instances, the gastric tear extends up into the esophageal mucosa. In the absence of gastric hiatal herniation, the intraluminal pressure is greatest in the distal esophagus, and disruption of the esophageal mucosa may occur. At extremely high intraluminal pressure, esophageal circular and longitudinal muscle layers may also tear, producing a full-thickness, emetogenic rupture called Boerhaave's syndrome. An unusual phenomenon observed in several patients suggests that an additional mechanism may contribute. During endoscopy, I have observed active retching that resulted in a transient "mushrooming" of the stomach into the esophagus as a kind of reverse intussusception. Mushrooming of the stomach more than 10 cm into the esophageal lumen was found in one patient with a large tranient hiatal hernia during retching. The tears that resulted were all in the cardia of the stomach. The larger portion of the mucosa on the greater curvature seemed to be mushrooming during retching. The preponderance of Mallory-Weiss tears along the lesser curvature may therefore result from relative immobility of that portion of the stomach and subsequent exposure to high-shearing forces and pressures during retching or vomiting.

The diagnosis of Mallory-Weiss tears can often be established on historical grounds alone. Vomiting or retching preceding the hematemesis is reported in over 50 percent of instances, whereas primary hematemesis that occurs without the documented antecedent emesis occurs in less than 40 percent. In approximately 5 percent of cases, melena is reported as the sole presenting symptom. Although alcohol use and/or abuse remains a common accompaniment of the Mallory-Weiss tear, it is important to recognize that any forceful retching may produce sufficient increases in intragastric pressure to produce the lesion. The resultant bleeding is often arterial and, in contrast to an emetogenic rupture, is painless in more than 60 percent of instances.

INITIAL MANAGEMENT

Our initial approach to the patient with Mallory-Weiss-related hematemesis is the same as for any patient with upper gastrointestinal hemorrhage and consists of an orderly sequence of resuscitation, diagnosis, and treatment. A clinical assessment of the magnitude of hemorrhage is made based on the patient's vital signs, including the presence or absence of orthostatic hypotension. A nasogastric tube is passed to confirm the presence of intragastric blood and to ascertain whether the patient is actively hemorrhaging at the moment. A large-bore intravenous catheter is inserted, and resuscitation with crystalloid solutions is begun. In patients suspected of major blood loss, a Foley catheter and a central venous pressure line are also inserted in order to monitor the status of volume replacement. Appropriate laboratory studies are obtained, including an assessment of the patient's bleeding and clotting status. This is especially important in patients with a concomitant history of alcohol abuse. Type-specific blood is also crossmatched. The presence of severe epigastric pain, difficulty in breathing, or shock out of proportion to the estimated amount of blood lost should alert one to the possible concomitant presence of a Mallory-Weiss tear and an emetogenic rupture, which is a rare event indeed.

DIAGNOSTIC STUDIES

Endoscopy

Despite the controversy that surrounds the use of early endoscopy in patients with upper gastrointestinal hemorrhage, it has been the policy in our institution to use this approach in (1) all patients suspected of having sustained a major gastrointestinal hemorrhage, and (2) any patient in whom even a minor bleed may have serious consequences; for example, those patients over 60 years old, those with a low admission hemoglobin, those who require three or more units of blood to achieve hemo-dynamic stability, and those in whom the nasogastric aspirate contains bright red blood. We have adopted this approach because of our inability to accurately predict, on clinical grounds alone, which patients in this high-risk category will require operation and because, if operation is undertaken, perioperative mortality is substantially increased in the absence of firmly established preoperative diagnosis, irrespective of the source of hemorrhage. With specific respect to Mallory-Weiss tears, the diagnosis is made by the presence of either active bleeding, a clot, or a fibrin crust over a mucosal tear immediately adjacent to the gastroesophageal junction. Patients with a non-bleeding linear lesion consistent with a Mallory-Weiss tear may also have another definite source of bleeding in the stomach and should be treated for that definite source of bleeding.

Early diagnostic endoscopy is highly accurate (90%) and can provide valuable information, including the location and length of the laceration and the presence or absence of any associated lesions such as esophagitis, gastritis, peptic ulcer, or esophageal varices. Indeed, such lesions are encountered in 40 to 70 percent of patients with Mallory-Weiss tears and are actually responsible for the major component of the hemorrhage in a sub-stantial number. The high incidence of concomitant acute gastric mucosal lesions (AGML), duodenitis, and esophagitis is thought to be due to ethanol ingestion. The incidence of esophageal varices (7.3%) also attests to the frequency of ethanol abuse in this patient population. The associated mucosal lesions may have induced the retching and/or emesis which produced the Mallory-Weiss laceration. An awareness of other potential bleeding sites is important in understanding the etiology of the Mallory-Weiss laceration, and in planning surgical or medical treatment. Furthermore, endoscopic visualization of the tear is of significant prognostic value. Those that are actively bleeding or demonstrate fresh clot may well continue to bleed or rebleed early, whereas those without active bleeding or with simple mucosal contusions (''ring'' and ''disc'' lesions) are unlikely to cause the patient any subsequent difficulty. Prior to subjecting the patient to endoscopy, the stomach should be lavaged copiously with saline through a large-bore orogastric tube. This maneuver not only removes intragastric clots, but it frequently acts as a therapeutic maneuver.

The majority of patients with Mallory-Weiss tears require only simple saline lavage and general supportive care. I have used endoscopic electrocoagulation with success, but have employed it less frequently in recent years since I have found that most bleeding stops spontaneously.

When indicated, a monopolar coagulating electrode is passed through the biopsy channel of the gastroscope and the area of the stomach or esophagus adjacent to the bleeding site is coagulated. Three or four applications are usually required, but no individual site is treated repeatedly. Our results have been quite good (initial control in 10 out of 12 patients), but the risk of producing transmural necrosis is real and requires careful adjustment of the duration and amplitude of the applied current. New endoscopic hemostatic methods such as bipolar electro-coagulation, laser, heater probe, and injection of dehydrated alcohol may obviate the need for surgery. Endoscopic hemostasis by submucosal injection of dehydrated ethanol was successful in two of the three patients in whom this was attempted.

Angiography

On rare occasions, the rate of hemorrhage is so brisk that endoscopic visualization of the bleeding site is impossible. In these instances, angiography may play an important role in the diagnosis and treatment. Angio-graphy, with either intra-arterial vasopressin infusion or arterial embolization, has been reported to be effective in treating persistently bleeding Mallory-Weiss tears. This procedure is accurate in more than 70 percent of patients with Mallory-Weiss tears. Extravasation of contrast medium is observed most commonly from the left gastric artery, but may also be seen from branches of the splenic or inferior phrenic arteries. In the presence of hemorrhage of this magnitude, it is possible to use the selectively placed catheter to initiate an immediate trial of angio-graphic pharmacotherapy. Vasopressin is infused selectively for 20 minutes at a rate of 0.2 U per minute, at the end of which time a repeat arteriogram is per-formed. If the bleeding has stopped, the infusion is continued at the same rate for 24 hours, then decreased to 0.1 U per minute for an additional 24 hours. If no bleeding ensues at this point, 5% dextrose in water is infused through the catheter for 12 hours and then removed. On the other hand, if bleeding continues after the initial infusion of vasopressin, the dosage is increased to 0.4 U per minute. If hemorrhage is still demonstrable after 20 minutes, operative therapy may be undertaken.

Vasopressin given in this manner is not innocuous. Systemic complications, including hypotension, arrhythmias, myocardial infarction, sepsis, and small bowel infarction, have been observed as well as local complications such as a false aneurysm and infection at the site of entry. The use of angiography in the presence of massive hemorrhage is probably justified, particularly in patients who present with the prohibitive operative risks of cirrhosis. Under less urgent circumstances, however, a more discriminating approach to selecting patients for pharmacotherpy is warranted.

Barium Studies

In contrast to endoscopy and arteriography, the use of barium studies as a diagnostic tool in patients with Mallory-Weiss tears is a fruitless exercise, having a diagnostic accuracy approaching zero. The tears are too superficial to be filled with barium. Furthermore, residual intraluminal barium precludes the use of diagnostic and/or therapeutic angiography in those rare instances in which this approach is required.

NONOPERATIVE MANAGEMENT

The clinical course of patients can be predicted on admission by observation of two factors: (1) the degree of bleeding at the time of endoscopy, and (2) the presence of liver disease. Patients in whom bleeding has stopped before endoscopy usually maintain a benign hospital course. By contrast, massive bleeding at the time of endoscopy can be a grave sign since massive bleeding was present in 11 of our 12 fatal cases; significantly, eight of these 12 were cirrhotic. Except in the following instances, initial therapy in patients with Mallory-Weiss tears should be relatively specific. In those in whom no active bleeding is detected at the time of endoscopy and in whom the tear is in a gastric location, the stomach is intubated in order to accomplish titration of intragastric content of a pH greater than 4. In most instances, the instillation of 30 to 60 ml of antacid on an hourly basis is sufficient to accomplish this. The gastric contents are aspirated hourly, their pH determined, and evidence of rebleeding sought. In those instances in which a non-bleeding tear is located in a junctional or esophageal position, intubation is omitted in order to avoid direct irritation of the laceration. Sixty milliliters of antacid are ingested every 2 hours while the patient is awake. Complications of antacid therapy are few and relatively easily managed. They include hypernatremia, hypermagnesemia, metabolic alkalosis, diarrhea, and, when aluminum-containing antacids are used, medication bezoars.

Cimetidine is also added to the regimen, 300 mg being given intravenously every 6 hours. In patients with severely compromised renal function, the dosage should be reduced in order to avoid potential complications of mental confusion and leukopenia. It should also be recalled that cimetidine impairs the activity of certain hepatic drug-metabolizing enzymes, most importantly those involved with the degradation of propranolol and diazepam.

Additional therapeutic measures include the correction of abnormalities in bleeding and clotting function and the administration of transfusions as necessary. Of the patients with hematemesis secondary to Mallory-Weiss lacerations, 75 to 90 percent require less than three units of blood to restore normal circulating blood volume. Even if active bleeding is identified at endoscopy, the same regimen is used. However, a nasogastric tube is placed, irrespective of the location of the tear, in order to assess the presence or absence of continued bleeding. Under either circumstances, the therapeutic watchword is "observation" combined with judicious transfusion. In more than 90 percent of cases, this approach is associated with cessation of hemorrhage, usually within a matter of hours. Rebleeding is uncommon (1% to 2%) and is usually manifested within 2 to 3 days. If no further hemorrhage is evident by this time, the nasogastric tube is removed, antacid consumption reduced, and the patient is gradually advanced to a regular diet.

Despite the measures just outlined, bleeding continues in approximately 10 percent of instances, necessitating additional therapeutic intervention. Such a circumstance is not uncommon in patients with severe liver disease and should be anticipated when more than one unit of blood is required every 6 hours in order to maintain hemodynamic stability. No more than two such 6-hour intervals should be allowed to pass before more aggressive action to control hemorrhage is undertaken.

Several options are available. Although reported experience is small, systemic (intravenous) vasopressin may be utilized to stop bleeding. Initially, 20 units are infused as a bolus over a 15- to 20-minute period. Subsequently, vasopressin is given as a continuous drip at a rate of 0.2 to 0.4 U per minute. The success of failure of this approach is usually evident within 1 to 2 hours. Some authors prefer systemic to selective (intra-arterial) vasopressin under these conditions because of similar efficacy (a 15% to 20% reduction in mesenteric blood flow) and because the catheter complications associated with intra-arterial infusion (thrombus formation with limb ischemia) are avoided. Furthermore, the other complications of vasopressin infusion such as ventricular arrythmias, depressed cardiac output, fluid retention, and, rarely, myocardial infarction seem to occur with equal frequency, irrespective of the route of administration. Vasopressin should be used with great caution in the presence of ischemic heart disease. Patients treated in this manner require simultaneous and continuous cardiac monitoring. Because of these potential problems, it has not been our policy to use systemic vasopressin in all patients with Mallory-Weiss tears as soon as the diagnosis is made—an approach that has been advocated by some.

Other potential therapies include the topical application of norepinephrine endoscopically and angiographic embolization of Gelfoam or autologous clot into the appropriate feeding vessel. I have had no experience with either of these modalities, and reported experience is both small and disappointing. Tamponade of the laceration by means of a Sengstaken-Blakemore balloon has been occasionally recommended. However, most series report a low success rate (25% to 30%), and several indicate that inflation of the gastric balloon may actually recreate the mechanism of injury and increase the size and depth of the tear.

OPERATIVE MANAGEMENT

Operative therapy should not be delayed once it is clear that alternative approaches have failed. Perioperative antibiotic coverage is recommended, and I prefer to use one of the newer-generation cephalosporins, giving the first dose preoperatively and two additional doses in the early postoperative period. Most lacerations are readily visualized through a high anterior gastrotomy by using a large diameter retractor while pulling upward on the nasogastric tube. This allows the cardia to be brought into view and exposes the folds at the esophagogastric junction. Occasionally, invagination of the cardia with a sponge forceps and/or placement of a traction suture in the distal end of the esophagus may be required to facilitate exposure. Rarely, lacerations may extend for a considerable distance into the esophagus. Under these conditions, downard traction on an inflated 30-cc Foley catheter placed into the distal esophagus usually reveals the entire extent of the tear.

Lacerations are successfully repaired with a variety of suture materials. I prefer continuous 3–0 silk, beginning the repair at the most distal portion of the tear. Operative mortality is low (5%), but postoperative morbidity can be considerable, especially in cirrhotics (40% to 60%).

Common complications include postoperative bleeding, wound infection, subphrenic abscess, pancreatitis, delirium tremens, renal failure, hepatic failure, cardiac arrhythmias, atelectasis, and pneumonia. Some believe that complications can be reduced by avoiding gastrotomy and have advocated full-thickness plication of the tear from the serosal aspect of the gastroesophageal junction, using intraoperative endoscopy to guide suture placement. I have not had experience with, or occasion to use, this technique. Recurrent bleeding following successful operative repair of a Mallory-Weiss laceration is uncommon, and the prognosis, especially for non-alcoholic patients, is excellent.

GASTRIC TUMOR

WALTER LAWRENCE, Jr., M.D.

Clinically significant gastric neoplasms include a few benign tumors and primary lymphomas, but the overwhelming preponderence are carcinomas of glandular origin. Variations of these carcinomas of the stomach comprise more than 90 percent of gastric tumors that become clinically evident. These will be addressed first.

ADENOCARCINOMA OF THE STOMACH

There are two well-recognized observations in terms of the epidemiology of gastric cancer. The first is that the incidence of this disease has been decreasing in the United States over the last 50 years. The second is that there is a great deal of geographic variation in mortality rates from gastric cancer. It remains a relatively common killer in countries like Japan, Chile, and Iceland, where the death rate is approximately five times that of this country. It is still an important disease for us, however, as there are 25,000 new cases each year in the United States.

Several physical problems have been associated with a higher incidence of gastric cancer. Patients with pernicious anemia, hypochlorhydria, or achlorhydria appear to develop this disease more frequently than others. Also, a number of studies have shown that a prior gastric resection with Bilroth II anastomosis leads to a higher incidence of gastric cancer, and vagotomy has been implicated by some. However, it is difficult to separate the importance of the usual mucosal factors associated with cancer (e.g., gastritis) from the postgastrectomy state since some gastritis is always present in the gastric remnant.

Clinical Presentation

With no truly diagnostic symptoms or signs for diagnosing early gastric cancer, or even curable gastric cancer for that matter, the physician must be aggressive in completely evaluating any patient over forty with the suggestion of an upper gastrointestinal disorder. In the last 20 years, fiberoptic gastroscopy has played a larger and larger role in the evaluation of patients with possible gastric disease (particularly peptic ulcer disease), and it has proved to have a great potential for proper identification of suspicious lesions or early gastric cancer, as well as providing an opportunity for accurate histologic diagnosis. The Japanese have identified a higher proportion of ''early'' and superficial cancers by this approach, but this has not been the trend in the United States.

Pathology

Adenocarcinoma is by far the most common cancer involving the stomach. Borrman described four gross presentations of this lesion in 1926 and his classification has been useful. The types are polypoid carcinoma (I), ulcerating carcinomas with sharply demarcated margins and no infiltration of significance (II), ulcerating and infiltrating cancers without a clear-cut margin (III), and diffusely infiltrating carcinomas (IV). Additional gross types have also been proposed, including superficial spreading carcinomas (large, favorable superficial lesions that are confined to the mucosa and submucosa of the stomach) and "early" gastric cancer (a pathologic entity singled out by the Japanese that does not extend beyond the submucosa). Although favorable "early" gastric cancers may constitute up to 30 percent of some Japanese series, these early cancers are seen in less than 10 percent of any American series. These various pathologic types of adenocarcinoma of the stomach have had prognostic significance after resection in that Borrman types I (polypoid) and II (ulcerocancer) are much more favorable than the more common type III (ulcerating and infiltrating). The gross type described as diffusely infiltrating carcinoma (IV) has the poorest prognosis of all and is rarely treated successfully by resection despite apparent localization of the process at the time of operation.

Staging

The staging of the patient with carcinoma of the stomach, as an aid in selecting treatment, is based on the clinical extent of the disease, as demonstrated by the physical examination and by roentgenographic and endoscopic studies (clinical-diagnostic stage). A more accurate staging classification for end-results reporting after operative treatment is based on the extent of disease found at the time of surgical exploration of the abdomen.

The findings of cervical lymph node metastases, liver metastases, peritoneal metastases, or metastatic lesions at less frequent sites establishes the clinical stage as stage IV, a category only suitable for a palliative approach. Often these adverse findings are not apparent until celiotomy is performed, although preoperative evaluations may allow proper categorization and treatment planning.

The principal factor affecting the TNM classification on postgastrectomy pathologic staging from the standpoint of the primary tumor (T) is the degree of penetration of the gastric wall by the carcinoma. The size or location of the primary tumor is of less significance in assigning T and estimating prognosis. The nodal involvement (N) is a significant prognostic factor in the staging process, and the level of the N ranges from no metastases to nodes (NO), to lymphatic spread to immediately adjacent nodes (N1), to nodes in the perigastric area often on both the lesser and greater curvatures (N2), or to more distant nodes (N3). Distant metastases to peritoneal surfaces, the liver, or other sites detected at operation are categorized as MI, a uniformly poor prognostic sign.

Operative Management

At present, and for the foreseeable future, surgical resection is the only truly effective method for the primary treatment of gastric cancer. Today, despite definite improvements in operative and postoperative management that have diminished operative mortality, the overall control rates after resection for gastric cancer remain low. If a regionally localized process in the stomach is found at the time of exploration, adequate resection of the primary neoplasm, as well as actual and potential regional lymphatic extensions, is performed. Less than 40 percent of patients who are "explored" for possible resection are able to undergo a resection with some hope for cure. Palliative resection does have a role, however, even if all the gross disease that is found cannot be resected.

Although the incidence of regional lymphatic spread varies with different gross and histologic types of cancer, the overall incidence of lymphatic spread from carcinoma of the stomach is high, approximately 60 percent. In addition, gross observations often do not reveal whether or not lymph node metastases are present. In designing a radical gastrectomy for patients with "curable" gastric cancer, one must include the removal of potential regional lymphatic extensions.

Choice of Operation

The major options for resection of gastric cancer are distal subtotal gastric resection, simple total gastrectomy, or "extended" total gastrectomy. The latter procedure includes resection of adjacent organs involved by the neoplastic process by local extension, such as the body and tail of the pancreas, liver, transverse colon, or, in rare instances, the head of the pancreas. Inclusion of extragastric organs in the resection is an infrequent consideration owing to the fact that there are usually additional signs of incurability when these organs are involved. This naturally discourages the surgeon from proceeding with a major multi-organ resectional procedure.

The specific operation employed is chosen in each patient by determining the extent of disease that is present. Total or extended total gastrectomy is no longer chosen "in principle" as we failed to show significant benefits from the routine and uniform application of these procedures to most gastric cancer patients back in the 1950s. Total gastrectomy is preferred to proximal subtotal resection of the stomach for proximal gastric cancers in most circumstances. An adequate margin for lesions in the area of the cardia often results in a relatively small distal gastric remnant of esophagogastric anastomosis if adequate margins are achieved. In addition, patients surviving long intervals after proximal gastrectomy usually have reflux esophagitis problems. Reservoir reconstruction after total gastrectomy probably leads to a better functional result for long-term survivors than is achieved by maintaining a small distal segment of stomach by esophagogastric anastomosis.

Reconstruction After Surgical Resection

After distal subtotal gastrectomy, continuity should always be restored by gastrojejunostomy rather than gastroduodenostomy. The former procedure avoids the problem of gastric outlet obstruction in patients should they develop recurrent carcinoma following attempted "curative" resection. Recurrence tends to manifest itself in the region of the pancreas in most instances and is more likely to obstruct a gastroduodenal anastomosis in the immediate region than an anterior gastrojejunostomy.

The weakest point in the reconstruction after total gastrectomy is the esophageal anastomosis, and this should be carried out as precisely as possible to avoid subsequent leakage in the postoperative interval. Because this requires excellent operative exposure, I prefer a thoracoabdominal incision when the choice of operation is total gastrectomy. Another precaution to be followed before completing the esophagojejunal anastomosis is performance of frozen section pathologic examination of the transected esophagus to ascertain that this site is cancer-free. The reason for this is that submucosal extension of the cancer often occurs beyond the gross margins of the lesion. The anastomosis itself is preferably completed with an inner row of interrupted silk sutures placed through all layers of the esophagus and the jejunum, with the knots tied within the lumen (Fig. 1). External buttressing sutures help to seal the anastomosis, but the full-thickness inner row is the crucial part of the anastomosis from the standpoint of avoiding leaks. Some surgeons have employed intraluminal stapling instruments for this anastomosis, with success.

Prior to restoring continuity by the end-to-side esophagojejunostomy, just described, I construct a double-lumen jejunal pouch (using a stapling device) in order to create a reservoir to substitute for the resected stomach.

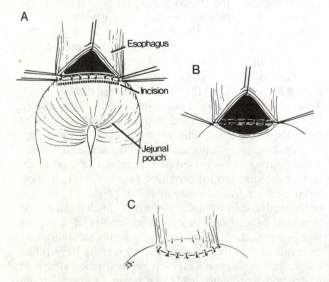

Figure 1 Esophagojejunostomy is accomplished by interrupted sutures through all layers of esophagus and jejunum. An outer row buttresses this anastomosis.

It is more convenient to accomplish this before the esophagojejunostomy, but it is not necessary to do so. A Roux-en-Y anastomosis of proximal jejunum to the loop of jejunum distal to the pouch prevents reflux into the esophagus and reduces the rate of outflow of foodstuff from the jejunal reservoir area (Fig. 2). This anastomosis is completed *after* the end-to-side esophagojejunostomy so that the surgeon is certain that the intestinal loops fit comfortably without angulation in the upper abdomen. This pseudopylorus tends to reduce both postgastrectomy "dumping" symptoms and nutritional problems. Other methods of reconstruction after total gastrectomy that attempt to achieve some form of reservoir substitute for the stomach may well be equal to this one, but the use of some form of reservoir construction has been shown to be clearly superior to simple esophagojejunal anastomosis without a reservoir of some type.

Palliative Gastrectomy

A significant number of patients with gastric cancer have unfavorable operative findings at the time of celiotomy, such as tiny serosal implants, liver metastases, ovarian metastasis, or metastatic disease in lymph nodes outside the range of a radical en bloc dissection. This is the finding in more than 60 percent of patients with gastric cancer who are subjected to operation with the hope that a curative resection can be accomplished. A palliative resection of the gastric cancer is always preferred under these circumstances if the procedure can be accomplished without resorting to total gastrectomy, without transection of gross tumor at the site of the planned anastomosis, and without major hazard to the patient. If these conditions are met, palliative resection provides significant relief of symptoms in the majority of patients and also appears to prolong survival. In carefully selected patients, even total gastrectomy may be employed for palliation, particularly if the patient has obstruction as a major problem or if extensive lymphatic spread is the only finding preventing a complete curative resection. Patients with nonresectable lymphatic spread have been shown to have a much longer survival interval after palliative resection than patients who are considered incurable because of liver or peritoneal metastases.

Complications of Gastrectomy for Carcinoma

Patients who have undergone high subtotal gastrectomy or total gastrectomy are prone to develop postprandial symptoms, the so-called dumping syndrome. This symptom complex inhibits intake and is the primary cause of nutritional problems when they occur. There is great variability among individual patients in this regard, but it seems wise to avoid hyperosmolar feedings (high carbohydrate) until the patient has established himself on a reasonable diet in the postoperative period and has recovered completely from the operation. It is my custom to gradually advance the diet offered to the postgastrec-

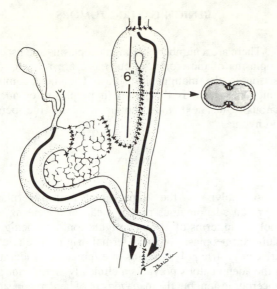

Figure 2 Diagram of a useful method of reservoir reconstruction after total gastrectomy.

tomy patient to a six-feeding, high protein, high fat, low carbohydrate diet (antidumping diet) and maintain him on this until convalescence has progressed to the point where weight gain has occurred and dietary experimentation can be considered. The possibility of anemia as a complication of gastrectomy must be borne in mind as well, and the most frequent early mechanism for this is decreased iron absorption. Inadequate absorption of vitamin B_{12}, through the loss of intrinsic factor, is a much later mechanism for anemia in patients undergoing total gastrectomy. It is not a major problem until 4 or more years after the operation because of the large liver stores of vitamin B_{12}.

Technical complications, such as anastomotic leak, rarely occur after partial gastrectomy, but the possibility of leakage at the site of an esophagojejunostomy is enough reason to maintain an external drain in the subdiaphragmatic area for a period of 8 to 10 days postoperatively. My approach is to gradually withdraw this drain after an esophagram has shown no anastomotic leak and the patient has successfully initiated oral intake. Although anastomotic leaks are rare with precise anastomotic techniques, adequate drainage of a small leak is accomplished via the drain site if a leak does occur, and the patient can be fed distal to this site through the "nasogastric" tube until the small fistula closes.

Role of Radiation and Chemotherapy in Gastric Cancer Management

Radiation therapy is rarely useful in the management of gastric cancer since the usual reason for nonresectability is the lack of localization of the malignant process. On the other hand, radiation therapy has been useful for palliation in selected patients for relief of a localized area of obstruction, particularly in the region of the cardia, and also for patients with chronically bleeding cancers that

cannot be resected. Some surgeons have been using intraoperative adjunctive radiotherapy in clinical trials, but this technique has not been studied long enough to allow a full evaluation.

Many chemotherapeutic agents have been employed singly for the palliation of gastric cancer with generally disappointing results. In one large review, approximately 22 percent of patients with advanced unresectable gastric cancer who were treated with 5-fluorouracil (5-FU) demonstrated transient evidence of improvement of a limited degree, with no definite increase in survival time. Many other single agents have been employed with minimal palliative benefit being noted, except possibly for the drug Adriamycin. However, there has been more enthusiasm for various combinations of agents for the palliation of patients with advanced gastric cancer. Agents in these combinations include 5-FU, nitrosoureas, mytomycin-C and Adriamycin. The specific combinations of 5-FU, Adriamycin and mytomycin-C (FAM), and 5-FU with methyl-CCNU, have been associated with objective response rates that are over 40 percent in prospective trials. Nevertheless, it is still uncertain whether overall survival is significantly increased as a result of this approach to palliative chemotherapy for nonresectable gastric cancer.

The overall results of operative resection for gastric cancer are dissatisfying enough to encourage aggressive clinical trials of adjuvant chemotherapy for patients undergoing so-called "curative" gastrectomy. A recent study from the Gastrointestinal Tumor Study Group appears to show a significant survival advantage at four years for gastric cancer patients treated within 6 weeks of gastrectomy with the combination of 5-FU and methyl-CCNU (compared to randomized control patients receiving no chemotherapy). A similar adjuvant study (from the Veteran's Administration) with a slightly different dosage of these same agents failed to show benefit. Currently, there are several prospective clinical trials comparing FAM with postoperative observation. The final results of these and future adjuvant studies are being eagerly awaited since combinations of agents appear to be effective in the palliative management of advanced disease, and our postsurgical results leave much to be desired.

Prognosis for Adenocarcinoma of the Stomach

At present, the overall outlook for patients with gastric carcinoma remains poor since two-thirds of the patients have either physical or operative findings at the time of diagnosis that completely eliminate the possibility of surgical "cure"; no more than one-third of the patients undergoing "curative" resection currently live 5 years or more after treatment. This postsurgical salvage of 10 to 15 percent of all patients with the diagnosis of adenocarcinoma of the stomach is discouraging. The majority of patients who develop regrowth of their gastric cancer usually do so within 3 years of their primary surgical treatment, and roughly 90 percent of patients reaching the 5-year mark remain cancer-free in most series.

There are some prognostic factors that modify these discouraging statistics somewhat, and these may be of some importance in determining the prognosis of individual patients with this disease. The various gross pathologic presentations serve as prognostic indicators, as described earlier. However, the presence or absence of lymphatic metastases is the most significant prognostic variable that has been noted in all series of patients subjected to "curative" gastric resection. Only a small proportion of patients with lymphatic metastasis (15%) enjoy long-term survival after radical gastrectomy even though this resection includes the regional lymph nodes. The patients without lymphatic metastasis who are suitable for curative radical gastrectomy are the only group with a reasonably good prognosis; approximately 50 percent of these patients enjoy long-term survival. Despite the lack of conclusive evidence from adjuvant chemotherapy as yet, this approach is still our major hope for possible improvement in these treatment results.

OTHER MALIGNANT TUMORS OF THE STOMACH

Malignant lymphoma is the second most common cancer arising in the stomach, accounting for up to 8 percent of all cancers of this organ. Although the disease present in the stomach may be just one manifestation of a systemic process in some patients (particularly patients with Hodgkin's disease), non-Hodgkin's lymphoma often has its primary and only site in the stomach. The second most common cancer of mesodermal origin is leiomyosarcoma, a lesion comprising 1 to 3 percent of all gastric cancers. With either of these diagnoses, the neoplastic lesion is often resected on the assumption that it is a carcinoma on the basis of gross evaluation. The unsuspected diagnosis of lymphoma or sarcoma is then only revealed after the operation, unless a preoperative endoscopic biopsy has correctly identified the lesion. In each instance, the general plan for resection is virtually identical to that for adenocarcinoma, and no harm is done by this delay in accurate diagnosis. One major difference, however, is that the prognoses for both leiomyosarcoma of the stomach and primary lymphoma of the stomach are considerably better than that for adenocarcinoma (5-year survival rates are approximately twice as high).

Although the primary objective of operation for these uncommon lesions is identical to that for adenocarcinoma, the relative radiosensitivity of lymphoma has led to the recommendation that all patients with primary lymphoma of the stomach be given adjuvant radiation therapy after surgical resection. Cases of non-Hodgkin's lymphoma of the stomach are too infrequent to prove the value of radiation therapy conclusively, but the dogma has a reasonable basis, particularly for patients with regional lymphatic metastases. The latter group are those for whom I carry out this treatment plan. Chemotherapy must be considered for this group as well as for patients with even more extensive disease.

BENIGN GASTRIC TUMORS

There are a number of benign neoplasms and pseudoneoplasms of the stomach, but these are rare in comparison to the malignant lesions. The most common benign neoplasm is the polyp (hyperplastic or adenomatous), the next most common being the benign leiomyoma.

Polyps

A "polyp" of the stomach may be a hyperplastic polyp, an adenomatous polyp, a cancer appearing as a "polyp" in terms of gross configuration, or a benign or malignant neoplasm of mesodermal origin. The relative rarity of gastric polyps seems to eliminate consideration of the adenomatous polyp as a clinically significant precancerous lesion, but the management of benign-appearing polypoid lesions of the stomach is still confused by differing concepts of their neoplastic potential.

The relationship between hyperplastic polyps and cancer is practically nonexistent. Two features suggesting some relationship between the adenomatous polyp and cancer of the stomach are the slightly increased incidence of adenomatous polyps in a stomach with an established cancer, and the high incidence of achlorhydria and atrophic gastritis both in patients with adenomatous polyps and in those with cancer. Although 15 to 20 percent of adenomatous polyps do develop cytologic atypism (carcinoma in situ), there is little evidence that this lesion frequently proceeds to clinical cancer. Fortunately, these cytologic changes have not been observed frequently in polyps smaller than 2 cm in diameter, a factor that allows us to develop a reasonable and logical treatment plan for these small polypoid lesions.

If single or multiple polypoid lesions of the stomach actually cause symptoms, such as bleeding or obstruction, surgical intervention is certainly indicated to eliminate these symptoms. A solitary polyp, or multiple lesions of limited extent, can be treated by conservative resection. If there are no symptoms, the polypoid lesion less than 2 cm in diameter can be safely observed by serial radiographic or gastroscopic examinations on the basis of data from a number of series. However, if a single lesion is larger than 2 cm, excision of the entire lesion in question is indicated. If there is diffuse polyposis (a rare situation), gastrectomy may be required to eliminate the abnormality, but there is no clear-cut evidence for a relationship of this process to cancer that is comparable to that of familial polyposis and colon cancer.

Leiomyomas

These are common lesions of the stomach at autopsy, but they do not come to attention clinically unless they reach a large size. The usual presenting symptom is blood loss from ulceration of the overlying mucosa. Some leiomyomas reach a huge size and retain the pathologic features of a benign lesion; some may become quite cystic. Some intramural lesions of this type are difficult to differentiate from the malignant variant, leiomyosarcoma. At times, this determination is finally made by the pathologist only in terms of the frequency of mitotic figures in the surgical specimen.

Treatment is usually adequate local excision of the leiomyoma. This entails full-thickness resection of a segment of the gastric wall involved with the neoplasm with a 2- to 3-cm margin. Formal gastrectomy with anastomosis is not usually required. The operative management of a low-grade leiomyosarcoma is similar to this since lymphatic spread is not an important feature of this neoplasm.

Other Mesodermal Tumors

Lipomas, neurogenic tumors, glomus tumors, accessory pancreas, and inflammatory tumors (eosinophilia granuloma or inflammatory polyps) are extremely rare and require only local resection of the lesion with repair of the stomach. Carcinoid of the stomach is a rare

lesion and is usually thought to be a carcinoma because of its gross features at the time of operation. Actually, this neoplasm is usually treated as a carcinoma, and this seems reasonable since some of these lesions are capable of metastasis.

One benign related lesion that may confuse both the surgeon and his surgical pathologist is ''pseudolymphoma.'' This diffuse or discrete lesion accompanies some benign gastric ulcers and, in these instances, undoubtedly represents an atypical inflammatory response in the region of the ulcer. Differentiating this lesion from true lymphoma at the time of operation is frequently a difficult problem for the surgical pathologist since lymphomas may also develop ulceration. Fortunately, most gastric pseudolymphomas present in the antropyloric region with sparing of the gastroesophageal region. It is the consensus that resection is appropriate management for this process, but the extent of resection would clearly be less than for cancer if a clear-cut diagnosis of pseudolymphoma can be achieved. Long-term follow-up of patients undergoing resection for pseudolymphoma is indicated because of the theoretical but unproven possibility of progression from pseudolymphoma to a truly malignant lymphoma.

GASTRIC RESTRICTIVE PROCEDURE FOR MORBID OBESITY

ANTHONY L. IMBEMBO, M.D.

The effects of obesity on health have been rather difficult to unravel over the years and even now are poorly understood. In the past, it was the mortality studies done by various insurance companies that constituted the most often quoted reason for viewing significant obesity as a serious disease correlating with a shortened life expectancy. In the 1959 tables issued by the Metropolitan Life Insurance Company, the mortality of obese patients weighing 20 to 30 percent more than the median for a given age group was several times the expected rate for control, nonobese individuals. The company has recently issued revised *Tables of Desirable Weights* which are higher than the 1959 standards, especially for short people. The new tables were compiled on the basis of traced mortality among 4.2 million individuals who applied for life insurance between 1954 and 1972. Below-average weights were still found to correlate with greater longevity. However, the data for obesity of a moderate degree are less definite than in the past. There are numerous difficulties in accepting such data as being accurate or representative as they have been drawn from a highly selected pool of individuals and, in all likelihood,

constitute an atypical population. In addition, outcomes are largely based on the vagaries of information collected from various imprecise sources, such as death certificates, which reflect a wide range of professional competence.

Of much more interest in determining the possible adverse effects of obesity on health are the various prospective studies that have been, or are being, carried out in an attempt to correlate obesity with various serious conditions, the incidence of which has been commonly assumed to be increased in an obese population. Hypertension now has been shown to be more common in the obese patient, although the severity of the hypertension usually is moderate and the degree of obesity may not correlate at all with the severity of the hypertension. In the Framingham study of cardiac and related diseases, hypertension developed ten times more often in patients who were 20 percent or more overweight. It has also been shown that the hypertensive obese patient has a greater risk of developing left ventricular hypertrophy and congestive heart failure than does an individual in the normal weight range. More recently, the Framingham group have also shown that obesity is an independent risk factor for development of significant cardiovascular disease.

The relationship of obesity to cerebrovascular disease is significant and seems to exist even in the absence of hypertension. Both obesity and significant weight gain are associated with a five- to tenfold increase in the incidence of cerebrovascular disease or stroke. Increasing body weight and increasing age are both associated with an increased incidence of diabetes mellitus. It has been estimated that the incidence of diabetes is five to seven times greater in individuals who weigh more than twice their ideal weight. In addition, 80 percent of patients with adult onset diabetes are significantly overweight. Weight loss often ameliorates glucose intolerance, although it is somewhat unclear whether all of the complications of diabetes are prevented by weight reduction.

A number of other conditions seem to occur with greater frequency in the massively obese patient. The incidence of deep venous thrombosis and chronic venous insufficiency seem to be increased, at least on the basis of retrospective data. This may be due to venous stasis from the relative immobility of these large patients or to the frequent finding of elevated plasma free fatty acid levels. Free fatty acids accelerate coagulation and may therefore be associated with the development of venous thrombosis. There is a clear association between chole-lithiasis and obesity, the incidence of gallstones being estimated as 30 to 40 percent in the obese population. Obesity does not seem to correlate specifically with hyper-lipidemia. Although cholesterol production is increased in obese patients, serum levels tend to be relatively normal as a result of increased cholesterol elimination in the stool. However, increased cholesterol synthesis may be partially responsible for gallstone formation. Orthopaedic problems seen with great frequency include degenerative arthritis of the lumbar spine, hips, and knees and intervertebral disc herniation.

Massive obesity is not only a medical problem, but also a social, psychologic, and economic one. Massively obese patients generally demonstrate low self-esteem, passive dependency, vulnerability to depression, marked self-consciousness, and a sense of helplessness or ineffectiveness. They usually have a markedly distorted body image and are relatively unresponsive to the usual internal cues controlling eating. They experience difficulty in interpersonal relationships, marriage, employment, and community acceptance. They frequently demonstrate a tendency to withdraw in an effort to avoid the risk of ridicule.

The treatment of choice for obesity remains a dietary program of caloric restriction. Unfortunately, this does not work very often. In several series from large centers, only 10 to 20 percent of patients were able to lose 20 pounds in patient populations consisting of individuals weighing more than 200 pounds. Even fewer patients were able to maintain weight loss for more than a few months, and one-quarter never returned to the clinic setting after the first visit. Over the years, numerous drugs have been advocated at various times for the management of obesity. Modifications of various sympathomimetic amines have been developed and aggressively promoted for use in weight control. When adequate trials of such medications were done, efficacy was found to be limited. About 50 percent of obese subjects showed no response at all to the medication; another one-third significantly reduced their food intake, but were unable to distinguish the drugs being tested from placebo. At present, drug therapy has no role in the treatment of obesity.

Various psychotherapeutic approaches have been applied with increasing frequency on the assumption that abuse of food is a behavior disorder and therefore a learned response. Research on the behavioral treatment of obesity has achieved popularity that may verge on faddism. Despite extensive study, it has been difficult to develop a clear picture of the clinical import of behavioral technologies because sample sizes in most studies are small, and treatment of necessity is restricted to short temporal intervals. Most behavioral modification programs work toward the development of self-monitoring and stimulus control techniques, emphasize slowing of the rate of eating, help to generate social support, and stress exercise coupled with dietary planning. The evidence suggests that the results are somewhat better than those obtained with most of the other forms of therapy. The weight loss tends to be modest, averaging between 10 and 20 pounds in individuals weighing more than 200 pounds. However, the losses tend to persist for at least a year following treatment. The patients generally are not able to achieve additional weight loss outside such a program. However, variability among patients is considerable.

Radical dietary programs are to be condemned. Serious adverse effects may result from such efforts. Diets that result in significant ketosis may precipitate hyperuricemia and gout, nephrolithiasis, and occasionally chronic renal failure. Hypotension can result from longstanding fluid and electrolyte losses. Cardiac function may be significantly impaired by ketosis, as well. Peripheral neuropathy and Wernicke's encephalopathy have also been reported to develop as a consequence of prolonged fasting.

INDICATIONS AND PATIENT SELECTION

The impetus for surgical treatment of massive obesity stems from (1) the assumption that obesity of considerable degree has an adverse effect on health and (2) the well-recognized observation that medical management is almost totally ineffective in the treatment of this problem. Two general types of procedure have been used for the surgical treatment of massive obesity. An extensive experience has been gained with the small bowel bypass of either the end-to-side or end-to-end variety. With these procedures, weight loss generally resulted both from the induction of a severe malabsorption state and from a variable, but fairly consistent, change in dietary intake secondary to anorexia. The majority of patients who have undergone small bowel bypass experience significant weight loss. However, the complication rates, particularly long-term, are excessive. Among the more significant complications are liver failure, arthritis, calcium oxalate renal stones, electrolyte abnormalities, pseudocolonic obstruction, and intractable diarrhea. As a result, the small bowel bypass has largely been abandoned.

More recently, various gastric restriction procedures have been under intense investigation in many centers. All of these procedures are based on the creation of a small proximal gastric reservoir. In addition, the outlet from the reservoir is severely restricted, usually measuring no more than 1 cm in diameter. With the gastric bypass procedure, the distal stomach and duodenum are totally excluded, a gastrojejunostomy being created to the small proximal gastric pouch. In the various, more recently described gastric partitioning procedures, the exclusion does not occur. Instead, the stomach is partitioned by means of stapling techniques of various types in order to create the small proximal reservoir with a severely restricted outlet. The success of any gastric restriction procedure depends on induction of early satiety following ingestion of small amounts of food. Significant behavior modification is also necessary relative to patterns of eating and food abuse. These patients must learn to avoid large meals and to adhere to a regular meal pattern rather than nibbling throughout the day. For example, it is well recognized that gastric restriction procedures can be rendered ineffective if the patient ingests high calorie foods in small amounts virtually throughout the day.

The indications for surgical treatment of massive obesity should remain highly restricted. The patient must be massively obese, weighing at least twice ideal weight, and the obesity should be totally refractory to conventional therapeutic efforts. It is my feeling that the procedure must be fully warranted as the techniques and approaches continue to undergo rapid evolution and remain somewhat investigational. I tend to insist on documentation attesting to failure of conventional therapy aimed at achieving weight loss. Such efforts should have been under physician or hospital direction. Correctable endocrinopathies must be ruled out. These are rather infrequent in obese patients presenting for surgical treatment. Nonetheless, thyroid function tests, diurnal study of cortisol secretion, and urinary corticosteroid studies should be obtained. The patient should be in relatively good health except for obesity. However, the presence of certain conditions that may be ameliorated by significant weight loss may constitute a partial indication for a surgical approach to weight reduction. Such conditions include diabetes mellitus, essential hypertension, hypercholesterolemia, Pickwickian syndrome, and sleep-apnea syndrome. Finally, social and economic considerations may play a role in deciding whether to proceed. For example, massively obese individuals may be employable only after significant weight loss has occurred.

Proper patient selection is essential for success. The patients are managed by a team consisting of the surgeon, a psychiatric support group, a dietitian, and a nurse clinician. Candidates for the procedure are seen by the operating surgeon for an initial evaluation, which includes a detailed medical history and complete physical examination. Emphasis is placed on weight history and dietary habits. The contemplated procedure is reviewed in detail, emphasizing both the possible benefits and the risks, including failure to lose weight. Detailed descriptive information regarding the structured postoperative dietary program is also provided. Emphasis is placed on adherence to the program in an effort to achieve behavior modification. It is stressed that the weight loss that occurs following a gastric restriction procedure depends, to a considerable degree, on patient cooperation, motivation, and understanding.

If deemed to be a potentially suitable candidate by the surgeon, the patient is referred for psychiatric evaluation. By means of multiple interviews, an attempt is made to determine whether the patient has the emotional stability, intelligence, and motivation to succeed should the gastric restriction procedure be performed. Particular efforts are made to uncover impulsive or addictive behavior, immaturity, and depressive tendencies. The family situation and available supportive resources are reviewed. The patient's spouse is expected to participate in the evaluation; spousal cooperation, support, and understanding are important for success. The patient is expected to participate in group interaction and therapy. The group consists of individuals being evaluated for the procedure and those who have undergone gastric restriction and are in the process of behavior modification. In this way, the preoperative patient is directly exposed to the postoperative program and comes to appreciate that considerable support will be available during the period of weight loss. Group participation also leads to increased understanding of the postoperative regimen. Meetings with the preoperative group permit further assessment of motivation and ability to comply with the established program. Acceptance for surgical treatment requires approval both by the surgeon and by the psychiatric support team. Prior to the patient's admission to the hospital, an upper gastrointestinal series is performed to rule out unsuspected conditions, such as a significant sliding hiatal hernia. Gastric restriction may worsen pre-existing gastroesophageal reflux or facilitate its development in the setting of a large hiatal hernia. In addition, preoperative pulmonary function studies are obtained to facilitate anesthetic management.

TECHNIQUE

At present, I perform gastric partitioning for the treatment of massive obesity. In many hands the gastric bypass has been found to be superior to gastric partitioning as regards weight loss. However, it is my feeling that by using the specific gastric partitioning technique (described below), coupled with careful patient selection and postoperative support, excellent results can be achieved with minimal operative risk.

In our institution, gastric partitioning is performed utilizing a left lateral thoracic approach. This approach has been developed in an effort to facilitate exposure of upper abdominal structures so as to easily and reproducibly create a small proximal gastric reservoir. Following placement of suitable venous access lines, the patient is positioned for a left lateral thoracotomy. The skin of the entire left chest and upper abdomen is prepared and draped. A true lateral thoracotomy skin incision is made. The dissection is carried down to the underlying latissimus muscle, which is divided completely. The electrocautery is used throughout to minimize bleeding. Once the latissimus has been divided, the ribs are counted from above. The eighth interspace is used to enter the thorax. Usually, the lateral incision provides excellent exposure and there is no need to divide posterior muscle groups. The intercostal muscles are divided and the pleural space entered. A large rib-spreading retractor is introduced, and by gentle patient traction, exposure is achieved.

A nasogastric tube must be placed before the patient is positioned. The position of the tube in the esophagus is confirmed. The spleen is easily palpated through the diaphragm. The diaphragmatic incision parallels the rib cage, thereby minimizing the risk of damage to branches of the phrenic nerve. The incision should be planned to begin fairly close to the esophageal hiatus and extend to a point just anterior to the previously palpated spleen. Traction sutures of 2–0 silk are placed in the diaphragm. These are used to elevate the diaphragm from the underlying intraperitoneal structures. The incision is then made, horizontal mattress sutures being used for hemostasis and traction.

The left triangular ligament of the liver may have to be taken down to facilitate exposure. The greater curvature of the stomach is mobilized from the level of the upper short gastric vessels to the diaphragmatic hiatus. It is usually unnecessary to separate the entire spleen from the stomach, except when the spleen is particularly large. Each of the divided short gastric branches is ligated with 2–0 silk. There are usually some filmy attachments between the posterior stomach and the peritoneum overlying the tail of the pancreas. These are taken down easily. Next, the lesser curvature of the stomach is cleared from the esophageal hiatus to a point approximately 5 cm distally. Usually the uppermost branch or two of the left gastric artery must be divided as it enters the wall of the stomach. There are corresponding anterior and posterior branches, each of which must be divided, clear this segment of lesser curvature. Care is taken not to disrupt the esophageal attachments so as to minimize the risk of subsequent gastroesophageal reflux.

The gastric staple line must be positioned so as to create a proximal pouch with a capacity of approximately 20 cc. For significant weight loss to occur, it is exceedingly important that a very small pouch be devised. The staple line generally extends from a point 2 cm distal to the gastroesophageal junction on the lesser curvature to a point 3 to 4 cm distal to the junction on the greater curvature. The partitioning usually is done with the TA-55 automatic stapler, utilizing 4.8-mm staples. The stapler should be introduced from the lesser curvature side. Before the partitioning is performed, three staples are removed on the greater curvature end of the cartridge. A Keith needle is helpful in removing the staples from the cartridge. Prior to the actual firing of the staples, the pouch should be calibrated. This procedure consists of closing the stapler at the point contemplated for firing and instilling saline through the nasogastric tube into the proximal pouch. If the pouch is deemed too large, the stapler is moved proximally to create a smaller pouch. Once a suitably small pouch has been designed, the stapler is fired. A single staple line is used. After the staples have been fired, the nasogastric tube is passed through the aperture on the greater curvature side into the distal stomach. Care must be taken to avoid bunching of the stomach wall within the jaws of the stapler prior to firing;

otherwise the staples do not completely occlude the stomach.

Various techniques have been designed and advocated to reinforce the staple line and to minimize the risk of early dilatation of the aperture between the proximal and distal stomach. In general, I believe that such reinforcement is not necessary. The technique of reinforcing the channel with Teflon pledgets is to be condemned. Such external pledgets enhance fibrotic ingrowth, and obstruction of the staple line is a frequent occurrence. A single Prolene suture placed on the lesser curvature side of the aperture adjacent to the nasogastric tube, which has been passed into the distal stomach, may be the only reinforcement occasionally necessary.

The wound is irrigated with an antibiotic-containing solution. Hemostasis is ensured. The diaphragm is closed with interrupted horizontal mattress sutures of 2–0 nonabsorbable material. A single No. 36 Argyle chest tube is placed and brought out through a separate stab wound inferior to the incision. The chest incision is closed in the standard way with pericostal sutures and running 1–0 Vicryl sutures to the various muscle layers. Since there is not a great deal of fat on the thoracic wall, even in the most obese patient, the subcutaneous tissue is easily closed with running 2–0 Vicryl sutures and the skin closed with sutures or skin clips.

Prior to the procedure, prophylactic antibiotics, effective against *Staphylococcus aureus* and the more common bowel organisms, are started. Antibiotics are continued for 2 days following the procedure. In addition, prophylactic subcutaneous heparin, 5,000 units every 12 hours, is started several hours prior to the procedure and continued until discharge. Subcutaneous heparin may help to minimize the incidence of postoperative venous thrombosis in these high-risk patients.

POSTOPERATIVE CARE

Intraoperative problems are minimal when the foregoing approach is used. The risk of splenic injury is almost eliminated since exposure is excellent. With superior exposure, it is possible to ensure creation of a very small gastric pouch, a step essential for success with gastric partitioning. In general, the patient's immediate postoperative course is benign. I have experienced no instance of leakage from the gastric suture line in over 50 patients. Wound infection is rare since the bowel in never entered. Patients tolerate the thoracic approach as well as an upper abdominal midline incision from a pulmonary standpoint. Pain is relatively modest and can be easily controlled by means of standard analgesic medications. The chest tube is removed as soon as drainage is minimal, usually on the first postoperative day.

Oral feedings are started once the adynamic ileus has resolved completely. Initially, the patient receives 30 cc of water or ice per hour. This is gradually increased until 60 to 90 cc per hour are tolerated by the patient. The patient is instructed to sip the fluid allotment slowly and not to ingest the entire amount at once. As soon as possible, the patient assumes responsibility for recording oral intake. The maintenance of a dietary log throughout the period of weight loss is an important behavior modification technique. Once water has been tolerated, clear liquids are introduced. The patient is then gradually advanced to a liquid diet, which includes soup and some blenderized foods. All foods must be thin enough to pass through a straw. The patient is instructed not to take more than 60 to 90 cc each hour. Any sense of fullness means that the patient should withhold oral intake for another hour. The patient's caloric intake is limited to 600 to 800 calories per day. A specific listing of permitted foods is provided. Liquids high in calories and sugar content are avoided; such foods include regular carbonated beverages, milkshakes, and whole milk. A liquid multivitamin supplement should be taken daily. Long-term metabolic complications of gastric partitioning are rare; however, there have been occasional reports of vitamin deficiency. An exclusively liquid diet is continued for a minimum of 8 weeks.

Long-term postoperative care is shared by the surgeon, psychiatric support team, and dietitian. The patient is scheduled for regular visits to the surgeon, as leader of the team. Every visit includes a review by the dietitian of the patient's dietary log and daily caloric intake. Once immediate postoperative problems have resolved, patients return to the clinic on a monthly basis. In addition, the patient begins participation in the postoperative group therapeutic program. As before, the group consists of both pre- and postoperative patients. This form of support has been found to be of great value in dealing with specific dietary problems and in providing emotional support. Individualized visits with the psychiatric team are also arranged as necessary to deal with any significant emotional problems that may arise.

On occasion, morbidly obese patients test the capacity of the gastric pouch by exceeding the amount of food allotted, causing a sense of fullness and/or moderately severe epigastric distress. Patients are urged not to test the suture line for fear of dehiscence or premature dilatation of the proximal pouch. After the 8-week liquid intake phase has been completed, soft foods are introduced. Patients again are urged not to ingest more than 2 to 3 ounces of solid food at a time. They are instructed to weigh portions and, again, not to ingest high caloric liquids at all. Caloric intake is restricted to 800 to 1,000 calories per day. Most patients do not reach the upper calorie limit. They are urged to introduce new foods one at a time to ensure adjustment and tolerance.

Following this procedure, approximately 85 percent of patients have an excellent result, defined as a weight loss greater than 25 percent at the 2-year follow-up point. Success depends on the technical details just described, proper patient selection, and consistent, careful, and understanding postoperative support. Failure to lose weight may result from a technical error. However, in most cases, it is due to inability to achieve significant behavior modification as regards eating. This emphasizes the importance of patient selection for success in management of this difficult problem.

PEPTIC ULCER

TZU-MING CHANG, M.D.
BRUCE E. STABILE, M.D.
EDWARD PASSARO, Jr., M.D.

Although there appears to have been no change in the way peptic ulcer disease presents, there is clear evidence that both in the United States and Europe there has been a decrease in the incidence of peptic ulcer disease. Moreover, the risk of acquiring the disease has been shown to be related to the individual's year of birth (the "cohort phenomenon"), with the relative risk being carried forward throughout life. As a consequence of the declining incidence, the average surgeon has had a correspondingly decreasing experience treating the disease while the individual patient is older and more difficult to manage by virtue of his age. In this chapter we present our current thoughts on the treatment of this disease based on a long experience at our hospital. Interested readers are directed to a recent monograph we have prepared (Current Problems in Surgery, Year Book Medical Publishers, Inc., January, 1984) for detailed reference material if desired.

A number of operations are now available to the surgeon who treats peptic ulcer disease. The choice of operation rests on a variety of considerations, and in each case the operation should be tailored to the individual patient's needs. Factors to be weighed in selecting a particular operation include the location of the ulcer; the indication for operation; the chronicity of the disease; the degree of suspicion of malignancy; the age, sex, and nutritional state of the patient; the presence of other serious illness; the clinical stability of the patient during surgery; and the experience and personal preference of the surgeon.

A singularly important concept in surgery for peptic ulcer disease is that clinical outcome is dependent on the operative indication. Both patient and surgeon should be aware that the results of operation to a large degree are determined by whether the operation is to be performed for pain, bleeding, perforation, or obstruction, or some combination thereof. Unfortunately, in many texts and individual reports of surgical experience, this observation is not always considered, making interpretation of the data difficult. Other important determinants of surgical outcome are the patient's clinical condition and the surgeon's abilities. With fewer surgeons accumulating an adequate experience, surgery for peptic ulcer disease may soon be relegated to those with a particular interest and experience in the disease. The complications attending failed surgery for peptic ulcer disease are formidable. Reoperation is often required and may be particularly difficult.

DUODENAL ULCER

Intractability

Although such pain was common in the past, few patients are now referred for operation for uncontrolled pain. However, about 8 percent of patients fail to heal their ulcers with conventional histamine H_2 receptor antagonists, e.g., cimetidine and ranitidine. On the other hand, most of these patients obtain prompt relief from their symptoms despite the presence of a persistent or recurrent ulcer on endoscopy. Repeated endoscopic examinations, therefore, are important in the evaluation of these patients. More commonly, patients fail therapy with these agents because of recurrence of both symptoms and ulcers following cessation of the medication.

Despite the fact that many American surgeons are not conversant with it, we consider parietal cell vagotomy to be the most appropriate procedure for intractability. The operation denervates only the parietal cell-bearing portion of the gastric mucosa and thus is not attended by the need for a drainage procedure as in the case of truncal (total abdominal) or selective (total gastric) vagotomy. Parietal cell vagotomy has a lower mortality (0.1% to 0.3%) than any other procedure for duodenal ulcer disease. This is appropriate for a complication which in itself is not lethal. Additionally, its low morbidity from either surgical complications (e.g., intra-abdominal sepsis) or late sequelae (e.g., dumping, gastric retention, or diarrhea) make it ideally suited to treat this complication. These advantages stem from the fact that the lumen of the gastrointestinal tract is not entered during the procedure, and that the antral-pyloric emptying function of the stomach is only minimally altered.

Procedures that combine more extensive vagotomy (truncal or selective) with emptying procedures such as pyloroplasty, gastroenterostomy, or antrectomy, which either ablate or bypass the antral pyloric pump, cause untoward sequelae (e.g., early satiety, weight loss, gastric retention, diarrhea, and dumping) much more commonly (20% to 40%) than does parietal cell vagotomy (5% to 10%). We consider the advantages of the latter procedure to so outweigh the alternative operations that parietal cell vagotomy is recommended as the only procedure for the intractable duodenal ulcer.

The wide experience of surgeons in Scandanavia with this procedure shows that ulcers located in the pyloric channel or in the prepyloric antrum should not be treated with parietal cell vagotomy. In these instances, ulcer recurrence rates of 20 to 30 percent have been noted. Ulcers in these locations, while behaving clinically like duodenal ulcers, are particularly refractory to both medical and conservative surgical management. They are best treated by truncal or selective vagotomy, antrectomy, and gastroduodenostomy.

The main disadvantage of parietal cell vagotomy is an ulcer recurrence rate of approximately 10 to 15 percent, which is not significantly different from that reported with truncal vagotomy and pyloroplasty. It has been clearly shown that the recurrence rate is a function of the operating surgeon so that surgeons less facile with the procedure have unacceptable recurrence rates of 20 percent or more. Necrosis of the lesser curvature of the stomach due to devascularization or direct operative injury has been noted in a number of cases and is associated with a 50 percent mortality. Thus, reperitonealization of the lesser curvature following the vagotomy is commonly done to avoid delayed necrosis and perforation. Perforation of the esophagus, as with any other form of vagotomy, is also a potential hazard.

Postoperative recurrent ulcers in the duodenum are best treated by a combination of truncal vagotomy, antrectomy, and gastroduodenostomy.

Perforation

The vagaries of a perforated ulcer are such that this complication provides a strong test of clinical judgment. Many papers have addressed the individual issues which have provoked continuing controversy on the optimal surgical approach. In this debate, too often the emphasis has been placed on a definitive operation whereas the overriding consideration is to get the patient through the immediate insult. In our experience, most patients with perforation require resuscitation and closure of the defect, and that all considerations for a definitive operation be deferred.

In young patients (under 30 years of age) with perforation, the history for duodenal ulcer disease tends to be short (less than 3 months) or nonexistent. In patients without a prior history of peptic ulcer disease, we recommend simple closure of the ulcer with a reinforcing omental onlay and subsequent close follow-up for recurrent disease. The majority of these patients (greater than 70%) require no further procedure.

Patients with an antecedant history of duodenal ulcer disease of 3 months or more should be considered for an initial definitive procedure. Studies have shown that up to 70 percent of these patients have subsequent serious ulcer complications if only a simple closure is done. Judgment is essential in ascertaining at operation whether a given patient should undergo a more extensive procedure. Important factors include duration of perforation, degree and extent of intra-abdominal contamination, degree of scarring of the duodenum, presence of other ulcer complications (e.g, bleeding), and the general condition of the patient. We consider parietal cell vagotomy and closure of the perforation to be the best procedure. There is an extensive experience both in this country and in Europe which attests to both its efficacy (90%) and its low morbidity and mortality. The operating time is slightly longer than for truncal vagotomy and pyloroplasty, and this may make it not applicable to all patients. The latter procedure, because of the rapidity with which it can be done by the experienced surgeon, is more suitable for the patient whose condition is unstable.

Patients who suffer a perforated duodenal ulcer while in hospital for other causes constitute an increasingly larger group that warrants special attention. Our exprience is that such patients tend to be diagnosed late since they have other serious medical and surgical problems to explain changes in their clinical course. As a consequence, the diagnosis is rarely considered by the primary physician. Moreover, because of medication and/or recent operation, the usual clinical picture of abdominal rigidity is not present, and the diagnosis is not made until abdominal distention and shock become apparent. Because of the complicating medical factors, we consider the treatment of such patients to be highly individualized. For example, let us consider a patient who remains in the surgical intensive care unit 4 days after a complicated procedure for extensive cancer. The patient is hemodynamically unstable with a perforation considered to be more than 24 hours old. We would reconsider nonoperative therapy. Water-soluble contrast studies would be made in an attempt to determine if the patient had sealed his perforation or if abdominal contamination continues. A clinical trial of nasogastric tube intubation, antibiotics, and histamine H_2 receptor antagonist therapy would be instituted. Patients who fail to improve with these measures require simple closure of the duodenal defect, often under local or regional anesthesia.

Finally, patients who present with perforated (anterior) duodenal ulcer, but also have a recent history or findings of gastrointestinal bleeding (blood in nasogastric aspirate, hematemesis, melena, or anemia), should be carefully explored at operation for the presence of an occult bleeding (posterior) ulcer. We have termed this condition "kissing ulcers," and in a group of eight such patients, we noted a mortality rate of 50 percent from postoperative bleeding from the unrecognized posterior ulcer following simple closure of the perforated ulcer. Patients having the condition of synchronous anterior and posterior ulcers are best treated by truncal vagotomy and antrectomy, recognizing the increased risk the procedure imposes. Lesser procedures are attended by an unacceptable mortality related to recurrent hemorrhage postoperatively.

Bleeding

Bleeding represents the most lethal complication of duodenal ulcer disease. The most important controllable factors in determining mortality are the timeliness and adequacy of preoperative transfusions and the timeliness of operative intervention. The plea, therefore, is for early involvement of the surgeon in the management of these patients, and particularly in the care of the elderly patient who is unable to withstand the insult of repeated episodes of hypotension. Considerations for operative intervention and preoperative evaluation vary considerably among hospitals. We endorse early endoscopic evaluation in patients suspected of having bleeding duodenal ulcer. Although early endoscopy has not been shown to reduce the mortality rate, it materially improves the management of the individual patient. Among its benefits are (1) confirmation of the diagnosis, excluding other lesions requiring specific forms of treatment, (2) cleansing of the stomach and duodenum, allowing subsequent bleeding rates to be accurately monitored, and (3) identification of patients who have factors predictive of ongoing bleeding or early rebleeding, i.e., the "visible vessels" in the base of the duodenal ulcer or fresh blood clot adherent to the ulcer. Early endoscopy, we feel, allows for a more ordered approach to the subsequent management of the bleeding patient, and we remain unconvinced that the subset of patients with hemorrhage requiring operative control are not benefited by the procedure.

Inasmuch as bleeding is the most lethal complication of duodenal ulcer, we consider truncal or selective vagotomy and antrectomy to be the operation of choice because of its indisputable effectiveness in curing the ulcer. Cure rates approach 98 percent or greater with this procedure, whereas lesser procedures are no more than 85 percent effective. Considerations of dumping, diarrhea, and the like are of secondary importance when faced with an immediately life-threatening lesion. Vagotomy and pyloroplasty with stick-tie of the ulcer is commonly employed (particularly in the elderly patient), but we are concerned about the high early rebleeding rate (15%) and recurrent ulcer rate (10%) associated with this operation. We reserve its use for the bleeding patient who is unstable on the operating table.

Obstruction

From the patient's viewpoint, obstruction is the most favorable indication for duodenal ulcer surgery since patient satisfaction after operation is greater than that achieved with any other indication. Factors that may contribute to the more favorable outcome include (1) the patient usually presents with a long history and the diagnosis is known, (2) initial treatment can be easily obtained by the patient (not eating, inducing vomiting for relief) or in hospital (nasogastric tube decompression), and (3) the problem is mechanical in nature, due to either duodenal scarring or antral dysfunction, and lends itself to remedy by mechanical surgical means. More than 90 percent of patients achieve excellent clinical results with operation, and physiologic derangements from the procedure such as dumping and diarrhea are characteristically less frequent than after surgery for other complications.

We consider truncal vagotomy, antrectomy, and gastroduodenostomy (Billroth I) to be the best procedure for obstruction due to chronic duodenal ulcer. The operation should include removal of the mechanical obstruction from scarring at the pyloroduodenal junction and removal of the antrum, which may be unable to adequately empty the stomach through a small but patent lumen. In our experience, most cases of obstruction are due to the latter.

The procedure demands that the surgeon be able to deal with a markedly scarred duodenum so that a Nissen closure of the duodenum or a Strauss exclusion of the ulcer can be accomplished.

Vagotomy and pyloroplasty, in our experience, is an inadequate and inappropriate procedure in the setting of obstruction. Pyloroplasty is often literally impossible in the patient with an extensively diseased pyloroduodenal junction. On the other hand, vagotomy and gastro-jejunostomy, although a procedure of second choice, can be used in the exceptional patient in whom massive inflammation in the pyloroduodenal region precludes a safe antrectomy.

Parietal cell vagotomy and dilatation of the pylorus and duodenum through a gastrotomy has been done in a small series of patients both in England and in the United States. Although the initial results were reported as favorable, the procedure's enthusiasts have not continued their series. We consider the procedure to be ill-advised for the truly fibrotic gastric outlet.

GASTRIC ULCER

The location of the ulcer in the stomch is an important determinant of how the ulcer should best be treated. Gastric ulcers in the pyloric channel or prepyloric antrum, as already noted, behave clinically like duodenal ulcers. These ulcers are best treated by a truncal or selective vagotomy and antrectomy. Selective vagotomy preserves the innervation of the abdominal organs other than the stomach and is associated with a lesser frequency and severity of postvagotomy diarrhea when compared to truncal vagotomy. Because of the failure to demonstrate a diminution in other postoperative side effects (e.g., dumping, bile reflux, early satiety) and the relative greater technical difficulty of the procedure, selective vagotomy is rarely performed in preference to truncal vagotomy in the United States.

The typical gastric ulcer occurring at or just proximal to the incisura or the lesser curvature or those in the corpus of the stomach are best treated by a distal hemigastrectomy which incorporates the ulcer. This empirical operation is extraordinarily effective in curing the ulcer, the recurrence rate being less than 4 percent. Ulcers at or near the esopha-gogastric junction are difficult to treat because of their location. When ulcer excision can be safely accomplished, this should be done along with a distal hemigastrectomy. If ulcer excision is unsafe, the lesion is best left in situ, and a distal hemigastrectomy (the Kelling-Madelener procedure) should be performed following adequate biopsy of the ulcer to ensure that it is nonmalignant. The majority of benign ulcers heal without incident within 6 weeks following the Kelling-Madelener procedure. Healing should be evaluated by follow-up endoscopic examinations.

Whenever possible, the complication of gastric ulcer (bleeding, perforation, obstruction) should be treated by definitive gastrectomy, which includes the ulcer. In particular, a bleeding gastric ulcer is less likely to stop without operation than is duodenal ulcer bleeding, and early surgery is strongly recommended to reduce the high mortality associated with this lesion.

RECURRENT ULCER

The development of another ulcer after a presumed successful operation for peptic ulcer is a particularly devastating and often clinically difficult problem to manage. In brief, occult endocrine causes (gastrinoma, hyperparathyroidism, retained excluded antrum) should be searched for, but most often some inadequacy of the initial operation, usually inadequate vagotomy, is responsible. Each operation for peptic ulcer disease has its own incidence of failure (recurrent ulcer formation) and its own time frame in which the ulcer is likely to appear. The range is an incidence of 0 to 2 percent for vagotomy and antrectomy occurring usually within 2 years, to a greater than 30 percent incidence after simple gastroenterostomy with a latency period of almost 20 years.

It is obvious that no single surgical approach will suffice for all cases. Endocrine causes should be removed when possible. Some postoperative uncomplicated recurrent ulcers can be managed with H_2 receptor antagonists. Excluding endocrine causes, the current surgical approach is directed at correcting inadequacies of the initial operation such as incomplete vagotomy (generally a missed right vagal trunk). In addition, a resection of the distal stomach, if not done initially, or higher resection of the gastric remnant along with the recurrent ulcer should also be done.

ZOLLINGER-ELLISON SYNDROME

CLIFFORD W. DEVENEY, M.D.

The Zollinger-Ellison syndrome consists of (1) acid hypersecretion (greater than 15 mEq H^+ per hour), (2) hypergastrinemia caused by non-beta islet cell tumors of the pancreas, and (3) virulent peptic ulcer disease. The syndrome was described by Zollinger and Ellison in three patients in the mid 1950s before the discovery of gastrin.

Subsequent discovery of the causative peptide, gastrin, and development of the gastrin radioimmunoassay, have enabled us to diagnose gastrin-producing tumors before the complete syndrome of virulent ulcer disease develops. It is desirable to diagnose a gastrin-producing tumor (gastrinoma) and begin appropriate therapy before complications of ulcer disease occur. Although peptic ulcer disease from gastrinoma is rare (fewer than 3% of patients with peptic ulcer disease), patients undergoing peptic ulcer surgery should have gastrinoma excluded before their operations.

CLINICAL CHARACTERISTICS

In many patients the peptic ulcer disease caused by a gastrinoma has no distinguishing clinical features, particularly if the disease is of recent onset. However, the patient with a gastrinoma often has some features that are not usually seen in ulcer patients without gastrinoma. Findings that should arouse suspicion of gastrinoma are listed as follows.

A Family History of Multiple Endocrine Adenopathy (MEN I). After parathyroid hyperplasia, gastrinomas are the most common tumor in the MEN I syndrome. In most series of gastrinomas, 30 to 50 percent of the patients have MEN I syndrome, and in series of MEN I patients, 50 to 70 percent of the patients have gastrinomas.

Severe Watery Diarrhea. Twenty to thirty percent of patients with gastrinoma have diarrhea, which is caused by acid hypersecretion and disappears when hyperacidity is controlled with H_2 receptor antagonists.

Characteristics on Upper Gastrointestinal Contrast Films. The presence of giant gastric rugal folds, multiple duodenal ulcers, and flocculation of barium all suggest gastrinoma.

Recurrent Ulcer After Previous Ulcer Surgery. Any patient with recurrent ulcer after an ulcer operation should be suspected of having Zollinger-Ellison syndrome. Although the diagnosis is suspected before ulcer operation in many patients with Zollinger-Ellison syndrome because of a family history or associated findings, some patients with the syndrome are discovered only because of recurrent ulcer after previous ulcer surgery. Since gastrin can be measured readily by radioimmunoassay, any patient about to have surgery for peptic ulcer disease should have serum gastrin measured.

DIAGNOSIS

The Zollinger-Ellison syndrome is caused by gastric acid hypersecretion stimulated by gastrin-producing tumors. Thus the two most important diagnostic criteria are gastric acid hypersecretion and hypergastrinemia.

Acid Secretion. In the unoperated patient, a basal acid output of greater than 15 mEq H^+ per hour is highly suggestive of gastrinoma. Because the stomach is being continually stimulated by gastrin, the pentagastrin-stimulated acid secretion is not much higher than the basal acid secretion. A ratio of basal to stimulated secretion of 0.6 or greater suggests gastrinoma. Twenty to thirty percent of patients with gastrinoma do not exhibit such

hypersecretion, and as many as 10 percent of patients without gastrinoma may have a basal acid secretory rate of 15 mEq H^+ per hour or more. Acid studies are not as reliable after ulcer operation, particularly gastric resections, but any patient who secretes more than 5 mEq H^+ per hour after ulcer surgery should be suspected of having gastrinoma. Although acid studies alone are not diagnostic, they are an essential part of the work-up and may be used to confirm or exclude the diagnosis of gastrinoma when combined with serum gastrin measurements.

Serum Gastrin Measurements. The serum gastrin level is less than 100 picogram (pg) per milliliter (50 picomole per liter) in the duodenal ulcer patient without gastrinoma as well as in normal fasting subjects. These values vary somewhat with different gastrin radioimmunoassays. Most patients with gastrinoma have basal gastrin levels greater than 500 pg per milliliter. Patients with gastrin levels in the range of 100 to 500 pg per milliliter require provocative tests for gastrin release to confirm the diagnosis.

Hypergastrinemia without acid hypersecretion occurs when gastric pH is chronically 5 or greater, after vagotomy when the antrum is not resected, and in patients with chronic renal failure. These causes of hypergastrinemia can be easily identified by gastric analysis, which yields less than 2 mEq H^+ per hour basally.

Hypergastrinemia with acid hypersecretion occurs after extensive small bowel resection, with gastric outlet obstruction, with retained gastric antrum, and in antral G-cell hyperplasia. The hypergastrinemia that follows small bowel resection usually resolves within several months, and when it is due to gastric outlet obstruction, it returns to normal after the stomach is decompressed. After antrectomy and Billroth II reconstruction, hypergastrinemia results if a substantial remnant of antrum is left with the duodenal stump. The resultant hypergastrinemia causes a syndrome of acid hypersecretion and recurrent ulcer similar to the Zollinger-Ellison syndrome. Fortunately, there is virtually never any problem in distinguishing antrum from duodenum, and the retained antrum syndrome is extremely rare.

Antral G-cell hyperplasia is manifested by the release of excessive amounts of gastrin from the antrum and causes hypergastrinemia with gastric acid hypersecretion. Antral G-cell hyperplasia is considerably less common than gastrinoma. It can be distinguished from gastrinoma by the secretin test and the gastrin response to a standard meal.

For gastrin levels between 100 and 500 mg per milliliter or nondiagnostic levels of acid secretion, the secretin test and the gastrin response to a standard meal can be used to confirm or exclude the diagnosis of gastrinoma.

Secretin Test. The hormone secretin is given as a bolus of 2 units per kilogram, and blood is taken for gastrin before injection and 2, 5, 10, and 15 minutes after the injection. A prompt increase in serum gastrin of 100 pg per milliliter or more is seen at 2 or 5 minutes after injection in patients with gastrinoma, but not in patients with other causes of hypergastrinemia. Although false-negative tests may occur in up to 10 percent of patients with gastrinoma, false-positive tests are rare.

Gastrin Response to a Standard Meal. The standard meal consists of two eggs, two pieces of bacon, and two pieces of toast. Coffee is not included. Blood is taken before the meal and at 30, 60, and 90 minutes postprandially. When postprandial gastrin values are expressed as a percentage of fasting gastrin, patients with gastrinoma have a less than 40 percent increase in serum gastrin, whereas those with hypergastrinemia from an antral source (i.e., antral G-cell hyperplasia) will exhibit an increase greater than 100 percent above fasting levels.

Results of the secretin test and the gastrin response to a standard meal are summarized in Table 1. It should be stressed that these provocative tests should be reserved for patients with both hypergastrinemia and acid hypersecretion whose serum gastrin values lie in a nondiagnostic range (100 to 500 pg per milliliter). Hypergastrinemia without acid hypersecretion is not caused by gastrinoma and does not require evaluation with provocative tests.

TREATMENT

Three modes of treatment of gastrinoma are (1) control of acid hypersecretion with H_2 receptor antagonists, (2) resection of the gastrinoma for cure, and (3) total gastrectomy.

Histamine H_2 antagonists effectively control acid hypersecretion for months to years and probably can be effective for longer periods. Patients with gastrinoma require significantly larger doses than patients with non-gastrinoma peptic ulcer disease. It is not unocmmon to require 5 to 10 g cimetidine daily or 1,200 to 2,000 mg ranitidine daily. Ranitidine, which is the preferred drug because it has fewer side effects at high doses, should be given in divided doses every 6 hours. To determine the effective dose, gastric analysis should be performed in the hour before the next dose is due because this is the time when the drug level is lowest. The dose used should maintain acid secretion below 10 mEq H^+ per hour.

After acid hypersecretion has been controlled with H_2 receptor antagonists, one should attempt to localize tumor and assess resectability. If the patient has MEN I, he will have multiple pancreatic tumors and can be excluded from curative resection. If it is unknown whether he has MEN I, a serum calcium determination is an excellent screening test. Virtually all MEN I patients have hyperparathyroidism by the time they develop gastrinomas. Thus, a normal serum calcium excludes MEN I.

Arteriography, CT scan, and transhepatic portal venous sampling are all used to localize gastrinomas preoperatively. Because arteriography localizes only about 30 to 50 percent of these lesions, it is not often used. Abdominal CT scans with intravenous contrast localizes most tumors greater than 2 cm in diameter and some tumors between 1 and 2 cm, but does not display the smaller lesions, which are more difficult to identify at

TABLE 1 Results of Tests for Zollinger-Ellison Syndrome

	RESPONSE (Increase in Gastrin)	
	Secretin Test	STD Meal*
Duodenal ulcer without gastrinoma	< 100	> 100%
Antral G-cell hyperplasia	< 100	±**
Zollinger-Ellison syndrome (gastrinoma)	> 100	< 40%

* Expressed as % of fasting level

** ± = Equivocal

operation. However, CT scans are safe and noninvasive, and should be obtained in all patients with gastrinomas to detect tumor.

Transphepatic portal venous sampling is the most sensitive method of localizing tumors. To perform this test, the portal vein is percutaneously cannulated in the liver and a catheter is guided through the portal vein into the veins draining the pancreas and duodenum. Samples are taken systematically along the splenic vein and small pancreatic tributaries, and gastrin levels are measured. An abrupt increase in gastrin at a single point or at multiple points suggests a gastrin-producing tumor in that area (i.e., head of pancreas, tail of pancreas). In experienced hands, this test has been accurate in determining the location and extent of gastrinomas in about 70 to 80 percent of patients.

Although acid secretion can be indefinitely controlled by H_2 receptor antagonists in the majority of patients, most experts recommend exploratory laparotomy to assess tumor resectability, unless preoperative tests have demonstrated unresectable tumor or the patient has MEN I, in which case the entire pancreas is involved. In patients without preoperative evidence of metastasis, resection for cure is possible in only 20 percent. The reasons for unresectability are malignant tumor with metastases, multiple tumors within the entire pancreas, or the inability to find the tumor. Although curative reseciton is possible in only a small portion of the patients, most physicians believe it is worth the attempt because is removes a potentially malignant tumor and it cures the syndrome.

Most gastrinomas reside within the pancreas or in the duodenal wall around the pancreas. Solitary tumors in the body or tail of the pancreas or in the duodenal wall are most easily resected for cure. Tumor within the head of the pancreas can often be safely enucleated. Most surgeons would not perform a pancreaticoduodenectomy (Whipple procedure) to resect this tumor because the morbidity and mortality rates of a Whipple procedure militate against its use for a tumor that is most often benign or of low-grade malignancy and in which gastric hyperacidity can be controlled with H_2 receptor antagonists or by total gastrectomy. Resection should be attempted only when it can be safely done with minimal morbidity. A parietal cell vagotomy is often performed whether or not tumor is resected because it facilitates subsequent control of acid secretion with H_2 receptor antagonists.

If tumor cannot be resected, patients should be treated initially with H_2 receptor antagonists. Most will require increasing doses to control hyperacidity. They should be studied periodically with gastric analysis to ensure that control of acid secretion is adequate. Patients who escape control or who develop ulcer complications during treatment with H_2 receptor antagonists should be treated with total gastrectomy. Patients tolerate this procedure surprisingly well and it eliminates acid secretion.

About half of all gastrinomas are malignant, as defined by lymph node and hepatic metastases or direct spread beyond the pancreas. If the tumor is malignant and has metastasized to the liver, the 5-year survival is only 40 percent; the cause of death is liver failure. If the tumor is found only in lymph nodes and pancreas, the prognosis is much better, and virtually none of these patients die from tumor. Streptozocin and 5-fluorouracil have been used to treat hepatic metastasis, but do not produce lasting remissions. Solitary hepatic metastases occasionally can be resected for cure, but unfortunately there is no effective therapy available for multiple hepatic metastases.

REMEDIAL OPERATION FOR POSTGASTRECTOMY AND POSTVAGOTOMY SYNDROMES

JOHN ALEXANDER-WILLIAMS, Ch.M., M.D., F.R.C.S., F.A.C.S.

Operations designed to give a permanent cure for peptic ulceration usually involved vagotomy or partial gastric resection or both. Operative treatment now has a low mortality and a high rate of success in curing the ulcer. Generally, operations that disturb physiology the least, such as highly selective (or proximal gastric) vagotomy, usually have the highest rate of recurrent ulcer. The more major operations, such as vagotomy and antrectomy or subtotal gastric resection, have the lowest risk of recurrent ulcer, but the highest risk of inducing new symptoms as a result of the altered physiology.

Since the advent of effective ulcer-curing drugs with few side effects, such as the histamine H_2 receptor blocking drugs, there have been three changes of emphasis in the selection of patients for ulcer curative surgery: (1) many fewer patients have been submitted to surgical treatment, (2) because the complication of recurrent ulceration can usually be managed readily by histamine H_2 receptor blockade, surgeons are becoming less obsessed by the risk of recurrence and more concerned about the risk of inducing other less easily managed postoperative problems; and (3) the decreased number of ulcer-curative operations has meant that surgeons in training, or in relatively small communities, cannot maintain a high degree of technical expertise from frequent practice of the latest operation. Therefore the technically more complicated operations, such as proximal gastric vagotomy, tend to be performed only in highly specialized and interested centers.

In my own practice, the need for gastric revisions for failed ulcer-curative operations has decreased considerably. Twenty to thirty years ago there was a change from gastric resection to truncal vagotomy, and more recently, a change from truncal to proximal gastric vagotomy. However, it remains true that about 80 percent of patients having ulcer-curative surgery are pleased with the results, whereas 20 percent or more continue to have symptoms sufficiently severe to warrant treatment. It is for this group of patients that remedial gastric surgery can be considered as one of the options of treatment.

A MULTIFACETED PROBLEM

Several distinct facets of the postgastrectomy and postvagotomy syndrome are recognized: dumping, gastric retention, bile vomiting, and diarrhea. Although these syndromes often can be separated clinically and accurately categorized with the aid of both simple and sophisticated measurements, most patients exhibit a combined symptom pattern that includes some aspect of one syndrome and some aspects of another. It is rarely possible to categorize a patient into one pure symptom group. Therefore, in the evaluation of these patients, it is necessary to assess all aspects of the various problems that can occur as a result of the altered physiology brought about by operations designed to cure chronic peptic ulceration.

It is not the scope of this chapter to discuss in detail the methods of assessment, but I would emphasize the need for a most exhaustive assessment, requiring the facilities of a well-equipped and research-oriented gastroenterology unit. I will refer here simply to the broad categories of tests that should be or could be performed before operation.

INVESTIGATIONS

X-ray studies should include oral cholecystography and a barium galactose meal to assist in the estimation of the rate of gastric emptying.

Endoscopy provides the best reliable evidence of recurrent or stomal ulceration. It also helps in the assessment of esophagitis and bile reflux gastritis.

Esophageal function studies are indicated only when special laboratory facilities are available and help to determine whether antireflux procedures should be incorporated with gastric reconstruction operations.

Acid secretory studies, with measurements of basal and gastrin analogue-stimulated peak acid output, are essential investigations before the planning of any gastric reconstructive surgery. They indicate whether a suspected ulcer is a true peptic recurrence and also indicate the need for vagotomy when bile reflux procedures are planned or when a previous vagotomy has been performed.

Gastric emptying can be estimated by the barium galactose meal pictures or by the presence of food residue on endoscopy. However, I always advocate radioisotopic scanning for the measurement of the rate of emptying of liquid and solid meals.

Duodenogastric reflux can be estimated crudely by appearances on endoscopy or by the aspiration of gastric contents, either as an early morning resting test or as a continuous 24-hour aspiration. The quantity of bile can be assessed by direct measurement or by measurement of the amount of radioactive-labeled marker excreted by the liver.

A noninvasive external measure of duodenogastric reflux can be obtained with the use of radioactive-labeled bile salt derivatives (HIDA).

Although such accurate measures are important in prospective research projects, the accurate quantitation of duodenogastric reflux is not essential to the planning of bile reflux procedures; a clear history of frequent bile-stained vomiting is a much better indication of the need for bile diversion.

Bacteriologic assessment of the aerobic and anaerobic organisms resident in the stomach are important before gastric reconstruction operations. The achlorhydric postoperative stomach is often teeming with pathogenic organisms, and appropriate antimicrobial prophylaxis is essential to minimize the high risk of septic complications.

Biliary and pancreatic investigation by retrograde cannulation and contrast radiology is indicated only when there is a strong suspicion of biliary or pancreatic disease.

The *irritable bowel syndrome* will often cause symptoms in patients after gastric operations that may be mistaken for postgastrectomy or postvagotomy syndromes.

Psychiatric assessment should be part of the sensible surgeon's data base before he or she considers reoperation. There are often many indications in the assessment history that indicate a strong likelihood of psychological factors. Although, in the past, I have had a specialist conduct psychiatric assessment of patients before operation, I now do the assessment myself. Keeping in mind that many psychotic patients with dyspeptic symptoms are easier to manage if their dyspeptic symptoms are relieved.

REMEDIAL REOPERATIONS FOR RECURRENT ULCER AND BILE REFLUX

It may seem strange to group these two indications together, but I have done so deliberately. There are few patients with recurrent ulceration after gastric resection who do not have some element of duodenogastric reflux, and all patients who require bile diversion are at risk of developing recurrent peptic ulceration unless we render them achlorhydric or hypochlorhydric. Therefore, my choice of operation for both these conditions is vagotomy (or revagotomy), antrectomy, and a Roux-en-Y anastomosis.

Recurrent Ulceration

The presence of a Zollinger-Ellison syndrome should always be excluded by appropriate acid secretory studies and serum gastrin levels.

Endoscopically proven recurrent ulceration in a patient who has been shown to be producing sufficient acids for peptic ulceration to occur (pH below 3.5) is usually best treated with effective anti-ulcer therapy. At present, the histamine H_2 receptor blocking agents have proved to be the most effective.

A few patients cannot control their recurrent ulceration by medical means either because of unreliability in taking medication or because of a particularly resistant ulcer diathesis.

When operative treatment is chosen, some advocate that the factor responsible for the recurrent peptic ulcer be determined and then treated individually. In other words, if a patient is found to have an incomplete vagotomy, they advocate simply completing the vagotomy, and for a patient who appears to have recurrent ulcer and a complete vagotomy, they treat only by antral resection. My own experience in trying to pursue this logical policy is that secretory tests are not always totally reliable, and the policy of simply completing the vagotomy has had a high proportion of failures. I therefore prefer the "belt and suspenders" policy of revagotomy and antrectomy.

Bile Reflux Gastritis

This represents a complex of abnormalities, which in its purest form is characterized by the vomiting of clear bile-stained fluid, but also includes esophagitis, fullness, and epigastric burning.

Medical therapy has little value, although many patients improve with time or learn to accept their symptoms. When the symptomatic consequences of duodenogastric reflux are severe, a bile diversion operation is indicated, but it is always worth waiting at least

2 years before reoperating to see whether spontaneous improvement occurs.

The anastomosis of the gastric remnant to the jejunum in bile diversion operations strongly predisposes to stomal ulceration unless acid secretion is abolished by vagotomy and antrectomy.

OPERATIVE TECHNIQUE

The operation is usually performed through the previous upper abdominal wound, which is excised if it is unsightly. In patients with a broad costal margin, I sometimes employ a transverse or bilateral subcostal incision.

Careful division of upper abdominal adhesions is essential, and for this I use a cutting diathermy current. It is particularly difficult to divide adhesions between the undersurface of the left lobe of the liver and the lesser curvature of the stomach. Great care should be exercised during this dissection to avoid unnecessary damage to the liver with possible subsequent bile extravasation.

The left coronary ligament of the liver is identified. This is then divided, and the left lobe of the liver retracted toward the right to give access to the esophageal hiatus (Fig. 1). If there is difficulty in identifying the esophagus because of adhesions, it is helpful to place a nasogastric tube to facilitate palpation. Careful dissection around the esophagus enables this organ and accompanying vagal nerve fibers to be isolated.

To avoid perforation of the esophagus during exploration, the operator's finger encircles the back of the esophagus from the left to the right. As the tip of the finger comes around to the right of the esophagus, the edge of the esophageal muscle fibers can be seen clearly and perforation thus prevented. The position of the major vagal trunks can usually be identified by palpation in the periesophageal tissues. The esophagus is encircled by a rubber tube and retracted forward. The major vagal fibers

are then divided, or if a vagotomy is already performed, a careful search is made for residual vagal strands. I do not find the vital staining of vagal nerve fibers of any value, but do find that careful palpation and "teasing" with a nerve hook allows detection of minute nerve fibers. I then destroy them with coagulation diathermy (Fig. 2). The lower esophagus is mobilized for about 6 cm from the cardia and has all the fibrous and nerve tissue dissected from it until it is soft and freely mobile. At this stage, an electrical test of vagal innervation (Vagorec test) can be used to ensure that the vagotomy is now complete.

The first part of the duodenum is then identified. If a pyloroplasty has been performed using thread sutures, this facilitates the identification of the pyloroplasty. If there is a recurrent ulcer at the site of the pyloroplasty, the dissection can be difficult. I do not hesitate to cut into the duodenum "free-hand" to facilitate identification of the ulcer; the color change at the junction between antral and duodenal mucosa can be seen clearly. It is essential to remove all the gastric mucosa from the duodenum to prevent the antral-exclusion syndrome.

When it is easy to mobilize the first part of the duodenum, I often occlude it with a stapler (Fig. 3).

Dissection of the lesser and greater curve between clamps allows an antrectomy to be performed, closing the proximal end of the stomach with a longer stapler (Fig. 4).

The stomach now has a complete vagotomy and antrectomy and should remain virtually achlorhydric. It is now safe for the stomach to be anastomosed to the jejunum, which is normally highly susceptible to peptic ulceration.

A proximal loop of jejunum is identified close to the duodenojejunal junction. A loop is held up to ascertain that it has sufficient mobility to be brought up and anastomosed to the gastric remnant. The mesentery is transilluminated to facilitate identification of the blood vessels in the mesentery. The gut is divided between fine noncrushing clamps. I prefer the handle-less Pace-Potts

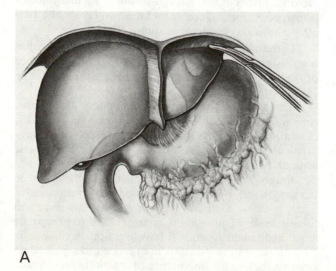

A

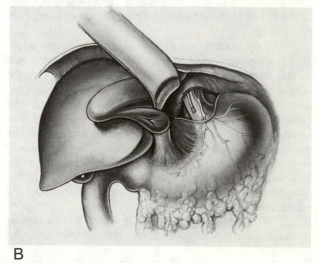

B

Figure 1 When the initial vagotomy has been performed below the left lobe of the liver, the best plan is to divide the left coronary ligament of the liver (A) and reflect the left lobe medially (B). The esophagus is then approached high in the esophageal hiatus. A previous incomplete vagotomy is noted.

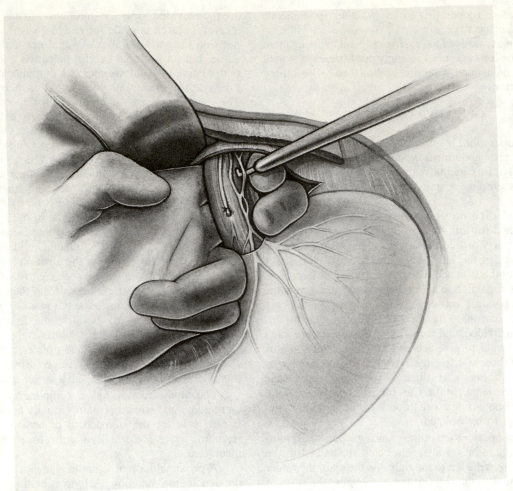

Figure 2 All the vagal fibers can then be identified and divided. To facilitate this, I have developed an insulated nerve hook which allows individual residual fibers to be picked out from within the muscle while the esophagus is held on the surgeon's fingers. The fibers are then destroyed by diathermy.

clamps, which facilitate passage of the distal end of the divided bowel through the hole in the mesocolon (Fig. 5 and Fig. 7).

The tip of the greater curve end of the gastric staple line is then amputated to provide a lumen of equal size to that of the cut end of the jejunum that has been brought up for anastomosis (Fig. 6). I usually employ soft non-crushing clamps to isolate the segment of bowel and then perform an open two-layer anastomosis. I employ a combination of interrupted stay sutures and continuous running sutures of 3–0 Vicryl. I like to avoid nonabsorbable sutures as these often become visible during postoperative endoscopic surveillance. Stay sutures ensure that the circular continuous stitch does not narrow the anastomosis.

The inner layer is then reinforced with an outer seromuscular continuous layer with a minimum of inversion.

The hole in the mesocolon is then closed with sutures to prevent internal herniation.

The proximal end of the divided jejunal loop is then anastomosed 50 to 60 cm "downstream" from the proximal anastomosis. An end-to-side "Y" anastomosis is then performed. Once again I use two layers of a running continuous absorbable suture (Fig. 7).

I generally do not drain the abdomen unless there has been a significant amount of damage to the undersurface of the liver, which I think might result in bile extravasation.

The wound is closed with continuous, large-bite, running nonabsorbable sutures, and the skin wound is closed primarily. The operation is covered with appropriate antibiotics, as determined by preoperative gastric aspirate culture.

Rarely, when technical difficulties make the operation hazardous and I anticipate many days of postoperative ileus, I employ a balloon catheter gastrostomy and a soft Silastic feeding jejunostomy, brought out through separate small abdominal wounds. I have used this technique in 84 patients with two deaths, both related to sepsis. Both occurred before the importance of antibiotic prophylaxis was appreciated. The results are satisfactory in about 70 percent of patients, but many remain severely symptomatic.

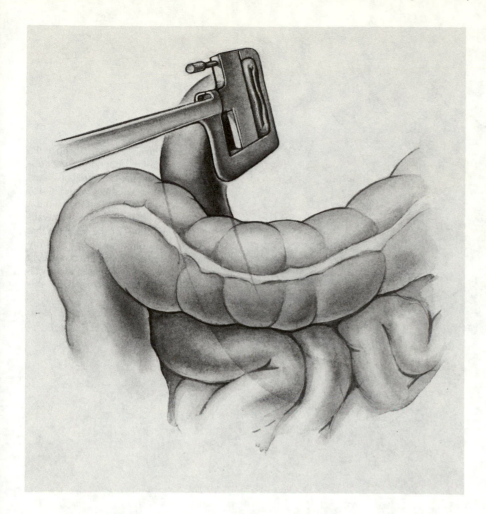

Figure 3 After the duodenum is mobilized, the duodenal stump is closed by means of a TA 55 Auto Suture stapling device. The duodenum is divided just proximal to the staple.

Figure 4 The antrum of the stomach is mobilized and divided from the body of the stomach either between clamps or, in the interests of speed and safety, by stapling the proximal end with a TA 90 Auto Suture stapling device. The staple line runs from the incisura angularis to the greater curve of the stomach.

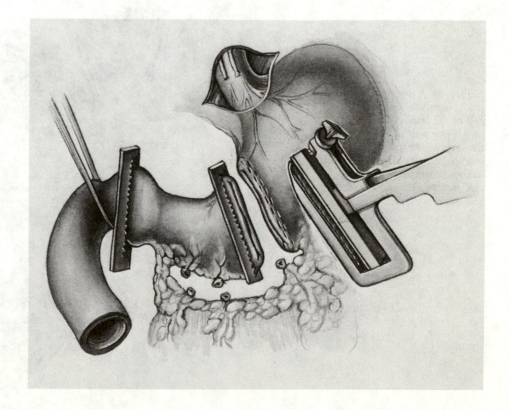

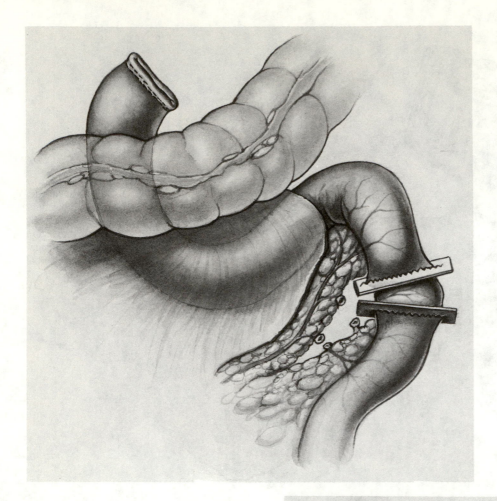

Figure 5 The first loop of the jejunum beyond the duodenojejunal flexure is isolated and a window made in the mesentery so that the jejunum can be divided. The first available loop of the jejunum that will allow sufficient mobility for the distal end to be brought up and anastomosed to the gastric stump is chosen for this purpose.

Figure 6 A clamp is now placed across the greater curve end of the stapled suture line of the stomach so that when the apex of the greater curve is amputated, it will leave a lumen approximately the same size as that of the small bowel (30 mm).

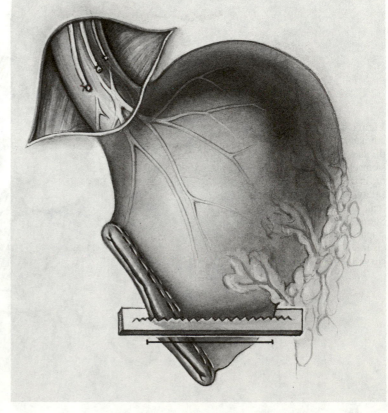

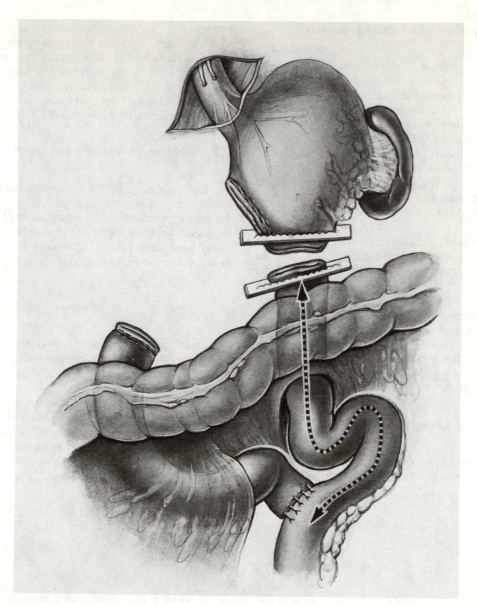

Figure 7 The distal end of the jejunum is brought up through a hole in the mesocolon so that it may be jointed end-to-end to the gastric remnant. Continuous absorbable sutures of Vicryl are used for the inner hemostatic suture and for the outer continuous serosa-to-serosa suture. The cut end of the proximal jejunum is then anastomosed to the side of the efferent loop 50 to 60 cm distal to the gastric anastomosis. To facilitate the accurate measurement of the length of this loop, a tape is cut to lay against the bowel.

Other Gastric Reconstruction Operations

Early dumping is a common complication of all gastric operations except proximal gastric vagotomy. Symptoms of dumping often accompany other syndromes such as bile vomiting or diarrhea. Most patients who complain of dumping in the early months after operation cease to complain as the months and years go by—because they learn to avoid the symptoms of dumping or because the body adjusts to compensate for the vasomotor changes or because the patients become tired of complaining.

In most patients, dumping can be controlled if they are advised to take small dry meals and to lie down after a large meal. Many can be helped by the administration of methoxypectin, which reduces the gastric emptying rate, or disaccharide inhibitors, which delay the absorption of sugars.

I believe that it is rarely ever necessary to perform a remedial operation for dumping; the results of such operations, although dramatically successful initially, are disappointing in the long term.

Taking Down of a Gastrojejunostomy

Patients who have been treated by vagotomy and gastrojejunostomy and who suffer from severe dumping usually also suffer from bile reflux. Taking down the gastrojejunostomy is an extremely simple and usually dramatically effective procedure.

The anastomosis is identified. I prefer to divide it free-hand with scissors, taking a little cuff of gastric mucosa off the stomach and suturing it with two layers of continuous Vicryl. The gastric mucosa is then trimmed off the jejunum, which is closed transversely with two layers of 3–0 Vicryl. I prefer hand-sewn anastomoses to staples.

I have performed this operation nine times and complete relief of symptoms resulted in every case. In the first four patients, I performed a pyloroplasty at the same time to ensure that there was no gastric retention because of previous vagotomy. However, I have since realized that pyloroplasty is unnecessary because the vagotomy, performed many years ago, produced only a temporary gastric paresis, which has now completely disappeared. Provided there is no duodenal stenosis, gastric emptying is usually unimpaired after the gastrojejunostomy is closed.

Pyloroplasty Reconstruction

It seems logical to try to reconstruct the pyloroplasty if patients have severe dumping after vagotomy and pyloroplasty. This operation entails dividing precisely along the suture line of the pyloroplasty, pulling the incision longitudinally, and reconstructing as it was before the pyloroplasty, using interrupted or continuous absorbable sutures. Although some have claimed good results from this operation, I have performed it on four occasions with disappointing long-term results. I do not advocate it.

Interposed Jejunal Loops and Pouches

I will not describe the techniques used to interpose pouches, isoperistaltic or retroperistaltic loops, between the gastric remnant and the duodenum. I have limited experience with this operation, it has uniformly bad results in my hands, and I have had to take down a number of these operations performed elsewhere by others.

Diarrhea

Diarrhea is particularly common after truncal vagotomy. It can usually be controlled medically and usually tends to improve with time, although occasionally it is disabling.

Some have advocated remedial operations such as the creation of an interposed jejunal loop or an interposed reversed ileal loop. These operations will not be described in detail because I do not think that they are ever justifiable in the long term. In my experience, they always cause more problems than they control.

SMALL BOWEL

SMALL BOWEL OBSTRUCTION

GREGORY B. BULKLEY, M.D., F.A.C.S.

Mechanical obstruction of the small intestine is one of the most common clinical problems faced by the general surgeon. It can be defined as a partial or complete anatomic blockade of the intestinal lumen, whether by an intrinsic or extrinsic lesion. This definition therefore excludes paralytic ileus, primary mesenteric ischemia, and similar conditions from which mechanical obstruction must often be distinguished clinically. The predominant cause of small bowel obstruction is adhesions from a previous laparotomy, but it can also be caused by a number of other lesions, benign and malignant (Table 1). Although the underlying lesion is often suspected, and should always be kept in mind, the appropriate approach to small bowel obstruction (SBO) is a more generalized one, based more on the degree of obstruction and the systemic status of the patient than on the primary cause.

DIAGNOSIS

The diagnostic approach to SBO should be systematic and readily lends itself to classification into four phases, which may be addressed sequentially (Fig. 1).

Recognition of Mechanical Obstruction

The first problem is to identify the patient as someone with SBO. In most cases, this is straightforward,

TABLE 1 Etiology of Small Bowel Obstruction

Cause	Approximate Incidence (%)
Adhesions	60
Malignant tumor (1/3 primary; 2/3 metastatic)	20
Hernia (4/5 abdominal wall; 1/5 internal)	10
Inflammatory bowel disease	5
Volvulus	3
Miscellaneous	2

based on the characteristic symptoms, physical signs, and the signs noted on flat and upright plain abdominal films. This aspect of the diagnostic problem of SBO is usually one of the lesser challenges in the management of patients with an acute abdomen. In most cases, this assessment should be completed within a few minutes of the first encounter with the patient, as it does not require waiting for laboratory tests or special diagnostic studies. Two types of patients may be particularly challenging in this regard, however. The first is the occasional patient who presents with a complete mechanical SBO and a gasless abdomen. This condition can be caused, for example, by a closed loop obstruction, although it is *not* a reliable diagnostic indicator thereof. In this situation, the absence of air to provide contrast on the plain abdominal roentgenograms precludes the recognition of dilated loops and air fluid levels. An inexperienced or cursory viewing of these films can sometimes result in failure to recognize the presence of SBO altogether. However, closer study should reveal a "ground glass" haziness in the midabdomen, or the effect of a central mass on adjacent, air-outlined structures such as the stomach, colon, and/or uninvolved small bowel. If serious question persists, a contrast study can be performed (to be discussed), although one should obtain an angiographic study first in those few cases in which there is serious suspicion of primary mesenteric ischemia. Patients who develop acute mechanical SBO in the postoperative period may also present a serious problem with respect to recognition (to be discussed).

Distinguishing Partial From Complete Obstruction

Because I believe that the management of complete SBO is primarily operative, whereas that of a partial obstruction is primarily nonoperative, this distinction is an important one, representing a major branch point in the approach to treatment. I therefore always try to assess the completeness of obstruction as definitively and as quickly as possible. A number of clues from the history and physical examination can be helpful, and the gas pattern on the plain abdominal film can be particularly useful. The correlation of the duration and degree of symptoms with the presence or absence of distal gas on the x-ray film is often the most helpful assessment. Although one can be fooled by the presence of colonic gas introduced

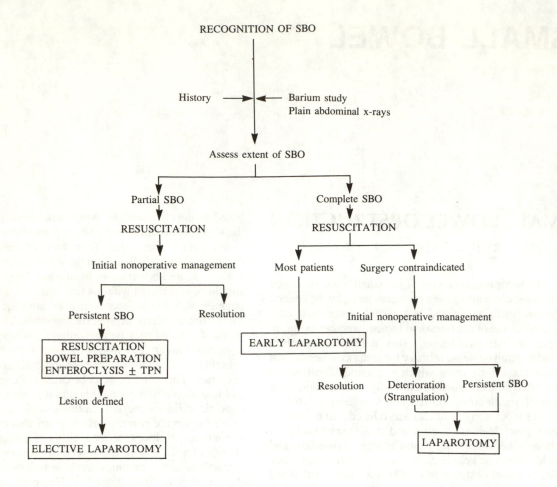

RECOGNITION OF SBO

History → ← Barium study
Plain abdominal x-rays

Assess extent of SBO

Partial SBO / Complete SBO

RESUSCITATION / RESUSCITATION

Initial nonoperative management

Most patients / Surgery contraindicated

Persistent SBO / Resolution

RESUSCITATION
BOWEL PREPARATION
ENTEROCLYSIS ± TPN

EARLY LAPAROTOMY

Initial nonoperative management

Resolution / Deterioration (Strangulation) / Persistent SBO

Lesion defined

ELECTIVE LAPAROTOMY

LAPAROTOMY

Figure 1 Management of acute small bowel obstruction.

by sigmoidoscopy, the introduction of air by a digital rectal examination of a patient in the supine or lateral decubitus position is a highly unlikely, and certainly unproven, proposition. Of great assistance here is the viewing of abdominal films, serially obtained, a few hours after the initial evaluation. This points up the importance of obtaining the initial roentgenograms as quickly as possible after the patient first presents for evaluation. As in the management of other patients with acute abdominal conditions, repeated examination by the same observer over a period of time remains one of the most reliable means of clinical diagnosis.

Despite the foregoing, many patients present a real diagnostic challenge with regard to this critical distinction of partial from complete SBO. For example, early complete obstruction is virtually indistinguishable from partial obstruction on the abdominal film. In these cases, I like to proceed rapidly to the use of contrast, often within an hour of initial presentation. This approach is rapid, cheap, readily available at any time, and safe when applied appropriately. It is therefore efficient. First, one must be confident that the patient does not have obstruction of the colon, and if serious doubt exists, a barium enema should be performed beforehand to rule out this

possibility. However, this is rarely necessary. Then 50 to 100 ml of dilute barium is introduced from above, usually via a nasogastric or intestinal tube in these nauseated patients. The tube is then clamped for an hour, or for a shorter period if the patient begins vomiting. Flat abdominal films are then obtained, and nasoenteric suction is resumed. Even if most of the contrast material is suctioned out, a sufficient residual almost always passes downward to reveal the degree and level of the obstruction. This progress can be followed with sequential films, often in conjunction with the positioning of an intestinal tube. With the exception of a few patients with a profound ileus, the answer is usually obtained within 2 or 3 hours of the initial evaluation; complete obstruction is recognized or ruled out definitively. Moreover, in patients with partial obstruction, the degree and level of obstruction is often indicated on these and subsequent films, and this assessment is most helpful in deciding whether to operate on these patients. Fluoroscopic examination is not necessary. Neither is it necessary to prepare the gastrointestinal tract for contrast studies. The recognition of these facts by both the surgeon and the radiology department does much to facilitate obtaining this study, which does *not* require the presence of a radiologist.

Despite a wealth of clinical experience, much of it published, with the use of barium in SBO, this approach remains controversial in some circles. Nevertheless, the safety of barium is undisputed in cases of *small* bowel obstruction. Unlike the colon, the small intestine is incapable of absorbing water to a degree that would create a proximal impaction. (It is important, however, to first preclude the possibility of colonic obstruction, as already discussed.) Moreover, there is no benefit to using larger volumes of contrast material, as this only tends to obscure the specific information sought. If large volumes are avoided, the risk of significant barium contamination of the peritoneum is minimal, even if there is an unintentional enterotomy at the time of subsequent laparotomy. Finally, I personally do not like to use water-soluble contrast media in this situation. It provides significantly poorer images, especially after the contrast has passed more distally and become diluted with secretions. Furthermore, it presents a substantially increased risk for pulmonary injury in the event of aspiration, from vomiting or when anesthesia is induced. Finally, its osmotic properties tend to increase the sequestration of "third space" fluid within the intestinal lumen and to stimulate peristalsis. This may increase the risk of perforation and certainly increases the level of the patient's distress.

Distinguishing Simple From Strangulation Obstruction

The early recognition of strangulation in patients with mechanical SBO has been a great source of controversy over the years. Perhaps because every surgeon has been indocrinated as to the classic signs of strangulation at some time during his training, the myth persists that such a distinction is possible, despite an overwhelming preponderance of evidence to the contrary. This issue has been greatly confused by the mixing of patients who have *partial* with patients who have *complete* obstruction. It is therefore essential to determine first, as already outlined, the degree of the obstruction. Except for the rare patient with a strangulated Richter's hernia that has not been detected on physical examination, any patient with partial obstruction can be considered to have a negligible risk for stangulation and managed accordingly (to be discussed).

However, patients with complete obstruction are at substantial risk for strangulation. In operative series, this risk has been consistently reported at 30 percent, but is probably lower in series that include patients managed nonoperatively. In patients with complete SBO, several retrospective and our own prospective study have demonstrated unequivocally that the accurate recognition of early vascular compromise is simply not possible on clinical grounds. Traditional criteria such as continuous (as opposed to colicky) pain, fever, tachycardia, signs of peritonitis, leukocytosis, or the elevation of any of a number of serum electrolytes (potassium, phosphate) or enzymes (alkaline phosphatase, AST, ALT, LDH, CPK) are simply not sensitive, specific, or predictive of strangulation. Moreover, there is no combination of these factors that can accurately predict vascular compromise. Most important, we found that the operating surgeon's preoperative impression of the presence of strangulation was equally unreliable: the diagnosis of simple obstruction (no strangulation) was correct only 70 percent of the time. When the overall incidence of strangulation (30%) was taken into account, this proved to be no better than would have been achieved by chance alone. Moreover, only one of the six patients with early reversible ischemia (viable intestine) were detected preoperatively. Retrospective series, including that of Silen, have reported a similar experience. This is not surprising in light of the fact that the signs that have been used to identify strangulation are a reflection of de facto tissue necrosis, or of the body's response thereto. Therefore, to wait for signs of strangulation is to wait for the presence of irreversible damage. This factor probably contributes substantially to the fact that the mortality for strangulation is more than double that of simple obstruction in most reported series. Therapeutic decisions (to be discussed) in patients with *complete* SBO must be based on the 30 percent chance of the presence of ischemic bowel despite the complete absence of the "signs of strangulation."

Identification of the Underlying Cause

In most situations, the decision for surgery is made on the basis of the factors already discussed, without regard to the suspected cause of obstruction. In other cases, however, important clues from the history and physical examination suggest an underlying lesion that may modify the therapeutic approach from the outset. Radiation enteritis, peritoneal carcinomatosis, incarcerated hernia, intra-abdominal abscess, and multiply recurrent adhesive obstruction are all lesions (to be discussed) that would influence the surgeon's approach to the obstruction. In most cases, however, the obstructive process is initially dealt with on its own terms, and underlying lesions are managed secondarily on an individual basis.

TREATMENT: GENERAL MEASURES

Systemic Considerations

Patients with SBO are invariably dehydrated due to a cessation of oral intake, vomiting, and the sequestration of fluid in the bowel lumen. This should be replaced aggressively with an isotonic saline solution such as Ringer's lactate, following standard guidelines for the replacement of deficits. Many patients require additional monitoring of intravascular volume with catheters in the superior vena cava, pulmonary artery, and/or urinary bladder. Because of the previous (deficit) and ongoing (abnormal losses) fluid requirements are often substantial, and it is important not to underestimate the fluid and electrolyte needs of these patients, particularly just prior to the induction of general anesthesia. I once gave over 30 liters of Ringer's lactate in an 8-hour perioperative period to a 30-year-old woman with normal cardiac and renal function who had acute, simple, uncomplicated SBO. Throughout this period, her central venous pressure and urinary output remained low. Not surprisingly, 3 days later, as her recovery progressed, she mobilized the "third space" load with a spontaneous urine output of over a liter an hour for 24 hours.

All patients with mechanical SBO are at risk for portal septicemia due to loss of the intestinal barrier to bacteria. This is true for patients with simple as well as strangulation obstruction. For this reason and because of the significant risk of the occult presence of ischemia (strangulation), I prefer to treat all patients with SBO with broad-spectrum antibiotics (penicillin, gentamicin, and clindamycin) until the condition has been resolved. This is not so much to prevent surgical wound infection as to prevent clinical sepsis in these already systemically compromised patients.

Tube Decompression

Virtually all of these patients benefit from the use of a nasoenteric tube to allow decompression of the gastrointestinal tract proximal to the obstruction. This provides symptomatic relief from the nausea and vomiting and, to some degree, the abdominal pain. It allows the administration of contrast material to these nauseated patients. It helps prevent aspiration at the time of the induction of anesthesia. It greatly facilitates the surgical exploration and the subsequent abdominal closure. In some cases, it may provide a splint to prevent recurrent obstruction (to be discussed). In some situations, it provides definitive treatment in lieu of surgery, particularly in cases of partial obstruction. However, the decision to use a decompressing tube should be made without regard to the decision for or against surgery, as the latter decision must be made on its own merits.

I much prefer the use of a Cantor tube with the apical bag filled with about 7 ml of mercury. I ignore the instructions on the package and pass the tube nasogastrically with the patient sitting upright. I then place the patient in the right lateral decubitus position and send him for a plain abdominal roentgenogram. (Often this film coincides with the 1-hour postbarium film already discussed.) I do this immediately to ensure placement of the tube tip in the distal antrum *before* waiting for it to pass through the pylorus. I continue to repeat these films and aggressively reposition the tube and/or patient until the mercury bag has passed the ligament of Treitz. (During this period, I leave the other end of the tube untethered and connected to straight drainage.) With this aggressive approach, the mercury bag almost always reaches the jejunum within an 8- to 12-hour period, which is often prior to surgery. Up to this point, decisions about the patient's position based on assumptions of tube position related to elapsed time are invariably wrong unless the patient is monitored radiologically. Thereafter, I attach the tube to low, intermittent suction and allow it to pass distally at its own rate, with films initially at 12-hour intervals, then at 24-hour intervals.

Although well-documented clinical experiences at some institutions have demonstrated equivalent decompression with a nasogastric tube, the presence of an intestinal tube greatly facilitates decompression at the operating table. When using a long intestinal tube, it is important to remember to separately evacuate the stomach with a nasogastric tube prior to the induction of anesthesia to avoid aspiration. When surgery must proceed prior to the passage of the Cantor tube into the intestine, and decompression is still required to facilitate anastomosis or abdominal closure, I try to avoid an enterotomy whenever possible. Sometimes the intestinal contents can be milked proximally into the stomach and evacuated therefrom by the anesthetist. Sometimes, following release of the cause of obstruction, this lumenal material can be milked distally into the colon where it presents less of a problem. When this is impractical, it is possible, with the help of an unscrubbed assistant at the head of the operating table, to pass a pediatric Leonard tube orogastrically and for the surgeon to manually guide it around the duodenal C-loop and ligament of Treitz, and into the distal small bowel. This semi-rigid tube, stiffened by a coiled spring, is not difficult to handle with practice, and its large lumen facilitates decompression. Its semi-rigid wall necessitates rather gentle curves, and it is therefore ideal for splinting the intestine in cases of recurrent adhesive obstruction. Following decompression, because of its size, the proximal end of this tube should be passed retrograde back into the oropharynx and brought out through the nose. This can be accomplished by passing a Levine tube prograde from the nose to the oropharynx, grasping the tip with endotracheal tube forceps and suturing it to the proximal end of the Leonard tube before pulling this back out through the naris. Usually the anesthetist is happy to oblige in these tasks while the operation proceeds.

Operative Versus Nonoperative Management

The most controversial aspect of this disease is the role of surgery in mechanical SBO. On the one hand, there is the substantial risk (already discussed) of delaying treatment of unrecognized, indeed unrecognizable, intestinal ischemia. On the other hand, there are numerous large series, albeit retrospective and often controlled poorly, if at all, that clearly document success with initial nonoperative management, with surgery reserved for selected patients who deteriorate or fail to improve.

This issue has been greatly confused by failure to distinguish partial from complete obstruction. Many of the aforementioned series include both types of patients, and therefore the real results are obscured. Clearly, patients with *partial* obstruction should be managed initially without surgery (to be discussed), and there seems to be little disagreement on this point. Patients with *complete* small bowel obstruction can then be considered separately, in light of the already discussed substantial risk of occult strangulation. Because of the aforementioned compelling figures, my primary approach to these patients is to proceed to laparotomy within 12 to 24 hours, after the patient has been rehydrated and has achieved therapeutic tissue levels of antibiotics, and decompression is well under way. I do not believe that an initial therapeutic trial of nonoperative management is justified or advantageous on a routine basis. On the other hand, there is frequently justification for a 12- to 24-hour delay while an unstable patient is resuscitated. Moreover, a number of special clinical circumstances justify serious consideration of a trial of primary nonoperative treatment. These include documented carcinomatosis, multiply recurrent adhesive obstruction, radiation enteritis, and a number of other conditions. This decision, therefore, not unlike any other difficult decision in clinical medicine, should weigh the risks and the benefits of the nonoperative approach against those of the operative. One of the major risks of nonoperative management that must be recognized is the substantial (30%) risk that one is delaying the treatment of occult intestinal ischemia. When the benefits of nonoperative management are great enough to justify this risk, this choice is a reasonable one. Under most circumstances, however, and particularly in patients with a routine presentation of acute complete SBO, this risk is simply not justified. On this basis, my own choice for the routine management of complete SBO is early laparotomy.

TREATMENT OF SPECIFIC LESIONS

Strangulation Obstruction

The preoperative diagnosis of strangulation has been addressed. When strangulated bowel is encountered at operation, the underlying cause is removed simply and easily by reduction, combined with lysis of the adhesion or repair of the hernia. A determination must then be made as to intestinal viability. Briefly, this can usually be determined quickly and accurately on clinical grounds alone, after at least 15 minutes following reduction of the strangulation. When the clinical evaluation of viability is equivocal, the use of the fluorescein technique is rapid, simple, and accurate, and usually obviates the need for a subsequent second-look laparotomy. This subject is discussed in more detail in the chapter on *Mesenteric Vascular Occlusive Disease*.

Viable intestine can clearly be left in situ, but nonviable bowel must be resected with (short) margins of intestine that are unequivocally viable. Unlike the situation in patients with primary mesenteric occlusion, this transition is usually discrete in these cases. Nevertheless, a primary anastomosis should not be attempted in bowel of questionable viability. In this situation, which should only arise when a massive resection is necessitated, it is better to exteriorize the questionable ends of the remaining intestine as stomata, with the intention of subsequent reanastomosis.

Adhesions

Patients with an initial presentation of acute SBO due to adhesions usually benefit from early operative lysis. Even patients with partial obstruction from this cause often require surgery (to be discussed). Although these procedures are facilitated by tube decompression, an enterotomy is rarely required and should be avoided if possible. No attempt should be made to formally splint or tether the bowel, although I usually arrange the loops in as gentle curves as possible, often facilitated by the Cantor tube.

Patients with multiply recurrent adhesive obstruction present an exceedingly difficult, but fortunately uncommon problem in management. I usually try to treat such patients nonoperatively whenever possible, for it is unusual for these patients to have the residual intestinal mobility to allow the formation of a closed loop obstruction. Moreover, there is less likelihood for a definitive cure to be effected surgically, although the majority of these patients do not suffer recurrence.

The prevention of recurrence is a more difficult proposition. Aside from normal measures of good surgical practice, which include gentle handling of tissue, hemostasis, avoidance of unnecessary dissection, avoidance of enterotomy, meticulous cleaning of starch from gloves, and avoidance of a separate suture line to close the peritoneum per se, there is no specific measure for the prevention of adhesions. Agents such as steroids, which inhibit adhesion formation, also inhibit healing and there is at present no practical way to approach this aspect of the problem. The surgeon must therefore focus on minimizing the additional serosal injury necessitated by his dissection and on trying to position the bowel to avoid kinking when adhesions do form. Plication procedures have not been demonstrated to be of benefit, and I rarely employ them. On the other hand, there is little reason not to try to arrange the bowel loops in gentle curves, splinted with the Cantor or Leonard tube (already discussed). Although this method has not been demonstrated to significantly reduce recurrence in clinical studies, it may be of benefit in some cases. Postoperatively, the splint (tube) should be left in place for about one week, even after its suction has been discontinued and the patient has resumed eating. It can then be removed, or cut off and allowed to pass per rectum if there is difficulty in pulling it out through the nose. Although I believe the risk of erosion and perforation from Cantor tubes has been greatly exaggerated, the stiffer Leonard tube should probably be repositioned at 8-hour intervals and removed after 24 to 48 hours.

Incarcerated Hernia

When an incarcerated abdominal wall hernia is the cause of obstruction, the obstruction itself can often be managed by simple reduction. After reduction of the hernia, these patients should always be admitted for observation, and this facilitates elective hernia repair a few days later if no signs of intestinal ischemia appear. They rarely require laparotomy.

Malignant Tumor

Small intestinal obstruction due to a primary malignant tumor is more often due to a lesion of another abdominal organ, often the colon. Management of these patients is the same as for patients with simple SBO, combined with resection of the primary lesion whenever this is feasible.

Patients with documented carcinomatosis present a more difficult problem, however, and are often managed successfully over the short term with tube decompression. When this is unsuccessful, I do not hesitate to offer laparotomy to all but the most severely ill patients. The benefits of local control of intestinal obstruction to avoid pain and an indwelling intestinal tube usually more than justify the discomfort of surgery, although the management of these patients should be individualized. At surgery, a bypass of the obstructed area is often preferable to a primary resection that would necessitate an extensive dissection.

Patients with a history of treatment of a prior malignant tumor, often of the breast or within the abdominal cavity, are sometimes assumed to have carcinomatosis as the basis for obstruction. This is an error, less common today than it was a decade ago, for about one-third of these patients have obstruction due to an unrelated lesion, and about two-thirds have a resectable or bypassable lesion. To write off a patient with a prior malignant tumor based on an unconfirmed diagnosis of carcinomatosis is inexcusable.

Crohn's Disease

Patients with primary inflammatory bowel disease of the small intestine can present with partial or complete SBO. These patients can often be managed successfully by tube decompression and a pharmacologic assault on the primary inflammatory process. This is particularly true when the obstruction is due to the acute inflammation, and an initial trial of nonoperative management here is usually justified. On the other hand, when the obstruction is due to scarring as the result of the body's attempt to heal a longstanding inflammatory process, primary resection is required in most cases. This policy does not preclude initial nonoperative management to effect decompression and perhaps reduce inflammation. In most cases, the obstructive component due to irreversible scarring proves to be only partial as the phlegmon resolves. In most of these situations, the patient can then undergo resection under elective circumstances, often after parenteral treatment of concurrent nutritional depletion.

Abdominal Abscess

An acute abdominal abscess can produce a clinical picture indistinguishable from complete, mechanical SBO,

although at surgery it is often found that the lumen is anatomically patent adjacent to the abscess. The mechanism is probably an intense local ileus, exacerbated somewhat by external compression. In any case, drainage of the abscess itself is often sufficient to relieve the obstruction, and in many cases, the patient does not require a full-scale laparotomy to effect this. If the obstruction persists, laparotomy can be performed later under more favorable clinical circumstances.

Radiation Enteritis

This horrendous disease is best managed by its avoidance, which can often be effected by well-trained radiotherapists who carefully design their ports, and who avoid treatment of abdominal malignant tumors for which there is little potential for benefit. Careful patient positioning and the assurance of small intestinal mobility prior to pelvic radiation is particularly important. In these situations, the surgeon can also be helpful beforehand by careful closure of the pelvic floor after the resection of a pelvic malignant tumor. When acute enteritis occurs within a few weeks of radiation therapy, it sometimes responds to steroids and tube decompression. In these situations, surgery can sometimes be avoided. More often, however, SBO due to radiation enteritis presents years after the completion of therapy, and at this point there is no effective treatment for the primary disease process. Moreover, this process is almost certain to progress. Some patients with partial obstruction can avoid surgery for a time, but most require laparotomy. The surgeon then has the choice of resection or bypass of the affected bowel. Contrary to the conventional approach, I prefer to resect when possible, particularly when a relatively short intestinal segment is involved. The dissection is sometimes not so difficult as anticipated, particularly when one realizes that there is no harm in injuring the intestine to be excised. Whether one resects or bypasses the involved area, it is essential to avoid the anastomosis of radiated intestinal tissue.

Partial Obstruction

When the barium study confirms the diagnosis of *partial* SBO, initial management generally consists of a trial of tube decompression, without surgery. In the majority of these cases, the obstruction is relieved, and usually does not recur, particularly if the underlying lesion is an adhesion. Surgery is reserved for patients whose obstruction is not relieved sufficiently to allow normal oral alimentation, and for those suffering from recurrent bouts of partial SBO.

In either group, the location, degree, and anatomy of the lesion can often be defined by an enteroclysis study. A Cantor tube should be passed down to a point as close to the obstruction as possible. Residual barium from previous studies should be evacuated as efficiently as possible, by suction from above and by enemas from below. A small volume of dilute barium is then introduced under fluoroscopic control by a radiologist experienced in this technique. The quality of the imaging obtained in the specific area of interest is often superb, greatly facilitating the decision for or against surgery at this admission, and often providing useful clues as to etiology. Once the decision has been made to proceed with surgical resection, the operative approach is no different from that for complete SBO and is influenced primarily by the nature of the underlying lesion.

Acute Postoperative Obstruction

Small bowel obstruction that appears in the immediate postoperative period presents a challenging and often mismanaged problem. In the first place, it is difficult to recognize, as its primary symptoms, pain and vomiting, can often be attributed to the incision and to postoperative ileus, respectively. A careful history that reveals colicky, as opposed to constant, aching pain, and that pays particular attention to the time course of symptoms, signs, and the abdominal films is often revealing. Here again, repeated evaluation by the same observer over a period of time is invaluable. When the diagnosis is suspected, it can be confirmed by barium contrast given through a nasoenteric tube (as already discussed) as long as there is no danger of proximal perforation or suture line leakage.

CROHN'S DISEASE OF THE SMALL BOWEL

VINCENZO SPERANZA, M.D., F.A.C.S.
MARIO SIMI, M.D.

Crohn's disease, a chronic, focal, transmural granulomatous inflammation, can occur in any part of the alimentary tract. It most commonly affects the distal ileal loop, either alone (terminal ileitis) or, less often, with limited continuous colonic involvement (right-sided ileocolitis). Many investigations, some revealing abnormalities in apparently normal mucosa, suggest that Crohn's lesions are a macroscopic expression of a latent panenteritis. The course of the disease is characterized by unpredictable relapse, often leading to life-threatening complications, and postoperative recurrence which, although often with mild or no symptoms, is almost ineluctable in the long run.

Once recognized, the management of acute postoperative SBO remains controversial. When partial obstruction is confirmed or strongly suspected, a trial of nonoperative management is clearly preferable. Even when the condition fails to resolve, the opportunity to temporarily stabilize the acute situation and delay surgery a short while further into the postoperative period is worthwhile.

Complete obstruction presents a more serious problem, however. Many surgeons cite this situation as one in which they prefer an initial trial of primary nonoperative management. This position, while understandable in light of the clinical situation, is based more on the surgeon's emotions than on scientific grounds. Several series of patients with SBO have reported a higher incidence of missed strangulation among postoperative patients than was found in the studied population as a whole. Consequently, I believe that *complete mechanical* SBO in the acute postoperative period, when confirmed as described, is a relatively clear indication for early re-exploration. As in other clinical situations, the concurrent presence of substantial risk factors is *not* a contraindication to surgery. It is simply a compelling obligation that the physician make the correct therapeutic decision, the one that maximizes benefit and minimizes what might be substantial risks. In many situations, the choice that optimizes this cost:benefit ratio is early surgery.

As the etiology of the disease is unknown, therapy is directed toward palliation, not cure. The aim of both medical and surgical treatment is therefore to improve the quality of life. The management of Crohn's disese is primarily medical, based mainly on corticosteroids (ileitis) and/or sulfasalazine (colitis). However, about 80 percent of these patients eventually require surgical treatment.

INDICATIONS FOR SURGERY

Complications of the disease and failure of optimal medical management are the indications for surgery (Table 1). However, only some complications, such as the rare free perforation into the peritoneal cavity, unremitting bleeding, abscesses, large-volume external fistulas, enterovesical fistulas, and severe obstructive uropathy, are absolute indications; all the others are relative indications, to be judged case by case.

TABLE 1 Indications for Surgery in Crohn's Disease of the Small Intestine

	% in other series (average)	% in our series (154 cases)
Acute obstruction (unremitting or repetitive)	39.4	41.5
Failure of optimum medical management	32.7	31.8
Unresponsiveness of symptoms (e.g., pain, relapsing obstructive symptoms, malnourishment, general toxicity)	--	25.3
Intolerance to drugs (mainly side effects of corticosteroids)	--	6.4
Fistula	12	16.2
Enterocutaneous	4	5.1
Enteroenteric	3.5	5.8
Enterovesical	2.9	5.1
Others (e.g., female genital tract)	1.6	0
Abdominal abscess	6.7	5.8
Generalized peritonitis (from free perforation or rupture of an abdominal abscess)	5	1.9
Bleeding (acute unremitting and/or relapsing)	2.8	2.5
Severe obstructive uropathy (usually right-sided)	1.4	0

Acute small bowel obstruction, being partial and intermittent because of its inflammatory nature, can usually be relieved by nonoperative management (nasogastric suction, parenteral nutrition, corticosteroid therapy, antibiotics, and intensive care). However, repetitive obstruction is generally due to established scarring and requires surgery.

One of the most controversial indications for operation is failure of medical treatment.

The decision to operate is based on a thorough analysis of various factors:

1. Severity of symptoms
2. Presence of complications
3. Site, extent, and type of lesions
4. Medical treatment, how it was followed, why it failed, including the possible side effects of the drug used
5. Patient's age and psychosocial status
6. Whether or not the case is a postoperative recurrence
7. Duration of the symptom-free period since the preceding operation, if any
8. Inherent risks (closed loop, free perforation, cancer) from a previous intestinal bypass
9. Risks of surgery now, and the expected long-term postoperative results

Once the pros and cons have been weighed, surgery is advisable only if it seems likely to offer a marked improvement in the quality of life. When surgery is contemplated because optimal medical treatment is not working, both the patient and his physician should be fully involved in the decision. In particular, the outlook regarding bowel movements and subclinical or clinical recurrence needs careful explanation.

Growth retardation and delayed puberty are no longer considered indications for surgery in their own right. Being manifestations of malnutrition, they may be reversed, if the patient is still in the age of puberty, with a daily caloric intake well above normal, that is, an average of 4,000 kcal per day, by total parenteral or enteral nutrition.

TIMING OF SURGERY

The aforementioned indications may require operative intervention in one of the following time frames: emergency, as soon as possible; urgent, within 24 to 72 hours; semi-urgent, later than 72 hours and within 2 weeks; or elective.

Excluding the rare generalized peritonitis, which undoubtedly requires an emergency operation, all other apparently urgent conditions such as intestinal obstruction, localized peritonitis with or without a tender abdominal mass, and severe bleeding should, whenever possible, be dealt with electively, or at least semi-urgently, after a period of intensive medical management. With medical measures such as (1) bowel rest enforced by peripheral total parenteral nutrition or central venous when necessary, or elemental diet, according to the severity of disease, (2) intravenous broad-spectrum antibiotics, and (3) intensive care, surgery may be postponed and thus performed under more favorable conditions. The main drawbacks of urgent surgery are obviously inappropriate preoperative care, omitted bowel preparation, and poor knowledge of the sites and extent of lesions. All of these contribute to an increase in postoperative morbidity and mortality.

The mainstay of such a "reasonable waiting" policy is constant clinical vigilance and reassessment. Should localized peritonitis or acute intestinal obstruction fail to subside or improve in a few days, early operative intervention is mandatory. The rare massive hemorrhage usually responds to blood transfusion, correction of clotting defects, and angiographic procedures; otherwise early surgery is necessary.

PREOPERATIVE MANAGEMENT

In preparing our patients for surgery, we try to accomplish the following:

Limit the Severity of Disease. If this can be done both locally and generally, surgery can be undertaken electively, as already discussed.

Correct Metabolic and Nutritional Defects. Disturbances in fluid and electrolyte balance, acid-base derangements, and anemia all need attention, but nutritional deficits are of prime importance. Malnutrition significantly increases the rate of postoperative morbidity and mortality. Assessment of the patient's nutritional status is therefore mandatory. Malnutrition may be reflected in weight loss (more than 25%), arm muscle circumference less than 70 percent of normal, reduced serum transferrin, and, in particular, serum albumin levels less than 3 g. Total parenteral alimentation or elemental diet is often indicated. Supplementary vitamins (C,D,A, and K), minerals (iron, zinc, magnesium, and copper), and transfusion therapy (blood, plasma, and albumin) are also necessary. Malabsorption is one of the causes of impaired nutritional status. Intestinal absorption studies for fecal fat and possibly the Schilling and/or D-xylose test, according to whether the distal and/or proximal small bowel is involved, may be useful in prognostic evaluation and may sometimes influence intraoperative decisions.

Assess the Extent of Disease Involvement and the Presence of Complications as Accurately and Fully as Possible. This is essential to the planning of the best treatment since intraoperative assessment is often difficult. In the x-ray examination of the small intestine, barium follow-through should be replaced by *small-bowel enema* through duodenal intubation, which provides far more detailed information regarding the type and character of lesions. One can thus demonstrate early aphthous skip lesions and judge whether a fistula is blind (that is, intramesenteric) or involves another organ. The degree of stenosis of a stricture may also be evaluated. Another important advantage of this technique is that it may be safely carried out even during an obstructive episode. The nature of the obstruction can thus be diagnosed, and unnecessary or untimely laparotomy in patients with unknown or unsuspected Crohn's disease may well be avoided. *Double-contrast enema* is mandatory to rule out colonic involvement. *Fistulography* is often advisable when an enterocutaneous fistula is present. The routine use of *contrast urography*, which is more complete than ultrasound investigation of the urinary tract, is justified by the appreciable incidence of urologic complications (25%) such as obstructive uropathy, often clinically unsuspected. Similarly, a routine *cholecystogram* or ultrasonic scan reveals gallstones in many cases. *Ultrasonic or CT scan* also helps one to determine whether a tender palpable abdominal mass is a solid inflammatory phlegmon or contains an abscess; the former may regress with medical treatment, whereas in the latter, corticosteroids should be used with caution and surgery is usually indicated. We always perform *gastroduodenoscopy* and *proctosigmoidoscopy*; colonoscopy also may be required in some cases.

Prevent Infective Complications. The best way to reduce the risk of postoperative sepsis is to improve the patient's nutritional status and thus strengthen his immunologic defenses. Preoperative bowel preparation and perioperative systemic antibiotic cover are also fundamental. As most patients undergo elective surgery, we usually administer oral antibacterial agents effective against aerobic and anaerobic organisms (paromomycin plus metronidazole) for 2 days before operation. Whole-gut irrigation with saline solution is carried out on the day before operation. Parenteral (IV) microbial cover is started immediately before entering the operative theatre and continued for 5 days postoperatively. The combination of choice is metronidazole with either ampicillin plus lactamase-stable cephalosporin or with mezlocillin.

Prevent Adrenocortical Insufficiency. Many patients will have been on cortisone therapy for months and, as a result, are at risk for adrenocortical insufficiency by virtue of surgical stress and abrupt drug withdrawal. Steroid dosages must therefore be continued during operation and tapered postoperatively to achieve gradual weaning.

Prevent Postoperative Thromboembolism. The appreciable incidence of postoperative deep vein thrombosis (5%) is principally due to increased platelet aggregation, as we have demonstrated by serum assay of platelet factor 4 (PF4). Correction of eventual clotting abnormalities is necessary. Prophylaxis with an anti-aggregation drug, such as dipyridamole, should be started several days before surgery and continued until the patient is fully ambulatory.

Prevent Hemorrhagic Gastritis. Cimetidine prophylaxis should be given in cases of severe sepsis and in patients who require emergency or urgent operation.

OPERATIVE STRATEGY

Through a wide midline (xiphopubic)laparotomy incision, we first explore thoroughly the abdominal cavity and the entire digestive tract from stomach to rectum. The spread and severity of disease are assessed from the serosal side, estimating the boundaries of the lesions from the thickening and rigidity of the bowel wall, hyperemia, mesenteric wrapping, and enlarged nodes. Meticulous dissection is often required before all the loops of bowel are separated. There is no doubt that resection of the diseased intestinal segment affords complete or nearly complete regression of symptoms. We have found, as have others, that when gross residual disease is left, as after bypass, readmissions or further operations are more frequent. If at all possible, we prefer not to leave gross residual disease, but we also endeavor to avoid creating or aggravating malabsorption, keeping in mind the likelihood of future surgery for recurrence.

After a preliminary stock-taking of the lesions, we measure the total length of small intestine along the antimesenteric border, unfolding it gradually without undue stretching, concentrating especially on the amount of healthy bowel rather than on the diseased portions. These measurements have proved useful for a correct evaluation of the functional results after surgery, serving as a prognostic yardstick. They may also facilitate certain intraoperative decisions (to be discussed). In follow-up functional studies measuring fecal fat (normal values less than 5 g per day), we have noted that, because of the wide individual variations in the length of small intestine (290 to 550 cm, average 420 cm), malabsorption correlates with the amount of small bowel left rather than with the amount resected. A moderate degree of malabsorption (fecal fat: 12 to 20 g per day), and sometimes a severe degree (more than 20 g per day), has been found in patients with residual small bowel of less than 2 m. Although this is not often of great importance clinically, being compensated for eventually, we thought it wise to consider this length as a safety limit. When we used to perform "radical" resection, this length was particularly important. In practice, however, in a first exeresis for classic terminal ileitis, far more bowel always remained.

Classic Terminal Ileitis or Right-Sided Ileocolitis. After assessing the extent of disease from the serosal side, we perform a preliminary resection of the affected segment, with about 10 cm of apparently healthy tissue above and about 5 cm below as recurrence is usually preanastomotic. Then, opening the surgical specimen, we check the mucosal side, and if there are any lesions near either of the section lines, we make a further resection of about 5 to 10 cm. This approach may seem somewhat arbitrary, but it is a reasonable compromise between the strictly "conservative" and the "radical" resection, which removes 15 to 20 cm of healthy bowel above and below the lesion. We abandoned "radical" resection about 2 years ago, when we concluded that it neither prevented nor significantly delayed postoperative recurrence.

We do not use frozen sections to evaluate the histopathologic status of resection margins; they are both misleading and useless. The quick intraoperative diagnosis thus obtained is often at variance with the definitive histologic report, and the persistence of microscopic lesions does not appear to influence recurrence. We make no attempt to widen removal of enlarged mesenteric nodes, principally because this might necessitate a greater unnecessary sacrifice of bowel.

We usually excise neighboring skip lesions en bloc with the diseased bowel. If they are further away, either single or two or three close together, we treat them by making one or two small additional resections with "naked-eye" margins uninvolved, even when these lesions are not obstructive.

In Crohn's ileitis, we perform an ileal resection with end-to-end anastomosis. Terminal ileitis is treated by ileocecal resection, sparing the ascending colon for absorptive and antidiarrheal purposes. Right hemicolectomy is carried out only if the right colon is involved. Even if the discrepancy in size between the ileum and the colon is not a major problem, the anastomosis is more frequently made side-to-side using absorbable material and standard technique.

Recurrent or Widespread Small-Bowel Crohn's Disease. The intraoperative anatomic patterns (extent of lesions, length of healthy small bowel) in recurrence often are not so different from those found in many cases of initial disease. For the sake of clarity, however, we include recurrent disease in the same paragraph as widespread disease because, as a general rule, both conditions require a more conservative surgical approach. We must resist the temptation to resect all grossly diseased bowel and wisely try to retain as much as possible for nutritional support. Taking this for granted, the following factors may help our decision: (1) topography, number, type, and extent of lesions; (2) preoperative absorption tests, in particular fecal fat; (3) intraoperative measurement of small bowel; and (4) the length of residual small bowel recorded during the eventual preceding operation. The last-mentioned is especially useful because the measurement during reoperation is often approximate, to avoid undue unravelling of the intestine.

If the residual small bowel is likely to be, or is already, less than 2 m and/or if preoperative functional studies have shown significant malabsorption, we resect only the small diseased portion that provided the indication for surgery. When there are multiple and diffuse skip lesions and/or ileojejunitis, an uncommon but not rare event, we only deal with the obstructed segment or, rarely, with that segment containing perforation or producing a stagnant loop syndrome or exudative enteropathy. As dilatation above the lesion has usually been relieved by preoperative preparation, it may be difficult to judge the degree of stenosis of a stricture by simple palpation between thumb and forefinger. If necessary, stenosis can be evaluated by means of a fiberoptic gastroscope, either by mouth or through the margin of the concomitant intestinal resection or through an enterotomy. In this case, the endoscope is guided by the surgeon as far as the stenosis. Alternatively, one may use internal balloon diameter measurement with a Foley catheter. Only strictures through which the endoscope cannot pass or those less than 2 cm in diameter are treated, leaving the others in situ. We prefer limited resection to bypass whenever possible, even sometimes ignoring inflammation or aphthous lesions found on the section margins. We have had no experience with longitudinal incision of strictures followed by transvere closure (stricturoplasty), as suggested by Alexander-Williams and Lee.

At the end of the operation we always leave abdominal drainage in place, using two Redon sumps. These are kept in place until any exudate from mesenteric lymph vessels have subsided, usually about 6 days. The abdominal wall is then properly closed with slowly absorbable suture material such as Vicryl or Dexon. Closure of the skin and subcutaneous tissue is deferred only if there has been heavy contamination at operation.

Special Cases

Fistulas are improved but not healed by total parenteral nutrition. They are usually associated with a certain degree of stenosis of the bowel, owing to fibrosis or a concomitant abscess. Fistulas do not spread Crohn's disease into an adjacent intestinal viscus (sigmoid colon, proximal small bowel) or into an extraintestinal organ such as the bladder or uterus. Treatment therefore consists of primary resection of the diseased segment after careful dissection from the target organ. A useful way to uncover a suspected sigmoid orifice after separation from the diseased ileal loop is to insufflate air through the rectum while the abdominal cavity is full of saline; to reveal an enterovesical orifice, the bladder may be filled with dye. The opening in the target organ is simply sutured. When the bladder is involved, a catheter is usually left in place, for safety, for one week after the operation. If the fistula communicates with the intestine, and there is marked inflammation or the opening is too wide to be sutured safely, or there are many openings, then the diseased part of the target organ should be resected as well. The enteroduodenal fistula, which may arise in a recurrence after right hemicolectomy, is an unusual case. As the ileotransversostomy lies on the second duodenal portion, juxta-anastomotic lesions may work their way back into the duodenum. A simple suture of the orifice in the duodenum, after dissection and new ileocolic resection, may lead to a postoperative duodenal fistula. It is therefore safer and more advisable to use the duodenal opening for a two-layer anastomosis with the jejunum, putting the omentum, if still present, around it.

The intraparietal tract of the enterocutaneous fistula has to be widely debrided and removed. The peritoneum is then closed from the inside with absorbable sutures, and the opening onto the skin is packed and left to heal by secondary intention.

Abscesses, which form through microperforations of the intestinal wall, may be superficial (intraparietal) or deep (mesenteric along the paracolic gutters, or pelvic). If these are merely drained, a fistula usually forms. Thus, deep abscesses absolutely require resection of the responsible bowel segment, and culture of pus is imperative.

Free perforation is an extremely rare event. After peritoneal lavage and debridement, primary resection and anastomosis can usually be accomplished. Suction drainage and continuous irrigation devices may be an important adjunct.

Obstructive uropathy is usually relieved by simple removal of the causative inflammatory mass. Ureterolysis is indicated only when there is severe retroperitoneal fibrosis causing ureter entrapment. However, in practice, the ureter should always be exposed and freed to make removal of the abdominal mass safer.

Gastroduodenitis is sometimes discovered. The stomach and/or duodenum is an uncommon but not rare site of disease, nearly always associated with the classic involvement of the terminal ileum or very occasionally with jejunoileitis. Surgery may be required for a complication arising from one or more of the foregoing sites, ignoring all other localizations without complications. The most common indication for surgery in Crohn's disease of the stomach and/or duodenum is obstruction. Bypass is the only suitable procedure. Gastrojejunostomy combined with selective vagotomy is indicated when the obstruction involves the gastric antrum or the proximal duodenum, duodenojejunostomy when it affects the third or fourth duodenal portion.

Ileitis mimicking appendicitis is sometimes detected at operation performed for a presumed appendicitis and may be acute or chronic. The acute form, being more often due to a *yersinia* infection, rarely progresses into the chronic form, that is, typical Crohn's disease. In both conditions, a simple appendectomy is recommended to avoid subsequent diagnostic problems except when there is gross involvement of the cecum with risk of fecal fistula, or when there is intestinal obstruction. If the cecum is involved, the abdomen must be closed without appendectomy. If there is intestinal obstruction, intestinal resection is obligatory.

Appendicitis from or in Crohn's disease may be found at operation in a patient with typical Crohn's disease. Removal of the acutely inflamed appendix is obviously indicated, but if the cecum is also diseased, intestinal resection is advisable.

Perianal suppurative lesions, such as skin tags, fissures, fistulas, and abscesses, are more frequent in Crohn's disease of the large bowel, but they are often associated with Crohn's ileitis, sometimes appearing before Crohn's disease itself is manifest. Aggressive surgical management is often followed by a high incidence of local recurrence and sometimes by anal stenosis or fecal incontinence. Therefore, in agreement with many surgeons, we advocate in these patients only conservative or minimal surgical treatment such as simple drainage of pus. However, these procedures should be done in the operating room under general or regional anesthesia, not in the office. We find complementary treatment with oral metronidazole extremely effective, even though some time after the drug has been withdrawn relapses are more frequent.

POSTOPERATIVE MANAGEMENT

This is basically a continuation of the pre- and intraoperative preventive measures already discussed, and these pertain primarily to postoperative sepsis. If infection occurs, in spite of antimicrobial therapy, the antibiotics must be substituted with those indicated by the cultures.

The nasogastric tube is left in place for 48 hours. Parenteral nutrition with 3,500 to 4,000 kcal per day is continued until intestinal transit is resumed. This usually happens on about the third or fourth postoperative day.

Daily monitoring of the usual postoperative parameters is indispensable, particularly hemochrome, hematocrit, and albumin determinations and fluid and electrolyte balance. The patient usually is discharged in about 12 days.

PROGNOSIS AND FOLLOW-UP AFTER SURGERY

Early Postoperative Morbidity and Mortality

Surgery for Crohn's disease carries a high morbidity rate, related both to location, particularly in colitis, and to the severity of disease. In small-bowel disease, the rate of early postoperative complications varies in the literature from 15 to 28 percent, and in our experience about 29 percent of patients were affected (18.8% in the last 10 years). As already mentioned, the principal causes of morbidity and mortality are malnutrition, emergency operation, and coagulation defects. The most common complications are infections, particularly wound and abdominal sepsis unrelated to the use of corticosteroid therapy (Table 2). Postoperative mortality ranges from 0 to 3 percent and is 2.5 percent in our series (1.1% in the last 10 years).

Postoperative Surveillance

After surgery our patients are seen about every 6 months by our gastroenterology staff. Clinical and laboratory tests are carried out regularly to follow disease activity and diagnose recurrence promptly. In recent years, in addition to the well-known activity indexes CDAI, NCDAI, and SI, we have used serum CEA assay in monitoring patients for recurrence.

The principal aim of postoperative surveillance is to begin pharmacologic therapy without delay in the event of a flare-up of disease. However, the drugs of proven efficacy in the active stage do not seem to be beneficial in the treatment of quiescent disease or in the prevention of recurrence.

Recurrence

The incidence of postoperative recurrence is directly correlated with the length of follow-up, statistical methods employed for analysis, and particularly with the criteria used to define recurrence. Symptomatic recurrence must be distinguished from radiologic recurrence and from that requiring operation.

In our opinion, the most appropriate definition of recurrence based on both clinical practice and speculative research is: clinical and laboratory findings of re-emergent disease confirmed by x-ray findings and/or endoscopy and/or histopathologic findings after the removal of all evident lesions. This view substantially agrees with the Cape Town classification.

Recurrence as defined above and calculated by actuarial analysis occurred 5 years after operation in 44 percent, 10 years after operation in 60 percent, and 15 years after operation in 78 percent of our patients operated on for ileitis and right-sided ileocolitis. The site of recurrence had been clearly conditioned by the initial location of disease. The most common site of recurrence was preanastomotic, but colonic involvement also seemed to favor postanastomotic recurrence.

In a recent retrospective study, the following prognostic clinical factors for recurrence were considered: sex, age, length of preoperative history, initial location, extent of lesions, indications for resection, and number of operations performed. Only a preoperative history of more than 5 years correlated directly with recurrence, although many other authors report opposite trends. Most important of all, no significant correlation appeared between the recurrence rate and either the length of macroscopically free resection margins or the histologic grading at the two section lines. This agrees with the findings of most authors and, even allowing for the limitations of a retrospective study, favors conservative resection to obtain merely grossly uninvolved margins.

Survival and Quality of Life

Follow-up of our patients from 2 to 21 years, median about 10 after operation, has also shown that the postoperative functional and health status has been fair or even good in most cases of recurrence (80%, Table 3). About 28 percent of patients required two operations and 4.4 percent three operations for recurrence. The postoperative rate of morbidity and mortality was not significantly different from that after the first operation. Some patients died because of the evolution of the disease itself quite apart from postoperative complications. The overall mortality in our series is therefore 6.4 percent. Our results confirm other authors findings. In con-

TABLE 2 Early Complications After Surgery for Crohn's Disease of the Small Intestine

	% in other series* (average)	% in our series* (over 154 operated cases)
Wound infection	10.1	10.3
Abdominal abscess	4	4.5
Thromboembolism	3.5	4.5
Deep thrombosis	2	2.5
Pulmonary embolism	1.5	1.9
Septicemia	3	1.2
Pneumonia	3	5.1
Anastomotic leak	2.8	0.6
Obstruction	2.5	--
Bleeding	1.6	1.9
Fistula	1.5	2.5
Wound dehiscence	1.5	0.6
Other (e.g., hepatitis, urinary infection, convulsion, heart failure)	2.4	2.5

* Several patients had two or more complications.

TABLE 3 Quality of Life After the First Exeresis for Terminal Ileitis or Right-Sided Ileocolitis (90 cases): Follow-up 2 to 21 yrs (average, 10 yrs)

	Pts without recurrence (33 cases)		Pts with recurrence (57 cases)	
	No.	%	No.	%
Good	28	86	27	47.5
Fair	5	14	20	34.4
Poor	--	--	10	18.1

p< 0.001

clusion, in spite of the tendency of Crohn's disease to recur, and even though survival in these patients is on the whole slightly lower than normal life expectany, sur-gery can, when there are suitable indications, significantly improve the quality of life.

TUMOR OF THE SMALL BOWEL

MOREYE NUSBAUM, M.D.

Small bowel tumors may be either benign or malignant. They are relatively uncommon. About 40 percent are benign and 60 percent malignant. The benign tumors of the small intestine are primarily adenomas, leiomyomoas, lipomas, fibromas, angiomas, pancreatic rests, and neurilemomas. The exact incidence of benign tumors is uncertain since the majority of them go unrecognized, and unless incidentally reported at the time of autopsy, their true incidence is not recorded unless clinical symptoms surface.

Neoplastic lesions of the small intestine represent only about 0.4 percent of all malignant tumors and about 2 percent of all intestinal tract malignant tumors. The most common malignant tumors of the small intestine are, in their order of frequency, adenocarcinomas (which constitute approximately 50% of recorded malignant lesions), carcinoids, lymphosarcomas, and leiomyosarcomas (Table 1).

TABLE 1 Classification of Tumors of the Small Bowel

Tissue of Origin	Benign	Malignant
Glandular epithelium	Adenomatous polyp, villous adenoma, Brunner's adenoma	Adenocarcinoma
Enterochromaffin cells		Carcinoid
Smooth muscle	Leiomyoma	Leiomyosarcoma
Lymphoid tissue	Pseudolymphoma	Lymphosarcoma
Fat	Lipoma	Liposarcoma
Connective tissue	Fibroma	Fibrosarcoma
Nervous tissue	Neurilemoma	Malignant schwannoma
Blood vessels	Hemangioma	Angiosarcoma
Lymph vessels	Lymphangioma	Not reported
Mixed	Peutz-Jegher's polyp	
Other		Metastatic lesions

EPITHELIAL BENIGN TUMORS

Of these tumors, adenomatous polyps are the most common in the small bowel, despite the fact that they are in themselves rare, but as in the large bowel, they can progress to carcinoma in many cases and therefore should be removed. They are rare in the duodenum and more common in the ileum; they can bleed and cause intestinal obstruction leading to surgery. The intestinal polyposis of Peutz-Jegher's syndrome are actually hamartomas and benign, but are associated with concomitant malignant tumors of the gastrointestinal tract in 4 percent of cases. They frequently present with intussusception. Gardner's syndrome is a variant of familial polyposis and is pre-malignant. Two cases of small bowel adenocarcinoma have been reported in this entity.

NONEPITHELIAL TUMORS

Nonepithelial tumors of the small bowel include leiomyomas and fibroleiomyomas. They represent 20 percent of all benign tumors of the small intestine. Mucosal erosion with hemorrhage is a common presenting symptom of these tumors. Two-thirds of these are malignant and 30 percent of them metastasize to the liver and to the regional lymph nodes. Fibromas are rare tumors of the small bowel and may just represent fibrous degeneration of small bowel polyps. Tumors of the nerve endings such as neurilemomas and neurofibromas are found on rare occasions. Lipomas are also found in the small bowel. They are rare and produce obstruction by intussusception or, occasionally, produce presenting symptoms of ulceration and hemorrhage.

ENDOCRINE TUMORS

Tumors of the gastrointestinal endocrine cells that involve the small bowel relate to the APUD cell line. In the small bowel there is one principal amine-secreting cell, the enterochromaffin cell, which is argentaffin-positive and is associated with 5-hydroxtryptamine production. It may also secrete bradykinin or other polypeptide hormones, but this has not been proved as yet.

Seventy percent of all carcinoids are found, usually incidentally, in the appendix of young adults and are completely benign. The remainder occur mostly in the low ileum, usually in the sixth or seventh decades of life; they are frequently multiple and can be associated with carcinoma elsewhere in the gastrointestinal tract. These chromaffin tumors are slow-growing, but often have lymph node and hepatic metastases at the time of surgery.

All carcinoids of the small bowel should be regarded as carcinomas of low-grade malignancy with a tendency to metastasize that relates directly to increase in their size. Clinically, patients with carcinoids present with small bowel obstruction, or intussusception, or with demonstrated mesenteric lymph node masses, as well as liver metastases that produce an associated carcinoid syndrome. Abdominal pain and episodes of diarrhea after meals without preceding pain are characteristic of this entity. The tumor is grossly bright yellow in color, and its metastases have an associated fibrotic consistency, which can impair the small bowel mesentery and the blood supply to the gut.

The other tumor of endocrine cell origin that occurs in the small bowel is the gastrinoma, which can occur in the duodenum. If found, they frequently can be managed by local enucleation or resection without necessitating major pancreaticoduodenal resection.

EPITHELIAL MALIGNANT TUMORS

Of the epithelial neoplasms of the small bowel, primary carcinomas constitute less than 1 percent of all intestinal carcinomas. It is equally distributed in the duodenum, jejunum, and ileum. In the duodenum, carcinoma of the ampulla of Vater is the most common. With these exluded, supra-ampullary and infra-ampullary duodenal lesions are equally common.

The presenting symptom of small bowel carcinoma may be bleeding, intussusception, or obstruction. It metastasizes to local lymph nodes and from there to the para-aortic nodes. There is an increased incidence of carcinoma of the small bowel associated with glutin-induced enteropathy and with Crohn's disease. Metastatic carcinoma to the small bowel can occur, but it is not common. Primary tumors that were reported to metastasize to the small bowel include those of the lung, adrenal, ovary, stomach, colon, uterus, cervix, and kidney, and occasionally melanomas. Metastatic lesions usually can be differentiated from primary lesions in the small bowel since they tend to localize to the serosa or submucosa and rarely cause mucosal ulceration.

MALIGNANT LYMPHOID TUMORS

Malignant lymphoid tumors of the small bowel include, most frequently, lymphosarcoma and Hodgkin's disease. Lymphoid tumors have a poor prognosis, the majority of patients surviving no longer than 2 years.

Primary lymphoma of the small bowel frequently involves the terminal ileum and presents with intussusception and small bowel obstruction. Lymphomas with pre-existing lymph node disease, such as alpha-chain disease or multiple lymphoid polyposis and gluten free enteropathy, may have a slightly better prognosis. Primary lymphomas elsewhere can spread to the small bowel, and 50 percent of such lymphomas do, in fact, metastasize to the small bowel. The majority of these are Hodgkin's disease and reticulum cell sarcoma. Occasional solitary plasmacytomas of the small bowel have been reported.

DIAGNOSIS

Symptoms include those of partial or complete small bowel obstruction, with or without volvulus. Hemorrhage, which may on rare occasions be massive, most often represents only microscopic blood loss in the stool or an unexpected iron deficiency anemia. Intussusception may occur, particularly with some of the intestinal benign polyps and more frequently with liposarcoma than with other malignant lesions. On rare occasions, perforation of the small bowel can occur as a result of tumor.

The prime diagnostic tool is a high index of clinical suspicion as a result of a careful history and physical examination. In retrospect, many of the symptoms are chronic and overlooked instead of being noted as indicators for specific diagnostic procedures and early surgical therapy. If there is any clinical indication of a small bowel tumor, a small bowel barium enema through a tube placed in the upper jejunum provides the best visualization of mucosal detail in the small intestine and thus is more helpful in the diagnosis of small bowel lesions than are routine progress meal or barium enema studies that reflux. Serial tagged red cell nuclear scans may help to localize bleeding to the small bowel. In the face of either acute or occult blood loss from the gastrointestinal tract, the use of arteriography may lead to earlier diagnosis of these lesions, particularly if magnification arteriography is used in areas of suspicion. Endoscopy of the small bowel is not clinically applicable except in the duodenum, although there is future promise of an endoscopic technique to evaluate the upper small bowel. Occasionally, colonoscopic techniques can allow for passage into the terminal ileum for evaluation of this area.

SURGICAL CONSIDERATIONS

The majority of patients with small bowel tumors present as surgical emergencies as a result of small bowel obstruction. At the time of surgical exploration, an occult small bowel tumor must be ruled out, particularly in patients who have not had prior surgery and have no obvious reason for their small bowel obstruction or volvulus. Early small bowel lesions also might be discovered by careful exploration of the small intestine at the time of laparotomy for any condition. Careful bimanual exploration of the small bowel, tumor such as a carcinoid, resection of which may result in cure. Although routine exploration of the small intestine should be an integral part of all abdominal explorations, it is frequently done in a cursory manner or, during the exigencies of surgery, completely omitted. By attending to this detail, I have been able to find and remove benign small bowel tumors such as polyps, pancreatic rests, neurilemomas, neurofibromas, and carcinoids.

If a small tumor is identified, its exact nature, if not obvious, should be confirmed by frozen section diagnosis. Certain small bowel tumors, such as carcinoma and carcinoids, have a characteristic appearance and may not require frozen section prior to surgical removal. Carcinoid of the small bowel is characterized by a yellow appearance, associated fibrosis of the mesentery, and firm lymph nodes. Adenocarcinoma of the small bowel characteristicaly penetrates and causes puckering of the serosal side and ulceration of the mucosal side. Surgery of benign small bowel tumors generally consists of an enterotomy and local resection, but occasionally a sleeve resection of the involved area may be advisable. Special problems may be encountered with benign adenomatous lesions of the ampulla of Vater, as well as the different portions of the duodenum. Unless extremely large, as in some cases of villous adenoma of the duodenum, these may be removed by local resection. In the case of an extremely large lesion of the duodenum, such as a villous adenoma, which is known to be a premalignant lesion, a pancreato-duodenal resection may be necessary for maximal removal of tumor provided the patient's potential for long-term survival and general medical condition will permit. For patients with malignant lesions of the small intestine, evaluation of the extent of disease is important. The presence of lymph node metastases, and certainly of hepatic metastases, reinforces the poor prognosis of a late lesion. If the lesion is confined to the small bowel, resection of the small bowel tumor with a 6-inch margin on either side and a wide wedge of mesentery is recommended. Suspected lymph nodes in the para-aortic area or the root of the mesentery should be evaluated by biopsy,

as should hepatic lesions. Lymph nodes should be included in the resection if their inclusion would not necessitate resection of a major portion of the small bowel, since lymph node involvement itself carries a poor prognosis. Since surgery under these conditions is primarily palliative, it is not reasonable to remove extensive yardage of small intestine. However, if these nodes can be removed, either by local resection without removing additional small intestine or with a moderate loss of small intestine, their removal may lead to improvement in palliation. This is particularly true of patients with malignant carcinoid tumors in whom the debulking process may allow for longer survival as well as better response to the chemotherapy programs currently available. My own approach is to remove as many of these lymph nodes as possible, although in the face of a malignant carcinoid the desmoplastic reaction in the mesentery surrounding these nodes may make their removal difficult as well as hazardous to mesenteric blood supply. If there is a limited number of easily accessible metastatic implants in the liver, these also should be removed locally in an attempt to further debulk the tumor, particularly if a functioning carcinoid syndrome is part of its presenting preoperative picture. In diffuse lymphoid tumors of the small bowel, a full-thickness biopsy should be done to adequately evaluate the lesion for future chemotherapy and radiation therapy. Despite the many studies available for the diagnosis of small intestinal neoplasms, because they are uncommon, it is difficult to obtain significant information relating to long-term survival and prognosis. Studies on surgically removed tumors, particulary the malignant ones, report high morbidity and mortality rates because these patients have presented with symptoms at a late stage in the course of their tumor history and require frequent operation for recurrent obstruction. The 5-year survival rate for adenocarcinoma of the small bowel is only 20 to 30 percent. Prognosis is better in carcinoid tumors, with 5-year survival rates of 45 to 65 percent in patients without metastases and 21 percent if metastases are present at the time of surgery.

SMALL BOWEL DIVERTICULAR DISEASE

JOHN M. KELLUM, M.D.

With the aging to the population, diverticular disease of the small intestine is becoming relatively more common. Although recent studies offer a better insight into the clinical relevance of these entitites, our understanding of the relationship of gastrointestinal symptoms and diverticula is still far from complete. Except for Meckel's diverticulum, most small intestinal diverticula are acquired, pulsion, or pseudodiverticula like their colonic counterparts. They tend to occur on the mesenteric aspect of the bowel, most often seen at the point where the mesenteric vessels pierce the muscular wall. As in colonic diverticular disease, surgery may be indicated for the rare complications, namely, inflammation, perforation, obstruction, bleeding, and fistulization. This chapter summarizes the current understanding and preferred management of duodenal, jejunoileal, and Meckel's diverticula.

DUODENAL DIVERTICULUM

The reported incidence of duodenal diverticula on upper gastrointestinal contrast studies varies from 1 percent to as high as 20 percent. Of these, 95 percent occur on the concave (or pancreatic) aspect, 70 percent residing within 3 cm of the ampulla of Vater in the second portion of the duodenum. Most are solitary, and there is a frequent association with diverticulosis coli. Those located on the convex aspect are more likely to be multiple.

Although most duodenal diverticula are acquired, the *intraluminal diverticulum* is a congenital anomaly, which is distinguished from the ordinary duodenal diverticulum by having a mucosal lining on both surfaces and by projecting into the lumen. It has been associated with Down's syndrome. Obstruction and hemorrhage are indications for excision.

It has been estimated that duodenal diverticula result in symptoms in less than 5 percent of cases. Postprandial upper abdominal pain, nausea, vomiting, eructation, diarrhea, flatulence, and weight loss have all been ascribed to diverticula. Recurrent cholangitis or pancreatitis, in a few rare instances, have been associated with demonstrated reflux into the choledochus or duct of Wirsung from a peri-Vaterian diverticulum.

Evaluation in patients with such symptoms should include careful contrast duodenography and fluoroscopy in anterior-posterior, oblique, and lateral planes. Early filling of the colon on such studies may indicate a duodenocolic fistula. In patients with acute abdominal pain, supine and lateral plain x-ray films may demonstrate retroperitoneal edema or emphysema associated with diverticular perforation. Upper gastrointestinal fiberoptic endoscopy, especially with the side viewing scope, may localize hemorrhage or inflammatory changes to a duodenal diverticulum.

Indications for operation include recurrent inflammation, hemorrhage, perforation, obstruction, recurrent pancreatitis or cholangitis, and fistulization into the colon, gallbladder, bile duct, or stomach. It has been reported that 50 percent of the diverticula associated with fistulas are the rare posterior or lateral diverticula located on the convex aspect of the second and third portions of the duodenum.

Duodenal diverticula in the second portion of the duodenum should be exposed by means of a generous Kocher maneuver. Diverticula located near the ampulla, and expecially those projecting into the pancreas, should be approached both externally and internally through a vertical duodenotomy in the anterior wall. A probe placed through a choledochotomy and passed through the ampulla keeps the surgeon constantly aware of the relationship of the diverticulum and the distal bile duct. After teasing it away from the pancreas, the surgeon gently inverts the diverticulum, excises it, and closes it with interrupted silk from the luminal aspect. In many cases, this should be combined with sphincteroplasty to ensure free drainage of the bile and pancreatic ducts. If the diverticulum cannot be excised without compromising the ostia of the ducts, simple inversion with repair of the defect in the muscular wall of the duodenum is an acceptable alternative. Diverticula that are neither projecting into the pancreas nor peri-Vaterian are best excised from the serosal surface with a two-layer closure.

Diverticula in the third or forth portion of the duodenum are best approached with full mobilization of the right colon and an extended Kocher maneuver. For diverticula located near the superior mesenteric vessels or their branches, adequate exposure may necessitate dividing the ligament of Treitz and the posterior duodenal attachments with delivery of the duodenum out from under the vessels. External excision with a two-layer closure is the treatment of choice. When left with a large, partially necrotic defect in the duodenum as, for example, after division of a duodenocolic fistula, the surgeon may use a serosal patch to lessen the risk of a lateral duodenal fistula. This patch consists of an incontinuity loop of proximal jejunum sutured with seromuscular sutures at 5-mm intervals to the duodenal wall around the defect using healthy duodenal tissue away from the edges.

JEJUNAL AND ILEAL DIVERTICULA

Like duodenal diverticula, those in the remaining small intestines are acquired, pseudo, or pulsion diverticula consisting of herniations of mucosa and submucosa through the muscularis of the bowel wall. They are multiple and occur along the mesenteric aspect of the bowel wall at sites of blood vessel penetration. There is a frequent association with colonic diverticulosis. Although they are frequently located in the proximal jejunum, myriad diverticula along the entire small intestine may be seen in some cases. They are more commonly seen in elderly patients and have a slight female preponderance. The overall incidence is estimated to be 1.3 percent.

Small bowel diverticula are best demonstrated on barium radiographic examinations of the small bowel. Barium retention may persist after jejunal emptying. Occasionally, plain abdominal films taken with the patient in the upright position reveal diverticula as local collections of gas, sometimes accompanied by fluid levels.

Most patients are asymptomatic. The most widely recognized complication of multiple small bowel diverticula is the malabsorption syndrome, induced by bacterial overgrowth and characterized by megaloblastic anemia, steatorrhea, and weight loss. This syndrome may be associated with intestinal pseudo-obstruction and has been associated with abnormal motility patterns in the small intestine both in areas with and in those without diverticula. Some patients have signs of progressive systemic sclerosis. Low doses of such antibiotics as tetracycline or metronidazole given on an intermittent or rotaing basis may control the malabsorption and steatorrhea. Recently reported long-term follow-up of patients subjected to segmental resection for malabsorption or pseudo-obstruction suggest a high incidence of recurrent symptoms, presumably from abnormal motility in the remaining small bowel.

It is not always possible to differentiate functional from mechanical obstruction. The latter may result from enterolith formation in diverticula, from intussusception, or from inflammation with intramural or mesenteric inflammatory masses. Segmental resection is indicated in such patients. Bleeding from diverticula may be difficult to distinguish from other gastrointestinal sources. The technitium blood-pool scan may indicate an upper small bowel source; this finding in conjunction with demonstrated diverticula on contrast roentgenographic studies would indicate resection.

If localization by blood-pool scanning is equivocal, selective mesenteric arteriography may be diagnostic if bleeding is brisk. Perforation is heralded by signs of peritonitis and pneumoperitoneum. Usually resection and primary reanastomosis are possible. Occasionally with gross feculent peritonitis or with delayed diagnosis of a perforating ileal diverticulitis, resection with ileostomy and creation of a colonic mucous fistula may be advisable.

MECKEL'S DIVERTICULUM

This congenital diverticulum is a result of a failure of closure of the vitelline duct. It is a true diverticulum in that it contains all three coats of the intestinal wall. It occurs on the antimesenteric side of the ileum and is usually about 5 cm in length. It is usually of broader diameter and neck than the appendix. It may be remembered as occurring in 2 percent of individuals and within 2 feet of the ileocecal valve. Of the complications requiring surgery, 60 percent occur in children under 10 years of age.

The most frequent complication in the pediatric age group is peptic ulceration and bleeding. About 50 percent of all Meckel's diverticula contain ectopic mucosa, usually gastric, but occasionally pancreatic, duodenal, jejunal, colonic, or biliary. Those containing gastric mucosa can be identified by means of ^{99m}Tc pertechnetate scanning, particularly after a pentagastrin injection (6 mg per kilogram subcutaneously) given 15 minutes before the scan to enhance uptake of the isotope by the gastric mucosa. Pretreatment with cimetidine to block excretion of the isotope from the gastric mucosa and glucagon to reduce motility and luminal excretion further increases the sensitivity of this test. The small bowel contrast radiographic series rarely demonstrates a Meckel's diverticulum.

The next most common complication in children and the most common in adults is intestinal obstruction, which may result from intussusception, volvulus, or internal hernia around an adhesion from the tip of the diverticulum to the abdominal wall. Diverticulitis is usually the result of inspissated material within the lumen and is frequently indistinguishable from appendicitis. Over half of these diverticula are perforated at the time of operation, highlighting the frequent difficulty of diagnosis. Occasionally, plain abdominal films demonstrate a calcified enterolith in an uncharacteristic location for the appendix.

Resection is the treatment of choice for all complicated Meckel's diverticula and for most discovered incidentally at laparotomy. Most can be successfully treated by wedge resection with suture of the defect in the wall of the ileum. Occasionally, in small children, the mouth of the diverticulum is so large along the longitudinal axis of the bowel that such closure would compromise the lumen. In such patients, a segmental resection of the ileum containing the diverticulum should be performed. In patients with hemorrhage, it is wiser to do an open inspection of the adjacent ileal mocosa prior to closure, since the peptic ulceration may be in adjacent ileum rather than in the diverticulum itself.

MESENTERIC VASCULAR OCCLUSIVE DISEASE

GREGORY B. BULKLEY, M.D., F.A.C.S.

Acute intestinal vascular insufficiency remains one of the most challenging clinical situations that the surgeon faces. Overall, our success rate is dismal, the reported mortality for major vascular occlusion ranging from 50 to 100 percent. For its most common and least lethal form, intestinal strangulation, the mortality rate is more than double that for mechanical small bowel obstruction. Its successful management requires the skillful setting of diagnostic and therapeutic priorities in a clinical setting that is invariably complex. For example, the delay of laparotomy is in some cases disastrous, in other cases essential to a successful outcome.

Acute mesenteric ischemia may be due either to the anatomic occlusion of a mesenteric vessel or to vasospasm of arteriolar beds that these vessels serve. Anatomic arterial occlusion is seen most commonly in the presence of atherosclerosis, where it is due either to the thrombosis of or hemorrhage into an existing atherosclerotic plaque or to embolization from a proximal site (Table 1). In a few patients, the slow, progressive stenosis of the mesenteric vessels may lead to chronic intestinal angina, characterized by postprandial pain and weight loss. Acute vascular insufficiency may also result from the disruption of one or more mesenteric vessels due to either exogenous trauma or a surgical procedure. Rarely, the primary vascular occlusion is venous thrombosis, precipitated by dehydration, a hypercoagulable state, portal hypertension, or polycythemia. In this situation, arterial insufficiency develops subsequently and somewhat more slowly, but with the same devastating effects. However, the most common cause of acute mesenteric vascular insufficiency is strangulation obstruction of the small intestine, which complicates about one-third of cases of *complete* small bowel obstruction. This may be due to a midgut volvulus, adhesions, or a strangulated hernia. Nonocclusive mesenteric ischemia (NOMI) is the result of a profound splanchnic vasospasm which can appear as an endogenous response to severe physiologic stress, such as shock, congestive failure, sepsis, and respiratory insufficiency. This condition may also be caused or exacerbated by the exogenous administration of splanchnic vasoconstrictors, including vasopressor agents and digitalis.

GENERAL PRINCIPLES OF MANAGEMENT

Early Diagnosis

The key to the successful management of all forms of intestinal ischemia is *early* diagnosis, which leads to prompt and definitive treatment. The high mortality associated with these diseases is not usually due to our inability to reverse the underlying vascular lesion. The surgeon is frequently able to reduce the strangulation or to anatomically revascularize. The radiologist can pharmacologically reverse the vasospasm underlying NOMI. Nevertheless, the patient often succumbs because this treatment is instituted only after irreversible intestinal tissue damage has taken place. This leaves the surgeon to choose between a massive bowel resection incompatible with a meaningful subsequent existence, or the ravages of uncontrolled ongoing sepsis. Furthermore, the high overall mortality of these conditions, and the frequently elderly and debilitated population that they strike, have led to a depressing therapeutic nihilism on the part of many otherwise aggressive clinicians. Although it is undoubtedly true that mesenteric ischemia, especially NOMI, can appear as an agonal conclusion to the overall downhill course of an unsalvageable patient, in most cases a

TABLE 1 Pathogenesis of Acute Mesenteric Ischemia

Condition	Primary Cause	Major Contributing Factors
Arterial thrombosis	Thrombosis of or hemorrhage into a preexisting atherosclerotic plaque	Dehydration, low cardiac output, hypercoagulable state
Arterial embolism	Embolus from heart (mural or valvular) or aorta	Atrial fibrillation, recent myocardial infarction, cardiac catheterization
Traumatic arterial disruption	Abdominal trauma; aortic surgery	Status of collateral flow
Venous occlusion	Venous thrombosis; trauma (including surgery)	Dehydration, hypercoagulable state, portal hypertension
Strangulation obstruction	Abdominal adhesions; hernia	Delayed laparotomy for small bowel obstruction
Nonocclusive mesenteric ischemia	Splanchnic vasospasm Endogenous: renin/angiotensin Exogenous: splanchnic vasoconstrictors	Shock CHF Sepsis, respiratory failure

retrospective review of the hospital course reveals that timely and aggressive intervention might well have resulted in the salvage of a meaningful life.

The major cause of this problem is the widespread conviction that the manifestations of intestinal ischemia are so devastating and dramatic that they are easily recognized. This misconception is often based on indelible impressions created by terminal patients with end-stage mesenteric vascular disease; indeed few clinical syndromes are as dramatic as late intestinal ischemia. What many fail to recognize is that the early, reversible, and hence treatable forms of mesenteric ischemia are often quite subtle in presentation and sometimes, as in the obtunded patient, provide no symptoms, signs, or laboratory abnormalities whatsoever as clues to the diagnosis. In fact, those signs and laboratory abnormalities that we most often associate with these diseases represent the local and systemic response to established bowel necrosis. The early signs of decreased mesenteric blood flow are often subtle and frequently masked by obtundation and by coexisting and predisposing conditions. Clearly, if one waits for evidence of advanced intra-abdominal sepsis to initiate treatment, the results of therapy will remain dismal, and this therapeutic nihilism will continue to appear justified. On the other hand, an aggressive approach, based on early diagnostic studies in patients at risk and suspected of having early mesenteric ischemia, appears to have improved survival in at least one large series reported by Boley and his colleagues from Montefiore Hospital in New York.

The major clinical features of each form of acute mesenteric ischemia are summarized in Table 2. The diagnosis can only be suspected on clinical grounds, however, usually by an alert physician with a high index of suspicion based primarily on the clinical setting. Once considered, the diagnosis must be eliminated or confirmed definitively by either angiography or laparotomy. It is a major error to depend on the passage of time to allow the diagnosis to become more obvious. The appearance of definitive physical signs and laboratory abnormalities inevitably indicate that irreversible bowel necrosis has appeared, that the opportunity for successful revascularization has been lost, and that overwhelming sepsis and cardiovascular collapse are imminent. Patients suspected of having mesenteric thrombosis, embolus, or NOMI should undergo immediate angiography of *all three* mesenteric vessels. It is essential that this be done *prior* to laparotomy. Only patients with intestinal ischemia secondary to strangulation obstruction should undergo exploration as the initial definitive step.

Management of Systemic Manifestations

The management of patients with acute mesenteric vascular disease can be considered with respect to the treatment of the underlying cause, correction of the specific anatomic lesion, and reversal or limitation of the systemic consequences (see Table 4). This last aspect can be dealt with in general terms, regardless of the particular anatomic lesion.

Dehydration and Hypovolemia

All forms of mesenteric ischemia are associated with some degree of hypovolemia as the ischemic insult produces a change in the permeability of the capillaries and the mucosal membrane. This fluid loss can be particularly striking in cases of venous thrombosis and in cases of intestinal strangulation in which the venous component dominates the initial occlusive process. It is therefore essential that the patient be monitored carefully, usually with at least a central venous pressure line and a Foley catheter, the latter to allow the hourly assessment of urine output. The serial measurements of blood pressure and pulse, although important, are simply not adequate in themselves. In patients with significant cardiovascular disease, it is best to monitor the pulmonary capillary wedge pressure with a Swan-Ganz catheter in the pulmonary artery. This also facilitates the measurement of cardiac output and the calculation of peripheral resistance, parameters that must be monitored to optimize the use of cardiotonic and vasoactive agents that may be required. Vasoconstrictors such as levarterenol (Levophed) and digitalis should be avoided if possible. Fluid losses should be replaced rapidly and aggressively, using lactated Ringer's solution and albumin. Although much of the albumin that is administered stays in the intravascular space only transiently, it helps to mitigate the transcapillary fluid losses that result from the disruption of the basic Starling relationship by the ischemic injury.

Sepsis

The predominant clinical feature of mesenteric vascular disease is the systemic sepsis that results initially from the loss of the mucosal barrier to bacteria and endotoxin, and later from the necrotic intestine itself. Probably because of the size of the bacterial inoculum and the dose of endotoxin, the sepsis engendered by intestinal ischemia may be particularly fulminant, especially at later stages of the disease. It is also remarkably resistant to antibiotics, probably because the process of inoculation continues until the underlying process has been reversed. It may be particularly devastating immediately following revascularization of an ischemic bowel segment by vascular bypass or, more often, by reduction of strangulation. All patients suspected of having ischemic bowel disease should therefore be given high intravenous doses of broad-spectrum antibiotics, which include specific anaerobic coverage. This specifically and emphatically includes *all* patients with mechanical small bowel obstruction. My preferences are penicillin, gentamicin, and clindamycin. It must be stressed that even the most vigorous antibiotic program provides only temporary support while definitive diagnostic studies and treatment are instituted.

Acidosis

Patients with mesenteric ischemia often manifest profound metabolic acidosis owing to sepsis, peripheral

TABLE 2 Diagnosis of Acute Intestinal Ischemia

Condition	Clinical Setting	Symptoms	Physical Signs	Laboratory Indicators	Definitive Diagnosis

Arterial thrombosis	ASCVD
	H/O intestinal angina
	Dehydration
	CHF
		Severe pain
		  Sudden onset
		  Crampy→continuous
		Nausea/vomiting
			Early:
			  Benign abdomen
			  Hyperactive bowel sounds
			  Abdominal distention
			  Stool + or − for blood
			  Often systemically stable
				Early: None
				Late:
				  Leukocytosis
				  Acidosis
					Angiogram
					Laparotomy

Arterial embolism	Atrial fibrillation
	Recent MI
	Recent cardioversion
	Cardiac catheterization
	Arteriogram
		Abdominal distention
		Transient diarrhea
		Bloody stool
			Late:
			  Diffusely acute abdomen
			  Ileus
			  Sepsis
			  Cardiovascular collapse
				Hemoconcentration
				Alk.phos./CPK	

Traumatic disruption	Abdominal trauma
	Postoperative:
	  Abdominal aneurysm
	  Bowel resection
	  Colostomy/ileostomy
		Usually none	Trauma: Intra-abdominal
			  hemorrhage
			Postoperative:
			  None
			  Ileus/distention/sepsis
				Trauma: Falling
				  HCT/Hgb
				Postoperative:
				  None
				  Leukocytosis
				  Acidosis
					Laparotomy
					±Angiogram

Strangulation obstruction	Previous abdominal
	  surgery
	Hernia
	H/O congenital defects
		Signs of "simple
		  obstruction"
		Severe pain
		Continuous pain
		Bloody stool
			Early:
			  Signs of "simple
			  obstruction"
			Late:
			  "Acute abdomen"
			  Sepsis
			  Cardiovascular collapse
				Early: None
				Late:
				  Leukocytosis
				  Acidosis
				  Alk.phos./CPK
					Laparotomy

Nonocclusive ischemia	Shock
	Sepsis
	Respiratory failure
	CHF
	Vasoconstrictor therapy
	Digitalis
	Recent cardio-
	  pulmonary bypass
		None (obtunded)
		Diffuse, continuous
		  pain
		Abdominal distention
		Nausea/anorexia
		Ileus
			Early: None
			Late:
			  "Acute abdomen"
			  Sepsis
			  Cardiovascular collapse
				Early: None
				Late:
				  Leukocytosis
				  Acidosis
				  Alk.phos./CPK
					Angiogram
					±Laparotomy
					(late)

Venous thrombosis	Dehydration
	CHF
	Polycythemia
	H/O thrombophlebitis
	Recent portal venous
	  surgery
		Subacute onset
		Abdominal distention
		Dehydration
		Transient diarrhea
		Bloody stool
			Early:
			  Abdominal distention
			  Dehydration
			  Ascites
			Late:
			  "Acute abdomen"
			  Sepsis
			  Cardiovascular collapse
				Early:
				  Hemoconcentration
				Late:
				  Leukocytosis
				  Acidosis
				  Alk.phos./CPK
					Angiogram
					  (venous phase)
					±Laparotomy
					  (late)

Ischemic colitis	Same as nonocclusive
	  ischemia
	Recent aortic surgery
	Recent cardio-
	  pulmonary bypass
		None
		Distention
			Early: None
			Late:
			  "Acute abdomen"
			  Sepsis
			  Cardiovascular collapse
				Early:
				  Hemoconcentration
				Late:
				  Leukocytosis
				  Acidosis
				  Alk.phos./CPK
					Sigmoidoscopy
					Colonoscopy

hypoperfusion, and toxic products from the bowel itself. This is best managed by the aggressive administration of sodium bicarbonate, with frequent monitoring of the arterial blood gases. An arterial line facilitates the frequent drawing of arterial blood samples and provides for optimal monitoring of blood pressure. Because of the massive losses of isotonic saline into the bowel wall and lumen, the sodium load associated with bicarbonate administration is rarely a problem in these patients. Nevertheless, some of the most severe cases can be better treated with THAM, a TRIS buffer designed for clinical use, which allows the administration of a large base buffer load in a relatively small volume and with a minimal sodium load.

Multisystem Failure

Patients with ischemic bowel disease often manifest the multisystem failure syndrome. Although the management of each aspect of this problem is beyond the scope of this chapter, it is worth noting here that often the most severe forms of organ-system failure can be reversed if the underlying lesion can be corrected and the septic source eliminated. In the meantime, the massive peripheral vasodilatation of septic shock can be confirmed by the measurement of peripheral resistance and treated primarily with volume support. The cardiogenic shock of late sepsis can be treated by optimizing the left atrial filling pressure and by infusing inotropic agents. Although there is no hard evidence that they are actually harmful in a clinical situation, vasopressors and digitalis are probably best avoided. Acute renal failure is managed appropriately, and in the face of oliguria or anuria, this presents serious problems of fluid balance as these patients still require large-volume infusions to replace gut losses, and body weight is useless as an indicator of intravascular volume in such patients. Here again, the central venous and pulmonary capillary wedge pressures, combined with measurements of cardiac output and peripheral resistance, are essential as guides to fluid therapy. Respiratory failure necessitating intubation and ventilation, hepatic failure, and central nervous system dysfunction (obtundation) frequently accompany the advanced stages of this syndrome. All are managed supportively until the underlying lesion can be dealt with definitively. However, optimal treatment of the multisystem failure syndrome consists primarily of avoiding it by diagnosing and treating intestinal ischemia at its early stages. All too often this syndrome represents the means by which the diagnosis is first seriseriously entertained, and at this stage the chances for success are small.

Timing of Surgical Intervention

In all salvageable cases of intestinal ischemia, except those caused by NOMI and ischemia colitis, early surgery offers the *only* means for definitive reversal of the ischemic lesion. It is therefore desirable that laparotomy proceed with a minimum of delay. Specifically, this means that about an hour or two, at most, should be spent setting up appropriate access for monitoring, starting intravenous antibiotics, improving the cardiac output, and angiography. It is a serious error to delay surgery in a misguided attempt to optimize systemic parameters, as one usually observes an initial improvement, a therapeutic plateau, and then a progressive deterioration as ongoing sepsis becomes overwhelming and the ischemic bowel lesion becomes irreversible. One should try to complete diagnostic studies and initiate laparotomy during this plateau period.

An essential legitimate cause for delay is the necessity for obtaining a preoperative arteriogram in patients with mesenteric vascular occlusion. This is important both as a means of definitive diagnosis and as an anatomic guide to bypass or embolectomy. In cases of suspected NOMI, initial angiography is essential both for diagnosis and for treatment. Surgery in these patients is reserved for the resection of unsalvageable bowel after perfusion has been maximized by vasodilator infusion. Patients with small bowel obstruction do not need preoperative angiography as the diagnosis of strangulation, so difficult to make preoperatively, is easily made at laparotomy.

Some cases of acute mesenteric infarction present in such a fulminant form and in such otherwise debilitated patients that consideration must be given to a nonaggressive approach that seeks only to ease the patient's demise. Although this decision must be an individual one, these patients have little to lose from an attempt at aggressive

therapy. In a conscious patient, the discomfort of an arteriogram or a laparotomy under general anesthesia is small in comparison to the agonizing pain of intestinal angina, peritonitis, and systemic sepsis. In an unconscious patient, the question is moot. I tend to be initially quite aggressive in the treatment of any patient whose previous existence had been meaningful, regardless of the severity of his condition. If I find an unsalvageable situation at laparotomy, I close rapidly and then focus only on easing the patient's discomfort with large intravenous doses of morphine.

Intraoperative Determination of Viability

After perfusion of the intestine has been optimized by vasodilator therapy in NOMI, by reduction of a strangulation, or by revascularization of an occlusion, an operative decision must be made whether to resect the injured intestine and to what extent. This decision is made by the assessment of viability: the prediction whether that section of bowel will maintain its structural integrity and heal. One should put aside, for the moment, the question whether a late stricture will form as this presents no immediate threat to survival and is better dealt with later, if necessary. Intestinal viability is assessed clinically by the observation of arterial pulsations, peristalsis, and the color of the segment in question. In most cases, the result is obvious. When the surgeon feels confident of this clinical assessment of viability, he is usually correct, as we have demonstrated in a controlled study. When he is unsure, the observation of the pattern of reperfusion under ultraviolet illumination with a standard (3,600 Å) Wood's lamp, following the intravenous administration of 1 g sodium fluorescein slowly over about 30 seconds via the intravenous line, is usually accurately discriminate. This technique allows rapid screening by observation of the entire area of bowel in question. Any area of nonfluorescence that is greater than 5 mm in diameter usually indicates impending infarction, although an occasionally overly pessimistic assessment is made, especially in cases of venous occlusion. It is important to be sure that small blood clots on the surface are not interpreted as areas of nonperfusion. The bowel must be laid out for observation prior to the injection of the dye, as the transudation of the dye across the serosa passively stains nonviable areas lying in a puddle of dye-laden peritoneal fluid. At present, it is only possible to use this technique once in a 48-hour period, and so it is important to choose that time when perfusion has been optimized. Other adjuvant methods for the assessment of viability either have proved too cumbersome for practical clinical use or, like the Doppler technique, have proved unreliable in controlled clinical trials. If doubt still exists as to viability, the abdomen can be re-explored at 24 to 48 hours to provide a second look. I have found this to be less necessary since we adopted the fluorescein technique, but it is occasionally useful, especially if the patient continues to deteriorate in the postoperative period. Contrary to the original counsel of those who introduced the second-look procedure, I do not feel the necessity of reoperating on a patient who is doing well after surgery. This is due to my confidence in the fluorescein method.

When intestinal viability is borderline at the margins of resection, it is better to avoid anastomosis of the cut ends, and these should be brought out as stomata. (This measure also permits the continued assessment of their viability). This is true whether the small or large bowel is involved. In cases in which a high small bowel fistula is created, it is possible to consider early anastomosis as the patient recovers from his systemic illness. In the meantime, it is important that optimal enterostomal therapy be provided to avoid skin erosion. This is greatly facilitated by the use of gentle, continuous suction on a small sump catheter and a surrounding stomal appliance secured with Stomadhesive or karaya. Fluid losses can be easily replaced if they are carefully monitored in this way. It is important to watch for the development of acidosis due to bicarbonate losses and to treat it appropriately.

Occasionally the extent of bowel resection required does not leave the patient with enough bowel to sustain survival by enteral alimentation. In these cases, the deci-

sion for long-term or even permanent parenteral alimentation must be considered. In general, I have eschewed this option in elderly patients with advanced atherosclerosis, but each decision must be made on an individual basis. Certainly younger patients, for example those with a congenital midgut volvulus, deserve serious consideration for long-term parenteral alimentation.

MANAGEMENT OF SPECIFIC ENTITIES

The management of acute intestinal ischemia from various causes is summarized in Tables 3 and 4.

Acute Arterial Occlusion

When intestinal ischemia is the result of the acute occlusion of a major mesenteric artery, the diagnosis is often obvious clinically (see Table 2). Accordingly, many of these patients are diagnosed earlier and hence are in more stable condition at the time of diagnosis. As soon as the

TABLE 3 Overview of Management of Acute Intestinal Ischemia

Condition	Underlying Cause	Specific Lesion	Systemic Consequences
Arterial thrombosis		Laparotomy Endarterectomy/thrombectomy Vascular bypass Assess viability Resect dead bowel ±Anticoagulation	Hydration Antibiotics Reverse acidosis Support cardiac output Ventilatory support Avoid vasoconstrictors
Arterial embolism	Anticoagulation Cardioversion Proximal thrombectomy Aneurysmectomy Valve replacement	Laparotomy Embolectomy Assess viability Vascular bypass Resect dead bowel	Hydration Antibiotics Reverse acidosis Support cardiac output Treat other embolic sites Ventilatory support Avoid vasoconstrictors
Venous thrombosis	Hydration—often massive Anticoagulation ± Portasystemic shunt	Anticoagulation ±Laparotomy ± Thrombectomy Assess viability Resect dead bowel	Hydration—often massive Antibiotics Reverse acidosis Support cardiac output Ventilatory support Avoid vasoconstrictors
Strangulation obstruction	Early laparotomy Reduce incarcerated hernia Lyse adhesions Detort volvulus	Nasogastric/intestinal suction Early laparotomy Assess viability Resect dead bowel	Hydration Antibiotics Reverse acidosis Support cardiac output Ventilatory support Avoid vasoconstrictors
Nonocclusive mesenteric ischemia	Hydration Support cardiac output D/C splanchnic vasoconstrictors ? Ablate renin/angiotensin axis	Intra-arterial vasodilators Delayed laparotomy Assess viability Resect dead bowel	Hydration Antibiotics Reverse acidosis Support cardiac output Ventilatory support Avoid vasoconstrictors
Ischemic colitis	Same as for nonocclusive ischemia	Delayed laparotomy Assess viability Resect dead bowel	Hydration Antibiotics Reverse acidosis Support cardiac output Ventilatory support Avoid vasoconstrictors

TABLE 4 Critical Points in Management of Acute Intestinal Ischemia

Condition	Early Diagnosis	Treatment
Arterial thrombosis	Angiography	Early vascular bypass Accurate assessment of viability
Arterial embolism	Angiography	Early embolectomy Anticoagulation Accurate assessment of viability
Venous thrombosis	Angiography Laparotomy	Anticoagulation Hydration Accurate assessment of viability
Strangulation obstruction	Early laparotomy	Early operative reduction Accurate assessment of viability
Nonocclusive mesenteric ischemia	Early angiography	Intra-arterial vasodilators Reversal of underlying systemic condition Delayed laparotomy Accurate assessment of viability
Ischemic colitis	Sigmoidoscopy	Reversal of underlying systemic condition Delayed laparotomy Accurate assessment of viability

patient's condition has been stabilized and monitoring capabilities secured, he should be transferred to the cardiovascular diagnostic laboratory and an arteriogram obtained of the celiac, the superior mesenteric (SMA), and the inferior mesenteric (IMA) arteries. This study establishes or rules out the diagnosis and sometimes distinguishes an embolus from a thrombus. If an embolus is suspected, particularly if there is a prior history of a recent myocardial infarction, cardiac catheterization, endocarditis, atrial fibrillation, cardioversion, or prior embolization, anticoagulant therapy with heparin is indicated, if not immediately, then in the postoperative period.

Laparotomy should then follow directly, the leg having been prepared to provide access to a saphenous vein. Embolectomy or thrombectomy is attempted through a longitudinal arteriotomy with a No. 3 Fogarty catheter. If free inflow (and backflow) is obtained, this may be sufficient. The artery usually is closed with a vein patch to avoid stenosis. If free inflow is not obtained, with or without the removal of an embolus, then a bypass probably is required. In cases of advanced atherosclerosis of the orifice of the SMA, with or without an embolus, an endarterectomy is rarely successful, and a bypass from the aorta below the renal arteries to the distal SMA may be necessary. Saphenous vein is the preferred material, but expanded polytetrafluoroethylene (Gortex) may also be used. Viability is then assessed at least 15 minutes following revascularization, and the appropriate resection performed if necessary. Most surgeons prefer to give heparin in the postoperative period or to at least use low-molecular-weight dextran.

Venous Thrombosis

This unusual condition occurs in the face of a predisposing factor such as severe, especially acute, portal hypertension, polycythemia vera, severe dehydration, and other hypercoagulable states. The diagnosis is suspected on the basis of the massive fluid losses and the more gradual onset of symptoms, in the presence of one of the predisposing factors. Following fluid resuscitation, the diagnosis can be confirmed by observing the venous phase of the mesenteric angiogram. For the most part, treatment is by anticoagulation; surgery is reserved for the resection of dead bowel at 24 to 48 hours. There is little rationale for early laparotomy as venous thrombectomy is rarely successful. In cases of acute portal hypertension, such as that due to the Budd-Chiari syndrome, a portosystemic shunt seems worth trying.

Strangulation Obstruction

Any patient with mechanical small bowel obstruction is at substantial risk of vascular compromise; about one-third of patients who undergo laparotomy for obstruction have strangulation. Furthermore, it is not possible to distinguish clinically patients with early strangulation from those with simple obstruction. This fact has been repeatedly demonstrated by retrospective studies and again recently in a controlled, prospective study in which the clinical assessments of strangulation and no strangulation were both incorrect in one-third of the cases. Therefore, the primary treatment of *complete* mechanical small bowel obstruction should be laparotomy, usually within 12 hours of presentation. Delay must be justified by clinical circumstances severe enough to justify the 30 percent risk of delaying treatment of acute intestinal ischemia. In my opinion, this delay should not be predicated on the absence of signs of strangulation. Intestinal strangulation causes both the m ost common and the most treatable form of mesenteric vascular disease. With prompt laparotomy, reduction of the strangulation, and judicious resection of only the nonviable bowel, recovery can usually be expected. In these cases, a primary anastomosis can usually be performed because the intestinal margins are abrupt and lie outside the area of strangulation.

Nonocclusive Mesenteric Ischemia (NOMI)

This condition represents selective vasoconstriction of the mesenteric resistance vessels in response to some form of severe physiologic stress. It is therefore essential to attempt to treat the underlying cause while addressing the disease itself. This usually includes optimization of the cardiac output with fluids and inotropic agents, but avoidance of vasopressor agents and digitalis glycosides. Sepsis, respiratory insufficiency, metabolic acidosis, and electrolyte abnormalities must be aggressively corrected. Unfortunately, as NOMI progresses, it contributes substantially to those very factors that have caused it in the first place, and a vicious circle ensues. Therefore, management of the systemic effects of bowel ischemia must be particularly aggressive.

This disease can only be diagnosed by angiography in those patients suspected of having it by an alert clinician. The appearance of abdominal pain, distention or ileus, associated with sepsis or cardiovascular deterioration in patients in the population at risk should immediately prompt an arteriographic study (see Table 3). Treatment consists of the selective intra-arterial infusion of a splanchnic vasodilator, usually papaverine, via the same catheter used to establish the diagnosis. A second arteriogram is obtained 15 to 20 minutes after the onset of infusion to demonstrate morphologic evidence of reversal of the previously demonstrated vasospasm. The patient is then returned to the intensive care unit, and the infusion is continued for 24 to 48 hours. If doubt exists as to the effectiveness of therapy, this can be reassessed at any time by repeated arteriography. The position of the infusion catheter can even be checked in the intensive care unit by injecting a bolus of dye at the time a flat portable film of the abdomen is taken.

Surgery should be delayed because it adds to the level of physiologic stress and because it cannot reverse the primary lesion. It is a grave error to operate on one of these patients without first establishing the diagnosis arteriographically. In such circumstances, the patient's abdomen should be closed and the patient transported directly to the catheterization laboratory. When a patient has received optimal vasodilator therapy for a day or two, and begins to show signs of increasing sepsis or of an acute abdomen, laparotomy is then appropriate to facilitate the resection of necrotic bowel. This delay also facilitates the assessment of viability because the initial laparotomy becomes, in effect, a second-look procedure.

Ischemic Colitis

Colonic ischemia may result from any of the aforementioned circumstances; the colon may even be involved in an intestinal strangulation due to cecal or sigmoid volvulus. Perhaps the most common cause of colonic ischemia is the division of the IMA during aneurysmectomy. The principles of management are essentially the same as those already outlined and should be guided by the particular etiology. A substantial difference is the availability of the colonic mucosa for direct observation, and all patients suspected of having ischemic bowel disease should undergo gentle proctosigmoidoscopy with minimal air insufflation. Recently, fiberoptic sigmoidoscopy or even colonoscopy has been found to be safe and helpful. Involvement of the colon in any diffuse ischemic process may indicate proximal small bowel involvement as well. The mucosa is more sensitive to ischemia than the muscularis, but the integrity of the muscularis determines ultimate viability; the mucosa regenerates if the muscular tube survives. One must therefore be careful not to overestimate the depth of the necrosis or to underestimate the length of bowel involved.

Unlike patients with other forms of mesenteric ischemia, many with ischemic colitis can be kept under observation, especially if the lesion is known to be limited to the colon. In these cases, the plain abdominal film is often helpful because gas in the lumen often provides contrast for images rivaling those of a barium enema. Patients with disease limited to the mucosa sometimes recover without surgery, although late strictures may form. Close followup is recommended; intervention is indicated only when there is evidence of sepsis or peritonitis.

Many patients with a necrotic colon require a total abdominal colectomy and usually resection of the necrotic rectum as well. In some cases, the collateral circulation of the rectum, via the inferior hemorrhoidal vessels from the systemic circulation, is adequate to allow it to be left as a Hartmann's pouch. Although it is rarely possible to use this segment to later restore a functioning rectum, avoidance of an abdominal-perineal resection in these severely ill patients is a distinct advantage. A preoperative proctoscopic examination is essential so that the extent of the resection required can be determined.

ENTEROCUTANEOUS FISTULA

JOSEF E. FISCHER, M.D., F.A.C.S.

Enterocutaneous fistulas remain a potentially dangerous and fatal complication. Mortality rates in referral institutions for patients with enterocutaneous fistulas may still be as high as 20 percent despite advances in parenteral or enteral nutrition, intensive care, antibiotics, and parasurgical care.

ETIOLOGY

Enterocutaneous fistulas often follow surgery as a result of the breakdown of anastomosis or due to abscesses surrounding anastomoses which result in anastomotic breakdown. Operations for inflammatory bowel disease or for cancer are especially prone to result in enterocutaneous fistulas. Spontaneous fistulas, which at present probably constitute less than 20 percent of the enterocutaneous fistulas seen, may be related to treatment of neoplastic disease by radiation or to spontaneous fistulas arising from inflammatory bowel disease.

As with any disease process with a 20 percent mortality, meticulous management and attention to detail are critical in attempting to salvage patients with this feared complication. Considering that coronary artery bypass surgery or elective abdominal aortic aneurysm operations can be carried out with a 1 percent mortality, the magnitude of the problem becomes clear.

CAUSES OF DEATH

The causes of death in patients with gastrointestinal cutaneous fistulas have historically been electrolyte imbalance, malnutrition, and sepsis. Malnutrition was in turn related to the degree of output from fistulas, with high-output fistulas defined as greater than 500 cc per 24 hours and associated in most major series with 100 percent malnutrition. A lesser degree of malnutrition was seen in moderate-output fistulas, defined as between 200 and 500 cc per 24 hours, and even less with low-output fistulas at less than 200 cc per 24 hours, corresponding to the fact that high-output fistulas were generally those of the small bowel and thereby compromised nutrition to a greater extent.

Although the problem of malnutrition has been largely eliminiated by enteral or parenteral nutritional support, persistent sepsis remains the major cause of death. Malnutrition may be a contributing factor in that substrate utilization in septic patients may be sufficiently impaired to interfere with adequate nutritional support, the result being hyperglycemia and/or lack of fat utilization. Indeed, inappropriate nutrition may still be prevalent in patients with overwhelming sepsis due to our lack of knowledge concerning the appropriate means of nutritional support.

Electrolyte imbalance, which should not exist given the easy availability of arterial blood gas and plasma electrolyte measurements, is nonetheless surprisingly frequent in most series of patients with fistulas.

GOALS OF TREATMENT

The purpose of surgical management of patients with fistulas is three-fold:
1. Most important is the control of sepsis, since this is the major cause of mortality, with antibiotics and/or drainage the principal tactic.
2. Malnutrition should be prevented by appropriate nutritional support, enteral or parenteral depending on preference or circumstances.
3. The fistula must be closed, in many cases by the control of sepsis and provision of adequate nutritional support. However, surgical resection and/or closure will be required in many instances. Meticulous surgical judgment and technique are essential to achieve good results.

MANAGEMENT

As with any difficult situation, it is helpful to divide patient management into various stages in order to focus on the principal challenges and therapeutic decisions of each stage. My own personal approach has been to use the following five phases.
1. Recognition/stabilization
2. Investigation
3. Decision
4. Definitive therapy
5. Healing phase

Phase 1: Recognition/Stabilization

Replacement of Deficits. The patient who develops a postoperative fisula, in most cases, has not done well for a period of 5 or 6 days following operation; ileus has persisted, there has been fever, and the patient has been toxic. A wound abscess appears and is drained, usually to be followed within 24 hours by intestinal contents. When such a fistula is recognized and/or the patient is received in transfer, established deficits of crystalloid, red cells, and albumin are usually present. The bowel has accumulated a deficit of 3 to 4 liters, which must be replaced by ample crystalloid. The anemia should be corrected to a hematocrit of approximately 35 to 37. Colloid osmotic pressure is depressed by a low serum albumin. Edema of tissues often makes healing difficult and interferes with bowel function. Transfusion of salt-poor albumin should be used liberally to bring the serum albumin up to a level of at least 3.3 g per deciliter.

Management of Electrolytes. Peripheral crystalloid infusions usually are not necessary for the management of electrolytes. Except for extremely high-output fistulas (more than 3 liters), most of the electrolyte management can be carried out via hyperalimentation or enteral nutrition solution. It is important, however, to be aware of the hypertonic nature of pancreatic secretion with respect to sodium and bicarbonate as compared with the plasma. The loss of 1 or 2 liters of pancreatic fluid is (in my experience) difficult to manage because of the large amounts of sodium required and the energy utilized in bringing plasma up to the hypertonic state of pancreatic secretions. Using supplements of sodium acetate, sodium chloride, and potassium acetate, it is usually possible to maintain electrolyte concentrations within normal limits. Magnesium may also be lost, and acid-base balance must be carefully monitored up to and including the provision of 0.1 N HCl (hydrochloric acid) in hyperalimentation solutions.

Control of Fistula Drainage and Care of the Skin. A number of preparations are useful in preventing skin maceration and breakdown. Healing of skin is essential if operation is necessary, since operation cannot be carried out through a badly damaged abdominal wall. Enlistment of an enterostomal therapist with experience in handling difficult stomas is invaluable to the provision of adequate nursing care for such patients. Karaya powder or seal, or ileostomy cement, honey, glycerin and Karaya powder slurries and/or ion exchange resin (which keeps the skin acidic and thus prevents activation of pancreatic enzymes requiring a basic environment) are all useful, but I find Stomadhesive to be the most useful. If Stomadhesive can be made to adhere around the fistula, it can be left on for a week or 10 days when properly applied, and the skin heals underneath.

The control of fistula drainage is generally carried out with a sump, one that remains soft so that it will not erode at body temperature and has a sufficient diameter to efficiently suck thick enteral drainage. I prefer a home-made sump in which an Intracath (14-gauge) is threaded down to the tip of a Robinson nephrostomy catheter made of brown latex. For thicker intestinal contents, such as colonic drainage, a larger catheter is required. The brown latex catheter remains soft at body temperature and does not erode the bowel. The sidearm vent, in this case a 14-gauge Intercath, can be irrigated with antibiotic solutions so as to break the suction. Such a sump may be attached to moderate or high gastrointestinal suction to narrow the tract around the tube and thereby allow healing of the fistulous tract.

Provision of Nutritional Support. Most patients have been starving for the several days of bowel preparation prior to operation and for the 5 or 6 days until the fistula is recognized. Thus, a substantial lean body mass deficit has already been incurred. However, provision of nutritional support, generally (at least initially) through hyperalimentation, is never an emergency procedure. Subclavian or internal jugular access demands an adequate venous pressure, and the patient should be well hydrated, relaxed, and supplemented with premedication (preferably Valium and Demerol intravenously in combination) with the assistance of a hyperalimentation team, including a nurse. Provision of nutritional support should only be delayed in the case of obvious abscesses which require

drainage, that is, abscesses pointing to the skin. It is useful to take advantage of such a situation prior to drainage by performing needle aspiration of the abscess, removal of some of the contents for both aerobic and anaerobic cultures as well as smear, and instillation of a water-soluble dye to delineate the abscess cavity. The advantages gained by this particular maneuver can rarely be achieved at any other time in the course of the fistula.

Conservative management with nutritional support is the preferred means of closing the fistula. A protein intake of 1.7 g protein equivalent per kilogram of body weight per day is desirable. This may be met by standard amino acid solutions, or in the case of overwhelming sepsis, some marginal advantage may be gained by the provision of a balanced branched-chain amino acid enriched solution. Calories should be supplied at approximately 35 calories per kilogram per 24 hours, of which 75 percent should be in the form of glucose and 25 percent in the form of a lipid emulsion to maximize hepatic protein synthesis. Trace metals, including magnesium, should be supplied in abundance (up to 32 mEq per 24 hours, and losses of zinc (probably up to 20 μg per 24 hours) should be replaced with zinc chloride. Additional trace metals are also important. B and C vitamins should be supplemented at 2 to 5 times the minimal daily requirement, and a minimal daily requirement of vitamins A, D, and E should be administered as well.

Enteral Versus Parenteral Nutritional Support. Respectable rates of fistula closure have been achieved by means of enteral support, although it is difficult to achieve adequate enteral support in the presence of a fistula because of lack of bowel function, and ileus and sepsis are usually present in these patients. Enteral support requires 4 feet of small bowel for efficient absorption of nutrients. The nutrients can be pumped into the stomach and drained through the fistula, provided there is 4 feet of bowel distal to the ligament of Treitz, or placed into the fistula if the bowel below the fistula is 4 feet in continuity. There is little question that enteral support will allow fistula closure. However, it generally takes 5 to 10 days to achieve caloric and nitrogen balance with enteral support, and in the interim the patient should be supported with hyperalimentation. Alternatively, a combination of both parenteral and enteral support is useful in maintaining hepatic protein synthesis. If the enteral solution is pumped into the stomach by continuous infusion, osmolality and then volume should be increased. If gut access is by catheter jejunostomy into the small bowel, volume should be increased first and then osmolality, inasmuch as, with jejunal feedings, hypertonic solutions may be poorly tolerated and full-strength enteral support may never be achieved. Whereas parenteral nutrition generally decreases fistula drainage, the introduction of enteral support is usually followed by an initial rise in fistula drainage.

Use of Nasogastric Tubes. Nasogastric tubes do not reduce fistula drainage and should be used only in the presence of intestinal obstruction and in the postoperative period. If intestinal obstruction is present, a long tube should be placed into the duodenum and passed down as far as it will go, preferably to the area of the fistula. If no obstruction exists, my practice is not to use a nasogastric tube. Indwelling nasogastric tubes encourage reflux of gastric contents into the esophagus, and I have seen six cases of late esophageal strictures following long-term indwelling nasogastric tubes in patients with fistulas. It is occasionally necessary to do a gastrostomy under local anesthesia to provide continuous gastric drainage. If the obstruction is relieved, the gastrostomy may be used for the provision of nutritional support.

Antibiotics. A review of large series of patients with fistulas has revealed that in a given course of therapy for fistulas, patients receive up to nine (generally between seven and nine) different antibiotics. Consequently, it is important to reserve antibiotics for times when they are needed, for example, perioperatively. Thus, unless the patient is septic, as evidenced by somnolence, high swinging fevers, and impairment of hepatic or renal function, antibiotics are not given. If sepsis is not controlled by antibiotics quickly, operative drainage is absolutely necessary. One may choose to carry out an entire refunctionalization (as proposed by Welch) in which all abscesses are drained, fistulas are resected, end-to-end anastomoses carried out, and intestinal continuity re-established. This concept was extremely important prior to the introduction of parenteral nutrition, when early restoration of intestinal continuity was the only means of ultimately providing adequate nutrition and preventing death by starvation. Early operation should be reserved only for sepsis and a localized abscess that can be drained.

Phase 2: Investigation

After approximately 7 to 10 days, when the patient's stamina has improved and the tract has matured so as to provide a vehicle for investigation, a collaborative effort is undertaken by the responsible surgeon and a senior radiologist. This is probably the single most important diagnostic step in the decision-making process. I prefer to use water-soluble dye placed in every available fistulous tract through a No. 5 pediatric feeding tube. It is essential that fluoroscopy be observed by both the surgeon and the radiologist, and that a number of films be taken, particularly spots of the early films when the dye is injected. This provides maximal information. What one looks for is the nature of the fistulous tract, the site of entry into the bowel, the nature of the adjacent bowel (whether damaged, strictured, inflamed), and the presence or absence of intestinal continuity (i.e., whether the fistula is a side fistula or represents complete disruption of anastomosis). It is important to try to visualize the passage of the dye to determine possible distal obstruction. The size of the adjacent abscess is important. If the abscess is too large, closure is less likely.

In general, it has not been necessary to utilize classic barium examinations, such as small bowel follow-through or barium enemas. They do not provide much information that cannot be gained through a well-executed fistulagram

and often do not demonstrate the fistula, especially if the bowel is in continuity and the fistula is a lateral fistula.

Phase 3: Decision

After viewing the fistulagram and observing the behavior of fistula drainage, it is possible, approximately 2 weeks after treating the fistula, to obtain some idea as to whether spontaneous closure will occur. Those signs previously enumerated concerning the site of the fistula, the nature of adjacent bowel, the presence of a large adjacent abscess, intestinal discontinuity, and distal obstruction will all influence the responsible surgeon in the decision that operative closure will be necessary. These signs notwithstanding, there are certain anatomic sites that are favorable as far as fistula closure is concerned. Esophageal (especially lateral esophageal) fistulas, lateral duodenal fistulas, biliary and pancreatic fistulas, and jejunal fistulas, as well as lateral colonic fistulas, tend to close in the absence of distal obstruction. For whatever reason, gastric fistulas and, in all series, ileal fistulas tend to be resistant. Fistulas of the ligament of Treitz, perhaps because there is insufficient mobility of the bowel to close the gap, also tend not to close. Patients with inflammatory bowel disease may close their fistula only to have it reopen. Thus, in the face of IBD, I allow the fistula to close with parenteral nutrition and then operate on the patient in a sepsis-free environment to resect the area of fistula. Patients with radiation damage, especially to the pelvis, often are difficult to treat because the abdominal wall is fibrotic. In addition there is often an encased mass from the center of which emanates a fistula, with sepsis and woody induration of surrounding tissues.

Based on the data of many authorities working in the field, if the fistula shows no signs of closing, i.e., drainage has not been dramatically reduced after 4 weeks of sepsis-free adequate nutritional support, the fistula is unlikely to close and operation should be planned.

If sepsis is uncontrolled and signs of renal or hepatic impairment occur, presaging multiple organ failure, it is essential that drainage of abscesses or phlegmon be carried out as soon as the patient can be stabilized and brought to the operating room. A fatal outcome is the alternative.

Phase 4: Definitive Therapy

If 4 weeks of sepsis-free, adequate parenteral or enteral nutrition has been carried out and only a small decrease in the drainage of the fistula is apparent, or if the anatomic considerations dictate operative closure, operation should be planned with meticulous attention to detail. These operations are long and tedious. Surgeons should not place themselves in a situation of having to do a rushed procedure. The operation should be performed through an adequately healed abdominal wall in which a secure abdominal closure above the anastomosis can be obtained. The patient should be prepared with the appropriate antibiotics, as determined by cultures performed preoperatively. The dissection should proceed from the ligament of Treitz up to, and freeing, all adhesions and identifying the entire length of small and large bowel. Intermesenteric abscesses should be drained and good bowel secured for end-to-end, two-layer, nonabsorbable suture anastomosis, which is my preference. All the major reviews of enterocutaneous fistulas have revealed that the best rates of closure and the lowest incidence of complications are obtained by definitive resection and end-to-end anastomoses, with bypass or staged resections running a poor second.

It is important to obtain an adequate abdominal wall to protect the anastomosis. In some patients in whom sepsis has destroyed a portion of the abdominal wall, and obtaining a secure closure requires complicated maneuvers, it has been my practice to involve a fresh plastic surgical team to close the abdomen. I believe this is prudent; these operations often last 5 or 6 hours, and a fresh team provides a more secure, sepsis-free abdominal closure more often than a fatigued surgical team trying to do a hurried abdominal wall closure. Musculocutaneous flaps are a new and effective means of obtaining such excellent closure.

Adjunctive procedures are important and useful. A gastrostomy renders unnecessary an indwelling nasogastric tube, which otherwise might be in place for 7 to 10 days, the period of ileus that usually follows such an extensive reconstruction. If the surgeon desires, the gastrostomy tube can be left on drainage for a prolonged period of time (up to 2 weeks), particularly in the presence of inflammatory bowel disease, until such suture lines are adequately healed with nutritional support. Jejunostomies, either needle-catheter jejunostomies or standard jejunostomies, may provide another means of supplying nutrition in the postoperative period. Above all, in this operative approach, meticulous attention to detail and dissection, accuracy of anastomoses, and careful planning, including adequate closed-suction drainage, are important to obtain the desired result.

Phase 5: Healing

Whether the fistula has closed spontaneously or closure has been obtained with resection, it is important to continue nutritional support as well as antibiotics well into the postoperative period. Newly laid down protein is mobilized during starvation if nutritional support is discontinued too soon. These patients are often anorectic and therefore some judgment is required to get them to eat. In general, the traditional liberalization program (clear liquids, full liquids, soft diet, full diet) may not be tolerated in the patient who has been without oral intake for as long as 6 weeks or 2 months, and it may be necessary to start the patient on something palatable (such as a soft diet) without passing through the preliminary steps.

Some of these patients remain anorectic and do not eat at all, or eat 1,500-calorie, which is the minimal amount necessary before hyperalimentation is discontinued. If this appears to be the case, my own practice is to leave the catheter in place, run normal saline (not containing dextrose) through the line, and allow the patient a trial of oral diet. In 2 or 3 days, sufficient oral intake usually occurs, allowing the hyperalimentation line to be discontinued. A gastrostomy may be useful to provide enteral nutrition after appropriate healing of the anastomoses.

LATE COMPLICATIONS

I have previously discussed esophageal stricture, which may follow indwelling nasogastric tube for a prolonged period of time. In general, this may become manifest 3 or 4 months after the fistula has been closed and the patient has been discharged from the hospital. Usually, these respond to dilation.

SHORT BOWEL SYNDROME

HERBERT E. GLADEN, M.D.

Physical or functional loss of intestinal absorbing capacity may lead to the malabsorption, steatorrhea, diarrhea, and weight loss that characterize short bowel syndrome. This loss of capacity is usually multifactorial, including elements of physical loss of length, mucosal disease, bacterial overgrowth, partial small bowel obstruction, motility disorders, and a host of secondary effects. Etiology of short bowel syndrome is similarly varied, differs with the age group considered, and commonly involves surgical resection. Jejunoileal bypass has provided, in a recent "experiment of nature," an exposition of the complications of short bowel syndrome. Effective therapy of short bowel syndrome mandates a thorough understanding of the underlying physiology.

TREATMENT BASED ON PHYSIOLOGY

Fluid Absorption and Secretion

Absorption and secretion are two sides of the same coin. Passive fluid flux is driven by gradients in solute and osmotic particle concentration. The intact stomach retains particles until they have been fluidized by combined chemical and mechanical action; particles larger than 1 mm in diameter are retained in the stomach and are emptied only by the especially powerful contractions that occur periodically during fasting. The fluid chyme is ordinarily metered precisely from the stomach at a rate the intestine can handle. Every effort should be made to avoid surgical disruption of this metering mechanism in patients who have or are likely (as by affliction with Crohn's disease) to develop short bowel syndrome. In a patient with short bowel syndrome, what would otherwise be a trifling postgastrectomy sequela can be an extremely serious complication. If complications of stomach surgery are suspected of contributing to the short bowel syndrome, a simple therapeutic trial of measures aimed at the gastric component may be beneficial. Rapid gastric emptying may be minimized by separating liquid and solid components of the diet, so that fluids taken with meals will not enhance rapid gastric emptying. Frequent small meals may be advantageous, since the rate of gastric emptying is related to the volume of fluid in the stomach.

By the time the intestinal content reaches the ligament of Trietz, its pH and osmolality ordinarily approach that of serum. Fluid is exchanged rapidly across the intestinal wall, and pancreatic, biliary, and intestinal secretions are added. As the chyme passes along the intestine, a relationship is struck between continued cleavage of foodstuff into smaller osmotically active particles and the continuous removal of these particles from the lumen. A considerable enterocirculatory cycle of water results; although 9 or 10 liters a day enter the upper small intestine to dilute the chyme into osmotic equilibrium, only 1 to 2 liters reach the ileocecal valve. Caffeine (and presumably other phosphodiesterase inhibitors such as aminophylline) increases the net fluid load delivered to the colon, and should be avoided if diarrhea is a problem. Gastric hypersecretion may be a concomitant to short bowel syndrome (discussed under *Endocrine Effects*). Sodium absorption, and hence that of water, can be greatly facilitated by the presence of glucose in the lumen. This principle underlies "cholera solution" oral fluid repletion therapies so crucial in less developed countries. The same concept may be used to increase net fluid absorption in short bowel syndrome.

Carbohydrates

Although glucose in the intestinal content is beneficial, the presence of lactose in the lumen frequently causes difficulties. The lactase enzyme system for cleaving milk sugar is evanescent in some genetic groups and fragile in all. Even patients who have previously tolerated milk products without difficulty may have trouble for a time after surgery, and milk products should therefore be added to the diet cautiously. Undigested lactose acts as an osmotic cathartic in the small bowel and may be fermented in the colon where it causes further mischief. Exogenous lactase supplements are now available which may be added to milk products immediately before consumption to mitigate this problem. Specific absorption mechanisms are to a degree inducible, which is one rationale for using reduced volumes and dilute solutions in restarting feedings in those with digestive abnormalities.

Proteins

Specific mechanisms exist in the small bowel for absorption of dipeptides and tripeptides as well as for amino acids. Polypeptide-containing solutions (Ensure, Isocal, Sustacal) often may be as efficacious as pure amino acid solutions and generally present a lower osmotic load and are more palatable than pure amino acid solutions. Here, as in many other aspects of short bowel syndrome, individualized treatment based on therapeutic trials is a recurrent refrain. Severe protein deficiencies may cause atrophic changes in the gut and subsequent "vicious-circle" malnutrition; parenteral nutrition may be used to break this cycle. Daily protein turnover in the body is normally several times the dietary intake. If there is a deficiency in specific essential amino acids available, more protein may be broken down than is synthesized. There is a heirarchy of amino acid use, with visceral protein defended at the expense of somatic protein. Sufficient exogenous calories must be provided, of course, to avoid use of body protein stores for energy.

Fats and Bile Acids

Absorption of fat is more complex and fragile than that of protein or carbohydrate, and a much greater length of intact intestine is required. Gastric hypersecretion may inactivate pancreatic lipase sufficiently to impair breakdown of complex fats, especially if pancreatic reserves are borderline from preexisting disease. Treatment with cimetidine and/or pancreatic enzyme supplements may be used to enhance fat digestion in this case.

Long-chain triglycerides in normal dietary fat require bile acids for chylomicron transport and efficient absorption. Loss of specific distal ileum absorbing sites for bile acids or bacterial deconjugation and precipitation (to be discussed) disrupts the normally 95 percent efficient enterohepatic cycle. Despite increased hepatic production, reduced bile-salt availability in the small intestine may cause steatorrhea. Breakdown and hydroxylation of fats in the colon can lead to a cathartic effect ("fatty-acid diarrhea"). Paradoxically, a low concentration of bile acids in the small bowel may be accompanied by too high a concentration of bile acids in the colon, where they, too, exert a laxative effect. Whether the main problem is "fatty-acid diarrhea," steatorrhea, or "bile-acid diarrhea" may be difficult to determine, and may vary from time to time and with time as adaption occurs. The most cost-effective way to determine the exact mix of these components in a particular patient is by a carefully controlled therapeutic trial. The treatment modalities for the different components are somewhat in conflict, and so there is a possibility that treatment aimed at bile-acid-induced symptoms may increase steatorrhea or vice versa.

Low-fat, high-fat, cholesterol supplemented, and medium-chain triglyceride-supplemented diets can all be used successfully at one time or another. Medium-chain triglycerides are now available in reasonably palatable form, and do not require bile acids for absorption, but are much more expensive than ordinary dietary fats. Oral administration of bile salts has not been useful in this setting.

A bile-acid binder, such as the resin cholestyramine (Questran), is most apt to be effective in the watery diarrhea that often accompanies a modest loss (less than 100 cm) of the small bowel. Cholestyramine therapy is expensive, may require as much as 16 grams (4 packets of Questran) a day given with meals, and has numerous side effects. Nausea, bloating, and even constipation may occur, and effective bile-salt binding interferes with absorption of fat-soluble vitamins (A,D,E,K), minerals, and medications such as digoxin, diuretics, and anti-coagulants. Mandatory concomitants of this therapy include regular laboratory tests, vitamin and mineral supplements as needed, and proper timing of medication doses to avoid their being bound by the cholestyramine. Psyllium (Metamucil) and aluminum-containing antacids are less potent binders of bile salts, but have fewer side effects than cholestyramine. Antacids vary widely in their bile-salt binding capacity, with magaldrate (Riopan) particularly efficacious. The cathartic tendencies of magnesium-containing antacids must be kept in mind when prescribing treatment for peptic symptoms (to be discussed). If a functional gallbladder is present, overnight accumulation of bile may be used to advantage. Ingestion of the majority of the days' fats at breakfast may reduce steatorrhea or fatty-acid diarrhea, while an early morning dose of bile-acid binder may have enhanced effect.

Endocrine Effects

Hypergastrinemia, increase in parietal cell mass, and gastric hypersecretion are reliably produced in animal models of short bowel syndrome. Although the evidence is not as clear, they probably contribute in many cases to human short bowel syndrome as well. Jejunoileal bypass, in contrast to resection, does not have the same result. Theories to account for this include the jejunum as a site for catabolism of gastrin, or the role of an entero-gastrone "humoral brake" to gastric secretion released by the jejunum. Proposed hormone candidates for this enterogastrone include cholecystokinin (CCK), vasoactive intestinal peptide (VIP), gastric inhibitory peptide (GIP), and serotonin; elucidation and treatment potential await

development of effective specific blockers. The intestinal fluid-absorbing capability may be overwhelmed by the increased volume of secretion; inactivation of pH-dependent pancreatic enzymes may contribute to fat malabsorption; and peptic disease or its treatment may exacerbate digestive complaints. Since consequences of hypersecretion may be so profound, and since measurement is simple, gastric analysis as a guide to therapy should be strongly considered in patients with short bowel syndrome. Effective medical treatment of gastric hyper-secretion is fortunately now available. Hormonal influences are also probably important in compensatory hypertrophy, but as yet no therapeutic intervention is available except provision of intraluminal nutrient as a stimulus.

Bacteriology

The bacteriology of the gut has been convincingly shown to be important in certain instances of short bowel syndrome. Preservation of the ileocecal valve is of great importance in mitigating effects of this disorder. It was once thought that the ileocecal region served as a partial obstruction and thereby slowed transit, with a resulting increase in absorption, but it now seems more likely that the main effect of the valve is to isolate colonic flora from ileal flora. There have been several instances of ileocecal valve reconstruction in man, with report of "good" results, and animal studies have been definitely encouraging, but this technique must be regarded as experimental. The "blind loop" syndrome in which bacterial overgrowth occurs in an area of intestinal stagnation is a model for this contribution of bacterial changes to short bowel syndrome. Anaerobic species such as Bacteroides have the enzymatic apparatus necessary to cleave the amide bond and deconjugate bile salts, interfering with their active reabsorption. These bacteria, when present in the ileum in sufficient numbers, may also interfere with absorption of vitamin B_{12} by several mechanisms. Even with an intact ileocecal valve, abnormally slow transit due to, say, diabetic enteroparesis or previous surgery may lead to bacterial overgrowth. Truncal vagotomy, but apparently not proximal gastric vagotomy, leads to marked changes in the gut flora. This may contribute to the troublesome diarrhea that sometimes occurs after truncal vagotomy, an additional argument against cavalier attack on this nerve.

Motility

Too-rapid transit through the gut impairs absorption. On the other hand, too-slow transit leads to bacterial over-growth, and may also shift the balance from absorption to secretion, resulting in the familiar syndrome of partial small bowel obstruction. Opiates increase the force of contractions while disordering their coordination. The exact mechanism and that of anticholinergics in control of motility and diarrhea remain controversial, and caution must be exercised to avoid overdose. Loperamide (Imodium) is another effective drug. It appears to have a direct effect on intestinal smooth muscle.

Adaption

Species differences are so profound that the extensive literature on intestinal adaption after massive resection must be applied cautiously to human work. Unlike the case in laboratory rodents, hyperplastic changes in the human villi progress for a year or more, and so physician and patient should not become discouraged by early difficulties. Intraluminal nutrients, endogenous secretions (especially biliary), and systemic factors all seem to play an important role in adaption. Since we do not yet have direct intervention to speed the process, enteral nutrition therapy must be advanced at Nature's rate. Fortunately, total parenteral nutrition (TPN) support now allows this luxury of time. It makes sense to establish early a long-term access route such as a "Hickman" type central venous catheter to decrease the complication rate. Most patients eventually are successfully restored to full enteral nutrition. This is fortunate, since the cost of even home TPN therapy may exceed $200 per day and in-hospital therapy costs are much higher.

Early in recovery, diarrheal losses exceed 2 to 3 liters per day, and the mainstay of nutrition must be parenteral. It does seem reasonable to include small amounts of oral glucose-and-electrolyte solutions to supplement this and to stimulate adaption. Antidiarrheal medications must be used with great caution, to avoid problems with overdose. Despite the availability of home TPN, most patients require a supervised environment during this period because of their unstable medical situation.

When diarrheal losses have begun to decrease, oral intake may be cautiously advanced. Paradoxically, poor appetite in the face of starvation has long been recognized in this setting. When and if enteral nutrition becomes sufficient while diarrhea is held below about 2 liters a day, the patient is weaned from parenteral support. Oral feedings should be kept simple at first:

1. Avoid ordinary fats (medium chain triglycerides may be used).
2. Avoid hyperosmolar feedings, especially if the stomach metering mechanism is not intact.
3. Avoid even moderate use of milk products until certain they are tolerated.
4. Remember that peptides may be absorbed as well or better than amino acids, and result in lower osmolality solutions for the same protein equivalent.
5. Monitor and supplement vitamins and minerals.

When it seems certain that the patient is tolerating a restricted diet, cautious liberalization, including addition of regular dietary fats, is undertaken. A good rule is to make only one change at a time.

Complications

Nutritional deficiency means more than just insufficient calories, protein, and fat. Dehydration remains an ever-present threat. Even those who are ordinarily able to maintain fluid balance may have so little reserve as to collapse from an otherwise trivial viral diarrhea. Malabsorption of fat-soluble vitamins such as A, D, and K results in night blindness, osteomalacia, and bleeding problems. Folate and vitamin B_{12} deficiencies are common, although vitamin B_{12} replacement usually is not necessary if less than 100 cm of terminal ileum is removed and the ileocecal valve is preserved, preventing adverse bacteriologic effects. It must be remembered that clinical vitamin B_{12} deficiency may take years to develop. Deficiencies of potassium, calcium, magnesium, iron, and trace elements such as zinc and possibly copper, chromium, and selenium may reach clinical significance. Proper supplementation and a low oxalate diet (to be discussed) may be required indefinitely. Close physician support and extensive patient education is essential at all stages. Remember that patients are subjected to great amounts of unwise advice, since nutrition superstition and quackery are so rampant.

Intestinal hyperoxaluria is a common problem in patients who have an intact colon. Fat malabsorption results in intraluminal formation of calcium soaps. Dietary oxalate, which would ordinarily be chelated with the calcium and excreted in an insoluble form, is instead reabsorbed in the colon. Jejunoileal bypass increases absorption of labeled oxalate from 10 percent of that ingested to 50 percent, and the formation of renal stones is facilitated by the chronic mild dehydration of many of these patients. Twenty percent or more of jejunoileal bypass patients develop symptomatic nephrolithiasis.

Symptomatic cholelithiasis is also unusually common in short bowel patients, especially in the pediatric population. Presumably the reduction in the circulating pool of bile salts increases lithogenicity of bile. Despite this, prophylactic cholecystectomy at time of original intestinal resection is not indicated, since the presence of a functioning gallbladder may be of more importance to a short-bowel syndrome patient than to others.

SURGICAL THERAPY

Preservation of Length

Whenever possible, it should be the practice at resection to measure the length of the small intestine remaining. The notorious inaccuracy of estimation as opposed to direct measurement (along the antiluminal border with a measured strand of suture) may be proved to any surgeon's satisfaction in a few moments in the operating room. If further resection is required at a later operation, the intestine may not be as amenable to measurement because of adhesions.

There has been a sort of dismal fad to pepper the literature with reports of survival with shorter and shorter lengths of intestine; with enteral support only, life can be maintained on what seems to be an impossibly short length of intestine. Remember that other conditions must be favorable, and the duodenum intact and in continuity if this is to be achieved. If such is the case, about half the jejunoileum can be resected without much disability; when only 25 percent remains, the defect is usually quite severe, especially if there has been resection of the ileocecal valve, or disruption of the gastric reservoir mechanism. The distal intestine seems more important length for length than the proximal jejunum, notwithstanding the importance of the ileocecal valve. The reason for this is not clear, but may be due to specific absorbing sites in the distal ileum.

Nutritional support has permitted a conservative approach to Crohn's disease. Since this disease is apparently systemic and incurable, indications for palliative surgery are limited to intractability and to severe complications such as obstruction, fistulas, debilitating perianal disease, toxic megacolon, or growth failure. No effort need be made to get extensive margins free from microscopic disease; if the intestine is clinically suitable for anastomosis, results should be as good as if greater lengths are resected.

There are several aids to allow surgeons to determine intraoperative viability of bowel that has suffered a vascular insult. Contractile activity is a poor indicator. If a sterile ultrasound doppler device is available, the ability to detect flow in the distal vessels is enhanced. Intravenous injection of one or two ampules of fluorescein with subsequent examination of the intestine under ultraviolet light (Wood's lamp) will demonstrate perfused areas. If there is any question of viability, or in desperate circumstances when no viable bowel is apparent despite restoration of blood flow, a "second-look" operation, performed 12 to 18 hours after the first exploration, can result in salvage of initially compromised bowel. With advances in anesthetic and support techniques, the risk of multiple operations even in critically ill patients has become more acceptable, especially when the benefit may be a substantial preservation of intestine of initially uncertain viability. The mucosa is much more sensitive to the adverse effects of ischemia than is the muscularis, but has considerable regenerative power. Substantial lengths of intestine can often be salvaged despite mucosal slough. Late strictures are not uncommon in the intestine that has survived a severe ischemic insult, and close observation should be carried out to permit early therapeutic intervention in these fragile patients.

Avoidance of Post-Gastric Surgery Complications

Dumping syndrome or postvagotomy diarrhea can severely exacerbate short bowel syndrome. The increased morbidity in this population mandates conservatism in gastric surgery. If surgery for peptic disease is forced by circumstances, the choice is often between the operation with lowest morbidity and mortality (proximal gastric vagotomy [PGV]) and the operation with the lowest recurrence rate (vagotomy and antrectomy [V&A]). This decision is made more difficult by the paucity of sound statistics on the clinical impact of ulcer recurrence since the advent of cimetidine. Use of the PGV should be strongly considered, since it is a remarkably safe procedure and burns fewest bridges. Necessity for reoperation following PGV is comparatively rare in this era of H_2 blockers. It must be remembered that *any* gastric vagotomy, including PGV, impairs the reservoir function to some extent. Recent linkage of high relapse rates following medical treatment of peptic disease with smoking suggests that cessation of tobacco use may be an extremely important part of peptic disease therapy. It should be strongly urged in all short bowel syndrome patients as a prudent, safe, inexpensive prophylactic measure.

Motility Measures

An incredible number of operations have been proposed to alter motility and enhance absorption in short bowel syndrome. This suggests that none of the operations has been clearly proved to be of great benefit. Recirculating loops, reversed intestinal onlay patches, reversed proximal segments, reversed distal segments, reversed proximal and distal segments, longitudinal muscle layer myotomies, and a host of more-or-less obstructive maneuvers have all been tried. The only procedure with substantial human exposure has been the distal reversed segment. In this procedure, a piece of small intestine, as far distal as practical, is transected, reversed, and reanastomosed so that its "peristalsis" will oppose the flow of intestinal contents. In addition to the risk of an additional anastomosis, it is difficult to choose a length that will be neither too short to be effective nor so long as to be obstructive, especially with the continuing effects of adaption. Current practice is to use a length of approximately 10 centimeters. Stasis and stagnation resulting from excessive length might be expected to contribute to bacterial overgrowth problems. An additional consideration is that the intestine apparently handles indigestible bits differently than it does fluids. Mall and Halstead at the Johns Hopkins Hospital observed in 1896 that dogs with reversed segments develop obstructing bezoars of indigestible materials in and proximal to the reversed segment. This has been confirmed in numerous animal studies, although not reported to date in man. If a reversed segment is employed as a desperate measure, the theoretic possibility of bezoar formation should be borne in mind during postoperative observation.

The Future

Intestinal transplantation is technically feasible, but maintaining immunosuppression while implanting a bacteria-laden organ presents formidable obstacles. I have no doubt that these technical details will eventually be overcome, but not soon.

Techniques based on the electrophysiology of the intestine appear closer to reality. As in the heart, contractile activity in the small intestine is under control of electrical signals that arise from a proximal pacemaker site and spread distally. In the small intestine, the pacemaker site is in the first part of the duodenum, and the electrical activity does not spread into the stomach or colon. As in the heart, electrical pacing techniques may be used to control the rate and site of origin of the waves of depolarization that spread over the organ. By placing electrodes distally on the small intestine, a portion of it may be driven backward. This serves as a controllable means of influencing the transit of digesta. Recent work done at the Mayo Clinic indicates that this can both increase absorption acutely and, more importantly, alter rate of weight loss in animals with short bowel syndrome. Work with this

technique on humans is just beginning and it is too early to know whether its use on humans will be possible or practical.

TEAM APPROACH

Because of the complexity, intensity, and long duration of short bowel syndrome treatment, it is unlikely that any one individual will have both the time and expertise to provide comprehensive care. The treatment team at one time or another may include gastroenterologists, surgeons, pharmacists, nurses, enterostomal therapists, dieticians, and many others. The team approach to treatment, however, must supplement and not supplant the patient-physician relationship that is so crucial for coordination and continuity of care, and for psychological support.

LARGE BOWEL

DIVERTICULAR DISEASE OF THE COLON

MALCOLM C. VEIDENHEIMER, M.D., C.M., F.R.C.S.(C), F.A.C.S.

Although Littre, in the early 1700s, commented briefly on diverticula in the colon, the understanding of diverticular disease of the colon is usually credited to Cruveilhier, who described it as a pathologic condition in 1849. However, clinical interest in the disease did not arise until the beginning of this century.

Diverticular disease occurs with equal frequency in men and women, but a change toward a preponderance of the disease in women has been suggested recently. The condition, frequently found in persons living in Western countries, usually becomes evident by the age 40 years and occurs in about 50 percent of the population in older age groups. An estimated two-thirds of 85-year-old persons in North America have diverticula of the colon. The reported incidence of inflammatory change associated with the presence of diverticula varies from 10 to 25 percent. Younger patients with diverticular disease tend to have more virulent attacks of acute diverticulitis and are prone to the development of complications in association with these attacks.

The pathophysiology of diverticular disease is a thickening of the circular and longitudinal muscle coats of the colon. However, histologic examination does not demonstrate true hypertrophy or hyperplasia of these layers of the bowel wall. The colon is shortened in the area involved with diverticular disease, and this causes a concertina-like appearance of the colon as the mucosa is thrown into transverse folds. Studies have shown an increase in intraluminal pressure and segmentation within portions of colon involved by diverticula. The increase in intraluminal pressure plays a role in the cause of herniation of the mucosa of the bowel where the blood vessels penetrate the muscular coat.

ACUTE DIVERTICULITIS

Bacteria-laden feces may become entrapped within the narrow-necked diverticulum and form a nidus for bacterial growth. Because the diverticulum on the surface of the bowel is covered by serosa only, a pericolic inflammatory reaction results, possibly involving the adipose tissue and the mesocolon, and a localized phlegmon develops. The clinical picture of acute pain in the lower abdomen, which is more severe on the left side than on the right, associated with tenderness, guarding, a palpable mass, and elevation of the leukocyte count, is well known.

The initial management of a patient with acute diverticulitis aims at resting the bowel. When symptoms are minor, intake of liquids is permissible, and broad-spectrum antibiotics are taken orally. When symptoms are severe, intake of liquids is restricted, and broad-spectrum antibiotics are administered intravenously. Occasionally, a patient may require nasogastric intubation to ensure that the intestine is at maximal rest. Symptoms are satisfactorily resolved in most instances with this management, but continued assessment of the patient's clinical picture and review of laboratory studies will demonstrate the success or failure of this course of action. When the symptoms subside, a barium enema study of the sigmoid colon is performed carefully to demonstrate the presence of diverticular disease and to elicit any radiologic evidence of localized perforation or obstruction. The mucosal detail differentiates between problems associated with diverticular disease and those associated with cancer of the sigmoid colon. A vigorous roentgenographic examination of the entire colon should not be undertaken at this time, and the surgeon should so inform the radiologist. Similarly, flexible endoscopic procedures should be avoided in the acute inflammatory phase of the illness.

In rare instances, when the diverticulitis remains acute, surgical intervention may be required. Unfortunately, the operative findings at early intervention are usually those of extensive local inflammation. It is considered unsafe to perform primary resection and anastomosis without an accompanying diversionary colostomy at this time. Should operative intervention be required during an acute phase of diverticulitis, I prefer to remove the diseased bowel, anastomose the healthy ends, and, when the inflammatory reaction has been intense, decompress the anastomosis by a diverting left transverse loop colostomy.

COMPLICATIONS

Because diverticular disease is primarily a pericolitis, the manifestations of the disease are found on the surface of the colon. As complications develop, adjacent structures may become involved. A phlegmon may evolve into a localized pericolic abscess, varying in size from microabscess to 15 to 20 cm in diameter. Free perforation may occur when the abscess bursts into the abdominal cavity, and then, depending on the amount of leakage from the bowel, feculent peritonitis of varying degrees will occur. The abscess may also burst into some adjacent structure, resulting in formation of a fistula into the bladder, vagina, small bowel, uterus, ureter, or out onto the abdominal skin. The phlegmonous response may cause such local swelling as to encroach on the lumen of the bowel causing obstruction. These major complications (abscess, perforation, fistula, and obstruction) are all part of the inflammatory reaction associated with diverticulitis. Hemorrhage, another major complication of diverticular disease, has a different pathogenesis, and its management will be discussed later in this chapter.

When one of the inflammatory complications of diverticular disease has occurred, urgent or even emergency operative intervention is required. The choices of operative procedure range from simple diversion to direct attack on the inflamed bowel by resection with or without an anastomosis. In general, I favor removal of the infective focus at the time of operation and perform resection even if a generalized peritonitis exists. This procedure relieves the patient of continuing sepsis, is more definitive than proximal colostomy and drainage of the site of the inflammatory reaction, and renders a second operation unnecessary. Resection with distal mucous fistula and proximal end colostomy is advocated by some surgeons, but in my experience foreshortening of the mesocolon, which is associated with complicated diverticular disease, seldom permits the mucous fistula to be brought out to the abdominal wall. The same criticism holds for the Mikulicz type of operation, which has been advocated.

Resection with closure of the distal rectosigmoid and formation of a proximal end colostomy is a standard procedure for complicated diverticular disease. This Hartmann type of operation is the one most commonly used and has the advantage of removing the diseased intestine without risk of compromising an anastomosis performed in an inflammatory area. The disadvantage of the Hartmann operation is that the rectosigmoid stump is now in the wall of the previously inflamed area or abscess cavity. Subsequent retrieval of the stump may be so difficult that ureters and pelvic vessels are at risk of being injured. However, much of this criticism is circumvented by the use of the end-to-end anastomosis (EEA) stapler (United States Surgical Corporation, Stamford, CT) to reconstitute the intestine after the Hartmann operation.

My choice is primary resection with direct primary anastomosis at the initial operation. The area of inflammation is thoroughly lavaged, and drains are placed into the area for at least 1 week. Irrigating drains should be inserted in a frank abscess cavity. The anastomosed intestine is not used in the presence of such an inflammatory reaction, but the fecal stream is diverted by a left-sided fully diverting loop transverse colostomy. The left-sided transverse colostomy allows the effluent to be better formed than that from a right-sided transverse colostomy. The stoma is situated close to the splenic flexure with no redundancy of colon between the efferent side of the stoma and the splenic flexure. This eliminates the potential for prolapse of the distal limb of the colostomy if the stoma remains in place longer than the anticipated 8 weeks.

The operative management of acute inflammatory changes associated with complicated diverticular disease need not be difficult. Tissue planes are often more clearly defined as a result of edema that has occurred around the inflammatory mass. When the peritoneum has been divided by sharp dissection, the phlegmonous mass of colon and abscess cavity can be mobilized from the left lower abdomen and pelvis by blunt finger dissection. The risk of injury to ureter and iliac vessels is greatly minimized. The phlegmon that fills the pelvic inlet should not deter the surgeon because of the availability of a short segment of uninvolved distal sigmoid colon always present above the pelvic peritoneal floor. This relatively blood-free mobilization is similar to that obtained in surgical management of acute gangrenous appendicitis and acute cholecystitis. In my opinion, the safety of resection is much greater at this time than when inflammatory tissues have become fibrotic and exposure of the ureter and iliac vessels requires sharp dissection with the attendant risk of injury.

The patient is discharged from the hospital and is studied in 8 weeks. Endoscopic examination should be performed with the rigid sigmoidoscope to visualize the anastomosis, and pressure applied to the perianastomotic region should bring into view any residual purulent discharge present at the suture line. A barium study is obtained through the anus while the patient's hand compresses the distal limb of the loop colostomy. The pressure within the left colon thus achieved demonstrates the presence or absence of distensibility and leakage at the anastomosis. When results of these studies are normal, the patient is admitted to the hospital for closure of the transverse colostomy. If a persistent leak is noted at this examination, the studies are repeated 8 weeks later.

In my experience, the results of this two-stage operative approach for complicated diverticular disease have demonstrated fewer complications and fewer deaths than follow the classic three-stage operation. In the presence of fecal peritonitis of more than a few hours' duration, I would choose the Hartmann operation over primary anastomosis with proximal colostomy because of its shorter operative time.

Hemorrhage results from erosion of a penetrating blood vessel by inflammatory reaction at the neck of a diverticulum. Although bleeding may occur from diverticula situated in any portion of the colon, the right colon or the sigmoid colon are the most common sites. In the young patient, bleeding tends to cease spontaneously. In the older patient, bleeding from a diverticulum tends to persist and may be massive. Angiography demonstrates the site of bleeding in these patients, and attempts are made to stop the bleeding by infusion of vasopressin (Pitressin) or by embolization. After bleeding has stopped in the young patient, a barium study is obtained 2 or 3 weeks later to confirm the presence of diverticula. The young patient with bleeding from a diverticulum does not require subsequent resection of that segment of bowel. Because older patients tend to have recurrent bleeding, administration of Pitressin is usually a temporizing measure to stop the bleeding and allows elective resection to be performed when the patient's hemodynamic status improves.

ELECTIVE MANAGEMENT

The management of the complications of diverticular disease results in a surgical mortality rate of about 10 percent. Surgical treatment of complicated diverticular disease is associated with a high rate of morbidity, and the patient may require several admissions to the hospital, losing considerable time away from work and leisure activities. For these reasons, I have adopted an aggressive approach to the surgical management of patients with diverticular disease. I believe that a person under 50 years of age who has one acute attack of diverticulitis should undergo elective resection of the colon, and a person over 50 years of age could experience two attacks of diverticulitis before elective surgical intervention is recommended. The clinical and roentgenographic features that justify elective resection are roentgenographic evidence of a leak at the time of barium study, clinical features associated with urinary tract symptoms at the time of the acute attack, clinical or roentgenographic evidence of obstruction that persists after the acute attack has settled, and difficulty in differentiating roentgenographically between diverticular disease and cancer. Elective resection should be performed 8 weeks after the acute episode has lessened. This period of time will permit subsidence of the major inflammatory reaction and afford the patient the best opportunity to undergo resection and primary anastomosis without accompanying colostomy.

The question always arises as to how much colon should be removed. Since I do not subscribe to the precept that all diverticula must be removed, I resect only the area that has caused the acute episode. The sigmoid colon is examined, with particular attention to the junction of the mesocolon with the mesocolic border of the bowel, to determine the extent of induration along the length of the intestine. Only the indurated section of bowel is removed, and primary anastomosis above the pelvic peritoneal floor maximizes the safety of the anastomosis. In about 150 consecutive patients undergoing elective resection, the average length of resected intestine was 17.5 cm.

I have not had a single death after elective resection for diverticular disease in more than 200 consecutive resections of colon. The morbidity rate after elective resection for diverticular disease is less than 5 percent. In a follow-up period of 10 or more years, none of these patients has required further operation for symptoms related to diverticular disease.

The safety of elective resection for diverticular disease has been demonstrated. Subsequent acute attacks may result in complications. Complicated diverticular disease is associated with sizable rates of morbidity and mortality. I believe that an aggressive approach toward early elective surgical treatment before the development of complications is justified.

CHRONIC ULCERATIVE COLITIS

JACOB C. HANDELSMAN, M.D.

Chronic ulcerative colitis is a surgically curable disease. This does not imply that every patient should undergo surgery, since the operations are rigorous and the mechanics of restoring defecation are intricate. Nevertheless, in many circumstances the surgeon assumes the responsibility for the cure, for presenting to the patient and his medical colleagues the surgical options, and for respecting the contraindications to certain procedures. His or her knowledge and attitudes may determine whether or not necessary surgery is carried out.

INDICATIONS FOR SURGERY

Life-threatening Hemorrhage. Although uncommon, hemorrhage is, without question, an indication for surgery.

Infection. Although perforation is unusual in ulcerative colitis, toxic dilatation of the colon is a relatively common, life-threatening complication. The colon, dilated and with compromise of the integrity of its wall, may leak or rupture, and this catastrophe is associated with a high mortality rate. In these circumstances, I try to limit the procedure to an abdominal colectomy, leaving the patient with an ileostomy and a defunctionalized rectum. This will get the patient through the crisis. Further planning is then possible.

Chronic Problems or Intractibility Under Medical Care. Continuous suboptimal health, impairing social and career performance, in the patient who is receiving good medical care is a definite indication for surgery. In the pediatric age group, failure to grow or develop may pose the problem. Therapeutic dilemmas, usually arising from sensitivity to sulfonamides or intolerance of steroids, may dictate the need for surgery. Even such a complication as serious perineal injury from the diarrhea may prove to be a block to medical success. Remote complications may involve the skin (pyoderma gangrenosum, erythema multiforme), musculoskeletal system (joint effusions, arthritis), eyes (iritis, uveitis), kidneys, or biliary tract. In general, the treatment for the remote manifestations of ulcerative colitis consists in addressing the intestinal disorder. When this is controlled, the nonintestinal manifestation subsides. However, there are two notable exceptions. One is ankylosing spondylitis. The second is cirrhosis and/or sclerosing cholangitis. Other hepatobiliary problems normally yield to surgical therapy to some degree.

The surgical treatment for these chronic manifestations of ulcerative colitis is total extirpation of the colon and rectum or its mucosa.

Cancer. The patient who has had ulcerative colitis for more than 6 or 7 years is particularly prone to develop colonic cancer of a vicious type, often multifocal. This incidence starts at about 6 percent at 7 years, rising by 2 percent annually. Those who seem to be most susceptible are patients who develop the disorder at an early age, have an explosive onset, get pancolitis, and are difficult to control. Apparent good health despite continuing colonic findings is no insurance against malignant change. If cancer occurs, immediate surgery is indicated. Total abdominal colectomy and resection of the rectum or its mucosa is basic, but the operation must be extended to encompass mesentery, nodes, and contiguous tissues as in any resection for cancer.

Threat of Cancer. Certain changes in the appearance of the colonic mucosa imply that the condition may be undergoing malignant change. Polypoid changes, especially villous, and changes in areas where flat and more normal mucosa meet are especially dangerous. Cellular changes in the nuclei or cytoplasm along with mucous depletion are among a group of changes termed "dysplasia." These are recognized premalignant changes. The colonoscope has made it possible to recognize these areas and to carry out systematic biopsies. The appearance of such changes in a patient under treatment mandates resection.

SURGICAL PROCEDURES

Four surgical procedures are available to the patient with ulcerative colitis. Three are curative: (1) proctocolectomy with Brooke (standard) ileostomy; (2) abdominal colectomy, mucosal proctectomy, and endorectal pull-through; and (3) proctocolectomy and continent ileostomy (Kock Pouch). These last two provide continence for the patient; no appliance is worn. In the endorectal pull-through procedure, the mucosa of the rectum is removed, and the terminal ileum is fashioned into a pouch that is nestled into the muscular shell of the rectum and anastomosed to the upper anus. A temporary diverting ileostomy is made above this. The patient defecates anally. The continent ileostomy operation fashions an internal reservoir and valve of the terminal ileum. The patient intubates this in order to defecate (Table 1).

A fourth procedure is not curative: A portion of the diseased rectum is intentionally left after the colectomy, and the ileum is sutured to it. This requires careful case

TABLE 1 Ileostomy Possibilities

A standard (Brooke) ileostomy may be converted to a Kock pouch.

A Kock pouch may be converted to a standard ileostomy.

An endorectal pouch anastomosis may be changed to a Kock pouch or standard ileostomy.

It is necessary to have a preserved anus to move from standard or continent ileostomy to an endorectal procedure.

selection and subsequent meticulous monitoring for cancer, dysplasia, or colitis. I continue to have reservations about this procedure. I have used it only sparingly and with the most energetic admonitions to the patient about his responsibilities in future follow-up.

Proctocolectomy

A few general remarks are in order regarding this well-established procedure: (1) I am not impressed that taking or leaving the omentum makes a difference; (2) no male patient has sexual dysfunction if the mesentery of the rectosigmoid and rectum is left behind after being divided close to the bowel wall; (3) perineal wounds are closed per primam. Suction tubes are introduced to the pelvis via stab wounds medial to the ischial tuberosities.

When definitive surgery is indicated, I recommend either endorectal pull-through or continent ileostomy unless there is a contraindication.

Clear liquids are prescribed for the 48 hours preceding surgery. Oral neomycin and erythromycin, 1 g each, are given orally 19, 18, and 9 hours preoperatively. Antibiotic enemas are given before surgery. Systemic antibiotics are given before and after the operation.

Endorectal Pull-through Procedure

This operation is designed to permit the ileostomy patient to defecate through the anus. A reservoir is made and the sphincter preserved.

The patient is positioned for combined synchronous resection. Following abdominal colectomy, the rectum is meticulously stripped of its mucosa for 4 to 5 cm proximal to the dentate line. This is carried out from below. Incision is made at the dentate line and dissection pursued between submucosa and muscularis by one of several techniques. During the operation, the rectum may be everted or left in normal position to facilitate dissection. If the mucosa is ravaged, this procedure may not be possible. In many cases, steroid enemas for 2 or 3 weeks before the operation improve the mucosa to a condition that permits dissection. At 5 cm above the anus, the rectum is divided, and the anus and the muscle of the denuded segment of rectum are left in place.

The terminal 25 cm of ileum are fashioned into a "J" shape. The antimesenteric borders are sutured with continuous 2–0 chromic catgut and the common wall open-ed. A two-layer anastomosis is completed with 2–0 chromic catgut. This pouch is nestled into the rectal muscular remnant, and the bottom of the "J" is incised and anastomosed at the dentate line with 3–0 Dexon. The pelvis is drained. Careful hemostasis is an important factor in avoiding infection.

A Brooke or Turnbull ileostomy is made in the right lower quadrant and remains for 3 months while the rectum heals. During this time the patient carries out sphincter exercises daily. I see my patients and carry out prophylactic dilation every 2 to 3 weeks. A contrast study of the new rectal apparatus is carried out before the ileostomy is closed.

After the ileostomy is closed, the patient is beset by liquid stools and a frequent urge to defecate. This may be ameliorated by thickening the stool with psyllium and by slowing peristalsis with drugs. I consider a result satisfactory if a patient has one movement nightly and five or fewer daily. Although most patients achieve this, it may require as long as a year. Patients retain good discrimination between gas and stool.

Results. The procedure is unsuccessful about 10 percent of the time. Poor sphincter function and fistulas from the pouch afflict some. Infection may lead to this. In some patients, unsatisfactory control at night spells failure. In these circumstances, conversion to a Kock pouch or standard ileostomy is possible (see Table 1).

Contraindications. Crohn's disease is a contraindication to this procedure because of the danger of activity in the ileum. A history of poor sphincter function or of anal abnormality is a warning of problems to come. When this question arises, I avail myself of rectal sphincter manometric studies. Patients who are too old, too young, or emotionally unstable may be unable to endure the necessary training.

Continent Ileostomy

This procedure permits the patient to do without an appliance and therefore to have an ileostomy low toward the groin and flush with the skin. This has obvious cosmetic advantages. The operation may be done in a patient whose rectum has been removed, or in a patient who desires conversion from a standard ileostomy. It is done in one stage.

The terminal 45 cm of ileum are used in this procedure. The proximal 30 cm are made into a pouch. Continuous 2–0 chromic catgut suture is used for this. Eight centimeters of the terminal ileum are then intussuscepted into the pouch and secured with silk sutures and staples. This base is secured with fascia. This makes a valve that is stool- and gas-proof. The remainder of the terminal ileum is made into an ileostomy. The ileostomy is led through the abdominal wall and the pouch secured behind it internally. The ileostomy is sutured flush with the abdominal wall. The patient defecates by emptying with a large-bore catheter three to five times daily. This catheter is left indwelling for 4 to 5 weeks postoperatively while

pouch and valve heal. The technique of intubation is easily learned.

Results. Two types of complication may occur. The pouch may leak in the postoperative period, but this heals on a regimen of hyperalimentation, suction to the pouch, and antibiotics.

Slippage of the valve may occur after months or years. This defeats the purpose of the operation. Usually a secondary procedure is required to reconstruct the valve. Although some 15 percent of patients may experience these complications, the eventual success rate is about 92 percent. If the pouch fails, it may be replaced by conventional ileostomy (see Table 1).

Contraindications. I regard Crohn's disease as a firm contraindication since it may develop in the pouch. Arthritis, extensive obesity, or inability to cope with the need for repeated intubation also contraindicate this procedure. I am wary of the patient under 13 or over 60 years of age.

POSTOPERATIVE COMPLICATIONS

Continent ileostomy and endorectal pull-through are both forms of ileostomy. As such they are subject to the dysfunctions that occur with the more usual ileostomies. Diarrhea, with rapid depletion of fluid and electrolytes, may occur. If quantities greater than the usual daily output of about 750 cc begin to appear, fluids must be forced. If this is not possible, the patient must be hospitalized.

As with conventional ileostomy, stricture (partial obstruction) may produce serious diarrhea (ileostomy dysfunction). In these pouch operations, the obstruction may be at the inlet or outlet of the pouch. If this is suspected, contrast radiography can establish the diagnosis accurately. Dilation may be completely successful in relieving this. I have used Foley balloons or Hegar dilators under general anesthesia for this purpose.

A syndrome of fever and diarrhea may afflict patients with a pouch, whether continent ileostomy or endorectal. This is known as "pouchitis." This clinical picture of diarrhea and fever probably comes about because the ileum is not normally required to act as a reservoir. It is difficult to demonstrate a common cause, but bacterial overgrowth and/or mucosal inflammation and ulceration are demonstrated in some patients.

Flagyl and tetracycline have proved useful in coping with this complication. I have given azulfidine to some patients to good effect.

Although the true incidence of this poorly understood complication is difficult to determine, 5 to 10 percent is probably an accurate assessment.

Although these newer surgical procedures have introduced certain new problems, they have also provided certain new insights. Increasingly, the rectum has been left in situ during emergency resections. This has been done to preserve for the patient the future opportunity for endorectal pull-through. Incidentally, however, it has given us the opportunity to observe that it is safe to retain the rectum for significant periods of time.

Another line of clinical research has been opened by procedures that utilize the ileum for reservoir purposes. In an effort to cause the ileum to dilate by partially obstructing it, an occluding device through which inter- mittent defecation can be accomplished has been devis- ed. It is being given clinical trials now to see whether it may also free one from the need for an appliance.

GRANULOMATOUS COLITIS

ARTHUR H. AUFSES, Jr., M.D.

Since the classic description of regional enteritis by Crohn, Ginzburg, and Oppenheimer in 1932, the illness now known as Crohn's disease has increased in incidence and prevalence throughout the world. Although the incidence of the disease may have reached a plateau in certain areas, in general its growth continues unabated. This is especially true of Crohn's disease involving the colon. Colonic involvement with regional ileitis (ileo- colitis) was first described by Colp in 1934, and at present about 45 to 50 percent of all patients with Crohn's disease have involvement of both the small and large bowel.

Crohn's colitis was first recognized as a distinct entity by Wells in 1952, but it remained for Lockhart-Mummery and Morson, 8 years later, to clearly separate granuloma- tous colitis from ulcerative colitis. Currently, approx- imately 15 percent of all patients with Crohn's disease have granulomatous colitis without other apparent intestinal involvement. As a relatively "new" disease, one might consider that better pathologic recognition and separation from ulcerative colitis is responsible for this increased incidence. However, the incidence of ulcerative colitis has remained stable, and since new cases of granulomatous colitis now outnumber new cases of ulcer- ative colitis, it is clear that there is an absolute increase in the number of patients with granulomatous colitis.

DIFFERENTIAL DIAGNOSIS

In order to plan proper management of any patient with colonic inflammatory bowel disease, a correct etiologic diagnosis is essential. Diagnostic criteria for granulomatous colitis based on pathologic, radiologic, and clinical criteria have been elaborated by Lockhart- Mummery and Morson, Cook and Dixon, Marshak et al, and Korelitz et al, and these have been well summarized by Roth.

The pathology of Crohn's disease is similar wherever it is found throughout the intestinal tract. The pathogno- monic finding in Crohn's disease is the epithelioid granuloma, but this is found in only about 50 percent of cases. Other histologic findings are those of a transmural inflammatory process with a marked increase in the submucosal layer, and fissuring of the bowel wall. Granulomas may be found in the regional lymph nodes as well. Macroscopically, the 1- to 2-mm sharply punched out aphthous ulcer is the earliest gross lesion detectable. These ulcers may heal or enlarge and then coalesce to form the longitudinal ulcer seen most commonly on the mesenteric border of the bowel. The cobblestone mucosa formed by intersection of longitudinal and transverse ulceration is characteristic. The creeping fat of Crohn's disease is seen in the colon in granulomatous colitis as are "skip lesions." The rectum is spared in about 20 percent of cases.

Radiologic examination utilizing conventional and/or double air contrast barium enema in Crohn's disease of the colon demonstrates the aphthous ulcers, larger ulcers, nodular defects, fissures, tracking, stricture formation, cobblestone mucosa, sinus tracts, and fistulas. The seg- mental nature of the disease may be apparent, and if the rectum is normal, the disease is almost certainly not ulcer- ative colitis. If, in addition to the colonic findings, there is typical Crohn's disease of the terminal ileum, the disease in the colon is granulomatous colitis. The ileal changes are usually readily distinguishable from the so- called backwash "ileitis" of ulcerative colitis.

The intermittent diarrhea, crampy abdominal pain, and fever of granulomatous colitis do not by themselves distinguish this illness from the other colitides. Perianal disease, however, is a frequent accompaniment of Crohn's colitis and may be present in as many as 90 percent of patients with severe rectal involvement by Crohn's disease. The occurrence of a perirectal abscess and/or fistula in childhood or adolescence, followed at a long interval by intestinal symptoms, should alert the clinician to the possibility of granulomatous disease. Occult bleeding is usual; massive bleeding may occur, but is rare. Extraintestinal manifestations of Crohn's disease are common, and although the uveitis, iritis, spondylitis, and erythema nodosum may not necessarily distinguish granulomatous from ulcerative colitis, these findings certainly go far to rule out other colitides.

Sigmoidoscopy should always be the first diagnostic test performed in any patient with intestinal complaints. In Crohn's colitis the aphthous ulcers can be identified as well as the normal islands of mucosa and the irregular ulcers. In ulcerative colitis the ulcerations are more likely to be pinpoint in size, and there is a marked hyperemia and friability of the diffusely involved mucosa. Biopsy of the latter is more likely to show only diffuse mucosal changes as opposed to the submucosal fibrosis and edema of Crohn's disease. The finding of one or more epithelioid granulomas would confirm the latter diagnosis.

If one excludes diverticulitis, approximately 80 to 85 percent of all patients with colonic inflammatory bowel disease have either ulcerative or granulomatous colitis. Other forms of colitis must be considered in differential diagnosis. Pseudomembranous colitis caused by *Clostridium difficile* and associated with prior antibiotic use may be confused with granulomatous disease. Other acute bacterial disorders of the colon, such as those caused by *Campylobacter fetus* subspecies *jejuni, Shigella,* or *Salmonella* may present a picture not dissimilar to granulomatous disease. Stool cultures are essential to rule out these lesions. The ''gay bowel'' syndrome seen in sexually transmitted disease is manifested by various forms of proctitis. In the older age group, the radiologic appearance of diverticulitis, ischemic colitis, or lymphoma may be similar to the findings in Crohn's colitis. After taking into account all of the foregoing causes of colitis, there remains about 5 percent of all cases of colonic inflammation which defy exact diagnosis and end up classified as ''indeterminate'' colitis.

MANAGEMENT

Toxic megacolon that does not respond to nonoperative management, unrelenting massive hemorrhage, and perforation with or without colonic dilatation represent emergency indications for surgery. In the absence of these catastrophic complications, most patients with granulomatous colitis are managed nonoperatively for varying periods of time. In general the patient with granulomatous colitis is operated on later in the course of disease than the patient with primarily small bowel involvement.

Medical Management

Nonoperative therapy includes symptomatic management as well as treatment with potentially disease-specific medication. Among the former are such measures as dietary manipulation, including both high and low bulk diets, antispasmodics, and antidiarrheal agents. Sulfasalazine is the drug most often given. The 5-acetyl salicylic acid component of this drug appears to be the active agent. Steroids are normally given, but are of greater value in small bowel disease. Metronidazole may produce marked improvement, especially in patients with perianal disease. Broad-spectrum antibiotics should be reserved for use in dealing with septic complications. Immunosuppressive therapy utilizing Imuran or 6-mercaptopurine has its advocates. Total parenteral nutrition may be of value in stabilizing an acutely ill or debilitated patient prior to surgery, but rarely provides permanent relief.

Surgical Management

The patient becomes a candidate for surgical management of Crohn's colitis when the aforementioned therapies, alone or in combination, fail to maintain an adequate quality of life. Unfortunately these patients, primarily adolescents and young adults, are never ''well,'' but manage to ''get along.'' The same is true of the adolescent who fails to thrive and suffers from growth retardation. If the latter group is to be allowed a period of growth, surgery must be carried out several years before epiphyseal closure and sexual maturation.

In addition to the ''medical intractability'' noted above, the specific complications of fistula, abscess, obstruction (relatively uncommon in Crohn's colitis), and perianal disease are the most common indications for operation.

Preoperative bowel preparation for elective surgery is, in general, no different than for colonic surgery for any cause. However, cathartics need not be used, and enemas should be given with caution. Oral antibiotics should be given for bowel sterilization, and prophylactic intravenous antibiotics may be employed preoperatively and perioperatively. I prepare the patient with oral neomycin and erythromycin base and give a cephalosporin intravenously 1 hour preoperatively and then every 4 hours for three or four doses. The severely debilitated patient may be brought to a more optimal state by a short period of preoperative total parenteral nutrition. The ability of TPN to restore positive nitrogen balance may make possible a definitive procedure as opposed to only a diversionary operation. If the patient has been receiving steroids, they must be continued through the postoperative period.

Although the extent of colonic disease usually has been well delineated by radiologic studies, I prefer to have patients examined by colonoscopy preoperatively. Although small bowel disease is readily apparent at the operating table, mild to moderately severe colonic involvement may be difficult to identify. The thickened colon with increased vascularity and ''creeping fat'' may not be obvious, especially in the transverse colon because of the attached omentum. In addition, the enlarged mesenteric lymph nodes may not be noted in the mesentery of the ascending or descending colon.

I perform the operation through a generous vertical midline incision to allow for wide exposure and ease of exploration. The entire bowel is visualized from esophagogastric junction to rectosigmoid. The small bowel is measured and note made of all diseased areas.

The preferred procedure for granulomatous colitis is resection of the involved colon. When the rectum is spared, subtotal colectomy and ileorectal anastomosis should be performed. If the terminal ileum is involved, it too must be removed. Patients with marked rectal involvement and severe perianal disease require total proctocolectomy. One must bear in mind that in the severely septic patient, diversion of the fecal stream alone allows the disease to come under control. Loop ileostomy, as described by Turnbull, is the preferred diversionary procedure. In combination with drainage of established abscesses, this measure eliminates the need for massive colonic resection in the face of severe illness. When there is severe perianal disease with sepsis, rectal resection should be delayed until diversion and adequate drainage allow for subsidence of the infectious process. In the technical performance of rectal resection, one must adhere to the principle of dissecting close to the wall of the bowel so as not to injure any of the pelvic or perineal nerves in order to preserve sexual function. In the absence of established infection, the perineal wound may be closed primarily with suction drainage of the perineum. In a patient undergoing total proctocolectomy and ileostomy, the site for ileostomy should be chosen with care before the patient is placed on the operating table to be sure that the stoma is in good position to handle an appliance without dificulty. The stoma is fashioned by the usual Brooke everting ileostomy technique. Although some groups are performing continent ileostomies with Kock's pouch, most surgeons in the field believe that these procedures are contraindicated in Crohn's disease because of the danger of recurrence in the pouch, necessitating sacrifice of large segments of small bowel. Mucosal proctectomy and ileoanal anastomosis are also contraindicated because the transmural nature of Crohn's disease makes mucosal stripping extremely difficult if not impossible.

The management of the catastrophic complications noted earlier deserves special comment. Angiography is indicated during massive bleeding in an attempt to localize the source of bleeding. In Crohn's disease it is usually from a single vessel, and knowledge of the site of bleeding may allow for a lesser procedure. Perforation must be handled by exteriorization or resection of the perforated segment, but no attempt should be made to perform an anastomosis in the presence of peritoneal infection. Toxic megacolon can most often be managed nonoperatively employing nasogastric suction or long intestinal tube intubation, intravenous fluids and antibiotics, and steroids. Frequent repositioning of the patient allows for redistribution of the gas and eventually leads to decompression in almost all cases. If the patient does not respond to these measures, subtotal colectomy and ileostomy should be performed. The Turnbull procedure of ileostomy and venting transverse colostomy has its advocates.

Postoperative complications in these patients are usually related to sepsis. A significant number of patients undergoing operation for Crohn's disease already have intra-abdominal or retroperitoneal infection or are immunosuppressed either by malnutrition or steroid administration, and infectious complications are frequent. If infection is present in the abdomen, delayed primary closure of the skin and subcutaneous fissure should be employed.

The ever-present possibility of recurrent disease is a burden that all patients with Crohn's disease have to bear. If any segment of the colon remains after surgery, such as after ileorectal anastomosis, the recurrence rate is significant. On the other hand, it may be many years before further surgery is needed if at all. Following total proctocolectomy, there is an incidence of recurrence in the terminal ileum, either at or just proximal to the ileostomy stoma, but the majority of these patients do very well indeed.

Despite the potential for recurrent disease, the vast majority of these patients are grateful for their surgery and, in the postoperative period, frequently wonder why it was not performed at an earlier time.

OBSTRUCTION OF THE LARGE BOWEL

FABRIZIO MICHELASSI, M.D.
GEORGE E. BLOCK, M.D., F.A.C.S.

NEOPLASTIC DISEASE

Cancer of the colon accounts for over one-half of all obstructions of the large bowel, the remaining cases being caused by volvulus (15%), diverticular disease (10%), hernia (4%), and such less common causes as intussusception, adhesions, carcinomatosis, ischemic strictures, foreign bodies, inflammatory bowel disease, and fecal impaction. Although malignant obstructing lesions may occur anywhere in the large bowel, they are most common in the descending colon and the rectosigmoid.

True large bowel obstructions occur in approximately 15 percent of all colorectal cancers, but the clinician must differentiate between an actual acute obstruction and the mere roentgenographic appearance of obstruction to retrograde flow of contrast media. The clinical presentation of large bowel obstruction is associated with a history of constipation, failure to pass gas or feces per rectum, abdominal pain, and distention. Nausea and vomiting occur late, if at all, and are secondary either to a dilated small bowel or to a reflex response to sudden colonic distention. An abdominal mass or localized tenderness occasionally may be elicited by palpation, and loud, high-pitched bowel sounds may be heard on auscultation. There is usually diffuse tympanism of the abdomen. Rectal examination rarely reveals a palpable obstructing carcinoma, but helps to rule out a fecal impaction as the cause of obstruction.

The patients are often anemic from chronic blood loss, but at the time of admission the anemia may be masked because of acute dehydration and hemoconcentration.

Proctosigmoidoscoy should be performed on all patients in whom a large bowel obstruction is suspected. In distal colonic and rectal obstruction, this procedure not only identifies the site and nature of the obstructing lesion, but also relieves the vast majority of obstructions caused by sigmoid volvulus. The flexible colonoscope permits visualization of lesions beyond the reach of the rigid proctoscope, but overzealous and protracted manipulation of the acutely ill patient suffering from colonic obstruction is to be avoided.

X-ray examination of the abdomen in the supine, upright, and decubitus positions should be obtained in all cases of suspected intestinal obstruction. These may demonstrate not only the location of the obstructing lesion by showing the most distal extent of the gas pattern, but also a pneumoperitoneum in patients who have a concomitant colonic perforation. Perforation is reported to occur in 2 to 18 percent of patients suffering from neoplastic obstruction of the colon; one-half of the perforations are at the site of the carcinoma and the remainder are in the cecum. Contrast studies help to localize and define the nature of the obstructive lesion and to rule out the possibility of pseudo-obstruction. The examination should be performed under the direction of the surgeon so that if barium is used as a contrast material, a large amount will not be forced past a partially obstructing lesion to convert it into a complete obstruction. If a diverticular abscess or a perforated carcinoma is suspected, a water-soluble contrast material should be chosen in preference to barium.

Immediate Treatment

Patients with colonic obstruction due to neoplasm are usually acutely and chronically ill and often elderly so that preoperate rehydration and volume repletion are essential. Nasogastric suction is instituted immediately in order to minimize abdominal distention and to prevent vomiting and aspiration. Systemic antibiotics appropriate for aerobic and anaerobic organisms should be administered prior to operation.

Operation for obstruction unaccompanied by a pending or actual perforation may be delayed until the patient is resuscitated and rehydrated and decompression has been attempted. However, if the patient has tenderness over the cecum, evidence of peritonitis, general sepsis, or a closed loop obstruction, operation should promptly follow a brief resuscitative effort.

For patients with right-sided carcinoma and an incompetent ileocecal valve, passage of a Cantor tube often decompresses the small bowel and proximal ascending colon, allowing for an elective rather than an emergency operation. In the case of left-sided lesion, a partially obstructing tumor may become acutely obstructing by the lodging of hard fecal material at the stenotic area. In these instances, an initial trial of nonoperative therapy by a series of gentle enemas is appropriate. However, these attempts to convert a complete obstruction into a partial obstruction are successful in fewer than 10 percent of the patients. If marked improvement has not occurred by the time the resuscitation of the patient is completed, the nonoperative approach must be abandoned in favor of operation.

Palliative Surgery

Almost half the patients with obstructing cancers of the colon are incurable when first seen. The limited life expectancy of the patient with an incurable lesion must be taken into account when determining the nature and extent of any palliative procedure. The mean survival time for patients with an unresectable carcinoma who are palliated by a colostomy is only 6 months; for patients undergoing a palliative resection of the primary lesion, life expectancy is approximately 10 months.

Palliative resection of the obstructing lesion is possible in the majority of patients with incurable disease and should be performed, if possible, to relieve the obstruction and to prevent future bleeding and perforation. For patients with unresectable disease, relief of obstruction may be achieved either by a proximal ileostomy or colostomy or by internal diversion of the fecal stream. Cecostomy is an unsatisfactory choice for palliation, and a proximal loop colostomy is often associated with prolapse.

"Curative Treatment" of the Right Colon

Fifty-five to sixty percent of patients with obstructing colorectal carcinomas have potentially curable lesions. Little controversy exists concerning the treatment of choice for the right-sided colonic lesions. These should be primarily resected by an appropriate cancer operation, sacrificing the branches of the superior mesenteric artery to the right side of the colon and ensuring an adequate lymphadenectomy. The decision whether to perform an immediate or delayed anastomosis depends on the general condition of the patient, the degree of distention, the amount of fecal material in the small bowel, and the presence or absence of sepsis. If the condition of the patient is unsatisfactory, if there is massive distention of the small bowel, if the small bowel is filled with odoriferous feces, or if there is localized or generalized peritonitis, a primary anastomosis should not be performed and an end-ileostomy chosen. The distal colonic segment may be exteriorized as a mucous fistula (the safer procedure) or closed and placed in the abdominal cavity. Secondary anastomosis is usually accomplished within 6 weeks following the initial procedure. If the condition of the patient and the condition of the proximal and distal segments of the bowel allow for primary anastomosis, it may be accomplished in either an end-to-end or end-to-side fashion. It must be emphasized that primary resection of the right-sided colonic lesions, if it is to have merit, must be based on an adequate cancer operation. Attempts at limited resections inappropriate for a cancer of the large bowel have been met with disappointing 5-year survivals.

"Curative Treatment" of the Left Colon

For left-sided lesions, a three-stage procedure involving primary decompression by colostomy followed by resection and finally by closure of the colostomy has long been the mainstay of operative treatment. However, the cumulative mortality and morbidity of the three procedures is high (up to 30% and 80% respectively), hospitalization is long, and about 40 percent of patients given a "temporary" colostomy retain the stoma permanently. Primary resection of the left-sided lesion is conceptually an attractive approach, but fell into disfavor after early attempts met with a uniformly high death rate. The deaths were directly attributable to an anastomotic failure in the unprepared bowel. Conversion of the primary resection thesis into a two-stage procedure has led to a very low hosptial mortality and a short hospital stay, and has the potential for an improved 5-year survival. In this operation, which is our choice, the left-sided lesion is resected by an appropriate cancer operation with early high ligation of the inferior mesenteric artery and excision of the primary lymph node basin for the left colon. The colonic lesion is then resected with adequate margins, and an anastomosis is not attempted. Rather, the proximal colon is brought out through a separate wound as an end-colostomy, and the distal bowel may be exteriorized as a mucous fistula or closed as a Hartmann pouch.

In certain instances, we elect to perform a near-total abdominal colectomy with an ileosigmoidostomy or ileoproctostomy. With this relatively safe and simple anastomosis, the distal bowel can be cleansed perioperatively. It is chosen for patients who are young and at risk for the development of further carcinomas, patients with lesions at or near the splenic flexure whose lymphatic drainage is potentially via both the inferior mesenteric and superior mesenteric nodal system, and for patients with multiple polyps and/or synchronous carcinomas. Carcinomas of the rectum large enough to obstruct the colon are rarely curable. Therefore, extended pelvic dissections via an abdominal-perineal dissection are almost never indicated for the acutely obstructed patient. For these patients, a primary resection is indicated without a pelvic or perineal dissection. If abdominal-perineal dissection is the only method of extirpating the tumor, the patients are best treated by a two-stage procedure employing an end-colostomy for immediate decompression to be followed, if appropriate, by an abdominal-perineal resection.

Results

Because of the variation in therapies for obstructing carcinomas of the colon, the operative mortality is reported to range from 5 to 38 percent. The operative mortality can be reduced to a minimum by adequate resuscitation, early operation, and the avoidance of a primary anastomosis in all cases of left-sided and unsuitable right-sided lesions. Predictably, the reported 5-year survivals from these carcinomas vary greatly. Factors contributing to the unfavorable prognosis of obstructing colorectal carcinomas include the large number of advanced tumors encountered at the time of diagnosis and the unacceptably high operative mortality rate when an inappropriate anastomosis is attempted. Comparison by stage of cancer shows that long-term survival does not differ significantly from that obtained with elective resections.

OTHER CAUSES OF LARGE BOWEL OBSTRUCTION

Complete obstruction of the colon occurs in about 10 percent of the patients suffering from diverticulitis and usually indicates an abscess formation with encroachment on the lumen or stenosis from repeated bouts of inflammation. The obstruction accompanying diverticulitis is rarely a cause for emergency operation as the obstructive symptoms usually respond promptly to nonoperative therapy. If complete colonic obstruction is not relieved within a few hours, however, operative therapy is indicated. If obstruction is caused by stenosis or a small, well-contained, and well-localized abscess, an immediate resection should be accomplished because the results are superior to those obtained by delayed resection. Primary anastomosis is to be avoided in the unprepared bowel or if there is generalized or severe localized peritonitis. If the obstruction is caused by a large intraperitoneal abscess, immediate resection is not accomplished. These patients are best treated by extraperitoneal drainage of the abscess, proximal diversion of the fecal stream, and appropriate adjuvant treatment including antibiotic therapy. The colon obstructed by diverticulitis occasionally (3%) harbors an occult carcinoma. In these instances, wide excision of the tumor-bearing segment of the colon and its lymphatic drainage must be accomplished.

Sixteen percent of all intussusceptions occur in adults. In the large bowel, the cause of obstruction is usually carcinoma and warrants an appropriate cancer resection.

VOLVULUS OF THE COLON

JOHN R. ANDERSON, M.B., Ch.B., B.Sc., F.R.C.S.(Edin.)

Acute volvulus of the colon accounts for 1 to 7 percent of all cases of intestinal obstruction in Western countries. Although uncommon, it is only exceeded by carcinoma and diverticular disease as a cause of large bowel obstruction. The sigmoid colon is involved in 65 to 80 percent of cases and the right colon in 15 to 30 percent. The transverse colon, in most large studies, is involved infrequently (2% to 5%) and only 20 patients with splenic flexure volvulus have been reported in the literature.

Volvulus is an axial rotation of part of the alimentary tract. The pathophysiology involves a closed-loop obstruction with its consequent risks of tension gangrene as well as torsion of the mesentery with possible embarrassment of the venous drainage and arterial supply to the involved loop. All cases of volvulus are therefore examples of strangulation obstruction, and this should be borne in mind when considering management. Gangrene occurs in about 10 percent of patients with acute sigmoid volvulus, but in a much higher proportion of patients with acute volvulus of the right colon (20% to 30%). The development of gangrene is probably related to the speed of onset of the twist, to the degree of torsion, and to the length of the mesentery as well as the quantity of fat within it. In the presence of peritonitis, the diagnosis of gangrene with perforation is straightforward, and the need for laparotomy obvious. When the gangrene is patchy, as frequently happens, it may be exceptionally difficult to determine the viability of bowel before undertaking treatment.

ACUTE SIGMOID VOLVULUS

The safest initial treatment of a patient in whom the bowel is thought to be viable is deflation per rectum using a long rectal tube passed through the rigid sigmoidoscope. This results in satisfactory deflation of the loop in 75 to 85 percent of patients. The rectal tube should be strapped to the buttock and left in place for 4 to 7 days to allow further assessment of the patient, many of whom are elderly with serious concomitant medical disorders. In the majority of patients, sigmoid colectomy should be carried out as a semi-urgent procedure to prevent further recurrence, but there is a small group of patients who are considered unfit for laparotomy, and in my experience, once a volvulus has been satisfactorily deflated via the sigmoidoscope, recurrent attacks can be subsequently deflated in the same way, often on numerous occasions. If, at the time of sigmoidoscopy, there is evidence of devitalized mucosa or if blood-stained fluid issues from the rectal tube, emergency laparotomy should be undertaken. Laparotomy also is necessary for patients suspected of having nonviable bowel.

At laparotomy the most important step is first to untwist the bowel and then determine its viability. Great care must be taken in assessing the short segment of colon at the neck of the twist as this may be the only part of the bowel that is nonviable. It is often bruised and its associated mesentery edematous, and the procedure of placing hot packs on this area, and leaving the final assessment for at least 5 minutes, has proved invaluable to me. When viable bowel is confirmed, a variety of surgical procedures are possible. Operative detorsion, with or without colopexy (simple suturing to the parietal peritoneum, or suturing the apex of the sigmoid loop to the transverse colon over a broad base), has a high recurrence rate. The postoperative mortality following detorsion, with or without fixation, is similar to that following other operative procedures, and to subject a patient to an operation that has a similar significant mortality but a higher recurrence rate is unacceptable. Mesocoloplasty (incising the sigmoid mesocolon longitudinally from its base through any fibrous bands to the apex of the loop and resuturing it transversely to shorten the long sigmoid mesentery and to broaden its base) has been used in a small number of patients with successful short-term results. Extraperitonealization of the sigmoid colon is also effective in preventing recurrence. I have had no experience with either of these procedures. In the majority of cases, resection is necessary to prevent long-term recurrence.

Before resection, I prefer to carry out on-table lavage and to primarily suture the anastomosis. After mobilization of the colon, the rectum is divided. A corrugated wide-bore tube is then inserted into the distal sigmoid colon and secured with two ligatures tied around the full circumference of the bowel. The distal end of the corrugated tube is tied into a large plastic bag and placed in a container on the floor of the operating room. The lavage is carried out by inserting a large latex urinary catheter into the cecum through one of the anterior tenia, and invaginating it with a double purse-string suture. Some authors advocate removing the appendix and inserting the catheter through the stump, but this may lead to kinking of the tube postoperatively. The colon is then lavaged with warmed Hartmann's solution until it is completely free of all fecal matter, and the effluent is clear. This adds 20 to 35 minutes to the length of the procedure and uses approximately 9 liters of fluid. The patient is given antibiotics perioperatively including doses 6 and 12 hours after surgery. If there is gross disparity between the ends of the colon, or if for any other reason the surgeon feels that primary anastomosis is unsafe, an endcolostomy and either a distal colonic mucous fistula or closure of the distal stump, as in the Hartmann procedure, is a satisfactory and safe alternative.

The Paul Mikulicz resection has been advocated by some authors as the procedure of choice, but has two disadvantages. First, the resection must include the neck of the volvulus, and when this is situated close to the rectum, extensive mobilization may be necessary to allow the distal limb of the colostomy to be brought up without tension and may in fact be impossible. If there is any tension at all on the distal limb, there is a risk of retraction, and if the resection is not carried below the neck of the volvulus, there is the risk of retrograde thrombosis and gangrene of the distal limb of the colostomy. The second disadvantage of this procedure is that when the colostomy is closed, especially if there is any evidence of a megacolon at the time of laparotomy, there is a risk of recurrence of the volvulus. For these reasons the Paul Mikulicz resection should be avoided in patients with acute sigmoid volvulus.

When the viability of the sigmoid colon is in doubt or when frank gangrene is present, resection is mandatory. When there is patchy gangrene, without evidence of perforation in an otherwise stable patient, resection with on-table lavage and primary anastomosis can be carried out. When there is extensive gangrene or frank perforation, an anastomosis should be avoided, and in this situation, Hartmann's operation would appear to be the procedure of choice. When the twist in the sigmoid loop is situated in the proximal sigmoid colon and where the distal limb after resection is long, an end-colostomy with a distal colonic mucous fistula allows easier restoration of gastrointestinal continuity at a later stage.

ACUTE VOLVULUS OF THE RIGHT COLON

The treatment of this condition should always be surgical. As with acute sigmoid volvulus, it can be difficult to determine whether viable bowel is present preoperatively, and in this situation, to carry out colonoscopy in an attempt to deflate the distended colon is potentially hazardous.

When viable bowel is found at laparotomy, the treatment options available to the surgeon are similar to those for acute volvulus of the sigmoid colon. Table 1 lists 11 series published since 1970. Some of the authors have included cases of intermittent or chronic right colon volvulus, and others have also included examples of the so-called cecal bascule. In this latter condition the cecum becomes folded anteriorly and superiorly over a fixed ascending colon, and although a closed loop obstruction develops, there is usually no mesenteric torsion. This therefore does not represent a true volvulus as defined earlier. In my experience, when the colon is viable a well-anchored tube cecostomy is all that is required in this situation. The treatment of intermittent or chronic right colon volvulus is to be discussed later in this chapter (see - *Intermittent Volvulus of the Colon*).

Simple cecopexy, suturing the cecum to the parietal peritoneum over a broad base, has become the preferred procedure of a number of surgeons. From the results shown, this is followed by recurrence in 17 percent of patients. Despite a broad fixation, the thin-walled, fluid-filled, heavy cecum may tear loose from some of these sutures in the immediate postoperative period. When there is massive cecal distention, I do not always find it possible to obtain a satisfactory position of the cecum in the right lower abdominal quadrant, and in this situation resection may be necessary. However, in the majority of cases, the addition of a tube cecostomy to decompress the bowel allows satisfactory positioning. The combination of tube cecostomy with cecopexy is effective in preventing long-term recurrence. The reasons for this appear to be rapid decompression of the dilated colonic segment (which helps to prevent the right colon from tearing free), together with fixation of the bowel in two planes at 90° to each other. Tube cecostomy alone also appears to be effective in preventing recurrence, but as already stated, this procedure may have been used more frequently in the studies quoted in cases of the so-called cecal bascule. Tube cecostomy itself is not without complications, including death as a result of massive gangrene of the anterior abdominal wall. It is my practice to invaginate the cecostomy tube with two purse-string sutures and then to carefully fix the cecum to the parietal peritoneum and transversus abdominis with a further three or four interrupted sutures, placed close to the exit point of the tube.

Resection in the presence of viable bowel also prevents long-term recurrence, but this more major procedure carries with it an increased mortality and morbidity when compared to the combination of tube cecostomy with cecopexy.

TABLE 1 Long-Term Results of Various Procedures for the Treatment of Acute Volvulus of the Right Colon (number of patients followed up/number of patients with recurrence)

Author	Resection	Cecopexy	Cecostomy	Cecopexy + Cecostomy	Detorsion	Mean follow-up (yrs)
Bystrom et al (1972)	10/0	20/5	--	--	6/0	*
Inberg et al (1972)	8/0	5/1	--	--	23/5	*
Meyers et al (1972)	5/0	3/3	--	--	1/0	4.9
Smith and Goodwin (1973)	3/0	2/0	9/0	7/0	--	*
Andersson et al (1975)	3/0	9/2	2/0	3/0	7/0	7.0
Halvorsen and Semb (1975)	8/0	5/1	--	--	7/1	1-25 (mean value not stated)
Rivas and Dennison (1978)	7/0	5/1	1/0	--	6/0	*
O'Mara et al (1979)	12/0	18/0	4/0	--	--	5.7
Howard and Catto (1980)	2/0	5/0	1/0	4/0	3/0	5.7
Author's series	24/0	15/3	3/1	10/0	1/1	8.2
Total	85/0	93/16	26/1	24/0	57/7	

* Not stated

TABLE 2   Management of 19 Patients with Gangrenous Right Colon Volvulus

State of Cecum	Resection and Primary Anastomosis		Resection with Ileostomy & Colonic Mucous fistula	
	No. of patients	No. of deaths	No. of patients	No. of deaths
Perforation	3	3	2	1
Confluent gangrene	2	2	2	1
Patchy gangrene	7	0	3	0

When nonviable bowel is present at laparotomy, resection is mandatory. Table 2 lists the 19 patients with a gangrenous right colon in my series, and relates the procedure carried out to the presence or absence of perforation, and to whether the gangrene was confluent or patchy. Although the numbers are small, the only patients to survive when perforation was present, or when confluent gangrene was found, were those undergoing resection with the formation of ileostomy and a distal colonic mucous fistula. In the presence of patchy gangrene, resection with primary anastomosis appears to be safe.

In the uncommon situation in which the right colon volvulus is secondary to a more distal obstructing lesion, I prefer, when possible, to carry out on-table lavage as described for acute sigmoid volvulus, with resection of the obstructing lesion and primary anastomosis. After completion of the anastomosis, the cecum and ascending colon are sutured to the lateral abdominal wall, and the cecostomy fixed, as previously described, to the anterior abdominal wall. When, at laparotomy, the right colon is found to be nonviable, resection is carried out from the cecum to beyond the obstructing lesion, and either an ileostomy or a primary ileocolic or ileorectal anastomosis is fashioned.

ACUTE VOLVULUS OF THE TRANSVERSE COLON AND SPLENIC FLEXURE

Diagnosis of these conditions in the emergency situation can be difficult and is usually made at laparotomy. The procedure of choice in all situations, whether the bowel is viable or nonviable, is resection. Various forms of colopexy have been tried, but as with acute sigmoid volvulus, the recurrence rates are high.

With volvulus of the transverse colon, it is my practice to carry out an extended right hemicolectomy with primary anastomosis, but when there is free perforation, consideration should be given to forming an ileostomy with a distal colonic mucous fistula.

With splenic flexure volvulus the colon is resected after on-table colonic lavage, and continuity restored with a primary anastomosis. The Paul Mikulicz resection has been used in this situation, but there is a high risk of recurrence following this procedure, and it cannot be recommended as an acceptable treatment for this reason.

THE ILEOSIGMOID KNOT

This rare condition occurs when a loop of small intestine descends into the left parocolic gutter and encircles the sigmoid colon. As the knot tightens, the bowel obstructs, forming a double closed-loop obstruction with rapid progression to strangulation. It probably represents a complication of primary volvulus of the small intestine rather than the colon. Radiologic examination of the abdomen prior to laparotomy may, on occasion, identify the condition, but in the majority of cases the diagnosis is made at laparotomy.

The operative management of this condition is straightforward. Excision of the knot intact should be carried out with primary small bowel anastomosis. Depending on the circumstances, the colon can be primarily sutured, possibly after lavage, or an end-colostomy and distal colonic mucous fistula fashioned. Some authors advocate unknotting of the distended loop, but this is frequently followed by irreversible shock, perforation, contamination of the operative field, or fistula formation and should be avoided.

INTERMITTENT VOLVULUS OF THE COLON

Intermittent volvulus of the colon at all sites tends to occur in a younger age group than that seen in patients presenting with acute volvulus. The diagnosis usually is suggested by the clinical history and is confirmed by barium enema examination.

In all situations, except intermittent volvulus of the right colon, the involved colonic segment should be resected as an elective procedure with primary anastomosis. In my experience, volvulus of the right colon can be dealt with effectively by means of a cecopexy of the peritoneal flap type. The right leaf of the mesentery attached to the cecum is incised along the border of the cecum and ascending colon, and the flap of peritoneum raised with its base laterally. The cecum and ascending colon are then positioned to the right lower abdominal quadrant, and the peritoneal flap replaced over the cecum and ascending colon and sutured to the anteromedial tenia with interrupted nonabsorbable sutures. In the elective situation with prepared bowel, the risks of the cecum tearing free are minimal, and the long-term results following this procedure are gratifying.

RECTAL PROLAPSE

HERBERT C. HOOVER, Jr., M.D.

The proper operative procedure for rectal prolapse remains controversial. At least 75 operative procedures have been described, and new ones appear regularly, giving good evidence for a lack of consensus concerning the appropriate surgical approach.

Although etiology remains somewhat controversial, most evidence supports an intussusception of the rectum or rectosigmoid upon itself as the most common cause of rectal prolapse. The sliding hernia and extended pouch of Douglas, which usually accompany the prolapse, are most likely secondary rather than primary. The question is not of great importance, for it is the symptomatic problem of intussusception of the rectum that requires the surgeon's attention.

The diagnosis can be readily made in most cases by an examination of a patient who is straining. The gloved hand can easily palpate all layers of the bowel wall which often prolapse as much as 10 to 15 cm outside the anus. Digital rectal examination as well as sigmoidoscopy and a barium enema are recommended for all patients because a tumor may (rarely) be the leading point of the intussusception.

THERAPEUTIC OPTIONS

Therapy should be surgical in all patients who present with symptomatic prolapse. Patients with complete rectal prolapse are often in a poor-risk category because of age, neurologic disorders, advanced cardiovascular disease, pyschiatric disorders, or other debilitating problems. The individual patient's requirements and risk factors should be uppermost in the surgeon's mind in deciding on the choice of operation. There is certainly no single approach that is advisable for all patients.

Many of the 75-plus procedures described are of historical interest primarily and should not be attempted by the inexperienced surgeon. The operative options include a variety of procedures involving a transabdominal approach alone, a combined abdominoperineal approach, and one-stage perineal approaches. Another variable relates to the resection or preservation of the redundant bowel associated with rectal prolapse. The trend in recent years has been to abandon the complex procedures that emphasize the repair of the pelvic floor defect. The currently favored approach is transabdominal, with the objective to reduce and prevent recurrent intussusception by fixing the rectum to the sacrum. Of all the operative procedures described, the Ripstein procedure, in which a Teflon sling is used to fix the mobilized rectum to the presacral space, has probably been the most widely used in good-risk patients. However, outside of Ripstein's own series, the recurrence rates are significant, and bowel management problems ranging from episodic abdominal pain to fecal impaction due to late strictures are not uncommon. In recent years, a number of authors have advocated an even simpler but similar abdominal approach that has become my preferred method of treatment for good-risk patients. The method involves a simple posterior rectopexy that appears to be as effective as more complex methods and is not associated with significant complications.

It is important to have an option for poor-risk patients who would not tolerate an intra-abdominal operation. The simplest (and probably the oldest) approach consists of encircling the distal anal canal with a constricting silver wire (Thiersch). It involves only the perineal approach and is the least traumatic, but also the least successful, method of controlling rectal prolapse. It is associated with a high rate of failure caused by breakage of the wire, development of fecal impaction, infection, or making the anal orifice too narrow or too wide. A variety of alternative materials such as polyethylene, Teflon, nylon, or polyester tape have shown no clear advantage over the silver wire. The procedure should be considered only for the rare patient who is such an extremely poor risk that a surgical procedure cannot be considered. In most poor-risk patients, however, a perineal rectosigmoidectomy, as popularized by Altemeier, offers an excellent approach. Both posterior rectopexy and perineal rectosigmoidectomy will be described here.

PREOPERATIVE PREPARATION

Patients with a protracted history of rectal prolapse are given a period of preoperative hospitalization of 3 to 7 days to detect, treat, and correct any associated diseases. A concentrated effort is made to reduce the prolapse and to decrease the associated edema, hyperemia, and superficial ulceration that may be present.

Three days preoperatively, the patients are given 1 or 2 oz of castor oil to empty the lower bowel. In addition, a daily, cleansing, warm soap suds enema is administered. A low residue diet is given, being changed to clear liquids one day before the operation. Preoperative oral antibiotics (neomycin and erythromycin) are given one day before the operation in all patients. Systemic antibiotic therapy is routinely started one hour preoperatively and followed by an intraoperative dose and two postoperative doses.

POSTERIOR RECTOPEXY

Either general inhalation anesthesia or a regional block may be used. After a foley catheter is placed, the abdomen is opened through a lower midline incision and carefully explored for concurrent problems. Trendelenburg's position facilitates packing the small bowel out of the pelvis. The peritoneum is incised on either side of the lower sigmoid mesocolon adjacent to the promontory of the sacrum, staying medial to the ureters. The rectum is mobilized from the sacrum down to the tip of the coccyx. The lateral ligaments and midrectal vessels are not divided, nor is the peritoneum in front of the rectum incised. Paired sutures of 2–0 silk or other nonabsorbable material are inserted deeply into the presacral periosteum on either side of the midline, starting at the lower sacrum and continuing every 2 cm until reaching the sacral promontory. The needles are left on the sutures, which are then placed through the serosa and musculature of the posterolateral rectal wall while the assistant firmly reduces the prolapse by upward traction. The mucosa should not be penetrated, but the needle should take a broad sector of the rectal wall. With properly prepared bowel, mucosal penetration should not cause undue concern. The sutures are tied from the lowest to the highest, firmly fixing the rectum inside the sacral concavity. A sigmoid resection is added only rarely in patients having such redundancy of the sigmoid that volvulus is considered a strong possibility. No sutures are placed in the levators, and the pouch of Douglas is not altered. The abdomen is closed without drainage. Ambulation is encouraged on the first postoperative evening. The Foley catheter is removed after 2 or 3 days. Oral alimentation can usually be started within 3 to 4 days, and the patient discharged from the hospital by day 7 to 10. Stool softeners are used the first month postoperatively.

PERINEAL RECTOSIGMOIDECTOMY (ALTEMEIER METHOD)

General or low spinal anesthesia is used. After a Foley catheter is inserted, the patient is placed in the lithotomy position with elevation and overhang of the hips at the end of the operating table. The head of the table is lowered 15 degrees to minimize venous oozing during the dissection.

The bowel is prolapsed and its apex grasped with Allis clamps. Gentle traction is applied to exteriorize the prolapse and to bring its mucocutaneous junction into view. The sliding hernia usually presents as a protruding mass bulging on the anterior surface. One must ensure that small intestine has not been trapped in this hernia sac. The four quadrants are then marked for traction and orientation with the insertion of four 3–0 silk sutures. A circumferential incision through all layers of the rectum is made 1.5 cm proximal to the mucocutaneous line, using electrocautery. The outer layer of the prolapse is then stripped from the inner layer, exposing the sac of the sliding hernia on its anterior wall. This sac is opened vertically throughout its full extent, exposing its posterior wall, which is the visceral peritoneum of the rectosigmoid colon. The excess peritoneal reflection is trimmed away to facilitate its eventual closure.

A cleavage plane is established between the rectosigmoid colon and its elongated and thickened mesentery. A Penrose drain is placed to encircle the bowel for lateral traction. Holding the bowel to the left, a progression of Kelly clamps is placed across the entire width of the mesentery. The mesentery is divided and carefully transfixed with suture ligatures. The rectosigmoid is thus mobilized until the redundant bowel cannot be pulled down any further. The hernia sac is then ablated by continuous 2–0 chromic catgut, making an inverted Y suture line.

The medial border of the levator ani muscles can then be easily identified and grasped with Allis clamps. They are approximated in the midline anterior to the rectum with three to four interrupted 1–0 chromic catgut sutures. This eliminates the defect in the pelvic diaphragm, and a sacral curve is imparted to the bowel to increase the effectiveness of the puborectalis muscle. The defect is narrowed to permit the passge of the bowel and to allow the insertion of the surgeon's index finger. If it is too tight, stricture or impairment of the blood supply may develop. A larger opening increases the likelihood of recurrence of the prolapse.

The exposed section of bowel can be divided into two lateral halves by anterior and posterior incisions carried to the level of the proposed resection. With interrupted 3–0 chromic catgut sutures, the anterior and posterior angles of the bowel can be anchored to the anal mucocutaneous border in the midline with alignment of the original anterior and posterior quadrant traction sutures. The bowel is totally transected and sutured progressively in quadrants with a series of interrupted 3–0 chromic catgut sutures. By carefully dividing the bowel obliquely, one quadrant at a time, one can correct the disparity between the narrower bowel and the dilated anal ring. All layers of the bowel wall and anal ring should be included in each suture, making a single anastomotic suture line. The anastomosis can be done even more expeditiously by means of an intraluminal stapling device. If this method is planned, the bowel should be transected 1 cm longer at both ends to allow for placement of the purse-string suture. Special care must be taken to avoid any tension or redundancy at the suture line. No drainage of the perirectal space or perineum is necessary. A Vaseline gauze wick is inserted into the new anal canal and removed in 48 hours.

Rectal examination, insertion of rectal thermometers, or other procedures are not permitted for the first 7 to 10 days postoperatively. Active exercises to contract the sphincter muscles are encouraged four times daily starting 2 weeks postoperatively, but the value of the exercises is doubtful.

Ambulation is discouraged for the first 2 to 3 days postoperatively to avoid tension on the suture line. Patients are kept NPO for 3 or 4 days, during which time appropriate intravenous therapy is given. A liquid diet is started thereafter, and the diet is advanced as indicated. Discharge from the hospital usually takes place within 12 to 15 days, depending on the presence of various associated debilitating factors requiring additional supportive treatment.

GENERAL COMMENTS

The posterior rectopexy procedure is simple to perform. It introduces no foreign material other than sutures and appears to be as effective as the more complex procedures. Most of the major series are relatively recent, but it is unlikely that the late recurrence rate will exceed that of other procedures. Altemeier's results with perineal rectosigmoidectomy have been excellent, but others have shown less success. It is a procedure not familiar to most surgeons and involves a significant learning curve. Complications after perineal rectosigmoidectomy include local abscess from anastomotic leaks, pelvic abscess, and incontinence due to anal sphincter damage and rectal stricture. Recurrences have been a significant problem in most series other than Altemeier's. However, the results are unquestionably better than anal encircling procedures in patients who are not considered candidates for an abdominal procedure.

One factor that limits the success of any procedure for prolapse is long-standing fecal incontinence. This may be based on an associated neurologic disorder or the presence of mental retardation. Stretching of the anal sphincter and the damage to its innervation by the downward displacement of the pelvic floor are probably contributing factors in many long-standing cases. None of the procedures for rectal prolapse directly solve the problem of incontinence. Many patients are improved significantly, and in some the problem is entirely solved. A long period of time may be required to regain sphincter tone; thus, secondary procedures for incontinence should be delayed for at least one year when possible. Given the physical and psychological problems associated with the rectal prolapse, many patients are so relieved to have the disorder corrected that a minor degree of fecal incontinence is tolerated by them.

SOLITARY RECTAL ULCER SYNDROME

KENNETH W. SMITH, M.D., F.A.C.S.

Although described in the literature by Cruveilhier one hundred and fifty years ago and labeled solitary rectal ulcer by Lloyd-Davies fifty years ago, this difficult problem has become somewhat more clearly understood only in the last fifteen years. Even giving a proper name to this entity is difficult since there is not always an ulcer to be seen, and when ulceration does occur the ulcer is not always solitary. As seen in Figure 1, solitary rectal ulcer shares an intimate relationship with several other medical conditions. The term solitary rectal ulcer syndrome (SRUS) is thus preferred by most authors and will be used here. A longstanding history of straining at stool and irregular or abnormal bowel habits, along with complaints of low abdominal or pelvirectal pain and pressure and some degree of rectal bleeding, should immediately suggest the possible existence of solitary rectal ulcer syndrome. Biopsies taken from patchy areas of intense hyperemia or ulceration of the rectal wall should show characteristic thickening of the lamina propria, replacement or obliteration of the lamina propria by fibroblasts and proliferating muscularis mucosa, hypertrophy of the muscularis mucosa, and misplaced glands within the submucosal layer. At this point, treatment is dictated by the associated physical findings.

PELVIC MUSCLE SPASM

It is my belief that SRUS begins with, or is intimately associated with, the vicious cycle that develops between pelvic muscle spasm (PMS) and straining at stool (SAS). The pelvic muscle spasm of which we speak is described in the literature under such terms as levator spasm, proctalgia fugax, and the old term coccygodynia without coccyx trauma; this spasm is responsible for much of the pain experienced with SRUS. Since the rectum is surrounded by this muscle system, the tenesmus produced by pelvic muscle spasm induces straining at stool against a relatively empty rectum, which in turn produces more muscle edema, inflammation, and irritability along with several other changes. Thus the vicious cycle of pelvic muscle spasm and straining at stool is established. Treatment at this stage therefore involves breaking this cycle at as many points as possible.

There are numerous primary causes for pelvic muscle spasm and straining at stool, and in any patient suspected of this syndrome, any and all such factors must be identified and treated. SRUS, especially the pelvic muscle spasm phase, is much more common in women for two major reasons: (1) the female gynecoid pelvis has a much larger surface area covered and supported by the pelvis muscle system alone without the secondary bony pelvic support; and (2) the various pelvic female organs may

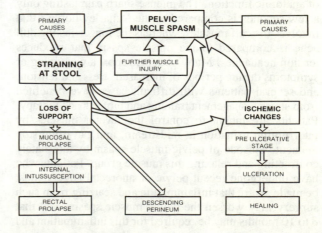

Figure 1 The PMS-SAS cycle and its consequences

serve as foci for numerous pathophysiologic processes that may generate pelvic muscle spasm. Thus a thorough evaluation of the gynecologic system in women, as well as the urinary tract and pelvic intestinal system in both sexes, must be carried out and all identified problems properly treated. Extraperitoneal, neuromuscular, and skeletal causes must not be forgotten. A complete work-up thus might include laboratory examinations, roentgenograms, contrast studies, sonograms, CT scans, endoscopy, and laparoscopy, depending on the patient's history and physical findings.

By the time most patients with SRUS are seen by the consulting surgeon, the primary factor initiating the pelvic muscle spasm is no longer present, having been successfully treated or having disappeared by virtue of its self-limiting nature. And yet the patient has become locked into the vicious cycle of pelvic muscle spasm and straining at stool. At this point, treatment must be directed toward alleviating the pelvic muscle spasm itself. The applications of heat remain one of the most effective ways to treat muscle soreness and irritability, and one of the simplest ways to apply heat to the pelvic area is a deep warm tub bath. The frequency of such tub baths is determined by the severity of symptoms, and the recommended time for each session is a minimum of 15 to 20 minutes. Transrectal digital massage of the pelvic muscle system has been advocated by Thiele, and electrogalvanic stimulation of the levator system using a rectally placed electrode has been advocated by Sohn, both of these methods being used within an office setting. Posture should be corrected, since "slouching" has been reported to increase the pelvic muscle spasm. Skeletal muscle relaxants, such as diazepam, may be used in acute short-term situations such as following anorectal surgery or lower urinary tract manipulation, but their use on a chronic basis is to be discouraged. Exercises that stretch the lower trunk muscles, especially walking, are often beneficial. Long periods of standing or sitting, especially long automobile trips, often worsen the muscle spasm, and patients are encouraged to change positions as necessary under these circumstances. Weight loss is encouraged in overweight individuals.

The patient should be educated regarding this aspect of anatomic function. The intense sharp pain lasting only a few seconds is compared to the "charley horse" that involves the calf muscles, whereas the longer-lasting dull ache is compared to the muscle spasm that produces tension headaches. Many patients report a worsening of symptoms during periods of increased stress and tension, and several patients with difficult cases have benefited from stress management training and biofeedback therapy. Patients are taught to control the levator muscles by interrupting urination in midstream, and can often stop the acute episode of pelvic muscle spasm by alternately contracting and relaxing this muscle group. Patients who have undergone recent pelvic or anorectal sugery must be made aware that inflammation and scarring from such surgery may worsen the pelvic muscle spasm, and that 8 to 10 months may be required for this inflammation and scar tissue to subside. Above all, patients must be encouraged, and reminded that the disappearance of symptoms, just like their appearance, is expected to be slow and gradual.

STRAINING AT STOOL

Although often unaware of the fact, most patients with SRUS have a habit of straining at stool. True constipation secondary to a redundant or hypomotile colon, sedentary life style, or lack of adequate dietary fiber and fluid is sometimes present. Parental training, demanding a daily bowel movement often at a specific time of day, may result in long periods of straining at stool. More often, however, this urge to repeatedly empty the rectum by straining is the direct result of changes produced by the cycle of pelvic muscle spasm and straining at stool.

Patients with SRUS have a high incidence of irregular bowel habits. Many patients complain of diarrhea, but on closer questioning this usually means multiple passages of small amounts of stool and mucus occasionally tinged with blood. Constipation usually means a feeling of rectal fullness or incomplete rectal emptying following a bowel movement, which induces continued straining attempts, but with little result. We believe that these are only different interpretations of the same tenesmus resulting from the PMS-SAS cycle. Treatment of the straining at stool component of this cycle involves a multifactorial approach. Patients are placed on a high fiber diet and encouraged to use a bulk agent of the psyllium hydrophilic mucilloid type, as well as to increase oral fluid intake. All forms of laxatives are strongly discouraged, and intestinal irritants (coffee, tea, colas, chocolate, beer, citrus and tomato products, hot spicy foods) are eliminated from the diet.

Patient education and reassurance, however, are the main aspects of treatment at this point. The basic mechanics of the PMS-SAS cycle are explained in such language that the interrelationship is understood. It is pointed out that rectal fullness, "gas cramps," or a sensation of incomplete evacuation following a "normal" bowel movement are part of the underlying process, and that forceful straining against an essentially empty rectum only worsens the condition. The use of an occasional small-volume (100 to 150 cc) tap water enema is suggested whenever complete rectal emptying is in doubt.

When seen relatively early in the PMS-SAS cycle, the patient with SRUS usually has minimal findings on physical examination. There may be tenderness on the inner aspect of the superior anterior iliac crest where portions of the pelvic muscle system take their origin. Pressure or traction on the levator muscles by the examining finger on digital rectal examination almost always reproduces the pain of which the patient complains. Endoscopic examination of the rectum may be entirely normal at this point. However, continuation of the PMS-SAS cycle produces further, more significant changes. Although these changes occur simultaneously, they will be considered separately for the sake of discussion.

LOSS OF SUPPORT

With a full rectum, the increased intra-abdominal pressure produced by normal straining efforts, coupled with relaxation of the puborectalis muscle, results in defecation. Against an essentially empty rectum, however, excessive straining produces stretching of the pelvic muscles along with the supportive and connective tissues of the rectum. Careful examination reveals certain physical findings, some of which have been described in the literature as separate clinical entities. In reality these represent particular stops along a progressive path of consequential events.

Mucosal Prolapse

The increased intra-abdominal pressure produced by excessive straining efforts is brought to bear on the posterior pelvic peritoneal reflection, located somewhere along the anterior wall of the lower or midrectum. Continuation of such pressure over a period of time results in prolapse of the anterior rectal wall beginning with the mucosal and submucosal layers. Inspection of the anal area often reveals a "pouting" of the anus with a somewhat edematous anterior skin tag or early mucosal prolapse. In addition to tenderness of the levator muscles, on digital examination one may find thickening of the anterior rectal wall, and straining efforts by the patient at this point may produce anterior prolapse, which can be felt by the examining finger. Treatment at this point again centers around breaking the PMS-SAS cycle, as already described. Once the excessive straining has ceased, these early changes usually regress and no definitive treatment is necessary. If bothersome skin tags or redundant mucosa remain, these may be treated with simple excision or rubber band ligation. Extreme caution must be taken to avoid even these simple surgical procedures prior to adequate resolution of the PMS-SAS cycle, since post-surgical edema and inflammation will only heighten the associated tenesmus and straining and may result in a nonhealing surgical wound.

Internal Intussusception

The mucosal prolapse already described undoubtedly represents a relatively early phenomenon in the loss of support changes that occur in SRUS patients, and indeed may represent only the leading edge of full-thickness prolapse of the anterior rectal wall. As the straining continues, this full-thickness prolapse involves an increasingly greater circumference of the rectal wall until internal intussusception of the rectosigmoid (first-degree rectal prolapse, internal rectal prolapse) eventually occurs. These patients often describe feeling "a ball in the rectum" or some similar description of a sense of obstruction of the rectum. Only the astute clinician will make the diagnosis of rectosigmoid intussusception when

presented with this history and these symptoms, and then only after careful examination. The intussusception is rarely found if the patient is examined in the usual knee-chest position, since the force of gravity must be overcome with the patient in this position. If the patient is asked to strain while in the lateral decubitus (Sims) or squatting position, the prolapsing segment of intestine can often be felt with the examining finger or seen with the rigid or flexible endoscope. Although somewhat embarrassing for the patient, digital rectal examination with the patient sitting on the commode after having evacuated a small volume enema is one of the best methods of palpating such a prolapse.

If the patient is seen in what is clinically judged to be a relatively early phase of development of internal rectal prolapse, treatment should be conservative and again directed at breaking the PMS-SAS cycle. If such treatment fails and the patient's symptoms are disruptive, and if the patient is a reasonable surgical risk, some form of transabdominal rectopexy, with or without sigmoid resection, is recommended.

Rectal Prolapse

Once internal rectosigmoid intussusception occurs, if the straining habit continues, it is usually only a matter of time until complete external rectal prolapse makes its appearance. The diagnosis and treatment of complete rectal prolapse is relatively straightforward and is dealt with in detail elsewhere in this book. My personal preference for the good-risk surgical candidate is transabdominal rectopexy, as described by Ripstein. If redundant sigmoid colon is present, I prefer to combine a generous sigmoid colon resection with fixation of the rectosigmoid colon to the sacral promontory. After mobilizing the posterior rectosigmoid colon from the sacral hollow, two or three sutures of 2–0 braided nonabsorbable material are used to secure the two lateral edges of the rectosigmoid to the periosteum of the corresponding lateral edge of the sacral promontory. The anastomosis of descending colon to the rectosigmoid is carried out just above this point of fixation.

In the poor-risk surgical patient, my procedure of choice is a Thiersch-type anal circlage utilizing a Silastic-Dacron band. This can be done under local, regional, or general anesthesia.

ISCHEMIC CHANGES

At some point in time, the loss of support produced by the forceful straining habit is usually associated with certain ischemic changes. These changes occur primarily within the mucosal and submucosal layers of the rectal wall and lead to the passage of blood. The pathogenesis of this process was eloquently described by Madigan and Morson in 1969 and Rutter and Riddell in 1975. It is the appearance of such rectal bleeding that usually brings such patients to the surgeon's office.

Preulcerative Stage

Authors of early papers on solitary rectal ulcer noted a group of patients whose history, symptoms, and physical findings were identical, but in whom no gross ulceration could be found. These patients were logically described as being in a preulcerative stage of solitary rectal ulcer syndrome. The only additional physical finding, as compared to patients seen earlier in the PMS-SAS cycle, is the presence on visual inspection of the rectum of one or more irregular areas of intense hyperemia of the rectal mucosa from which small amounts of bright red blood can occasionally be seen to ooze. Biopsy of these areas reveals microscopic ulceration as well as the classic findings associated with SRUS, as described earlier. The patient seen at this stage is often given a diagnosis of "nonspecific proctitis," but the astute physician should carefully search for anterior rectal wall prolapse or internal intussusception when presented with these findings.

Treatment is directed at the PMS-SAS cycle and toward correction of any associated prolapse. The instillation of steroidal or nonsteroidal suppositories, creams, foams, or enemas into the rectum seems to be of little benefit.

Ulceration

If the ischemic changes become severe enough, the mucosal layer is sloughed, and the classic solitary rectal ulcer makes its appearance. This ulcer is not unique to the rectum, and may be found in the intestinal tract wherever such ischemic changes occur. It is most commonly found at the leading edge of any segment of intestine involved in prolapse or intussusception. It therefore becomes mandatory for the physician who discovers a solitary rectal ulcer to search carefully for a hidden or occult rectal prolapse, a point well made in the literature.

Treatment of the patient with solitary rectal ulcer is the same as that already described for the preulcerative stage. If the straining habit ceases, the ulcer should heal, unless recurrent prolapse is present. The ulcer itself should not be excised or electrocoagulated since the underlying ischemia will prevent healing, and the result will be an ulcer even larger than the one originally treated.

Healing

The ulcer may heal either spontaneously or as a result of proper treatment. Since ulceration is superficial, the deeper portions of mucus-secreting glands may become entrapped in the submucosa and be covered by regenerating mucosa. This histopathologic picture has been labeled *colitis cystica profunda*. These entrapped glands may continue to secrete mucus, which collects in pools beneath the regenerated mucosal lining, thus giving rise to a sessile mass at the site of the original ulcer. If symptomatic to the patient or worrisome to the examining physician, this nodular mass can be excised transanally and closed primarily.

If the rectal ulceration is diffuse or circumferential, over a period of time enough scar tissue may be formed to cause a rectal stricture. If seen relatively early in its formation, such a stricture may be dilated with the examining finger or with the rigid proctosigmoidoscope. An unyielding stenosis must be approached surgically. If the area of involvement is low enough, this may be done transanally. Under the anesthesia of choice and with adequate exposure, multiple radial incisions are made around the circumference of the stenotic area. These are gradually deepened until the scar tissue begins to yield to the dilating instrument. Contrast x-ray studies of the rectum should be done preoperatively to ensure that the stenotic segment is not excessively long. Hazards of this approach are excessive bleeding and free perforation of the rectum. Injection of the stenotic area and surrounding mucosa with a solution of ephinephrine, 1:200,000, and judicious use of electrocauterization usually prevent excessive bleeding. If the stenotic segment is below the peritoneal reflection, free perforation is less likely. The stenotic area that is too high or too long to be approached transanally is treated by transabdominal low anterior resection.

The successful treatment of any given patient with SRUS depends first of all upon the physician's understanding of the interrelationships among the various elements of the syndrome itself. If attention is focused too narrowly on only the most bothersome symptom or the most obvious physical finding, there will be little chance of curing the patient. There is no standard outline of treatment because there is no standard mold into which the patient fits. Resolution of the problem depends not only on age, sex, symptoms, and physical findings, but also on physical health, mental well-being, and the ability of the patient to understand and carry out his or her part of the treatment program. The PMS–SAS cycle must be carefully explained and successfully treated, for continuation of the straining habit will inevitably lead to progression of the syndrome. The successful treatment of SRUS also demands a close physician-patient relationship built upon mutual trust, understanding, and above all patience, because some cases may resolve in weeks, some in years, and some may never completely resolve.

RADIATION ENTERITIS AND PROCTITIS

AMANDA M. METCALF, M.D.
ROBERT W. BEART, Jr., M.D.

Serious intestinal injury occurs in 1 to 10 percent of patients treated with abdominal or pelvic irradiation. The incidence of such complications is primarily dependent on the radiation dose and the volume of bowel irradiated. Other factors that have been demonstrated to increase the risk of developing such injury include previous abdominal operation, pelvic inflammatory disease, asthenic habitus, coexistent vascular disease, and concomitant use of chemotherapy with radiation therapy.

The anatomic location and relative frequency of the malignant disease treated with radiotherapy determine the relative frequency with which specific injuries are encountered. In most series, the majority of injuries occur after radiation therapy for carcinoma of the uterine cervix and prostate; therefore, injuries to the ileum and rectum are most frequent, followed in order of decreasing frequency by injury to the rectosigmoid, sigmoid, cecum, transverse colon, and jejunum. It is important to recognize that these injuries are frequently coexistent and that symptoms of urinary tract injury are also present in as many as 15 percent of cases.

Symptoms of chronic radiation injury typically occur at a mean of 33 months after completion of radiation therapy, but they may occur as early as 3 weeks or be delayed as long as 25 years. Although insidious in onset, such symptoms tend to be chronic and progressive in nature, paralleling the underlying pathophysiology of obliterative endarteritis and submucosal fibrosis. The most frequent signs and symptoms of chronic radiation enteritis reflect an underlying obstructive process; fistulas, pain, perforation, and massive bleeding are less common.

Radiation proctitis or proctosigmoiditis most commonly presents as rectal bleeding, diarrhea, or tenesmus. Rectovaginal fistulas are also relatively common. Colovesical fistulas are less common, as is rectal pain associated with deep rectal ulceration.

Because surgical intervention carries a significant risk of postoperative morbidity and mortality, minor symptoms are not an indication for operation. Medical treatment that may be of benefit includes dietary manipulation, antispasmodics, steroids or other anti-inflammatory drugs, or antibiotics. We have found metronidazole to be of help in controlling the pain of rectal ulceration. In our patient population, 90 percent of patients are adequately treated medically and 10 percent require operation.

PREOPERATIVE EVALUATION AND MANAGEMENT

Preoperative evaluation should include contrast studies of the small and large bowel and urinary tract, colorectal endoscopy, and cystoscopy. X-ray studies of fistulas are useful. Formal nutritional assessment should be performed in all patients with a history of significant weight loss, and identified deficiencies should be corrected. Patients in whom a diverting stoma may be necessary should have sites of optimal stoma placement marked preoperatively. Radiation-damaged skin should be avoided. Visitation with an enterostomal therapist is valuable. If bowel preparation is possible, this should be performed. Vaginal irrigation should be considered in female patients. Prophylactic intravenous antibiotics should be used and continued in the immediate postoperative period.

OPERATIVE MANAGEMENT

Radiation Enteritis

The most frequent indication for operation in patients with radiation enteritis is obstruction. In rare instances, obstruction is found to be clearly secondary to adhesions, in which case careful enterolysis is indicated. In most cases, however, obstruction is secondary to intestinal stenosis. On gross inspection, the obstructing segment is grayish white, with thickened walls and serosal telangiectasis. Adjacent bowel, although more normal in appearance, frequently has also sustained significant radiation injury. Surgical options in this situation are either bypass or resection of the involved segment. Considerable controversy exists as to which is the optimal procedure. Most surgeons would agree that when multiple loops of small bowel are caught in the pelvis, bypass is preferable to extensive dissection with its attendant risk of injury to bowel and other pelvic viscera. With isolated segmental involvement of small bowel, we prefer to carry out a wide resection of the involved area with primary anastomosis. Our anastomotic leak rate in this situation has been less than 10 percent. Regardless of the procedure chosen, the frequent involvement of the terminal ileum and cecum makes anastomosis in this region unreliable, and anastomosis to the mid or distal transverse colon is preferable.

Small bowel fistula or perforation requires treatment with either wide resection or diversion with complete exclusion of the involved segment. We prefer to use wide resection if possible, but we have noted a 20 percent anastomotic leak rate when this was combined with primary anastomosis. Temporary proximal diversion or exteriorization might well be wise in this situation. In the rare patient with recurrent or massive gastrointestinal bleeding as the primary indication for intervention, we have relied on preoperative angiography to identify likely sources of bleeding and have excised those segments identified. This has been successful in preventing further significant blood loss in this small group of patients.

Colorectal Injuries

Rectosigmoid or rectal stenosis is the most common radiation-induced colorectal injury requiring surgical intervention. Construction of a diverting colostomy, with either the transverse or descending colon, is the safest procedure in this situation. The frequent involvement of the sigmoid colon makes a sigmoid colostomy less desirable because stenosis and necrosis of such a stoma often occurs (50%). Occasionally, rectosigmoid or rectal stenosis improves with time, and intestinal continuity can be restored without resection of the involved segment. More often, progressive stenosis occurs, which may be further complicated by the development of fistulas to adjacent pelvic viscera. Restorative procedures for rectosigmoid or rectal stenosis are fraught with complications, especially when marked pelvic fibrosis or serious concomitant injury to other intra-abdominal viscera is present. These are relative contraindications to restorative attempts. Recurrent or residual malignant disease is an absolute contraindication to a restorative procedure.

Several surgical options have been proposed for the good-risk patient who strongly desires restoration of intestinal continuity. Isolated rectal ulcers secondary to implant therapy, with normal surrounding mucosa, can be treated by wide local excision. For isolated rectosigmoidal injuries with rectal sparing, anterior resection with descending colorectostomy and temporary proximal diversion is reasonable. Mobilization of the splenic flexure usually is necessary to ensure a tension-free anastomosis with minimally radiated descending colon. Low anterior resection or pull-through (colo-anal) type procedures for mid or low rectal stenosis have occasionally been successful in the absence of pelvic fibrosis.

The procedure described by Bricker appears to be the best option for mid or low rectal stenosis. In this approach, the rectum is not mobilized from the presacral space, and the rectosigmoid is generally left in situ. The proximal uninvolved colon is divided and either is used as an antiperistaltic vascular pedicle graft for "patching" the area of stenosis or is anastomosed to the anterior wall of the rectal ampulla. The overall success rate for rectal stenosis is reported to be 84 percent with this procedure, with an operative mortality of 8 percent.

Rectovaginal fistulas are the second most common indication for surgical intervention, and these are usually associated with low or midrectal stenosis. Approximately 80 percent of patients obtain symptomatic relief with diversion alone, although such fistulas rarely heal spontaneously. Local repairs are usually unsuccessful, even when proximal diversion is used. Again, the procedure described by Bricker is probably the best-tested option. In his report of nine patients with radiation-induced rectovaginal fistulas, all achieved successful repair, although 30 percent required multiple procedures.

Rectal ulceration (usually of the anterior rectal wall) with severe rectal pain is a relatively uncommon radiation sequela, but one that is often refractory to therapy. Recurrent carcinoma should be ruled out by computed tomographic scan of the pelvis. Ulcer biopsy may be necessary to rule out metachronous rectal carcinoma, but should be performed carefully because it may lead to fistula formation. Occasionally, patients obtain symptomatic relief with orally administered broad-spectrum antibiotics such as metronidazole. Response to diversion alone is unpredictable in terms of symptomatic relief, as are more extensive procedures. Presacral nerve block has been reported to be of benefit in a small number of patients and should probably be attempted prior to extensive pelvic procedures.

Proctitis without stenosis rarely requires surgical intervention. Seventy percent of patients with symptoms refractory to medical management obtain relief of tenesmus and bleeding with diversion. Forty percent of patients subsequently are able to have intestinal continuity restored without resection, with satisfactory functional results. Patients with persistent rectal bleeding may benefit from laser therapy with the yttrium-aluminum-garnet laser. Insufficient data are available to document the role of this modality. Abdominoperineal resection for radiation injury carries a high risk of morbidity and should not be undertaken lightly.

Rectovesical fistulas are rare in our experience. Traditionally, complete diversion has been necessary to control symptoms. More extensive procedures such as anterior or complete exenteration have been associated with a high incidence of morbidity and mortality.

Significant radiation injury to the gut occurs infrequently, but once manifest, it often requires surgical intervention. Enteritis may be treated by either resection or bypass. Radiation-induced injury to the rectum and sigmoid usually requires multi-stage procedures for definitive correction, with a significant risk of postoperative morbidity and mortality. Serious consideration should be given to diversion alone to provide symptomatic relief.

ISCHEMIC COLITIS

DONALD L. KAMINSKI, M.D.
VIRGINIA M. HERRMANN, M.D.

Ischemic colitis is a recently recognized disease process, having been initially described in 1963 by Boley. It is defined as the development of hemorrhagic necrosis or coagulation of the colonic wall, of varying thicknesses and involving varying lengths of colon, owing to impairment of blood flow. Blood flow impairment may be occlusive, nonocclusive, or both.

Information has accumulated suggesting that the colonic circulation predisposes the colon to ischemia in the presence of decreased cardiac output and regional anatomic occlusion, while the remainder of the gastrointestinal circulation remains adequate. The colon has less blood flow per 100 grams of tissue than does the remainder of the gastrointestinal tract. Peristalsis and nutrient absorption in the small intestine are associated with increased blood flow, whereas in the colon, these functional changes are associated with decreased blood flow. These blood flow characteristics explain the occurrence of colonic ischemia in the absence of involvement of the remainder of the intestinal tract and when mesenteric arterial occlusion is absent. Additionally, sterilization of the bowel protects its integrity in the presence of marginal circulation. Conversely, the colonic bacterial flora may enhance its susceptibility to damage when blood supply is inadequate. The small intestine becomes necrotic primarily only in the presence of major mesenteric vascular occlusion. The colon becomes ischemic in a wide variety of circumstances spontaneously and in association with many disease states (Table 1).

Since 1974, we have treated 47 patients with ischemic colitis, including 35 undergoing colon resection. In many cases, spontaneous ischemic colitis is a self-limited disease process that does not require operative intervention. The disease is now well recognized and anticipated, the symptoms distinct, and endoscopic and radiographic diagnosis readily obtainable. It is estimated that only 20 percent of the patients with spontaneous ischemic colitis will require operative intervention for full-thickness gangrene or stricture. The disease involves primarily the left side of the colon.

Shock-associated ischemic colitis is primarily a disease of the right colon. The presentation is much less distinct and the diagnosis difficult. Treatment is operative, and the mortality, related to sepsis in a patient with significant associated illness, is high.

The basis of our experience includes 22 patients with spontaneous ischemic colitis and 25 patients with shock-associated ischemic colitis. We will not consider further iatrogenic ischemic colitis produced by direct colonic devascularization (see Table 1).

SPONTANEOUS ISCHEMIC COLITIS

The relevant clinical characteristics of the 22 patients with spontaneous ischemic colitis are outlined in Table 2.

Presentation

The typical patient with spontaneous ischemic colitis is 60 to 80 years old, although the condition has been described in young women who are taking oral contraceptives. Our youngest patient was a 47-year-old man. Sixteen of our patients had no relevant discernible associated illness and were functional individuals prior to the development of their colonic disorder. The patients develop relatively acute abdominal pain, usually left-sided. They usually come to the hospital because of the onset of bloody diarrhea. The pain is mild initially and tenderness is present over the involved colon. Peritoneal irritation correlates with the degree of colonic necrosis.

TABLE 1   Factors Predisposing to the Development of Ischemic Colitis

Spontaneous factors
  None
  Intestinal vascular atherosclerosis
  Emboli
  Congestive heart failure
  Digitalis toxicity
  Collagen vascular disease
  Hypercoaguable states

Shock-associated factors
  Multiple trauma
  Cardiopulmonary bypass
  Ruptured ectopic pregnancy
  Upper gastrointestinal hemorrhage
  Pancreatitis
  Cerebral vascular accident
  Sepsis (renal, pulmonary)
  Cardiopulmonary arrest
  Renal transplantation
  Status epilepticus

Iatrogenic factors
  Abdominal aneurysmectomy
  Aortoiliac reconstruction
  Gastrectomy

Ten of the patients in this series with spontaneous ischemic colitis presented with evidence of an intra-abdominal catastrophic event, four with free intraperitoneal air. These patients required vigorous resuscitation pre-operatively and were usually operated on without a diagnosis of ischemic colitis.

It seems unreasonable to attempt to classify the severity of the disease other than as partial-thickness ischemia or full-thickness gangrene. Patients with bloody diarrhea and abdominal pain should undergo contrast colonic radiographic studies or endoscopic evaluation of the colon. Both studies are diagnostically useful. Contrast studies should be performed with water-soluble media if the patient has signs of peritoneal irritation. Flexible sigmoidoscopy or colonoscopy may be useful in decompressing the colon if it is distended. Acute ischemic colitis with mucosal necrosis results in the characteristic roentgenographic picture of submucosal edema with thumb-printing and saw-toothed mucosa. The endoscopic changes, in our opinion, are less diagnostic. The mucosal surface is hemorrhagic and bleeds easily, and the bowel is less distensible. In some cases in our series, we were able to discern this as diseased colon; however, it could not be determined whether the changes were inflammatory, malignant, or ischemic.

Precautions have been proposed concerning the use of contrast studies and colonoscopy in patients with compromised colonic blood flow. The precautions are based on the theoretic dangers of decreasing blood flow associated with increased intraluminal pressure. Distention of the colon and increased intraluminal pressure to 30 mm Hg significantly decrease colonic blood flow in animal experiments. Although the theoretic hazards of increased intraluminal pressure should be considered by the radiologist or endoscopist, the potential dangers should

TABLE 2 Clinical Characteristics of Twenty-Two Patients with Spontaneous Ischemic Colitis*

Primary Presenting Symptoms	X-Ray Findings	Endoscopy	Indications for Operation	Colon Involved	Treatment
Abdominal pain or peritonitis (8)	Submucosal edema (11)	Mucosal necrosis (5)	None (7)	Right colon (3)	Right colectomy and ileocolostomy (3)
Melena (7)	Colonic distention (7)		Peritoneal signs (7)	Left colon (16)	Observation (7)
Abdominal distention (6)				Splenic flexure (7)	Left colectomy and anastomosis (2)
Diarrhea (1)	Free air (4)		Perforation (4)	Sigmoid (9)	Left colectomy and colostomy (7)
			Distention (3)		
			R/O cancer (1)		Subtotal colectomy and anastomosis (1)
					Subtotal colectomy and ileostomy (2)
				Total abdominal colon (3)	

* Values in parentheses indicate the number of patients.

not dissuade physicians from performing these procedures and obtaining a diagnosis.

Treatment

Patients with abdominal pain, bloody diarrhea, and an endoscopic or roentgen diagnosis of ischemic colitis are given general supportive care. Withheld oral intake, intravenous fluids, nasogastric intubation and suction, and parenteral antibiotics are generally recommended. However, there is no evidence to indicate these interventions influence the course of the disease.

Careful in-hospital observation is indicated until pain disappears and intestinal function becomes normal. Although the mucosal ischemia may progress to full-thickness gangrene while the patient is being observed, the frequency of the progression is unknown and, in our experience, has been unusual. The condition of the patient presenting with full-thickness necrosis worsens during the period of observation, and the indications for operative intervention become increasingly evident.

Two agents are available for pharmacologic enhancement of colonic blood flow in a patient with ischemic colitis: papaverine (0.6 mg per minute) and glucagon (2 μg per kilogram per hour). The latter is more specific and is not associated with generalized vasodilation. There have been occasional reports of glucagon administration in ischemic colitis, and we have given the drug to two patients with no adverse effects. In such a commonly self-limited disease, it would be difficult to document benefit associated with increased colonic blood flow produced by glucagon. Support of the systemic circulation and maintenance of optimal cardiac output are much more important than considerations for locally increasing colonic blood flow.

The role of mesenteric arteriography in the diagnosis and management of the disorder seems to be minimal.

Atherosclerosis and narrowing of small arteries and arterioles is possibly a factor in the development of the ischemic process. The eponyms of "nonocclusive colonic ischemia" and "reversible ischemic colitis" suggest that the disease may be unassociated with arteriographically identifiable major mesenteric vascular occlusion.

The decision to operate on a patient is based on clinical evidence of possible full-thickness gangrene. It has been postulated that mucosal ischemia results in submucosal edema and luminal narrowing, whereas death of the muscle is associated with loss of integrity and dilatation. We identified no pathologic dilatation of the involved intestine in 40 percent of the colon specimens that were gangrenous.

Operative therapy for spontaneous ischemic colitis includes colonic resection. The amount of colon to be resected and whether to perform a primary anastomosis are the difficult questions. Obviously, all grossly involved colon should be removed. The opened specimen may show mucosal necrosis while the serosal surface appears normal. Histologic evaluation by frozen section can confirm the presence of necrosis at the margins of resection. Unfortunately, skip areas can occur, and information obtained by contrast studies, endoscopy, and gross examination must be evaluated to ascertain the amount of colon to be removed. There seems to be limited indication for proximal colostomy without resection in a patient with necrosis of the intestine. If the gangrenous process involves both the right and left colon, we ordinarily perform a subtotal colectomy.

If we are confident that all the ischemic colon has been resected, we perform a primary anastomosis when the resection involves the right colon. A left-sided colectomy with an end-colostomy and mucous fistula or Hartman's pouch will usually be performed for left-side involvement. Colon resection in extremely ill patients with severe intra-abdominal contamination should be associated with an ileostomy or colostomy rather than a primary anastomosis.

Outcome

Seven of our patients with spontaneous ischemic colitis recovered without operative therapy; one developed a later stricture. All these patients should have a follow-up barium enema 6 months following an episode of ischemic colitis that abates without operative treatment. There has been no recurrence among our patients or reported in the literature.

Of the 15 patients requiring colon resection for spontaneous ischemic colitis, nine died from the disease (60% mortality). Of the five patients who had partial-thickness necrosis, one died. Ten patients who underwent resection for gangrene of the colon had an 80 percent mortality.

SHOCK-ASSOCIATED ISCHEMIC COLITIS

The relevant clinical characteristics of the 25 patients with shock-associated ischemic colitis are presented in Table 3.

Presentation

The development of colonic ischemia in patients who are acutely ill from other unrelated diseases is a different process from that of spontaneous ischemic colitis. Patients with an acute severe illness potentially may develop (1) alveolar-capillary pulmonary membrane damage, (2) acute tubular necrosis of the kidney, (3) acute gastric mucosal lesions, (4) acalculous cholecystitis, and (5) ischemic colitis.

The colon does not autoregulate blood flow as well as the rest of the gastrointestinal tract, and oxygen extraction at low perfusion pressures does not increase significantly to provide adequate tissue oxygenation. We assume that these characteristics result in the development of gangrene of the colon while the remainder of the intestinal tract is viable.

Patients with shock-associated ischemic colitis are identified 2 to 3 days following the development of their primary illness, their initial clinical characteristics being (1) evidence of sepsis with an elevated temperature and leukocytosis and (2) decreased intestinal activity. Bloody diarrhea may be absent and hematochezia is unusual, but melena does occur. The intra-abdominal source of sepsis is suspected because of abdominal distention and pain. The patient's subjective symptoms depend on the patient's neurologic status and degree of consciousness.

Plain films of the abdomen demonstrate large and small bowel distention consistent iwth an ileus pattern. By day 4 to day 7, the patient generally undergoes abdominal exploration for intra-abdominal sepsis, and the ischemic colon is identified. At St. Louis University Hospital, we performed preoperative contrast studies in five severely ill patients who underwent resection for ischemic colitis, and submucosal edema was identified. None of these patients suffered colonic perforation. To obtain contrast films of the colon in seriously ill patients, some of whom require respirator therapy, is challenging, and results are less than ideal. To add to the difficulty of diagnosis, spontaneous ischemic colitis with mucosal necrosis is a left colon process and is more readily diagnosed by endoscopy than is shock-associated ischemic colitis, which requires pancolonoscopy to identify areas of necrosis in the cecum in an acutely ill patient in the intensive care unit. Therefore, the diagnosis of this disease process will continue to be made in the operating room during exploratory laparotomy for suspected intra-abdominal sepsis.

Preoperative preparation requires that the patient's intravascular volume be correctly expanded and ascertained by measurement of central filling pressures. Coagulopathy should be corrected, if present. Broad-spectrum antibiotics should be administered if not already

---

TABLE 3   Clinical Characteristics of Twenty-Five Patients with Shock-Associated Ischemic Colitis*

Primary Presenting Symptom	X-Ray Findings	Indications for Operation	Colon Involved	Treatment
	Ileus (10)			
Abdominal pain (9)	Colonic distention (9)	Peritoneal signs (13)	Right colon (17)	Right colectomy and ileocolostomy (12)
Sepsis (6)	Submucosal edema (4)	Sepsis (6)		Right colectomy and ileostomy (5)
Melena (5)		Abdominal distention (4)	Left colon (4)	Left colectomy and colostomy (3)
Abdominal distention (5)		Melena (2)		Subtotal colectomy and ileostomy (1)
	Nonspecific (2)		Total abdominal colon (4)	Subtotal colectomy and anastomosis (2)
				Subtotal colectomy and ileostomy (2)

* Values in parentheses indicate the number of patients.

begun. If the patient has pathologic distention of the cecum and melena, and the suspicion of ischemic colitis exists, we do not recommend that preoperative cleansing of the colon be attempted. Bowel preparation in acutely ill patients with an ileus may be unsuccessful, and oral hyperosmotic agents and enemas may result in large amounts of retained intracolonic liquid material that increases the operative problems.

Operative Therapy

The gross pathologic findings in shock-associated ischemic colitis characteristically are different from those in spontaneous ischemic colitis. The bowel in shock-associated ischemic colitis generally has patchy areas of gangrene confined to a portion of the bowel, ususaly the cecum and ascending colon. In spontaneous ischemic colitis, a segment or large portion of the bowel is inflamed and edematous with mucosal necrosis, but obviously gangrenous in a confluent manner with full-thickness necrosis.

The entire colon should be evaluated at the time of exploration. The serosal surface of involved bowel has patches of bowel that are black and exudative. The anterior surface of the cecum may appear to be minimally involved, and the surgeon may be tempted to perform some form of local excision or inversion of the area. We recommend instead that he or she open the lateral peritoneal reflection and examine the posterior surface of the right colon. We have found the retroperitoneal right colon to be the most common and severely involved area in shock-associated ischemic colitis.

We have not encountered shock-associated ischemic colitis without patchy areas of gangrene on the serosal surface and recommend extirpation of the involved segment, usually by means of a right colectomy or subtotal colectomy. Only three of our 25 patients were treated with a left-sided colon resection.

Because the ileum and left colon are relatively healthy in this disease, we perform an ileocolostomy with a functional side-to-side stapled anastomosis, utilizing well-vascularized transverse colon or sigmoid colon. This technique ensures maximal anastomotic blood flow.

Utilization of intestinal stoma creation or primary anastomosis needs to be individualized. Hemodynamically unstable patients with severe intraperitoneal contamination are more safely managed without an anastomosis. On the other hand, an ileostomy is difficult to manage in a patient with severe concomitant illness.

Outcome

Ten years ago we treated a young trauma patient with a closed head injury who died of sepsis. At autopsy, the patient was found to have a necrotic right colon. In 1970, Montessori and Leipa, in the Canadian Medical Association Journal, described the findings of 20 patients with colonic necrosis identified at autopsy. Two-thirds of these patients had a precipitating catastrophic event or major operative procedure. Only an increased awareness of the possibility of colonic necrosis in such patients will enable us to suspect the problem and treat it appropriately.

All 25 patients with shock-associated ischemic colitis had full-thickness gangrene. Eleven patients died following operative treatment, and assuredly intra-peritoneal sepsis was an important factor in the death of many of those patients. One of the last six patients, since our published report on this disorder in 1981, has died. Earlier diagnosis and treatment, related to an increased degree of suspicion, is the single most important factor in improving the dismal outlook for patients with shock-associated ischemic colitis.

COLORECTAL POLYPOSIS

THOMAS L. DENT, M.D.
STEVEN G. HARPER, M.D.

A *polyp* is a mass that protrudes into the lumen of the colon or rectum. It may be a benign or malignant mucosal neoplasm, a hamartoma, an inflammatory lesion, or one of a variety of intramural growths. Generally, polyps produce no signs or symptoms, but occasionally cause overt or occult rectal bleeding and, rarely, colonic obstruction or intussusception. Polyps are usually detected by screening digital examination, sigmoidoscopy, or barium enema.

Prior to the development of snare polypectomy through a flexible fiberoptic colonoscope in the early 1970s, polyps within the reach of the rigid proctoscope could be removed endoscopically, but those above the reach of the proctoscope required laparotomy and either colotomy or colectomy. The ability to endoscopically visualize and treat the vast majority of colonic polyps has simplified the surgical approach to polypoid disease. Treatment now follows a straightforward sequence: endoscopic classification, excisional biopsy (adequate treatment for most small or pedunculated benign lesions), and operative therapy (necessary for large or malignant lesions). In addition, most polyps now can be treated on an outpatient basis with decreased morbidity, mortality, and total dollar cost. In treating patients with polypoid

TABLE 1   Microscopic Classification

Mucosal
  Non-neoplastic
    Hyperplastic
    Hamartoma
    Inflammatory
  Neoplastic
    Tubular adenoma
    Tubulovillous adenoma
    Villous adenoma
    Polypoid carcinoma
Nonmucosal
  Lipoma
  Carcinoid
  Lymphoma
  Leiomyoma

disease, today's surgeon should be as skillful with a colonoscope and snare as with traditional operative techniques.

THERAPEUTIC PRINCIPLES

Macroscopic Classification

Traditionally, polyps have been classified *microscopically* (Table 1). Mucosal polyps may be either non-neoplastic (hyperplastic, hamartomatous, or inflammatory lesions) or neoplastic (tubular adenomas, tubulovillous adenomas, villous adenomas, or polypoid carcinomas). Nonmucosal lesions are uncommon and include lipomas, carcinoids, lymphomas, and leiomyomas. We have found, however, that an initial classification of polyps based on *macroscopic* morphology as seen endoscopically (Table 2) facilitates diagnosis and therapy. Regardless of the means of detection, *all* polyps should be visualized endoscopically and classified macroscopically before a specific treatment is chosen. Ninety-eight percent of patients have single or scattered mucosal polyps; the remaining 2 percent have nonmucosal polyps, multiple polyps, or polyposis syndromes. Treatment of single or scattered polyps is first directed toward the individual polyp(s) as determined by the configuration; treatment of multiple polyps, toward the affected segment of colon; and treatment of polyposis syndromes, toward the entire colon.

Polyp-Cancer Sequence

There is an excellent body of evidence that most, if not all, cancers of the colon arise from benign adenomatous epithelial polyps. The incidence of malignancy increases in direct proportion to the size of a polyp. Since the early detection and complete removal of colonic polyps should provide excellent prophylaxis against colon carcinoma, all colonic polyps should be removed entirely unless serious disease furnishes a contraindication.

Excisional Biopsy

Current diagnosis and subsequent therapy require complete excisional, rather than fractional, biopsy. Negative fractional biopsies are frequently misleading because invasive cancer can exist in areas of otherwise benign neoplastic polyps, as happens in up to 6 percent of pedunculated tubular adenomas and up to 30 percent of sessile villous adenomas. By definition, *invasive* cancer of the colon is penetration of the muscularis mucosa by neoplastic cells. Lack of such penetration means that the lesion—regardless of whether it is an adenoma, a severely dysplastic lesion, or even carcinoma in situ—may be regarded as clinically benign. Examination of the entire intact polyp is the best means of deciding whether or not invasion has occurred. If the lesion is benign, excisional biopsy has provided not only definitive diagnosis but also adequate therapy. If, on the other hand, invasive malignancy is seen histologically, further therapy is usually indicated.

Clearing Colonoscopy and Follow-up

Clearing colonoscopy, the colonoscopic search and eradication of additional neoplastic lesions, is an essential part of the treatment of all neoplastic polyps and provides a neoplasm-free colon as a baseline for subsequent surveillance. Additional polyps in areas distant to the index polyp are found in at least 20 percent of patients with one neoplastic polyp; more importantly, 2 percent of patients with a neoplastic polyp harbor a coexistent invasive cancer elsewhere in the colon. Although the time interval between follow-up examinations has not been established, we perform colonoscopy every 2 to 3 years because of the 20 to 30 percent incidence of subsequent (metachronous) development of polyps or cancer in other areas of the colon. Any additional neoplasms discovered during these examinations are treated by snare excision or hot biopsy forceps cauterization.

SINGLE OR SCATTERED MUCOSAL POLYPS

Diminutive Polyps of the Colon and Rectum

Polyps less than 5 mm in diameter are frequently hyperplastic, occasionally adenomatous, and almost never

TABLE 2   Macroscopic Classification

Single or scattered mucosal polyps
  Diminutive
  Pedunculated
  Sessile

Nonmucosal polyps

Multiple polyps

Polyposis syndromes

contain cancer. If biopsy reveals only hyperplastic cells, no further diagnostic studies, treatment, or follow-up are indicated. If biopsy reveals adenomatous mucosa (with its increased risk of coexistent neoplasm), colonoscopy is indicated both to eradicate these small adenomas with hot biopsy forceps and to identify coexistent larger polyps or cancers.

Pedunculated Polyps of the Colon and Rectum

Fortunately, more than 90 percent of mucosal polyps have stalks, which facilitate endoscopic removal by means of an electrocautery snare. Following clearing colonoscopy, the entire polyp, with approximately half its stalk attached, should be snare-excised, and the entire specimen should be submitted for complete histologic examination.

If the polyp is clearly benign or even contains carcinoma in situ, polypectomy can be considered adequate therapy. If the lesion is a true polypoid cancer with poor histologic differentiation, lymphatic invasion, or involved excisional margins, radical colectomy is indicated. However, there is considerable controversy about treatment if only a focus of invasive cancer occurs within the head of an otherwise benign adenoma, as occurs in about 6 percent of patients with pedunculated polyps. Some surgeons advocate radical colectomy in such patients because of the risk, albeit small, of residual tumor or regional lymphatic metastases. Others feel that polypectomy and close follow-up are sufficient because they believe the operative mortality of colectomy (1% to 2%) exceeds the risk of residual tumor or regional lymphatic metastases. Since the reported incidence of metastases from such lesions varies, we base our choice of treatment on both the patient's operative risk and the tumor's location. In a relatively young, healthy patient with a polyp above the rectum, colectomy is probably wise. In an old or relatively poor-risk patient, we recommend polypectomy alone.

For pedunculated rectal polyps within the reach of the scalpel, those with a small focus of invasive cancer can be locally re-excised if residual tumor is suggested by histologic examination. Follow-up is facilitated because digital examination and rebiopsy of the polypectomy site should identify early recurrence. The slight increase in the possibility that metastatic lymph nodes are overlooked by this method is counterbalanced by the increased hazard of an abdominoperineal resection and the lessened quality of life with a colostomy.

Sessile Polyps of the Colon

Stalkless polyps present a greater therapeutic challenge. Initial treatment, again, depends on gross morphology. The apparent absence of a stalk, as identified only by barium enema, should be verified by colonoscopic visualization because apparent sessile polyps may actually have stalks, allowing snare polypectomy. If the attach-

ment to the colon wall is narrow (less than 1 cm) or if the polyp is small and a pseudostalk can be created, snare polypectomy may be possible. If histologic examination of the entire specimen fails to reveal invasive carcinoma, polypectomy can be considered adequate therapy; recurrence of benign sessile polyps, however, is common and requires more frequent follow-up. Since there is no stalk to provide an additional excision margin of safety, radical colectomy is indicated if invasion through the muscularis mucosa is demonstrated.

Sessile polyps with broad attachments are generally unsuitable for snare polypectomy and require partial colectomy. Although piecemeal polypectomy has been enthusiastically reported, we think its role is limited because of the high incidence of perforation and bleeding, high risk of local recurrence, and difficult orientation of biopsy fragments for complete histologic examination. There is no longer any place for colotomy and local excision of a polyp with frozen section examination when partial colectomy with mesenteric lymph node excision carries no greater operative risk and would be the appropriate therapy if the lesion were malignant.

Sessile Polyps of the Rectum

Because of their accessibility to both finger and scalpel, treatment of sessile polyps of the lower rectum (up to 8 cm from the dentate line) is easier than treatment of those in the upper rectum (8 to 16 cm from the dentate line). Once again, macroscopic classification is of great importance. If digital examination reveals a *soft* tumor, transanal excision in the submucosal plane including a margin of normal mucosa (Parks) is followed by a careful histologic search of the specimen for invasive malignancy. Even large lesions, up to 70 percent of the rectal circumference, can be removed by this technique, which does not require full-thickness rectal wall excision. The resultant defect can be closed primarily, aided by plication of the rectal circular muscle if necessary, or even left open to heal by secondary intention. We occasionally employ electrodesiccation for small sessile polyps; however, recurrence is common, and a margin of surrounding normal mucosa must be coagulated. Electrodesiccation also can be used to control larger lesions in poor-risk patients. *Firmness* in a lower rectal lesion strongly suggests invasive malignancy. Forceps or incisional biopsy of the firm area usually demonstrates this invasion, and the appropriate cancer operation, partial coloproctectomy with coloanal anastomosis or complete coloproctectomy with colostomy (Miles), then should be performed. Occasionally, full-thickness excisional biopsy of small lesions is required to determine the presence and extent of neoplastic invasion and may be considered definitive therapy in a poor-risk patient with a small, mobile cancer.

We have found posterior proctotomy (Kraske) rarely necessary with current improvements in transanal retraction. Occasionally, the transsphincteric approach (York Mason) is indicated for particularly large or difficult benign lesions of the lower rectum. Both the Kraske and York Mason approaches have the theoretic disadvantage of implanting malignant cells outside subsequent radical excision planes if cancer is found.

Sessile polyps of the upper half of the rectum are similar to sessile polyps of the rest of the colon in their inaccessibility to excisional biopsy. Even if fractional biopsies are reported to be benign, adequate diagnosis and definitive therapy must be obtained by low anterior resection of the rectosigmoid colon, usually with colorectal or coloanal anastomosis by either hand-sewn or stapled techniques. Therefore, whether or not the lesion turns out to be histologically malignant, the appropriate radical operation has already been performed.

NONMUCOSAL POLYPS

Nonmucosal polyps also require excisional biopsy. If direct endoscopic visualization and biopsy of a colonic mass reveals it to be covered by normal mucosa, the firmness of the lesion should be determined. Invariably, soft lesions that can be indented with the biopsy forceps are lipomas and rarely require surgical therapy. If the tumors are solid, surgical excision is indicated. Despite several reports to the contrary, it is our view that no submucosal lesion should be snare-excised because of the great danger of colonic perforation. Segmental resection for solid tumors of the intraperitoneal colon is generally indicated, but local excisional biopsy of submucosal tumors of the rectum will avoid a colostomy if the lesion is benign; subsequent therapy depends on the histologic interpretation.

MULTIPLE POLYPS

Multiple polyps are defined as 10 to 100 neoplastic mucosal (adenomatous, tubulovillous, or villous) polyps. This condition combines elements of both single polyps and polyposis syndromes. Although the therapeutic principles for each individual polyp are the same as for single mucosal polyps, multiple polyps must be approached differently because of their distribution and number.

Depending on the endurance of the patient and the endoscopist, the individual polyps can be treated by snare polypectomy alone. This can be done during one or several colonoscopic examinations until all the polyps (usually up to 10 to 20) have been excised. If the polyps are clustered in one area of the colon, as verified by total colonscopy, segmental colectomy should be considered. Subtotal colectomy with an ileoproctostomy is indicated in any of the following circumstances: more than 10 to 20 polyps scattered throughout the colon, a mixture of pedunculated and sessile lesions, or an inability to eliminate all polyps by snare polypectomy. Follow-up for multiple polyps includes more frequent colonoscopic examinations—possibly as often as once a year—because these patients logically would have a higher incidence of colon cancer.

POLYPOSIS SYNDROMES

Juvenile Polyps

Usually pedunculated, juvenile polyps are hamartomas, composed of vascular tissue with cystic spaces lined by mucus-secreting epithelium. They are by far the most common type of colonic polyp in infants and children. Juvenile polyps are single in 70 percent of the patients and multiple in the rest. Rectal bleeding is the most frequent symptom and leads to demonstration of the polyp(s) by barium enema or sigmoidoscopy. Occasionally, juvenile polyps prolapse through the anus or may be discovered in the stool following autoamputation. Diagnosis, therapy, and elimination of the bleeding source can be accomplished by snare polypectomy. Patients with multiple juvenile polyps who have a firm histologic diagnosis made by removal of the largest or lowest polyp can be treated expectantly since the other polyps will autoamputate or regress during the teenage years. In patients without a family history of juvenile polyposis, the polyps are not thought to be associated with an increased incidence of malignancy, and colonoscopic or radiologic follow-up after removal is not indicated.

Adenomatous Polyposis Syndromes

These include familial polyposis, Gardner's syndrome, and Turcot's syndrome, and have two features in common: the presence of hundreds or even thousands of neoplastic (tubular, tubulovillous, or villous) polyps and the inevitable development of colon carcinoma if left untreated.

Familial polyposis, the prototype of a hereditary precancerous condition, is transmitted as an autosomal dominant trait. It occurs in one of every 7,000 to 10,000 births, affecting males and females equally. The polyps can be either pedunculated or sessile, vary in size from microscopic to 3 to 4 cm in diameter, begin during puberty, and produce symptoms of diarrhea and hematochezia at about age 20. If untreated, invasive carcinoma of the colon inevitably follows between 10 and 15 years later. The diagnosis can be established by the endoscopic and/or barium enema demonstration of polyps carpeting the colon and rectum. Biopsies demonstrate a spectrum of neoplastic epithelium. Exclusion of coexisting malignancy by barium enema or colonoscopy may be difficult because of the distorted colonic lining. The only reported extracolonic manifestations of familial polyposis are occasional gastric and duodenal adenomas. The neoplastic polyps of Gardner's syndrome occur in association with osteomas (skull, mandible, and long bones) and soft tissue tumors (epidermoid cysts, sebaceous cysts, fibromas, lipomas, and desmoids). The neoplastic polyps of Turcot's syndrome occur in association with brain tumors.

The treatment for patients with these premalignant syndromes should be individualized and should be instituted as soon as diagnosis is made and prior to the development of invasive carcinoma. For a patient with less than 20 rectal polyps, we prefer abdominal colectomy with creation of an ileorectal anastomosis and fulguration of the rectal polyps. The reported incidence of adenocarcinoma developing in the remaining rectum ranges from 4 percent at 30 years (Bussey, St. Mark's Hospital) to 50 percent at 20 years (Moertel, Mayo Clinic). Therefore, although the need for an ileostomy is eliminated, the potential for developing adenocarcinoma in the retained rectum still exists, necessitating proctoscopic examination at least every 6 months with fulguration of all newly arising polyps. For a patient with more than 20 rectal polyps or for one who is unwilling to submit to such rigorous follow-up, we favor a total colectomy, a mucosal proctectomy, and an ileoanal anastomosis. We recommend that *all* family members of patients with these polyposis syndromes have a thorough colonic examination by either air-contrast barium enema or colonoscopy and be followed on a regular basis.

COLORECTAL TUMOR

PAUL H. SUGARBAKER, M.D.

ETIOLOGY

The cause of large bowel cancer, and of most human cancers, is unknown. Epidemiologic data suggest a low rate of spontaneous mutation that leads to malignant degeneration of the epithelial surface of the colorectum. This low rate of malignant degeneration can, it seems, be regulated up or down, depending on a number of different dietary and environmental factors. Factors tending to increase the rate of malignant transformation in a population may be from the oral ingestion of saturated fats, from carcinogens in food contaminated by industrial waste, or from carcinogens resulting from the bacterial action on food. Other components of the diet may down-regulate the rate of malignant change in the large bowel. Addition of wheat or citrus fiber to the diet may absorb carcinogens, absorb bile, or change the bacterial flora so that there is less production of bacterial byproducts with carcinogenic potential. It is possible that a more rapid stool transit time that results from bulk in the diet may merely decrease the exposure time of the large bowel epithelium to carcinogens. There are also dietary supplements that may down-regulate the rate of malignant transformation. Selenium and vitamin A have been suggested as "chemopreventors" of colon cancer. At present, it is safe to say that the large bowel works best when it is asked to move a bulky stool through its lumen. A stool that is rich in fiber improves the bowel motility, lessens the incidence of functional (psychogenic) problems, and, as a final bonus, may diminish the rate of malignant transformation.

SCREENING

The screening tests available for colorectal malignant disease are listed in Table 1. Screening for large bowel cancer is effective because this disease, detected at an early stage, is nearly 100 percent curable by simple surgical procedures. Even more importantly, if a premalignant precursor of large bowel cancer, the adenomatous polyp, is detected and removed by snare polypectomy, the polyp-to-cancer transition can be interrupted. The stool test for occult blood has been moderately successful in screening for large bowel cancer. Unfortunately, most polyps do not bleed, and therefore Hemoccult can never be the optimal screening tool. Endoscopy is the screening method of choice. Experience reported by Gilbertson and Nelms from the University of Minnesota suggests that patients kept polyp-free by repeated sigmoidoscopic examination will be kept cancer-free. Also, Shinya in New York City compared two populations of patients who had colon or rectal cancer removed. One group had regular colonoscopy following surgery and the other group had routine follow-up care. Approximately 30 percent of patients who underwent colonoscopy every 6 months had polyps removed; no cancers developed in this group of patients. Eight cancers occurred in the control population of patients. Again, based on the concept that patients kept polyp-free remain cancer-free, one speculates that large bowel cancer is a preventable disease.

Endoscopy of the large bowel is the most promising screening technique for large bowel cancer. Figure 1 shows the extent of the colorectal lumen that is visualized by sigmoidoscopy, by fiberoptic sigmoidoscopy, and by colonoscopy. Automated advancement of the fiberoptic colonoscope is currently being pursued as a screening tool to visualize polyps and early cancers throughout the large bowel.

TABLE 1 Screening Tests for Colorectal Cancer

Digital rectal examination

Stool test for occult blood

Rigid sigmoidoscopy

Flexible sigmoidoscopy

Colonoscopy

CEA blood test

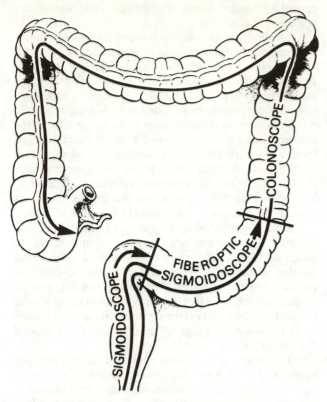

Figure 1 Extent of visualization of large bowel with endoscopes.

DIAGNOSIS

Most patients with large bowel cancer have symptoms when first seen by the physician. Unfortunately, these symptoms represent bowel dysfunction that occurs relatively late in the natural history of this disease. Table 2 shows the symptoms frequently present with rectal, left colon, and right colon cancer. Blood on the stool is the most frequent complaint in patients with rectal cancer; with colon cancer patients most frequently complain of pain. Pain in left colon cancer is often colicky, whereas the pain in right colon cancer is ill-defined. The difference in symptomatology between rectal cancer, left colon cancer, and right colon cancer occurs because of differences in the caliber of the colon lumen and differences in the character of the stool (liquid verses solid).

If a patient complains of symptoms compatible with large bowel cancer, the work-up should include a sigmoidoscopic examination plus a double-contrast barium enema or a colonoscopy. Some physicians prefer to recommend both radiologic and endoscopic evaluation of the large bowel. Barium enema and colonoscopy should not be thought of as competing in their diagnostic potential, but rather as complementary. If symptoms of colonic disease persist despite a negative work-up, the work-up should be repeated. The large bowel is a large and redundant organ and errors in diagnosis, both radiologic and endoscopic, are frequent. Other diagnostic tests indicated are a complete physical examination, urinalysis, rectal examination, and a stool test for occult blood.

If a patient is found to have a lesion within the large bowel, other tests are indicated prior to surgery. CEA levels greater than 5 ng per milliliter are associated with a poorer prognosis. Also, a computerized tomogram of the abdomen using both intravenous and oral contrast is indicated. This examination may suggest hepatic metastasis, reveal retroperitoneal lymph adenopathy, show the position of right and left ureters, diagnose extrarectal spread in patients with rectal cancer, show the functional status of both right and left kidney, and may hint at primary tumor involvement of the adjacent organs or structures within the abdominal cavity, especially the bladder. Other tests such as bone scan, full lung tomography, and liver and spleen scan may be done as baseline examinations to be used in the future for comparative studies, but in and of themselves do not give sufficient clinical information to be recommended.

In the postoperative period, a baseline CEA examination should be obtained. If an elevated preoperative CEA level fails to fall to within normal limits in the absence of liver disease, the patient carries an extremely poor prognosis.

POLYPS

Colonoscopy has dramatically changed the approach to the treatment of large bowel polyps. All mucosal abnormalities detected within the large bowel should be subjected to biopsy. Lesions 1 cm or greater should be removed by snare polypectomy technique. The risk of polyp removal in experienced hands is so low that virtually

TABLE 2 Comparison of the Five Most Frequent
Symptoms in Rectal, Left Colon, and Right Colon Cancer

Rectum and Rectosigmoid (258 Patients)	Left Colon (99 Patients)	Right Colon (984 Patients)
Melena (85%)	Abdominal pain (72%)	Abdominal pain (74%)
Constipation (46%)	Melena (53%)	Weakness (29%)
Tenesmus (30%)	Constipation (42%)	Melena (27%)
Diarrhea (30%)	Nausea (25%)	Nausea (24%)
Abdominal pain (26%)	Vomiting (23%)	Abdominal mass (23%)

From Postlethwait RW. Malignant tumors of the colon and rectum. Ann Surg 1949; 129:34–36.

TABLE 3 Construction of a "Surgical Equation" for Treatment of Cancer in Colonic Polyps Removed by Colonoscopic Polypectomy

Is the excised polyp sessile or pedunculated?

Is the focus of carcinoma in situ or invasive?

Was the margin of resection clear?

Is the focus of carcinoma poorly differentiated?

Is lymphatic invasion present?

What is the patient's operative risk?

Will close endoscopic follow-up be possible?

no polyp should be left in the bowel. A problem frequently arises when adenocarcinoma is found in a polyp that has been removed by snare electrocautery. The surgical equation helpful in deciding whether or not resection of the involved portion of the bowel is indicated is shown in Table 3.

RESECTION OF COLORECTAL CANCER

The surgical procedure used to remove a colon or rectal cancer depends on the natural history of the disease and the anatomic pathways of spread of this tumor. As the mucosal abnormality, usually arising in an adenomatous polyp, undergoes continuing malignant degeneration, it first invades through the muscularis mucosa. If confined to the muscularis mucosa, the malignant process is in situ and is not in danger of metastasizing. Continued growth of the malignant tumor takes place through the bowel wall to encounter lymphatic channels that course richly between the inner circular and outer longitudinal muscle layers. These lymphatics encircle the bowel lumen in a segmental fashion. As bowel wall lymphatics become infiltrated by malignant cells, the tumor constricts the bowel lumen and obstructive symptoms develop. Penetration of tumor through the bowel wall may continue so that tumor adhesions between the primary tumor and adjacent organs or structures can occur to small bowel, female internal genitalia, bladder, abdominal wall, or any other intra-abdominal structure. As penetration of the bowel wall progresses, the likelihood of lymphatic metastases to lymph nodes and hematogenous metastases to the liver parenchyma or lung increases. Distant hematogenous metastases from large bowel cancer in the absence of local lymphatic spread are unusual. Lower rectal cancer may metastasize to the lungs in the absence of hepatic spread because of direct venous drainage into the systemic circulation through the middle and inferior hemorrhoidal vessels. Lung metastases in the absence of hepatic metastases from colon cancer rarely occur.

The tendency of tumor to encircle the bowel wall in a segmental fashion by invading along lymphatics accounts for the fact that most large bowel tumors are wider (extend further around the bowel) than they are long (along the course of the bowel). This accounts for narrowing of the colon lumen and the obstructive symptoms so frequently seen with colorectal cancer and the minimal longitudinal

spread of tumor within the bowel wall beyond the epithelial abnormality.

Treatment is designed to remove the primary tumor with generous lateral margins as well as all lymph nodes and lymphatic channels that can be safely extirpated. Because of the segmental nature of cancer spread, the margin of normal bowel distal to the tumor, especially rectal cancer, need not be extensive. A margin of only 3 to 5 cm of normal bowel distal to the lower edge to the primary tumor is not associated with increased rates of local or systemic failure. Longitudinal spread more than 1 cm beyond the tumor mass is extremely unusual and, if it occurs, is due to retrograde lymphatic metastases. This is associated with tumor recurrence either locally or distally, regardless of the surgical procedure selected.

Rather than focusing on extensive proximal or distal margins of resection, the surgeon should strive to maximize the lateral margins of resection. The perirectal fat that surrounds a rectal tumor should be carefully preserved on the specimen. The soft tissues of the retroperitoneum that are adherent to a right colon tumor should be carefully dissected off the right ureter and right kidney so as to preserve a generous mass of soft tissue around the primary tumor.

The extent of lymphatic resection for the primary tumor is greatly variable between different groups of surgeons. For example, some surgeons excise the entire left colon for a sigmoid lesion; others perform only a segmental resection. Data to support one procedure over the other are lacking. However, most large series that retrospectively compare hemicolectomy with segmental resection show a 4 to 7 percent improvement in survival with the radical procedure. Perhaps those few patients with one to four positive nodes who will recur following segmental resection constitute this small proportion of patients who may have improved survival with radical surgery. Further studies on this issue need to be performed.

CANCER OF COLON AND UPPER THIRD OF THE RECTUM

The standard treatment for colon cancer and cancer of the upper third of the rectum is resection and anastomosis (Fig. 2). With careful preparation of the patient and with meticulous surgical technique, the results

TABLE 4 Five-Year Survival of Patients Following Surgical Treatment of Colorectal Cancer

Classification	Description	5-Year Survival
Dukes A	Disease limited to the bowel wall with no demonstrated metastases	80%
Dukes B	Disease extending through the bowel wall with no demonstrated metastases	70%
Dukes C	Disease in the bowel wall with lymph node metastases present	30%
Dukes D	Disseminated disease	1%

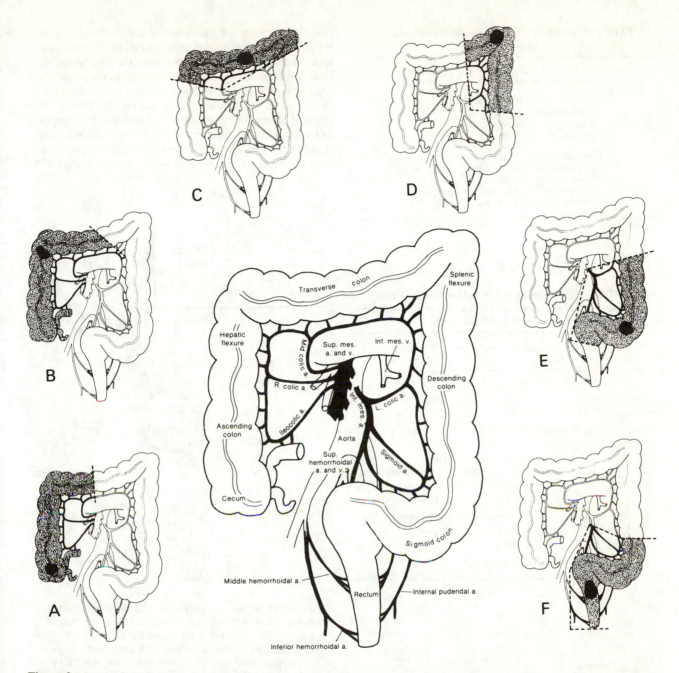

Figure 2 Anatomic resections commonly employed for cancer at different sites within the large bowel. (From Sugarbaker PH, MacDonald J, Gunderson L. Colorectal cancer. In: DeVita V, Helman S, Rosenberg SA (eds). Cancer: Principles and Practice of Oncology. Philadelphia: Lippincott, 1984.)

of these anatomic resections are usually good when one considers the poor prognosis for most patients with cancer. The expected survival of these patients is shown in Table 4. These improved statistics over those of the past are probably due to screening programs, earlier diagnosis, more efficient selection of patients for curative surgery by radiologic tests, and improved surgical technique.

CANCER OF LOWER TWO-THIRDS OF THE RECTUM

The treatment options for carcinoma of the rectum, based on the segment affected, are presented in Table 5

and Figure 3. Tumors in the upper third of the rectum are treated by low anterior resection. Even small tumors in this area have a certain low percentage of lymph node metastases, so that all lesions except polyps with small foci of malignant degeneration should be removed by low anterior resection. The key principle by which patients with cancer in the middle and lower third of the rectum are treated is selection (Table 6). About 10 percent of cancers in the middle or lower third of the rectum can be safely removed by local procedures. The majority of tumors should be removed by abdominoperineal resection with sacrifice of the anal sphincter. Primary radiation therapy by the Papillion technique is a reasonable alterna-

TABLE 5 Surgical Options in the Treatment of Colorectal Cancer

Cancer of colon and upper third of rectum
   Resection and anastomosis

Cancer of lower third of the rectum
   Abdominoperineal resection
   Local excision or fulguration
   Primary radiation therapy

Cancer of middle third of the rectum
   Abdominoperineal resection
   Low anterior resection
   Local excision or fulguration
   Primary radiation therapy

TABLE 6 Selection of a Local Procedure Versus Abdominoperineal Resection for Cancer of the Middle and Lower Thirds of the Rectum

	Local Treatment Favored	Abdominoperineal Resection Favored
Size	Small < 3 cm	Large > 3 cm
Configuration	Polypoid	Ulcerating
Mobility	Mobile	Tethered or fixed
Circumference of bowel involved	< 25%	> 25%
Grade	Well-differentiated	Poorly differentiated
CT scan	Normal	Extrarectal involvement
Consistency	Soft consistency	Hard consistency
CEA level	Normal	Elevated
Age	> 70	< 70
Cardiopulmonary status	Compromised	Good

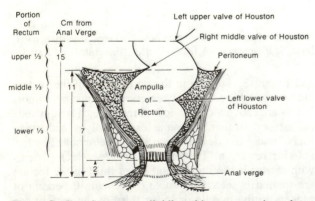

Figure 3 Rectal anatomy dividing this structure into three surgically important portions. (From Sugarbaker PH, MacDonald J, Gunderson L. Colorectal cancer. In: DeVita V, Helman S, Rosenberg SA (eds). Cancer: Principles and Practice of Oncology. Philadelphia: Lippincott, 1984.)

tive in treatment of the selected early rectal cancers. Fulguration is also a treatment option. However, I favor local excision. With this procedure, the histopathologic examination of the resected specimen gives the physician a great amount of information about this tumor that is destroyed in fulgurating or irradiating the tumor. The depth of invasion through the bowel wall and the adequacy of the margins of resection can be determined accurately if local transanal excision is used. A successful technique for local removal of rectal tumor is shown in Figure 4.

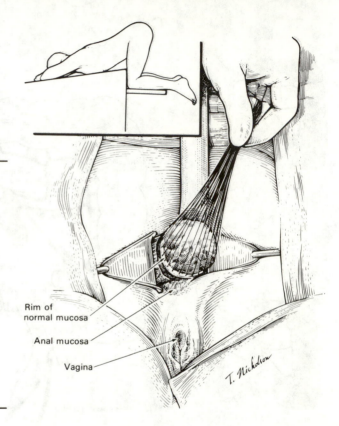

Figure 4 Transanal full-thickness excision of the rectal wall to remove selected rectal tumors located below the level of the peritoneal reflection. The inset shows the patient in the knee-chest position, which should be used if the rectal tumor is located on the anterior rectal wall. If the tumor is on the posterior rectal wall, the patient should be placed in the lithotomy position. In performing the transanal excision of the rectal tumor, one must obtain good exposure by wide dilation of the anal sphincter and careful placement of a self-retaining retractor. Silk stitches are placed through the full thickness of the rectal wall approximately 2 mm beyond the shoulder of the tumor. These silk sutures allow the surgeon to place traction on the tumor so that tissues to be transected are placed on stretch. The line of excision is approximately 2 mm beyond the silk sutures and should be full-thickness rectum down to perirectal fat. As the tumor is removed, the rectal wall should be reapproximated so that at the completion of the excision of the rectal tumor, the full-thickness closure of the rectal wall will also be finished. As soon as the specimen is released, the downward traction on the rectum is lost, and the excision site disappears from view. (From Sugarbaker PH, MacDonald J, Gunderson L. Colorectal cancer. In: DeVita V, Helman S, Rosenberg SA (eds). Cancer: Principles and Practice of Oncology. Philadelphia: Lippincott, 1984.)

TABLE 7 Selection of Low Anterior Resection or Abdominoperineal
Resection for Cancer of the Middle Third of the Rectum

	Low Anterior Resection Favored	*Abdominoperineal Resection Favored*
Sex (exposure within the pelvis)	Female	Male
Position of tumor	Tumor in upper portion of mid-rectum	Tumor in lower portion of mid-rectum
Size of tumor	Small	Large
Mobility of tumor	Mobile or tethered	Tethered or fixed
Distant disease	Distant disease present	Distant disease absent
Body build	Asthenic	Mesomorphic
Prior anorectal disease	No anorectal problems	Prior anorectal surgery

ABDOMINOPERINEAL RESECTION VERSUS LOW ANTERIOR RESECTION FOR CANCER OF MIDDLE THIRD OF RECTUM

The surgeon often must decide whether to perform an abdominoperineal resection or a sphincter salvage procedure for carcinoma in the middle third of the rectum. The segmental nature of the lymphatic and blood supply to the colon and rectum makes the sphincter salvage procedure reasonable with a minimal distal margin of resection. The question that one must ask is "What is a reasonable distal margin of resection?" The studies of Wilson and Beahrs at the Mayo clinic suggest that a 2-cm margin as compared to a 5-, 10- or 15-cm margin of resection on a rectal cancer does not adversely affect survival. The lateral margins of resection are more important than the distal margin of resection in the prevention of local recurrence. Large tumors that penetrate through the bowel wall may be difficult to excise with surrounding perirectal fat if a low anterior resection is done. With an abdominoperineal resection, this tissue may be more easily sharply dissected from the surrounding sacrum and levator ani muscles. The other criteria that may lead a surgeon to select an abdominoperineal resection or a low anterior resection for a midrectal cancer are shown in Table 7.

ADJUVANTS TO SURGERY

A large number of cytotoxic drugs and drug combinations have been used in the surgical adjuvant treatment of large bowel cancer; 5-fluorourocil, mitomycin C, and methyl CCNU all have response rates of approximately 20 percent. Unfortunately, combinations of drugs are no more effective than single agents, either in reducing bulk disease or as adjuvants. Radiation therapy has been used as an adjuvant for rectal cancer. It appears to be effective in reducing the incidence of pelvic and perineal recurrence, but has not been convincingly shown to translate into improved survival. At present, chemotherapy or radiation therapy used as a surgical adjuvant to colon or rectal cancer resection should only be recommended in a protocol setting.

FOLLOW-UP

The follow-up schedule for patients with surgically treated large bowel malignant tumor varies greatly between individual surgeons. Some believe in frequent follow-up visits so that recurrent disease can be detected early and dealt with definitively by further surgery. Others believe that the results of reoperation are so dismal that careful and expensive follow-up is not indicated. Recent studies on the use of serial CEA postoperatively as a guide to reoperation suggest that approximately 10 percent of patients who have this aggressive follow-up are salvaged for the long term by reoperative surgery. This is true not only for local regional recurrence, but also for isolated hepatic metastases. The disease-free survival following hepatic resection of one to three metastases in the liver from colorectal malignant disease is approximately 30 percent. Therefore, surgery becomes its own adjuvant in the treatment of patients with malignant tumor of the large bowel.

ANAL CANCER: SQUAMOUS CELL CANCER AND MELANOMA

VICTOR W. FAZIO, M.B., B.S., F.R.A.C.S., F.A.C.S.
IAN T. JONES, M.B., B.S., F.R.A.C.S., F.R.C.S.(Eng.)

Carcinomas of the anal canal and anal verge are uncommon lesions that account for only 2 percent of all colorectal malignant tumors. Most are seen in the sixth and seventh decades of life. Lesions of the anal canal are more common in women and outnumber anal verge or perianal lesions in a ratio of three to one. Predisposing factors for squamous cell cancers include prior irradiation, chronic fistula, inflammatory conditions such as condylomata acuminata and granuloma inguinale, and perhaps eczema and pruritus ani. The intraepidermal carcinoma, Bowen's disease, may progress to become a frankly invasive squamous cell cancer.

Lesions of the anal canal and anal verge behave and are treated differently so that a practical understanding of the anatomy of the region is essential. Although there is some variation in the terminology used in the literature, we define the anal canal as the terminal portion of the alimentary tract continuous with the rectum above and the anal verge below (Fig. 1). In that part of the anal canal lying above the dentate line, the mucosa is of a transitional type between the columnar epithelium of the rectum above and squamous epithelium below the dentate line, and several different cell varieties are present. This area represents the embryologic cloaca or junction of the hindgut and ectoderm. Distal to the squamous epithelium of the anal canal is the anal opening or anus and the external skin; this area is called the *anal verge or perianal region*. While it has no precise anatomic demarcation, its outer limit is arbitrarily set at 6 cm from the anus. The squamous epithelium of the anal verge can be histologically differentiated from that of the anal canal by the presence of the epidermal appendages such as hair follicles, sebaceous glands, and sweat glands found in normal skin elsewhere.

Cancers of the anal canal arise from the unstable cell population of the transitional zone and always involve the dentate line. These tumors come to resemble one of the multiple cell types found in this zone so that a number of histologically different tumor types have been described in the area with a profusion of names including squamous, cloacogenic, transitional, and basaloid carcinomas. Despite this, experience has shown that all can be treated as variants of squamous cell carcinoma. They present with bleeding, discharge, discomfort after defecation, or a mass, but these symptoms may be trivial in nature and presentation may be delayed. Occasionally, the diagnosis is made in an asymptomatic individual as an incidental finding after histologic examination of a hemorrhoidectomy specimen. Rarely, an adenocarcinoma is seen in this area, possibly as a result of direct extension of a low-lying rectal cancer or of implantation from a proximal colorectal primary into a chronic fissure or hemorrhoidectomy wound, but this group of tumors is not discussed in this chapter.

At the anal verge, well-differentiated squamous cell carcinoma is the usual tumor encountered, although in rare instances a basal cell carcinoma, Bowen's disease, or extramammary Paget's disease is seen. Squamous lesions of the anal verge are smaller, grow more slowly, and have a better prognosis than those of the anal canal. They present as a small lump or ulcer that fails to heal, and signs of regional spread are unusual.

CARCINOMA OF THE ANAL CANAL

Despite the relative rarity of these lesions, their treatment has been the subject of considerable discussion over recent years. It is appropriate to briefly mention new developments in this field to qualify our own approach.

Although cancers of the anal canal differ from rectal cancer in that they are highly radiosensitive and that their lymphatic drainage is to the inguinal lymph nodes as well as the presacral and pelvic nodes, traditionally their treatment has been the same, i.e., abdominoperineal resection. There were some good results following treatment of anal canal cancers by radiotherapy in the 1930s, but the use of this modality was frequently associated with a high incidence of severe radionecrosis and fibrosis that destroyed anorectal function. On the other hand, abdominoperineal resection, which offers a reasonable chance for cure with 5-year survival rates ranging from 35 to 68 percent, suffered the inherent disadvantages of permanent colostomy and possible bladder and sexual dysfunction. Even so, it has become the standard against which all other treatments are compared.

In Europe, however, some centers continued to treat these tumors by irradiation, and with modern equipment, morbidity was dramatically reduced. Using a combination of external beam irradiation and interstitial iridium-192

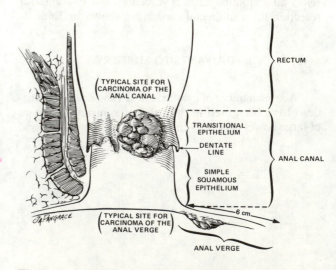

Figure 1 Anatomy of the anal canal and the anal verge

needle therapy, Papillon of Lyon, France has achieved a 65 percent 5-year survival rate for patients with lesions considered to be surgically resectable, and three-fourths of these patients have normal anal function.

At Wayne State University, Nigro has pioneered the use of combined chemotherapy and radiation therapy in the treatment of squamous cancer of the anal canal. External beam radiotherapy and chemotherapy given before surgery led to significant tumor reduction, and indeed most resected specimens were found to be tumor-free at pathologic examination. Nigro now reserves abdominoperineal resection for patients with residual or recurrent tumor found after primary treatment by combined chemotherapy and radiation therapy. In his recent review of 104 patients treated by this combination 79 percent were alive and disease-free after 2 to 11 years of follow-up.

We have been encouraged by this experience and, with the assistance of colleagues from the departments of radiotherapy and oncology at the Cleveland Clinic, have been treating patients with anal canal cancer in a similar fashion.

When these patients are first seen, it is imperative to have an accurate assessment of the tumor by thorough examination and representative biopsy. Frequently, this is best performed under anesthesia. Because of the anatomic structure of the region, Dukes' classification is not appropriate to define these lesions, but a clear description of size, site, and quadrant involved; cephalad and caudad limits of tumor extension; fixation to underlying sphincters; and evidence of involvement of vagina, rectovaginal septum, and pelvic lymph nodes are all essential to the administration of treatment and the monitoring of tumor response. If inguinal lymph nodes are enlarged or if there are other suspicious lesions, these also require biopsy.

In the usual situation in which tumor is confined to the anal canal, treatment by combined chemotherapy and radiation therapy is indicated. There are no absolute contraindications to this treatment. External beam irradiation is delivered by high energy linear accelerator to the primary lesion, the low pelvic area, and the inguinal lymph nodes. Nigro urges that the total radiation dose should not exceed 3,000 rads, as the chemotherapy with its known enhancing effect on radiation therapy may cause unwanted morbidity. We and other workers favor a higher dose, averaging 4,000 rads given in daily 200-rad fractions.

On the day that radiation is commenced, chemotherapy is also given as a continuous infusion of 5-fluorouracil, 1,000 mg per square meter per day for 4 days, and is accompanied by a single bolus of mitomycin-C, 15 mg per square meter. Four weeks later, the infusion of 5-fluorouracil is repeated.

The patients are followed to ensure that total resolution of the tumor occurs and to exclude later recurrence. It is usual to see evidence of actinic changes at the site of the tumor or even for a little induration to persist. We do not practice routine scar excision, but any suspicious lesion is managed by examination under anesthesia with multiple needle biopsies. If the presence of residual or recurrent tumor is confirmed histologically, the patient is submitted to abdominoperineal resection.

Inguinal metastases, when present at the time of initial presentation, are generally a sign of poor prognosis. We would avoid the inconvenience and morbidity of node dissection in this group, but treat them with additional radiation dosage to the involved area. Metachronous inguinal node metastases, however, are frequently associated with long-term survival, and we would perform a superficial inguinal node block dissection on these patients, although there is accumulating evidence to suggest that irradiation may be just as effective in this situation. Despite the rich lymphatic and vascular pathways supplying this region, the disease tends to remain localized, and only 10 percent of patients show evidence of distant metastases. For these patients, we endeavor to use nonsurgical treatment whenever possible.

The 16 patients we have treated in this manner represent the majority of new cases of anal canal cancer presenting to us over the last 5 years. Twelve patients have shown a complete response and remain disease-free. Two patients developed recurrent disease in the anal region during the second year after therapy: one of these has been disease-free for a further 11 months after abdominoperineal resection and another patient, who refused this surgical option, is currently disease-free seven months after further radiotherapy. Two patients have disease present: one failed to attend for follow-up and was seen elsewhere with apparently incurable local disease; another patient with locally recurrent disease also refused abdominoperineal resection, and has not been controlled with further treatment by irradiation.

Morbidity has been confined to a single radiation fissure cured by temporary loop colostomy and a case of myelosuppression, which resolved spontaneously. This experience, supported by that of Nigro, has led us to adopt combined chemotherapy and radiation therapy as the preferred method for managing squamous cell carcinoma of the anal canal.

CARCINOMA OF THE ANAL VERGE

As previously stated, cancers of the anal verge are much less aggressive than anal canal cancers. They can be adequately managed in most cases by local excision with a clearance of 2.5 cm of normal tissue on all sides. Occasionally, part of the lowermost fibers of the sphincters are excised in the specimen, but these defects heal well after skin grafting, and continence is preserved if less than half the anal circumference is excised. It is unusual for these lesions to show signs of lymphatic metastases, but if present, these can be dealt with by superficial inguinal node dissection or external beam irradiation.

In 1979, we reviewed our experience at the Cleveland Clinic with cancer of the anal verge. *Ten patients* were treated primarily by us with local excision and skin grafting. *Five* were cured (after 5 to 20 years of follow-up); *three* developed local recurrence, two of whom were cured by repeat local excision, but one developed further recurrence after abdominoperineal resection and died; *one* patient had disease present at the time of study, and *one* died of myocardial infarction but disease-free 15 months after surgery (this being the only non-five-year survivor in this group).

Seven patients were sent to us with recurrence after local excision performed elsewhere. *Three* of these were treated by further local excision and electrocoagulation: two were cured, but the third died of further recurrence. *Two* were managed by abdominoperineal resection and were disease-free 9 years later, and *two* who had advanced disease when first seen by us were treated palliatively and died.

PREOPERATIVE BOWEL PREPARATION

ISIDORE COHN, Jr., M.D., M.Sc.(Med.), D.Sc.(Med.)

Forty-six years have passed since the first serious planned evaluation of the preoperative use of modern antibacterial agents for intestinal antisepsis. The very durability of an argument on a topic that would seem to be so easy to resolve attests to the argumentative nature of surgeons, their reluctance to accept new ideas that have less startling effects than the introduction of x-rays or antibiotics, or a reluctance based on some ungrounded fears that change in an approach to an age-old problem might endanger their historically accepted solution to that problem. Unfortunately, the infection rate following either elective or emergency procedures on the large bowel demonstrates clearly that the time-tested answers have not been satisfactory. In all fairness, it must be admitted that within the past few years there has been greater acceptance of the use of antibiotics to help control the bacterial flora of the colon, but there are still significant members of the profession who profess not to find antibiotics useful in most of their elective cases.

The evidence is overwhelming for the following points:

1. The flora of the large bowel is enormous and is more concentrated than anywhere else in the normal human body.
2. Anaerobic organisms are the major component of the colonic flora.
3. Antibiotics can reduce significantly the flora of the bowel lumen.

MELANOMA

This rare lesion of the anorectum has a deservedly sinister reputation. It is derived from ectodermal tissue and may advance rapidly to attain a very large size. Even if the primary lesion is small when the patient is first seen, distant metastases are probably already present as there is early dissemination of these tumors by the lymphatics and blood stream.

Response to radiotherapy or chemotherapy is not seen, and abdominoperineal resection of the anorectum offers the only and, admittedly, small chance for cure. Our experience with this depressing disease parallels that of other workers in the field, and 5-year survival is seen in fewer than 10 percent of cases. It is important, when possible, to avoid the added burden of a colostomy in the patient with incurable disease, and appropriate palliative treatment only should be offered.

4. Antibiotics have demonstrated their ability to protect bowel deprived of some or most of its normal blood supply, and therefore antibiotics should be of value in the questionable intestinal anastomosis or in the bowel with a compromised blood supply.
5. Mechanical cleansing of the bowel is essential prior to any elective surgical procedure.
6. The infectious complication rate following surgery of the colon is higher than that following procedures on other parts of the gastrointestinal tract.
7. Antibiotics are no substitute for either proper surgical technique or adherence to basic surgical principles.
8. Age, obstruction, inflammatory disease, perforation, and other noncolonic concomitant problems increase the risk of operation.

Some areas in which there is not so much agreement would include the following:

1. Do antibiotics lower the rate of wound infection?
2. Which antibiotics are best?
3. Should preoperative antibiotics be administered by the oral, parenteral, or combined routes?
4. How long a period of preoperative preparation is necessary?
5. Do "prophylactic antibiotics" lead to dangerous emergence of resistant strains?
6. How long should antibiotics be continued in the postoperative period?
7. Are the effects of orally administered antibiotics due to their action within the bowel or to their effects following systemic absorption?
8. What is the preferred method of mechanical cleansing?

Let us concentrate first on those areas in which there is no universal agreement and try to find some rationale for the answers that seem appropriate.

The real objective of antibiotic use in large bowel surgery should be to reduce the incidence of bacterial complications, and this would be manifest most commonly in wound infections, presuming careful surgical technique is used in the colonic anastomosis. If antibiotics do not lower the frequency of wound infections, the answers to most of the rest of the questions would be academic. The basic question should not be how, but whether, antibiotics do indeed lower this complication rate. While some individual authors continue to maintain that there are no real justifications for the use of antibiotics in carefully performed surgical procedures, the weight of evidence is clearly against them, and it is now easy to cite the evidence. One very careful survey of clinical trials from 1965 to 1980, in which patients given various antibiotics prior to elective surgery of the large bowel were compared with patients prepared with mechanical cleansing only, concluded that "the issue of antibiotic prophylaxis versus simple mechanical preparation of the colon is now resolved" in favor of the use of antibiotics. One cannot ignore such a detailed, statistically validated study of all the prospective trials reported during the selected interval. Thus question 1 must be answered in the affirmative: antibiotics *do* lower the rate of wound infection.

For question 2, there is no clear agreement, and this is probably the major remaining source of argument in the field. Each author has his own particular agent that seems to be the most effective in his hands, and this is the one he recommends. Even after the appearance of a variety of statistically evaluated studies, which often have differing results, they continue to advocate their own favorite. My own particular preference continues to be kanamycin because of a large experimental and clinical experience with it and its satisfactory performance under a variety of conditions. Some base their dislike of this agent on in vitro studies of the sensitivity of colonic organisms. Our experience, both in the laboratory and in the clinical setting, suggests that some of the so-called resistance found in vitro may not be valid for the clinical setting. The level of antibiotic in the colon may be a thousand times as high as that in the usual laboratory sensitivity test, and therefore the two are not comparable. However, it would be inappropriate not to mention some of the other agents that are available, are good bacteriologically, and have been recommended for this purpose, and they are summarized in Table 1.

TABLE 1   Recommended Drugs

Drug	Regimen*
Erythromycin-neomycin or	Neomycin (1 g) and erythromycin base (1 g) orally at 1 PM, 2 PM, and 11 PM 1 day preop.
Kanamycin or	1 g every hour for 4 hours, then q6h for a total of 72 hours
Metronidazole	750 mg q8h for 72 hours

* Mechanical cleansing and low residue diet required

There is almost as much discussion about the route of antibiotic administration as there is about the choice of agents. Solid data are not easy to find, though one can summarize quickly the arguments on each side. The choice of the oral route for a poorly absorbed agent provides maximum concentration of the antibiotic in the large bowel where it should be most effective. This choice also minimizes the patient's risk of developing antibiotic-resistant strains outside the colon and diminishes the risk that the patient may develop some resistant strains as a result of prior medication for some other purpose. With the possible exception of those institutions with an unusually large volume of elective large bowel surgery, there is little risk of developing a hospital-based flora that is resistant to an antibiotic chosen in this fashion. In favor of the parenteral route is the simultaneous systemic level of antibiotic that is obtained and the beneficial effects this may have on lowering the incidence of infection in the wound. However, the excretion of antibiotic directly into the lumen of the colon with its primary effect there is diminished by choice of this route. There does not seem to be any real justification for the combined route of administration. The arguments cited in favor of the oral route are among the reasons kanamycin has been a continuing selection of ours.

The duration of preoperative antibiotic preparation depends, to a certain extent, on the answers to question 8, and thus questions 4 and 8 will be answered together. There is bacteriologic evidence that the colonic flora can be reduced to extremely low levels within 24 hours after initiation of combined mechanical and antibiotic therapy. However, the control of the bacterial flora is not so uniformly achieved in this short time, and mechanical cleansing by most of the standard techniques is not reliable. Without adequate mechanical cleansing, oral antibiotic therapy is irrelevant, and therefore this is an absolute prerequisite of therapy. My earlier studies showed that *reliable* reduction in bacterial flora could be achieved with the combination of 72 hours of mechanical and antibiotic therapy, and therefore this has been my own choice. Effective bacterial control may be achieved in 24 hours in many patients, but one never knows which patient has had good control and which one has not, and it has seemed that this was a risk it was not necessary to take.

In recent years, the standard method of purgation and enemas has been challenged by those who recommend a variety of other means of mechanically cleansing the colon. Osmotically effective agents have been used to bring large quantities of fluid into the gastrointestinal tract and thereby cause its evacuation. A more distinct departure has been the intestinal lavage approach, which uses a continuing flow of a large quantity of fluid administered by nasogastric tube with the patient sitting on a toilet so that fluid can be expelled as quickly as it is administered and thus cleanse the entire gastrointestinal tract. Advocates of this approach claim that it is easier on patients than other methods of cleansing, although this is difficult to accept on first approach. The problems inherent in this technique relate mostly to individuals in the older age group and those in whom the danger of fluid overload would be significant. It should be emphasized that the

TABLE 2   **Author's Preferred Program for Intestinal Antisepsis**

Mechanical cleansing for 3 days
  Patient hospitalized
  Purgatives by oral route
  Daily enemas
  Last enema given night before operation until clear
Low residue or elemental diet for 3 days
Kanamycin 1 g every hour for 4 hours, then q6h for 72 hours

original promise that a low residue or nonresidue diet would be adequate by itself has not been realized. Even though such a diet should be a part of the standard technique of bowel preparation, it is not sufficient in itself.

"Prophylactic antibiotics," when used properly, do not lead to the emergence of resistant antibiotic strains, and therefore this concern about preoperative preparation should be eliminated. If antibiotic administration is limited to the necessary period of preparation, or even extended for another few days because of some unexpected delay, there is little or no danger of resistant strains developing, and this is even clearer if orally administered poorly absorbed agents are used.

Oral antibiotic administration should be discontinued at the time of operation. Parenterally administered agents, if used for "prophylaxis," should be continued no more than 3 days in the postoperative period, but then would be used for their control of wound infection rather than for their effect on the colonic flora. If perioperative antibiotics are to be used systemically as a means of controlling wound problems, they should be started in the immediate preoperative period and given for only 1 to 3 days following operation, assuming there is no evidence of a specific infection, which would require treatment rather than prophylaxis.

There does not appear to be any clear-cut study that determines whether the beneficial effects of orally administered antibiotics result from their action reducing the bacterial flora within the colon or from the level of circulating antibiotic that combats bacteria in the wound during and after operation. With the exception of those nonabsorbed, orally administered agents, there does not seem to be any way to resolve this problem at the moment. However, there does not seem to be any indication for the simultaneous use of both oral and parenteral antibiotics if one is going to use an absorbable agent for the oral route. If the choice is for a nonabsorbed agent, parenteral antibiotics might be used in the immediate preoperative and the immediate postoperative periods, particularly when there has been undue contamination during the procedure, regardless of the cause of that contamination. Such perioperative antibiotic administration should be limited to the period before the operation that would be required to obtain adequate circulating and wound concentrations and continued only for 1 to 3 days following the operation. If the agent chosen for intestinal antisepsis is one that is absorbed from the gastrointestinal tract, systemic antibiotic administration should be reserved for cases in which there is undue contamination or in which

some other factor convinces the surgeon that there is an increased risk. Even then such usage should be limited to the perioperative period as just described.

With the background of both an extensive experimental experience and an even longer and larger clinical experience, I have continued to use the program in Table 2 for preoperative intestinal antisepsis.

There are times and conditions when this program should be modified, and it is important to be aware of these limitations: (1) intestinal obstruction, (2) inflammatory disease of the bowel, (3) pre-existing colostomy, (4) emergency procedure of any kind, and (5) age, debility, and major medical complications.

In patients with intestinal obstruction, there is not time to prepare them properly as for an elective procedure, and in any case the obstructing element, no matter what it is, will prevent proper cleansing of the bowel proximal to the point of obstruction where the cleansing is needed most. Time should not be wasted on efforts to clean the colon under these conditions, and the patient is better served by an earlier attempt to relieve the obstruction and do whatever other procedure is necessary.

If the bowel is inflamed, as in diverticulitis or ulcerative colitis, further purgation is both dangerous and unnecessary. In either such condition, the naturally increased peristalsis provides cleansing of the bowel, and the danger of perforation from the increased pressure of enemas or laxatives is too great to warrant their use. Oral and/or systemic antibiotics may be a major part of therapy, but more as a means of controlling any inflammatory component of the disease than as a means of reducing the flora of the colon.

In the presence of a pre-existing colostomy, the usual means of cleaning the bowel will not suffice. If the planned procedure may involve segments of the bowel proximal and distal to the colostomy, oral administration of antibiotics and laxatives is indicated, along with instillation of antibacterial agents into both limbs of the colostomy and irrigation of both of these plus the rectum. If it is clear that all of the operation will be distal to the colostomy, and closure of the colostomy is not planned, attention can be limited to the distal limb of the colostomy and the rectum. However, operative findings often change these plans, and it is wiser to have both sides of the colostomy prepared to avoid having to abort a procedure because of inadequate preoperative planning.

Emergency procedures, by their very nature, preclude the possibility of any planned preparation, regardless of whether this be a perforation due to intrinsic disease, trauma, acute obstruction, hemorrhage, volvulus, or other condition. In these situations, maximum care must be taken to avoid or minimize spillage of colonic contents, to tailor the procedure to the conditions found, and to use antibiotics as wisely as possible to prevent further complications. In my experience, irrigation of the colon during the operative procedure has led to spillage into the peritoneal cavity and wound more often that it has prevented trouble, and I have not found it valuable. Even the instillation of an antibacterial substance into the lumen of the colon has not been effective in my hands, and I prefer to proceed with the operative procedure and avoid delay by maneuvers that may be counterproductive.

In the presence of major noncolonic disease that contributes to risk, the various factors must be weighed against one another. The aged patient tolerates complications less well than the younger one, but also tolerates

less well the effects of a stringent program of preparation. The method of whole gut lavage must be used with caution in the patient with cardiac or renal dysfunction. A careful assessment of the patient's overall condition should help to determine what modification of the plan would be in the patient's best interests.

ACUTE APPENDICITIS

DAVID L. DUDGEON, M.D.

Appendicitis remains a diagnostic challenge, despite almost a century of successfully applied surgical therapy. This surgical dilemma is illustrated by a decreasing mortality rate for nonperforated (0.1%) and perforated appendicitis (3.0%), while the overall occurrence rate of the advanced, perforated form of appendicitis (35%) remains unchanged over the past 40 years. The patient with perforated appendicitis has a significantly higher morbidity rate, resulting not only in physical and mental anguish, but also in an increased duration of hospitalization, with an average of 4.5 days for nonperforated appendicitis and 11.4 days for the perforated disease. An earlier diagnosis and subsequent improved morbidity rate for acute appendicitis can only be accomplished by an increased awareness on the part of the public and physicians.

DIAGNOSIS

The classic description of the diagnostic symptoms and signs of appendicitis includes initial periumbilical crampy pain, which becomes a more constant pain and migrates to a right lower quadrant position. Nausea with or without vomiting, anorexia, and low-grade fever are common accompanying symptoms in the progression of the disease. The most pertinent physical finding is the presence of localized point tenderness near "McBurney's point" in the right lower quadrant, which usually is present within 24 hours of the onset of symptoms. A few laboratory studies, usually a CBC with a total white blood cell count and differential, urinalysis, and occasionally a chest and/or abdominal roentgenogram can support, but should never alter, your clinical diagnosis of acute appendicitis. More complex diagnostic studies are indicated only in the presence of other potentially complicating systemic conditions, such as diabetes, sickle cell anemia, and cardiac failure.

The disease occurs most commonly in the prepubertal period and through the second decade of life. The differential diagnosis of acute appendicitis is extensive; however, a careful history and physical examination and, if necessary, close observation with repeated examinations by the same

physician should result in the correct preoperative diagnosis in more than 80 percent of cases. More sophisticated adjunctive diagnostic procedures such as abdominal sonography, computerized tomography and/or colon contrast roentgenographic studies have recently been touted as ways to expedite and improve the accuracy of the diagnosis of appendicitis. Although these procedures are occasionally helpful, I have noted both false-positive and false-negative results and consider them to be of limited value.

PREOPERATIVE PREPARATION

Preoperative preparation for the otherwise healthy patient with acute appendicitis is minimal, but the patient with a known perforated appendix and peritonitis requires vigorous therapy. Unfortunately, among patients at opposite ends of the age spectrum, i.e., children under 2 years of age and the elderly, there is an increased incidence of perforated appendicitis at presentation. The mortality and morbidity rates in these and all other appendicitis patients who present with signs of generalized peritonitis and sepsis are improved by meticulous attention to preoperative preparation. This includes intravenous rehydration, using Ringer's lactate, as a bolus injection of 10 ml per kilogram, until a urine output of 1 to 2 cc per kilogram per hour is obtained. A fever higher than 38.5°C or 101.5°F, particularly in children, should be reduced by means of rectal acetaminophen suppositories and exposure to room temperature. Alcohol sponging for a fever is deleterious because it may precipitate shivering thermogenesis.

Preoperative antibiotic therapy is used selectively. If systemic signs or physical findings point to appendiceal perforation, intravenous broad-spectrum antibiotics, including an effective anti-anaerobic agent, are given so that effective tissue/blood levels are achieved preoperatively. Intraoperative antibiotic therapy is begun for the unexpected appendiceal perforation discovered during laparotomy. The anaerobic agent is discontinued in 3 to 5 days, and the other antibiotics stopped 7 days following surgery. Antibiotics are also indicated for patients who have no evidence of preoperative appendiceal perforation if they have underlying physical conditions that predispose them to complications of bacteremia (e.g., infants less than 6 months of age and patients with congenital or acquired cardiac anomalies or diabetes). These prophylactic agents are discontinued 48 hours after surgery.

SURGICAL TECHNIQUE

Anesthetic management is important, since aspiration during induction and/or endotracheal intubation is a real hazard. The pediatric patient who has not vomited and may have a stomach full of secretions is a prime candidate for this potentially lethal complication.

Once the patient is anesthetized, the relaxed abdomen should be re-examined for evidence of a palable mass or thickening due to the underlying appendiceal phlegmon or abscess. If this mass is located at a distance form McBurney's point, it may influence the positioning of the abdominal incision. Most patients require a curvilinear skin and subcutaneous incision located over McBurney's point and lateral to the rectus sheath. There is some advantage in placing the incision higher, slightly above the level of the anterior superior iliac spine, in the male. In the female, who has a wider pelvis, a lower incision at or below the level of the anterior superior iliac spine permits sufficient access and results in an improved cosmetic result. The muscular abdominal wall is incised by means of the muscle-splitting or "gridiron" technique. The fascia of the external oblique is incised along the course of its muscle fibers, and then the muscle is split bluntly by instrumentation or finger dissection, depending on the size of the patient. The internal oblique and transverse abdominis muscles are split in the same way. The peritoneum is freed of the transverse abdominis muscle, elevated, and opened under direct visualization to prevent damage to the underlying bowel. Peritoneal fluid may be encountered at this time and should be sampled for a Gram stain examination as well as aerobic and anaerobic cultures. A simple abdominal wall retractor, i.e., a Richardson retractor, is used to facilitate digital localization of the inflamed appendix. In many cases, by a gentle sweep of the finger around the cecal border laterally and inferiorly, the surgeon encounters the appendix and breaks down the surrounding loose inflammatory adhesions, allowing mobilization of the cecum and appendix into the wound. Dense adhesions may require sharp division of these lateral and inferior bands before the cecum can be elevated. Underlying vessels (e.g., iliac artery) and/or the right ureter may be firmly attached to the dense inflammatory reaction of the ruptured appendix and must be carefully avoided during mobilization of the cecum and appendix. Identification of the appendix may be difficult owing to dense fibrinous adhesions or a retrocecal appendiceal position. Identification of the anterior taenia coli of the cecal wall with retrograde visualization of this structure to the tip of the cecum will lead to the base of the appendix. If mobilization of the appendix is not possible because of inflammatory reaction, separation and ligation of the mesoappendiceal vessels progressing from the appendiceal base to its tip will afford hemostasis and a safe appendiceal excision. The vessels should be ligated with absorbable ligatures, using larger-diameter material for secure occlusion if the mesoappendix is indurated.

In most patients with appendicitis, the freely mobilized appendix can be lightly grasped with a Babcock forceps and the mesoappendiceal vessels individually ligated and divided, proceeding from the tip to the base of the engorged organ. If a localized abscess or generalized peritonitis is noted or if the patient is less than 2 or 3 years of age, I prefer not to invert the appendiceal stump. Cecal wall induration makes stump inversion difficult and results in excessive loss of cecal diameter. Stump inversion in a small child places the child at risk for a stump-related colo-colic intussusception. In these patients, I doubly ligate the stump approximately 1.0 cm below the cecal base and excise the appendix. When there is no local contamination or excessive cecal wall induration, I use a cecal wall purse-string suture of 3–0 material approximately 1 cm from the appendiceal base. The appendix is squeezed gently with a straight clamp to force any underlying fecalith either into the cecum or distally into the appendix. An absorbable 2–0 or 3–0 ligature is applied around the appendix 1 to 2 cm below the cecum and tied. The appendix is excised distal to this suture, and the mucosal lining of the stump is electrocauterized to destroy any mucous glands. The stump is inverted, and the purse-string secured.

Before the cecum is replaced and the incision closed, the mesoappendix is again inspected to ensure hemostasis, and a local saline irrigation is used. Intraperitoneal drains are used only for well-defined abscess cavities with thick fibrinous walls. Generalized peritonitis is not an indication for prophylactic intraperitoneal drains. An intraperitoneal drain is usually placed through a separate skin incision caudad to the laparotomy incision and secured to the skin by a suture; the distal end is tagged with a sterile safety pin.

The incision is closed in layers with a running absorbable suture approximating the peritoneum and transversalis fascia. The internal and external oblique muscles are independently closed with 2 or 3 interrupted absorbable sutures. If this is a nonperforated, nongangrenous appendicitis, the subcutaneous tissue is approximated with interrupted absorbable sutures and the skin closed with a 4–0 absorbable continuous subcuticular suture. In the elderly or immunocompromised patient with perforated appendicitis, the subcutaneous tissue and skin are kept open for local wound care, to be closed secondarily with Steri-Strips when the wound has a clean granulating base, approximately 5 to 10 days postoperatively. Children with perforated appendicitis and peritonitis can have a subcutaneous drain placed and the skin gently approximated with interrupted monofilament, nonabsorbable 4–0 sutures. The drain is removed on the fourth postoperative day, rendering unnecessary the use of open wound dressings in children with well-vascularized tissues. Minimal dressings are used, i.e., occlusive Steri-Strips with collodion for noncontaminated wounds and light gauze dressings and tape for open wounds, wounds with external sutures, or those with exiting drains.

POSTOPERATIVE CARE

In cases of nonperforated appendicitis, the nasogastric tube is removed in the operating room, and maintainence intravenous fluids are given until resumption of intestinal activity, 24 to 48 hours after surgery. These patients are usually discharged from the hospital on the second to fourth postoperative day.

Patients with perforated appendicitis require nasogastric tube drainage for 3 to 4 days postoperatively. Antibiotic coverage is maintained as previously noted, along with maintenance intravenous therapy until resumption of enteral feeding. The drains are removed in 4 to 5 days unless drainage is excessive. All drains are removed by 7 to 10 days.

ALTERNATIVE MANAGEMENT OF PERFORATED APPENDICITIS

Young patients may present with a history compatible with perforated appendicitis and a palpable mass in the lower abdomen. If the patient has had these symptoms longer than 5 days, but is tolerating orally administered fluids, a trial of intravenous broad-spectrum antibiotic therapy can be considered. The antibiotic therapy should be effective against both aerobic and anaerobic organisms, and any accompanying symptoms of fever should defervesce within 36 hours after therapy is instituted. Likewise, abdominal pain should rapidly resolve and the mass soften, become nontender, and decrease in size after 2 to 4 days of therapy. Treatment with orally administered antibiotics is started after 7 to 9 days of intravenous therapy, and the patient is then discharged and followed as an outpatient for 6 weeks. Oral antibiotics are discontinued after the third week of therapy. An interval appendectomy is subsequently performed in all patients to prevent a recurrence of appendicitis with perforation and generalized peritonitis.

Occasionally, a well-defined abscess cavity can be drained extraperitoneally without a primary appendectomy. A second operation for appendectomy through a clean field 6 weeks following the drainage procedure is indicated. This is an unusual regimen and is generally reserved for elderly septic patients.

A normal-appearing appendix at the time of laparotomy warrants further intra-abdominal inspection. This includes examination of the distal 3 feet of terminal ileum for evidence of inflammatory bowel disease or, in rare instances, Meckel's diverticulitis. In older patients, right colon diverticular disease is a possibility. In females, even in the pre-adolescent age group, the pelvis, ovaries, and fallopian tubes must be examined for cysts, torsion, or inflammation. In most children, a medial extension of the transverse incision suffices; however, in adults, it is preferable to close the limited right lower quadrant incision and proceed with a second, vertical midline approach.

Even with proper preoperative assessment and observation, a normal appendix is found at laparotomy in approximately 10 to 15 percent of cases. Other diseases can closely mimic the signs and symptoms of acute appendicitis and result in a "false-positive" preoperative diagnosis. Certain systemic diseases, such as Henoch-Schoenlein purpura, hemolytic uremic syndrome, nephrotic syndrome with primary peritonitis, sickle cell disease, diabetic ketoacidosis, and the so-called right lower quadrant syndrome that occurs in the immuno-incompetent patient, can all produce right lower quadrant pain and tenderness. Consideration of these entities in the appropriate patient could prevent an unnecessary operation.

COMPLICATIONS

The most common complications of acute appendicitis are intra-abdominal or wound infections. Wound infections are more common in adult patients with or without a preceding appendiceal perforation. Localized increased wound pain, induration, and erythema herald the underlying, usually subcutaneous, abscess. Sutures should be removed from the suspected wound, which should be opened to facilitate drainage and early healing by second intention. Intra-abdominal abscess should be suspected following surgery for appendiceal perforation if the patient develops temperature spikes, mucous diarrhea, and abdominal pain and/or tenderness. Physical examination, particularly the digital rectal examination, can be diagnostic. More obscure symptoms or a normal physical examination warrant an abdominal sonographic or computerized tomographic study for evaluation. I routinely perform a rectal examination in these patients, even if they are asymptomatic, just before they are discharged from the hospital. Children in particular can have indolent lesions that are palpable only as an induration of the rectal wall, then become clinically apparent as an abscess after hospital discharge. Transvaginal or rectal drainage of an abscess is performed only when the abscess is about to rupture spontaneously, both to avoid the inadvertent transgression of an intervening loop of intestine and to reduce the bleeding of an incised immature phlegmon. Postoperative intra-abdominal abscesses should be drained extraperitoneally, if possible.

Prolonged postoperative ileus and an occasional early bowel obstruction are treated by nasogastric decompression, usually without long, small bowel tubes. Parenteral nutrition should be instituted after 5 to 7 days in most patients with prolonged ileus, but even earlier in the debilitated or young patient.

Appendicitis is no longer the "killer" it once was, but morbidity is still high among patients who suffer appendiceal perforation.

HEMORRHOIDS

WILLIAM A. WALKER, M.D.
STANLEY M. GOLDBERG, M.D., F.A.C.S.

Although a number of definitions of hemorrhoids have been proposed over centuries, current understanding of anorectal anatomy and physiology indicates that hemorrhoids are composed of multiple elements, not just dilated venules. These elements include venous sinuses, arterioles, smooth muscle, and connective tissues that comprise the anal cushions. The classic positions for these cushions are right anterior, right posterior, and left lateral, although variations are common. Redundancy of tissue formed by these cushions allows the anal canal to accommodate the passage of feces without tearing. These cushions also contribute to continence by aiding in a complete closure of the anal canal. These anal cushions are normal and should be preserved.

When increased straining occurs, most commonly because of the hard stool seen with the constipating low fiber diet common to the western world, these cushions become engorged and stretched, allowing a gradual elongation and dilation of the hemorrhoidal tissue which finally results in prolapse or symptomatic hemorrhoidal disease. This situation is exacerbated by a concurrent descent of the rectal mucosa in many cases. In addition to hard stool, other contributing factors include heredity, obstruction of venous outflow (pregnancy or portal hypertension), anal stenosis, and diarrheal states. Undoubtedly the gradual degeneration of connective tissue seen with increasing age plays a role in the development of symptomatic hemorrhoidal disease.

Hemorrhoids are a normal part of every anal canal and are significant *only* when symptomatic. There certainly exists a population of individuals who have what appear to be significant hemorrhoids, but who are completely asymptomatic. These individuals require no therapy. Likewise, there is a large group of patients who present with bleeding, pain, prolapse, pruritus, and discharge who do require therapy of their hemorrhoidal disease.

DIAGNOSIS AND CLASSIFICATION

Patients who complain of "hemorrhoids" may actually be suffering from other lesions, and the presence of other disorders should be excluded. Patients should be specifically questioned regarding the exact details of their symptoms. This will allow differentiation of other disorders such as rectal mucosal prolapse, hypertrophied anal papillae, skin tags, condyloma, fissure, fistula, polyp, or neoplasm. Fleeting anal pain is also seen with levator ani muscle spasm in the proctalgia fugax syndrome.

Examination of the patient who complains of hemorrhoidal symptoms requires excellent lighting and the use of a proctoscopy table. The principles of physical diagnosis should be adhered to, including inspection and palpation. These simple techniques can often reveal the presence of anal fissure, which would cause bleeding or pain, or a fistula, which might cause discharge. Following inspection and digital examination, the anus is examined with the anoscope. The David modification of the Ives anoscope is a small, comfortable anoscope that allows adequate examination even in the most apprehensive patient. After the anoscope is introduced, the patient is asked to strain, push, or bear down so that rectal mucosal prolapse and the magnitude of the hemorrhoids can be evaluated. In evaluating any patient who complains of hemorrhoidal disease, the distal colon should also be examined, preferably with a flexible proctosigmoidoscope. Any symptoms that are not absolutely attributable to hemorrhoidal disease demand complete evaluation of the colon, either by air-contrast barium enema or total colonoscopy.

Once the presence of hemorrhoidal disease has been established, a classification of the degree of hemorrhoids is necessary to provide consistent therapy and evaluation. Initially, internal and external hemorrhoids must be differentiated. External hemorrhoids are derived from the external hemorrhoidal plexus and drain into the systemic venous circulation. These hemorrhoids are most often located at or distal to the anal verge. External hemorrhoids almost always present with acute thrombosis. Bleeding is rare unless rupture occurs. Skin tags are the sequelae of thrombosed external hemorrhoids. Internal hemorrhoids are derived from the normal anal cushion and drain via the portal venous system. Internal hemorrhoids present with bleeding that is usually painless and, rarely, anal pain. Asymptomatic hemorrhoids are also commonly associated with thrombosis or prolapse. The classification of internal hemorrhoids is based on these symptoms. First-degree hemorrhoids are characterized by painless, bright red bleeding, usually with a bowel movement. When seen through the anoscope, they bulge into the lumen slightly. Second-degree hemorrhoids prolapse beyond the anal verge with straining or defecation, but spontaneously reduce. Third-degree hemorrhoids prolapse with straining, but must be manually reduced. Fourth-degree hemorrhoids cannot be reduced and are permanently prolapsed.

OFFICE MANAGEMENT OF HEMORRHOIDS

The vast majority of patients suffering from hemorrhoids can be managed without operation. The mode of treatment in these patients is determined by the degree of hemorrhoidal disease. Simple first-degree hemorrhoids, characterized by painless bleeding, can often be managed with dietary measures alone. This consists of increasing the amount of fiber in the diet, usually by adding one-third to one-half cup of raw unprocessed bran to the diet daily. For patients who have persistently hard stools, a lubricating suppository may also be beneficial. The use of hydrocortisone ointments, suppositories, or over-the-counter ointments or suppositories is not indicated. In the occasional case in which the patient continues to have bright red blood after being on an adequate diet, these small first-degree hemorrhoids can be treated by either sclerotherapy or rubber band ligation. For first-degree hemorrhoids, however, this should only be done after an adequate trial of dietary manipulation. Sclerotherapy is accomplished by injecting 3 to 5 ml of a solution of 5% phenol in vegetable oil into the submucosa directly above the hemorrhoids. This causes submucosal scarring with obliteration of the bleeding site. Sclerotherapy is reserved for patients with minimal redundancy of the hemorrhoidal tissue, a condition that could make rubber banding difficult. For patients with sufficient tissue for the application of a rubber band, the rubber banding technique is employed.

The patient who presents with uncomplicated bleeding hemorrhoids of the second and third degree is an ideal candidate for rubber banding. Fissure or other causes of pain or bleeding *must* be excluded prior to the application of the rubber bands. The patient is placed in the knee-chest position on the proctoscopy table and the Hinkel-James anoscope introduced. This anoscope allows access to the rectal mucosa above the hemorrhoidal tissue. The redundant rectal mucosa above the hemorrhoid is grasped with forceps, and at this time, should the patient complain of any discomfort, the forceps should be moved higher in the anal canal. This will prevent inclusion of somatically innervated anoderm in the rubber band, which causes intense pain. The hemorrhoid itself is not included in the rubber band since the pathophysiology of hemorrhoid disease is based on the concept of prolapse rather than enlargement of the hemorrhoidal plexus. The most redundant segment is chosen for the application of the rubber bands, and two rubber bands are simultaneously applied with the banding gun (Fig. 1). Should significant redundancy exist elsewhere, multiple bands may be employed. The patient may complain of an aching sensation, and this can be resolved by injection of a local anesthetic in the pedicle formed by the rubber bands. The

patient is asked to return in 6 to 8 weeks, at which time the anal canal is reinspected and further quadrants banded if indicated. Up to six to eight banding sessions may be required for the complete resolution of symptoms. Banding should be continued until all symptoms disappear.

Several other modalities have been advocated in the treatment of hemorrhoidal disease. These include cryotherapy, infrared photocoagulation, laser therapy, sphincterotomy, and forceful dilation of the anal canal. Although sclerotherapy is occasionally useful, its lack of precise control makes it less attractive than rubber banding. Cryotherapy no longer has a place in the treatment of hemorrhoidal disease. This technique is characterized by prolonged wound healing with a foul smelling discharge and is in no way better than rubber banding. Although infrared photocoagulation of hemorrhoids has been accomplished elsewhere, this technique is no more effective than rubber banding and adds substantial equipment costs. Sphincterotomy is performed only in the presence of a concomitant fissure. It is of no use for the treatment of hemorrhoids alone. Dilation of the anal canal is practiced by Mr. Lord in Great Britain, but has not been successful in other practitioners' hands. Although lasers have been utilized in many areas of medicine, treatment of hemorrhoids with laser therapy results in an open wound similar to that of cryotherapy, and its use should not be continued. Although banding is preferable, it is certainly not without complications. Instances of bleeding occur with the slough of tissue, especially in patients who have been taking aspirin or other anticoagulants. Rare instances in which infection results in a fulminant perineal gangrene have been reported. Any patient who complains of pain following rubber banding should be examined without delay to ensure that infection is not developing. Occasionally, banding may precipitate thrombosis, which also causes pain. This may require formal hemorrhoidectomy as an emergency procedure. Rubber banding has no role in the therapy of external hemorrhoids.

Patients who present with symptoms of hemorrhoidal disease and who are found to have thrombosed external hemorrhoids fall into two groups: those who present between 1 and 4 days after the onset of pain and those who present after 4 days. Should the patient present with an acute episode within 4 days of onset, excision is the preferred method of therapy for external hemorrhoids. This includes an ellipse of skin overlying the external hemorrhoid so that the entire venous plexus is excised. Simple incision and drainage of a thrombosed external hemorrhoid is often ineffective because multiple channels become thrombosed. The patient is placed in the knee-chest position on the proctoscopy table, and local anesthetic (1% lidocaine with epinephrine) is injected. A very slow injection through a 30-gauge needle results in a nearly painless induction of local anesthesia in most cases. One should remember that about 5 minutes must elapse before the full effect of the epinephrine and local anesthetic is realized. Once the thrombosed hemorrhoid has been excised, cautery can be employed to stop small bleeders in the submucosa. A sufficient amount of skin should be excised to prevent premature closure. If any

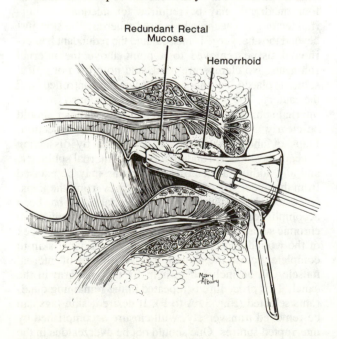

Redundant Rectal
Mucosa

Hemorrhoid

Figure 1 Rubber banding technique

question exists as to the extent of the thrombosis, which might result in the need for a more extensive procedure, the patient might better be handled in an outpatient surgical suite or operating room.

Should the patient present after 4 days, conservative therapy should be employed consisting of sitz baths, bulk agents, and nonconstipating analgesics (Fig. 2).

Occasionally, a patient may present in whom the hemorrhoid has become acutely ulcerated due to necrosis of the overlying skin with spontaneous drainage of the clot. Should this be the patient's first episode of external hemorrhoidal disease (without pain at the time of the visit), no further therapy is required. However, should the patient relate recurrent symptoms of external hemorrhoidal disease, excision of the skin surrounding the open external hemorrhoid and debridement of the base may prevent future recurrence.

OPERATIVE THERAPY

Hemorrhoids requiring operative management are characterized by pain, prolapse that has failed to respond to banding, and persistent bleeding that has also failed to respond to banding. Occasionally, prolapse with acute thrombosis and necrosis may occur, also necessitating hemorrhoidectomy.

The preoperative evaluation of the patient should be the same as that of patients who are seen in the outpatient setting. Concomitant processes such as fistulas or fissures should be ruled out, and patients should undergo flexible proctosigmoidoscopy. Any patient with other than classic hemorrhoidal symptoms requires a more thorough evaluation of the colon. Extreme caution should be used in selecting for operative hemorrhoidectomy patients who suffer from incontinence, diarrhea, or Crohn's disease or patients who are elderly. Operative hemorrhoidectomy in these patients may lead to unacceptable complications (particularly incontinence) and every effort should be made to avoid operative therapy of their hemorrhoidal disease. Occasionally, rectal prolapse may confuse the unwary examiner and lead to a needless anesthetic and

potential operative complication. Prolapse of the rectum can be distinguished from hemorrhoidal disease by the presence of concentric rather than radial folds in the tissue.

In the acute setting of prolapsed, thrombosed, and perhaps strangulated hemorrhoids, the patient should be immediately admitted and prepared for surgery. There is no place for conservative therapy in such cases. Suppositories are contraindicated. Endoscopic examination can be deferred until the time of surgery or postoperatively because of the acute pain and discomfort suffered by these patients. Similarly, enemas are not necessary.

Ordinarily, the patient is admitted on the morning of surgery and taken to the operating room where he will be placed in a prone jackknife position with a roll beneath his iliac crest. A moderate degree of Trendelenberg position aids visualization of the anal canal. Similarly, a headlight provides excellent illumination of the canal. The patient should not be shaved since this merely induces itching in the postoperative period and serves no purpose in aiding surgery. The patient should have received one prepackaged enema prior to being taken to the operating room.

Local anesthesia is preferred. Marcaine (0.25%) with 1:200,000 epinephrine is used, and this can be supplemented with lidocaine if the patient suffers undue discomfort during the injection of Marcaine. Similarly, elective use of diazepam as an adjunct is useful in many patients. Should the patient refuse local anesthesia, either regional anesthesia or general anesthesia is acceptable.

With the buttocks taped apart, the anal area is prepped with povidone-iodine. No dilation of the anal canal is performed. A Pratt bivalve or Fansler operating anoscope is introduced to examine the anal canal and select the quadrants for hemorrhoidectomy. Usually the left lateral, right anterior, and right posterior quadrants are selected. This is variable and sometimes only two or as many as four quadrants may be required for adequate hemorrhoidectomy. A technique is used whereby the skin just beyond the anal verge is incised, and the redundant hemorrhoidal tissue removed to a point above the internal sphincter. No clamps are used, and no crown or apical suture is placed. Submucosal bleeders are controlled with the cautery. The hemorrhoidal tissue is removed from the internal sphincter muscle. The internal sphincter should be clearly evident on the completion of the dissection. Flaps of anoderm should be developed by dissecting beneath the anoderm and on top of the internal sphincter, and any additional hemorrhoidal tissue may be excised from the underside of the anoderm by everting the flaps. Once complete removal of hemorrhoidal tissue has been accomplished, the wound is closed with a running 3–0 chromic suture on a taper-cut needle, beginning at the apex of the wound and continuing out to the perianal skin to completely close the wound. The small bites of internal muscle can be included to help fix the anoderm in the canal. This procedure is repeated in the remaining quadrants selected (Fig. 3, A to F). If desired, skin tags can be removed transversely, with closure accomplished by interrupted sutures. One should not be overzealous in the removal of these skin tags, however, since they may

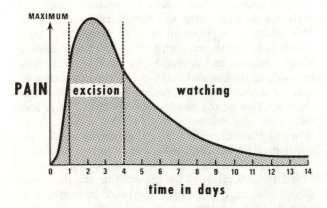

Figure 2 Pain levels with thrombosed hemorrhoids, both within 4 days of onset (*excision*) and beyond that point (*watching*)

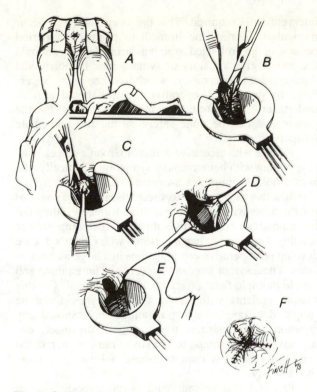

Figure 3 Surgical hemorrhoidectomy (see text)

contribute to the accommodation of stool during defecation. Similarly, anoderm should be preserved to prevent anal stenosis. This is easily accomplished when using the Fansler anoscope, which maintains a constant diameter of 3.5 centimeters.

Usually the most prominent hemorrhoid is excised first to allow a better estimation of the amount of anoderm remaining. Should any question of the amount of anoderm remaining exist, hemorrhoids may be removed by making a simple incision over the hemorrhoid and then excising the hemorrhoidal plexus beneath the anoderm, thus preserving the anoderm present.

In the case of acutely prolapsed and thrombosed hemorrhoids, which may be strangulated, the procedure is begun with the largest hemorrhoid first and then continued to subsequent regions in order of decreasing size. This approach results in preservation of anoderm and complete removal of thrombosed hemorrhoidal tissue without compromising the width of the anal canal.

On completion of the hemorrhoidectomy, the anal area is cleaned, but no packing or dressing is applied. A

TABLE 1 Tenets of Hemorrhoidectomy

No shaving
No dilation
No clamp
No crown or apical stitch
No packing or dressing
No open wound

final inspection of the suture lines is made, and should any residual bleeding be present, this is easily controlled with simple figure-of-8 stitches. This is rarely a problem, however, if adequate hemostasis is obtained with a cautery during the initial dissection. By performing a completely open dissection with the patient in the prone position, one avoids inadvertent injury to the external or internal sphincter and is assured complete visualization of the procedure. This prevents excessive excision of anoderm, which may result in anal ectropion or anal stenosis. The tenets of hemorrhoidectomy are listed in Table 1.

Should the hemorrhoidal disease be complicated by the presence of an anal fissure, a left lateral sphincterotomy can be accomplished while the left lateral hemorrhoidal mass is being removed. This in no way requires any adaptation or alteration of the technique previously described. Should a degree of anal stenosis be present, similar division of the fiberotic band can be accomplished in the same quadrant. At no time, however, should the anal canal be forcefully dilated.

At the completion of the procedure, no packing or other dressing is required. Throughout the case, the administration of intravenous fluids should have been limited to 100 ml or less. This contributes greatly to the prevention of postoperative urinary retention. For the same purpose, intravenous fluids are discontinued in the recovery room. A regimen of high fiber diet and psyllium seed is begun immediately postoperatively. Sitz baths are taken at the patient's discretion. Narcotic analgesics may be required for the first 24 to 48 hours, but on discharge the patient is supplied with a non-narcotic analgesic to prevent constipation. Should the patient fail to have a bowel movement by the third postoperative day, a prepackaged enema is generally administered, and the patient is then discharged wtih instructions to return to the office in 2 weeks for the routine postoperative examination.

Complications following closed hemorrhoidectomy have not been significant. Table 2 lists complications observed in 500 consecutive closed hemorrhoidectomies. Bleeding, which occurred in 4 percent of these cases, usually is noted about the tenth postoperative day and usually is minor. However, should any question as to the

TABLE 2 Complications Following 500 Consecutive Closed Hemorrhoidectomies

Complication	% of Cases
Abscess formation	0.0
Fistula-in-ano	0.4
Anal fissure	0.2
Anal stenosis	1.0
Incontinence	0.4
Skin tags	6.0
Fecal impaction	0.4
Thrombosed external hemorrhoid	0.2
Acute urinary retention	10.0
Bleeding	4.0

TABLE 3 Suggested Plan of Hemorrhoid Management

Extent of Disease	Treatment
First-degree hemorrhoids	
Asymptomatic	No treatment
Symptomatic	Exclusion of other causes of bleeding, high fiber diet, rubber band ligation, sclerotherapy
Second-degree hemorrhoids	Rubber band ligation
Third-degree hemorrhoids	Rubber band ligation, closed hemorrhoidectomy
Fourth-degree hemorrhoids	Closed hemorrhoidectomy
Prolapsed strangulated hemorrhoids	Emergency closed hemorrhoidectomy
Thrombosed external hemorrhoids	
Painful	Excise: local anesthesia
Painless	Observe
Perianal skin tags	Excise under local anesthesia if symptomatic
Hypertrophied anal papillae	
Asymptomatic	No treatment
Symptomatic	Excise

magnitude of the bleeding exist, the patient should be admitted for observation and bed rest. In the vast majority of cases, the bleeding stops spontaneously, and no further therapy is required. Occasionally, however, the patient continues to bleed and has to be returned to the operating room for identification and suture-ligation of the bleeder. Abscess formation does not seem to be a problem. Fistula and fissure formation may occur and may require therapy if symptomatic. If skin tags are observed postoperatively and are symptomatic, they can be removed under local anesthesia in the office at the convenience of the patient and the surgeon. Once again, however, care should be taken to minimize removal of anodermal and perianal skin since some redundancy is necessary to accommodate the passage of stool. A rational plan for the management of hemorrhoidal disease is presented in Table 3.

SPECIAL CASES

Occasionally, hemorrhoidal disease occurs simultaneously with pregnancy, inflammatory bowel disease, portal hypertension, leukemia, or lymphoma, or combined with other disease processes such as fissure or fistula.

Hemorrhoidal symptoms occurring during pregnancy can be treated conservatively unless the hemorrhoids prolapse and thrombose acutely, in which case operative intervention is required. This has been known to occur particularly during the immediate postpartum period because of the prolonged straining during delivery. Should the patient give a history of symptomatic hemorrhoidal disease prior to pregnancy, which has then been exacerbated by pregnancy, operative therapy should also be undertaken. This provides considerable relief for the patient and can be done safely during the immediate postpartum period.

Patients with ulcerative colitis or Crohn's disease may also present with hemorrhoidal symptoms. Typically, the hemorrhoidal symptoms are made much worse by the diarrhea that is common to these diseases. It is safe to treat patients with ulcerative colitis surgically if they fail to respond to conservative therapy, including rubber banding. On the other hand, patient's with Crohn's disease develop postoperative complications in a large number of cases. These symptoms can be severe and unremitting and lead to multiple fistula tracks which fail to heal. For this reason, patients with Crohn's disease should not be subjected to operative hemorrhoidectomy. Should any question exist regarding the diagnosis, the most conservative therapy should be employed rather than risk the complications of Crohn's disease following hemorrhoidectomy.

Patients who present with portal hypertension in hemorrhoidal disease should also be managed conservatively. Should their symptoms become intolerable or should marked bleeding occur, they are best managed by simple oversewing of the hemorrhoidal plexus. Should any question exist as to the magnitude of the procedure, careful preoperative evaluation regarding coagulation status and the status of liver function should be determined. In patients with cirrhosis and poor liver function, local anesthesia is preferred.

Patients with leukemia or lymphoma or other patients who are immunosuppressed represent a population at high risk for complications following hemorrhoidectomy. The compromised status of the immune system can lead to fulminant and life-threatening infection. Occasionally, what is felt to be hemorrhoidal disease may actually represent local leukemic or lymphomatous infiltration, and operative excision of these lesions can lead to severe complications with infection and nonhealing wounds. Should the patient present with acute strangulated hemorrhoids, however, the best course is operative removal since debridement of the necrotic tissue, establishing a clean wound, is more conducive to proper wound healing.

When patients with hemorrhoidal disease present with fissure or fistula, the addition of fistulotomy or internal sphincterotomy does not significantly increase the morbidity of the procedure.

ANAL FISSURE, ANORECTAL ABSCESS, AND FISTULA-IN-ANO

RONALD H. FISHBEIN, M.D.

ANAL FISSURE

Anal fissure is a common condition for which the symptoms of pain and discomfort would appear to be out of proportion to the anatomic disturbance noted on physical examination. In or near the posterior midline, one may find a superficial split in the anoderm below the level of the pectinate line. This longitudinal crack in the tissues is only rarely found on the lateral or anterior wall of the canal. It is not likely to heal spontaneously and, in some individuals, tends to recur in spite of treatment. If measures are not taken early to effect a cure, the fissure will deepen to expose the lower fibers of the internal sphincter muscle. Often a sentinal tag or reddened nodule of skin develops at the lower end of the fissure, and this is painful and tender.

Whether this spectrum of acute superficial to chronic deep fissure is, in every case, the result of sudden distention of the anal canal by a bulky stool is difficult to document. Trauma would seem to be responsible in most cases. Although a fissure may be accompanied by the passage of small quantities of bright red blood, it is the symptom of pain that makes the condition unbearable. The pain is due in part to the general sensitivity of the area and in part to the phenomenon of sphincter spasm, which agonizingly follows each evacuation.

In its early stages, when the disruption of the anoderm is superficial, simple measures may suffice to cure the condition. Strategies directed at relieving constipation by softening and increasing the bulk of the stool have been helpful. The employment of high fiber diet supplemented by a psyllium seed product and a prodigious daily fluid intake is appropriate. Although much has been written recommending manual forceful dilation of the anal sphincter under anaesthesia, most authors would agree that this form of uncontrolled trauma often damages the sphincteric mechanism and may result in permanent partial incontinence. Contrasted with a traumatizing 6- to 8-fingerbreadth dilation masked by an anesthetic, the gentle, gradual introduction of index and middle fingers into the well-lubricated anal canal for 2 to 3 minutes often relieves the spasm of an acute fissure. Combined with the use of a proprietary topical anesthetic ointment and stool softening agents, daily dilation by physician or patient usually results in gradual relief and healing.

Because sphincter spasm is so universally thought to perpetuate the course of anal fissure, interruption of the spasm by sphincterotomy, with or without debridement of the chronic wound, is considered appropriate. Before one proceeds with the surgical correction of a medically unresponsive anal fissure, care must be taken to rule out other more specific causes of anal fissure or ulceration. Inflammatory bowel disease, anal malignant disease, tuberculosis, or syphilis may cause fissures that mimic the more common post-traumatic variety.

After local, regional, or general anesthesia is administered and with the patient positioned in dorsal lithotomy or prone jack-knife position, a posterior partial internal sphincterotomy may be performed. The edges of the fissure are trimmed or curetted, the sentinal tag excised, and through the base of the wound the lowest portion of the internal sphincter muscle fibers are sharply divided. Several milliliters of 0.5% bupivacaine are injected into the surrounding tissue to take advantage of its long-acting anesthetic effect.

Although satisfactory relief of pain and a low incidence of recurrent anal fissure may be anticipated by this operation, the occasional occurrence of moderate degrees of perineal soilage following the operation may render it undesirable. The cause of this soilage is thought to be a cleft that develops at the site after healing. Commonly referred to as a "key-hole deformity," it sabotages the best efforts of the sphincteric mechanism by allowing gas and liquid to escape.

Less likely to lead to this unpleasant sequela is the lateral subcutaneous sphincterotomy, an operation of no greater magnitude than a posterior sphincterotomy. After the anesthetic of choice is administered and with the patient in the dorsal lithotomy position, the intersphincteric groove is palpated, usually on the left side of the anal orifice. This groove marks the interval between the lower border of the internal sphincter and the inner rim of the subcutaneous portion of the external sphincter. A short incision, perhaps only 0.5 cm, is performed. An unopened straight clamp is bluntly introduced into the wound approximately 2 cm between the layers of internal and external sphincter muscles. Once this is achieved, the clamp is removed and a narrow scalpel blade is introduced with the cutting edge facing the lumen of the anal canal. With the index finger of the other hand within the anus and serving as a guide, the fibers of the lower portion of the internal sphincter are divided. Care is taken to withdraw the scalpel blade before inadvertently incising the anoderm. The tip of the index finger that has served as a guide is now used to place pressure against the lateral wall of the canal to prevent hematoma formation. The skin incision is then loosely approximated with a single absorbable suture. One may debride the posterior fissure and trim the sentinal pile.

ANORECTAL ABSCESS

Anorectal abscesses are thought generally to have their origins within the crypts of Morgagni at the dentate line, for it is there that the mucous-secreting anal glands are located. Opening into the depths of the crypts, these mucosa-lined compound glands arborize, sending branches across the submucosa and through the smooth muscle bundles of the internal sphincter. It has been postulated that particulate matter lodging in a crypt may lead to inflammation and cryptitis, with development of a cryptoglandular abscess. In this manner, a microabscess is conducted through the rectal wall, where it expands and further develops within the intersphincteric plane. With the passage of time, an intersphincteric abscess is capable of extending along one or more avenues cephalad, caudad, laterally, or circumferentially. With this tendency to extend along natural planes or directly through vital structures, tissue necrosis proceeds until the abscess is properly drained.

Though prompt treatment is indicated when a diagnosis of anorectal abscess is established, certain caveats are to be observed. Sepsis in the perineum may also be caused by inflammatory bowel disease, tuberculosis, venereal diseases, suppurative hydradenitis, sacrococcygeal pilonidal disease, periurethral abscess secondary to urethral stricture, Bartholin's gland abscess, anal gland carcinoma, and trauma. It is also important to provide adequate anesthesia to ensure proper drainage while avoiding injury to critical structures. Finally, it is essential that the three-dimensional anatomy of the region be thoroughly understood since edema and the mass effect of an abscess can distort ordinarily familiar landmarks.

A cryptoglandular abscess, having penetrated the internal sphincter, may descend to the fibrofatty tissue and there expand to appear as a painful, erythematous mass at the anal verge, the common perianal abscess. A second pathway for a primal intersphincteric infection is to continue laterally through the longitudinal muscle fibers as well as the deeper portion of the external sphincter to enter an ischiorectal fossa. Here it may expand enormously and even travel posteriorly around the rectum to invade the contralateral ischiorectal fossa. Pain, tenderness, and a more diffuse swelling to one or both sides of the anal verge is characteristic.

Immediately prior to operation, the administration of antibiotics is advisable to protect against the inevitable bacteremia that follows surgical manipulation. A broadly effective cephalosporin as well as a penicillin is indicated. Although the use of local anesthesia may be tempting, the patient's comfort is best served by regional or general anesthesia. Following the induction of anesthesia, the patient should be placed in the dorsal lithotomy position and a speculum examination of the anorectal canal performed. The internal opening of the abscess may be visible, making treatment of an anticipated fistula possible. an incision is then made directly into the mass beside the anal orifice. After it is drained, the cavity is gently but thoroughly explored. It is this assessment that allows one to distinguish a simple perianal abscess from a unilateral ischiorectal or even a bilateral ischiorectal horseshoe abscess. The latter also requires a contralateral incision. If the internal orifice has been identified and the abscess cavity is relatively small, the intervening anoderm, sphincter, and skin may be cleanly incised. This should destroy the diseased crypt and prevent the subsequent development of a chronic fistula-in-ano. It is generally believed that in one-third to one-half of all cases of drained anorectal abscesses, the cavity will shrink to a narrow chronically discharging tract between the internal orifice and the perineal skin, a fistula-in-ano.

An abscess that has originated in an anal gland at the dentate line may dissect beneath the mucosa to form a submucosal accumulation. However, it may ascend the intersphincteric plane and develop into a mature abscess between the inner circular and outer longitudinal muscle coats of the rectum. Deep rectal pain, fever, chills, and painful evacuation without an external mass or tenderness may be the presentation of a submucosal or high intermuscular abscess. If spontaneous drainage of pus per anum has not already occurred, digital examination discloses the characteristic painful mass in the wall of the rectum. With optimal anesthesia, exposure, and lighting, the mass is first aspirated with syringe and needle. Once pus is recovered, a scalpel or cautery is used to further evacuate the cavity. A small Penrose drain is inserted into the interior, secured with an absorbable suture to the cut edge of the mucosa, and the free end led through the anal orifice.

An infrequently encountered abscess is one that develops above the levator muscles. Whether originating from an abdominopelvic source or by extension from an originally intersphincteric location, the pelvirectal abscess may defy identification. Occasionally a transabdominal exploration is necessary for localization and evacuation and to establish the etiology. A pelvirectal abscess otherwise may be discovered in the course of drainage of an ischiorectal abscess that has intruded on the supralevator space. A generously sized drain should be inserted to guard against premature closure of the surgical wound.

FISTULA-IN-ANO

In more than 90 percent of cases of suppurative anorectal disease, fistula-in-ano represents the chronic residual of an acute abscess. Perhaps because of the ease with which a serious and permanent injury can be caused by imprecise surgical treatment, the literature on the subject of fistula-in-ano has focused on the spatial relationships between the various types of fistula and the normal anorectal anatomy. Historically, descriptive classifications of the pathways taken by suppuratively induced fistulas seem to eclipse the accounts of surgical techniques for cure. As with anorectal abscesses, already described, a fistula-in-ano usually originates in an anal crypt and terminates at one or more locations in the perianal area. Between these points, a simple direct pathway or a circuitous route may develop. The track may traverse only the subcutaneous tissues or it may pass through the circular sphincteric mechanism, either low or high within the anal canal, before emerging on the skin of the perineum. The fistula may pursue a circumferential course from the involved crypt to gain access to either or both ischiorectal fossae before necessitating through the perianal skin. A fistula may be complex, with secondary offshoots ending blindly in the perirectal tissues. Rarely, a fistulous track ascends outside the anorectal ring.

At the time of examination, one-third of all fistulas-in-ano would appear to lack an internal opening while often the point of emergence on the perineal skin appears only as a nodule of granulation tissue. An untreated fistula is prone to develop into a recurrent acute anorectal abscess or, rarely, a squamous cell carcinoma. A fistula-in-ano may result from or be confused with a number of inflammatory or infectious conditions already mentioned in the discussion of anorectal abscess. Once the etiology of the fistula is understood, operative treatment should follow. Should chronic ulcerative colitis or Crohn's disease be responsible for a fistula, the appropriate medical or surgical therapy directed at the control of the inflammatory bowel disease is primarily indicated. If the more common cryptoglandular infection is the basis for the fistula, an operation should be planned which would either unroof or totally excise the entire track with its ramifications.

Nothing less than complete familiarity with the anatomy of the anorectum will ensure safety for the patient. This must be supplemented with a careful examination and assessment under regional or general anesthesia prior to starting the operation. A thorough search for the internal orifice of the fistula should be made. The tissues must be palpated in an attempt to locate the induration associated with a chronic track or an undrained septic focus. The anorectal ring should be identified. It is the palpable junction of the puborectalis sling with the upper borders of the internal and external sphincters. The anorectal ring is recognizable through the lateral and posterior walls of the anorectum. It must be remembered that division of the anorectal ring in the course of treating a high fistula causes a disasterous loss of fecal and gas control. Also, simultaneous division of the internal and external sphincters at more than one location leads to a profound and lasting incontinence.

Following administration of the anesthetic, the anal sphincter is dilated. To establish the course of the fistulous track, several drops of methylene blue in 4 or 5 cc of hydrogen peroxide, injected with a blunt needle through the external orifice, usually identifies the internal opening. A malleable probe or grooved director may then be inserted. By means of a scalpel or electrocautery, the overlying bridge of tissue is incised. As the fibrous tube of the chronic fistula is approached, a decision should be made whether to excise the entire structure or to simply incise into the track. The choice is determined by the complexity of the course that the fistula takes. If simply a fistulotomy is performed, the granulation tissue lining the track should be curetted and submitted for microscopic examination. If an internal opening is not found, the track should be traced as close to the pectinate line as possible. Side branches must be exposed and excised or unroofed. Multiple external orifices require probing and must be connected with one another by incising the intervening bridges of skin and subcutis. It may be necessary to excise a narrow strip of skin to prevent premature closure of the wounds. In the case of a posterior horseshoe fistula, the internal opening is usually found to one side of the posterior midline at the level of the crypts. After connecting the internal and ipsilateral external openings with an incision across the sphincter muscles, the external orifices are connected by an incision outside the margin of the external sphincter.

Whether fistulotomy or fistulectomy is selected, the resulting wounds may be treated by allowing them to granulate while assiduously cleansing the wounds daily and inserting a light gauze wick. However, a simple direct track may be totally excised, following which the sphincterotomy may be repaired and the wound sutured and allowed to heal per primum.

ANAL STRICTURE (STENOSIS)

HERAND ABCARIAN, M.D.

Anal stricture or stenosis is among the most common anorectal conditions encountered by physicians and surgeons. Anal stricture (i.e., abnormal narrowing) may be due to intrinsic or extrinsic causes. Each of these major groups can be classified into benign or malignant conditions (Table 1).

Benign intrinsic lesions are most common. Congenital anomalies, when mild and left untreated or, as in the case of low imperforate anus, treated with "cut-back" procedure, often lead to anal stricture in adult life. Inflammatory causes of stricture include ulcerative colitis and, especially, Crohn's disease. Crohn's strictures may occur in 5 to 10 percent of patients with this disease. Tuberculosis, actinomycosis, lymphogranuloma venereum, amebiasis, and other rare diseases can produce anal stricture in advanced cases. Disuse strictures are normally due to long-term use of oil or saline laxatives; the resultant liquid stools preclude normal dilation of the anal canal and gradual anal stenosis follows. Trauma, especially due to prior anorectal surgery, may be the most common cause of all strictures. Anal stricture following hemorrhoidectomy occurs in 5 to 10 percent of patients postoperatively. In chronic neglected anal fissures, a low-lying anal stenosis can often be demonstrated even after the anal spasm is overcome with anesthesia. Circumferential suture lines secondary to coloanal or ileoanal anastomoses can result in stricture with an even higher incidence rate (10% to 20%). Strictures of the anal canal can also occur as a result of sepsis (extensive horseshoe fistula-in-ano). However, ischemic and radiation injuries of the anorectum usually result in stricture of the low or middle rectum rather than the anal canal.

Malignant intrinsic strictures are usually due to low-lying rectal or anal cancer, especially cloacogenic (basaloid) squamous cell cancers and melanomas.

TABLE 1 Etiology of Anal Strictures

Intrinsic (Common)
  Benign: congenital, inflammatory, disuse, trauma (post-
      hemorrhoidectomy), anal fissure, anal sepsis.
  Malignant
Extrinsic (Rare)
  Benign: endometriosis, pelvic abscess.
  Malignant: prostatic cancer.

Benign extrinsic lesions are fairly uncommon. Perianal and perineal endometriosis may lead to anal scarring and stenosis. Malignant extrinsic lesions are also rare and are usually due to circumferential encasement of the lower rectum by an aggressive prostatic cancer. These strictures are usually located just above the anal canal.

SYMPTOMS AND SIGNS

Most patients complain of constipation, need for laxatives, feeling of incomplete evacuation, and decrease in the caliber of stools. With increased straining, the patients complain of anal pain and bright red rectal bleeding.

Careful examination of the anorectum is usually diagnostic. If this is not possible owing to the patient's discomfort or resistance, examination under anesthesia should be planned both for diagnostic and therapeutic purposes. A small anoscope or proctosigmoidoscope (stricture scope) should be used to examine the entire stenosed segment. Any mucosal lesions of inflammatory or neoplastic origin should be subjected to biopsy. Occasionally, the definitive treatment can be performed at the same time. Obviously, in addition to examination and biopsy under anesthesia, other diagnostic modalities such as barium enema, CT scan, skin tests for tuberculosis and lymphogranuloma venereum (LGV), and complement fixation test for LGV and amebiasis can aid in diagnosing the rarer causes of anal stricture.

TREATMENT

The treatment of a stricture depends on the etiology, location, and extent of stenosis. Most short and low-lying strictures, which allow insertion of the examining finger and cause only mild symptoms, can be managed by placing the patient on a high fiber diet and laxatives. As long as soft stools pass comfortably through the stenosed segment, no surgery is necessary. However, severe strictures causing rectal pain and bleeding with each bowel movement may have to be operated on, and any attempt at continued conservative treatment only prolongs the patient's misery.

Nonoperative Treatment

The medical management of an anal stricture includes use of high bulk diet, psyllium products, detergents (di-

octyl sulfosuccinates), lactulose (Chronulac), or lubricant laxatives. Glycerine suppositories or even small quantities of saline or phosphate enemas may be helpful in urgent situations. Dilation of anorectal strictures can be performed digitally or by means of dilators such as Hegar's gynecologic dilators, Young's anal dilators, anoscopes, or stricture sigmoidoscopes. Dilation with the aid of a Foley balloon catheter has also been described.

By and large, the results of anal dilation, except for a small minority of cases, are disappointing. Anal dilation in the office is painful and results in splitting of the scar and the anoderm, and the subsequent healing by fibrosis causes further cicatrization and stenosis. Dilation under anesthesia, although painless at the time, results in a similar unfavorable outcome. As a rule, a definitive procedure must be done to correct the stenosis. Finally, not all anal stenoses need to be corrected either by dilation or by surgery. For example, in an elderly patient with longstanding cathartic abuse who has disuse anal stenosis, gradual deterioration of the sphincter mechanism may result in partial anal incontinence. Under these circumstances, a relative anal stenosis may act as protection for the individual, and dilation or anoplasty may result in worse functional results, i.e., total anal incontinence.

Surgical Management

The surgical procedure selected depends on the nature and extent of the anal stricture. The procedures will be discussed in order of increasing complexity.

Lateral Internal Sphincterotomy

This is the simplest method and is associated with a high success rate and few complications. It can be performed with no bowel preparation, under local anesthesia, and on an outpatient basis. It is most suitable for low-lying strictures, i.e., secondary to anal fissure, mucocutaneous strictures following hemorrhoidectomy, and strictures due to ileoanal or coloanal anastomosis. Briefly, the procedure consists of an incision in the lateral wall of the anal canal, beginning at the dentate line (mucocutaneous junction) and extending to 2 cm beyond the anal verge. This incision, of necessity, divides the scar tissue present in this area. The internal sphincter is then dissected free and its distal half (caudad to dentate line) is divided in its full thickness. The external sphincter is left undisturbed (Fig. 1).

Midline Sphincterotomy and Anoplasty

Indications for this procedure are the same as for lateral internal sphincterotomy. Actually, prior to the early 1970s, when lateral sphincterotomy was described by Notaras, midline sphincterotomy and anoplasty was the most commonly used procedure for anal fissure and stenosis. This operation also may be performed under local anesthesia and with no bowel preparation.

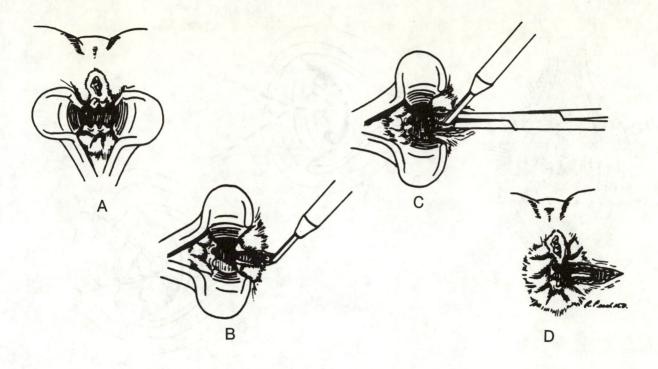

Figure 1 Lateral internal sphincterotomy: *A* Typical posterior midline fissure; *B* Incision of anoderm; *C* Division of the internal sphincter distal to the dentate line; *D* The completed procedure. The external sphincter is left undisturbed.

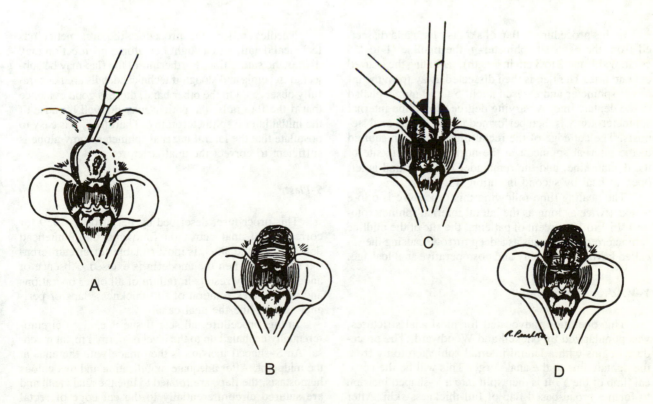

Figure 2 Midline sphincterotomy and anoplasty: *A* Posterior incision surrounding midline anal fissure; *B* The skin, including the fissure is excised just proximal to the dentate line; *C* Midline internal sphincterotomy to correct the stenosis; *D* Rectal mucosa sutured to the internal sphincter.

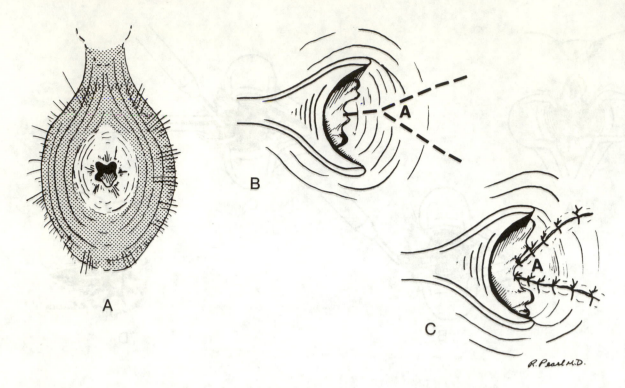

Figure 3   Y–V advancement flap: *A* Anal stricture; *B* Y-shaped incision in lateral anal wall; *C* Completed Y–V advancement flap.

In this procedure, a flap of skin is raised and dissected from the external sphincter in the midline (1 to 1.5 cm in width and 2 to 3 cm in length), including the scarred dentate line. The flap is then dissected away from the internal sphincter and excised about 5 to 10 mm cephalad to the dentate line. A varying degree of midline internal sphincterotomy is then performed to correct the anal stenosis. The cut edge of the rectal mucosa is then sutured to the internal sphincter at the normal anatomic site of the dentate line, and the remainder of the wound is left open to heal by second intention (Fig. 2).

The healing time following this procedure is 6 to 8 weeks (twice as long as the lateral internal sphincterotomy). In 5 to 10 percent of patients, the site of the midline sphincterotomy remains as a deep furrow, causing the so-called keyhole deformity and postoperative anal leakage.

Y–V Advancement Flap

This operation, advocated for most anal strictures, was popularized by Nickell and Woodward. The procedure begins with a lateral internal sphincterotomy from the dentate line to the anal verge. This will be the vertical limb of the Y. It is then split into a V-shaped incision to form a broad-based flap of full-thickness skin. After adequate undermining to avoid tension at the suture lines and careful hemostasis, the tip of the V is extended cephalad and sutured to the proximal portion of the vertical limb of the Y to complete the Y–V plasty (Fig. 3).

Needless to say, this procedure requires meticulous technical detail, and a slight hematoma or infection may disrupt the suture line. Furthermore, the flap may be subject to ischemia and slough if technical details are not carefully observed. On the other hand, there is good evidence that if the flap fails, the patient may do well because of the initial lateral sphincterotomy. Therefore, it is easy to postulate that the lateral internal sphincterotomy alone is sufficient to correct the anal stricture.

S–Plasty

This procedure, described by Ferguson in 1959 for correction of anal ectropion following the Whitehead deformity of the anus, is most suitable for circumferential strictures when the anoderm is excised. Absence of anoderm usually results in failure of all other operations and necessitates rotation of full-thickness flaps of perianal skin to line the anal canal.

In this procedure, all scar tissue is excised circumferentially cephalad up to the level of normal rectal mucosa. An S–shaped incision is then made with the anus at the midpoint. After adequate mobilization and meticulous hemostasis, the flaps are rotated to line the anal canal and are sutured circumferentially to the cut edge of rectal mucosa, anchoring each suture to the internal sphincter to avoid disruption of suture lines or ectropion. The lateral open defects on the buttocks are left open to heal by second intention (Fig. 4).

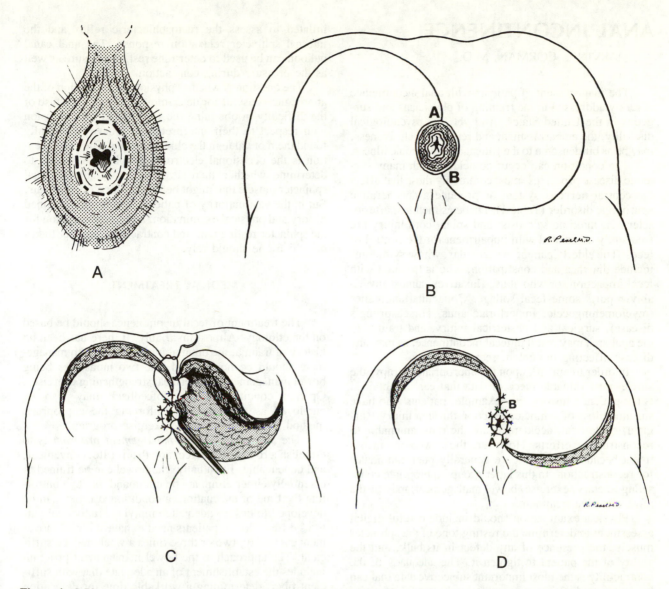

Figure 4 S-Plasty: *A* Strictured anus: circumferential incision to excise scar tissue up to normal rectal mucosa; *B* S-shaped incision on buttocks; *C* Rotation of flaps, suturing skin to rectal mucosa; *D* Completed S-Plasty. Note 180° rotation of medial flap margins.

Obviously, in addition to meticulous technical detail, bowel preparation and antibiotic coverage are mandatory. Delayed absorbable sutures (polyglycolic acid or polyglactin) are usually used. Careful postoperative care of the wound, bowel management, and prolonged follow-up are essential.

Resection

When a low stricture in the rectum is somewhat above the reach of sphincterotomy or plastic procedures, a pull-through or very low coloanal anastomosis with the EEA stapler (with a distal purse-string suture placed through the anus) may be the procedure of choice. These very low anastomoses are usually protected with a diverting colostomy.

In cases of severe anorectal stricture due to Crohn's disease, conservative treatment usually is not effective, and most of these patients need either proctectomy or proctocolectomy, depending on the extent of colonic involvement.

ANAL INCONTINENCE

MARVIN L. CORMAN, M.D.

The management of patients with anal incontinence is rarely addressed in the training of physicians and surgeons in the United States. And yet, the psychological disability, the embarrassment and resultant reclusiveness, may be as burdensome to the patient as any chronic illness.

The condition can occur coincident with many systemic disease processes, most commonly those that affect the central nervous system or produce a degenerative neurologic disorder (Table 1). Diabetes mellitus, arteriosclerosis, multiple sclerosis, and spinal cord injury are frequently associated with impairment for the control of feces. The elderly patient in particular, whose symptoms include diarrhea and constipation, who is troubled with fecal impaction, or who abuses laxatives, almost invariably reports some fecal soilage. Congenital anomalies (myelomeningocele, imperforate anus, Hirschsprung's disease), surgical and obstetrical injury, and trauma to the anal area may result in fecal incontinence, as may any disease affecting the colon, rectum, or anus.

In order to embark upon the appropriate therapy, the single most valuable piece of data that can be obtained is the patient's history. For example, patients who have sustained loss of sphincter function through injury (surgical, obstetrical, accidental) are the most amenable to reconstructive efforts. However, those who are incontinent because of disease are generally poor candidates for reconstruction. In this latter group, appropriate counseling (dietary, exercise, bowel management) may be the most effective treatment.

Physical examination should include careful digital assessment to determine the resting tone of the sphincter muscle, the presence of any defect in its bulk, and the ability of the patient to tighten it. The adequacy of the contractility is the most important subjective data that can be determined. Sensory examination by means of a pinprick may reveal diminished perception and suggest a neuropathic etiology for the incontinence.

Anoscopy and proctosigmoidoscopy should be performed to identify any synchronous lesions. Barium enema examination is warranted in the older patient, again to look for associated disease. However, this study may be limited by the patient's impaired control.

Physiologic tests have been advocated to objectively quantify the degree of impairment and to identify the muscular groups involved. The two investigations employed for evaluating pelvic floor physiology are electromyography (EMG) and anorectal pressure determination. Electrical activity is assessed by inserting a fine-needle electrode in the puborectalis muscle and in the subcutaneous external sphincter. Maximal contraction of the sphincter produces an electrical response that can be correlated with the normal presence or with the reduction of action potentials.

Anorectal manometry usually involves insertion of either a balloon-tipped catheter connected to a transducer or an open-tipped catheter. A balloon in the rectum is inflated to assess the rectosphincteric reflex and the internal sphincter relaxation response. The anal canal balloon can be used to determine resting pressure as well as the pressure during contraction.

The question is whether physiologic evaluation of the anorectum is useful for determining therapy. Because of the difficulty in obtaining the studies and the confusion with respect to their interpretation, I have not usually found them of value in the clinical setting. The one exception is the occasional electromyographic study used to determine whether there is indeed available residual sphincter muscle that might be utilized for a direct repair. But in the vast majority of patients, a carefully obtained history and physical examination, and an appreciation for the sphincter resting tone and contractility, are the studies on which one should rely.

MEDICAL TREATMENT

The treatment of fecal incontinence should be based on the etiology. Almost invariably, if there has been no history of trauma, the optimal initial approach to management should be nonsurgical, the two modalities being bowel management and perineal strengthening exercises. Operant conditioning or biofeedback may also be employed as a means of reinforcing the appropriate method for carrying out the exercise program.

The aim of the *bowel management program* is to establish a routine for defecation that is safe, convenient, and dependable. Eventually, the bowel can be trained to essentially either eliminate on command, or, by controlling the time of evacuation, a conditioned reflex can be developed to ensure adequate emptying. Individual patterns differ. Not all patients need to have a bowel movement every day; two or three times a week may be sufficient. The approach to the bowel management program includes the establishment of an adequate diet with sufficient fiber, determining a workable time for defecation (usually in the morning right after breakfast), and the use

TABLE 1   Causes of Fecal Incontinence

Trauma
   Surgical (fistulectomy, hemorrhoidectomy,
            sphincterotomy, sphincter stretch)
   Obstetrical
   Accidental

Congenital anomalies (spina bifida, myelomeningocele,
           imperforate anus, Hirschsprung's
           disease)

Neurogenic diseases (multiple sclerosis,
           arteriosclerosis, diabetes)

Colorectal diseases (hemorrhoids, rectal prolapse,
           inflammatory bowel disease)

Miscellaneous
   Laxative abuse
   Chronic diarrhea
   Fecal impaction
   Encopresis

From Corman ML. Colon and Rectal Surgery. Philadelphia: JB Lippincott, 1984.

of a stimulant laxative, suppository, or small retention enema. Instructing the patient to massage the abdomen can also be helpful to stimulate complete evacuation.

Perineal strengthening exercises are helpful in the medical management of the patient with fecal incontinence. Muscle bulk and voluntary contractility of the external sphincter, puborectalis sling, and levatores can be improved significantly by such exercises. By simply asking the patient to pretend that he is holding in a bowel movement while counting to 10, a number of times during the course of the day, the efficacy of the contractile function can be improved. Dramatic muscle strength should not be expected overnight, but given sufficient time, the patient should note an improvement in voluntary control.

The exercise regimen can be more effective by the use of operant conditioning. This involves the placement of a balloon-tipped catheter in the rectum, connecting it to a transducer, and reading a measurable response to sphincter contraction on a polygraph. By positive or negative verbal reinforcement, the patient is able to sense rectal distention and learn that the stimulus is a cue to initiate sphincteric contraction.

In summary, therefore, exercise, in combination with a bowel management program, can in most instances ameliorate difficulties with control. However, if these methods fail, and if the patient has a condition amenable to reconstruction, a surgical approach is indicated.

SURGICAL TREATMENT

There are in essence two methods of surgical treatment for anal incontinence: (1) direct repair of the existing musculature, and (2) repair designed to supplement the sphincter mechanism. Table 2 contains a list of the various approaches.

Apposition and *overlapping* of the external sphincter are the best approaches that can be employed if the defect can be corrected by these means. Fistula surgery, lacera-

TABLE 2 Types of Anal Incontinence Repairs

Anorectal muscle repairs
  Apposition of sphincter muscles
  Overlapping of sphincter muscles
  Reefing of sphincter muscles
  Narrowing the anal canal
  Use of perineal muscles other than the sphincter muscle
  Puborectalis repair (postanal perineorrhaphy)
  Pubococcygeus repair

Use of other muscles
  Gluteus
  Vastus internus
  Adductor longus
  Gracilis

Anal procedures
  Fascia lata
  Thiersch procedures (wire, Teflon, Marlex, catgut, Dacron-impregnated Silastic mesh)

From Corman ML. Colon and Rectal Surgery. Philadelphia: JB Lippincott, 1984.

tions, impalement, and birth canal injuries are often ideally suited to one of these techniques. Usually a curvilinear incision is used in the region where the defect is present, extending it as necessary to permit exposure of the cut ends of the sphincter (Fig. 1). It is usually preferable to permit eschar to remain on the sphincter to hold the sutures when the ends are apposed, but as illustrated here, all fibrous tissue has been debrided. Repair of the sphincter muscle is then performed. My particular preference is to use a long-term absorbable suture (e.g., 1–0 Dexon or Vicryl). When sufficient sphincter muscle remains, an overlapping technique is preferred. Further length can be achieved by undermining the skin and by freeing the muscle for 1 or 2 cm at each end. With this technique, breakdown of the repair is less likely. However, care must be taken not to narrow the anal canal, particularly if the overlapping technique is employed.

Usually external sphincter repair is combined with a *reefing* maneuver, a puborectalis plication. This is a procedure involving plication of the deep portion of the external sphincter and puborectalis sling and is commonly employed transvaginally for rectocele repair. As illustrated in Figure 2, reefing may be performed anteriorly or, as shown in Figure 3, it may be done posteriorly. However, these maneuvers fail to increase the actual strength of the muscular contraction. What they do accomplish is to change the anorectal angle and, to some extent, narrow the anal orifice.

POSTOPERATIVE CARE

All patients who undergo sphincter repair should have a bowel-confining regimen instituted, at least in the immediate postoperative period. This consists of a clear-liquid diet, with the addition of "slowing" medications (e.g., Lomotil, deodorized tincture of opium, and codeine). The duration of this program depends on the amount of surgical trauma and may vary from 3 to 7 days. In women, an indwelling catheter is useful until defecation is permitted. Systemic antibiotics may be appropriate for varying periods of time, depending on the amount of surgical manipulation and degree of contamination.

Local care includes gentle cleansing of the wounds with antiseptic solution three times daily and the application of a topical antiseptic ointment. Patients are encouraged to perform perineal strengthening exercises immediately after the operation. When the patient is able to take a regular diet, a stool softener and a bulk laxative preparation containing psyllium are also advisable.

SUPPLEMENTING THE SPHINCTER MECHANISM

As suggested, when there is sufficient residual sphincter, direct repair usually produces a satisfactory result. Unfortunately, when muscle tissue has been lost as a result of trauma or disease, such an approach is usually unsuccessful. In such instances, surgical reconstruction designed to create an artificial sphincter by sup-

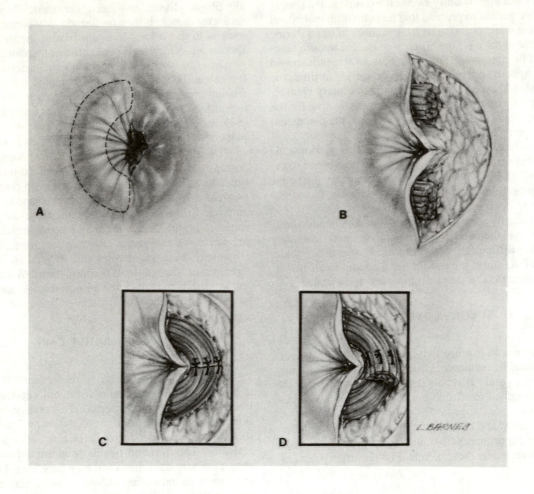

Figure 1 Technique of direct sphincter repair. *A*, Residual sphincter is outlined by a dashed line; tissue loss is demonstrated on the opposite side. *B*, Ends of the divided sphincter are identified. Eschar has been debrided. *C*, Technique of apposition. *D*, Technique of overlapping. (From Corman ML. Colon and Rectal Surgery. Philadephia: JB Lippincott, 1984.)

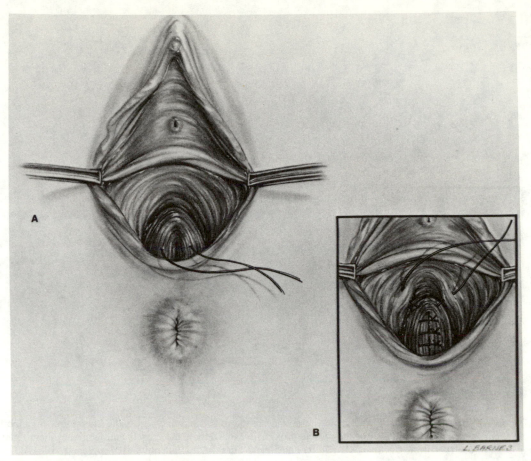

Figure 2 The reefing procedure as performed anteriorly in women. *A*, Vaginal mucosa has been elevated and the sphincter identified. *B*, Sphincter is reefed, and the perivaginal fascia is used to complete the repair. (From Corman ML. Colon and Rectal Surgery. Philadelphia: JB Lippincott, 1984.)

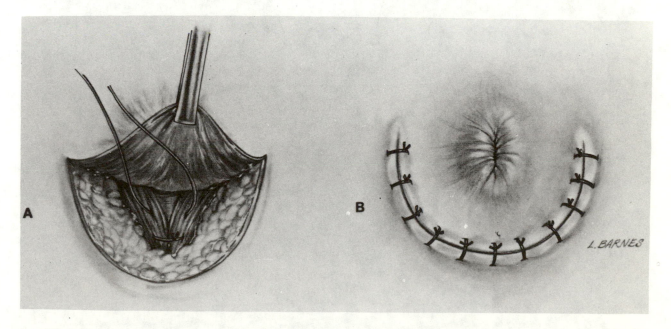

Figure 3 Posterior reefing procedure. *A*, Curvilinear incision exposes the sphincter posteriorly. Sphincter is plicated posteriorly. *B*, Closure. (From Corman ML. Colon and Rectal Surgery. Philadelphia: JB Lippincott, 1984.)

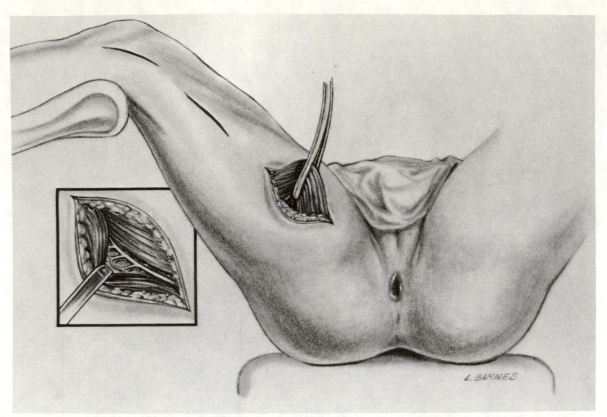

Figure 4 Gracilis muscle transposition. Two incisions are made in the thigh, and one across the knee joint, for mobilizing the gracilis muscle. Penrose drain is placed around the muscle proximally; this tethers the muscle and facilitates identification of the neurovascular bundle (*inset*). (From Corman ML. Colon and Rectal Surgery. Philadephia: JB Lippincott, 1984.)

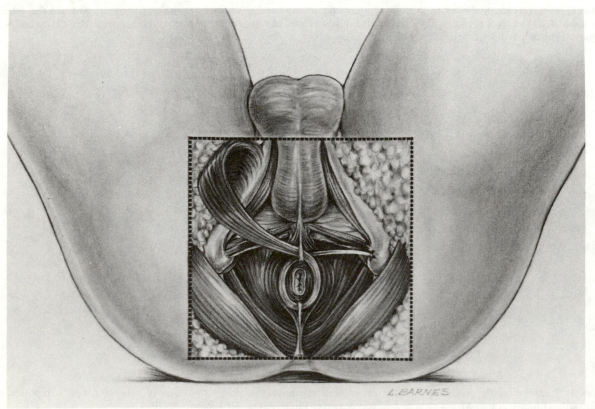

Figure 5 Gracilis muscle transposition. Final position of the transposed muscle. (From Corman ML. Colon and Rectal Surgery. Philadephia: JB Lippincott, 1984.)

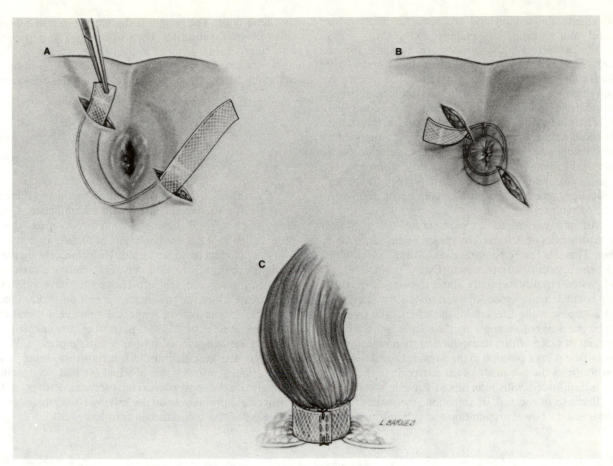

Figure 6 Elastic fabric sling. *A*, Dacron-impregnated Silastic sheet is passed through the two incisions. *B*, Sheet is passed circumferentially around the anus and sutured in place. *C*, Final position of the sheet. (From Corman ML. Colon and Rectal Surgery. Philadelphia: JB Lippincott, 1984.)

plementing the sphincter mechanism may have some merit.

The procedure that I prefer under such circumstances is the gracilis muscle transposition. The gracilis muscle is the most superficial muscle in the medial aspect of the thigh. It is broad in the upper thigh, becomes narrow, and tapers to a tendon that inserts below the tibial tuberosity. The major blood supply enters proximally so that division at the insertion and mobilization of the muscle to the proximal neurovascular bundle do not compromise viability.

Technique

Patients are placed in the perineolithotomy position in order to expose both the thighs and the anus. The side utilized for transposition is draped so that it can be removed easily from the stirrup.

Three incisions are employed on the medial aspect of the thigh—in the proximal thigh, in the midthigh, and across the knee joint (Fig. 4). After the entire muscle and tendon have been freed, the tendon is divided as distally as possible. It is most important to preserve maximal length of the tendon.

Attention is then turned to the anal dissection. A curvilinear incision is made approximately 1.5 cm from the anal verge anteriorly and posteriorly. A tunnel is developed between the proximal thigh incision and the anterior perianal incision, and the muscle is pulled through. A tunnel is then developed in the extrasphincteric space on either side of the anal canal. The tendon is passed clockwise if the right gracilis muscle is being transposed, or counterclockwise if the left gracilis muscle is used. After the tendon is passed 360 degrees and *behind* the muscle, an incision is made over the contralateral ischial tuberosity. Three monofilament nonabsorbable sutures (Prolene) are placed in the gluteal fascia and held in place. The tendon is pulled through a tunnel developed between the ischial incision and the anterior perianal incision. At this point, the leg from which the gracilis muscle was taken is removed from the stirrup and adducted. This is an extremely important maneuver because it releases tension on the muscle. If the tendon were to be anchored without adduction, the substitute sphincter would be loose, and the results would be unsatisfactory. With maximal adduction the surgeon pulls the tendon taut. It should be snug when the finger is inserted in the rectum. Too tight an orifice may be corrected by dilation. The sutures are placed into the tendon and secured. All incisions are closed, and no drains are employed (Fig. 5).

Postoperatively, the bowels are confined for one week. The patient is kept at bed rest for 48 hours, after which gradual ambulation is permitted. The wounds are gently cleansed three times daily, and a topical antiseptic ointment is applied in a manner previously described.

The goal in the postoperative period is to establish a workable time for defecation. By using a suppository immediately after breakfast, complete evacuation can be promoted. This, in addition to dietary measures, and occasionally the use of laxatives or perhaps "slowing" medications, inevitably results in continence in properly selected patients.

An alternative to supplementing the sphincter mechanism can be achieved by means of an *elastic fabric sling*. This is a Dacron-impregnated Silastic sheet which has been appropriately trimmed (Dow Corning #501-7) and passed circumferentially about the anus (Fig. 6). A strip is cut 1.5 cm wide. An overlap of 1 cm is created, and a stapler is used to secure the edges. The diameter can be checked before applying the stapler by holding the material in place with a hemostat and then returning the sheet to the proper position in the wound. Digital examination confirms the adequacy of the narrowing. The suture line is reinforced with interrupted Prolene sutures.

Because of the risk of infection, the patient should be placed on a bowel preparation and systemic periopera-tive antibiotics. The patient is discharged in 3 to 5 days, when bowel function has been restored. The particular advantage of this material is that it can stretch, and on rectal examination it is difficult to distinguish the sensation of the sheet from that of the normal, intact anal sphincter.

RESULTS

It is difficult to evaluate the relative merits of different operations in the treatment of fecal incontinence. Generally, the best results are obtained if direct repair is possible. Much depends on the judgment of the surgeon and the type of defect to be corrected. Unfortunately, neither of these variables is readily apparent when one searches the literature on the subject. Those who have suffered obstetrical injury or sphincter laceration from other traumatic events can be expected to have a good-to-excellent result in perhaps 90 percent of cases as long as there is adequate residual sphincter muscle present. With respect to the gracilis muscle transposition, those who have sustained prior trauma or who have had a congenital anomaly are the most successfully treated. Patients with a neurologic problem or an underlying bowel disorder as the cause of the incontinence fare less well.

PILONIDAL SINUS AND CYST

W. JOHN B. HODGSON, M.D., M.S., F.R.C.S., F.A.C.S.

Pilonidal sinus is an acquired, common, recurring problem with a high cost to the population in terms of days of hospitalization, discomfort as an outpatient, and loss of both earning and productive capacity. These sinuses consist of granulation tissue-lined spaces, often containing broken hair shafts and lacking any evidence of epithelium, sweat glands, sebaceous glands, or normal hair follicles. There is a suggestion that distorted hair follicles may be present in these cases. However, hair is present in only half the cases.

The exact etiology is uncertain, but it does involve breakdown of the skin either by friction or by tricofollic-ulitis, which leads to the development of a microabscess and hence a minute cavity within the dermis, which then tends to extend downward. Communication with the outside may subsequently be lost, but when hairs are seen in the sinuses, they are always dead, with their pointed ends directed to the blind end of the sinus, and appear to have been sucked in from the outside.

The appearance of the condition in the hands of hair dressers and reports of sinuses in the umbilicus, axillae, or external genitalia, and the time of presentation with a peak incidence between the ages of 15 and 30 years all argue against a congential origin in this condition.

Once referred to as "jeep drivers disease," it is no longer appropriate to describe a typical bearer of this affliction as a swarthy hirsute caucasian male, since a sizable proportion of the patients are now female and/or black. In general, therefore, this disease occurs in a youthful population and is difficult to manage.

MANAGEMENT OF ACUTE ABSCESS

In many cases, the onset of a sacrococcygeal pilonidal cyst is sudden. The patient becomes increasingly aware of a soreness or aching while seated. As the pain continues to escalate rapidly, an exquisitely tender, erythematous mass develops either in the natal cleft or to one side. This is an acute pilonidal abscess. It cannot be reversed by antibiotics at this point. Naturally, the offending organisms are usually one or more varieties of gram-negative rods. On occasion, as the abscess ripens, a marked degree of associated cellulitis and erythema may arise, leading to a generalized febrile condition that requires treatment with antibiotics. However, the real treatment is incision and drainage, which should be done as rapidly as possible after the diagnosis has been made. A large amount of malodorous pus may be obtained, mixed with old and clotted blood. The response is usually dramatic, and the process subsides rapidly. If this is the patient's first experience with this condition, incision and drainage can be successfully carried out in the outpatient department under local anesthesia. However, the larger abscesses are better drained under general anesthesia, and the patient is kept in the hospital for a few days thereafter. Various techniques are used to keep the skin open long enough for deeper healing to occur, and gentle packing is as easy a technique as any. Sitz baths can be taken on a daily basis in the hospital, and more often once the patient is discharged. Healing usually occurs within 2 to 3 weeks.

About one-third of the patients have no further trouble. The others, however, represent a continuing problem. Some may return with additional acute abscesses, whereas others may have continuing drainage from a sinus tract that seems to be associated with an unhealed drainage procedure following the first presentation. In this latter subgroup, if the sinus tract is superificial, cauterization with silver nitrate in the office may be all that is required for complete cure.

Some patients may not be aware that their pilonidal sinus is draining and may even seek advice for chronic rectal bleeding and soilage of underclothes, or even for an unexplained wetness or odor emanating from the perianal region. In these patients, pain is not a prominent feature. Patients who have such a problem or who have recurrent abscesses clearly need an elective curative procedure.

OPERATIVE MANAGEMENT

A great many techniques have been devised that are intended to effect a cure of chronic sacrococcygeal pilonidal disease. Some are attractive because they permit treatment on an amublatory outpatient basis. Other techniques offer the lure of minimal cutting or dissecting. However, some forms of treatment cause considerable discomfort. Some require the prolonged restriction of physical activity and even the curtailment of bowel function. Some require long periods of wound care and dressing changes. Most result in distressingly high failure rates. A procedure that is not uncomfortable, results in a closed wound that heals per primum, requires minimal restriction of activity, and carries a favorable cure rate would seem to be ideal.

Historically, surgical treatment has always been incision and drainage or marsupialization, because these are simple procedures and are sometimes effective. The shortcomings of these procedures have been recognized, particularly, the problems of recurrence and the fact that healing in these cases is by second intention. Furthermore many patients who seek assistance have pilonidal cysts that have been unsuccessfully treated in the past. They have scars and draining sinuses, and to fully excise such scar tissue as well as the cyst and the multiple tracts can leave a large soft tissue deficiency. Since the buttocks

move independently upon sitting and create a friction that forces hairs into minute abrasions or scars in the skin of the natal cleft, the operative procedure should be aimed at eliminating this shearing force. It should also be able to excise the unhealthy tissue and sinuses and allow a primary closure of the wound.

The one technique that gives the highest rate of healing without further recurrence is the Z-plasty method of Monro and McDermott. Our study comparing results of this technique with those of incision and drainage or marsupialization showed that 60 percent of patients in the latter group suffered recurrence. None of the patients in the Z-plasty group demonstrated recurrences, and all of these patients were satisfied with the results of their surgery. We also found that the natal cleft was flattened in the Z-plasty group and that a strong transverse scar was produced. Clearly this technique has all the attributes of the ideal technique for the management of pilonidal sinus and cyst.

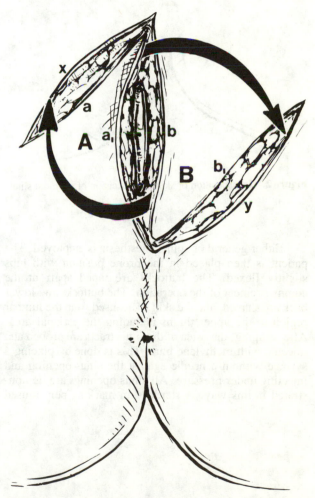

Figure 1 Excision of pilonidal sinus and first stage of Z-plasty. *A*, Left inferior flap. *B*, Right superior flap. *a*, Lateral edge of inferior flap. *a1*, Left excision line of sinus. *b*, Right excision line of sinus. *b1*, Lateral edge of superior flap. *x*, Line of incision of left buttock. *y*, Line of incision of right buttock.

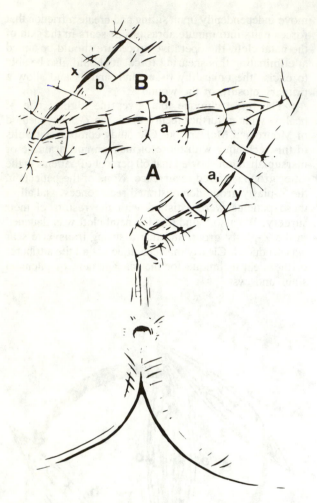

Figure 2 Transposition of skin after excision of pilonidal sinus.

Either general or spinal anesthesia is employed. The patient is then placed in the prone position with hips slightly flexed. The buttocks are taped apart at the commencement of the operation. The buttocks and lower back are shaved, and the skin is cleansed from the lumbar region to the upper thighs including the perianal area. After draping, the ostea of the sinus tracts are probed and injected with methylene blue. This is done by placing a syringe without a needle against the sinus opening and injecting under pressure. All sinus openings are demonstrated in this way. A sterile skin marking pen is used to indicate the tissue to be excised and this area is included within an elipse. The excision is then extended to form a Z (Fig. 1) so that transposition can take place once the skin and fat are undermined (Fig. 2).

A scalpel is used for the skin incision and the electrocutting cautery for the deeper tissues to help reduce unnecessary bleeding. The depth of the excision is taken down to the level of the postsacral fascia only. Care must be taken to avoid undercutting the skin. Again, using the electrocautery, the flaps are developed, taking the subfascial plane in order to expose the bare fibers of the gluteus muscle. A closed drainage system, such as a Hemovac, is inserted, and the 3–0 Vicryl sutures are used to begin closure from the bases of the flaps toward the apices. These sutures also serve to stitch the bases of the flaps down onto the muscle. When the general shape has been achieved, interrupted skin stitches are placed with 4–0 Ethilon. It should be noted that the lower edge of the incision nearest the anus is curved away slightly from the anus in order to prevent the development of a pit at this point (see Fig. 2), which could become another pilonidal sinus. Great care is taken in the closure to ensure that the skin edges fit together perfecty.

POSTOPERATIVE CARE

After full recovery from the anesthesia, the patient is allowed to walk, sit, or stand. I do not encourage these patients to lie in bed unless they lie on their side. A normal diet is provided, and a normal bowel evacuation is encouraged. Analgesics are given, and in most cases, discomfort continues for 3 to 4 days, during which time the dressing is held in place by broad strips of adhesive tape. The wound catheters are removed when no longer functioning, which is usually on the fourth or fifth postoperative day. By this time, it is possible to eliminate the dressing and to allow the patient to shower. Skin sutures are usually retained until the tenth or twelfth postoperative day.

I have not had problems with wound edge separations unless a simple stitch was placed when a mattress should have been used. Nor have there been problems with accumulation of serum under the flap because of the care taken to suture the base of the flap down to the postsacral fascia.

Because the closure is done without tension, the postoperative course is straightforward; the scar soon softens and within a few weeks is not noticed by the patient.

THE LIVER

LIVER ABSCESS

HENRY A. PITT, M.D.

Proper treatment of liver abscesses depends on the clinician's ability to establish the diagnosis and to determine the etiology and type of abscess. In the United States, both pyogenic and amebic liver abscesses are relatively uncommon disease entities. As a result, one or more liver abscesses are not always considered when a patient presents with fever, upper abdominal pain, or multiple organ failure. However, the physician who includes liver abscesses in his differential diagnosis is now able to employ several diagnostic modalities that were not generally available even a decade ago.

Fortunately, the widespread availability of ultrasound (US), computed tomography (CT), newer radionuclides, and CT- or US-guided percutaneous aspiration has resulted in earlier diagnosis and improved survival of patients with liver abscesses. The choice among these various options to identify one or more space-occupying intrahepatic lesions may be somewhat dependent on local expertise. In diagnosing pyogenic abscesses, however, computerized tomography has the advantages of being able to (1) detect lesions as small as 0.5 cm, (2) view the whole liver as well as the remainder of the abdomen, and (3) provide the surgeon or radiologist with an excellent anatomic guide for drainage. Ultrasound, on the other hand, may be ideal for following the progress of larger abscesses and for detecting amebic abscesses which, generally, are of moderate size at the time of presentation.

PYOGENIC VERSUS AMEBIC HEPATIC ABSCESS

The type of liver abscess that a clinician is likely to encounter is also dependent on where he is practicing. In most northern American states, pyogenic abscesses account for the vast majority of liver abscesses. In southern and southwestern states and some northern cities, however, recent immigration trends have resulted in an increased prevalence of amebic hepatic abscesses. As a result, in these areas pyogenic and amebic liver abscesses are now being seen with nearly equal frequency. The physician practicing in these regions also needs to rely on serologic testing to confirm his suspicions of an amebic liver abscess. Many serologic tests are now available that can provide accurate data in 24 to 48 hours. Therefore, each physician should check with his own laboratory to determine the accuracy of the tests available to him.

In addition to sophisticated scans and serologic tests, several other clinical and laboratory markers may help in differentiating pyogenic from amebic abscesses. In a review of 82 patients with liver abscesses seen at UCLA from 1968 through 1983, 42 patients were found to have pyogenic abscesses whereas 40 had amebic liver abscesses. The clinical characteristics differentiating these two groups of patients are presented in Table 1. Patients with pyogenic abscesses were significantly more likely to be older than 50 and to present with jaundice, pruritus, septic shock, or a palpable mass. On the other hand, patients with amebic abscesses were more likely to have been of Mexican descent, to have recently traveled to or from an endemic area, or to present with abdominal pain, diarrhea, or hepatomegaly. In this analysis, patients with pyogenic abscesses were also significantly more likely to have abnormal liver function tests or plain abdominal films. Except for serologic findings, laboratory data did not differentiate these two types of liver abscesses.

In this retrospective study extending back to the late 1960s, both radionuclide scanning and ultrasonography were quite accurate in diagnosing liver abscesses. Some authorities have also suggested that ultrasound can differentiate amebic abscesses by demonstrating (1) a smooth wall, (2) internal echoes that are less dense than surrounding normal liver, (3) contiguity with the liver capsule, and (4) slight distal sonic enhancement. Another method that we have employed to ensure accurate diagnosis is CT- or US-guided aspiration. However, this

TABLE 1 Distinguishing Clinical Characteristics in Patients with Hepatic Abscesses

Pyogenic	Amebic
Age >50 years	Mexican descent*
Jaundice	Recent travel*
Pruritus	Abdominal pain
Septic shock	Diarrhea
Palpable mass	Hepatomegaly

Adapted from Conter R, Pitt H, Tompkins R, Longmire W Jr. Differentiation of pyogenic from amebic hepatic abscess. Surg Gynecol Obstet 1985. (In press)
* To or from an endemic area.

153

technique has been reserved for patients in whom (1) serologic data are nondiagnostic, (2) there are concerns about secondary bacterial contamination of an amebic abscess, or (3) differentiation of an abscess from a cyst or primary or secondary tumor cannot be made by less invasive studies. In our hands, this technique has been safe and helpful in difficult cases.

TREATMENT OF PYOGENIC ABSCESS

When not diagnosed and appropriately treated, pyogenic hepatic abscesses are almost always fatal. For many years, the hallmarks of treatment have included prolonged antibiotic administration, direct surgical drainage of the liver abscess, and appropriate treatment of the underlying cause of the abscess. In recent years, however, suggested treatment options have included (1) percutaneous aspiration and (2) drainage of the abscess or biliary tree. As a result, treatment must now be individualized on the basis of many factors, one of the most important of which is the cause of infection. Etiologic categories include (1) *biliary obstruction* with ascending cholangitis, (2) *pylephlebitis* secondary to intra-abdominal infections such as appendicitis or diverticulitis, (3) *septicemia*, as with endocarditis, (4) *direct extension* from a contiguous disease process, (5) *trauma* from penetrating or blunt injuries, or (6) *cryptogenic*, when no primary source of infection is found even after abdominal exploration or autopsy. Further details of management options will follow a discussion of antibiotic choices.

Antibiotic Treatment

More than half the patients with pyogenic hepatic abscesses have positive blood cultures at the time of presentation. Therefore, early institution of antibiotic therapy is extremely important. The antibiotic regimen chosen should be based on knowledge of the spectrum of organisms likely to be isolated from pyogenic hepatic abscesses. Two-thirds of these patients harbor gram-negative aerobes, with *Escherichia coli* and *Klebsiella* and *Proteus* species being isolated most often. Streptococcal species are found in approximately 35 percent of patients. Approximately 20 percent of patients have aerobic streptococci, half of which are enterococci. Anaerobic and microaerophilic streptococci are isolated from approximately 15 percent of patients. The next most commonly cultured anaerobes include *Bacteroides* (10%) and *Clostridia* (3%) species. Thus, anaerobes are found in nearly 30 percent of patients.

Since many pyogenic abscesses harbor multiple organisms, broad-spectrum antibiotic coverage is indicated until specific bacteria have been isolated and sensitivities are known. With the proliferation of newer antibiotics, many antibiotic combinations are now capable of providing antibacterial coverage against organisms that are likely to be isolated from a pyogenic liver abscess. Various possible combinations of currently available antibiotics are listed in Table 2. Each of these options provides a broad spectrum against the gram-negative aerobes, streptococcal species including enterococci, and anaerobes including *Bacteroides fragilis*. In patients who are allergic to penicillin, the combination of vancomycin, an aminoglycoside, and either clindamycin or metronidazole also gives broad coverage. Metronidazole has the additional advantage of providing treatment for *Entamoeba histolytica* and should be included in the intial antibiotic regimen whenever there is suspicion of an amebic abscess.

One disadvantage of some of the proposed antibiotic regimens is that they include potentially toxic agents. Many patients with pyogenic hepatic abscesses are already at increased risk for developing renal failure because of advanced age, sepsis, jaundice, or preexisting renal disease. Therefore, whenever an aminoglycoside is used, serum levels should be carefully monitored. Moreover, if bacterial sensitivities demonstrate that less toxic antibiotics will suffice, the aminoglycoside should be discontinued. Because prolonged antibiotic administration may be required, less nephrotoxic agents have been suggested. However, these possibilities include either newer expensive agents or chloramphenicol with its potential for hematologic toxicity.

The duration of antibiotic therapy should be individualized on the basis of the number of abscesses, the clinical response, and the toxicity of the required antibiotic regimen. Patients with multiple biliary abscesses should probably receive at least 4 to 6 weeks of antibiotic therapy. In comparison, a shorter antibiotic course may suffice for a small solitary abscess that has been adequately drained. Initially, antibiotics should be administered parenterally. In patients who require a prolonged course of antibiotics, appropriate oral agents may be used after 2 to 4 weeks of parenteral therapy. In patients with liver abscesses of biliary origin, high biliary excretion of an antibiotic is a theoretical advantage. However, biliary excretion is markedly diminished with extrahepatic obstruction and with external drainage. In these situations, adequate serum and liver antibiotic levels are more important than high biliary excretion.

Aspiration

Over the past 30 years, scattered reports of small numbers of patients have suggested closed-needle aspira-

TABLE 2   Antibiotic Combinations for Initial Management of Pyogenic Abscesses

Ampicillin + clindamycin or metronidazole + aminoglycoside
Newer broad-spectrum penicillin + aminoglycoside
Newer broad-spectrum penicillin + third-generation cephalosporin
Ampicillin + third-generation cephalosporin (with good anaerobic spectrum)
Ampicillin + chloramphenicol

tion as an alternative to the generally accepted method of surgical drainage for pyogenic hepatic abscesses. The good results reported in these series confirm that closed-needle aspiration in combination with systemic antibiotic treatment can be successful in carefully selected cases. Patients who may tolerate this form of therapy include patients with a solitary abscess or a small number of abscesses who are relatively young, otherwise healthy, and have no other source of intra-abdominal infection. However, these are the very patients who would tolerate a laparotomy without difficulty. Theoretically, open surgical drainage of these patients should provide more adequate and dependent drainage and, therefore, result in more rapid resolution of the abscess. As already mentioned, however, CT- or US-guided aspiration can be useful in differentiating pyogenic abscesses from cysts, tumors, or amebic abscesses. Thus, when the diagnosis is in doubt, we have used needle aspiration for diagnosis, but have proceeded directly to abscess drainage if the Gram stain of aspirated fluid demonstrates bacteria.

Percutaneous Drainage

Several recent reports suggest that percutaneous drainage of pyogenic liver abscesses can be successful in 70 to 90 percent of selected patients. It must be remembered, however, that these are reports of *selected* patients, that the authors stress that adequate drainage must be achieved, and that this method may not be suitable for many patients with pyogenic abscesses. The categories of patients in whom percutaneous drainage should *not* be used include those with (1) multiple abscesses, (2) a known intra-abdominal source of infection that requires surgery, (3) an unknown etiology for the abscess, (4) ascites, (5) abscesses that would require transpleural drainage, and perhaps (6) underlying biliary disease requiring surgery. One or more of these categories, unfortunately, apply to most patients with pyogenic hepatic abscesses.

Another question that remains unanswered is whether percutaneous transhepatic biliary drainage (PTBD) is an appropriate method for managing patients with multiple pyogenic abscesses of biliary origin. Recent reports of small numbers of patients suggest that 30-day morbidity is moderately high and mortality may be 15 to 20 percent when patients with severe cholangitis and multiple liver abscesses are managed with PTBD. It must be remembered, however, that these patients with multiple abscesses of biliary origin do not fare well when treated with surgical decompression of the biliary tree. At present, my opinion is that if the underlying biliary disease is known and will eventually require surgery, operative decompression should be performed initially to avoid the added risk of two procedures. However, if the cause of biliary obstruction can safely be managed nonoperatively, PTBD of the septic patient may be acceptable if *experienced* radiologists are available.

Surgical Drainage

Prior to the introduction of antibiotics, the extraperitoneal approach to drainage of hepatic abscesses was recommended because of fear of contamination of the peritoneal or pleural cavities with transperitoneal or transpleural operations. These approaches are best suited for patients with a solitary abscess in whom the etiology is known and has been adequately treated. However, absolute certainty of these two conditions is a rarity. As already mentioned, these selected cases may be appropriate for percutaneous catheter drainage, which now makes extraperitoneal drainage nearly obsolete.

With systemic antibiotic coverage and proper surgical technique, transperitoneal surgical drainage can be performed safely. Transperitoneal surgical exploration has the advantage of providing (1) adequate exploration of the entire abdomen, (2) excellent exposure of the entire liver, (3) assessment of the best drainage site, and (4) access to the biliary tree for cholangiography or common duct exploration. These advantages are extremely important because the high mortality frequently associated with pyogenic hepatic abscesses has often been the result of failure to appreciate an underlying intra-abdominal source of infection or to adequately decompress an obstructed biliary tree.

Once the abdomen has been explored and the primary focus of infection has been managed, the liver should be carefully palpated. In most instances, preoperative CT or ultrasound will have been performed and greatly aid the surgeon in the localization of abscesses. Intraoperative ultrasound also may be extremely helpful if localization of an abscess becomes difficult. Once localized, the abscess should be aspirated with a needle, and pus should be placed directly into anaerobic culture media. Aspirated material should also be examined by a Gram stain and examined for amebae.

After carefully protecting the adjacent peritoneal cavity with laparotomy pads and having adequate suction available, the surgeon should then drain the cavity dependently. If the abscess is multiloculated, an attempt should be made to open into the various pockets, but further disruption of the abscess cavity may be tempered by the degree of hemorrhage. A biopsy should also be taken of the abscess wall to rule out a necrotic, infected tumor and to search further for amebic trophozoites. Moreover, biopsy of another area of the liver that appears uninvolved should be done to rule out multiple microscopic abscesses. Multiple drains, including Penrose, and soft sump tubes are then placed into the cavities and adjacent perihepatic spaces and are brought out through separate stab incisions.

In patients with multiple microscopic abscesses, no formal liver drainage is required, but a careful search for a biliary or intra-abdominal source should be undertaken. When a biliary source is found, choledochotomy with T-tube insertion is necessary because cholecystostomy alone does not provide adequate decompression of the biliary tree. The extent to which the biliary tree should be explored and the decision whether to increase intrabiliary pressure with choledochoscopy or completion cholangiography must be individualized on the basis of the biliary disease and the patient's intraoperative stability.

TREATMENT OF AMEBIC ABSCESS

In 1890, Sir William Osler first reported the presence of amebae in both the stool and liver abscess of the same patient. For the next 30 years, open surgical drainage was recommended for both pyogenic and amebic liver abscesses. However, in 1923, Manson-Bahr reported his experience in treating British troups in India with emetine and closed aspiration. Simultaneously, Ludlow published his results of the same treatment regimen in 100 Korean patients. Both of these investigators reported mortality figures that were dramatically better than those previously achieved with open drainage. During the past 30 years, advances in serologic testing and in noninvasive radiologic techniques, as well as the introduction of newer amebicidal drugs, have led to earlier diagnosis, avoidance of the need for aspiration in many cases, and improved survival.

Amebicidal Agents

For many years, emetine was the only effective drug available for treatment of amebic hepatic abscesses. Unfortunately, both emetine and dehydroemetine are cardiotoxic. The next amebicidal agent effective against extraintestinal amebiases to be introduced was chloroquine, which became available in 1948. For the next 20 years, treatment of an amebic hepatic abscess consisted of emetine or chloroquine or both. One problem with both of these agents, and particularly chloroquine, is relapse after an initial response. To avoid this problem, and the cardiac toxicity of emetine, lower doses of emetine plus chloroquine have been recommended and have resulted in cure rates of 90 to 100 percent. A further problem with these agents, however, is that neither emetine nor chloroquine will clear the intestines of amebae. Therefore, when using emetine and/or chloroquine, an intestinal amebicide such as diiodohydroxyquin, diloxanide furoate, carbarsone, or tetracycline must be added.

In the late 1960s metronidazole (Flagyl) was introduced for the treatment of amebic liver abscesses. Metronidazole has the advantages of being highly effective, less toxic, and able to treat both intestinal and extraintestinal amebiasis. Subsequently, comparative studies of metronidazole, 750 mg three times a day for 10 days, and chloroquine, 500 mg daily for 10 weeks, have shown that both regimens are highly effective, but that metronidazole has the advantage of a shorter course of treatment. Thus, metronidazole has become the agent of choice for treatment of amebic liver abscesses. However, not all patients respond to metronidazole, and in these patients a prolonged course of chloroquine or the combination of this agent with emetine or dehydroemetine may suffice.

Aspiration

The main reasons for aspirating an amebic liver abscess are (1) to establish a diagnosis and (2) to reduce the likelihood of rupture of a large abscess. Even before the advent of CT- or US-guided aspiration, most experts found diagnostic needle aspiration of amebic liver abscesses to be safe. However, as reliable serologic tests, which can yield results in less than 24 to 48 hours, have become available, the need for diagnostic aspiration has been questioned by several investigators.

Advocates of therapeutic aspiration list several indications including (1) persistence of symptoms despite adequate medical management, (2) large abscesses in the left lobe adjacent to the pericardium, (3) suspicion of bacterial superinfection, and (4) the presence of a large abscess in which previous aspiration has yielded more than 250 ml of pus. In one study, however, resolution time was unchanged by therapeutic aspiration, which may also increase the chance of bacterial superinfection. For these reasons, I would recommend that therapeutic aspiration be reserved for very large amebic abscesses, especially those on the left, which are likely to rupture into the pericardium, and for those that do not respond to conventional therapy.

Percutaneous Drainage

Although percutaneous catheter drainage of selected cases of pyogenic hepatic abscesses is being reported with increasing frequency, the application of this technique to patients with amebic abscess has not gained widespread popularity because (1) most patients respond to amebicidal therapy and (2) there are concerns about bacterial superinfection. Moreover, the fluid within amebic abscesses is often thick and viscous, making adequate drainage with relatively small percutaneously placed catheters difficult. Larger catheters, on the other hand, increase the risk of hemorrhage from the liver's parenchyma.

Surgical Drainage

Since most patients with an amebic abscess respond to amebicidal drug therapy with or without therapeutic needle aspiration, open surgical drainage has generally been reserved for patients with complications. Other reasons for avoiding surgical drainage include concerns about secondary bacterial invasion and the morbidity of a chronically draining sinus tract. Most authorities agree that surgical drainage is indicated in patients with rupture into the peritoneal cavity. On the other hand, no clear consensus exists regarding the need for surgical drainage in patients whose abscess has ruptured into the pleura, lung, or pericardium. In fact, some authorities recommend that patients with amebic pericarditis be treated with needle aspiration of both the pericardium and the liver abscess.

TABLE 3 Results of Treatment*

	Pyogenic Abscess		Amebic Abscess	
Treatment	No. Patients	% Mortality	No. Patients	% Mortality
None	4	100	1	0
Antibiotics only	12	100	32*†	0
Catheter drainage	4	0	1	0
Surgical drainage	22	5	6	0

Adapted from Conter R, Pitt H, Tompkins R, Longmire W Jr. Differentiation of pyogenic from amebic hepatic abscess. Surg Gynecol Obstet 1985. (In press)
* Or antiamebicides in patients with amebic abscesses.
† Three patients also had therapeutic aspiration.

Considerable variation exists among reported series in the percentage of patients requiring open surgical drainage. A recent analysis of 40 patients seen over a 15-year period at UCLA revealed that 29 patients (72.5%) responded to antiamebicides, whereas three patients (7.5%) required needle aspiration, one (2.5%) catheter drainage, and six (15%) surgical drainage. This relatively low percentage of surgically drained patients results from a policy of operating on patients who (1) fail to respond to antiamebicides, (2) present with a ruptured abscess, or (3) are thought to be at risk for rupture from a large, left-sided abscess.

RESULTS

Over the past 30 years, mortality rates for patients with pyogenic hepatic abscesses have varied from 24 to 88 percent, whereas those for amebic abscesses have varied from 0 to 34 percent. These large ranges can be explained to some degree by differences in patient populations and forms of treatment. With pyogenic abscesses, the number of abscesses, the etiology, and the form of therapy are critical to outcome. With amebic abscesses, however, outcome is more dependent on the presence of a major complication such as rupture into the peritoneum or pericardium.

The analysis of 82 patients (42 pyogenic and 40 amebic) from UCLA typifies recently reported mortality figures with rates of 40 and 0 percent for patients with pyogenic and amebic abscesses, respectively (Table 3). Mortality was 100 percent among four patients with pyogenic abscesses receiving no treatment and 12 patients treated only with antibiotics. However, many of these patients also had end-stage malignant disease, and an active decision had been made not to treat them aggressively. The four highly selected patients (10%) with pyogenic abscesses managed with percutaneous catheter drainage responded well to treatment. Moreover, only one of 22 patients (5%) treated by surgical drainage died of liver failure following left hepatic lobectomy. Thus, this series is typical of the good results now possible when a proper diagnosis of pyogenic hepatic abscess is established and both appropriate antibiotic therapy and adequate drainage are achieved.

In the UCLA series, none of the 40 patients with amebic abscesses died. These excellent results are a reflection of physician awareness of the problem, prompt diagnosis, and individualized therapy, which includes surgical drainage in only a minority (15%) of cases. Thus, this analysis suggests that the majority of patients with both pyogenic and amebic liver abscesses who have a diagnosis established and in whom appropriate therapy is initiated are now surviving. Although overall mortality rates for patients with pyogenic abscesses remain high, patients who do not survive tend to be those with end-stage malignant disease or severe immunodepression.

LIVER CYSTS

R. SCOTT JONES, M.D.

SOLITARY CONGENITAL NONPARASITIC LIVER CYSTS

Solitary cysts of the liver may be unilocular or multilocular, and they are uncommon. The development and the current widespread application of sensitive imaging techniques, such as ultrasound and computerized tomographic scanning, will probably lead to the detection of larger numbers of liver cysts ante mortem.

Pathology

Liver cysts may vary in size from a few millimeters in diameter to massive lesions occupying large volumes of the upper abdomen. The largest reported liver cyst contained 17 liters of fluid. Liver cysts tend to occur more commonly in the right lobe anteriorly and inferiorly, although they may occupy virtually any site in the liver. The surface of liver cysts is usually smooth and frequently exhibits a bluish hue. Microscopically, cyst walls possess three distinct layers. The inner layer is usually of columnar or cuboidal epithelium; however, tall columnar epithelium, mucus-producing epithelium, ciliated epithelium, and squamous epithelium have been observed in cyst walls. Vascular elements comprise the middle layer, while collagen, muscle fibers, bile ducts, and compressed hepatocytes form the outer layer. Islands of biliary ductular epithelium within the cyst wall are referred to as von Meyenburg complexes. The vast majority of liver cysts are benign and innocuous. In rare instances, however, malignant change may occur in liver cysts to produce adenocarcinomas, squamous cell carcinomas, and sarcomas.

Diagnosis

Solitary liver cysts can be detected at any age from infancy through later decades of life. Most cases are discovered between the fourth and sixth decades, and there is a slight female preponderance. Most patients having solitary cysts are asymptomatic. When clinically evident, liver cysts exhibit an upper abdominal mass, perceived by the patient or the examining physician, or hepatomegaly. Some patients experience upper abdominal pain or a sense of pressure or fullness. In most cases, liver function is entirely normal and remains so throughout the patient's life, unless other diseases develop to impair liver function. Jaundice is an infrequent manifestation of congenital cystic disease, occurring in approximately 9 percent of affected patients. Several reports ascribed the jaundice to external compression of the bile ducts by the cyst. However, I recently noted the occurrence of a benign bile duct tumor associated with liver cysts in two patients and collected several additional cases from the literature. It seems prudent to suspect bile duct tumors in jaundiced patients with solitary liver cysts, and careful cholangiography should be accomplished in those patients. Simple liver cysts exhibit other clinical manifestations such as spontaneous or posttraumatic rupture, internal fistula formation, and torsion, although these cases are rare.

The diagnosis of liver cyst can be suspected in a patient who has an upper abdominal mass and a history of vague upper abdominal discomfort or pressure. Plain films may disclose an upper abdominal mass or displacement of other organs. Ultrasound examination is extremely sensitive in revealing cystic lesions within the liver and is highly accurate in detecting solitary liver cysts. Computerized tomographic scanning may be less effective in determining whether a lesion is cystic or solid, but probably provides more accurate anatomic localization and definition of anatomic relationships to the cysts than does ultrasound. When arteriography is performed in patients with liver cysts, it reveals an avascular area corresponding to the cyst. Careful cholangiography is an important step in evaluating patients with liver cysts who have jaundice to determine whether biliary obstruction is present and, if so, whether it is due to physical compression by the cyst, by ductal tumor, or by some other disease such as common duct stones.

The differential diagnosis of a solitary congenital liver cyst may include parasitic cysts, neoplastic cysts, and abscess. With available clinical information, laboratory testing, and imaging studies, the diagnosis becomes evident in most cases. If a solitary liver cyst is detected by clinical findings and imaging studies, and if the patient is asymptomatic, no treatment is required. If the patient experiences symptoms, ultrasound-directed needle aspiration has been suggested, but recurrence of cysts treated in that manner is highly likely. Therefore, if symptoms are ascribed to the liver cyst, surgical treatment is indicated. If a liver cyst is detected incidentally during an abdominal operation and if the lesion is 5 cm or less in diameter, it should be left undisturbed. If it is between 5 and 10 cm in diameter, one may aspirate the cyst to confirm the nature of its contents, and that procedure should be followed by excision of the cyst. Lesions 10 cm or greater should be aspirated; then cystograms can be obtained by injecting radiographic contrast material into the cyst to confirm that the cyst does not communicate with the biliary ductal system (they usually do not). Then the cyst should be totally excised if possible. One must use judgment in attempting total excision of a large cyst because a portion of the cyst wall may be adjacent to large hepatic veins or other important structures that should not be injured. Total excision is desirable, but should not be carried out at the risk of damaging vital structures. Lobectomy is rarely indicated for solitary liver cysts. During any treatment of solitary liver cysts, one must always bear in mind that the lesions are usually benign and generally do not adversely affect the patient's longevity. The risk of the treatment clearly should not exceed the risk of the disease.

Recurrent Liver Cysts

I have treated two patients who developed recurrent solitary liver cysts after surgical treatment. Both patients were referred to me because of severe abdominal or back pain that occurred 2 to 3 months after the operation described as excision of the cyst. In both patients, imaging studies revealed the recurrent cyst. Reoperation and complete excision of the cyst eliminated the cyst and the symptoms in both patients.

ADULT FIBROPOLYCYSTIC DISEASE

Adult fibropolycystic disease of the liver is also relatively infrequent. It is inherited as a mendelian dominant trait and is usually detected during adulthood. Grossly, the liver is diffusely involved with multiple cysts, varying from microscopic lesions to masses 20 to 30 cm in diameter. Larger cysts are less common, however. The cysts may be thin-walled and are often so numerous that they seem to have destroyed much of the liver parenchyma. Histologically, there are variably sized cystic spaces lined with cuboidal epithelium. About one-third of the patients with adult fibropolycystic liver disease have associated polycystic kidneys. One-half to three-quarters of the patients with polycystic kidney disease have polycystic liver disease. Patients with adult polycystic liver disease may also exhibit cystic disease of the pancreas, the spleen, and, in rare instances, the lung. There is an increased incidence of intracranial aneurysms in patients with polycystic liver disease. Women are more commonly afflicted with this disease than men, and the age of detection may range from early adulthood up to the eighth decade. Patients are commonly asymptomatic, but may exhibit upper abdominal pain or gradually enlarging abdominal mass. Jaundice in polycystic disease can be due to extrinsic pressure on the bile duct by the cyst or concomitant ductal stones. Physical examination discloses a palpable mass in three-quarters of the patients. In the absence of obstructive jaundice, liver function is almost entirely normal, despite seemingly complete replacement of hepatic parenchyma by cysts. In addition, liver function is ordinarily maintained within normal limits throughout the patient's life. The natural history of this disease is usually dictated by the renal function, which is often impaired and may lead to chronic end-stage renal failure in some patients. Imaging studies such as ultrasound and computerized tomographic scanning disclose cystic lesions in the kidneys and in the liver. These findings, combined with impaired renal function, normal liver function, and, particularly, a family history of renal failure, should confirm the diagnosis. If there are no symptoms, no treatment of polycystic liver is necessary. If the patient is experiencing pain and discomfort, operation should be recommended. The appropriate treatment is to unroof as completely as possible those cysts located adjacent to the surface of the liver, then to create communication between the more deeply seated lesions and the peritoneal cavity by breaking down the septa. Careful cholangiography should be accomplished in patients exhibiting jaundice. Because polycystic liver diseae is rarely responsible for death, one must exercise extreme caution in its treatment.

CHILDHOOD FIBROPOLYCYSTIC DISEASE OF THE LIVER AND KIDNEY

Childhood fibropolycystic disease of the liver and kidney is transmitted as an autosomal recessive trait. There are three general categories, usually dependent on the relative severity of the renal and liver disease: perinatal, neonatal, and infantile. The perinatal disease is usually evident at birth. There may be mild liver involvement with some fibrosis and some dilated ducts. These patients usually exhibit severe renal disease and die in the neonatal period. The neonatal disease is usually detected when the patient is about one month old. There is some-

what more involvement of the liver, but somewhat less involvement of the kidney, than in the perinatal form. These patients usually die of progressive renal failure within a year. The infantile form is usually detected when the children are 3 to 6 months of age, when they develop renal failure. These patients experience renal failure throughout childhood, may develop hepatic fibrosis, and in some cases develop portal hypertension. The treatment consists of managing the renal failure. If bleeding esophageal varices develop, portal systemic decompression may be effective.

CONGENITAL HEPATIC FIBROSIS

The childhood-type polycystic kidney disease associated with congenital hepatic fibrosis has an autosomal recessive inheritance, although sporadic cases do occur. This disease is characterized by hepatosplenomegaly and portal hypertension with well-preserved hepatocellular function. It is encountered principally in children and is detected in them around age 10. Histologic examination reveals bands of fibrous tissue containing abnormal intralobular bile ducts and portal vein hypoplasia with intervening normal parenchyma with preserved architecture. The diagnosis is established by findings of impaired renal function, enlarged cystic kidneys, normal liver function, and fibrous bands in the liver on biopsy. Treatment of the disease depends on the predominant lesion. If the patient can be managed conservatively through childhood and adolescence, it is possible that the portal hypertension may improve and the bleeding esophageal varices may decrease as collaterals develop. But for patients who have repeated life-threatening upper gastrointestinal bleeding, portosystemic shunting should be carried out. There is controversy concerning the risk of hepatic encephalopathy following portosystemic shunting for congenital hepatic fibrosis. Renal transplantation may be necessary for the management of renal failure in these patients.

NEOPLASTIC CYSTS

Although neoplastic cysts of the liver are rare, they do occur. There are reports of cystadenomas and cystadenocarcinomas developing in the liver. A recent interesting report described functioning cystic endocrine neoplasms occurring in the liver and the pancreas. These lesions produced hypergastrinemia and were associated with manifestations of Zollinger-Ellison syndrome.

POSTTRAUMATIC CYSTS (PSEUDOCYSTS)

Posttraumatic cysts of the liver are extremely rare. They occur when an uninjured liver capsule accompanies a central or subcapsular liver fracture. The resulting hematoma may liquefy, and often there is communication of the cavity with bile ducts, with the result that posttraumatic liver cysts may contain bile. Posttraumatic liver cysts are usually caused by blunt abdominal trauma, and the patients are young. Pseudocysts have been detected days or months after injury. The lining of the pseudocyst is comprised of granulation tissue plus dense fibrous tissue. The clinical findings are abdominal pain with radiation to the back or shoulder, accompanied by an upper abdominal mass, which follows severe blunt abdominal trauma. Treatments described include external drainage or excision of the pseudocyst. The only pseudocyst we have treated was detected several years after the causal injury and was easily managed by excision.

PARASITIC CYSTS, HYDATID DISEASE

Hydatid cysts, the most common parasitic cysts of the liver, are caused by the cestode *Echinococcus granulosis*. Hydatid disease is prevalent in South America, the Far East, Southern and Eastern Europe, and Australia. This disease is rare in the United States, but may occur in Alaska and in the southern United States. *Echinococcus granulosis* is disseminated when the offal of infested sheep or swine is fed to dogs. The dogs' feces contaminate the ground or water around dwellings, and humans ingest the ova. After digestion, the ova unencyst to pass through the intestinal epithelium into the portal blood and thence to the liver. Although other organs including the lung can be involved, the liver is the most commonly affected site. Sixty to seventy percent of cysts arise in the right lobe, about 20 percent arise in the left lobe, and in 20 to 30 percent of cases, both lobes are diseased. Echinococcal cyst of the liver is a chronic disease that affects both sexes

equally and may occur at any age. The cyst may be asymptomatic for long periods and may be detected incidentally. Some patients may experience upper abdominal discomfort or may detect a mass. Approximately one-third of the patients experience the following complications in a decreasing order of frequency: (1) rupture into the bile ducts, (2) abscess, (3) intraperitoneal rupture, and (4) hepatobronchial fistula. Rupture of an echinococcic cyst into a bile duct causes colicky abdominal pain, jaundice, and fever. Plain films of the abdomen may reveal calcification in the cyst wall. Ultrasound is probably the best test for the diagnosis and delineation of an echinococcal cyst. One author stated that the ultrasound finding of the cyst with demonstrable daughter cysts was pathognomonic. CT scans delineate an echinococcic cyst with 98 percent accuracy. False-negatives occur in patients with fatty livers. Immunologic testing may be employed. In one study, the intradermal skin tests (Casoni test) were 69 percent positive; however, some authorities recommend that the Casoni test be abandoned. Immunoelectrophoresis is probably the test of choice. Echinococcic cysts require surgical treatment. Several authors recommend evacuation of the cyst and the application of a scolecidal agent (either 0.5% silver nitrate or 1% cetramide). Formalin should not be used because it can cause bile duct sclerosis or death. When cysts rupture into the bile ducts, common duct exploration and choledochostomy should be performed. There is controversy concerning the treatment of echinococcal cysts. Some recommend excision of the cyst; others advise hepatic lobectomy. Resection must undoubtedly be required on occasion. The cyst fluid is antigenic, and intra-abdominal leakage of the fluid may cause anaphylactic shock.

LIVER TUMOR

SHUNZABURO IWATSUKI, M.D.
THOMAS E. STARZL, M.D., PH.D.

With widespread application of sophisticated radiologic (CT scan, ultrasonography, and angiography) and chemical (CEA and alpha-fetoprotein) diagnostic methods, liver tumors are being detected more often and more accurately than before. Although asymptomatic mass lesions, found incidentally by radiologic examination, are more often benign than malignant, they should be considered as the latter until proved otherwise.

Some benign and malignant tumors have characteristic radiologic features, but the findings are by no means pathognomonic. A small piece of tissue obtained by needle biopsy is often inadequate to establish a definitive diagnosis, particularly in differentiating adenoma from low-grade hepatocellular carcinoma. If the diagnosis is uncertain, the lesion should be excised without delay with an adequate margin. The high mortality follow-

ing major hepatic resections which existed in the past has been minimized in recent years at many major centers. At our institution, the operative mortality has been less than 3 percent.

In planning how large a resection will be required, a CT scan is most useful to assess the extent of the tumor, but it can be misleading when a large tumor distorts normal anatomic boundaries. If resectability is uncertain after extensive preoperative investigations, the examining physician should refer the patient to a surgeon who is experienced in major hepatic resections instead of subjecting him or her to exploratory celiotomy by someone who is unprepared to undertake a definitive procedure.

BENIGN LIVER TUMORS

Cavernous Hemangioma

Hemangiomas are the most common benign tumors of the liver. They are usually small (less than 4 cm in diameter) and solitary. Occasionally, they are, or grow to be, very large. By convention, lesions larger than 4 cm are called giant hemangiomas. Most hemangiomas are asymptomatic and are found incidentally. However, giant hemangiomas can cause various disabling pressure symptoms and pain. Life-threatening spontaneous rupture of a hemangioma is uncommon, but this complication has been reported many times. The usual cause of a massive hemorrhage is an ill-advised percutaneous needle biopsy.

Symptomatic cavernous hemangiomas should be excised surgically. The majority of giant hemangiomas require lobectomy or trisegmentectomy, but some, those that are located on the surface of the liver or those that are pedunculated, can be enucleated along pseudocapsular margins without significant loss of normal tissue. We have resected 60 giant cavernous hemangiomas without any deaths.

Diagnostic uncertainty seldom is the indication for surgery because CT scan with contrast infusion usually gives unequivocal images, and angiographic diagnosis is even more definitive.

Adenoma

Many adenomas are large and cause disabling pressure symptoms, pain, and/or hemorrhage. Some adenomas are multiple and can, in rare instances, involve all four segments of the liver. It is not only the large adenoma that can rupture, bleed internally, and cavitate. Even a small adenoma can rupture and cause life-threatening intraperitoneal hemorrhage. The histologic distinction between adenoma and minimum deviation hepatoma is often dificult, particularly from a small needle biopsy specimen.

Most authorities agree that adenomas require resection in all but exceptional cases. A conservative approach carries too great a risk of rupture or hemorrhage, or of missing a malignant lesion. Reports of tumor regression after discontinuance of birth control pills are countered by an even greater number of failures with this approach, or of complications of tumors that enlarged during or after pregnancy. Anatomic hepatic resection is usually advisable, but smaller adenomas can be excised locally with adequate margins. Contraceptive pills should be discontinued as soon as the diagnosis of adenoma is entertained.

We have had two young female patients with multiple adenomas that occupied all four segments of the liver, causing hemorrhage and disabling pain. They were treated successfully with orthotopic liver transplantation.

Focal Nodular Hyperplasia

Focal nodular hyperplasia, a non-neoplastic mass lesion of the liver, is usually less than 5 cm in diameter and asymptomatic. The lesion rarely bleeds, and it does not predispose to malignancy. Unfortunately, the radiologic diagnosis of focal nodular hyperplasia by ultrasonography, CT scan, and angiography cannot be made with certainty. However, a needle biopsy usually confirms the diagnosis because of the characteristic histology. Rare large focal nodular hyperplasias cause disabling pressure symptoms and pain, necessitating hepatic resection.

Cysts

Congenital simple cysts of the liver that have an endothelial-like lining have been referred to as "spring-water cysts." They are usually asymptomatic and can safely be observed.

Simple cysts lined with cuboidal epithelium sometimes become large and multilocular. The lining may become fibrous, proliferative, papillary, or mucin-producing. They often communicate with the biliary system, bleed internally, or become infected. These symptomatic congenital cysts should be treated surgically. Although it is tempting to aspirate or drain the cystic fluid percutaneously, those procedures are often diagnostically equivocal and therapeutically ineffective, and may involve risks of introducing infection and of implantation of neoplastic cells or parasites, if used unwisely. Some advocate that the solitary cysts with clear fluid be unroofed and drained into the peritoneal cavity, and that cysts with bile-strained fluid be drained with a Roux-en-Y jejunal limb. We recommend resection of all symptomatic cysts, whenever possible. They can be locally excised or removed by anatomic resection. Although malignant change in the cyst wall is uncommon, we have treated three patients whose cyst lining developed squamous cell carcinoma; two of the three had been previously operated on with Roux-en-Y internal drainage techniques.

A cystadenoma of the liver should be totally excised because of the possibility of malignant degeneration and because it may not be distinguishable histologically from a cystadenocarcinoma. Small lesions may be excised locally with adequate margins, but larger ones should be removed by anatomic resections.

The pressure symptoms of polycystic disease of the liver can sometimes be palliated with multiple needle aspirations. Operative marsupialization, incisional drainage, or aspiration of large cysts cannot relieve the symptoms more effectively than simple percutaneous needle aspirations. Therefore, operative procedures for polycystic disease are rarely justified. However, there are occasional patients who have a dominance of normal tissue in the left lateral segment of the liver. We have treated two such patients by right trisegmentectomy and the result was prolonged symptomatic relief. We have used orthotopic liver transplantation to treat a woman whose huge liver caused uncontrollable pain and multiple rib fractures. She has been pain-free and off narcotics since the transplantation.

Other Benign Lesions

Rare benign tumors, such as fibroma, rhabdomyoma, leiomyoma, fibrous mesothelioma, and myelolipoma, cannot be easily distinguished from malignant tumors without pathologic examination. If the diagnosis is uncertain, the tumor should be excised with an adequate margin for detailed histologic examination.

MALIGNANT TUMORS

Primary Hepatic Malignant Tumors

Various types of primary malignant tumors develop in the liver; hepatocellular carcinoma (hepatoma) is the most common, followed by cholangiocarcinoma, hepatoblastoma, and various cell types of sarcoma. As long as the lesion is localized in three of the four segments of the liver, curative subtotal hepatectomy theoretically can be performed. Many hepatomas found in noncirrhotic livers grow slowly, and even very large tumors sometimes spare one segment of the normal liver. Results after major hepatic resections justify the efforts, because the 5-year survival rate is 40 to 50 percent for noncirrhotic patients.

However, hepatoma developing in a cirrhotic liver is a different therapeutic problem. The patients with well-compensated cirrhosis (no jaundice, no ascites, and serum albumin greater than 3 mg per deciliter) can usually tolerate a lobectomy, but the operative mortality is as high as 30 percent. Both the progressive nature of underlying cirrhosis and the multiplicity of malignant tumors in cirrhotic livers contribute to a grim prognosis.

The role of orthotopic liver transplantation for primary malignant tumors of the liver is limited. Our experience with 50 such patients, as well as the experience of others, has shown that primary malignant tumors of the liver that cannot be removed by conventional subtotal hepatectomy cannot be cured by total hepatectomy and liver replacement. The tumors have almost always recurred if the patients lived long enough. However, good palliation has been achieved for many patients for a year or two.

In contrast, cure usually has been achieved of tumors found incidentally in livers removed for other end-stage hepatic disease.

Metastatic Tumors

The liver is one of the organs most commonly involved by metastatic tumors. An aggressive approach with the resection of hepatic metastases is warranted because long survival has been regularly achieved, particularly when isolated or regional hepatic metastases have been from colorectal primaries. Our usual approach to metastatic liver tumors has been with anatomic resections rather than excisions. We have performed more than 80 major anatomic hepatic resections for metastatic tumors without any mortality and have found unexpected small additional metastases in the resected specimens in nearly 10 percent of the cases. The large size of the lesion, a multiplicity of metastases, or a short interval between resection of the primary and appearance of secondary lesions can adversely affect the survival rate after resection, but not enough to let any of these factors dissuade us from proceeding. Five-year survival after resection among our 50 patients with metastatic colorectal cancer is approximately 50 percent.

TECHNICAL REFINEMENTS IN HEPATIC RESECTION

Incision

A bilateral subcostal incision with an upper midline extension usually gives adequate exposure for any type of resection, especially if the xiphoid process is removed. In many cases the left subcostal extension is not necessary, particularly for right-sided resection. If a thoracic extension is decided upon, a right seventh intercostal incision is connected to the midportion of the right subcostal incision. The thoracic extension almost never is required, even in physically well-developed adults.

Right Lobectomy and Right Trisegmentectomy

The steps of the operation may vary, depending on the location and size of the lesion. Usually the right triangular ligaments are incised, and the bare area is entered. This allows the right lobe to be lifted into the wound and retracted to the left. Inability to mobilize the liver safely at this time and difficulty in visualizing the area where the right hepatic vein enters the inferior vena cava are the main reasons for considering a thoracic extension.

Before the hilar dissection is begun, anatomic variations of the hepatic artery must be looked for. In the "normal" situation, the common hepatic artery originates from the celiac axis and lies in the left anterior portion of the portal triad. However, the right hepatic or even common hepatic artery may originate from the superior mesenteric artery, and if so, the anomalous vessel will lie posterior to the portal vein. The left hepatic artery can originate from the left gastric artery or separately from the aorta; in which case it will be found in the middle of the gastrohepatic ligament, running toward the umbilical fissure.

The hilar dissection is begun by ligation and division of the cystic duct and artery. The right branches of the structures of the portal triad are isolated. The right hepatic artery is sacrificed first. Arterial anomalies are so numerous that ligation should never be performed without preliminary test occlusion and without being sure that during this occlusion there are pulsations distally in the region of the umbilical fissure.

At a more superior level, the right branch of the portal vein is detached and the stump is tied or closed with sutures. After dividing the right hepatic artery and the right portal vein, a line of demarcation is evident between the true right and left lobes, passing through the gallbladder bed and directed toward the vena cava.

Almost invariably, the hepatic bile duct is the hilar structure with the most superior bifurcation, and sometimes the division is within the substance of the liver. The right duct is ligated and divided where it comes off almost like the crossbar of a T. Dissection of the hilum at this point is completed for a true right lobectomy.

As the right lobe is retracted, dissection and encirclement of the right hepatic vein is now begun. The vein is doubly clamped with angled vascular clamps, divided, and sewn shut on both sides with continuous vascular sutures. This maneuver is potentially dangerous because the hepatic vein is extremely short and because a tear during the dissection would create a defect in the side of the vena cava. Sometimes the right hepatic vein is better dealt with from inside the liver during the actual transection of the liver. This is particularly important if a tumor is posteriorly located, bulky, or invading the diaphragm.

In performing a true right lobectomy, the liver is split at the exact line of color demarcation. The Glisson's capsule can be incised with electrocautery. Knife handles, clamps, and/or fingers can be used to crash down to interlobar strands, which are swiftly but carefully ligated and divided. For a true right lobectomy, the middle hepatic vein is left intact since it drains both the right and left lobes.

In order to perform a right trisegmentectomy, further hilar dissection is required. Before beginning this phase of the operation, the exact location of the umbilical fissure must be determined. The left branches of the triad structures are freed from the inferior surface of the medical segment of the left lobe. Small portal vein branches, arteries, and ducts that enter the liver surface must be handled meticulously.

In addition to the additional hilar dissection required for right trisegmentectomy, a number of small hepatic veins entering the anterior surface of the retrohepatic vena cava should be ligated and divided. If the caudate lobe is to be totally excised, all vena caval tributaries except the left hepatic vein are ligated and divided.

A crucial final step in the actual transection for right trisegmentectomy is the identification of the complex of arterial portal venous and duct structures that originate in the umbilical fissure and feed back from the main trunks to the medial segment of the left lobe. Although these so-called feedback structures originate in the umbilical fissure, they are not dissected there, but are found just to the right of the falciform ligament, usually within the substance of the liver. Only with the occlusion of the feedback vessels does the medial segment of the left lobe become cyanotic. The actual liver transection begins just to the right of the falciform ligament. Near the vena cava, the middle hepatic vein is ligated. It either enters separately into the inferior vena cava or, more commonly, joins the left hepatic veins to form a short common trunk. A common trunk must not be mistaken for a middle hepatic vein.

Left Lateral Segmentectomy, Left Lobectomy, and Left Trisegmentectomy

The ligamentum teres hepatis is ligated and divided, and the falciform ligament is incised superiorly into the suprahepatic bare area in which lie the main hepatic veins and suprahepatic vena cava. The left triangular ligament is incised, fully exposing the anterior surface of the left hepatic vein and the entry of the left phrenic veins.

If only the left lateral segment is to be removed, the hilar dissection should be kept to the left of the falciform ligament and umbilical fissure to avoid injury to the arterial, portal venous, and ductal structures feeding back from the fissure to the medial segment of the left lobe. As the parenchymal transection approaches the diaphragm posteriorly, the middle hepatic vein joining the left hepatic vein must be identified and preserved.

For a true left lobectomy, the lateral segment is lifted anteriorly and retracted toward the right. With this maneuver, the principal left lobar branches of the portal triad structures can be safely approached from their posterolateral aspect. The posteriorly located left portal vein is encircled first, ligated, and divided. The more anteriorly positioned left hepatic artery and left hepatic duct can then be more easily seen, dissected, and divided. If the caudate process to the left of the inferior vena cava is to be removed, the left hilar structures should be ligated at their origin. If this left portion of the caudate lobe is to be spared, the ligatures usually should be distal to the posteriorly directed first branch. When those maneuvers are completed, the true left lobe becomes cyanotic. With continuous traction of the left lateral segment anteriorly and to the right, the posterior incision of the eventual specimen is developed through the liver capsule. If a decision has been made to preserve the left part of the caudate lobe, the parenchyma of the liver is entered along the natural line of the obliterated ductus venosus. Alternatively, the caudate lobe can be removed with consequent complete visualization of the anterior and left lateral surface of the retrohepatic vena cava. The elected posterior line of transection is continued superiorly until the left hepatic vein is encircled, transected, and either ligated or sewn closed with vascular sutures. Earlier attempts to encircle the left hepatic vein may be dangerous because of posteriorly located tributaries which can be thereby injured. At this point, a left lobectomy is completed by transecting at the lobar plane defined by the color demarcation.

The additional requirement of a left hepatic trisegmentectomy is to remove the anterior segment of the right lobe. The main difficulty is to identify the correct intersegmental plane. There are two points at which this intersegmental plane can be properly entered. Some livers have a natural groove near the base of the gallbladder, which delineates the plane between the anterior and posterior segments. This groove, if present, is an excellent landmark. However, the search for this intersegmental plane is best begun superiorly, anterior to the right hepatic vein. With blunt dissection, the superior end of the previously defined line of posterior parenchymal incision is deepened near the diaphragm, using the point of the transected left hepatic vein as the starting point. The dissection finger is first brought anteriorly, then turned at right angles so that it can be swept transversely in the coronal plane. The fingertip emerges just anterior to the right hepatic vein. The middle hepatic vein is encountered and must be transected and ligated or sutured if this has not already been accomplished. Intraparenchymal tributaries to the right hepatic vein are ligated as encountered.

The superior to inferior scalping maneuver is continued, now aided by downward traction of the specimen. A resistant-free plane is sought, and all strands encountered are clamped or ligated. Inferiorly, the dissecting finger should emerge near the base of, and at right angles to, the gallbladder bed. Since the anterior segment retains its portal venous and hepatic arterial inflow almost until the specimen is out, the blood loss may be excessive. If so, the portal triad can be temporarily cross-clamped safely (the Pringle maneuver) for about one hour.

When the dominant natural transverse groove near the base of the gallbladder is present, the scalping process can be started at the hilum, ligating the arterial, portal venous, and ductal strands which run anteriorly, while protecting the vital residual posterior structures from injury.

The frontally presenting cut surface of the posterior segment after removal of the specimen permits precise visualization of residual bleeding joints and bile leaks. The extent to which ducts are exposed is greater than with other kinds of anatomic resections. An intraoperative cholangiogram through a T-tube should be obtained to check the integrity of the bile duct system before the closure.

Drainage and Other Care

The importance of adequate drainage of the subphrenic space after major hepatic resection cannot be overemphasized. Multiple closed-system suction drains can be placed in the huge, dead space, or open drainage can be used with multiple one-inch Penrose drains.

T-tube biliary drainage is not necessary unless the biliary system has been injured, except after left trisegmentectomy. After left trisegmentectomy, a T-tube should be left in with its upper limb passing into the remaining posterior segmental duct, which tends otherwise to become angulated.

Prophylactic antibiotics are started preoperatively and continued for a few days. Intraoperative correction of coagulopathy is important when a large amount of blood transfusion is required. Fear of hypoglycemia has been overemphasized. Usually, a maintenance infusion of 5% glucose and electrolyte solution is sufficient to maintain an adequate glucose level during and after operation. Transient jaundice and depression of multiple hepatic function tests are often seen after trisegmentectomy, but even after an 85 percent resection, relatively complete recovery can be expected within 1 to 3 weeks.

HEPATIC ARTERY LIGATION AND ARTERIAL INFUSION CHEMOTHERAPY

Hepatic artery ligation or radiologic embolization of hepatic artery has been used to treat nonresectable hepatic malignant tumors. The effects are usually temporary, and both procedures carry significant mortality and morbidity.

More recently, infusion chemotherapy through the hepatic artery by an implantable pump has been under investigation. Superiority of this hepatic artery infusion chemotherapy over conventional systemic intravenous chemotherapy is still uncertain. Various complications related to infusion catheter and implantable pumps have been reported at an incidence of 10 to 25 percent.

COLORECTAL CANCER METASTATIC TO THE LIVER: RESECTION

MARTIN A. ADSON, M.D.

Most of what has been learned clinically about the resective treatment of hepatic metastases has had to do with colorectal cancers because these primary lesions (1) are so common, (2) usually can be removed widely along with regional lymphatic spread, and (3) so often give rise to resectable hepatic metastases that *appear* to be the only sites of residual or recurrent growth. Also, most of what has been learned about metastases from colorectal cancers can be aplied clinically to the management of other visceral cancers that (1) are well differentiated, (2) originate where primary and regional growth can be removed, and (3) can spread to the liver through the portal vein.

What is known about the effect of removing hepatic metastases from such lesions is surprising: about 25 percent of patients so treated survive for 5 years or more! Removal of such *secondary* sites of tumor growth is more effective than the resective treatment of some *primary* visceral cancers because of biologic and anatomic factors that are poorly understood. It is true that some other cancers are poorly differentiated and inclined to early regional and distant spread that cannot be resected widely or dealt with in any other way. But these are just observations, not reasons; and there *are* good reasons to be surprised that resection of hematogenous metastases from colorectal cancer has any worth at all.

To remove metastases from the liver seems at first to be absurd when most malignant tumors have such a head start on the surgeon. Most visceral cancers can invade the blood stream after twenty doublings when they are just 1 mm small. Therefore, the capacity to shed, to spread and grow in the liver, lung, or bone *precedes* detectability of the primary tumor by many months or even years. Also, given so much opportunity for seeding of many, many cells, it seems unlikely that there ever would be just one site of distant spread.

This knowledge should discourage surgeons from removing metastatic tumors from the liver. However, some of what now looks like caprice or whimsy has been partially explained by the fact that cancer also has its vicissitudes. Half the patients who die from colorectal cancer do *not* have hepatic metastases. This failure of some tumors to spread to fertile soil relates to the inability of most single shed cells to survive, and to the need for cells to aggregate to achieve neovascularity and weather host defenses to live away from home. Even then, continuing proliferation involves only a fraction of this clump of cells, and many striving cancer cells do not survive at all.

It is the unpredictable outcome of the contest between the cancer and its host that accounts for some small success of surgeons who try to contend with hepatic metastases. Also, it is this unpredictability that accounts for failure, frustration, and the need to treat so many patients who will not be helped by a second major operative procedure. One-fourth of patients who have metastases removed are rid of troubling lesions for 5 years or more, but surgical success is precluded three times in four by the presence of metastases that could not be seen. Long-term survival is not determined by lesions that are seen and taken out, but rather by occult metastases that were left behind.

The problem involved in removing hepatic metastases is the same problem that limits effectiveness of all resective surgery done for cancer. As surgeons, we cannot see what is really going on. Therefore, as surgeons we either overtreat or undertreat three-fourths or more of most cancers, because most often we are ignorant of a cancer's real stage. We know a lot about patterns of growth and spread, but we do not know exactly what has happened to a specific tumor or its host when we try to treat the host who looks to us for help.

The disparity between what can be observed and what is really happening is likely to be resolved by improvement of techniques for detecting micrometastases. If we could see the occult metastases that are now the major cause of therapeutic failure, a proper choice of surgical therapy would be possible. But for the present, our choice of therapy must be based on *determinants of prognosis* evident in treated patients and upon the survival rates determined by the *natural history* of untreated disease.

DETERMINANTS OF PROGNOSIS

When the major determinants of prognosis (occult metastases which account for therapeutic failure in three patients out of four) are not evident, the study of observable determinants of survival of patients treated by resection has limited value. The facts derived from such studies are few and are not useful clinically in the choice of therapy for individuals; however, they are all we have for guidance at present.

Analysis is complicated by the multiplicity of factors. Kevin Hughes, working with Paul Sugarbaker and others, has offered a protocol for prospective study which involves recognition of 12 preoperative and eight operative factors that may have prognostic significance. The proposed study requires multifactorial analysis of 65 subgroups (derived from these 20 factors), to be correlated with four postoperative factors (with nine subgroups).

The study should be, as Huckleberry Finn described *Pilgrim's Progress*: "interesting but steep." Such a study is worthwhile if only because it involves observation of patterns of failure that have not been studied well, particularly sites of recurrence inside or outside the liver. I do have concern that much of what can be learned by analysis of our current blindness will be made irrelevant by the development of new techniques for imaging that will define a tumor's real stage. Nevertheless, it is much better to treat patients in a way that is planned for learning than to rely entirely on blind compassion with the wish that, as E. Starr Judd, Jr., said, "hope might triumph over judgment."

My colleagues and I have studied this aspect of choice of therapy by trying to see if surgical success or failure could be foretold by retrospective analysis of treated patients. The study involved 141 patients who had hepatic metastases from colorectal cancer removed between 1948 and 1982. Mean age of patients was 56 years, and 60 percent were men. Size of metastatic lesion (mean 4 cm) as well as site determined the extent of resection. More than half the lesions could be removed by simple wedge resection, but nearly one-third required removal of half or more of the liver. In three-fourths of the cases, solitary lesions were resected; in the rest, multiple lesions were removed from one or both lobes. More than half had Dukes' class C primary lesions, and 18 percent had extrahepatic metastases resected—extensions of tumor away from the primary and regional sites of growth.

Overall, 3- and 5-year survival rates of treated patients were 40 percent and 25 percent, respectively (Fig. 1). Enough is known about the natural history of untreated patients that 5-year survival rates can be used as evidence of surgical success. However, having found again that most patients were not benefitted, we studied the determinants of improved survival of these treated patients.

This analysis involved univariate and multivariate analysis of eight factors with 18 subgroups that might correlate with prognosis. We found that location and grade of the primary tumor and the time of removal of metastases (synchronous versus metachronous) were not

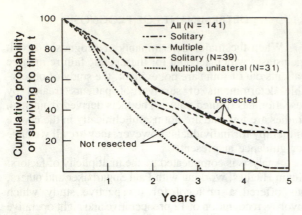

Figure 1 Survival curves of 141 treated patients compared with patients who had biopsy-proven metastases that were not resected.

significant determinants of survival. Also, size of lesions considered as a single factor and extent of resection had significance only in relation to operative mortality: none of the 74 patients who had minor resections done died from operation, but 4 percent of the 67 patients who had one-third or more of the liver removed died from such operations.

Three determinants of favorable prognosis were identified in our study. The first has to do with gender. In our initial study of the first 60 patients in this series, we found that all patients who survived 5 or more years after resection of hepatic metastases were women. Extended observation of our total group is confirmatory to some extent. Being female has some advantage that has borderline statistical significance (P equals 0.054).

The second determinant of favorable prognosis has to do with the extent of the primary lesion. The 5-year survival rates of patients who had restricted primary tumors removed (B Duke's, if hepatic metastases are ignored) were nearly twice that of patients whose resected primary tumors involved regional lymphatic nodes more extensively. This difference may be determined either by unresectable residual regional metastases or by the hematogenous dissemination that is more likely to occur from tumors that have invaded lymphatic pathways.

The third favorable determinant of prognosis is the absence of extrahepatic metastases, in that the presence of extrahepatic metastases that were removed when the liver metastases were resected precluded long survival. No patient who had metastases removed outside the liver survived for 5-years, and the 5-year survival rate of their counterparts who had no evidence of extrahepatic metastases was 30 percent. The influence of this factor was even more apparent in our separate study of the 67 patients who had metastases so large as to require major hepatic resection: when patients who had extrahepatic metastases removed along with the large metastatic liver lesions were excluded, the 5-year survival rates of their counterparts who had no evident extrahepatic metastasis was 46 percent. This latter finding must relate to the time required for hepatic metastases to grow so large as to require "major" hepatic resections, time that also should

allow some previously "occult" extrahepatic metastases to become evident.

The results of Fortner's multivariate analysis of 75 patients who underwent resection of hepatic metastases from colorectal cancer are much the same as ours. He found that age, sex, location of primary tumor, size, and whether metastases were synchronous or metachronous were *not* significant determinants of survival; he also found preoperative liver function tests and CEA assays to have no prognostic significance for patients who had liver metastases removed. Additionally, Fortner correlated results of resective treatment with the "extent" of disease. Postoperative survival rates of patients who had stage I disease (tumor confined to the resection portion of the liver without invasion of major intrahepatic vessels or bile ducts) were twice those of patients who had stage II and stage III disease (tumor rupture, direct extension to adjacent organs, histologically positive margins of resection, direct invasion of major vessels or bile ducts, lymph node metastases, or other extrahepatic spread). Unfortunately, except for his description of involved margins of resection, I could not learn from his report whether or not other described extensions of tumor were removed. His system of staging (stage I) based on large tumors (median 6 cm) that can be removed cleanly, but have not invaded major intrahepatic vessels or bile ducts is unclear to me when major structures are undefined.

Fortner found also, as Foster did so long ago, that the *number* of unilobar metastatic hepatic deposits removed was not a determinant of prognosis. This is one other observable determinant of prognosis—multiplicity of metastatic liver lesions—that has not been studied well. Correlations of survival with the number of metastases found and removed may be misleading when the *size, site*, and *pattern* of resected lesions are not considered as well. Multiple metastases may come from the primary tumor or may develop as secondary satellites arising adjacent to such a "primary" metastatic growth. In fact, Willis concluded that "the majority of hepatic growths are probably local intrahepatic descendants, generations removed from the pioneer metastasis."

Differentiation between these two phenomena should be made evident by careful study of gross patterns of multiplicity. Foster and Paul Sugarbaker have shown bilobar multiplicity to be unfavorable, but beyond that, most authors have not studied the size and disposition of metastases within a single liver lobe. "Clumped" or satellite multiplicity of lesions must have prognostic significance different from that of scatteredd lesions within a lobe, and the size of lesions must relate in some way to the *time* required for a few lesions to become large without successive generations of primary micrometastases becoming evident.

Sugarbaker has found that more than three metastases cannot be treated well, but has not yet studied the patterns of such multiplicity. Cady and McDermott also have studied *number* of liver lesions, along with some aspects of size and time, as determinants of prognosis of 23 patients who had multiple metachronous metastases removed. Having found (as Sugarbaker did) that patients

TABLE 1 Relationship of Size and Multiplicity of Hepatic Metastases to Survival Rate*

Survival, yr	Small Lesions				Large Lesions			
	Synchronous		Metachronous		Synchronous		Metachronous	
	1(n=27)	>1(n=2)	1(n=24)	>1(n=16)	1(n=4)	>1(n=1)	1(n=43)	>1(n=18)
3	37	50	56	21	25	0	30	50
5	26	50	33	0	0	0	18	37
10	11	0	22	0	0	0	18	0

* Values expressed are percentage of patients who survived. Small lesions were less than 4 cm, and large lesions, 4 cm or larger. 1 indicates solitary lesions, and >1, multiple lesions.

(5) who had more than three metastases removed did poorly, they have seen in this magic number a "unique biologic, not temporal" event which transcends most other determinants of prognosis, even though the four or more resected lesions were "clustered" in one "anatomic area."

In my own study of multiplicity of metastases, I found survival rates of our total sample of 104 solitary and 37 multiple resected lesions to be identical, but then found that large size (greater than 4 cm) of multiple metachronous metastases was a favorable determinant of prognosis (Table 1). Unfortunately, having stumbled upon this seeming paradox, I failed to study precise numbers and patterns of metastases in a proper way, but am working on that now.

In the future, our efforts to find evidence for biologic phenomena in anatomic observations of multiple hepatic metastases must involve not just *number*, but also *size*, *patterns* of metastasis, and *time*.

Something has been learned about determinants of prognosis: three or four subgroups of patients who can be offered resective liver surgery with more chance of success have been identified. However, we still do not know enough to deny such effort to many other individual patients.

EVALUATION OF RESULTS; THE NATURAL HISTORY OF UNTREATED DISEASE

Analysis of the effectiveness of resective treatment is made difficult by the small size of most treated samples and by limited periods of postoperative observation, incomplete observations upon which *estimates* of survival are based. Although use of such analytic methods is now widespread, the accuracy and actual clinical value of results so recognized still relate to sample size and to the length of observation of portions of the treated sample.

Enough is known about the natural history of untreated hepatic metastases to consider 5-year survival after resection as evidence of surgical success. However, it is difficult to know whether survival for 2 or 3 years has been provided by resection or by nature. Therefore, there is still need to know more about the natural history of resectable metastases that are not removed.

Unfortunately, most published observations of natural history involve advanced unresectable hepatic metastases

and, as such, are really terminal studies of demise. Such clinically evident harbingers that foreshadow death have some usefulness for the assessment of systemic therapies, but are surgically irrelevant. In these studies, the fate of untreated patients who might have been helped by resection is hidden by statistical analyses of samples wherein criteria for resectability have not been well defined.

Therefore, we have tried to study natural history in a more selective way. Prospective trials that involve observation rather than removal of resectable tumors cannot be justified, and even less structured studies of natural history are difficult today when so little is left to nature. Therefore, we studied retrospectively 252 patients (1946 to 1976) who had biopsy-proven hepatic metastases that appeared to be the major determinant of their survival. The process of excluding patients who had uncontrollable primary lesions or residual tumor elsewhere that might compromise survival was the same method used now to select patients for resection of their metastatic liver lesions. This is the best we could do in our search for historical controls.

One hundred and eighty-two of the 252 patients had widespread bilateral unresectable metastases. However, 39 patients (15%) had unresected solitary lesions, and 31 (12%) had unilobar multiple metastases that now would be considered resectable. Thus, 70 lesions (27%) probably could have been removed but, for reasons determined by individual surgeons, had not been taken out.

The survival curves of the patients who had "resectable" solitary (39) and multiple unilobar (31) lesions that were not resected are shown on Figure 1 along with overall survival rates of our 141 patients who had hepatic metastases removed.

The most important thing learned from this comparison is that resection has therapeutic value that is statistically significant (P is less than 0.0001). Furthermore, it can be seen that patients who have resectable hepatic metastases that are not removed do live longer than we used to think they could. Median survival rates of patients with resectable but unresected solitary or mulitple unilobar lesions were 21 and 15 months respectively, and more than 20 percent of patients who had solitary lesions left behind survived 3 years or more.

Most interesting, however, it the fact that median survival rates of both treated and untreated patients are grouped by nature in the middle of all curves. These observations of natural history, however crude, should be considered by clinical practitioners who wish to publish prematurely and by statisticians who are unacquainted with disease.

RESECTIVE SURGERY IN PERSPECTIVE

There is need to consider the benefits and limitations of hepatic metastasectomy in broad perspective by looking critically at all patients with liver lesions to see how many of them might be helped by resective surgery. Our retrospective study of natural history summarized above involved a total of 466 patients who had histologically proven metastases. Fifty-six patients were excluded from our study of natural history of untreated metastases because metastases had been resected. Thus, of the 466 patients who had hepatic metastases, 56 underwent resection and 70 had either solitary (39) or multiple unilobar lesions (31) that probably could have been removed. If our assessment of theoretical resectability is reasonably correct, we can conclude that 126 (27%) of the 466 patients had metastases that we would now consider to be resectable. Even if our view of resectability of multiple unilobar lesions is faulted in some way, 56 metastases were resected, and descriptions of unresected solitary lesions gave good evidence for their resectability. Thus, at least 20 percent (56 + 39 = 95) of the total sample of patients had resectable hepatic metastases that were the only evidence of residual disease.

This view of resectability can be used to update efforts that Foster, Fortner, and Sugarbaker have made to consider the potential value of hepatic metastasectomy on a national scale. Of 120,000 patients who develop colorectal cancer each year, half will develop recurrence after treatment, and half of these will have hepatic metastases. If about 25 percent of these patients have resectable hepatic metastases that appear to be the major determinants of survival, then there are, each year, 7,500 patients who might be candidates for hepatic resective surgery.

Intuitively, I think that this projection is faulty in some way, and most surgeons and oncologists are likely to consider this an optimistic view. However, even this view can be considered pessimistic in a realistic way because of the 7,500 "candidates" for hepatic metastasectomy, only 1,875 really would be benefitted by selective and resective procedures available today. Unfortunately, 5,625 patients would be subjected to the risk, discomfort, and expense of major operative procedures without receiving benefit, and efforts to perform such operations on as grand a scale are likely to involve unwanted risk.

I am uncomfortable with this hypothesis, but have offered it for comparative perspective. I am told by surgeons who deal mostly with trauma that one-half of the 45,000 deaths from motor vehicle accidents could be prevented if drunken drivers could be kept off the road, and that about one-fifth (5,000) of dead sober motorists might have been saved by reasonable seat-belt legislation.

This reductio ad absurdum may be justified or not, but gives me pause to consider several other things. First of all, it does seem that competence (as a hepatic resectionist) may beget inconsequence of a sort, that there is need for improved techniques for finding small hepatic and extrahepatic metastases to stage tumor systems that we now treat blindly, and that the greatest need is for effective biologic manipulations of cancer for use as primary treatments or as adjuvants to our surgical therapies.

Techniques now available for "imaging" lesions in the liver are wondrous in a way, but have limitations that beget expense and clinical embarrassment that is hard for all to bear. Each diagnostic modality available clinically today (radionuclides, computed tomography, ultrasonography, and magnetic resonance scans and angiography) can show large metastatic hepatic lesions that may be surgically attractive. However, micrometastases from colorectal cancer are not made evident by use of any of these techniques. Moreover, the comparative effectiveness of these five "tests" depends on the availability and affordability of new improved machines and on the interest and ability of their users. Therefore, the clinician who is looking for small lesions often is moved by conscientiousness, indecision, or need for procrastination to "order" two or three of these costly tests—in an ascending order determined by the fact that cheaper tests most often show the least. The fiscal embarrassment that relates to this competitive ineffectiveness of tests can be justified only by the fact that the clinical and cost-effectiveness of surgical evaluation used to reveal an untreatable condition is nil.

The usefulness and limitations of each of the five tests used to look at livers cannot be considered here. But having worked closely with many good radiologists who worked well with all techniques, I think that computed tomography done properly with prompt bolus or delayed enhancement and using a "best" machine will show the clinician as much or more than use of other techniques will show.

We are left now with our clinical embarrassment born of ignorance of each tumor's real stage. Until micrometastases (or solid avascular lesions smaller than 1 cm) can be seen within or outside the liver, we must choose our surgical therapies half blind. When use of biologic markers can be combined with a refined technique for imaging, we will be able to recognize patients who should be offered hepatic resections and thereby we will identify their more common counterparts, the patients who should be spared a needless surgical procedure.

Even now, the limitations of resective surgery done for metastases to the liver are all too clear. In the future, such operations can be offered to patients who are most likely to benefit from surgery alone, whereas many others are spared our ineffective efforts. Ultimately, the control of such tumors will come with better understanding of the biology of the cancer and its host. I do hope that oncologic surgeons will have to fade away gracefully for good reasons.

COLORECTAL CANCER METASTATIC TO THE LIVER: INFUSION CHEMOTHERAPY

JOHN C. BOWEN, M.D., F.A.C.S.
JOHN S. BOLTON, M.D.

The treatment of advanced colorectal cancer remains a challenging and vexing problem. The bloom of hope that accompanied the advent of chemotherapy in the 1960s had by the middle 1970s withered from the vine. For approximately 15 years, 5-fluorouracil (5-FU), administered both intravenously and orally, was the treatment of choice. However, under careful scrutiny, the best 5-FU could accomplish was a transient shrinkage of tumor mass in a small minority of patients—in most studies only 15 to 20 percent. This fact led Dr. Charles Moertel of the Mayo Clinic to write in 1975:

> There is not one shred of believable evidence that 5-FU contributes to the overall longevity of gastrointestinal cancer patients, regardless of the stage at which it is used.

Others argued that the treatment of the advanced stage of the disease did not give 5-FU a fair trial. Alterations of dosages and schedules of 5-FU and its nucleoside derivative, floxuridine (FUDR), have at times produced favorable reports only to be invalidated later by prospective randomized trials. Mitomycin-C was shown to have a response rate of 12 percent, but the duration of response was short, and complications, including hemtologic toxicity and chronic painful skin ulcerations caused by infiltrating the tissues, were all too common.

These unsatisfactory results led to experimentation with the use of intra-arterial chemotherapy in the 1960s. Because the liver is the most common site of distant metastases, the natural tendency has been to seek ways to treat the liver metastases as a starting point to control metastatic colorectal disease. The major rationale for the use of heptatic arterial infusion rather than systemic therapy for heptaic metastases is based on the observation that malignant lesions in the liver derive most of their blood supply from neovascular connections with the hepatic arterial circulation. Normal hepatocytes, however, are supplied predominantly by the portal circulation. Selective arterial infusion of a drug into the hepatic artery would be expected to deliver a higher concentration of the drug to the tumor bed. Furthermore, since the liver extracts and metabolizes drugs to a varying extent, selection of chemotherapeutic agents with a high rate of hepatic extraction would be expected to minimize systemic toxicity. Approximately 80 percent of fluorouracil and 95 percent of floxuridine are extracted on the first pass through the liver. Because 5-FU and FUDR are cell-cycle-specific drugs, continuous infusion (versus bolus) would seem desirable because their mechanism of action should produce a greater tumor kill as more cells progress through the vulnerable period in their cell cycle. On the other hand, because only 4 to 18 percent of mitomycin-C is extracted and its mechanism of action is cell-cycle-nonspecific, there is a greater rationale for giving it by pulsed infusion.

Although the first successful attempt to deliver a drug via the hepatic artery was reported in 1950, it was not until 1964 that Sullivan et al introduced chemotherapy by continuous intra-arterial infusion and noted "tumor regression" in 13 of 16 patients. Initial attempts to treat via a percutaneously placed catheter led to technical problems with the catheters, and the duration of treatment was necessarily brief.

Placement of catheters by laparotomy avoided some of the problems, but others remained. The catheters were attached to external pumping devices, and although response rates reported ranged from 32 to 83 percent, the utility of this approach was limited by technical problems and poor patient acceptance; therefore, duration of treatment was highly variable. Thus the problems of administering intra-arterial chemotherapy to the liver by an external pumping device and the questionable results raised doubts as to the future of intra-arterial chemotherapy for hepatic colorectal metastases.

Renewed impetus was given to the application of intra-arterial infusion therapy by the development of a totally implantable infusion pump by Blackshear and colleagues at Minnesota.

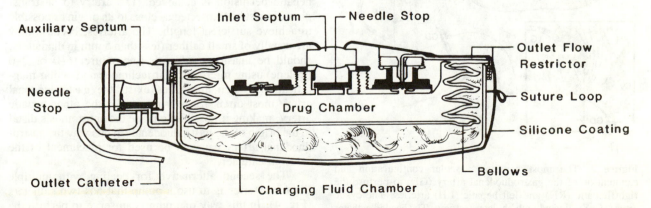

Figure 1 Diagram of the implantable constant infusion pump.

The currently available constant infusion pump (Model 400, Infusaid Corporation, Norwood, MA) is a remarkably simple device having only one moving part (Fig. 1). It relies on the physical concept that a vapor in equilibrium with its liquid phase exerts a constant vapor pressure at a given temperature (in this case body temperature) regardless of volume. The pump has two chambers, the outer one containing a fluorocarbon in a liquid-vapor combination. The inner chamber, containing the infusate, is periodically (usually every 2 weeks) refilled by percutaneous penetration of the self-sealing silicone rubber septum in the center of the pump.

Flow is predetermined by the manufacturer by inserting more or less resistance tubing in the pump. A side-port communicates directly with the tubing so that drugs or fluids can be injected by bolus as well. For example, a cell-cycle-nonspecific drug such as mitomycin-C can be administered through the side-port during an office visit.

The indication for regional FUDR therapy via the indwelling pump is the presence of multiple hepatic metastases of colonic origin which are deemed not resectable for cure. The presence of extrahepatic disease has been a contraindication to the use of the pump. In addition, the liver should not be more than 50 percent replaced by tumor, or at least the patient should be stable and not show biochemical evidence of liver failure.

An essential part of the preoperative evaluation is a selective angiogram of the celiac and superior mesenteric arteries. In about 15 to 20 percent of cases, the right hepatic artery is replaced and arises from the superior mesenteric artery or some other source. In a recent retrospective review of 200 angiograms by Daly and colleagues, only 70 percent were found to have the usual hepatic artery anatomy with the common hepatic artery

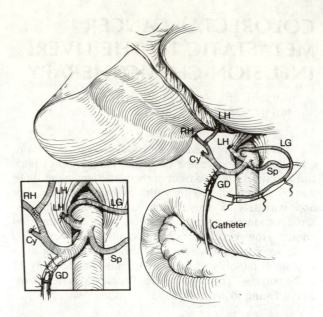

Figure 3 The left hepatic artery (LH) implanted into the right hepatic artery (RH) distal to the origin of the gastroduodenal artery (GD).

arising from the celiac artery and with the gastroduodenal artery branching before the bifurcation of the right and left hepatic arteries (Fig. 2). Furthermore, because of complications resulting from the perfusion of other organs with cytotoxic drugs, it is essential that all branching vessels to adjacent viscera be ligated.

During the early experience with pump implantation in patients with multiple anomalous arteries to the liver, it was necessary to implant two pumps to achieve complete perfusion. However, this practice was expensive, and it was technically difficult to find suitable branching vessels. Direct cannulation with relatively large tubing into a small right or left hepatic artery was technically difficult and no doubt resulted in thrombosis of some vessels. Now there are at least two methods to solve the problem of multiple blood supplies. The first and preferable method is to transplant either the right or left hepatic artery into its counterpart distal to an arterial branch (usually the gastroduodenal) that can be cannulated and ligated (Fig. 3). In this way only one catheter is employed and total hepatic perfusion is achieved. The artery to be transplanted must be transected as close to its origin as possible to achieve sufficient length. The arteries, because they are usually of small caliber (less than 5 mm in diameter), should be anastomosed with fine suture (6–0 or 7–0 Prolene) using microvascular technique and ocular magnification. When anomalies exist, the gastroduodenal artery most often arises from one or the other hepatic artery, making it possible to place the anastomosis distal to the origin of the gastroduodenal. In this way the gastroduodenal artery can still be used for placement of the infusion catheter.

The second alternative for dealing with multiple hepatic arteries is to use a pump that has two catheters (Fig. 4). In this way one pump can serve to perfuse the entire liver. However, because only one of the hepatic

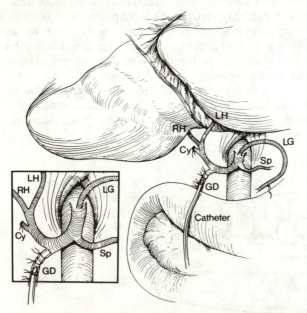

Figure 2 The most common vascular configuration and cannulation of the gastroduodenal artery (GD) to perfuse the right hepatic (RH) and left hepatic (LH) arteries. The cystic artery (Cy) is ligated with cholecystectomy. The beaded catheter is secured between sutures.

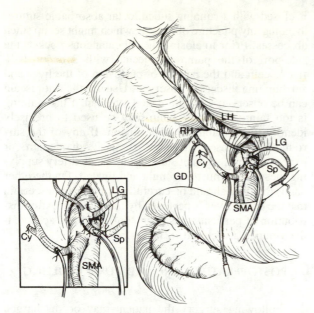

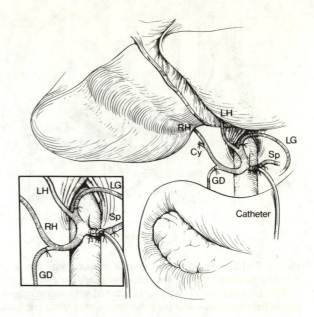

Figure 4 Use of double catheters. The larger catheter is used to cannulate the splenic artery (Sp) which can be ligated, and the smaller catheter is used to cannulate the right hepatic artery (RH) using a purse-string technique. All other vessels are ligated to prevent perfusion of adjacent organs.

Figure 5 Cannulation of the splenic artery (Sp) to achieve perfusion of both lobes of the liver. Gastroduodenal (GD), left gastric (LG), and cystic (Cy) arteries have been ligated.

arteries is likely to have a suitable branch, it may be necessary to directly cannulate the other artery. For this purpose, a smaller-bore tubing can be connected by a metal joint to the standard catheter. The smaller artery can then be directly cannulated and the tubing secured with a fine purse-string suture of 6–0 Prolene.

In other cases it may be necessary to cannulate the splenic artery in a retrograde direction to perfuse the common hepatic artery (Figs. 5 and 6). In this case it is necessary to ligate all other branches distal to the catheter tip that may perfuse adjacent viscera.

PUMP IMPLANTATION

Cephalosporin antibiotics are prophylactically given before the operation. Laparotomy is done, usually through an old midline incision, and the extent of disease is ascertained. If the disease is limited to the liver and the volume of the liver appears to be replaced no more than 50 percent, the decision to implant the pump is made. To implant the pump, it is first primed in the operating room by instilling a mixture of water and heparin to fill the inner chamber. Next, it is warmed by immersing it in warm water to induce flow through the Silastic catheter. The pump is implanted in the subcutaneous tissue of either the right or the left lower quadrant, preferably through a separate transverse incision. To secure it, suture rings in each of the four quadrants should be sutured to the underlying fascia to prevent rotation or flipping of the pump. This is done with a monofilament suture. It is important to orient the pump so that the central septum and the side-port can be easily palpated through the skin and so that

the overlying skin is free of scar tissue or other impediments to easy access. The orientation of the side-port should be noted in the chart for future reference.

Using the preoperative arteriogram as a guide, the common hepatic artery and right and left hepatic arteries or their anomalous counterparts are then dissected, and the branch arteries from each of these are identified. In approximately 70 percent of cases, the gastroduodenal artery can be used to gain access to the common hepatic

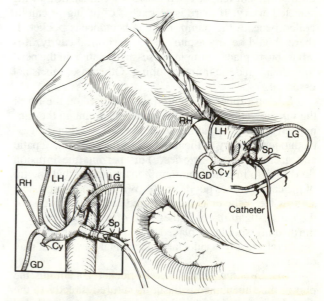

Figure 6 Cannulation of the splenic artery (Sp) because the gastroduodenal (GD) arises at the bifurcation of the right and left hepatic arteries. The left gastric (LG) artery is ligated to prevent perfusion of the stomach.

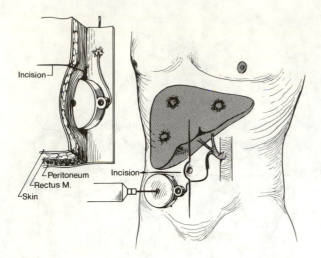

Figure 7 Infusion pump placed in a subcutaneous pocket in the right lower quadrant. The side-port can be oriented in any convenient direction. The pump is secured with suture rings to the underlying fascia, and the infusion catheter is tunneled into the coelomic cavity as shown.

artery or to the right or left hepatic arteries (Fig. 7). The gastroduodenal artery must be isolated between nonabsorbable sutures and prepared for cannulation. If there are any major branching arteries distal to the gastroduodenal artery that supply adjacent viscera, these branches must be ligated. After the site of cannulation has been chosen, the tubing from the pump is tunneled in a cephalad direction between the subcutaneous tissue and the anterior abdominal fascia to the right upper quadrant where the fascia of the anterior abdominal wall and the peritoneum are penetrated, and the catheter enters the coelomic cavity at a level just caudad to the hepatic artery (Fig. 8). The catheter is pulled through the peritoneum until sufficient length is available for cannulation of the selected artery. If there is an excess of tubing, it can be coiled beneath the pump in the subcutaneous pocket. If there should be any ascites in the peritoneal cavity, it is advisable to place a simple purse-string suture in the peritoneum around the infusion tubing. Otherwise, this is not essential.

Silicon rubber beads are manufactured on the tip of the infusion catheter to help secure the tubing in the cannulated artery. The tubing should be advanced in the gastroduodenal artery to the junction of the common hepatic and gastroduodenal arteries. This permits the infusion fluid to drip into the common hepatic artery, but the tip of the catheter does not protrude. With two nonabsorbable sutures the catheter is then sutured in place with one of the suture ligatures on either side of a silicone bead. A third suture should be placed distally to further secure it and to relieve any accidental or incidental tension that may occur.

To close the subcutaneous pocket containing the pump, the subcutaneous tissue is sutured directly to the underlying fascia so that the pump is completely sealed from the incision itself. Then the transverse incision is closed in the usual fashion, using layers of absorbable sutures to close the dead space in the wound, and the skin

is closed with a running subcuticular absorbable suture, avoiding any puncture of the skin which might set up stitch abscesses. Prior to closing the subcutaneous pocket, the side-port of the pump is injected with 2 cc of 10% fluorescein and the pattern of perfusion of the liver and surrounding viscera is observed. Usually the fluorescein can be observed with the naked eye, but if the staining is too faint, a Wood's lamp may be used to precisely identify the distribution of perfusion. If any of the surrounding organs such as the stomach, duodenum, or pancreas shows signs of staining, a branch artery supplying these areas must be sought and ligated. On the other hand, the liver should be carefully inspected to ascertain that the entire liver is perfused by the catheter. After distribution of perfusion has been confirmed and accepted, the wounds are closed in layers.

POSTOPERATIVE CARE AND PUMP REFILLING

Following surgery the patient may be discharged when clinically recovered. It is not necessary to continue antibiotic coverage. The patient is asked to return on the tenth to the twelfth postoperative day for a check of the wounds, and on the fourteenth day after surgery the pump is refilled. This is an important visit because at this time the exact infusion rate for the pump will be determined, providing information necessary for the calculation of the concentration of drug in the perfusate.

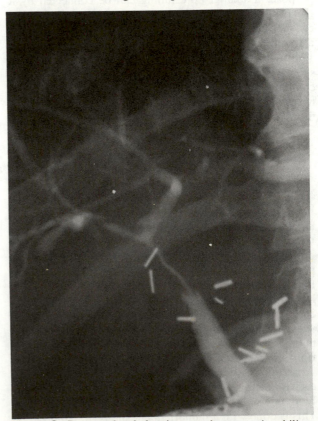

Figure 8 Retrograde cholangiogram demonstrating biliary strictures caused by constant infusion of FUDR via the indwelling pump.

To recharge the pump, the skin is prepared with povidone-iodine solution under aseptic conditions. The special Huber needle is connected to a 50-cc syringe with a stopcock. The needle is then inserted percutaneously into the pump septum at an angle perpendicular to the skin until the needle drops through the septum into the chamber and strikes a metal plate. After 14 days, sufficient pressure should remain in the drug reservoir to force the infusate into the empty syringe barrel. When the backflow into the syringe barrel ceases, the stopcock between needle and syringe is closed, and the residual volume in the syringe is noted. The residual amount is subtracted from the amount instilled at surgery (usually 50 ml), and the flow rate per day is calculated by dividing the residual amount by the number of days since instillation. Then a new solution containing FUDR is prepared which will deliver 0.3 mg per kilogram per day at the calculated flow rate. The drug is infused for 2 weeks and alternated with a saline infusion for 2 weeks. Each time the chamber is refilled, the infusion rate is rechecked and the dose of FUDR is determined on clinical grounds and recalculated.

RESULTS

To judge the efficacy of hepatic artery infusion chemotherapy in the treatment of colorectal carcinoma metastatic to the liver, two questions must be considered: (1) Is hepatic artery infusion chemotherapy better than no therapy? (2) Is it better than currently available systemic chemotherapy? The information available at present permits tentative answers to these questions.

The natural history of colorectal carcinoma metastatic to the liver is not yet accurately defined. Older series, including patients from the 1950s and 1960s, documented a poor median survival of 5 to 9 months. In these series, the liver metastases were for the most part detected clinically, and radionuclide scans and liver function studies were used as confirmatory evidence. In addition, no systemic effort was made to exclude the presence of extrahepatic metastases. The poor survival rates reported in these studies cannot be extrapolated to patients whose diagnosis was made at an earlier stage in the progression of their disease and in whom careful evaluation confirms that the metastases are limited to the liver.

Several recent series evaluating the natural history of colorectal cancer metastatic to the liver bear out the inadequacy of earlier studies. These newer studies suggest a median survival of 13 to 24 months for patients with limited liver involvement, as judged by such indices as normal liver function tests, normal liver size, good performance status, and fewer than four nodules visible on liver scan. In these series, the patients either were given no treatment or received various systemic chemotherapy programs. Occasional patients with very long survival (up to 67 months) were reported. Even in these series, no systemic efforts had been directed at early recognition of liver metastases, and the patients were not subjected to laparotomy to determine whether the metastases were confined to the liver.

In the present era, follow-up efforts in patients with colorectal carcinoma usually include serial CEA determinations. A rising CEA level triggers a sophisticated work-up, including an ultrasound or CT scan of the liver. If liver metastases are confirmed, additional testing is done to exclude the possibility of extrahepatic metastases. If this evaluation is negative, hepatic artery infusion chemotherapy is considered. If the patient is of good performance status, an exploratory laparotomy is performed to stage the extent of disease and to determine the applicability of intra-arterial infusion therapy. This protocol inevitably selects patients with early disease and good performance status. There has been no comparable series of such carefully selected patients, subjected to laparotomy and staging, and then observed without treatment. Thus, comparison of the survival of patients given hepatic artery infusion chemotherapy to "historical controls," even if matched by mathematical predictive models, is inherently biased and must be discounted.

Since no comparable untreated control group exists, the best criteria of efficacy from the phase II trials of hepatic artery infusion chemotherapy are the response rate, the duration of response, and the duration of survival. Table 1 summarizes the response rates in several series, ranging from 29 to 88 percent, with a response duration ranging from 6 to 13 months. The most optimistic reports, such as those of Balch et al and Niederhuber et al, have employed more loosely defined response criteria, such as a decrease in the CEA level by one-third or more. Those series with more stringent response criteria have a lower response rate. Median survival from the time of pump implantation is also summarized in Table 1 and has ranged from 12 to 18 months, probably owing to different selection factors among the series.

TABLE 1   Response Rates and Survival: Hepatic Artery Infusion for Colorectal Cancer Metastatic to the Liver

Study	No. Patients	Response Rate	Median Survival*	Criteria of Response
Daly	34	52%	NS	≥ 50% decrease in measurable lesions
Shepard	62	32%	17 months	≥ 50% decrease in measurable lesions
Weiss	21	29%	13 months	≥ 50% decrease in measurable lesions
Niederhuber	50†	83%	18 months	Scan, physical exam, CEA
Balch	81	88%	Approx 12 mos‡	Decrease in CEA by ≥ 33%

* From time of initiation of HA infusion chemotherapy.
† Patients with extrahepatic metastases excluded.
‡ 53% alive at 12 months.

In the absence of properly matched, untreated controls, it is difficult to put in perspective the reported 12- to 18-month median survival from pump implantation and initiation of hepatic artery infusion chemotherapy. Certainly this appears to be a modest improvement, if any. One effect that has been noted has been a shift in the immediate cause of death away from that of liver failure. However, in many cases, this allows the patient to die of progressive disease in extrahepatic sites.

The evaluation of the efficacy of hepatic artery infusion chemotherapy versus systemic chemotherapy is also fraught with difficulties. No comparable series of patients, matched for location and extent of disease, exists to compare the efficacy of hepatic artery infusion chemotherapy with systemic chemotherapy. The Central Oncology Group attempted such a comparison between intravenous chemotherapy and hepatic artery infusion chemotherapy using a randomized prospective format. The response rates and survival were not significantly different between the two arms. However, the hepatic artery infusion chemotherapy was given for a period of only 3 weeks, and thus the duration of treatment was not comparable to that of hepatic artery infusion chemotherapy delivered via the indwelling pump.

Most phase II trials of single-agent or combination chemotherapy for metastatic colorectal carcinoma report response rates of approximately 20 percent. However, one recent study of continuous infusion 5-FU reported a response rate of 40 percent, not markedly different from that reported with the use of hepatic artery infusion chemotherapy in the series utilizing the generally accepted criteria for judging response rates.

Several prospective randomized studies comparing hepatic artery infusion chemotherapy to systemic chemotherapy are in progress. All have suffered from slow accrual of patients, probably owing to the ready availability of hepatic artery infusion therapy in hospitals not participating in these studies. At least two of the studies, however, provide preliminary data. In these studies, all patients have metastases only in the liver as determined by preoperative evaluation and laparotomy. Laparotomy had been performed prior to randomization so that the two treatment groups are evenly matched. The results of these studies are summarized in Table 2. In neither study does it appear that hepatic artery infusion chemotherapy confers significant benefit. Of note is the fact that any increase in the reponse rate of the liver metastases to the hepatic artery infusion chemotherapy appears to be offset by a higher rate of distant failure. Thus, although some protection against progressive liver metastases and liver failure may be afforded by the hepatic artery chemotherapy, this regional approach does not adequately address the systemic component of the disease. These prospective randomized studies are still in progress, but major benefit from hepatic artery infusion chemotherapy is not anticipated.

COMPLICATIONS

Complications of the implantable infusion pump placement and hepatic artery infusate chemotherapy include the anesthetic and surgical complications incident to a major laparotomy for hepatic artery cannulation and pump implantation. Catheter-related problems, such as thrombosis, migration, or erosion, have occurred in less than 5 percent of cases in most series. Pump pocket infection is also uncommon, and pump pocket seroma, while still an occasional problem, can be largely prevented by closure of the peritoneum around the catheter. When it occurs, the seroma may be treated by percutaneous aspiration until it resolves.

In addition to the aforementioned problems, a variety of complications can ensue from the infusion of high concentrations of FUDR into the hepatic artery. Peptic ulcer disease has occurred in up to 29 percent of patients in various series; its reported incidence depends in part on how carefully it is looked for. The occurrence of peptic ulcer disease can be lessened, but not eliminated, by ligation of all branches of the hepatic artery supplying the distal stomach and duodenum, and perhaps by prophylactic use of cimetidine and antacids. Chemical hepatitis, reflected by increases in SGOT, SGPT, LDH, alkaline phosphatase, and GGT enzyme levels, occurs in the majority of patients at some time during the course of treatment. Chemically induced hepatitis may progress to an actual clinical syndrome of malaise, nausea, vomiting, anorexia, and jaundice. It is treated by reduction or temporary cessation of hepatic artery infusion chemo-

TABLE 2   Randomized Prospective Studies: Hepatic Artery Infusion vs Systemic Chemotherapy for Colorectal Cancer Metastatic to the Liver

Study	No. Patients	Study Design	Response Rate	Distant Failure	Morbidity
Kemeny	34	IV FUDR	40%	0%	Diarrhea
		HAI FUDR	41%	33%	Ulcer, biliary sclerosis
Stagg	48	IV FUDR	20%*	20%	Diarrhea
		HAI FUDR	41%*	35%	Biliary sclerosis

* Not a statistically significant difference

TABLE 3 Hepatic Artery FUDR Infusion: Incidence of Biliary Sclerosis

Study	Incidence of Biliary Sclerosis
Daly	2/41 (5%)
Hohn	7/35 (20%)
Bowen	2/20 (10%)
Total	11/96 (11%)

therapy and usually resolves within 2 to 4 weeks. Treatment is best interrupted when the enzyme levels are develops. The onset of chemical hepatitis is the dose-limiting factor in the majority of patients receiving hepatic artery infusion chemotherapy.

Biliary sclerosis is a unique complication of hepatic artery infusion of FUDR, and its reported incidence is rising with more frequent and prolonged use of hepatic artery infusion chemotherapy (Fig. 8). It is apparent that mild biliary sclerosis accounts for at least some of the reported incidence of "chemical hepatitis" and that in these cases the enzyme changes of chemical hepatitis represent bile stasis on the basis of biliary sclerosis rather than hepatocellular injury. The reported incidence of biliary sclerosis from several series is compiled in Table 3; these data represent clinical disease, and it is likely that clinically silent biliary sclerosis would be detected more often if sought with routine cholangiography. It is not clear yet whether biliary sclerosis is a specific complication of FUDR infusion or whether it would occur generally with a variety of chemotherapeutic agents given by this route.

Biliary sclerosis can be a difficult clinical problem. Its onset may be suspected when a patient develops progressive jaundice and pruritus accompanied by marked elevations of the alkaline phosphatase and GGT. Initial management is by prompt interruption of drug infusion. If the jaundice cannot be ascribed to tumor progression, and if it persists for more than 2 weeks, endoscopic retrograde cholangiography should be done. If biliary sclerosis is documented, prolonged cessation of treatment may be necessary. Often the jaundice resolves over a period of 6 to 8 weeks. Early surgical, endoscopic, or radiographic intervention should be avoided as these lesions are high, often multifocal, and difficult to bypass, stent, or dilate. Early intervention may compound the problem by causing cholangitis, and the preferred initial management is simple observation in the hope that the biliary sclerosis will remit.

PORTAL HYPERTENSION

PORTAL HYPERTENSION

W. DEAN WARREN, M.D., F.A.C.S.
J. MICHAEL HENDERSON, M.B., CH.B., F.R.C.S., F.A.C.S.

Bleeding from gastroesophageal varices is the major complication of portal hypertension requiring surgical management. Broadly, the surgical decisions have two distinct phases, first in the emergent situation with ongoing active bleeding, and second in the elective case when further life-threatening bleeding must be prevented. Bleeding can be stopped or recurrence prevented by surgical decompression of varices, but whether or not the patient survives is governed by the underlying liver disease. Cirrhosis, primarily alcoholic, is the leading cause of variceal bleeding in the United States, but on the worldwide scene other etiologies such as nonalcoholic cirrhosis, schistosomiasis, and portal vein thrombosis often have better preservation of hepatocyte function, the ultimate determinant of survival. Selection for surgery, the timing of operation, and the choice of procedure thus become the critical variables in overall patient management. This chapter will define our current views of overall patient management for this problem.

ACUTE VARICEAL BLEEDING

This phase of management is the same regardless of the underlying etiology of the variceal bleeding. The aim is to stop the bleeding and stabilize the patient for elective work-up, with minimum further compromise to the impaired liver.

Patient resuscitation differs from the standard measures applied to all bleeding patients in some important aspects. Blood loss requires blood transfusion; coagulation deficits require fresh frozen plasma and/or platelets. Saline and Ringer's lactate should be avoided because they increase ascites. Hepatic encephalopathy should be anticipated, and measures taken to minimize this risk. Sedation should be used with caution, blood should be rapidly cleared from the gut with enemas or mild purgatives, electrolyte status carefully monitored, and risks of infection minimized.

Early, accurate diagnosis of the bleeding site should be made by endoscopy. Iced gastric lavage may be required to clear the stomach for adequate visualization. Exclusion of peptic ulcer disease is important at this stage. Gastritis bleeding in patients with portal hypertension should be considered and managed as variceal bleeding.

Specific measures for control of acute variceal bleeding that has not stopped in the early resuscitative phase should sequentially follow these steps:

1. *Pitressin* should be given intravenously, 20 μ in 200 ml of 5% dextrose in water over 20 minutes, to be followed by a continuous infusion of 0.4 μ per minute. This may then be tapered, if bleeding is controlled, by 0.1 μ per minute every 6 to 12 hours. Control of bleeding is achieved in 50 to 70 percent of cases.

2. *Endoscopic sclerosis* has made a major impact in reducing the early mortality of acute variceal bleeding, reportedly controlling bleeding in 80 to 90 percent of cases. This rate does not appear to be altered by the method, whether rigid or flexible endoscope; the site of injection, whether intra- or paravariceal; or the sclerosant, of which there are many. In this situation our own preference is for flexible endoscopy with intravariceal injection of 2.5% sodium morrhuate.

3. *Balloon tamponade* should be reserved as a temporizing method for massive bleeding, while other treatment modalities are being arranged. It is no longer the initial treatment of acute bleeding. Attention to detail in management of the patient with a Sengstaken-Blakemore tube will minimize the risks of perforation, ulceration, and aspiration.

4. *Transhepatic embolization* provides diagnostic information as well as potential therapy for some patients. Initial control in 45 to 90 percent of patients having coronary vein embolization is followed by a high rebleeding rate of 25 to 86 percent within days to months. Complications, such as intra-abdominal bleeding (20%), and portal vein thrombosis (20% to 30%), limit the application of this method.

5. *Emergency surgery* should be considered in two settings. First, the good-risk patient (Child's A or B) whose bleeding is not controlled by the aforementioned methods should be considered for emergency selective shunt. Second, the patient with massive continuing bleeding, regardless of risk group, may be a candidate for a "salvage" portacaval H-graft shunt.

ELECTIVE MANAGEMENT OF VARICEAL BLEEDING

The priorities in the management of patients who have survived their acute bleeding episode must place equal emphasis on preventing further life-threatening bleeding, and on the preservation of residual hepatocyte function. The currently available methods for treating patients in the elective situation are selective shunt, total porto-systemic shunt, devascularization procedures, endoscopic sclerotherapy, and pharmacologic reduction of portal venous pressure. This plethora of methods speaks to the lack of satisfaction with one method for treating all patients with variceal bleeding. The aim, as yet not achieved, must be to define which therapy will best control bleeding and maintain hepatic function for each individual patient.

The important clinical and laboratory findings and investigative measures useful in deciding the timing and type of therapy will be briefly discussed.

Clinical Findings. Nutritional status should be considered prior to elective operation. Malnutrition should be corrected prior to surgery if bleeding is stabilized, and if it cannot be improved, the decision to operate should be reconsidered. Ascites frequently occurs following resuscitation from an acute variceal bleed; diuresis, with sodium restriction and aldactone, should be achieved prior to elective operation. Hepatic encephalopathy likewise is frequently precipitated by an acute bleed. Provided it clears rapidly with treatment of the precipitating factors, it is not an absolute contraindication to operation.

Laboratory Findings. Data that may necessitate delay in elective surgery are a bilirubin higher than 3 mg per deciliter, albumin less than 3 g per deciliter, a pro-thrombin time more than 4 seconds longer than control, and increased SGOT. Such values suggest decompensated liver disease or active hepatitis, and portend an increased operative mortality.

Investigative Measures. These studies should include a liver biopsy and hepatic angiography. Bio-chemical studies do not always indicate the true state of the hepatocyte, and hence we advocate biopsy prior to elective surgery. Active hepatitis should be treated, and surgery delayed pending stabilization of the process. Angiography, with the emphasis on venous phase visual-ization of the splenic and portal veins, is primarily done as a road map to aid in shunt surgery.

In our own practice we conduct quantitative measure-ment of hepatocyte function (galactose elimination capacity), liver and spleen size (CT scan), and hepatic (low-dose galactose clearance) and systemic (radionuclide angiocardiography) hemodynamics in all patients having elective shunt surgery. Such studies allow careful categor-izing of patients according to the severity of their cirrhosis, but are not essential parts of the work-up in everyday clinical practice.

Distal Splenorenal Shunt

The distal splenorenal shunt (DSRS) is the prototype for selective variceal decompression. Intravariceal pres-sure is reduced by transsplenic shunting to the splenorenal anastomosis. Hepatopedal portal flow, the vital factor in maintaining hepatocyte function, is maintained. It is important to emphasize that this is not a portal systemic shunt; portal hypertension must be sustained.

The major technical points of emphasis are:

1. Mobilization of the pancreas. This must be complete, is approached through the lesser sac, and is facilitated by taking down the splenic flexure of the colon.
2. The splenic vein must be dissected on the vein. It is easier to dissect the posterior before the anterior surface. This dissection should be from the superior mesenteric vein to the splenic hilus, as complete dissection of the vein from the pan-creas improves the selectivity by reducing portal to splenic vein collaterals at late post-shunt follow-up.
3. The anastomosis must be performed without tension or kinking. We use a continuous posterior suture, but interrupt the anterior row to avoid a purse-string effect.
4. Disconnection must interrupt the coronary, pan-creatic, splenocolic, and transgastric collateral pathways.

Perioperative Management

Fluid Management. We advocate monitoring with a Swan-Ganz catheter, arterial line, and Foley catheter perioperatively and for approximately 48 hours in the ICU postoperatively. Effective plasma volume should be main-tained with colloid rather than crystalloid. Fresh frozen plasma is used if the coagulation values are abnormal; otherwise 5% albumin is given. Normal saline solution and Ringer's lactate are more likely to precipitate ascites. Most cirrhotics are mildly hyperdynamic perioperatively (cardiac output (CO) = 6 to 10 L per minute), and main-tain or increase this in the first 48 hours.

Medications. Pain should be relieved with repeated small doses of morphine as required. Perioperative anti-biotic coverage should be used. We preload the hepato-cytes with steroids; dexamethasone, 40 mg IV, is given 6 hours prior to surgery and continued for 24 hours. In the postoperative period, aldactone should be started as soon as gastrointestinal function returns: the dosage should be adjusted to block renal sodium reabsorption, as measured by daily urine sodium and potassium determina-tions. Care must be exercised not to further impair renal function as judged by a rising BUN and creatinine.

Diet. The strict perioperative intravenous fluid sodium restriction is followed by a diet containing 2 g sodium and 30 g fat. The fat restriction is instituted because of the risk of chylous ascites in the first postopera-tive month, and can then be eased.

The regimen of fluid management, aldactone, and dietary restriction, as just outlined, serves to minimize the major immediate postoperative complication of ascites. If ascites occurs in the face of such management, diag-nostic paracentesis should be performed. Chylous ascites (fluid triglyceride greater than serum triglyceride) should be managed by tapping the abdomen dry and reinstituting the regimen just described. Occasionally this may need to be repeated. A LeVeen valve is rarely (2% of cases) required in the postoperative period.

Angiography. Shunt catheterization and SMA angiography should be done at one week. At catheterization, pressures should be measured in the splenic vein, left renal vein, inferior vena cava (IVC) at the renal vein. The most common problem at this time is renal vein hypertension, with a pressure gradient greater than 10 mm Hg from the left renal vein to the IVC in approximately 20 percent of cases. This may be associated with gastritis or frank variceal bleeding in up to 20 percent of those with a high gradient, but provided shunt patency is documented, these cases should be managed nonoperatively. A gradient across the anastomosis indicates a technical failure, which may necessitate reoperation or dilation.

Results

In the 18 years since its introduction, over 30 centers have reported data on the DSRS. These are summarized in Table 1. Not every study has reported all the listed statistics in detail, but the same generalizations hold. Specific points of emphasis are (1) good- to moderate-risk patients have been operated on with an acceptable mortality and good bleeding control; (2) long-term survival is governed more by the disease etiology than by the operation: nonalcoholics have a better long-term survival rate than alcoholic cirrhotics; and (3) the quality of life is significantly improved compared to that previously seen after total shunts: encephalopathy rates are low, and usually this complication is easily controlled.

Six prospective randomized trials have been instituted to compare DSRS to a variety of total portosystemic shunts. The salient features of these are summarized in Table 2: time to reporting has ranged from 6 months to 10 years. Encephalopathy is significantly lower after DSRS in all studies except one. Bleeding is equally well controlled by both types of shunt, but interposition Dacron shunts have a higher late occlusion rate. Quality of life assessment was significantly better in both the Emory

TABLE 1 Summary of Reported Worldwide Experience with DSRS from 30 Centers

Number of patients	> 1,000
Etiology	60% Alcoholic cirrhosis 40% Nonalcoholic etiology
Child's class	A = 46% B = 40% C = 14%
Operative mortality	9% (range 1%–19%)
Survival rates	3 year, 60%–75% 5 year, 50%–60%
Shunt patency	90%
Encephalopathy	10% (range 0%–18%)

(10-year follow-up) and Toronto (5-year follow-up) studies. No significant difference in late survival has been shown in these predominantly alcoholic cirrhotic populations.

Data on hemodynamic and hepatic function prior to, and following, DSRS are summarized in Table 3. These studies, in different groups of patients, show that portal perfusion is best maintained in those with portal hypertension of nonalcoholic etiology. At one year all groups show no significant loss in their hepatocyte function as measured by galactose elimination capacity (GEC). However, all the cirrhotic groups show a significant reduction in their liver volume. This change is also seen in similar patients having endoscopic sclerosis and suggests progress of their liver disease.

Total Portal Systemic Shunts

Total shunts control variceal bleeding, but accelerate hepatic failure by totally diverting all portal venous flow away from the hepatocytes. The classic end-to-side portacaval shunt irrevocably interrupts portal flow by dividing the portal vein and, in our opinion, is rarely indicated. Side-to-side shunts, including the wide variety of interposition shunts (portacaval, mesocaval, mesorenal, central splenorenal), all have the potential of occlusion, with restoration of portal flow, if incapacitating encephalopathy or hepatic failure occurs. We advocate short H-graft interposition portacaval shunt in the emergency situation with massive continued bleeding.

Results of total shunts, first in prophylactic studies and later in therapeutic randomized trials, have all shown no difference in survival between medically managed and shunted patients. The 95 percent control of bleeding was offset by the accelerated liver failure, giving a 30 to 40 percent 5-year survival rate after such shunts and a 30 to 50 percent incidence of encephalopathy and liver failure. Some have attempted to predict, on the basis of preoperative assessment, the 20 percent of patients who will do well in the long term following total portal systemic shunts, but these have been unsuccessful.

Recently, Sarfeh and his group have suggested that partial portal decompression with an 8- to 10-mm interposition portacaval H-graft may decompress the portal hypertension sufficiently to control bleeding, but not enough to totally divert all prograde portal flow. This principle is difficult to accept hemodynamically and requires further evaluation at this time.

Devascularization Procedures

The extent of such surgery in the treatment of variceal bleeding may incorporate some or all of the following: splenectomy, esophageal transection, gastric transection, gastric and esophageal devascularization, coronary vein ligation. They may be performed totally by an abdominal approach or by a combined thoracoabdominal approach. In our practice, the place for such operation is limited to

TABLE 2   The Summarized Status of Six Prospective Randomized Trials Comparing DSRS to a Variety of Total Portal Systemic Shunts

	Total Number of Patients	Operative Mortality	Late Mortality	Encephalopathy	Shunt Occlusion
DSRS	143	9.8%	35%	21%	6.3%
Total shunts	147	9.5%	43%	40%	9.6%

patients in whom selective variceal decompression cannot be performed because of unsuitable or thrombosed vessels. We believe this is preferable to a total shunt procedure unless there is exsanguinating bleeding. We limit devascularization to a totally abdominal operation and advocate follow-up endoscopy and sclerosis if varices are still visible.

The reported results of devascularization procedures are varied. The Japanese have had greatest success with fewer than 10 percent of patients rebleeding after extensive devascularization. Most other workers have reported a 20 to 50 percent rebleeding rate within 2 years. The major advantage is that portal venous flow and hepatic function are maintained after such procedures.

Endoscopic Sclerotherapy

The role of longitudinal sclerosis in the prevention of recurrent variceal bleeding has still to be defined, despite its major impact on acute bleeding. At present many patients are being treated by repeated sclerosis, usually done at serially increasing time intervals after their acute bleed. A fiberoptic, flexible endoscope is used, the aim being to obliterate varices. Instead of the intravariceal injection used to treat acute bleeding, many workers use a paravariceal injection method in order to induce fibrosis in the esophageal wall. The multitude of different sclerosant solutions and combinations speak to the lack of an ideal.

Our own use of longitudinal sclerosis is increasing in the treatment of poor-risk patients and those with significant concomitant diseases, in whom there would be a significant operative risk. The role of sclerotherapy needs to be carefully defined, and to that end we are currently conducting a prospective randomized study whereby this therapy is compared to selective variceal decompression. We use flexible endoscopy, sodium morrhuate, and paravariceal injection, based on an initial course of 2 to 3 sessions in the first 10 days, followed by monthly sessions until obliteration is achieved.

Reported results show some common trends. Rebleeding occurs in 20 to 60 percent of patients within the first year, the risk appearing to lessen over time. The failure rate (i.e., when further sclerosis fails to control the recurrent bleeding episodes) is between 10 and 20 percent. Prospective randomized studies comparing sclerosis to medical therapy have shown significant improvement in survival at 2 years with sclerotherapy. Longer follow-up and comparison to other forms of therapy (e.g., selective shunt) are required.

The question is frequently asked whether multiple sclerotherapy sessions make subsequent shunt surgery more difficult. In our experience, the dissection of the

TABLE 3   Quantitative Liver Function, Mass and Hemodynamic Data Prior to and One Year After DSRS in Patient Subgroups (Ten patients managed by chronic endoscopic sclerosis are included for comparison.)

	No. of Patients	GEC (mg/min)	Liver Volume (cc)	Liver Blood Flow (ml/min)	Portal Perfusion	Cardiac Output (l/min)
Normal		500 ± 50	$1,493 \pm 230$	$1,378 \pm 218$	1	5
Cirrhosis, alcoholic	16					
Preoperative		$337 + 99$	$2,113 \pm 600$	$1,133 \pm 265$	2.0	6.9 ± 1.7
1 year		305 ± 69	$1,836 \pm 637^*$	$1,339 \pm 406^\dagger$	3.5^*	$10.0 \pm 3.5^*$
Cirrhosis, nonalcoholic	8					
Preoperative		362 ± 98	$1,489 \pm 433$	$1,045 \pm 269$	2.0	6.9 ± 1.7
1 Year		324 ± 93	$1,311 \pm 487^*$	964 ± 169	2.0	7.3 ± 2.8
Portal vein thrombosis	6					
Preoperative		378 ± 57	966 ± 253	979 ± 192	1	--
1 Year		353 ± 83	$1,028 \pm 310$	924 ± 169	1	--
Endoscopic sclerosis	10					
Preoperative		333 ± 58	$1,963 \pm 502$	$1,286 \pm 651$	1.5	6.3 ± 1.2
1 Year		353 ± 86	$1,646 \pm 418^*$	$1,150 \pm 391$	1.4	6.4 ± 1.6

Significant pre- to 1-year change: $^* p < 0.05$; $^\dagger p < 0.07$.

splenic vein for selective variceal decompression is harder in patients who have had sclerotherapy because of retroperitoneal and perivascular thickening.

Pharmacologic Control of Variceal Bleeding

Propranolol reduces portal venous pressure in patients with portal hypertension. The extensive studies of Lebrec and his co-workers show that this is associated with reduced pulse and cardiac output, but not with reduced liver blood flow. The dose of propranolol required to give the desired effect (judged by a pulse reduction of 25%) depends on the severity of liver injury and shunting. Although they have shown a significantly improved survival in good-risk alcoholic patients treated with propranolol, others have not been able to produce such results. Undoubtedly the hemodynamics can be manipulated; this may be of benefit in some patients at some stages in their disease, but we would not advocate the widespread use of propranolol to treat all patients with variceal bleeding. More studies and a better understanding of which patients may benefit and which patients may be adversely affected are required before the role of propranolol can be stated.

ENDOSCOPIC SCLEROTHERAPY FOR ESOPHAGEAL VARICES

CRAIG A. JOHANSON, M.D.

Dissatisfaction with the high rate of morbidity and mortality associated with emergency portacaval shunt has led to a renewed interest in endoscopic variceal sclerosis (EVS) as a method of controlling acute esohageal variceal hemorrhage. Thirty percent of patients with cirrhosis of the liver and varices bleed from their varices, and 70 percent of this group then have a second bleeding episode. Many of these acutely bleeding patients have a diminished hepatic reserve which places them in a high-risk group for emergency surgical intervention. Most series now document a greater than 50 percent mortality for Child's class C patients undergoing emergency portacaval shunt. This fact, coupled with the high degree of efficacy of EVS, has made this procedure the first choice of therapy for acutely bleeding esophageal varices.

DIAGNOSIS

A disgnosis of acute variceal hemorrhage is best made endoscopically. Numerous studies have demonstrated the superiority of endoscopy over radiographic techniques in ascertaining the etiology of upper gastrointestinal bleeding. Since endoscopy now also offers us the opportunity of making therapeutic as well as diagnostic interventions, the initial endoscopic examination should be carried out with an instrument and examiner capable of performing EVS if bleeding varices are present.

Arteriographic techniques have no place in the diagnosis or therapy of esophageal varices, although they may be useful in the management of gastric varices. Barium contrast studies are to be avoided in the management of the acute gastrointestinal bleeder since the presence of barium in the upper gastrointestinal tract will interfere with any further diagnostic or therapeutic maneuvers by the endoscopist or the arteriographer.

PROCEDURE

Patients with upper gastrointestinal hemorrhage should be admitted to an intensive care unit, and cardiorespiratory and circulating blood volume status should be evaluated initially. Resuscitation with packed red blood cells, colloid, and crystalloid as indicated should be initiated. Appropriate laboratory evaluations including CBC, liver function tests, and clotting parameters should be obtained.

The initial endoscopic examination is then carried out with a dual-channel or large (3.5 mm) single-channel flexible fiberoptic instrument. Rigid endoscopes were intially used for EVS, and some surgeons continue to use them in the acutely bleeding patient because of their definite advantage of high volume suction and their less well-documented advantage in postinjection variceal tamponade. The disadvantages of rigid instruments, however, seem to outweigh their advantages. Chief among these is the need for general anesthesia with the rigid scopes and the uncommon but serious complication of esophageal perforation.

Immediately prior to endoscopy, the posterior pharynx is anesthetized with a topical lidocaine spray or gargled antihistamine solution in the "caine" sensitive individual. Intravenous sedation with diazepam, meperidine, or a combination of the two is then given to the point of comfort. An anesthetist usually is not required, but the patient's blood pressure, pulse, and respirations must be closely monitored by someone other than the endoscopist throughout and after the procedure. A high incidence of aspiration pneumonia in heavily sedated or even encephalopathic patients undergoing endoscopic procedures has led some surgeons to recommend nasotracheal intubation prior to EVS. This is usually unnecessary, except for patients with pulmonary decompensation of any degree.

With the patient in the left lateral recumbent position, the endoscope is then advanced into the esophagus, stomach, and proximal duodenum under direct vision. Frequent suctioning through the endoscope (and of the oropharynx by separate means) is necessary in the acutely bleeding patient. An adequate and forceful means of washing the mucosa through the scope is also helpful in dislodging clots, which may be obscuring the field but are not usually promoting hemostasis. If a bleeding esophageal or gastric varix is encountered, or if varices are present in the absence of another potential bleeding lesion (peptic ulcer, gastritis, Mallory-Weiss tear, neoplasm), EVS is performed immediately.

TECHNIQUE

A flexible sheathed needle is inserted through the endoscope and the needle tip advanced out of the sheath. Several types of injecting needles are available commercially which differ primarily in their degree of flexibility. There seems to be little advantage of one over the other, and they all assume a fairly rigid character if the entire unit does not protrude several centimeters out of the endoscope during injection. The importance of the rigidity factor is that rapid movements by the patient with the needle implanted in a varix may result in a laceration if the needle unit is stiff. The best protection against this complication is rapid withdrawal of the needle back into the endoscope at the first sign of patient movement. With rapid operator reaction, I have seen no complications of esophageal laceration using even the most rigid needle produced. This needle has the advantage of reusability and greater economy as well as less potential for damage to the inner channels of the endoscope.

With the needle tip (usually 23 to 25 gauge) unsheathed, the needle is advanced by the endoscopist to pierce the target varix at an oblique angle. Sclerosant solution is then injected intravariceally. An attempt should be made to tamponade the varix after injection with the deflected tip of the endoscope. If the actual bleeding site can be identified either by the presence of blood streaming from the rupture orifice or by the presence of a ''punctum, black spot, or cherry red spot,'' injections should be made at, and 1 cm proximal and distal to, this site. If an active or recent bleeding site is not identified, EVS should begin by injecting each varix at the cardioesophageal junction and also 3 cm proximal to it. Since there are usually three to five varices present, this results

in six to ten injections at the first sclerotherapy session.

The type of material used as a sclerosing solution as well as the volume injected have varied widely in the published series. In the United States two agents, sodium morrhuate, derived from cod liver oil, and sodium tetradecyl sulfate, have been used most extensively. Thrombogenic activity is excellent with either agent, but both have the capacity to produce deep esophageal ulceration on occasion. This ulcerogenic potential is an inherent property of an effective sclerosing agent, demonstrating the potent irritative, inflammatory action necessary to promote venous thrombosis. I have generally used sodium morrhuate because of its ready availability and the more extensive experience with this agent. More recent experience with sodium tetradecyl sulfate has revealed it to be easier to inject through small-bore needles because of its lower viscosity. It also lacks the disagreeable fishy odor of morrhuate and is reported to be less toxic if inadvertently splashed into the eye from a poorly fitted syringe-injector coupling. However, this problem can be essentially eliminated by Luer-lock fittings and careful technique.

The volume of sclerosant injected is usually 3 cc at each site, with a maximum of ten sites injected per session for a total volume of 30 cc. This volume would represent the most aggressive approach in a patient who is actively bleeding and not responding to a smaller number of injections, or a patient with multiple large varices in whom an early response is mandatory.

The frequency of injection is usually a compromise between the realities of cost-effectiveness and theoretic consideration. Ideally, injections probably should take place no more frequently than every 7 to 10 days. Initiation and subsidence of the inflammatory, thrombogenic process could be expected to occur in this interval. Repeat injections could then be performed with safety, even in close proximity to prior sites, without the danger of additive effects and potential ulceratin. However, since I generally perform an initial series of three injections, a hospital stay of up to 3 weeks would be necessary. This is seldom practical at present, and so instead I generally perform the first two injection sessions 4 to 5 days apart if the patient's condition is stable, and then discharge him to return on an outpatient basis for the last session. Follow-up sessions are then scheduled exclusively on an outpatient basis at one month, and then every 3 to 4 months until the varices are obliterated. Interval bleeding is treated emergently and places the patient back at the beginning of the treatment protocol. Generally, it has been my experience that rebleeding episodes are much less difficult to manage in patients who have had some previous sclerotherapy than in those treated by previous surgical or medical methods.

Immediate postinjection bleeding occurs so frequently that it probably should not be considered a complication. Usually it is limited to a slow oozing, which ceases spontaneously within a few minutes of injection. If it continues or is brisk, repeated injections at or distal to the initial injection site usually bring it under control, particularly if combined with endoscopic tamponade. Rarely, a tamponade balloon (Sengstaken-Blakemore) must be utilized.

Only the gastric portion of the balloon should be inflated in this situation.

The injector needle enters the varix tangentially because of the anatomic relationship between the esophageal wall and the forward-viewing endoscope tip. This relationship is altered when varices are located in a hiatal hernia sac, or in the stomach where the needle may enter a varix at right angles. In these locations, special care must be taken to prevent transmural penetration by the needle (which extends 3 to 5 mm beyond the sheath tip) and injection into muscularis or the serosa. The depth of needle penetration can be reduced by limiting extension from the sheath or repositioning the endoscope to offer a tangential approach to the varix.

At each follow-up session, all varices are re-injected if they are not thrombosed residuals, which may persist for as long as 3 to 4 weeks following EVS, or if they are not ulcerated or covered by a white exudate. The presence of a thrombus in a varix can be determined by color (pale rather than bluish), consistency (hard rather than soft), and the resistance to injection exhibited by a thrombosed vessel. Back-bleeding does not occur when a thrombosed varix is injected.

RESULTS

Endoscopic variceal sclerosis is now generally conceded to be effective in controlling acute variceal hemorrhage in 90 to 95 percent of patients. The incidence of rebleeding is more difficult to assess and probably reflects the vigor with which a follow-up re-sclerosis protocol is pursued. My experience over a 5 year period suggests that re-bleeding occurs in 30 percent of the sclerotherapy patients during the first year of follow-up versus 70 percent in medically managed patients and less than 10 percent in patients treated by surgical shunt. The benefits of the surgical approach as measured by this parameter must be balanced against the increased mortality (greater than 50%) and morbidity (encephalopathy) with surgical shunt.

Obliteration of varices can be accomplished in virtually all patients if follow-up according to the described protocol can be accomplished. Unfortunately, in the group of patients under study, this is often difficult and accounts for the erratic and unsatisfactory results reported in several series. Nevertheless, the acute results themselves seem to justify EVS when one considers the benefits of decreased blood transfusion during the initial hospitalization and the ability to manage the patients, after the first several days, outside an intensive care unit.

COMPLICATIONS

Morbidity associated with EVS is usually transient and minor. Mild-to-moderate substernal pain, occurring immediately after injection and lasting 36 to 48 hours, occurs in 20 percent of patients and may represent esophageal spasm. More severe pain, occurring 24 to 36 hours after injection, probably represents chemical mediastinitis in its early stages. It does not correlate well with two other signs believed to represent mediastinitis, pleural effusion (20%) and fever (40%). Since fever is so frequently present postinjection and is most common with the sodium morrhuate agent, I believe that it must often represent a pyrogenic property of the sclerosant.

Adult resiratory distress syndrome has occurred with EVS in the presence of alveolar infiltrates on the chest film coupled with arterial oxygen desaturation. This has been attributed to the transport of slcerosant to the pulmonary circulation after EVS, producing an alveolar capillary leak by biochemical action rather than by the mechanism of fat emoblization, which has not been demonstrated. The differentiation of this syndrome from aspiration pneumonia is difficult, however, particularly in view of the frequency of aspiration in the setting of hematemesis and upper gastrointestinal endoscopy. As mentioned previously, these pulmonary complications have led some authors to recommend endotracheal intubation for all patients undergoing EVS. At present I reserve intubation for obtunded or comatose patients, and those with moderate-to-severe pulmonary insufficiency. Esophageal ulceration and subsequent stricture occur with a frequency of 20 and 10 percent respectively, and again reflect the number and frequency of sclerotherapy sessions as well as the amount of sclerosant injected at each site. The endoscopic appearance of postsclerotherapy esophageal ulcers is not dissimilar from the appearance of a coagulated serum exudate, which appears almost universally at the site of injection and may account for an ulceration rate reported as high as 50 percent. This exudate is a benign and probably necessary consequence of the injection of an irritating substance. Nevertheless, deep ulcers do occur and usually heal over a period of 7 to 10 days. These ulcerated areas, which are usually on or adjacent to a varix, should not be re-injected until they heal. In some cases this may necessitate postponing an EVS session. Rarely, an ulcer may erode into the varix with massive bleeding that usually requires an emergency portacaval shunt, or the ulcer may perforate causing severe mediastinitis, empyema, or tracheoesophageal fistula, often with fatal outcome.

Transient bacteremia is probably fairly common after EVS and has been variously reported in 5 to 50 percent of cases studied. In most cases it does not appear to be of clinical significance, and antibiotic prophylaxis is not indicated except in patients with valvular heart disease or implanted prosthetic devices.

Esophageal stricture occurs in 10 percent of patients following EVS and usually follows in patients who are more vigorously treated. The strictures are located at the sites of injection and often are multiple. They develop 4 to 8 weeks postinjection and generally respond readily to gentle bouginage. These strictures often occur at areas of previous ulceration, and vigorous dilation has resulted in perforation. Tight or resistant strictures should be managed with fixed-diameter balloon dilation rather than with metal olives.

PROPHYLAXIS

The question of prophylaxis EVS is currently being evaluated at centers in the United States, Europe, and Africa. Initial reports are encouraging. Coupled with new information that suggests that the hemorrhagic potential of a varix may be predictable based on endoscopic appearance, prophylactic EVS may offer us a powerful new tool in the management of this highly lethal complication of chronic liver disease, mesenteric vascular thrombosis, and parasitic infestations.

Currently EVS should be the first choice of therapy for the patient with actively bleeding esophageal varices. Whether EVS has a role in the definitive therapy of variceal hemorrhage is less certain, although evidence is

ASCITES

HERBERT B. GREENLEE, M.D.

The maldistribution of extracellular fluid resulting in ascites has been recognized since the Greco-Roman period. Other than sporadic attempts at paracentesis, little progress was made in achieving an understanding of the pathogenesis and treatment of ascites until the last several decades. "Intractable" ascites, which persists in spite of diuretics and dietary sodium restriction, has led investigators to focus attention on a mechanical solution for this problem. Surgical attempts to correct this problem were directed initially at *increasing absorption of ascitic fluid*. Fixation of the omentum and/or spleen to the abdominal wall, often in combination with extensive abrasion procedures, was attempted to increase portosystemic drainage. Eversion of a segment of ileum (ileoentectropy) was suggested as a means of increasing the absorption of ascitic fluid. None of these methods has achieved clinical acceptance. Another approach designed to *reduce portal pressure* by a side-to-side portacaval shunt is effective in relieving ascites, but is complicated by a high in-hospital, as well as late, mortality and morbidity in this poor-risk group of patients.

The most successful approach to date for the surgical management of ascites involves *translocation of ascitic fluid directly into the venous system*. Initial attempts were hampered by technical problems related to shunt patency with the flow-activated values then available. A significant breakthrough was achieved by LeVeen who developed a highly competent value activated by a pressure gradient of 2 to 4 cm of water. Flow is initiated by the pressure gradient between the intrathoracic great veins and the abdominal cavity and can be increased by encouraging inspiration against resistance or by the application of an abdominal binder. Flow should decrease or stop as the central venous pressure increases and thus minimize the likelihood of pulmonary edema. Two new shunts now commercially available—the Denver and the

accumulating that this may be so. Certainly it is the only procedure to be considered in the high risk, Child's class C patient, and I feel that it is a highly effective option for those patients with good hepatic reserve, who, for various reasons, are reluctant to undergo portacaval shunt. Survival data are now beginning to show a trend towards improved survival in patients sclerosed rather than shunted and if this trend continues EVS would be favored as a definitive procedure. Even now financial factors favor EVS by a significant degree even when the long-term follow-up necessary for variceal obliteration in some patients is considered. At present this long-term follow-up must be considered to be the only major disadvantage to EVS in acute and long-term management of bleeding esophageal varices.

Cordis-Hakim shunts—have incorporated pumping mechanisms designed to clear the valve mechanism and minimize the chance of occlusion. Some object to these methods, citing the theoretic flushing of debris into the pulmonary circulation, but this has not been recognized as a frequent or significant problem.

INDICATIONS FOR PERITONEOVENOUS SHUNT

Intractable Ascites Secondary to Cirrhosis

The major indication for peritoneovenous shunt (PVS) is to relieve disabling ascites in the approximately 5 percent of cirrhotic patients with ascites who fail to respond to dietary sodium and water restriction and administration of diuretics. Failure of medical therapy is defined as the persistence of disabling ascites after aggressive and diuretic therapy in the hospital for a period of at least 2 to 4 weeks. The feasible limits of medical therapy have been reached if diuresis and fluid restriction have reduced glomerular filtration rate by one-half or more (twofold or more increase in serum creatinine concentration) without amelioration of the ascites. Patients selected for shunts must have stable or improving liver disease.

Malignant Ascites

In selected patients requiring repeated paracenteses for symptomatic ascites secondary to malignant disease, PVS may be used to control this disabling complication. It is most beneficial in patients whose primary neoplasm is in the breast or ovary, and a relatively long-term survival can be expected. In contrast, malignant ascites in patients with gastrointestinal or pancreatic cancer usually appears in rapidly advancing disease, and survival rarely exceeds 2 months. The palliation achieved by repeated paracenteses in these patients must be balanced against the morbidity of PVS. Thus far, there is little evidence to implicate PVS in acceleration of the course of malignant disease. Results suggest symptomatic relief in carefully selected patients with little, if any, effect on survival.

Hepatorenal Syndrome

The role of PVS for the ''hepatorenal syndrome'' remains controversial. The argument centers partly about the adequacy of the diagnosis. In many patients reported to be successfully treated, reversal of the azotemia by intravascular volume repletion has not been attempted. Medical treatment has resulted in prolonged survival in a small fraction of this group of patients. This observation has also been noted following PVS in a few well-documented instances. Results of a prospective, randomized, clinical trial comparing the effects of these alternative methods of treatment on survival are not yet available.

Ascites in Patients on Maintenance Hemodialysis

Although the pathogenesis of ascites in occasional patients with end-stage renal disease on maintenance hemodialysis has not been established, PVS is a helpful adjunct in the control of ascitic fluid collection for these patients.

Postoperative Ascites

Ascites occurs occasionally after an intra-abdominal operation, e.g., portosystemic shunt for bleeding esophageal varices. PVS has effectively controlled this problem, but it is recommended that insertion of the shunt be delayed for a period of approximately 2 weeks, not only to permit spontaneous resolution of the ascites, but also to minimize occlusion of the valve by fibrin and debris that are present during the early postoperative period.

Pancreatic, Chylous, and Cardiogenic Ascites

There are anecdotal reports indicating occasional benefits from PVS in these patients, but in general, treatment for these conditions is aimed primarily at correction of the etiologic factors.

RISK FACTORS FOR PERITONEOVENOUS SHUNT

The presence of certain coexistent medical problems are relative contraindications to PVS since they significantly increase morbidity and mortality. The risk-benefit ratio of PVS must be weighed carefully in the presence of the risk factors to be discussed here.

Severe, Active Liver Injury with Encephalopathy and Recurrent Coma

Peritoneovenous shunt may succeed in establishing an initial diuresis in these patients, but the downhill course frequently resulting in death does not appear to be altered and, in fact, may be accelerated if complications occur.

Infected Ascitic Fluid

The presence of sterile ascitic fluid must be confirmed by cultures and cell counts of aspirated peritoneal fluid 1 to 2 days prior to PVS. If infection is found, the operation should be postponed in order to avoid the disaster resulting from the rapid infusion of infected ascitic fluid into the systemic circulation. The patient should be free of infection at any site before insertion of a PVS, preferably for at least one month.

Coagulation Abnormalities

The presence of overt or subclinical coagulopathy identifies patients at high risk for postshunt bleeding. Coagulation derangements may be secondary to deficient hepatic synethesis of coagulation proteins, thrombocytopenia, and/or increased consumption of clotting factors. A search for occult sepsis should be made and corrected, if present. Infusion of fresh frozen plasma and/or platelets prior to shunting minimizes intraoperative and postoperative bleeding. In my experience, failure of the prothrombin time to correct to less than 2.5 seconds over control has resulted in a high incidence of overt postshunt coagulopathy with bleeding.

Large High-Pressure Hydrothorax

A large hydrothorax accompanying tense ascites may prevent successful shunt function because of the difficulty in achieving proper pressure gradient between the abdomen and the intrathoracic great veins. Usually, fluid enters the chest through a hole in the diaphragm. However, the flow may not be bidirectional. If the pleural effusion is small, it usually disappears following abolition of the ascites with PVS. With large fluid collections in the chest, insertion of a chest tube followed by sclerosis of the pleural surfaces prior to placement of the PVS may reduce the fluid accumulation in the chest sufficiently to permit satisfactory shunt function. Another option involves the use of a shunt with a pumping mechanism (e.g., Denver) so that the ascitic fluid may be ''pumped'' into the right atrium in spite of high intrathoracic venous pressure, which ordinarily would not permit spontaneous flow. In my experience, the combination of a large high-pressure hydrothorax and tense ascites has been a formidable challenge to treatment. The options just discussed have been used singly or in combination with variable success.

Primary Cardiac Failure

The presence of cardiac failure is a relative contra-indication to PVS if the failure is not secondary to the effects of ascites. Satisfactory shunt function is difficult to achieve owing to high intrathoracic venous pressure, and there is significant risk of initiating or aggravating pulmonary edema.

Organic Renal Failure

In the presence of oliguria that fails to respond to volume expansion and diuretics, PVS is contraindicated unless it is combined with postshunt hemodialysis.

TECHNIQUE OF OPERATION

The key features in operative management and the individual steps in the performance of the operation are to be discussed here.

General Preparation

The patient is placed in the supine position with the neck sligtly extended and a blanket roll under the shoulders. Local anesthesia is preferred, particularly if cirrhosis is the cause of the ascites. Standby anesthesia personnel monitor vital signs and provide appropriate sedation. Swan-Ganz monitoring is not routinely used unless congestive heart failure is present or anticipated. Intraoperative antibiotics are begun 2 hours before operation and continued for 24 hours. A urinary drainage catheter is placed just before the start of the operation. A wide skin prep from the mandible to the midabdomen is necessary to provide the surgeon with adequate flexibility in selecting suitable neck veins for insertion of the outflow tubing and in implanting the valve at an appropriate abdominal site.

Management of Ascitic Fluid

Some uncertainty still exists as to how much ascitic fluid (AF) should be removed at operation. The advantages of discarding little or none are that AF protein is salvaged and vital organ arterial perfusion rapidly improves secondary to expansion of the plasma volume. On the other hand, the rapid infusion of AF into the systemic circulation may contribute to the development of postoperative coagulopathy. A vigorous diuresis must be initiated to avoid postoperative fluid overload, and the resulting potassium depletion requires correctly calculated replacement. In a patient with minimal or moderate ascites

and minimal coagulation derangements, I favor saving as much AF as possible. In a patient with tense ascites, I empirically discard a portion of the AF at operation (up to 5 liters). If other factors have led to the decision to operate in spite of a relatively severe preoperative coagulopathy, most of the AF should be removed intra-operatively. Normal saline solution, 2 to 3 liters, is then placed into the peritoneal cavity to "prime" the shunt apparatus.

Key Steps in Technique

The technique of placing the LeVeen PVS apparatus is to be described here. (Denver shunt placement is similar except that the pumping mechanism must be placed so that it can be compressed against the rib cage.) Isolation of an appropriate neck vein is the initial step of the operation. I prefer the right internal jugular vein (IJV), although a suitably sized external jugular or cephalic vein is an acceptable alternative. Regardless of the site of entry chosen for the venous outflow tubing of the shunt, it is mandatory at the completion of the operation to verify by x-ray examination that the catheter tip is in the distal superior vena cava or right atrium. An abdominal incision is then made over the rectus muscle 4 to 6 fingerbreadths below the costal margin on the same side of the body as the cervical incision once the isolation and suitability of a neck vein has been verified. A pocket is prepared in the rectus sheath for the valve mechanism. A stab wound is made in the posterior rectus sheath and peritoneum, and the desired quantity of AF is discarded. The inflow portion of the shunt apparatus is then inserted through the stab wound into the abdominal cavity and anchored by a previously placed nonabsorbable purse-string suture. The venous outflow tubing is then passed subcutaneously from the abdominal incision to the cervical incsion using a tunneling rod. The tubing, after it is removed from the tunneler, is passed in a gentle curve behind the clavicular head of the sternocleidomastoid muscle toward the IJV. At this point, the appropriate length of tubing is selected to permit the tip to lie in the distal superior vena cava or right atrium from its entrance into the IJV. The excess tubing is removed and preparations made for insertion of the tube into the vein. I prefer ligation of the IJV and a controlled venotomy inferior to the ligature. A purse-string suture in the anterior wall of the IJV is an acceptable venotomy alternative. Free flow of ascitic fluid must be verified prior to insertion of the outflow tubing into the vein. Radiographic verification of proper placement of the tip of the outflow tubing is documented in the operating room on completion of the operation.

EARLY POSTOPERATIVE CARE AND PROBLEMS

Fluid Volume Overload

If no AF has been discarded in a patient with moderate or tense ascites, a properly functioning PVS results in a rapid increase in intravascular volume, cardiac output, and renal blood flow. Despite these changes, there is minimal spontaneous diuresis. However, these patients do become much more sensitive to diuretics. Generally, 20 to 60 mg of furosemide (Lasix), four to six times per day, are required during the first several days after operation to maintain a marked diuresis of at least 200 ml per hour. This rate of urine output minimizes the risk of pulmonary edema and of increased portal pressure, which may precipitate variceal bleeding. If some of the AF was discarded at operation, diuretic therapy need not be so aggressive. Significant potassium losses occur consequent to the diuresis and require replacement as necessary to avoid hypokalemia. The magnitude of potassium loss can be decreased by the continuation of preoperative spironolactone (Aldactone, Spiractone), 200 mg per day. Exogenous fluid intake during the early postoperative period is limited to one liter per day.

A different postoperative management approach is required following intraoperative removal of a large volume of AF as the intravascular volume will not be expanded as rapidly. The presence of severe coagulopathy is the usual indication for removal of large amounts of AF. In these patients, the intravascular volume should be expanded by the liberal intravenous infusion of fresh frozen plasma to replace discarded AF protein and to correct coagulation derangements insofar as possible. A portion of the discarded AF is replaced by several liters of isotonic electrolyte solution to permit prompt activation of the shunt. An elastic abdominal binder is applied immediately after operation to encourage flow of fluid through the shunt. This is in contrast to the patient with large amounts of remaining AF in whom application of the abdominal binder is postponed for approximately one week, by which time the AF volume and high intra-abdominal pressure has been reduced secondary to the vigorous diuresis during the first several days after operation. The precise quantity and composition of administered intravenous solutions depend on the severity of the coagulopathy, urine volume, and creatine clearance determinations. Diuretics are necessary to stimulate urine flow in the oliguric patient, but output need not be increased above 1,000 to 1,500 ml per day.

Postshunt Coagulopathy

The occurrence of coagulopathy after PVS may simply represent (1) a "pseudo DIC" consisting of an anticoagulated state secondary to infusion of AF containing no fibrinogen but large quantities of anticoagulant preformed fibrin degradation products, and (2) dilution of clotting elements in the blood secondary to volume expansion. On the other hand, "true DIC" leading to intravascular coagulation and consequent exhaustion of clotting elements may occur in an occasional patient. A mild coagulopathy usually can be controlled by the infusion of fresh frozen plasma, but severe coagulopathy with overt bleeding may require temporary occlusion of the shunt. The occurrence of this complication can be

minimized by postponement of PVS in any patient with a recent or current infection, marked derangement of coagulation parameters, or severe active liver injury.

Infection

The preoperative identification and treatment of any infection, intraoperative antibiotic coverage, meticulous sterile technique, and early postoperative removal of intravenous and urinary catheters will minimize the occurrence of this problem during the early postoperative period.

Nondiuresis

Failure of the expected postshunt diuresis to occur may be due to unrecognized organic renal failure or to a misplaced or occluded shunt.

LATE POSTOPERATIVE PROBLEMS

Recurrent Ascites

In a patient who has undergone successful diuresis, recurrent ascites usually indicates shunt malfunction. A chest roentgenogram following injection of contrast material into the outflow tubing on the anterior chest wall demonstrates sites of obstruction. A clot at or near the venous tip usually can be demonstrated with outflow obstruction, and ascitic fluid can be aspirated easily if the valve is patent. If inflow obstruction is present secondary to valve or inflow tubing obstruction, the dye does not clear (or disappears slowly) from the tube. In the presence of tense ascites and with a properly functioning shunt, dye is cleared from the tubing in less than one minute. It can then be decided whether only the obstructed portion of the shunt or the whole apparatus needs to be replaced. In an occasional patient, the severity of the ascites may have decreased sufficiently so that medical management controls accumulation of abdominal fluid in spite of complete shunt obstruction.

Intestinal Obstruction

A fibrous peel of thickened and fibrotic peritoneum may envelop and kink the bowel, causing obstruction in an occasional postshunt patient. A trial of conservative management with an indwelling tube is recommended as intial management. If this is unsuccessful, it is necessary to strip this peel at operation to free the trapped loops of bowel.

Gastrointestinal Hemorrhage

There is no definitive evidence that PVS predisposes to variceal bleeding in the absence of overt coagulopathy and if diuretic therapy is adequate to control overexpansion of the circulating plasma volume. The usual diagnostic and treatment choices available for the nonshunted cirrhotic population are utilized as necessary for the management of cirrhotics with this complication after PVS.

Infection

In both shunted and nonshunted patients with cirrhosis, peritonitis frequently is responsible for morbidity and mortality. Aggressive antibiotic therapy without removal of the shunt is successful in many cases if the diagnosis of "spontaneous" peritonitis is made early. Appropriate diagnostic evaluation is necessary to rule out an intra-abdominal catastrophe, e.g., perforated viscus, as the cause of the peritonitis. In this latter group of patients, aggressive surgical therapy is warranted in an attempt to avert almost certain death.

Incidental Intra-abdominal Operations

In a patient with a functioning PVS who requires an inta-abdominal operation, the outflow tubing of the shunt should be occluded to eliminate the risk of an air embolus. Several liters of saline solution are placed within the peritoneal cavity prior to closure to expel residual air before the shunt is reopened.

Abdominal Wall Hernias

I try to avoid repairing abdominal wall hernias at the same time the PVS apparatus is placed in order to avoid increasing the risk of wound hematomas in the event of severe postshunt coagulopathy. The hernia(s) may be repaired electively at a later date in a stable patient with minimal ascites. I have not occluded the shunt during the repair of abdominal wall hernias, although care is taken to keep the inflow portion of the shunt under residual or added fluid.

BENEFITS OF PROCEDURE

The rapid resolution of ascites following PVS improves physical mobility, nutrition, and renal function, although the hypothesis that life is prolonged by this operation remains unproved. Unfortunately, significant numbers of these cirrhotic patients continue to drink alcohol and remain vulnerable to a variety of life-endangering complications. The short-term benefits that result from resolution of the ascites may be partially or completely nullified by these subsequent catastrophes.

HEPATIC ENCEPHALOPATHY

LAYTON F. RIKKERS, M.D.

Hepatic encephalopathy is a psychoneurologic syndrome that may include changes in the level of consciousness, intellectual deterioration, changes in personality, and neurologic findings such as the characteristic flapping tremor, called asterixis. Symptoms may appear suddenly and rapidly progress to coma (fulminant hepatic failure) or develop insidiously over weeks or months (stable chronic liver disease). There is considerable evidence that the altered mental state that accompanies fulminant hepatic failure may differ, in both etiology and response to treatment, from the intermittent encephalopathy that frequently complicates the course of chronic liver disease. Because surgical intervention is common in patients with cirrhosis (variceal hemorrhage, ascites, gallstones, peptic ulcer disease), the latter syndrome is the one most frequently encountered by surgeons.

PATHOGENESIS

The exact pathogenesis of hepatic encephalopathy remains obscure. However, either hepatocellular dysfunction or portasystemic shunting must be present for the syndrome to develop. In most situations, both of these underlying factors apply. Portasystemic shunting may develop spontaneously secondary to portal hypertension or be surgically induced by one of a variety of portasystemic shunt operations.

Central to most theories regarding hepatic encephalopathy is the fact that nitrogenous cerebral toxins are intestinally absorbed and bypass hepatic detoxification through anatomic or functional shunts. For many years, ammonia has been the leading candidate toxin. Several factors incriminate ammonia as an important causative agent: (1) most patients with encephalopathy have an elevated blood ammonia; (2) administration of ammonium salts to cirrhotic patients may reproduce the entire neurologic syndrome; and (3) therapies that lower blood ammonia are beneficial to patients with encephalopathy.

Detracting from ammonia as the sole cerebral toxin are the findings that (1) blood ammonia concentration fails to correlate with the severity of encephalopathy in most studies and (2) 10 percent of patients with encephalopathy have normal blood ammonia levels. Other purported cerebral toxins include (1) mercaptans, which are metabolic products of methionine and responsible for the sweetish, musty odor to the breath (fetor hepaticus) in patients with liver failure, (2) certain short-chain fatty acids, (3) gamma aminobutyric acid, which is a physiologic inhibitory neurotransmitter, and (4) methane thiols. Many investigators now believe that not one, but several, of these candidate cerebral toxins act synergistically to cause the psychoneurologic changes of encephalopathy.

The false neurotransmitter hypothesis has recently been advanced to explain the pathogenesis of encephalopathy. According to this theory, the high ratio of aromatic to branched-chain amino acids present in the serum of patients with chronic liver disease leads to high concentrations of brain aromatic amino acids and interference with brain catecholamine metabolism. The result is an overproduction of the weak neurotransmitters, octopamine and tyramine, and depletion of the normal brain neurotransmitters, norepinephrine and dopamine. At present there is conflicting evidence regarding this hypothesis.

Encephalopathy develops spontaneously in less than 10 percent of patients. Usually one or more of the following factors is responsible for inducing an episode of encephalopathy: excess dietary protein, gastrointestinal hemorrhage, excessive diuresis, azotemia, constipation, sedatives, and infection. Since most of these precipitating factors cause hyperammonemia, they lend further support to ammonia as an important cerebral toxin in the syndrome.

THERAPY

General Measures

Treatment of encephalopathy begins by identification and elimination of any precipitating factors that are present.

Dietary protein should be reduced commensurate with the severity of encephalopathy. Patients with mild encephalopathy usually tolerate a 40- to 60-g protein diet. It appears that vegetable protein is better tolerated than meat protein. Oral intake should be eliminated for patients with severe encephalopathy to prevent aspiration and to further reduce dietary nitrogen. In this situation, it is essential to provide sufficient parenteral nutrition so that catabolism of endogenous protein is minimized. If it is expected that oral intake will resume in 1 to 3 days, a peripheral intravenous infusion of 10 percent dextrose in water should suffice. If a longer period of parenteral nutritional support is anticipated, central intravenous hyperalimentation should be initiated. Parenterally administered amino acids are generally better tolerated than oral protein in encephalopathy-prone patients. Standard amino acid solutions, diluted to reduce the nitrogen concentration, are satisfactory for most patients. If encephalopathy persists or worsens during nutritional support with a standard amino acid solution, a branched-chain-enriched amino acid solution may be used, but the efficacy of this more expensive amino acid mixture has not yet been clearly established. Once encephalopathy abates, oral nutrition with gradually increasing protein content is reinstituted until a maintenance diet containing 60 to 80 g of protein is attained.

Gastrointestinal hemorrhage, usually variceal in origin, is a particularly potent inducer of encephalopathy. In fact, mental status changes, which suddenly develop in an unshunted patient with varices, frequently herald the onset of hemorrhage prior to alterations in vital signs or the onset of hematemesis or melena. Gastrointestinal hemorrhage may cause encephalopathy via several mechanisms: (1) every 100 ml of blood contains 15 to 20 g of protein; (2) hypovolemic shock compromises hepatic and cerebral function; and (3) bank blood contains a considerable amount of ammonia. Obviously, successful treatment of encephalopathy secondary to gastrointestinal hemorrhage is dependent on control of hemorrhage, restitution of vascular volume, and aggressive intestinal catharsis.

Excessive diuresis may result in contraction of circulatory volume, hyponatremia, prerenal azotemia, and hypokalemic alkalosis, all of which may impair psychoneurologic function in susceptible patients. Diuresis can be safely achieved in over two-thirds of patients with cirrhotic ascites by simple dietary salt restriction alone or in combination with spironolactone in a dosage of 100 to 300 mg per day. More potent loop diuretics, such as furosemide, are more likely to cause hypokalemic alkalosis and volume depletion and therefore should be used only when these safer measures have failed. Hypokalemic alkalosis can be corrected in most patients by administration of intravenous potassium chloride. Azotemia, either spontaneous or diuretic-induced, probably contributes to encephalopathy because of the conversion of urea nitrogen to ammonia by intestinal bacteria.

Constipation contributes to encephalopathy because it results in increased contact time between bacteria and nitrogenous substances in the intestine. Prophylactic stool softeners should be prescribed for patients who have had episodes of encephalopathy in the past, and intestinal catharsis should be a component of the management of all encephalopathic patients.

Infection can be a potent inducer of encephalopathy because it leads to tissue catabolism and an increased endogenous nitrogen load. Therefore, infections should be promptly recognized and aggressively treated with antibiotics and surgical drainage when indicated in patients with chronic liver disease. Since spontaneous bacterial peritonitis may have an insidious onset in patients with ascites, paracentesis should be included in the diagnostic work-up of such patients when infection is suspected.

Specific Measures

Intestinal Sterilization. Oral neomycin, 4 to 6 g per day, is a time-honored and effective treatment for acute encephalopathy. The presumed mechanism of action is reduction of the colonic microflora, which are responsible for generation of ammonia and possibly other cerebral toxins. Neomycin is also effective when administered by enema. The disadvantages of neomycin therapy include nephrotoxicity, ototoxicity, and intestinal malabsorption. Therefore, other therapies are generally preferred for long-term treatment.

Lactulose. Lactulose is an important therapeutic advance for the treatment of both acute and chronic encephalopathy because it is just as effective as neomycin and has minimal associated toxicity. Lactulose acts both through its cathartic effect and by colonic acidification, which inhibits absorption of ammonia and other nitrogenous compounds. In acute encephalopathy, lactulose should be given every 1 or 2 hours in a dose of 20 to 30 g until mild diarrhea ensues. The dose is then adjusted (usually increased to twice or three times a day) to provide two or three soft stools daily. For comatose individuals, lactulose retention enemas at 6-hour intervals have generally been effective.

Branched-Chain Amino Acids. Normalization of the plasma amino acid profile by enteral or parenteral administration of nutritional formulations enriched in branched-chain amino acids has resulted in positive nitrogen balance and improvement of mental status in some controlled trials. Other studies have failed to demonstrate a beneficial effect of these solutions. At present, the enteral formulations should be reserved for the occasional patient (rare in my experience) who is chronically intolerant of more than 40 g protein per day. Parenteral nutritional mixtures enriched with branched-chain amino acids should be used only when standard hyperalimentation solutions diluted to deliver the equivalent of 60 g protein per day result in persistent encephalopathy. Therapy with either the enteral or parenteral formulations should be initiated only after aggressive lactulose treatment has failed to improve symptoms. More widespread use of this therapy awaits documentation of a beneficial effect in further controlled trials.

L-Dopa and Bromocriptine. L-dopa is a precursor of the normal brain neurotransmitters, norepinephrine and dopamine, and bromocriptine is a dopamine receptor agonist. Although both these agents have been effective in certain subgroups of patients with encephalopathy, neither has been efficacious in controlled trials including unselected patients.

Surgical Therapy. In isolated cases, restoration of hepatic portal perfusion by surgical interruption of a totally diverting portal-systemic shunt (e.g., interposition shunt) has resulted in improvement of cerebral function. Colonic exclusion and total colectomy have resulted in resolution of severe encephalopathy in some patients. However, the significant morbidity and mortality that follow such operations in patients with advanced liver disease have prevented overall benefit from such an approach.

BUDD-CHIARI SYNDROME

JOHN L. CAMERON, M.D., F.A.C.S.

The Budd-Chiari syndrome is an unusual form of portal hypertension resulting from outflow obstruction of the hepatic veins. In the far east, this is frequently secondary to a congenital vena caval web that partially obstructs the hepatic veins. In this country, however, the vast majority of patients with the Budd-Chiari syndrome have thrombotic occlusion of their three major hepatic veins. Since this leaves no route of egress for portal venous and hepatic arterial blood, the liver becomes massively congested. Such patients present with massive ascites, secondary to their congested liver. The natural history of this disorder is not well known. However, most data suggest that the majority of patients are dead within one year, and perhaps 80 to 90 percent are dead within 2 years of liver failure and/or bleeding esophageal varices.

DIAGNOSIS

The Budd-Chiari syndrome should be considered in any patient presenting with massive ascites. Although the entity can be idiopathic, in a significant percentage the disease is associated with polycythemia vera, paroxysmal nocturnal hemoglobinuria, cirrhosis, estrogen ingestion, or other hypercoagulable states (Table 1). Diagnosis of the Budd-Chiari syndrome can be made in a variety of ways. Perhaps the easiest and most definitive way of making the diagnosis is by hepatic vein catheterization. Either the hepatic veins are seen to be spider-like in configuration, representing recanalization of a thrombosed vein, or the angiographer is not able to engage the thrombosed orifice of the hepatic vein. A liver biopsy demonstrates the characteristic central venous congestion and hepatocyte necrosis. However, in a patient who has had the diagnosis confirmed by hepatic vein catheterization, a liver biopsy probably is not necessary. A superior mesenteric arteriogram should also be performed since in some patients with the Budd-Chiari syndrome, the thrombotic process also involves the mesenteric system.

MEDICAL MANAGEMENT

In the past, medical management of the Budd-Chiari syndrome has consisted of the administration of diuretics and anticoagulants. The majority of patients with the Budd-Chiari syndrome in this country are totally refractory to diuretics. Although anticoagulation may prevent extension of thrombus from the hepatic veins, it cannot be expected to result in improvement in the pathologic or clinical picture. In recent years, several patients have been managed effectively with streptokinase administration. For streptokinase to be effective, it has to be administered within several days of the thrombotic event. Most patients with the Budd-Chiari syndrome present with a gradual clinical picture, and the diagnosis generally is not made until months after hepatic venous occlusion has occurred. Therefore, the majority of patients with the Budd-Chiari syndrome are not candidates for streptokinase therapy.

SURGICAL MANAGEMENT

Virtually all patients with the Budd-Chiari syndrome should be managed surgically. The treatment of choice, conversion of the portal vein into an outflow track, can be accomplished by means of one of a variety of portasystemic shunting procedures. In a recent review of the English literature, 27 patients with the Budd-Chiari syndrome were reported to have undergone a side-to-side portacaval shunt, 10 had undergone a splenorenal shunt, and 9 had undergone a mesocaval shunt. Among these 46 patients, there were 18 long-term survivors. In most instances, however, portasystemic decompression had been delayed until the patient's clinical status was such that surgery could not be tolerated. In those patients who underwent operation early, while in a stable clinical state, long-term survival was achieved.

Our experience at The Johns Hopkins Hospital with the Budd-Chiari syndrome started about a decade ago, and at that time a side-to-side portacaval shunt was clearly the procedure of choice. However, our experience soon

TABLE 1   Diseases Associated with Budd-Chiari Syndrome: The Johns Hopkins Hospital Experience (15 Patients)

Disease	No. of Patients
Polycythemia vera	4
Cirrhosis	2
Paroxysmal nocturnal hemoglobinuria	1
Estrogen ingestion	3
Occult tumor	1
Idiopathic	4

demonstrated that this procedure can be technically difficult to perform in patients with the Budd-Chiari syndrome. The caudate lobe drains separately into the inferior vena cava via several small branches that are often not involved in the thrombotic process of the major three hepatic veins. Thus, the caudate lobe venous drainage is normal, and this lobe undergoes hypertrophy in response to the loss of functional liver mass in the right and left lobes. This hypertrophy can make approximation of the inferior vena cava and the portal vein difficult, if not impossible. For this reason, we prefer to perform the mesocaval "C" shunt. This operative procedure can be performed well away from the congested and enlarged liver and removed from the hypertrophic caudate lobe.

Mesocaval "C" Shunt

This operative procedure is performed through a midline abdominal incision extending from the xiphoid to midway between the umbilicus and pubis. These patients frequently have massive ascites, and we have removed as much as 26 liters on entering the peritoneal cavity. The transverse colon and mesocolon are reflected in a cephalad direction, and the root of the transverse mesocolon is dissected. The enlarged superior mesenteric vein is dissected free on top of the third portion of the duodenum and on top of the uncinate process to the point where it passes behind the neck of the pancreas. A 6-cm segment is isolated. The distal second and proximal third portion of the duodenum are then mobilized and the inferior vena cava identified. The inferior vena cava is partially occluded with a Satinsky clamp and an ellipse removed from its anterior surface. Utilizing a woven 18-mm Dacron graft, an end-to-side anastomosis is performed with a continuous suture of 5–0 Prolene. The graft is brought inferior to the third portion of the duodenum and then anterior to it, on top of the uncinate process, and is anastomosed obliquely to the anterior surface of the superior mesenteric vein near the point at which it passes posterior to the neck of the pancreas. Before this anastomosis is performed, the superior mesenteric vein is occluded proximally and distally with Cooley clamps. Major branches of the superior mesenteric vein are controlled with vessel loops. An ellipse of superior mesenteric vein is *not* removed, but a longitudinal venotomy is performed. This anastomosis is also carried out with a continuous suture of 5–0 Prolene. The superior mesenteric venous clamps are then removed while the Satinsky clamp is still in place. Air is removed from the prosthesis via a 19-gauge needle. The caval clamp is then removed. Generally, the congested liver can be seen to decompress within 15 or 20 minutes after the shunt is opened (Fig. 1).

BUDD-CHIARI SYNDROME WITH THROMBOSIS OF THE INFERIOR VENA CAVA

Unfortunately, not all patients with the Budd-Chiari syndrome are candidates for the mesocaval "C" shunt.

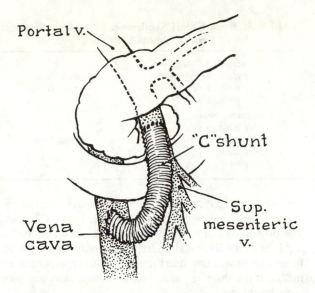

Figure 1 The mesocaval "C" shunt is performed using an 18-mm Dacron graft. The prosthesis is anastomosed to the anterior surface of the superior mesenteric vein, above its branches, at the point just before it passes posterior to the neck of the pancreas.

In some patients, the inferior vena cava at the level of the hepatic veins is also involved in the thrombotic process and is completely occluded. Thus, the infradiaphragmatic inferior vena cava either is occluded or has a pressure that approaches portal pressure and is not usable as a receptacle for a portasystemic shunt. In our experience, this complication occurs in as many as 50 percent of patients with the Budd-Chiari syndrome. Therefore, in the work-up of a patient suspected of having the Budd-Chiari syndrome, *an inferior venocavagram should always be performed* in search of either thrombosis of the inferior vena cava or compression by the hypertrophic caudate lobe. If either is present, a mesocaval shunt cannot be performed. In this instance, a mesoatrial shunt is the procedure of choice.

Mesoatrial Shunt

The mesoatrial shunt is performed by two teams. The abdomen and right anterior thorax are prepped and draped appropriately. The operative procedure is started in the abdomen as if a mesocaval shunt were to be performed. The superior mesenteric vein is dissected free for a 6-cm or 8-cm segment on top of the third portion of the duodenum and on top of the uncinate process of the pancreas. When it is completely dissected free, the chest is opened through a right anterolateral thoracotomy through the fifth interspace. This is performed by a second team so that much of the procedure can be overlapped. The total length of the operation does not exceed that of a mesocaval "C" shunt. The pericardium is opened and a tunnel is made from the abdomen, just beneath the xiphoid and sternum, into the anterior mediastinum, and through the mediasti-

nal pleura into the right chest. A mesoatrial prosthesis is then positioned. The mesoatrial prosthesis that we are currently using is a 16-mm Goretex graft with polyethylene support rings every 5 mm to prevent external compression. In addition, that portion of the mesoatrial prosthesis that passes on top of the left lobe of the liver and under the sternum is supported with a Silastic cuff to avoid the considerable pressure that is applied as the prosthesis passes into the mediastinum and right chest. The prosthesis passes from the mediastinum anterior to the stomach, into the lesser sac through the greater omentum, and through the base of the transverse mesocolon. At this point it is anastomosed end-to-side to the superior mesenteric vein, which has been occluded proximally and distally with straight Cooley clamps. Major side branches are controlled with vessel loops. The anastomosis is performed with a continuous suture of 5–0 Prolene. Once this anastomosis has been completed, the atrial anastomosis is performed with a continuous suture of 4–0 Prolene. With the superior mesenteric venous clamps left in place, the atrial clamp is removed and air is removed from the prosthesis with a 19-gauge needle. The superior mesenteric venous clamps are then removed. As with the mesocaval "C" shunt, hepatic decompression can be seen grossly within 15 or 20 minutes of opening the shunt.

THE JOHNS HOPKINS HOSPITAL EXPERIENCE

Over approximately a ten-year period, 15 patients with the Budd-Chiari syndrome were operated on and had their superior mesenteric vein converted into an outflow track. These 15 patients varied in age from 14 to 64 years, with a mean of 40 years. Thirteen were female and 2 were male. Eleven were white, 3 were black, and 1 was Asian. In most patients, the liver function tests were only mildly deranged at the time of admission. Bilirubin levels are generally only minimally elevated until end-stage disease develops. Transaminases are only 1½ to 2 times normal, and the alkaline phosphatase is only mildly elevated (Table 2). All 15 patients had inferior venacavography. In six patients, the inferior vena cava was patent with a normal pressure. In eight patients, the inferior vena cava was occluded with thrombus, and in the final patient, the cava was open but compressed and had a markedly elevated pressure. Thus, six patients were suitable candidates for a mesocaval "C" shunt, and the remaining nine patients underwent mesoatrial shunts. From this group of

TABLE 2 Budd-Chiari Syndrome: The Johns Hopkins Hospital Experience—Admission Liver Function Tests

Fourteen patients	
Bilirubin	2.1 mg%
SGOT	44 IU/L
SGPT	25 IU/L
Alk. phos.	176 IU/L
One patient	
Deeply jaundiced	
Hepatic coma	

patients, we have had seven long-term survivors who are ascites-free, with angiographically demonstrated patent shunts and, in many instances, a complete return to normal liver architecture and histology (Table 3). Our longest survival time is 7 years and 8 months; a second patient has survived for more than 5 years. Liver regeneration, which does not occur in the face of hepatic venous outflow obstruction, proceeds with a remarkable rapidity once the liver is decompressed. We have seen remarkable repopulation of the central venous area as early as 7 or 8 days following decompression of the liver via the superior mesenteric vein.

FOLLOW-UP

All of our patients with the Budd-Chiari syndrome who have left the hospital have had shunt patency verified via arteriography before discharge. More recently,

TABLE 3 Budd-Chiari Syndrome: Mesenteric-Systemic Venous Shunts Survivors

Mesocaval "C" shunt	
1 patient, 7 yr 8 mos	Normal liver
1 patient, 5 yr	Normal liver
1 patient, 1 yr	
Mesoatrial shunt	
1 patient, 5 yr	
1 patient, 3 yr	Normal liver
1 patient, 3 yr	
1 patient, 1 yr	

however, with patients who have undergone a mesoatrial shunt, shunt patency can be demonstrated via a CT scan. The prosthesis can be identified as it passes on top of the left lobe of the liver and under the sternum. If a CT scan is performed without, and then with, intravenous contrast media, if the shunt is patent, opacification can clearly be seen following injection.

GALLBLADDER AND BILIARY TREE

ASYMPTOMATIC CHOLECYSTITIS

JOEL ROSLYN, M.D.
RONALD K. TOMPKINS, M.D., M.Sc., F.A.C.S.

Gallstone disease continues to be a major problem in the United States. Approximately 20 million, or 10 percent, of all Americans have gallstones, and each year 1 million new cases are diagnosed. It has been estimated that up to 50 percent of these patients have asymptomatic gallstones. The question of how best to manage the patient with asymptomatic stones is not a new one, and the answers have long been a source of controversy. Sir William Osler believed that most gallstones caused no symptoms and, as such, did not merit surgical extirpation of the gallbladder. In contrast, William Mayo suggested in 1911 that the notion that gallstones were "innocent" was a myth, and that the presence of gallstones mandated cholecystectomy. The debate continues today and has been the subject of a few prospective studies as well as many editorials by both internists and surgeons. Currently available data are insufficient to accurately determine what the ideal treatment is for patients with asymptomatic gallstones. The first issue that must be resolved is to satisfactorily define when a patient with cholelithiasis is truly asymptomatic.

DEFINITION

Although something of a misnomer, biliary "colic" remains the primary manifestation of cholelithiasis. It has been well recognized that patients with gallstones exhibit a wide variety of additional symptoms, including fatty food intolerance, dyspepsia, and vague epigastric discomfort. Unfortunately, many of these symptoms are also present in patients without gallstones and therefore cannot be relied upon as absolute criteria to determine whether or not an individual is truly symptomatic.

Cholecystectomy is usually curative for patients who are plagued by biliary colic. Gallstone patients who complain of nonspecific dyspeptic symptoms without biliary colic are reportedly less likely to have a satisfactory result from cholecystectomy. However, the fact that up to 70 percent of such patients derive significant benefit from cholecystectomy suggests that these nonspecific symptoms are frequently due to gallstones, and therefore these patients should not be considered as having asymptomatic or silent gallstone disease. Furthermore, it is not clear what percentage of this subset of patients will ultimately go on to develop either biliary colic, cholecystitis, cholangitis, jaundice, or other complications of gallstone disease. Until such time as these data are readily available, we believe that the designation of asymptomatic or silent gallstones should be reserved for those selected patients who have neither abdominal pain nor vague, nonspecific complaints and who are found to have gallstones during screening examinations or by chance.

MANAGEMENT OPTIONS

Currently, there are three major therapeutic alternatives for the management of patients with asymptomatic or silent gallstones. These include (1) early cholecystectomy, (2) expectant management, in which cholecystectomy is performed only when biliary symptoms or complications develop, and (3) medical dissolution with oral agents. The ultimate decision as to which of these three avenues of treatment will be pursued by an individual patient is usually based on the physician's personal experience and bias. Until recently, data necessary to determine the treatment of asymptomatic stones was unavailable except in bits and pieces from several studies. These data include the rate at which symptoms develop in patients with asymptomatic stones; the rate at which complications such as acute cholecystitis, cholangitis, pancreatitis, and gallbladder carcinoma develop; the morbidity and mortality rates for early cholecystectomy; and the cost of treatment, whether it be early cholecystectomy, expectant treatment, or medical dissolution. Recently, groups from both the United States and Europe using theoretic models, have attempted to analyze the expected morbidity and mortality, and cost for each of the three therapeutic options currently available. Unfortunately, these statistical analyses reached conflicting conclusions so that it is still not clear which of these options is safest and most economical.

DISCUSSION OF ALTERNATIVES

Should individuals with truly asymptomatic gallstones undergo early cholecystectomy? (We prefer the term "early cholecystectomy" to that of "prophylactic cholecystectomy" as the latter properly refers to removal of the gallbladder prior to the formation of the disease, i.e. gallstones.) Should oral stone dissolution agents be tried, or should a period of watchful waiting be instituted? Although definitive answers are not currently available, the significance of these questions and their implications is underscored by the vast number of patients with asymptomatic gallstones as well as by the staggering medical costs that would be engendered by undertaking active therapy for this multitude of patients.

Physicians who recommend watchful waiting or expectant treatment point to the frequency with which gallstones are found at autopsy, suggesting that many patients live with silent gallstones. However, such studies are of little benefit in establishing the natural history of silent gallstones in living patients. Another argument in support of expectant treatment derives from recent, prospective linear studies, which attempt to trace the natural history of asymptomatic gallstones in well-defined populations. Although these studies suggest that only a small percentage of patients with asymptomatic stones develop serious complications, several factors indicate that these data may not be representative of the general population. In the most widely quoted study, only 13 of 123 patients studied were women. Furthermore, 35 patients in this group with supposedly asymptomatic gallstones decided to have an early cholecystectomy so that the real study population consisted of only 88 patients, and the vast majority were men. Direct extrapolation of this study to the general population may not be valid.

The medical dissolution and prevention of gallstones has been a goal of clinicians dating back to ancient times. Throughout the years, numerous agents have been employed in an attempt to dissolve cholesterol gallstones. The present era of gallstone dissolution was initiated in the early 1970s by studies that suggested that the administration of a primary bile acid, chenodeoxycholic acid (CDCA), was effective in dissolving gallstones. Since then, numerous studies have examined the efficacy and safety of this substance as well as a related bile acid, ursodeoxycholic acid, as agents for dissolution. The most recent and complete study was a randomized, prospective, double-blind study of over 900 patients. In this study, there was complete gallstone dissolution in less than 14 percent of patients receiving high-dose CDCA while partial dissolution was observed in an additional 27 percent of patients. The efficacy of both chenodeoxycholic acid and ursodeoxycholic acid is dependent on careful patient selection. We believe that there are few indications for use of dissolution agents in the management of patients with asymptomatic cholelithiasis. The long-term therapy that is required and the high recurrence rate when the drug is discontinued makes this therapeutic modality undesirable in most instances.

The major issue remains as to whether patients with asymptomatic gallstones should have early cholecystectomy or cholecystectomy only after the development of either biliary symptoms or complications. The cost, both in terms of real dollars and resources, for recommending early cholecystectomy for all patients with asymptomatic gallstones is prohibitive. Linear studies indicating that the actual incidence of biliary complications occurring in patients with asymptomatic gallstones is less than previously believed suggest that an individualized approach to decision making for patients with asymptomatic gallstones is both feasible and desirable.

Advocates of early cholecystectomy, even for so-called silent gallstones, point out that the operative mortality rate for elective cholecystectomy for patients under 50 years of age is 0.3 percent. In sharp contrast is the 5 percent mortality rate which has been observed in over 25,000 patients aged 65 years or older who have undergone elective cholecystectomy. Generalizations from available data regarding morbidity and mortality associated with cholecystectomy in patients with asymptomatic gallstones are not reliable because of the heterogeneity of the populations. The recognition that there are specific risk factors which enhance the morbidity and mortality of cholecystectomy provides further incentive to develop an algorithm for dealing with patients who have asymptomatic or painless gallstones.

RISK FACTORS

Risk factors are classified on the basis of increased incidence and risk of complications arising from gallstone disease. The best-known and perhaps the most common risk factor is diabetes mellitus. Several early studies suggested that diabetics with gallstones were more likely to develop acute cholecystitis with a greater associated incidence of complications. This concern has been somewhat tempered in view of a recent prospective study of 175 diabetic and nondiabetic patients undergoing cholecystectomy in which the incidence of gallbladder perforation, wound infection, and overall morbidity and mortality were not significantly different between the two groups. However, this study was not controlled for timing of operation, and it may well be that because of concern about diabetes in patients with biliary tract disease, these patients underwent earlier cholecystectomy with perhaps different antibiotic coverage. This study did not directly compare diabetic and nondiabetic patients with acute cholecystitis. Previous studies have indicated that in the presence of acute cholecystitis, diabetic patients have a much higher morbidity and mortality than nondiabetic patients. Therefore we continue to recommend that early cholecystectomy be strongly considered in diabetics with cholelithiasis whether or not they are symptomatic.

Recent studies have demonstrated a 40 to 45 percent incidence of cholelithiasis in both children and adults being maintained on long-term total parenteral nutrition (TPN). Although most of these patients are symptomatic, the diagnosis of biliary traact disease may not be readily apparent because of the complex underlying gastrointestinal disorder often present in many of these patients. In a recent study of 36 patients undergoing operation for TPN-associated gallbladder disease, 40 percent required emergency cholecystectomy for acute cholecystitis. In these very ill patients, the associated morbidity rate was 54 percent and the mortality rate was 11 percent.

Our expanding medical technology has led to the recognition of a third group of patients who are at great risk for developing complications from gallstone disease. These are patients who are immunosuppressed as a result of (1) steroid therapy for inflammatory bowel disease, collagen vascular disorders, or related autoimmune diseases, (2) malnutrition, or (3) disseminated neoplasm. The immunocompromised patient often presents without significant temperature elevations or physical findings until the disease is far advanced. In this setting, acute cholecystitis can be devastating. Strong consideration should be given for early cholecystectomy in immunocompromised patients with gallstones.

In addition to these three clinical settings, specific subgroups of patients with asymptomatic gallstones who are at increased risk of developing complications have also been identified. These include patients who have nonvisualization of the gallbladder during oral cholecystography, those who have gallstones greater than 2.5 cm in diameter, and those with calcified gallbladders. The last two subgroups have been associated with an increased risk of gallbladder carcinoma.

RECOMMENDATIONS

The management of patients with asymptomatic or painless gallstones continues to be a controversial area. This is due in part to the lack of a precise definition for asymptomatic patients, as well as the unavailability of well-controlled, prospective, randomized studies which have specifically addressed this question. Currently, we believe that the medical dissolution of gallstones is not a reasonable alternative for an individual with asymptomatic disease and should not be considered in most situations. Neither is routine, early cholecystectomy recommended for all otherwise healthy adults with asymptomatic gallstones. This admonition is based on the findings of several studies which suggest that the morbidity and mortality from cholecystectomy, as well as the cost, are at least equal to or in excess of that which results from expectant therapy.

We recommend early cholecystectomy for patients with asymptomatic gallstones in certain selected instances. Early cholecystectomy should be offered to any patient with asymptomatic gallstones who is overly concerned about developing a subsequent complication from his biliary tract disease (if that patient is otherwise a good operative risk). We believe that early cholecystectomy should be performed in patients who have increased major risk factors unless contraindicated because of general poor medical condition. Based on the likelihood that diabetics who develop acute cholecystitis have a greater associated incidence of complications, we continue to recommend elective cholecystectomy in this group of patients with asymptomatic cholelithiasis. The 40 percent incidence of emergency cholecystectomy observed in patients with TPN-associated gallbladder disease coupled with the significant operative morbidity and mortality in this group of patients, has led us to recommend frequent screening by ultrasound and early cholecystectomy in such individuals when stones first appear. Furthermore, cholecystectomy should be considered in patients without stones who are committed to a long-term course of TPN and who are to undergo laparotomy for other reasons. Like other gastrointestinal inflammatory disorders, acute cholecystitis is a potentially life-threatening complication when it occurs in an immunosuppressed patient. For this reason, we have come to recommend early cholecystectomy in this group of patients who have asymptomatic cholelithiasis and who are undergoing laparotomy or major organ transplant.

ACUTE AND CHRONIC CHOLECYSTITIS

ROBERT E. HERMANN, M.D.

Acute and chronic cholecystitis are common surgical problems in the United States, since gallstones are present in approximately 15 to 20 percent of the adult population. These problems are less common in young adults, but increase steadily with age. The frequency of gallstones and cholecystitis is also greater in women than in men in all age groups.

Of the entire group of patients who have gallstones, it is estimated from several studies that 40 to 60 percent have no symptoms and an approximately equal number, 40 to 60 percent, are symptomatic. Of that portion of the group with symptoms, approximately 20 percent develop acute cholecystitis; 10 to 15 percent have complicated cholecystitis (jaundice, cholangitis, or pancreatitis), and about 65 to 70 percent have symptoms of chronic cholecystitis or mild, vague symptoms difficult to interpret.

Factors that appear to increase the overall risk of the disease include the presence of acute inflammation or infection; common bile duct stones with jaundice, cholangitis, or pancreatitis; age over 65 years; and the presence of other coexisting illness, especially vascular disease and cirrhosis of the liver. There is evidence that patients with small stones in the gallbladder are more likely to develop complications of cholecystitis since these stones may pass into the common bile duct.

The treatment of cholecystitis is varied, depending on the mode of presentation of the disease.

THE ASYMPTOMATIC PATIENT WITH GALLSTONES

Controversy continues about the most appropriate therapy for the asymptomatic patient with gallstones found incidentally. Some surgeons believe that the presence of gallstones is always an indication for cholecystectomy. I have been guided by recent studies which show that only 20 to 30 percent of patients with gallstones develop symptoms during a follow-up period of up to 20 years. I now believe it is safe to follow most patients with asymptomatic gallstones, as long as they are advised about the relative risk of developing cholecystitis. At present, there is no way to determine which patients will develop symptoms during a period of follow-up observation.

I continue to believe that elective cholecystectomy should be recommended for young patients with small gallstones because of the greater risk of these stones passing into the bile duct and causing jaundice or other complications, and for insulin-dependent diabetic patients, since there is evidence that the diabetic patient has a higher risk of developing gangrenous cholecystitis with perforation and a lower tolerance for the inflammatory (infectious) aspect of cholecystitis than the nondiabetic. Since the risk of mortality from acute and chronic cholecystitis increases dramatically in patients older than 65 years of age, it seems reasonable to prophylactically remove the gallbladder when stones are found in all younger patients. Accumulating data on the natural history of gallstone disease, however, does not support this recommendation at present. If only 20 to 30 percent of patients develop cholecystitis during a 20-year follow-up, it is difficult to recommend cholecystectomy prophylactically for all young patients. For patients age 50 years or older with asymptomatic gallstones, especially males, present data would indicate that a policy of advising a low fat diet and follow-up observation would be the optimal advice.

ACUTE CHOLECYSTITIS

I believe that all patients with acute cholecystitis should be admitted to the hospital, and during the first 24 to 36 hours after admission, an attempt should be made to modify their inflammatory disease with medical therapy. Fluids are given intravenously to replace those lost by vomiting or into the area of inflammation; pain relief is obtained by meperidine hydrochloride (Demerol), 100 mg intramuscularly; antibiotic therapy is begun using a broad-spectrum antibiotic, usually a third-generation cephalosporin; and a nasogastric tube is passed in patients who have been vomiting or have gastric distention.

During this initial period of treatment, basic diagnostic studies are obtained. An ultrasound scan of the liver and biliary system is our first choice to identify gallstones, a dilated gallbladder or dilated bile ducts, a thick-walled gallbladder, or a small shrunken gallbladder, all of which indicate the presence of biliary disease. A technetium-99 scan (HIDA, DISIDA, or PIPIDA scan) is obtained to confirm that there is no visualization of the gallbladder while the liver, common bile duct, and duodenum are visualized. The nonvisualized gallbladder confirms the diagnosis of acute cholecystitis, indicating cystic duct obstruction or inflammation with passive dilation of the gallbladder. I no longer use the oral cholecystogram in patients with acute cholecystitis.

During this first 24 to 36 hours, the risk of an operative procedure is assessed by studying cardiorespiratory function with an electrocardiogram and pulmonary function studies; liver function is assessed by appropriate blood studies; renal function is checked by a creatinine or blood urea nitrogen level; and a serum amylase level is obtained to rule out pancreatitis.

For most patients with acute cholecystitis, I perform cholecystectomy 24 to 48 hours after their admission to the hospital, when the disease or inflammatory process have been modified and partially controlled, after diagnostic studies have confirmed the diagnosis, and after a general assessment of operative risk with correction of any risk factors found. If the patient with acute cholecystitis has a palpably dilated gallbladder (hydrops of the gallbladder) or shows evidence of increasing infection or sepsis during the first 48 hours, I would move ahead quickly to perform an urgent cholecystectomy. If, on the other hand, severe risk factors are identified which cannot be quickly or easily corrected, such as a recent myocardial infarction, severe renal failure, or pneumonia, I would continue medical therapy for the cholecystitis and delay the operative procedure.

If acute gallstone pancreatitis is identified, depending on other risk factors present and the severity of the pancreatitis, I would probably perform cholecystectomy within the first 48 to 72 hours after admission. If the patient shows evidence of severe pancreatitis, however, with shock, hypocalcemia, or other evidence of toxicity, further intensive medical therapy may be necessary to treat these additional problems prior to performing cholecystectomy and probable common bile duct exploration. In patients with severe gallstone pancreatitis, I am now combining cholecystectomy and common bile duct exploration with endoscopic sphincterotomy, to remove any gallstones impacted in the distal bile duct, thereby shortening the operative procedure. The optimal method of treating this severe problem has yet to be determined.

Cholecystectomy is a safe operative procedure when performed within the first 48 to 72 hours after the onset of acute cholecystitis, provided all risk factors are identified and appropriately treated. The technical aspects of the operation are not difficult during this early period of edema and inflammation. If the operation is performed after 4 or 5 days of acute inflammation, however, it becomes technically more difficult as chronic induration and fibrosis progress. Therefore, an early cholecystectomy performed electively, after the diagnosis is confirmed and medical therapy has been instituted, is, I believe, the safest and most cost-effective way to manage the patient with acute cholecystitis.

CHRONIC CHOLECYSTITIS

Most patients with chronic cholecystitis are seen in the office setting. They give a history of recurrent or intermittent episodes of right upper quadrant abdominal pain which frequently radiates into the back or subscapular area, is related to fried foods or heavy meals, and subsides over a period of several hours. Sometimes the episodes of abdominal pain are atypical, being located in the epigastrium or even the left upper quadrant of the abdomen, without relationship to fried foods or heavy meals, or with vague symptoms of gaseous distress, bloating, indigestion, or nausea.

An ultrasound examination of the gallbladder should be obtained to look for gallstones, thickness of the gallbladder wall, distention of the gallbladder, or other pathologic findings. A radionuclide scan is not a sensitive or accurate examination for patients with chronic cholecystitis. For these patients I continue to order an oral cholecystogram, double-dose study, to look for nonvisualization of the gallbladder or identifiable gallstones. In the patient with atypical symptoms, other diseases of the upper abdomen should be ruled out, including peptic ulcer disease, renal problems, and diverticulitis. When the diagnosis of cholecystitis can be made by history and confirmed by radiographic studies, the patient is scheduled electively for a cholecystectomy.

TECHNIQUE OF OPERATION

Since cholecystectomy is such a commonly performed operation, it must be performed safely. I prefer a subcostal incision for most patients. A midline longitudinal incision is used only for very thin patients or those with a narrow costal margin. The dissection is carried down through the subcutaneous tissue, and the rectus abdominis muscle is divided. The peritoneal cavity is opened, and wound liners or protective drapes are used to protect the incision from contamination. A general abdominal examination is performed to rule out any other disease in the abdomen. The right upper abdomen is then isolated and walled off by placing a large intra-abdominal laparotomy pad lateral to the duodenum, to depress the hepatic flexure of the colon. Retractors are placed against the liver to expose the subhepatic space, and another laparotomy pad is placed on the duodenum for traction downward.

A clamp is placed on the fundus of the gallbladder, and the gallbladder is dissected from the liver bed, from the fundus toward the cystic duct-common bile duct junction in all patients. I believe this to be the safest technique

for cholecystectomy as it starts the surgical dissection in a safe area and carries it down toward the potentially difficult or hazardous region of the cystic duct-common bile duct junction. As traction is placed on the gallbladder, gently pulling it away from the liver bed, the peritoneal reflections to the liver can be dissected and any small bleeding vessels coming from the liver to the gallbladder cauterized and controlled. Another laparotomy pad can be placed over the raw surface of the liver from which the gallbladder has been dissected and a large, flat blade retractor placed over this pad for further exposure.

With traction on the fundus of the gallbladder, as the dissection is carried down to the cystic duct, the cystic artery stands out as a taut cord. When it is identified, it can be clamped, divided, and ligated with a silk ligature. The cystic duct is then dissected down to the common bile duct, any stones in the duct are milked back into the gallbladder, and a ligature is placed on the upper cystic duct. The cystic duct is then partially divided and opened, and a flexible catheter or tubing is placed within the cystic duct to obtain an operative cholangiogram. Operative cholangiography should be a routine part of all cholecystectomies. It provides visualization of the entire biliary system for the surgeon so that he can be certain that he has not missed any unsuspected pathologic entities (stones, tumors, sclerosing cholangitis, congenital abnormalities) in the common bile duct. In a review of my own cholangiograms, an unsuspected stone or other disease was found in 7 percent of patients having a cholecystectomy.

Once the operative cholangiogram has been satisfactorily completed, the cystic duct is clamped approximately 0.5 cm from its junction with the common bile duct, the cystic duct is divided, and the gallbladder specimen removed. After the gallbladder specimen is removed, the gallbladder is opened and the bile is cultured in all patients. The cystic duct stump is tied with a silk ligature. The subhepatic space is then irrigated with sterile saline; the gallbladder bed on the liver is inspected for any further bleeding; and the porta hepatis and common bile duct are inspected for any evidence of bleeding, unusual thickening, palpable bile duct stones, tumor, or other pathologic conditions. As soon as the surgeon is assured that all bleeding is controlled and that no other disease is present, and when the operative cholangiograms are returned, reviewed, and seen to be normal, preparation for closure of the abdomen can be undertaken. If the operative cholangiogram shows a bile duct abnormality or if palpation and inspection of the bile duct or liver show any additional problems, the bile duct should be opened and explored or a biopsy obtained of the additional abnormality.

I close the abdomen primarily, without a drain, in all patients having elective cholecystectomy for chronic cholecystitis. In patients having cholecystectomy for acute cholecystitis, I continue to leave a subhepatic drain in place for 1 or 2 days postoperatively or until all drainage ceases.

The use of prophylactic antibiotics to cover all patients having cholecystectomy, including those having elective cholecystectomy for chronic cholecystitis, is controversial. I have begun to use antibiotics to cover the operative experience, started preoperatively and continued for the operative day only, in all patients having cholecystectomy, since it is known that approximately 15 percent of patients have common bile duct stones, placing them at high risk for the development of infection. Since the presence of bile duct stones cannot always be predicted preoperatively and since the use of antibiotics to cover the day of operation appears to do no harm and is not expensive, I now provide antibiotic coverage for all patients having cholecystectomy for both acute and chronic cholecystitis. Antibiotics are discontinued after 24 hours for patients operated on for chronic cholecystitis. For patients who undergo cholecystectomy for acute cholecystitis, antibiotics are continued for approximately 5 or 6 days postoperatively.

COMMON DUCT EXPLORATION

KENNETH W. WARREN, M.D., F.A.C.S.

Common duct exploration is a delicate operation that often is not performed when indicated and occasionally is carried out when it could and should have been avoided. Furthermore, it unfortunately is not always executed with the care, precision, and deftness that it deserves and requires.

The usual reason for exploring the common bile duct is to determine the presence or absence of common duct stones and to remove them completely when present. It is important that stones in the common duct not be overlooked at the time of cholecystectomy. This may occur from failure to explore the duct containing stones or from failure to remove all the stones from the ductal system despite exploration.

Although it is a truism that injury to the common duct during its exploration is a catastrophe, it is my observation that injury to the common bile duct coincident to cholecystectomy might have been avoided in some instances by a properly performed choledochotomy before division of the cystic artery and cystic duct. This observation, perhaps unrealistically, presumes that the surgeon will recognize the potential hazard to the common bile duct because of subtle circumstances involving anomalous ductal anatomy or, more frequently, by obvious pathologic changes seen in Charcot's triangle, which demand special vigilance during this intimate dissection.

INDICATIONS

Exploration of the common duct is indicated in patients who have a palpable stone in the common duct,

The overall mortality for cholecystectomy, in all age groups, is now approximately 0.5 percent. This mortality increases in patients with acute cholecystitis to approximately 3.5 percent. In all studies, the operative mortality for patients having elective cholecystectomy for chronic cholecystitis is approximately one-fifth that of patients having cholecystectomy for acute cholecystitis. The other major factor that affects operative morality is the age of the patient. There is almost no mortality rate for patients under the age of 50 years who undergo elective cholecystectomy for chronic cholecystitis, but operative mortality climbs as high as 12 percent for patients over 65 years of age who undergo cholecystectomy for acute cholecystitis.

who are or have been jaundiced recently, and whose common duct is dilated, measuring 10 mm or more in diameter. A rare but urgent indication for ductal exploration is the presence of suppurative cholangitis.

Currently available imaging techniques including ultrasound, computed tomography, endoscopic retrograde cholangiography, and transhepatic percutaneous cholangiography may establish the presence of a stone or stones preoperatively. I prefer to avoid percutaneous transhepatic cholangiography except in rare instances.

Relative indications for common duct exploration include a remote history of jaundice in a patient whose common duct is moderately dilated, the presence of small stones in the gallbladder where the caliber of the cystic duct is greater than the diameter of the stones in the gallbladder, a pale thickened common duct, and the presence of pancreatitis associated with a calculous gallbladder.

Most sphincteroplasties are performed without a choledochotomy because the papilla of Vater can almost always be identified by inspection and palpation through a properly placed duodenotomy. If the sphincter of Oddi is stenosed, however, it is safer to open the common duct and insert a No. 3 Bakes dilator into the intrapancreatic portion of the common bile duct and, with gentle pressure, project the papilla into view. The sphincter is then divided at the 11 o'clock position by incising it against the metal tip of the dilator.

I have described a relative indication for choledochotomy that will protect the common bile duct from injury during a difficult cholecystectomy as in the presence of a contracted gallbladder with dense scarring in Charcot's triangle. The choledochotomy is made in the supraduodenal region. A Bakes dilator of appropriate size is advanced cephalad with the bulbous end of the dilator in the region of the cystic duct and artery. With this precaution, it is difficult to apply a clamp to the common duct. The surgical literature is replete with the recommendations that in such a situation operative cholangiography protects the common duct, an assertion that I do not find convincing.

INCISION

The incision should be generous and properly placed. In analyzing the incisions employed for cholecystectomy in which serious injury to the common duct had occurred elsewhere, some generalizations could be made. If a vertical incision was used, it frequently was too short, too low, and too lateral. If a subcostal incision was made, it frequently was too oblique, too short, and too lateral. The falciform ligament and ligamentum teres are divided in all except very thin persons.

OPERATIVE CHOLANGIOGRAPHY

Conventional surgical teaching insists that operative cholangiography be performed in every patient undergoing cholecystectomy for calculous cholecystitis. I have no objection to this principle although I do not practice it routinely.

In most instances the gallbladder is removed before the common duct is explored. Exposure of the common duct is achieved by retracting the right lobe of the liver upward and displacing the duodenum downward. Sufficient countertraction should be exerted to stretch the common duct.

Cholangiography is performed by inserting a ureteric catheter into the common duct through a small incision in the cystic duct. When the end of the catheter has been inserted into the common duct, the ligature around the cystic duct is tightened, the diluted contrast material (Renografin-30) is injected into the common duct, and the film is exposed. I prefer that the film be overexposed from the standard setting by 25 percent. Some surgeons prefer that two films be taken at intervals after injection of 3 ml and 7 ml of contrast material. I read the films myself before the radiologist has read them or at least before I know what the radiologist's opinion is.

Does pre-exploration cholangiography reveal stones that might otherwise have been overlooked? Does it lower the incidence of negative and hence unnecessary explorations of the duct?

It has been estimated that routine operative cholangiography detects stones in the common duct in 4 percent of patients undergoing cholecystectomy that would have been missed if only conventional clinical indexes had been used, and it leads to a reduction in the number of ducts explored. The latter observation is important, but it should be emphasized that a negative exploration of the common duct at the time of cholecystectomy, in my experience, does not increase the mortality over cholecystectomy alone.

The operative cholangiogram, in addition to showing the presence or absence of stones, may reveal anomalies of the ductal system or other ductal disease.

CHOLEDOCHOTOMY

When proper exposure of the common duct has been achieved, the peritoneum overlying the duct is incised. The duct is aspirated with a 22-gauge needle, and the bile obtained is sent to the laboratory for culture and sensitivity studies. If the duct is large, an incision is made at an appropriate level that will best facilitate exploration of the ductal system both cephalad and distally. Since the junction of the cystic duct with the common duct is so variable, I do not relate the position of the choledochotomy to this anatomic landmark. Guy sutures of 3–0 silk are placed on each side of the choledochotomy. The length of the choledochotomy is about 2 cm.

EXPLORATION

If stones are seen when the choledochotomy is made, they should be removed immediately with ductal forceps. The common hepatic duct and the right and left hepatic ducts are explored with ductal forceps and with appropriate ductal scoops. The commercial ductal scoops, in my opinion, are inadequate for proper exploration of the ductal system. I have special silver scoops of my own design that I find invaluable in exploring the hepatic and extrahepatic ducts.

Exploration of the ducts using a combination of forceps and scoops is adequate for the removal of almost all stones within the major bile ducts. I do not believe the proper use of an appropriate ductal scoop poses any danger to the ductal mucosa. All instrumentation should be used in the manner for which the instrument was designed, and this includes the Bakes dilators. The Bakes instruments were designed to calibrate and not dilate the sphincter of Oddi. I routinely calibrate the sphincter of Oddi when I explore the common bile duct. If one prefers, French catheters may be used for this calibration. The Fogarty catheter may be decisive in the removal of fragments of a stone wedged in the distal common duct.

IRRIGATION OF THE DUCTAL SYSTEM

Dealing as I do with large numbers of patients with multiple recurrences of intrahepatic duct stones due to recurrence of common duct strictures and to primary recurrent intraductal stones, I have learned the value of hydrostatic pressure in the management of intrahepatic stones. Patients in this category may have hundreds of stones that cannot be removed by conventional or, at times, by sophisticated instrumentation.

After thorough exploration of the ductal system with forceps and scoops, I irrigate the ducts with a copious volume of saline solution. Recently, I have found that use of the Water Pic (Zimmer), with its pulsatile injection of saline solution, is an excellent way to irrigate the bile ducts. It is especially effective in removing multiple small stones and biliary mud.

CHOLEDOCHOSCOPY

Since the value of choledochoscopy apparently depends to some degree on irrigation attendant on this procedure, I will describe this procedure in the words of one of its leading advocates, Dr. Leon Morgenstern.

Choledochoscopes are either rigid or flexible; both have their uses. For most purposes the rigid choledochoscope is more versatile and provides images of superior quality. If I had to choose between the rigid and the flexible choledochoscope, I would choose the rigid one, but prefer to have both to cover all situations. The flexible choledochoscope is more useful for the long and tortuous ducts. The rigid choledochoscopes, of which the best is the Storz scope, employing the Hopkins rod-lens optical system, come in two sizes, one with a horizontal limb of 4 cm and the other with a horizontal limb of 6 cm. Of the two, the shorter is more useful and more easily handled.

Cholangioscopy is performed within the fluid-filled bile ducts. The fluid (saline) is delivered under 300 mm of water pressure to distend the ducts for accurate viewing. The choledochoscope is introduced distally first, bringing to view not only stones in the interior of the duct, but also signs of cholangitis such as edema and reddening of the duct wall, with shreds of mucoid and fibrinous material waving in the current of irrigative fluid. The end point of the distal exploration with the choledochoscope, which has a telescopic lens, is the visualization of the sphincter of Oddi and the observation of its opening and closing. If the sphincter of Oddi is not seen, the exploration is incomplete. If an impacted stone is seen, it may be grasped with an accessory instrument attached to the choledochoscope, or a Fogarty catheter may be passed under direct vision beyond it for retrieval.

I believe that exploration of the duct is best done with the operator on the left side of the patient. Visualization of the distal duct is also aided by kocherization of the duodenum and downward traction on the duodenum as the choledochoscope is passed distally. This renders the distal duct taut and permits a good telescopic view of the duct's interior. Inexperienced operators often claim that instead of a view of the ducts, they see a succession of red circles. This indicates that the viewing end of the choledochoscope is pressing against the duct wall rather than projecting its viewing angle through the fluid-filled medium within the duct. With practice, good visualization of the duct can be obtained within a few minutes. The rhythmic opening and closing of the fishmouth-shaped sphincter at the distal extremity of the duct is the endpoint of the distal examination.

The choledochoscope is then directed cephalad. To keep the fluid from escaping from the incisional aperture as the duct is being filled, the guy sutures may be crossed around the choledochoscope, making the system relatively closed, although some fluid continues to escape and must be continually suctioned. The landmark for the proximal ductal exploration is the sharp, carina-like spur between the right and left ducts. Frequently, as the instrument is passed in a cephalad direction, secondary and tertiary ducts may be seen, particularly in the widely dilated ducts of more advanced obstruction. Stones floating in the recesses of the higher ducts may be retrieved either by using auxiliary forceps or by passing the Fogarty catheter under direct vision just beyond the stone and withdrawing it with the stone pulled before it.

Currently the best flexible choledochoscope is that made by the Olympus Company. It has an outer diameter of 5 mm. Visualization is good, albeit not so sharp as with the rigid scope. I use the flexible scope when the stone is beyond the reach of range of visualization of the rigid instrument owing to extreme length, tortuosity, or anomaly of the duct.

Having done the standard exploratory maneuvers with Randall forceps and Fogarty catheter, as well as correct inspection of the duct interior with the cholangioscope, the surgeon has completed the exploratory maneuvers and is ready for insertion of the T-tube.

INSERTION OF T-TUBE

Despite some excellent reports of satisfactory results after primary closure of the duct, I invariably use a T-tube after common duct exploration. The caliber of the T-tube used varies according to the diameter of the common bile duct, but the size usually is a 14 or 16 F. The duct is closed with interrupted 3–0 chromic catgut sutures. Closure is tested by injecting the T-tube with saline solution.

Completion cholangiography is performed. Since the previous manipulation within the distal duct may have caused the sphincter to go into spasm, I inject 7 or 8 ml of the contrast solution into the T-tube. I compress the proximal limb of the T-tube with my left thumb and index finger as another 7 or 8 ml of the radiopaque solution is injected, thus ensuring visualization of the distal end of the common duct and ensuring the appearance of the contrast solution in the duodenum when results of cholangiography are normal.

The external limb of the T-tube is brought out through a lateral stab wound and anchored to the skin with a 3–0 nylon suture. The intraperitoneal course of the external limb of the T-tube must be on a direct line from its emergence from the bile duct to the anterior abdominal wall. This precaution is important to ensure access to the common duct by the radiologist or the endoscopist if a stone has been overlooked. With properly performed completion cholangiography, a retained stone should be an exceptionally rare event. An appropriate sump drain is inserted into Morison's pouch, and the abdominal incision is closed.

MANAGEMENT OF T-TUBE

The T-tube is attached to gravity drainage. My curiosity about the amount of daily bile drainage is not very acute. I am distressed if no drainage occurs, which implies some debris, blood clot, or a kink in the tube.

I am also concerned if a large amount of biliary drainage persists, but these events are so rare that I do not rush to obtain a cholangiogram. If either event occurs in the absence of acute symptoms or signs, the problem usually disappears spontaneously. The T-tube is left to gravity drainage for 7 days. The tube is then clamped around the clock if no symptoms occur.

Again, it is conventional surgical teaching to obtain another cholangiogram about the tenth postoperative day. If results of cholangiography are normal, the T-tube may be removed. In the elderly or debilitated patient or one whose postoperative course has been complicated, the T-tube should be left in place. I frequently discharge such

RETAINED COMMON DUCT STONES

DONALD W. WEAVER, M.D., F.A.C.S.

Few areas in surgery have changed more in the last two decades than the management of common bile duct stones. Prior to invasive radiology and the development of endoscopic methods to assess and manipulate the common bile duct, retained bile duct stones following cholecystectomy nearly always required reoperation. At present, most common bile duct stones can be removed without additional surgery.

Gallstones gain access to the common bile duct through a patent cystic duct and, except in unusual cases, when found later, were missed at the time of cholecystectomy. Often these stones, when small, spontaneously pass through the ampulla of Vater into the gastrointestinal tract without clinical sequelae. When the stones fail to pass and slowly become larger within the common bile duct, recognizable symptoms ensue. The most common clinical findings are intermittent pain and jaundice, but when the bile becomes secondarily infected, the classic triad of Charcot is completed with fever and chills.

Prior to the development of intraoperative cholangiography, indications for bile duct exploration rested on clinical criteria and operative findings. The presence of a palpable stone in the common bile duct or enlargement of the common bile duct to more than 2.0 cm in diameter were considered absolute indications for duct exploration. A previous history of jaundice, acute pancreatitis, and the finding of multiple small stones with a patent cystic duct were relative indications for bile duct exploration. Table 1 shows the incidence with which the common bile duct stone could be expected based on these clinical criteria.

Since operative cholangiography has been perfected, the decision to explore the common bile duct is often made on the basis of a positive cholangiogram. The ease of this procedure and the approximately 4 to 6 percent missed,

patients with the T-tube in place and remove it later in the office.

Drainage of bile from the T-tube tract rarely occurs. If it persists, a search for distal obstruction must be made. The danger of exploration of a small common duct should be mentioned. A 3- or 4-mm duct in an adult almost never requires exploration, and attempts to explore such a small duct may invite serious injury to the duct.

In the hands of a well-trained surgeon, exploration of the common duct should be associated with a mortality of less than 1 percent. With carefully performed intraoperative cholangiography, the incidence of a retained stone in the duct should not exceed 2 percent.

unsuspected common bile duct stones have justified the routine use of intraoperative cholangiography by many surgeons. Others, however, advocate selective use of intraoperative cholangiography and cite the added cost of the procedure, as well as the approximately 3 to 4 percent incidence of unnecessary common bile duct exploration associated with false-positive cholangiograms. Although I do not perform routine intraoperative cholangiography with uncomplicated cholecystectomy, before opening the common bile duct I always obtain a pre-exploration cholangiogram. Several points concerning the cholangiogram should be made. After isolating the cystic duct and surrounding it with a ligature, I ligate the cystic artery and remove the gallbladder from the liver bed. I then gently palpate the cystic duct, taking care to massage its contents toward the gallbladder. A silk tie is then placed at the junction of the gallbladder and the cystic duct to prevent stones from escaping through the cystic duct during the cholangiogram. A small transverse incision is then made in the cystic duct, and a cholangiocath is advanced into the common bile duct and tied in place. The cholangiocath has been previously filled with saline and a three-way stopcock placed on the end. Occasionally it is difficult to advance the cholangiocath through the cystic duct because of obstruction from the valves of Heister. Slight traction on the cystic duct and changing of the entry position usually allows the cholangiocath to advance.

TABLE 1   Reliability of Indication for Common Bile Duct Exploration

Indication	% Positive
Palpable stone	98
Cholangitis with jaundice	94
Pancreatitis	50
Positive preexploratory cholangiogram	50
Jaundice alone	35
Dilated duct	14
Small stones	10

Gentle aspiration on the syringe attached to the three-way stopcock confirms proper position when bile is seen in the catheter. The cholangiogram is obtained by instilling Renografin-30, or Renografin-60 which has been diluted one to one with saline, into the common bile duct. The use of Renografin-30 is important since a denser dye may obscure small stones. Before the initial film, I inject 7 to 10 cc of contrast medium. Another 10 cc is then added before obtaining the second film. The initial film usually shows good filling of the common bile duct and hepatic radicles, and the follow-up film shows passage of contrast medium into the duodenum. Occasionally, the left hepatic system is difficult to visualize with the patient in a standard supine position. When it is essential to visualize the left intrahepatic radicles and the standard cholangiogram has been inadequate, the patient should be rotated to the left from the supine position and contrast medium reinjected to allow filling of the left side of the liver. The rather midline anatomic position of the common bile duct may lead to bony interference with the cholangiogram by the spinal column. A small pad placed under the patient's right side prior to draping for the surgical procedure slightly rotates the patient and allows the common bile duct to be "lifted" roentgenographically from the spine. When the volume of the common bile duct is large and the amount of injected contrast material inadequate to fill the entire ductal system, the left hand can be inserted under the common bile duct through the epiploic foramen and gentle pressure applied with the index finger and thumb above the cystic duct while injecting contrast medium. Another cholangiogram is then obtained which will outline the lower part of the common bile duct and show flow into the duodenum. Once the cholangiogram is obtained and found to be satisfactory, the cholangiocath is removed, and cystic duct ligated, and the operation completed. In rare instances, despite the best and most persistent manipulation of the cholangiocath, it cannot be passed into an acceptable position to obtain a cholangiogram. Many factors influence the decision whether to persist in obtaining additional studies. If judged essential, a reliable cholangiogram can be obtained by sticking a No. 25 butterfly catheter, attached to a connecting tube, directly into the common bile duct and then injecting dye. I have had no personal experience in the use of intraoperative ultrasonography for the detection of common bile duct stones.

COMMON BILE DUCT EXPLORATION

The primary value of a pre-exploratory cholangiogram is to give the operating surgeon an indication of the number and location of the common bile duct stones. The Bakes dilators, stone scoops, and forceps are a traditional part of the instrument set-up for common bile duct exploration, but in recent years, I have largely abandoned their use because the risk of common bile duct injury is greater with their use than with the use of the Fogarty balloon-tipped biliary catheters. Occasionally I use a small Bakes dilator as a "sound" to see whether there are impacted stones in the distal common bile duct. Following choledochotomy, I pass the biliary Fogarty into both the right and left hepatic radicles successively and gently inflate the balloon, drawing it toward the choledochostomy. It is important to avoid overinflating the balloon in order to prevent rupture injury to ductal mucosa. The Fogarty catheter is then passed toward the ampulla and usually slips easily into the duodenum. The balloon is then inflated and its intraduodenal position confirmed by manual palpation. Next the catheter is gently pulled back until the ampulla is encountered, at which time the balloon is deflated and then inflated again once the ampulla is passed. Several passes with the catheter both proximally and distally usually result in complete clearing of the biliary tract of calculi. Following extraction of stone with the biliary catheter, I routinely perform choledochoscopy using a rigid right-angle choledochoscope. This provides an excellent view of the common bile duct, common hepatic duct, and hepatic bifurcation. A flexible choledochoscope that can be gas sterilized is also available and has the additional advantage of allowing luminal visualization all the way to the duodenum.

Although the surgeon obviously does not plan to leave stones behind, placement of the T-tube following common bile duct exploration can facilitate retrieval of these stones should they later be discovered. I cut short side arms on the T-tube and either remove the entire back wall of the side arm or cut a "V-shaped" defect in the back wall at the entrance of the long arm. This facilitates removal of the T-tube through the tube tract at a later date. I use the largest possible T-tube so that the tract formed to the skin may be a usable port of entry for the invasive radiologist should the removal of a duct stone be required. A minimum size 14 F T-tube is required in order to use the extracting baskets currently available. A specially designed T-tube catheter with a 12 F short arm and an 18 F long arm is available, but we have not used this. If the common bile duct is small and a larger tube tract desired, a segment from a red Robinson catheter can be cut to fit snugly over the long arm of the T-tube. This enlarges the access tract. The T-tube is brought out to the skin toward the lateral aspect of the wound in the most direct fashion so that the bile duct might be as accessible as possible. The T-tube is then secured within the common bile duct by means of interrupted 4–0 Vicryl sutures and secured at the skin with a 3–0 Nylon suture.

APPROACHES TO TREATMENT OF RETAINED COMMON DUCT STONES

There are several techniques that can be used to remove common bile duct stones: (1) dissolution with various litholytic agents, (2) extraction with stone basket, (3) endoscopic papillotomy, (4) spontaneous passage, and (5) reoperation. The approach to treatment of the retained stone in any individual patient depends primarily on the availability of the aforementioned techniques. In addition, chemical composition of the stone is an important factor in the decision to use litholytic therapy.

Dissolution

Various solutions have been used to dissolve retained common duct stones, but are effective only for cholesterol stones. Ether, choloroform, and other such organic solvents are not safe and should not be used. Although heparin has been used, in vitro studies and in vivo experience have not confirmed its effectiveness. Two solutions are in current use—monooctanoin (Capmul) and sodium cholate. Monooctanoin is the preferred solution for the dissolution of cholesterol common duct stones.

Monooctanoin is a medium-chain diglyceride of capric acid and caprilic acid. It is a good solvent for cholesterol and soluble in water. At present, this substance is an investigational drug and is approved for use only by a limited number of investigators. It is an effective solvent, and if the stones are high in cholesterol, a 90 percent success rate can be expected. Generally the stones dissolve in 3 to 7 days. If there is no significant change in the size of the stone after one week of infusion, it is unlikely that the cholesterol content is sufficiently high to dissolve the stones. The advantage of monooctanoin over the standard solution of 150 mM sodium cholate is the rapidity of action of monooctanoin compared to the 2 to 3 weeks of infusion required for cholate. To infuse monooctanoin, a Harvard infusion pump is calibrated with a 30-cc syringe to deliver 3 to 5 cc per hour. The syringe is filled with monooctanoin and placed in the pump. The tubing from the syringe leads to a stopcock, which is connected to the patient and a manometer (Fig. 1). The manometer is broken off at the 30-cm mark to prevent overpressurizing the bile duct. All three stopcock ports are opened, and the infusion is begun once the zero mark on the manometer is at the level of the patient's common bile duct. There are two possible side effects to which the patient and nursing staff should be alerted. One is due to increased pressure in the bile duct, which results in pain, chills, and fever. This occurs when stones migrate to obstruct the outflow of the common bile duct and the port in the stopcock to the manometer is inadvertently closed. If this happens, the infusion should be stopped and the T-tube attached to straight drainage. The other side effect is related to the rate of infusion. When the solution is infused at rates between 5 and 10 cc per hour, the patient may complain of cramping abdominal pain due to the increased volume of monooctanoin emptying into the duodenum. This problem is easily remedied by stopping the infusion until the symptoms subside and then resuming the infusion at the proper rate. Cramping is unusual at infusion rates between 3 and 5 cc per hour. The pressure on the manometer is recorded by the nursing staff every 2 hours, and the volume of infusion and any bile output is recorded every shift. The infusion is stopped and the T-tube is attached to gravity drainage at meal times. After eating, the patient is instructed to exercise by walking for 30 to 40 minutes. The patient may turn and kink the connecting tubing, resulting in an abnormally high pressure registered on the manometer. Not only does the manometer monitor the infusion pressure, but it also serves as a safety valve should a stone migrate and obstruct the distal common bile duct. Once the pressure in the bile duct exceeds 30 cm water, the solution overflows the top of the manometer. This is a necessary and important safeguard for the patient.

Daily SGOT, alkaline phosphatase, bilirubin, and amylase determinations are made and a cholangiogram obtained every third or fourth day. If there is no change in the size or number of stones by the seventh day, the infusion is discontinued.

With a low infusion rate, stones in the proximal part of the common bile duct or in the hepatic ducts may not have good contact with the solution since the solution is generally flushed distally by normal bile flow into the duodenum. In special cases with proximal stones and stones in the hepatic ducts, a small polyethylene catheter can be placed through the T-tube tract into the bile duct proximal to the stone, and the monooctanoin infused through this tube with the T-tube used as an exit port.

Extraction

This technique was popularized by interventional radiologists and has been highly successful in removing retained common bile duct stones through the T-tube tract. When a common bile duct stone has been confirmed

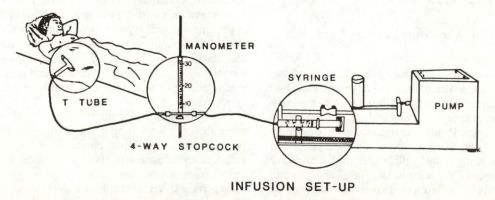

Figure 1 The equipment and connections used to infuse litholytic solutions into the common bile duct to dissolve cholesterol stones. The manometer is 30 cm in height and the 4-way stopcock permits continuous communication between the infusion, the manometer, and the patient.

following choledochotomy, I leave the T-tube in place for a minimum of 4 weeks to ensure an adequate tract. The patient is then sent to the radiology suite as an outpatient where intravenous sedation is given and the T-tube removed. Under fluoroscopic guidance, a Dormia basket is inserted into the common bile duct through the T-tube tract, and the stone is trapped in the basket. Gentle traction on the basket wire then usually results in dislodgement of the stone from the common bile duct. If the stone is large or faceted, it may not be easily removed. Often the patient experiences some nausea and abdominal discomfort when traction is applied to the stone within the common bile duct. If the stone is too large to be removed through the tract, crushing forceps can be inserted through the tract and the stone broken into small pieces. These pieces may then be individually extracted. In some cases this procedure has to be repeated in order to clear the common bile duct entirely. Once the procedure is completed, another cholangiogram is obtained, and a red Robinson catheter is inserted back through the T-tube tract to maintain patency until it is certain that all the stones have been removed. Patients undergoing biliary tract manipulation should be treated with parenteral antibiotic therapy prior to the procedure. Stone extraction requires more technical expertise than does dissolution. However, these skills are generally available in most radiology departments. These extraction techniques are difficult to employ when the T-tube tract is small or tortuous and the stones are large or impacted.

Endoscopic Papillotomy

In recent years endoscopic papillotomy has gained widespread acceptance in the management of retained common bile duct stones. This procedure requires a skilled endoscopist and is accomplished through the same side-viewing endoscope used to perform endoscopic cholangio-pancreatography. A specially devised cautery wire is passed through the endoscope into the common bile duct and the cautery wire bowstringed within the ampulla, cutting a variable depth depending on the duration and power of current applied. Once the sphincter is disrupted, small balloon catheters or endoscopic baskets can be placed up the common bile duct and stones extracted into the duodenum. In my experience, occasionally both endoscopic sphincterotomy and manipulation of the stone from above via the T-tube tract at different times may be required to remove the most difficult impacted stones. Although perforation and bleeding are potential complications of papillotomy, in the hands of a skilled endoscopist, this risk is small, and I believe the procedure has great promise as the skills to perform it become more widespread.

Other Approaches

When the stones are small, spontaneous passage often occurs. It is estimated that perhaps 20 percent of stones pass without specific therapy, usually within 2 to 3 months following choledochostomy. A longer wait usually is not justified. When a reoperation is required to remove a retained bile duct stone, I prefer to perform a choledocho-duodenostomy if the common duct is dilated. When a stone is impacted at the ampulla, a transduodenal sphincterotomy may be necessary to free the stone.

PRIMARY COMMON DUCT STONES

COLIN G. THOMAS, Jr., M.D.
ROBERT D. CROOM III, M.D.

Primary common duct stones are calculi that have undergone nucleation within the intra- or extrahepatic bile ducts. Those formed within the gallbladder and reaching the common duct through the cystic duct or a fistula are "secondary" stones. Primary common duct stones differ in composition from the more common cholesterol and mixed stones arising in the gallbladder in that they are composed primarily of bilirubinate salts and contain minimal amounts of cholesterol. Primary stones may be visually subdivided into "earthy" and "tarry" stones based on morphologic appearance. Earthy stones lack a crystalline interior, are usually brownish yellow to dark chocolate brown, and are easily crushed into granular, "earth-like," pasty fragments. Earthy stones are considered to be primary in that they arise within bile ducts. In many cases a variable amount of sludge or biliary mud is present with this type of stone. Tarry stones are black, shiny amorphous concretions that are likely to be associated with hyperbilirubinemic states (chronic hemolysis). In contrast to cholesterol and pigment stones, earthy and tarry stones are less readily differentiated by appearance.

Differentiation of primary and secondary stones is of more than academic importance, since the treatment of primary stones demands correction of the underlying pathogenic mechanism to avoid recurrence. Furthermore, stone composition may also influence postoperative management of retained common duct calculi and the likelihood of their dissolution by chemical agents.

The role of partial common duct obstruction in the genesis of choledocholithiasis has not been sufficiently emphasized (Table 1). Although most common duct stones form in the gallbladder, once within the common duct they may provoke spasm, edema, and ultimately fibrosis at the distal end of the common duct and the papilla of Vater. The resulting obstruction and bile stasis may be an important factor in both primary and recurrent choledocholithiasis. Bile stasis is commonly associated with a positive culture of bacteria indigenous to the gastrointestinal tract, in particular, *E. coli.*. These bacteria liberate beta glucuronidase, thereby deconjugating soluble bilirubin diglucuronide to form insoluble bilirubinate salts. Simply removing stones from the common duct without consideration and resolution of the etiologic mechanism(s) is no more appropriate than cholecystolithotomy in the management of cholelithiasis.

Clinical manifestations of choledocholithiasis are those of cholangitis, i.e., right upper quadrant pain, fever, and jaundice (Charcot's triad). Of these, pain is the most common (88%), followed by jaundice (50%) and fever (37%). A small number of patients (3%) may be asymptomatic. The natural history of common duct stones is not a benign one, and cholangitis (and its sequelae), pancreatitis, and variable scarring of the bile duct and papilla of Vater result from untreated choledocholithiasis. If the diagnosis of choledocholithiasis is made, removal of calculi and an appropriate operation to minimize the risk of recurrent disease should be performed in virtually all patients.

DIAGNOSTIC MEASURES

Laboratory studies that are helpful in the diagnosis are liver function tests (alkaline phosphatase, GGT, total and conjugated bilirubin, SGOT, SGPT) and serum amylase determination. Evaluation of coagulation parameters (PT, PTT) is advisable prior to invasive diagnostic tests, especially in jaundiced patients and thoe with abnormalities of liver function.

Precise localization of common duct stones and knowledge of the anatomy of the biliary tree are requisite to the appropriate management of choledocholithiasis. Although this information may be procured by intra-

operative cholangiography, such evaluation is best carried out preoperatively, thereby permitting optimal definition of pathologic changes and operative planning. Ultrasonography, CT scan, and radionuclide scans may delineate the size of intra- and extrahepatic bile ducts, but these imaging techniques do not identify calculi. Endoscopic retrograde cholangiopancreatography (ERCP) is the most valuable diagnostic procedure for determining bile duct size, presence and number of calculi, existence of ampullary stenosis and/or stenosis of the common duct, and presence of a choledochal cyst, cystic duct remnant, or Caroli's disease. Furthermore, it provides an opportunity to carry out papillotomy and retrieval of common duct stones in selected patients who have obstruction secondary to stenosis at the papilla.

Percutaneous transhepatic cholangiography (PTC) may provide similar information, but at a slightly greater morbidity. This diagnostic test is indicated when there is complete obstruction at the papilla or when ERCP has failed to provide adequate information. Additionally, PTC with either internal or external biliary drainage via an indwelling catheter may be an adjunct in the preoperative preparation of the patient with complete common duct obstruction or severe derangement of hepatic function from longstanding obstruction. Antibiotic prophylaxis should be employed in both ERCP and PTC to minimize the likelihood of cholangitis during manipulation of the biliary tract.

OPERATIVE MANAGEMENT

Selection and use of preoperative sedatives and anesthetic agents should avoid those tending to enhance sphincter activity (e.g., morphine sulfate, fentanyl, and other opiate and synthetic narcotics) at the distal common duct.

Operative management of primary common duct calculi includes careful examination of the liver, external bile ducts, duodenum, and pancreas. The presence or absence of cirrhosis should be determined. If cirrhosis is present, a wedge or needle biopsy of the liver may prove helpful as a baseline for correlation with altered hepatic function. The common duct, duodenum, and pancreas should be examined for associated neoplastic or inflammatory changes, and biopsy with frozen section examination obtained if warranted. Incision along the lateral aspect of the second and third parts of the duodenum (Kocher maneuver) permits mobilization of the duodenum, distal common duct, and head of the pancreas in a bloodless plane, thereby facilitating palpation of the common duct, region of the ampulla of Vater, and the pancreatic head and uncinate process. Findings on palpation should be correlated with those disclosed by the preoperative cholangiogram. If there are serious discrepancies, e.g., absence of a palpable stone, an intraoperative cholangiogram via a 21- or 23-gauge needle or a hepatopedally directed catheter in the common duct is advisable. Measurement of the common duct pressure (normally less

TABLE 1 Pathogenesis of Primary Biliary Tract Stones

Stasis with or without prior cholelithiasis
  Aging patient
  Secondary common duct stones with obstruction
  Stenosis of the duodenal papilla of Vater or
    postoperative common duct stricture
  Neoplasm
  Choledochal cyst
  Caroli's disease

Alcohol (+/− cirrhosis)

Parasites

Unknown

than 15 to 18 cm of water) by means of a venous manometer provides an estimate of the degree of obstruction and stasis. This initial measurement may be particularly valuable if there is no evidence of distal common duct obstruction at the time of choledocholithotomy. An elevated pressure supports the need for ensuring adequate common duct drainage via choledochoduodenostomy or sphincteroplasty.

Intraoperative cholangiography is advised in all patients with common duct calculi before common duct exploration unless there has been clear delineation of ductal anatomy preoperatively by either ERCP or PTC. The merits of cholangiography prior to choledochotomy relate to defining the anatomy of the biliary tree and any associated area(s) of stenosis, size of the common duct, filling defects in intra- or extrahepatic ducts, and characteristics of the ampulla of Vater. If the gallbladder is present, cholangiography is carried out through the cystic duct using a Cholangiocath with its tip in the midportion of the common duct. An adequate cholangiogram requires two radiographs, the first after injecting 3 to 5 ml of 25% Hypaque with the patient in a supine position with slight rotation (15°) to his left. A second injection of contrast agent, 8 to 20 ml depending upon the size of the common duct, is carried out with the patient in 10° to 15° of the Trendelenberg position. Both radiographs are made while the anesthesiologist produces a temporary arrest of ventilation. The first film should demonstrate filling of the common duct with a minimum of contrast entering the duodenum. This should provide a precise outline of the distal common duct and ampulla of Vater without obscuration by contrast agent within the duodenum. The second film should demonstrate filling of the intrahepatic ducts. Particular attention must be paid to the left hepatic duct in which (due to its anatomic characteristics) intrahepatic calculi are most commonly located. The operative cholangiogram should be interpreted independently by the surgeon and radiologist. If there are ambiguities or differences in interpretation, the surgeon should request personal consultation with the radiologist in the operating room and obtain additional radiographs. An alternative, double-contrast technique may be helpful in equivocal cases. This involves filling the duct with 50% Hypaque and then withdrawing all contrast and obtaining a roentgenogram to demonstrate contrast-coated and/or -impregnated calculi.

SURGICAL PROCEDURES

The optimum location for choledochotomy is at the junction of the common duct and duodenum or immediately proximal to an area of stricture or stenosis in the common duct. The duodenum is dissected and elevated from the underlying common duct for a distance of 1 to 2 cm. Choledochotomy in this area provides the option for performance of a subsequent choledochoduodenostomy following choledocholithotomy. Such an incision also permits a more direct approach to stones impacted in the distal duct.

If the common duct is of normal caliber, it should be incised longitudinally between stay sutures. Either a longitudinal or transverse incision may be used in a dilated duct. Bile culture should be obtained. Stones are removed by combining palpation with the use of stone forceps or a Fogarty biliary catheter and by gentle irrigation with warm saline. Retrieved stones should be characterized visually and representative calculi saved in the event their solubility needs to be determined for dealing with retained calculi.

We have had insufficient experience with cholangioscopy to determine its role. However, the choledochoscope has been found by others to be a useful adjunct to common duct exploration and has been used without increasing morbidity of the operation. In some cases it should reduce operative time by eliminating the need for blind and prolonged exploration and repeated cholangiograms. This approach would seem particularly applicable when multiple calculi have been demonstrated by cholangiography.

Following removal of calculi, an operative cholangiogram is mandatory to ensure completeness of choledocholithotomy. Even in experienced hands, calculi are retained or overlooked in 5 to 8 percent of patients, being primarily located in the smaller intrahepatic ducts. The "closing" cholangiogram may be procured via a Foley catheter inserted through the choledochotomy prior to duct closure, through a T-tube positioned within the common duct through the choledochotomy or through a catheter placed in the cystic duct stump.

Common Duct Drainage, Choledochoduodenostomy, and Sphincteroplasty

Since most "primary" common duct stones are associated with stasis, consideration must be given to correction of the underlying obstruction. If no obstruction exists to passage of a 3-mm Bakes dilator at the ampulla following choledocholithotomy and there is no significant dilatation of the common duct, only a T-tube needs to be placed. This provides immediate decompression of the common duct and also a later route for mechanical removal or dissolution of retained calculi. More commonly there is a dilated common bile duct that requires a drainage procedure even if a 3-mm dilator passes easily. We do not advocate the use of a Bakes dilator to "dilate" a stenotic papilla of Vater. Disruption of a scarred sphincter of Oddi by this technique further damages the delicate muscle fibers of the sphincter, induces sphincter spasm, and has been a direct cause of severe pancreatitis in several patients referred to our care. We favor judicious use of the 3-mm Bakes dilator to probe for sphincter patency, anticipating easy passage through a normal papilla of Vater. In the absence of an impacted stone, both choledochoduodenostomy and sphincteroplasty are effective in relieving distal choledochal obstruction and afford good drainage of the common duct. In our experience, choledochoduodenostomy has been associated with a lower morbidity. In view of the foregoing and the technical considerations of each approach, choledocho-duodenostomy is preferable in patients in whom (1) difficulty exists in identifying the papilla of Vater, (2) obesity or other factors make exposure difficult, (3) the length of the common duct stenosis contraindicates sphincteroplasty, (4) the presence of suppurative cholangitis makes duodenotomy and manipulation near the ampulla unduly hazardous, or (5) there is a perivaterian diverticulum. Transduodenal sphincteroplasty is the procedure of choice in patients with (1) an impacted stone(s) in the ampulla of Vater, (2) a small common duct making choledochoduodenostomy technically difficult, (3) stenosis of the papilla of Vater, and (4) the possibility of an ampullary tumor causing obstruction.

In many individuals either operative procedure achieves the desired relief of obstruction, and the selection ultimately must be determined by the ease of technical performance and the experience of the surgeon. In the performance of these operations, the surgeon must recognize the essentiality of avoiding unnecessary instrumentation of the bile ducts with its attendant hazards of cholangitis from inherent bactibilia or pancreatitis. Both procedures have the advantage of avoiding the need of tube drainage of the common duct with its associated foreign body reaction contributing to infection, stasis, sludge deposition, and stone formation.

Preparation for choledochoduodenostomy entails mobilizing the duodenum with a Kocher maneuver and reflecting the posterior wall of the duodenum from the anterior wall of the common duct for a distance of 1 to 1.5 cm. Extensive stripping of fibroareolar tissues from the common duct should be avoided to maintain good vascular supply and prevent ischemic necrosis. After placing two traction sutures on either side of the proposed choledochotomy, a stab incision is made in the common duct with a No. 11 knife blade, and the choledochotomy is carefully extended, by means of scissors, over a 1.5- to 2.5-cm distance. Placement of the choledochotomy should allow maintenance of the relationship between duodenum and common duct without tension or distortion after completion of the anastomosis. Choledocholithotomy is performed, and the region of the ampulla is carefully examined to ensure removal of all calculi and the absence of neoplasm. Excision of a 1- to 2-mm rim of common duct from the margin of the choledochotomy creates a wide oval opening in the subsequent anastomosis. A complementary incision is made through the duodenal wall, and the pouting and redundant duodenal mucosa is trimmed. A single-layer anastomosis using full-thickness through-and-through, inverting sutures of fine silk (3–0 or 4–0) is created; sutures are so placed that all knots are on the outside of the completed anastomosis. T-tube drainage of the common duct is usually considered unnecessary. Closed suction drainage of the subhepatic space is advisable in all patients.

Choledochoduodenostomy results in a segment of common duct between the anastomotic stoma and the papilla of Vater that theoretically would drain poorly. Although "sump syndrome" has been reported due to accumulation of duodenal contents within this "blind" segment, this complication develops infrequently and should not be considered a contraindication to choledocho-duodenostomy. Stenosis of the anastomotic stoma also may occur with resulting stasis and recurrence of common duct stones. This risk can be minimized by making the stoma of maximal size, i.e., the diameter of the dilated common duct.

Transduodenal sphincteroplasty is performed after localization of the sphincter of Oddi by the gentle passage of a biliary probe or biliary Fogarty catheter through the duodenal papilla via the cystic duct stump (coincident with cholecystectomy) or the site of choledochotomy, or by palpation of a stone lodged in the ampulla. The duodenum is mobilized and incised transversely overlying the site of the papilla through one-third to one-half of its circumference. A traction suture placed through the duodenal wall from within and immediately caudad to the papilla provides stability and enhances accessibility of the sphincter. Traction sutures are placed through the relatively tough sphincter, and it is transected at its superolateral margin for a distance of 1.5 to 2.0 cm. The incision must be long enough to ensure complete division of the area of stenosis and open the common duct to the point of dilatation. Superolateral incision avoids damage to the medially located major pancreatic duct (Wirsung). Excision of a sliver of one margin of the transected sphincter for biopsy is advisable to determine the histopathologic nature of the obstruction and to avoid overlooking an occult carcinoma. Stones located proximally in the bile duct usually can be extracted without need for a separate choledochotomy. In order to avoid stricture at the site of sphincterotomy, the duodenal mucosa is sutured to the incised common duct with a single layer of interrupted absorbable sutures (5–0 or 6–0 Dexon or Vicryl). The duodenal incision is closed with a single layer of inverting seromuscular (Lembert) sutures of fine silk (3–0 or 4–0). Drainage of the common duct by a catheter through the cystic duct stump or by a T-tube was carried out previously. More recently, such drainage has been regarded as not only unnecessary but undesirable because of foreign body reaction promoting stasis and infection. In debilitated or elderly patients, a temporary gastrostomy may be advisable.

Complications related to sphincteroplasty include pancreatitis, bleeding, and duodenal fistula. These occur infrequently, but their overall incidence and associated morbidity are higher than for the alternative procedure of choledochoduodenostomy.

Prophylactic antibiotics are begun preoperatively (we prefer cefoxitin [Mefoxin], 1 g every 6 hours) and are continued in the absence of clinical evidence of cholangitis for three doses postoperatively. Any catheter left in the common duct is connected to sterile gravity drainage.

Acute suppurative cholangitis is a potential complication of common duct calculi and is an indication for emergency decompression of the common duct. In the past, this invariably required emergent choledocho-lithotomy for patients who usually are elderly, critically ill, and poor operative risks. Decompression and drainage by insertion of a percutaneous catheter (PTC) into the common duct, in association with intravenous antibiotics and other supportive measures, usually achieve improvement in the patient's overall status and allow choledocholithotomy and choledochoduodenostomy to be performed electively.

ACUTE CHOLANGITIS

JOHN L. CAMERON, M.D., F.A.C.S.

Cholangitis comes from the Greek words "chole" meaning bile and "angeion" meaning vessel or duct. Therefore, literally, acute cholangitis means inflammation of the bile ducts. However, cholangitis as we know it clinically refers to a systemic infection resulting from infected bile within the biliary tree. The entity was first described by Charcot in 1877. His clinical triad of abdominal pain, chills and fever, and jaundice is referred to as Charcot's triad. Interestingly, he described the disease as "intermittent hepatic fever" and the pathogenesis as being secondary to stagnant bile from either gallstones or a stricture. Not much more is known of the pathogenesis of acute cholangitis today.

To develop acute cholangitis two conditions have to be present: (1) the patient has to have infected bile, and (2) there has to be an increase in biliary pressure. The presence of one without the other does not result in the clinical syndrome of cholangitis. The source of the responsible organisms has not been identified with certainty. It has been suggested that they (1) ascend from the duodenum, (2) reach the bile by a portal vein bacteremia, (3) spread via the lymphatics, or (4) come from the gallstones themselves. Probably in different clinical situations all four represent possible sources of the responsible pathogens.

CLINICAL PRESENTATION

Even though acute cholangitis is usually secondary to gallstones, and gallstones are more common in the female, most series of patients with acute cholangitis have a male preponderance. In a series of 78 patients from The Johns Hopkins Hospital, 40 were male and 38 were female. Acute cholangitis tends to occur in a somewhat older age group than the usual age for calculous biliary tract disease. The mean age of the 78 patients in the Hopkins series was 61 years, with a range of 30 to 87 years. Although the classic case of acute cholangitis is characterized by Charcot's triad, in most series all three components of the triad are present in only 50 percent of the patients at the time of admission (Table 1). In the Hopkins series, only 65 percent of the patients were febrile

Endoscopic Sphincterotomy (Papillotomy) With Choledocholithotomy

This technique is gaining wider application as clinical experience increases. The procedure seems especially applicable for the poor-risk patient with stenosis at the papilla of Vater and associated choledocholithiasis.

on admission, although all had a history of fever. Seventy-nine percent had abdominal pain on admission, but in most instances this was mild. Sepsis and severe abdominal pain should suggest diagnoses other than acute cholangitis. Finally, only 79 percent of the 78 patients in the Hopkins series were clinically jaundiced. Although virtually all patients had hyperbilirubinemia, in many instances it was mild.

Sixty-three of the 78 patients had abdominal tenderness. In most instances, however, the abdominal tenderness was mild. Once again, if severe abdominal tenderness is present, other diagnoses such as acute cholecystitis, acute pancreatitis, or other intra-abdominal catastrophes ought to be seriously considered. Severe abdominal pain and marked abdominal tenderness are not common findings in acute cholangitis. Peritoneal signs were not present in the majority of patients on physical examination at admission. Only 19 of the 78 patients had guarding in the right upper quadrant, and 16 had rebound tenderness. The majority of patients (66 out of 78) had normal bowel sounds.

Laboratory data demonstrated abnormalities in liver function tests in virtually all patients. Ninety-two percent of the patients had hyperbilirubinemia on admission. Eighty-six percent had an elevated serum alkaline phosphatase, 93 percent had an elevated SGOT, and 97 percent had an elevated SGPT. Even though abnormal liver function tests are not specific for the diagnosis of acute cholangitis, if liver function tests are not abnormal, one can almost completely exclude the possibility of this entity. In one-third of the patients from the Hopkins series, hyperamylasemia was present. This highlights the fact that

TABLE 1   Clinical Presentation of 78 Patients in The Johns Hopkins Hospital Series

Symptom	No. of Patients	Charcot's Triad
Fever	51/78	65%
Abdominal pain	62/78	79%
Abdominal tenderness	63/78	
Peritoneal signs		
Guarding	19/78	
Rebound	16/78	
Bowel sounds	66/78	
Jaundice	62/78	79%

most patients with acute cholangitis have partial obstruction of the biliary tree from gallstones.

The majority of patients with acute cholangitis have normal abdominal films. A few may demonstrate an ileus or a sentinel loop, and some may have radiopaque gallstones. However, most patients have no detectable abnormality. In the past, intravenous cholangiography was a study performed frequently in the work-up of a patient with acute cholangitis. Now, however, intravenous cholangiography is a diagnostic anachronism and is rarely, if ever, indicated. Among the 78 patients in The Johns Hopkins Hospital series, 48 had common duct stones. Interestingly, in 40 percent of the patients presenting with gallstones, prior cholecystectomy had been performed, and the stones were primary or recurrent common duct stones. This accounts in part for the older age group of patients presenting with acute cholangitis. Malignant strictures were present in 12 patients and benign strictures in 9 patients. There were miscellaneous causes of the biliary tract disease in the remaining nine patients.

BACTERIOLOGY

Blood cultures were positive in 40 percent of the patients presenting with acute cholangitis. In 45 percent, the organism was *E. coli*; in 40 percent, *Klebsiella*; in 5 percent, *Streptococcus faecalis*; and in 5 percent, *Bacteroides fragilis*. At the time of common duct exploration, bile cultures were positive in 100 percent of instances. Multiple organisms were common and occurred in 60 percent of patients. Again the most common organisms were *E. coli* (74%), *Klebsiella* (40%), and *Streptococcus faecalis* (36%).

In a recent bacteriologic study performed at The Johns Hopkins Hospital, the role of anaerobes in biliary tract infections was highlighted (Table 2). In a separate study of 73 patients presenting to The Johns Hopkins Hospital with common duct stones, bile cultures were evaluated. Forty of the 73 patients presented with common duct stones and jaundice, without signs of infection. The remaining 33 patients presented with common duct stones and cholangitis. Thirty-two percent of the patients with common duct stones and no cholangitis were male, whereas 45 percent of the patients with common duct stones and cholangitis were male, highlighting the increased incidence of males in cholangitis series. In addition, the mean age in the patients with common duct stones alone was 48 years; in those with common duct stones plus cholangitis, it was 61 years. The bacteriology was interesting in that anaerobes were cultured from the bile at the time of surgery in 5 percent of those patients presenting with common duct stones only. In contrast, 27 percent of the patients presenting with common duct stones and cholangitis had anaerobes cultured. Thus, when one considers the organisms that should be covered with antibiotics in managing a patient with acute cholangitis, they are *E. coli, Klebsiella,* and *Streptococcus faecalis,* and more recent data on anaerobes suggests that *Bacteroides fragilis* should also be included.

INITIAL MANAGEMENT

The spectrum of severity of disease is broad in patients with acute cholangitis. Some patients present with mild fever, but with otherwise stable vital signs and clearly are not severely ill. Other patients, when first seen, are comatose in septic shock. All patients should be managed initially with intravenous antibiotics. The large majority of these patients demonstrate an initial response to intravenous antibiotics and supportive care and improve clinically; thus surgical intervention for their biliray tree disease can be delayed until the procedure can be elective or semi-elective. Only 20 percent of the patients in the series from The Johns Hopkins Hospital had to undergo operation within the first 48 hours. The remaining patients experienced rapid defervescence, and their surgery was performed electively. The choices of antibiotics to be used in managing acute cholangitis are multiple. If the sepsis is not life-threatening and the vital signs are stable, it is current practice to use a second-generation cephalosporin such as cefoxitin. Other comparable antibiotics are used and are acceptable, but cefoxitin is commonly used and is effective. It is secreted in high concentrations in the bile and provides reasonable coverage for *E. coli, Klebsiella,* and *Bacteroides fragilis*. An antibiotic that has been used frequently in the past, and is still used by some, for biliary sepsis is ampicillin. This drug is totally unsatisfactory as it does not cover most *E. coli* strains and does not cover *Klebsiella*. It is ineffective against anaerobic organisms and only in high concentrations is effective against *Streptococcus faecalis*.

If the sepsis is life-threatening, the currently accepted regimen consists of an aminoglycoside to cover *E. coli* and *Klebsiella*, clindamycin or Flagyl to cover anaerobic organisms, and high-dose penicillin or ampicillin to cover *Streptococcus faecalis*. Other regimens are also used and are probably effective, but the triple-drug therapy just described is the most widely used regimen.

Appropriate supportive care should be administered, and if the patient is in septic shock, a Swan-Ganz catheter should be inserted. The majority of patients respond rapidly to this regimen. Once the patient is stabilized and has had several days of antibiotic therapy, either percutaneous transhepatic or endoscopic retrograde cholangiography should be performed to accurately delineate the biliary

TABLE 2 Patients with Common Duct Stones in The Johns Hopkins Hospital Series

	Common Duct Stones	Common Duct Stones and Acute Cholangitis
Number of patients	40	33
Age	48 years	61 years
Male	32%	45%
Bile culture positive	65%	88%
Gram-negative organisms	38%	76%
Gram-positive organisms	45%	45%
Anaerobes	5%	27%

tree disease. Then, generally within the first week of admission, most patients are ready for elective biliary tract surgery to correct the disease that led to their acute cholangitis.

CLINICAL COURSE

Mortality among the 78 patients presenting to The Johns Hopkins Hospital with acute cholangitis was 14 percent (11 out of 78). Three of the 11 deaths were from shock, which was unresponsive following admission to the hospital. One patient died from aspiration that occurred during the initial resuscitation, one patient died from anesthetic complications, but the majority of patients, 6 out of 11, died of recurrent sepsis after their initial biliary tract surgery. In all six instances, the operating surgeon felt that the biliary tract disease had been corrected at the time of surgery. In all six patients, however, inadequate stenting of a stricture, or a retained stone led to recurrent sepsis, which eventually took the patient's life. This highlights the fact that accurate cholangiography should be performed preoperatively in all patients presenting with acute cholangitis, so that the disease can be adequately managed at the time of surgery.

The most serious complications that occur in patients with acute cholangitis are liver abscess and renal failure. Ten patients in the Hopkins series developed a liver abscess (13%), and 4 of these 10 patients (40%) died. Acute renal failure developed in 20 of the 78 patients, although in most it was mild and easily managed.

ACUTE TOXIC CHOLANGITIS

Occasional patients with acute cholangitis do not experience immediate defervescence with intravenous antibiotics and remain septic. In the past, these patients were said to have acute suppurative cholangitis. However, even though some of these patients may have gross pus in their biliary tree at the time of exploration, many others have normal-appearing, but infected, bile. Therefore, the term suppurative cholangitis is not an accurate description and these patients are better said to have acute toxic cholangitis. Within a 6-hour period, if the patient has not shown considerable improvement and is in shock, emergency biliary decompression should be performed. In the past, this has always meant an emergency operative procedure, with biliary decompression carried out via the insertion of a T-tube. More recently, however, the same biliary decompression has been accomplished without the need for anesthesia and surgery—by percutaneous transhepatic decompression. A series of 18 such patients at The Johns Hopkins Hospital was recently described. Fourteen

of the 18 patients were men, and the age range was from 48 to 98 years. The mean serum bilirubin was 12 mg per deciliter. All patients had been treated with an aminoglycoside, clindamycin, and penicillin without adequate response. All patients were treated by percutaneous transhepatic decompression. In 9 of the 18 patients, gross pus was obtained. In the remaining 9 the bile was not suppurative, but was infected. Fifteen of the 18 patients were successfully managed for a survival of 83 percent. The remaining patients did not respond and died. However, this compares favorably to the 50 percent survival obtained in the past when such patients were treated by operative decompression via a T-tube. Most patients, after being managed by percutaneous transhepatic decompression, require subsequent surgery for correction of their biliary tract disease. However, the use of percutaneous transhepatic decompression allows the patient to be stabilized so that the diagnostic evaluation and operative procedure can be managed electively.

OVERALL MANAGEMENT OF ACUTE AND ACUTE TOXIC CHOLANGITIS

All patients presenting with acute cholangitis, no matter how mild or severe, should be administered intravenous antibiotics. If the disease is mild, cefoxitin is adequate. If the patient presents with life-threatening sepsis, an aminoglycoside, clindamycin or Flagyl, and penicillin or ampicillin should be administered. Most patients respond quickly. After the sepsis has been controlled, and the patient has been covered with antibiotics for several days, percutaneous or endoscopic retrograde cholangiography should be performed to accurately delineate the biliary tree disease. Elective surgical intervention should then be carried out. In some patients with primary or recurrent common duct stones, whose gallbladder has already been removed, the disease may be correctable by endoscopic papillotomy and stone extraction without the need for surgery. In patients who have strictures at biliary enteric anastomoses, the disease may be managed effectively with percutaneous Gruntzig dilation. However, most patients require surgical intervention.

If the patient does not respond rapidly and, therefore, by definition has acute toxic cholangitis, immediate biliary decompression is required. If a catheterization laboratory is available with the expertise, this should be carried out percutaneously. If it is not available, operative intervention with T-tube insertion should be carried out. Thereafter, while the patient is receiving intravenous antibiotics, appropriate diagnostic cholangiography should be performed to accurately delineate the disease. Elective surgical correction should then be performed, unless the clinical situation allows management via endoscopic or percutaneous techniques.

BILIARY STRICTURE

LAWRENCE W. WAY, M.D.

With few exceptions, biliary strictures result from operative injuries of the common bile duct during performance of a cholecystectomy. The injuries consist of ligation, transection, or excision of a portion of the duct. If the duct is completely occluded, the patient becomes jaundiced within a few days of surgery. If the duct is open, bile ascites or a bile fistula develops.

It is often advisable to refer patients with bile duct injuries to the care of a surgeon who specializes in such problems. Except in referral centers, few surgeons acquire a large experience with these lesions, and even though the precepts of management can be found in the literature, the outcome of care in an individual case depends more on details of surgical technique than anything else, something not readily learned by reading.

The cause is failure of the surgeon to see the common duct or his mistaking it for the cystic duct or an unimportant accessory duct. A common error is to take a portion of the common duct wall after tenting it up by traction on the cystic duct. In most cases, the operation does not include a common duct exploration. Although one might think that distortion of the biliary anatomy from disease such as acute cholecystitis would be a common predisposing factor, more often the injury occurs during an elective operation. Morphologic anomalies are also uncommonly present. In fact, it is more common for the surgeon to conclude incorrectly that the ductal pattern is abnormal, which then leads to deliberate transection of the common or right hepatic duct on the assumption that it is some other structure. Many injuries could probably be avoided if operative cholangiograms were performed early whenever the anatomy is thought to be abnormal or confusing.

ACUTE INJURIES

Injuries noted by the surgeon during the operation should be repaired immediately. If the duct has been transected, it should be reanastomosed end-to-end by means of fine (e.g., 5–0 or 6–0) interrupted sutures. Every effort should be made to construct a precise watertight closure using the same exacting technique required for repairing a small blood vessel (e.g., the radial artery). A T-tube should be inserted through a separate choledochotomy above or below the site of injury.

When a segment of duct has been damaged or excised, reconstruction requires a Roux-en-Y hepaticojejunostomy. With this type of injury, a primary anastomosis between the two ends of the duct is inevitably under tension even if the duodenum is mobilized. Although an anastomosis between a small (i.e., normal) common duct and the intestine is difficult, if it is performed without haste and with fine suture material, late stricture formation is uncommon.

INJURIES RECOGNIZED IN THE POSTOPERATIVE PERIOD

The management of injuries discovered in the immediate postoperative period offers special challenges. The surgeon must set aside the natural frustration from having caused an injury and not let it affect decisions. If the signs of injury are ignored, measures may be taken that delay diagnosis and complicate treatment. In particular, the surgeon must recognize the significance of excessive bile drainage, jaundice, or cholangitis postoperatively. Two to three hundred milliliters of bile per day from drains following an elective cholecystectomy is outside the limits of what is expected in an uncomplicated case. Drainage of this magnitude should suggest either that the ligature has slipped off the cystic duct or that a rent has been made in one of the hepatic ducts or the common duct. The drains should not be removed on the theory that they may be contributing to the high output. This just converts a bile fistula into a subhepatic abscess, which eventually must be redrained. If output continues to be higher than expected for a week or so, an ERCP should be performed, which usually elucidates the problem.

Because it is less invasive than transhepatic cholangiography, ERCP is the technique of choice for investigating suspected injuries within the first few weeks of cholecystectomy. Sometimes a common duct stone is found to be responsible for the symptoms, and endoscopic sphincterotomy can be performed as treatment. If months or years have passed since the last biliary operation, and if stricture is thought to be the best explanation for the findings, transhepatic cholangiography is the preferable method of studying the duct. The advantage of THC is an ability to provide superior opacification of the ducts on the hepatic side of the lesion, information that is of great help in planning the subsequent operation.

Transhepatic Balloon Dilation

Transhepatic balloon dilation has recently come into vogue as a method of treating biliary strictures. Although it may seem to be a simple solution to an otherwise complex problem, balloon dilation is not a panacea for biliary strictures. A strategy of using dilation routinely as the first treatment and saving surgical repair for the failures may be attractive at first glance, but is unsophisticated. Dilation is time-consuming, expensive, and risky, and it has a disappointing rate of prolonged success in primary injuries of the duct as opposed to stenotic choledochoenterostomies. Balloon dilation should be reserved for patients who have had a previous repair of the duct and who either have higher than average risks for laparotomy or special factors that militate against obtaining a good result with a surgical repair. The latter include the presence of portal hypertension, recent severe subhepatic infection, and restricturing after repair by a surgeon with extensive experience in treating this condition. Using these

211

guidelines, dilation is indicated in about 10 percent of cases.

Timing of Repair

The timing of surgery after a recent operation is an important consideration. If at all possible, subhepatic infection should be eliminated, and it usually is advisable to wait for several months after draining a subhepatic abscess before intervening surgically. During this period, a biliary fistula can be managed by a catheter in the fistulous tract (or common duct), collecting the bile in a bag. Cholangitis usually can be kept under control with antibiotics. Complete or nearly complete ductal obstruction is the only compelling reason for early reoperation. Late strictures present as recurrent cholangitis or, less commonly, as painless jaundice.

Technical Considerations

The most common type of injury results in a focal stricture at or above the place where the cystic duct meets the common duct. The higher the stricture, the more difficult the operation. The success of the repair depends on the surgeon's ability to cleanly dissect out the stricture and about 1 cm of duct proximal to it. More extensive mobilization of the duct runs the risk of making it ischemic. Failures are more often due to imperfect dissection than to any other factor. Usually there is a fairly abrupt transition from the thick-walled stricture to relatively normal duct, and the stricture should be excised with the line of transection in the normal tissue. An end-to-end anastomosis is almost never appropriate in these late cases. The tissues have become firm and more fixed in position, and attempts at spanning even a short gap result in an anastomosis under tension. Roux-en-Y hepaticojejunostomy and hepaticoduodenostomy are the procedures most commonly used. It is best to begin the operation planning to perform a Roux-en-Y reconstruction, since a Roux-en-Y limb can be brought up into the liver hilum and positioned with no tension. This is not always possible with the duodenum. If, after the dissection is complete, it is seen that a hepaticoduodenostomy could be performed comfortably, this procedure is acceptable.

Following these guidelines, a majority of cases will be repaired with the Roux-en-Y technique.

The anastomosis is performed between the end of the duct and the side of the intestine. I usually use a two-layer technique, the outer layer being 4–0 or 5–0 silk and the inner layer 4–0 Dexon. The type of suture is not so important as the general principles, however. These include the necessity of using precise technique, keeping nonabsorbable suture material out of the lumen, and using fine suture material with small ducts. The second outer row of sutures does not fold the anastomosis inward as it does with an intestinal anastomosis, but brings bowel up and around the sturdier duct, inverting the duct into a short tunnel of bowel wall.

Biliary Stents

A transhepatic stent (a Silastic tube) should be placed across the anastomosis, either with the U-tube technique or with the abdominal end of the stent in the intestinal lumen. The U-tube method is really only appropriate for Roux-en-Y repairs. There has been a running debate for years regarding how long to leave the stent in place. The answer is that it depends on the quality of the repair. For the most difficult reconstructions, it should be left in place for 6 months or more, but in the average case it can be removed in a month or two. Remember, stents are never used for easy biliary anastomoses when the duct is dilated (e.g., during a Whipple procedure). In other words, there is nothing about biliary anastomoses per se that mandates prolonged stenting.

Results

The results are excellent in 90 percent of cases. The ease of operation, which can usually be predicted from findings on the preoperative cholangiograms, correlates with the outcome. Whenever there is 1 cm or more of dilated common hepatic duct above the stricture, surgery should be curative. Strictures involving the bifurcation of the common hepatic duct are more challenging and the results less predictable. Seventy percent and 95 percent of recurrences are clinically manifest within 2 and 7 years of surgery, respectively.

POSTCHOLECYSTECTOMY SYNDROME

JEREMY N. THOMPSON, M.A., F.R.C.S.
LESLIE H. BLUMGART, B.D.S., M.D., F.R.C.S.

Following cholecystectomy, at least 5 percent of patients suffer from significant persistent or recurrent

symptoms which require further careful assessment. These patients, in particular those with upper abdominal pain, are said to have the "postcholecystectomy syndrome." This is an inappropriate name for a heterogenous group of conditions (Table 1), many of which are well understood while others still lack clear pathophysiologic definition. The surgical management may be straightforward, but is frequently difficult and time consuming.

We make no apology, even in a book devoted to surgical therapy, for describing in some detail the

TABLE 1 Possible Causes of the Postcholecystectomy Syndrome

Primary biliary causes
  Choledocholithiasis
  Gallstone-related pancreatitis
  Periampullary or bile duct tumors
  Papillary stenosis
  Inflammatory bile duct stricture
  Cystic duct problems
  ?"Biliary dyskinesia"

Postsurgical causes
  Bile duct stricture
  Choledochoduodenal fistula
  Papillary stenosis
  Intra-abdominal adhesions
  Wound neuroma
  Incisional hernia

Other causes
  Pancreatitis
  Peptic ulceration
  Esophagitis
  Irritable bowel syndrome
  Diverticular disease of colon
  Ischemic heart disease
  Spinal disorders

assessment and investigation of these patients. As in many other surgical conditions, an accurate diagnosis is an essential prerequisite to successful management. Laparotomy without such a preoperative diagnosis is destined to give disappointing results.

ASSESSMENT AND INVESTIGATION

Patients with continuing problems after cholecystectomy present a wide spectrum of symptom severity which will influence the extent of investigation considered necessary in any particular case. However, abnormalities of initial biochemistry or noninvasive investigations (e.g., ultrasound scanning, plain abdominal films) may prompt further assessment of patients with relatively minor symptoms. Routine assessment includes a full history with particular attention to the relationship of current symptoms to the previous surgery. In our experience, the most common presentation is with symptoms unchanged by previous cholecystectomy, suggesting either previously unrecognized biliary tract disease or a nonbiliary condition. New symptoms appearing immediately after cholecystectomy point to an iatrogenic cause, although some postsurgical complications only become symptomatic many months or even years after operation. The timing, location, and nature of the upper abdominal symptoms may suggest causes other than biliary tract disease, but a history of jaundice, pruritus, or rigors is a strong indication of further biliary problems. Our experience is somewhat selected, reflecting largely cases referred to a specialist Hepatobiliary Surgical Unit. The predominant referral problem in a consecutive series of 151 of our cases is shown in Table 2. The previous medical history and present medication (especially analgesic) requirements may give useful guides to the severity of the symptoms and to possible nonbiliary causes. Although some patients may seem anxious and neurotic, it is often difficult to know whether this is primarily the cause of their symptoms or secondary to unidentified continuing organic problems. It is unwise to let such factors unduly influence the assessment of these cases. A full physical examination is also important, although it is not often helpful. A careful examination must be made of the wound for evidence of an incisional hernia or localized area of tenderness suggesting a neuroma, and the lumbar region for evidence of spinal disease.

A careful scrutiny of previous patient records, operation reports, x-ray films including operative and T-tube cholangiograms, other investigations, and pathologic specimens is essential and occasionally leads to a previously unsuspected diagnosis. Multiple small gallstones, or previous ductal exploration in the absence of good postexploratory cholangiography or complete choledochoscopy, suggests the possibility of retained ductal calculi. Nonabsorbable sutures in the biliary tract occasionally act as the nidus for stone formation. A history of difficulty in removing distal bile duct stones or passing rigid instruments through the papilla, or a transduodenal transpapillary ductal exploration, leads us to suspect iatrogenic damage to the lower common duct or papilla. Failure to perform an operative cholangiogram, which gives useful anatomic information may have led to bile duct injury or retained ductal calculi. A history of intraoperative hemorrhage or postoperative peritoneal biliary drainage strongly suggests bile duct injury and stricture. The report of biliary tract, ampullary, or pancreatic disease at previous operation may be helpful, although they sometimes pass unnoticed at cholecystectomy. A cause of symptoms is less commonly identified following cholecystectomy at which no gallstones were found than in those patients with original calculous disease.

Routine hematologic investigations, including liver function tests and serum amylase, plain abdominal films, and an ultrasound scan of the liver, bile ducts, and pancreas are the usual initial investigations on our unit. CT scanning of the upper abdomen occasionally adds additional information, particularly with respect to pancreatic disease, but does not form part of our routine work-up. Whether or not these initial investigations have

TABLE 2 Presenting Complaints of Patients with Postcholecystectomy Syndrome

Predominant Problem on Referral	Number of Patients	%
Pain similar to that present before cholecystectomy	57	36
Episode of jaundice	57	36
New pain thought to be biliary on clinical grounds	26	17
Pain with elevated amylase	14	9
Other	3	2
Total	157	100

revealed abnormalities suggestive of biliary tract or pancreatic disease, we usually go on to perform endoscopic retrograde cholangiopancreatography (ERCP), which is the most valuable investigation in the assessment of this group of patients. Even with solid ultrasound or cholangiographic evidence of common bile duct calculi, we always perform preoperative duodenoscopy to carefully examine the papilla because on several occasions we have seen ductal calculi related to bile stasis and infection caused by unsuspected periampullary tumors. Thorough inspection of the upper gastrointestinal tract to exclude peptic ulceration or other disease is an essential part of endoscopic assessment, although the finding of such an abnormality should not prevent the imaging of both bile and pancreatic ducts as concurrent disease may occur. A careful inspection is made to identify any previous operative damage including the presence of a choledocho-duodenal fistula and stenosis of the papilla or previous surgical biliary-enteric anastomosis. Biopsies and cytology specimens are taken when there is suspicion of a periampullary, bile duct, or pancreatic tumor. In all patients an attempt is made to outline both biliary and pancreatic systems, even if an obvious abnormality is seen in the first duct cannulated. The diagnostic yield from endoscopy and ERCP is very high when there is a history of jaundice, cholangitis, or pancreatitis. The results in other patients, especially those with symptoms unchanged by cholecystectomy, are less helpful. The majority of symptomatic postcholecystectomy patients in our series of over 200 cases have been found to have abnormalities within the biliary or pancreatic ductal apparatus. Residual bile duct calculi, unrecognized pancreatic disease, and bile duct strictures were the more common causes found, whereas papillary or bile duct tumors and choledocho-duodenal fistulas accounted for most of the remaining abnormalities. Occasionally, failure to cannulate the bile ducts at ERCP necessitates fine-needle percutaneous transhepatic cholangiography, particularly if symptoms are troublesome.

TREATMENT OF BILIARY TRACT DISEASE

Bile Duct Stones

There seems little doubt that ductal stones should be removed even when they are not causing symptoms because of the risk of serious complications, although some patients may harbor calculi for years without any problems and the overall natural history is not well documented. Percutaneous stone extraction via a T-tube tract is the treatment of choice if bile duct stones are seen on postoperative T-tube cholangiography, but this is usually not an option in these patients. Medical therapy has little to offer at present, and the therapeutic choice for residual bile duct calculi therefore usually lies between endoscopic sphincterotomy followed by stone extraction and surgical re-exploration of the biliary tract. Endoscopic sphincterotomy and complete clearance of ductal stones

is achieved in about 85 percent of cases in expert hands, with a morbidity of 8 to 10 percent and a mortality of approximately 1 percent. Success rates for stones larger than 2 cm in diameter are much lower. Reported series contain a substantial proportion of patients who are considered to be high operative risks, and thus are not directly comparable with most surgical series. Because endoscopic techniques have only been used in recent years, limited follow-up data are available. The incidence of recurrent stones and papillary stenosis ranges from 5 to 10 percent in most of the recent endoscopic series, but may be expected to increase steadily with further follow-up. Although the results of surgical duct clearance at initial exploration are probably better, the results of surgical re-exploration are more comparable with endoscopy. The mortality and morbidity for surgical re-exploration of the biliary tract are comparable with those for endoscopic techniques in most patients, and it is our current practice to reserve endoscopic sphincterotomy for elderly and unfit patients who are regarded as high surgical risks (Table 3). In other patients we usually perform a re-exploration via a supraduodenal choledochotomy and avoid unnecessary instrumentation at the papilla. Both pre-exploratory cholangiography (either as ERCP or via a needle into the common bile duct at surgery) and a postexploratory study or choledochoscopy are essential aids to complete bile duct clearance. For postexploratory cholangiography, we use two small pediatric urinary catheters, one positioned with the balloon above and the other with the balloon below the choledochotomy, and usually combine this with choledochoscopy. By the careful use of these techniques, the incidence of retained bile duct calculi has been reduced to a low level. The occasional older patient who has a large (more than 15 mm in diameter) duct containing multiple friable stones is a candidate for side-to-side choledochoduodenostomy, which gives good results provided the anastomosis is at least 2 cm in length. Care must be taken to ensure that the common bile duct is used for anastomosis; we have seen two patients with recurrent symptoms following anastomosis of a large tortuous cystic duct remnant to the duodenum. A transduodenal exploration, which carries a higher operative morbidity and mortality, is occasionally necessary for impacted distal common bile duct stones. When this is performed, we use a sphincteroplasty technique with mucosa-to-mucosa

TABLE 3 Treatment of Postcholecystectomy Choledocholithiasis

Method	Indications
Supraduodenal surgical re-exploration	Treatment of choice except as below
Choledochoduodenostomy	Older patients with large duct and multiple friable stones
Transduodenal surgical re-exploration	Impacted distal bile duct stone which cannot be removed easily via choledochotomy
Endoscopic sphincterotomy and stone extraction	Elderly and infirm patients

suturing of the bile duct to the duodenum in an attempt to reduce the incidence of late papillary stenosis, which is a further hazard of this approach.

Bile Duct Stricture

The surgical treatment of benign bile duct strictures is covered elsewhere is this book, and so we shall not describe our approach in detail. Suffice it to say that our experience with over 100 postcholecystectomy strictures suggests that a direct mucosa-to-mucosa hepaticojejunostomy Roux-en-Y is nearly always possible and gives very good results, provided longstanding biliary tract obstruction has not already produced irreversible hepatic damage. Endoscopic or percutaneous dilation of benign postcholecystectomy bile duct strictures occasionally proves helpful in high-risk patients (e.g., those with portal hypertension) or in the management of some carefully selected failures of surgical treatment. However, caution should be adopted in the use of these techniques as incomplete relief of obstruction may improve symptoms, but allow continued chronic infection and progressive liver fibrosis.

Tumors

Periampullary or bile duct tumors occasionally present following cholecystectomy and are managed in the same way as lesions presenting primarily. Accurate preoperative staging is performed, including complete cholangiography and angiography. We then proceed to appropriate resectional or palliative surgery. In patients who are at high surgical risk, especially those with unresectable lesions, we sometimes make use of endoscopic sphincterotomy for periampullary lesions or percutaneously inserted endoprosthetic stents for bile duct tumors.

Other Biliary Disease

Occasionally, stones within a cystic duct remnant may cause symptoms and necessitate surgical re-exploration. Such stones may even migrate into the common duct and cause intermittent biliary tract obstruction. However, we have not had occasion to reoperate solely for an uncomplicated cystic duct remnant. Sphincter of Oddi incompetence following surgery or endoscopic sphincterotomy usually leads to duodenobiliary reflux and bile infection. Although most patients remain asymptomatic, common duct debris may accummulate and cause recurrent pancreatitis or cholangitis. In such patients, choledochojejunostomy with a long (70 cm) Roux loop reduces the incidence of ascending infection and reflux. Although we have performed biliary-enteric bypass to the common duct for papillary stenosis secondary to choledocholithiasis or previous surgery, we have not seen a patient with primary papillary stenosis.

TREATMENT OF NONBILIARY DISEASE

When diseases outside the biliary tree are identified, they are treated medically or surgically on their own merits. Wound problems may be responsible for postcholecystectomy symptoms. Incisional hernia requires surgical repair. When a patient has an area of localized wound tenderness, probably related to neuroma formation, without any other detectable abnormality, we attempt subcostal local anesthetic injection in the region of the related intercostal nerves. If such an injection repeatedly improves symptoms, we proceed to permanent nerve block. Intra-abdominal adhesions are almost uniformly present following cholecystectomy, but are only occasionally the cause of persistent postoperative symptoms. However, in the absence of any other cause found on investigation, a history suggestive of small bowel colic, especially when supported by an area of localized tenderness close to the wound or radiologic evidence of partial intestinal obstruction, is sufficient to justify reoperation for division of adhesions.

Patients with pancreatitis following cholecystectomy require very careful assessment to exclude residual biliary ductal stones or operative injury to the papillary region, particularly in the absence of excessive alcohol intake or other causal factors, although in some cases the gallstones may have been incidental to a presenting episode of pancreatitis. Peptic ulceration, esophagitis, irritable bowel syndrome, and other extrabiliary conditions are usually managed medically in the first instance and only occasionally require specific surgery.

PATIENTS WITH NO IDENTIFIED CAUSE

A thorough assessment of these patients leaves a significant proportion in whom no organic cause can be found. These patients have long been the subject of surgical study, and a variety of pharmacologic provocation tests have been used to justify surgical or endoscopic procedures, particularly on the sphincter of Oddi. The large placebo effect that may be observed in this group makes careful interpretation of reported results mandatory and the use of double-blind studies highly desirable. A few centers are now reporting encouraging results using endoscopic manometric pressure studies of the sphincter of Oddi, or ultrasound measurement of pancreatic duct dilatation in response to secretin as indicators of the symptomatic response to subsequent endoscopic sphincterotomy or surgical sphincteroplasty. Although these results are encouraging, and may represent important advances in the pathophysiologic understanding of this relatively small group of patients, they require further validation before being widely adopted. We have no personal experience of these techniques and at present avoid intervention, preferring simple symptomatic and supportive therapy whenever possible. There is, in our opinion, little place for exploratory laparotomy.

BILIARY CYSTS: CHOLEDOCHAL CYST AND CAROLI'S DISEASE

L. WILLIAM TRAVERSO, M.D., F.A.C.S.

When a patient with the biliary tract symptoms of obstructive jaundice and/or cholangitis is evaluated, cysts of the extrahepatic and intrahepatic biliary tract should be considered. Preoperative diagnosis of biliary cyst is more frequent today because of ultrasonography, computed tomography, and preoperative cholangiography. The preoperative diagnosis of biliary cyst, knowledge of the anatomy, and improved operative techniques have combined to greatly decrease the surgical morbidity and mortality of this disease. The preferred operative management has evolved toward cyst resection rather than internal drainage because of an improved understanding of the etiology and pathogenesis of the cyst. This discussion considers only macroscopic bile duct cysts and not microcystic liver disease (congenital hepatic fibrosis), simple liver cysts, polycystic disease, or echinococcal cysts.

Extrahepatic biliary tract cysts are termed choledochal cysts. The abnormality characterized by intrahepatic biliary tract cysts is termed Caroli's disease. When both intrahepatic and extrahepatic biliary cysts occur in the same patient, the combined abnormality is still designated Caroli's disease.

ANATOMIC CLASSIFICATION

Based on the original description of biliary cysts by Alonso-Lej, five anatomic types have been identified, each of which has been subdivided by various authors into many more types. However, the only anatomic distinction used for treatment decisions is the location of the cyst, whether intra- or extrahepatic. If all biliary cysts were considered together, 50 percent would be totally extrahepatic, whereas only 10 percent would be totally intrahepatic. The remaining 40 percent would be combined extrahepatic and intrahepatic cysts. Although choledochal cysts were believed to be the most common cyst of the biliary tract, the incidence of Caroli's disease (intrahepatic cyst) combined with a choledochal cyst in the same patient also appears to be a common disorder.

For completeness and reference to published reports, the anatomic classification is summarized here. The type I cyst is a choledochal cyst. Type II is a congenital choledochal diverticulum, a rare disorder. Type III is a terminal common bile duct choledochocele, another rare disorder. Type IV is a combined extrahepatic choledochal cyst with some form of intrahepatic Caroli's disease. Type V is solely intrahepatic cystic disease. Types I, IV, and V are the common disorders and are really just varieties of extrahepatic, intrahepatic, or combined cystic disease. The treatment for all types is surgery. My principles of surgical therapy for types I, IV, and V (to be discussed) are derived from the natural history and the anatomy of the disease. Type II cysts are excised by applying the principles of cholecystectomy. Type III cysts have been treated successfully by endoscopic papillotomy.

RATIONALE FOR CURRENT SURGICAL TREATMENT

Historically, treatment of the extrahepatic choledochal cyst has been internal drainage by a cyst-to-enteric anastomosis. The results from this experience favor resection because (1) an unacceptable incidence of complications follows internal drainage, (2) an increased risk for the development of bile duct carcinoma occurs with an unresected cyst, and (3) an abnormality of the pancreaticobiliary duct associated with biliary cysts favors resection.

Various internal drainage methods for choledochal cysts have resulted in a 34 to 58 percent reported incidence of one of the following complications: anastomotic stricture, biliary stasis and stones, recurrent cholangitis, and acute pancreatitis. In addition, various reports have indicated that carcinoma of the bile duct is 20 to 100 times more frequent in patients with biliary cysts than would be expected in the general population. In fact, an increased risk of developing carcinoma in a portion of the biliary tract below the choledochal cyst has been noted. An intriguing observation and a clue to the etiology of the disease is found when only intrahepatic biliary cysts are present and an extrahepatic bile duct carcinoma develops. It appears that the etiology for carcinoma may be arising from, or passing into, the extrahepatic biliary tree. To further emphasize this point, when both intrahepatic and extrahepatic cysts are present in the same patient, 60 percent of bile duct carcinomas develop in the extrahepatic tree. If all cases of bile duct carcinoma developing in patients with biliary cysts are examined, 80 percent of the carcinomas occur in the extrahepatic biliary tree. In addition, an intrahepatic carcinoma has not been observed in the absence of intrahepatic cystic disease.

With the advent of endoscopic cholangiography and pancreatography plus transhepatic cholangiography, a particular abnormality of the biliary tree was noted to be more frequent in patients with biliary cysts, namely, an anomalous junction of the bile duct to the pancreatic duct (Fig. 1). The pancreatic duct and bile duct joined inside the pancreas, outside of the duodenum and control of the sphincter of Oddi. This arrangement resulted in a long common channel, and because of the lack of sphincter control, the possibility of reflux of pancreatic juice into the bile duct existed. In addition, reflux in the opposite direction was also possible, and explained why a small percentage of biliary cyst patients presented not with symptoms of biliary tract obstruction but rather with acute pancreatitis. In several small series, this anomalous

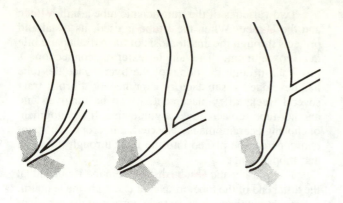

Figure 1 Schematic views of the pancreaticobiliary junction. From left to right: normal, common bile duct enters the side of the pancreatic duct, and pancreatic duct enters the side of the common bile duct. The latter two anomalous arrangements are associated with biliary cysts in 90 percent of cases in which the distal biliary tree was visualized by contrast studies. Shaded area represents wall of duodenum.

junction has been noted in 30 to 60 percent of patients with choledochal cysts. In a choledochal cyst survey, now completed in Japan, this anomalous junction was found in 90 percent of 457 patients who had a thorough examination of the biliary and pancreatic ducts during treatment for biliary cysts (information courtesy Professor Komi, Tokushima, Japan; in press, Surgical Gastroenterology). In addition, amylase has been found to be elevated in choledochal cyst bile of over one-fourth of these patients. Several studies of this anomalous junction in choledochal cyst patients have shown that pressure in the pancreatic duct is higher than in the bile duct during biliary manometry. It seems clear that *the reflux of pancreatic juice and the combination of bile and pancreatic enzymes could destroy portions of the biliary tree.* The observation that biliary cysts are more common in the extrahepatic biliary tree increases the credibility of this hypothesis. It also seems reasonable to extrapolate that internal drainage of a cyst would not interrupt this reflux mechanism and would lead to the complications observed after internal drainage, i.e., anastomotic stricture, biliary stasis and stones, recurrent cholangitis, and pancreatitis. It does not seem unreasonable to implicate the chronic inflammatory process as a predecessor for carcinoma of the bile duct, which, as discussed previously, is also more common in the distal portions of the biliary tree. The etiology of carcinoma could be related to the presence of pancreatic enzymes in the extrahepatic biliary tree. This possibility would favor the consideration of disconnecting the biliary tree from its normal pathway into the duodenum. Excision of a cyst accomplishes this goal while removing tissue at risk for carcinoma. It is not clear if the cyst would remain at risk for carcinoma if the flow of bile were diverted from the cyst while the cyst remained in place. The hypothesis concerning reflux of pancreatic juice would suggest that disconnecting the biliary tree from the cyst would interrupt the *formation* of biliary cysts, however.

SURGICAL OPTIONS: EXTRAHEPATIC CYSTS

For the foregoing reasons, excision is the treatment of choice for cysts of the extrahepatic biliary tract. In the largest reported series of biliary cyst patients, by Flanigan (955 cases), the operative mortality from internal drainage during the three decades after World War II appeared to be much lower than that of excision. Therefore a large experience with drainage was obtained. When the results of various internal drainage procedures were compared, the specific drainage procedure of Roux-en-Y choledochocystojejunostomy appeared to have the lowest incidence of perioperative morbidity and mortality and the lowest reoperation rate. The success of this best of internal drainage procedures was still low, with rates of 18 percent morbidity and 17 percent mortality. The reoperation rate was 13 percent. This was compared to the results of choledochocystoduodenostomy—55 percent morbidity and 38 percent reoperation. It seems clear that if an excision procedure is not possible because of pericholedochal cyst inflammation or the patient's condition, a Roux-en-Y choledochocystojejunostomy is the internal drainage procedure of choice. An alternative compromise would be to disconnect the biliary tree from the cyst, construct a choledochojejunostomy, and then marsupialize the cyst and oversew the distal biliary connection. This procedure would interrupt the pathogenetic mechanism, as described previously, and prevent complications of internal drainage of the cyst. Choledochal cyst tissue at risk for carcinoma would remain, but this may not be significant once the chronic inflammatory process is interrupted.

Lilly reported a modified choledochal cyst excision technique, which left a portion of the posterior cyst wall on the portal vein and hepatic artery, thereby decreasing the potential for major vascular complications. This dissection through a plane of the posterior cyst wall allowed resection of the entire choledochal cyst mucosa as well as the majority of the choledochal cyst wall. Lilly's technique reduced mortality rate for cyst removal from as high as 40 percent to less than 5 percent. In the first 83 cases reported for the Lilly excision technique, the morbidity was 8 percent, and the reoperation rate was 0 percent. Reasons for using the excision technique are (1) to remove the tissue at risk for carcinoma and (2) to disconnect the biliary tract from the pancreatic duct, thereby breaking the proposed vicious cycle of pancreatic juice reflux. Frequently the extrahepatic choledochal cyst extends down into the pancreas. After removal of as much cyst as possible, the remaining cyst should be oversewn. There are no reported cases of bile duct carcinoma developing in an oversewn remnant of choledochal cyst, probably because the flow of bile has been interrupted through this remaining portion of the distal common bile duct that still is exposed to pancreatic juice. Since choledochal cysts are diagnosed at an earlier stage today, a larger number of patients can have the entire cyst removed without using the Lilly technique because chronic inflammation and fibrosis are less extensive than in the patients of the past several decades. This has been the impression from several medical centers with choledochal cyst experience.

SURGICAL OPTIONS: INTRAHEPATIC CYSTS

Excision is the treatment of choice for extrahepatic cystic disease. When Caroli's disease is present, it is not commonly found unilaterally. This unfortunate situation does not allow for the hepatic resection that would totally remove the cysts, applying the same principles as those applied to an extrahepatic cyst. There are only 15 reported cases of hepatic lobe resection for unilateral Caroli's disease. The cystic dilatations have been in the left lobe in all of these patients. This limited resection experience has been associated with remission in 87 percent of these patients. The results of unilateral hepatic cyst treatment are in contrast to the treatment results for the typical Caroli's disease patient with bilateral intrahepatic cysts. Patients with this more common form of the disease present with life-threatening cholangitis and intrahepatic abscesses. A palliative drainage procedure is advisable. Ultimately the disease progresses to biliary cirrhosis, portal hypertension, and death from gastrointestinal hemorrhage or hepatic failure. The surgical objective is intrahepatic bile drainage of as much liver tissue as possible. While the prognosis and life expectancy of these patients is grim, recent successes in a limited number of patients indicate that placement of transhepatic U- or J-tubes may be helpful.

Bile stasis is associated with any biliary cyst. Chronic inflammation promotes cyst outlet narrowing and results in a vicious cycle of more stasis, stones, and cholangitis. The goal of transhepatic intubation is to bypass internally as many as possible of the anatomical or functional obstructions that occur along the major intrahepatic ducts.

The transhepatic tube courses through the right or left hepatic duct, up through the dome of the liver; then the tube passes into the peritoneal cavity, down over the dome of the liver to below the costal margin, and is brought out through the skin (Fig. 2). The tube is pulled into position after choledochotomy. A No. 3 Bakes dilator is passed to the end of the right or left hepatic duct and then pushed through the liver parenchyma to exit the liver dome anterior to the diaphragmatic attachments. A large silk suture is tied to the dilator and pulled through the liver and out the choledochotomy. The transhepatic tube is then tied to either end of the suture and pulled into position. The distal end of the transhepatic tube passes out of the liver through the common hepatic duct or distal edge of extrahepatic bile duct resection (if an extrahepatic chole- dochal cyst has been removed in the combination type of disease). The lumen of the tube provides drainage of bile through cyst outlet obstructions via an extensive number of fenestrations in the tube. Only the intubated cysts are drained, while cysts in the secondary and tertiary bile ducts that are not directly drained continue to develop biliary stasis and stones. These develop around the tube as well. Daily irrigation with saline is necessary. Frequently drainage is not totally effective, but the tube can be adjusted or changed under fluoroscopy until adequate drainage is obtained. Persistent attention to tube drainage has been beneficial in cases in which the intrahepatic bile stasis and infection have been previously uncontrollable.

Two varieties of the transhepatic tube are the J-tube and the U-tube. When the J-tube is used, its distal end projects through the anastomosis of the extrahepatic bile duct to jejunum. The single exterior connection is proximal through the dome of the liver. Once the tube has developed a satisfactory suprahepatic fibrous tract several weeks after placement, it can be removed and another tube replaced over a guidewire. If development of cholangiocarcinoma is suspected, a fiberoptic choledo- choscope can be placed into the liver through this tract and biopsies taken.

The transhepatic U-tube differs from the J-tube in that the distal end of the tube, instead of ending in the jejunum, is brought out through the enteric portion of the hepatico- jejunostomy and then through the abdominal wall. The two ends of the U-tube are exteriorized on the patient's abdomen. The U-tube was the first devised transhepatic conduit and could be easily changed by attaching a new tube to the indwelling tube. As the old tube was removed, the new tube was pulled into position. This was the initial reason for using the U-tube, but now that it has been determined that the J-tube can be easily replaced over a guidewire, the U-tube is being used less frequently, allowing the patient to have only one tube exteriorized per transhepatic tube placed.

As much of the intrahepatic biliary tract as possible should be drained with transhepatic tubes. This usually requires two tubes, but on occasion three or four tubes may be necessary. Since multiple tubes exit into the extra- hepatic biliary tree, consideration must be given to avoid- ing an iatrogenic extrahepatic obstruction. The normal extrahepatic bile duct can become mechanically obstructed

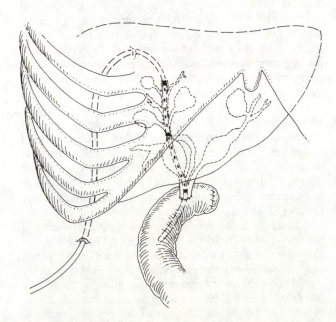

Figure 2 Schematic view of the transhepatic J-tube. The multiple fenestrations are placed to allow bile drainage inside the tube and bypass strictures or stones. Use of the three radiographic markers outlines the section of the tube with fenestrations.

by multiple tubes, and bile flow in this area is dependent on patent tube lumens. Daily irrigation is mandatory. If saline is not available, the patient can temporize with tap water.

The length of this extrahepatic area of intubated and normal bile duct is usually short because a choledochal cyst has been excised and a choledochoenteric anastomosis was constructed. However, a normal extrahepatic bile duct is present with Caroli's disease in 10 percent of biliary cyst cases. Placement of multiple transhepatic J-tubes results in the distal tubes ending in the extrahepatic bile duct. This portion of the tube should be cut as short as possible. Placement of transhepatic U-tubes without choledochoenteric anastomosis requires a tube exit site from the common hepatic duct below the holes of the U-tube. These tubes need to be changed frequently. In my experience, a small amount of bile surrounds the tubes in the extrahepatic bile duct and forms stones and sludge that lodge at the bile duct exit site. Bile preferentially follows the tube lumens and does not enter the duodenum. The solution is to prevent this mechanical obstruction and return bile to the intestine by constructing a choledocho-jejunostomy whenever a U-tube is placed.

The transhepatic tube is manufactured on a custom-order basis by the Mentor Corporation, Goleta, California. A circle nephrostomy tube made of silicone rubber was modified to produce the characteristics of the tube necessary for transhepatic use. The length of the tubing was increased to 100 cm, and the silicone rubber wall was thickened to allow for circumferential external attachment sutures without collapsing the tube. The commerical product is available in sizes 12, 16, and 20 F, but we prefer the smaller tubes, especially when placing multiple tubes.

Multiple fenestrations have been placed 4.5 cm above and below a central circular radiopaque marker to provide the most drainage holes possible without weakening the tube. The diameter of the fenestrations is 3 mm, and the perforations are placed 5 mm apart throughout the 9-cm segment of fenestrated tube. Radiographic markers are also placed at each end of the fenestrations. To ensure intubation of as many cysts as possible, the tube is pulled out of the liver dome until the top marker is observed and then replaced several centimeters back into the liver.

Since a tract forms slowly around the silicone rubber tube and bile may leak around the hepatic dome exit site of the catheter, adequate drainage of the suprahepatic space and the anastomotic site for at least one week is recommended. The drains can be removed when a transhepatic cholangiogram reveals no extravasation along the tube. Irrigation of the transhepatic tube should begin on the first postoperative day, and if the supra- and subhepatic areas have been well drained, the incidence of abscess formation should not increase. Chronic oral antibiotic administration is necessary for several months after transhepatic tube placement. Trimethoprim (80 mg) and sulfamethoxazole (400 mg) taken twice per day are helpful.

Occasionally the surgeon finds need for a transhepatic tube during an intraoperative biliary tract exploration for biliary cystic disease or bifurcation carcinomas. The transhepatic tube just described may not be available. However, an alternative transhepatic tube provides good temporary results. A red rubber 16 F nasogastric tube can be placed, and the commerical silicone rubber tube can then be ordered. To use the latex tube, several holes are cut in it intraoperatively. Care is taken not to weaken the tube, as it must be removed in the postoperative period. The tube is exteriorized as described for the standard transhepatic tube. The latex of a nasogastric tube stimulates a greater reaction than silicone rubber, and therefore the fibrous tract from the dome of the liver to the abdominal wall is formed faster. Three weeks later, using a guidewire and fluoroscopic control, the surgeon can substitute the silicone rubber tube for the latex tube through the well-developed fibrous tract.

GALLSTONE ILEUS

GEORGE L. NARDI, M.D.

Gallstone ileus is a form of small bowel obstruction that results from the passage of a biliary calculus through a bilio-enteric fistula into the intestine. It accounts for approximately 2 percent of all mechanical intestinal obstruction.

ETIOLOGY

Biliary fistulas may be external (cutaneous) or internal. There are numerous causes for such fistulas, but those involved with gallstone ileus are internal fistulas, over 80 percent of which result from long-standing cholecystitis. The chronically inflamed gallbladder becomes adherent to an adjacent viscus, and a fistula results secondary to pressure and erosion by the contained calculi.

The most common fistula of this type is cholecysto-duodenal. The next most frequent are cholecystocolic and choledochoduodenal; in the latter, peptic ulceration may play a role.

SYMPTOMS

This condition is most frequently seen in obese elderly women without a history of previous biliary disease.

Presenting symptoms are those of mechanical obstruction. Careful inquiry may reveal intermittent bouts of obstruction as passage of the stone down the intestine occurs. Eventually, if the stone is not passed, complete obstruction, requiring surgical relief, occurs.

DIAGNOSIS

Gallstone ileus should be suspected in an older woman with small bowel obstruction who gives a history of previous biliary colic.

Abdominal films may reveal not only the typically dilated loops of small bowel, but the obstructing calculus as well. This occurs when the stone contains calcium. If the stone is not opaque, it may sometimes be identified by a halo of surrounding air. Gallstones may also be identified in the gallbladder.

A careful scrutiny for air in the biliary tree should be made. This is pathognomonic.

TREATMENT

Immediate surgery is indicated after the patient's condition has been stabilized and antibiotic therapy initiated.

A vertical right-sided incision usually allows the best access for examination of the biliary tract and extraction of the stone, which is usually in the ileum.

The gallbladder should be quickly evaluated to confirm the presence of gallstones and the nature of the fistula.

Attention should then be directed to the small bowel, carefully inspecting and palpating it throughout its length to avoid missing multiple calculi and to locate the offending calculus, which is usually single.

When the impacted stone is identified, it should be gently milked upward into a segment of intestine that has not been compressed and removed through a longitudinal incision on the antimesenteric border. The bowel is closed in conventional fashion and care is taken to avoid narrowing the lumen.

On rare occasions the stone may be firmly impacted and cannot be dislodged. Under these circumstances, it may be safer to perform a limited resection of the bowel containing the stone rather than cutting through compromised bowel over the stone.

In poor-risk or elderly patients, nothing more need be done, and despite residual biliary disease, recurrent episodes are unusual. However, in younger, good-risk patients, correction of the primary biliary disease can be undertaken. This should be particularly considered if there is evidence of choledocholithiasis or if the patient gave a history of biliary colic or cholangitis.

The gallbladder should be mobilized, the fistula identified and divided, and the intestinal defect sutured. A cholecystectomy is then performed and the common duct explored if indicated.

SCLEROSING CHOLANGITIS

KENNETH W. WARREN, M.D., F.A.C.S.

Sclerosing cholangitis is an uncommon disease of unknown etiology. It represents a special pathologic reaction of the biliary tract in which marked narrowing of the lumen is caused by intense subepithelial fibrosis. Usually, the entire extrahepatic biliary tree and almost the whole intrahepatic biliary tree become involved. Not uncommonly, the process is limited to only a section of the biliary system. As a result of progressive sclerosis of the bile ducts, patients with sclerosing cholangitis run the gamut of progressive biliary obstruction and its sinister sequelae.

It is recognized that localized stenosis can occur. The operative findings in a series of patients reported by me indicated the varied anatomic distribution of this bizarre disease (Table 1). These anatomic variations have a decisive impact on the choice of a surgical procedure (to be discussed). Jaundice and pruritus are the most common clinical features, but abdominal pain, fever, and weight loss also occur. The clinical features in 84 patients are summarized in Table 2.

Although the cause of sclerosing cholangitis is unknown, its frequent association with chronic ulcerative colitis and, less frequently, with Crohn's disease, chronic thyroiditis, and retroperitoneal fibrosis cannot be ignored.

CHOLANGIOGRAPHY

Today, endoscopic retrograde cholangiography is the safest and most reliable preoperative documentation of the presumptive diagnosis of sclerosing cholangitis. This test,

TABLE 1 Operative Findings in 84 Patients with Sclerosing Cholangitis

Area Involved	Number
Total involvement of biliary tract	45
Involvement of region of ductal bifurcation	22
Diffuse involvement of extrahepatic ducts only	5
Distal common bile duct only	5
Diffuse involvement of intrahepatic ducts only	4
Others	3

TABLE 2 Clinical Manifestations in 84 Patients with Sclerosing Cholangitis

	Number of Patients	Percentage of Series
Clinical features		
Jaundice	78	93
Pain	58	69
Weight loss	53	63
Anorexia and malaise	50	59
Chills and fever	42	50
Pruritus	41	48
Nausea and vomiting	40	45
Colitis	27	32
Physical findings		
Jaundice	48	57
Liver enlargement	37	44
Local tenderness	29	34
Ileostomy	5	6

however, while valuable, does not differentiate sclerosing cholangitis from sclerosing carcinoma of the bile ducts. If endoscopic retrograde cholangiography is not successful, operative cholangiography is imperative.

Cameron studied the cholangiograms of 36 patients with sclerosing cholangitis and found the hepatic duct bifurcation to be the most severely affected area in 24 of 36 patients. He emphasized that proximal ductal dilatation above the stricture may not occur in this disease, and the significance of the obstruction at the hepatic duct bifurcation might not be appreciated in the selection of an appropriate operation.

TREATMENT

Medical Treatment

No effective medical treatment for sclerosing choledochitis exists. Attempts at medical management have emphasized corticosteroids and antibiotics. Choleretics, cholestyramine, azathioprine, and penicillamine have been tried. If any one or a combination of these medications were effective in the treatment of this disease, I would not be writing this chapter.

Unfortunately, the varied surgical procedures employed in the management of this disease are far from satisfactory.

Surgical Procedures

Surgical progress, in almost any anatomic area, is a halting, unsteady, unpredictable climb, frequently frustratingly slow and never achieving the aspirations or ambitions of the pioneers who strive to conquer the difficult or the impossible. Sclerosing cholangitis is such a challenge.

Early Surgical Experience. Forty years ago, before endoscopic retrograde cholangiopancreatography

or percutaneous transhepatic cholangiography (because of the small caliber of the intrahepatic ducts, the latter procedure usually is not applicable to the diagnosis of sclerosing cholangitis), the diagnosis and the delineation of the ductal anatomy in sclerosing choledochitis were made only at operation.

The choice of the incision was less important than its dimensions. Since at least 85 percent of patients had had a previous operation on the biliary tract, I insisted only that the incision be generous, be sufficiently high, and be sufficiently medial to permit easy access to the entire extrahepatic ductal system. If the common duct was difficult to identify, a classic Kocher maneuver was performed, exposing at least 1 inch of the left renal vein. If multiple attempts at aspiration identification of the common bile duct were unsuccessful, transduodenal identification of the common bile duct through the papilla of Vater was performed.

The common bile duct was then opened in the supraduodenal area, and an operative cholangiogram was obtained. With the anatomy of the intrahepatic and extrahepatic ducts demonstrated, a surgical strategy was devised. The common duct was opened. All calculi were removed with scoops, with stone forceps, and finally by hydrostatic pressure.

A biopsy taken of the ductal wall and mucosal scrapings, particularly at the site of a major stricture, were submitted to frozen section analysis to exclude carcinoma. Gentle dilation of the major ducts was performed with Bakes dilators. After the ductal system was irrigated, a T-tube, Y-tube, modified Y-tube, or transhepatic tube was placed in the ductal system.

If the distal common bile duct was markedly narrowed and associated with proximal dilatation of the biliary tree, a bypass procedure was performed. Cholecystoduodenostomy, cholecystojejunostomy, choledochojejunostomy, and hepaticojejunostomy have been selectively used.

Current Surgical Practice. Currently, more aggressive surgical procedures have been applied. The group at the University of California at Los Angeles Medical Center performed hepaticoenteric or choledochoenteric anastomosis on patients who had either a major area of extrahepatic blockage or primary involvement of the extrahepatic bile ducts. Some form of biliary bypass is definitely the proper operation for patients with this anatomic involvement, but the percentage of patients in whom this operative approach is possible varies from one reported series to another.

Cameron found that 24 of 36 patients had severe restrictive disease at the hepatic duct bifurcation and devised an operative procedure to remove the site of the most severe involvement and halt further progress of intrahepatic disease. This procedure consisted of excision of the entire extrahepatic biliary tree, including the hepatic duct bifurcation, dilatation of the intrahepatic biliary tree, insertion of bilateral transhepatic Silastic stents, and bilateral hepaticojejunostomy.

This operation has been performed on 20 patients. Results have been reported for the first 11. The mean age for these 11 patients was 41.9 years. Eight patients were men, and three were women. Among the 11 patients, 10 were white, and 1 was black. Diagnosis was made by the demonstration of multiple areas of beading and stenosis of the intrahepatic and extrahepatic biliary tree on cholangiography. The diagnosis was further confirmed at operation and by pathologic examination in all 11 patients. Six of the 11 patients had inflammatory bowel disease with a mean duration of 17 years. Marked hyperbilirubinemia was the indication for operation in 10 patients and sepsis in 1 patient. The 11 patients had symptomatic sclerosing cholangitis for a mean duration of 3.6 years before operation. Percutaneous cholangiography was carried out preoperatively to confirm the diagnosis and to determine the extent of disease. Ring catheters were left in position to aid in identification of the biliary tree at operation and to assist placement of the transhepatic stents. Patients were treated with gentamicin and either ampicillin or penicillin before cholangiography and operation. If necessary, the timing of the operation was delayed until the nutritional status of the patient improved.

A right subcostal incision is made, and the biliary tree is exposed. The extrahepatic biliary tree is easy to identify because it is firm and fibrotic. A cholecystectomy is performed if the gallbladder is present. The common bile duct is divided distally. The proximal biliary segment is separated from the portal vein and reflected in a cephalad direction. This assists exposure and dissection of the hepatic duct bifurcation. The bifurcation is mobilized, and the right and left hepatic ducts are divided at the points where they enter the hepatic parenchyma. Both hepatic ducts are carefully and slowly dilated with Bakes dilators to accommodate at least a No. 6 for a distance of at least 4 to 5 cm. Since the ducts are narrow and fibrotic and have multiple strictures, this is difficult to do. After dilation, a stone forceps is passed up into the biliary tree and out the superior surface of the liver. A stent is attached to the tip of the instrument and drawn back through liver parenchyma, through the intrahepatic biliary tree, and out the porta hepatis. Stents are placed in both the right and left ductal systems. These stents are made of silicone rubber and are 6 mm in outside diameter and 60 cm in length. Forty percent of the length contains multiple side holes. This portion of the stent is positioned in the liver and in the Roux-en-Y loop. A Roux-en-Y jejunal loop is constructed, and bilateral hepaticojejunostomies are performed around the stents, placing the distal ends of the stents in the Roux-en-Y loop. The proximal ends of the stents are brought out through abdominal wall stab wounds and connected to gravity bile bag drainage. Penrose drains are left at the site of the anastomosis. Silastic sump drains are left at the exit sites of the stents on the superior surface of the liver. Stents are changed on an outpatient basis every 3 to 4 months to prevent accumulation of sludge.

Because of the great variation in the degree and location of the ductal involvement in sclerosing cholangitis, it is obvious that the choice of the operative procedure must be individualized. Biliary-enteric anastomosis should be performed when the anatomic situation permits, even when excision of the extrahepatic segment of the ductal system with intrahepatic bilateral anastomosis is necessary.

Since the disease is usually relentlessly progressive, I prefer permanent, changeable stents in far-advanced sclerosing cholangitis. The unpredictable nature of the natural history of the disease, however, is indicated by an observation in one of my patients who had an excellent result for 19 years after choledochojejunostomy, but who now has terminal liver failure with end-stage biliary cirrhosis and bleeding esophageal varices.

PROGNOSIS

In the series of 84 patients reported by me in 1966, the average survival from the time of diagnosis was 6 years, the prognosis being worse in patients with associated chronic ulcerative colitis.

Only 13 percent of patients had no further problems after operation; about 25 percent continued to have sporadic mild episodes of cholangitis. For more than half the patients, the results of treatment were unsatisfactory; these patients continued to have cholangitis progressing to biliary cirrhosis, liver failure, and portal hypertension. Operative mortality was 8 percent; a further 20 percent of patients died of the disease during the average follow-up period of 37 months. Early postoperative complications included bacterial cholangitis (12%), biliary fistula (7%), postoperative gastrointestinal bleeding (7%), subphrenic abscess (6%), hepatic coma (3%), and septic shock (3%). The problems confronting these patients during the follow-up period were numerous; 34 percent had biliary cirrhosis, 15 percent had portal hypertension, 9 percent bled from esophageal varices, and 21 percent were troubled by recurrent biliary infection. The operative mortality rate currently is less than 2 percent.

Despite the grim prognosis, a positive surgical attitude is warranted. Many patients have benefited from multiple operations, and the relentless progression of the stenosing process may be delayed in the future by permanent changeable stents and by balloon dilation of major strictured areas by interventional radiologists.

LIVER TRANSPLANTATION

Despite the improving results of liver transplantation, the indication for this procedure in treating sclerosing cholangitis remains obscure. Physicians and surgeons are reluctant to recommend this procedure until the end stage of the disease has been reached, and by this time the procedure may be extremely hazardous. The technical demands of the operation are increased by multiple previous operations on the bile ducts.

BILE DUCT TUMOR

HENRI BISMUTH, M.D.
JEAN EMOND, M.D.

Neoplasms involving the biliary tree are nearly always malignant and arise from the biliary mucosa in either the gallbladder or the extrahepatic biliary tree. Because of their strategic location, unpredictable clinical course, and resistance to systemic modes of therapy, they remain a formidable challenge to the clinician. The surgeon is faced with patients for whom both curative and palliative treatments require a high level of clinical judgment and technical skill.

ADENOCARCINOMA OF THE GALLBLADDER

These highly malignant lesions are the most common biliary tumors, comprising between 50 and 80 percent of the cases. These tumors are thought to arise in diseased biliary mucosa as there is a high degree of association with cholelithiasis. Most patients are female (70%) and in the sixth decade. Although 15 percent of the tumors are well-differentiated papillary forms, most patients have infiltrative forms. Since the gallbladder bed is in the principal fissure between the right and left lobes, both venous and lymphatic drainage permit bilateral dissemination. Lymphatic spread also occurs toward the nodes of the hepatic pedicle.

Patients who present with symptoms usually have far-advanced disease. Nonspecific right upper quadrant pain is common, and 50 percent of patients present with obstructive jaundice. The diagnosis is usually made at surgery although the gross appearance can be misleading and confused with an inflammatory process.

The extent of disease determines the therapeutic approach to the patient. A tumor strictly localized to the mucosa discovered incidentally by the pathologist after cholecystectomy does not require further treatment. If there is invasion to the muscularis, further treatment is required. In the absence of metastases, we perform resection of segments 4 and 5 (Fig. 1) as these hepatic segments are contiguous with the gallbladder bed and susceptible to local invasion. A node dissection in the hepatic pedicle should also be performed. Extended right hepatic lobectomy is not a logical procedure for gallbladder cancer since an almost entirely normal right lobe is removed in the case of localized lesions, and there is essentially no chance of cure in cases of more advanced lesions.

If there is extension with obstruction of the biliary tree, a palliative measure is necessary to relieve the jaundice. If a reasonable life expectancy is anticipated, intrahepatic cholangioenteric anastomosis provides the most durable relief of the jaundice. In advanced cases, transtumoral intubation should be performed with either T-tube or U-tube drainage (to be discussed).

The overall prognosis for patients with carcinoma of the gallbladder is extremely poor. Patients with small tumors removed incidentally at operation for cholelithiasis comprise most of the 5-year survivors. Limited experience with radiation and chemotherapy has been reported with few favorable responses.

BILE DUCT CARCINOMAS

Bile duct cancers have been divided into three groups based on the level of biliary obstruction (Table 1). This classification has both prognostic and therapeutic importance since the approach is entirely different at each level.

Tumors of the Biliary Confluence

Adenocarcinomas of the junction of the main hepatic ducts are the tumors described by Klatskin and are part of a larger group of malignant tumors involving the hepatic hilus. Klatskin tumors comprise 50 percent of our series of hilar cancers, which present with a similar clinical picture and pose the same mechanical problems for the surgeon. The hilus can be invaded by neighboring liver or gallbladder cancers or else by nodal metastases from other gastrointestinal tumors, all of which can present with obstructive jaundice. Klatskin tumors tend to produce symptoms earlier in their course than the other hilar tumors. They are generally infiltrative in character, and although they metastasize late, local growth is inexorable.

Mid-Duct Tumors

This is the least common localization of adenocarcinoma of the bile duct.

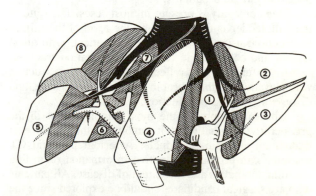

Figure 1   The anatomy of the liver as described by Couinaud is widely used in Europe and the Orient. The segments are based on the branches of the portal vein providing a logical approach to hepatic surgery. Segments 2, 3, and 4 are perfused by the left branch of the portal vein and comprise the left liver. Segments 5, 6, 7, and 8 comprise the right liver. Segment 1, the caudate lobe, is an independent structure with its own portal and hepatic venous system.

223

TABLE 1   Treatment of Bile Duct Tumors*

| Location | Surgical Treatment | | Nonsurgical Treatment |
	Curative	Palliative	
Proximal third (hilar tumors)	Resection of biliary confluence and proximal common duct ± hepatectomy	Intrahepatic cholangioenteric anastomosis or intubation (U- or T-tube)	Endoscopic or percutaneous intubation
Middle third	Pedicular resection of confluence and common duct	Proximal hepaticojejunostomy	Intubation
Distal third	Radical cephalic pancreatico-duodenectomy	Hepaticojejunostomy and gastrojejunostomy	Intubation

* Schema of the anatomic classification of biliary tumors and its relationship to the therapeutic possibilities at each level. It should be noted that both curative and palliative measures require an approach that is one level proximal to the disease.

Distal Duct Tumors

Adenocarcinomas of the distal duct have the best prognosis because of their favorable location. They invade within the head of the pancreas, and both curative and palliative measures are more readily accomplished.

BILE DUCT CANCERS: DIAGNOSIS AND CLINICAL FINDINGS

Bile duct cancers are slightly more common in men (60%). Intense, painless jaundice is the most common presenting complaint. Pruritus is sometimes present. Associated biliary infection is rare in patients who have not received previous treatment. Fifty percent of the patients have received some form of incomplete therapy prior to referral. The tumors are localized in 20 percent of patients, but this figure is less than 10 percent in previously treated patients.

Hepatomegaly is present in most cases. The state of the gallbladder is determined by the level of the biliary obstruction; it is tense and dilated in patients with distal lesions and collapsed in cases of proximal obstruction.

Liver function tests reflect the presence of obstruction with elevations of the bilirubin, alkaline phosphatase, and disturbance of the coagulation.

Ultrasonography is the most important test in the preoperative evaluation as it establishes the presence of dilated intrahepatic bile ducts. Arteriography and CT scanning can provide adjunctive information regarding vascular anomalies and the extent of disease. All patients who are surgical candidates should be explored since the only chance for cure is resection. The cholangiogram should be delayed until surgery to avoid introducing infection into a segment of liver that will not be amenable to drainage. Preoperative biliary drainage, which has not been proved to improve the results of treatment, reduces the size of the biliary ducts and can complicate the performance of biliary anastomoses.

TREATMENT OF BILE DUCT CANCERS

Resection represents the ideal treatment as it relieves symptoms while providing a chance for cure. Although some have advocated it as a palliative treatment, we reserve it for patients in whom there is no evidence of dissemination of disease. On the basis of strict criteria based on frozen section biopsies, less than 20 percent of the patients are candidates for resection. If curative therapy is not possible, palliative treatment of the jaundice is indicated as it improves short-term survival and the patient's comfort.

At operation, the level of the obstruction is determined and a complete cholangiogram is obtained at a level proximal to the obstruction. In cases of hilar tumor, this necessitates puncture of the liver.

Distal common duct tumors can be resected for cure by radical cephalic pancreaticoduodenectomy. The biliary tree and the pancreas are anastomosed to a single defunctionalized loop of jejunum. We generally do not stent either anastomosis. If resection is contraindicated by extension of the disease, hepaticojejunostomy and gastrojejunostomy are performed as a palliative measure.

Tumors of the midportion of the common duct can be resected for cure with skeletonization of the portal vein and the hepatic artery and reconstruction by hepaticojejunostomy. Palliation of the jaundice is performed by hepaticojejunostomy above the lesion or by intubation.

Hilar tumors represent a much more difficult surgical problem and have been the source of controversy. Curative treatment involves resection of the confluence and the proximal common duct with reconstruction by bilateral hepaticojejunostomy. Local invasion of the liver is treated with en bloc hepatic resection, as is unilateral involvement of a secondary biliary confluence. In a similar fashion a primary hepatocellular carcinoma that has invaded the hilus can be resected in the absence of dissemination. The biliary reconstruction is performed by means of mucosal anastomosis to a defunctionalized jejunal limb. If the anastomosis is small, a stent is placed through it and exited through the jejunum.

In most cases, palliative therapy is appropriate. We have attempted to avoid intubation and thus avoid the morbidity associated with chronic biliary intubation. Apart from the discomfort of living with tubes and dressings, external biliary fistulas, cholangitis, and obstruction with debris all result in repeated hospitalizations.

Because of these problems we perform intrahepatic cholangioenteric anastomosis as the treatment of choice in the palliation of hilar cancers. It provides the following advantages:(1) a mucosa-to-mucosa anastomosis is performed which assures prolonged patency without the use of indwelling biliary stents, and (2) the anastomosis is placed away from the seat of the tumor to delay the recurrence of the jaundice.

Since the intrahepatic biliary tree is more accessible on the left, the anastomosis is usually placed on the bile duct of segment 3 of Couinaud (see Fig. 1). Although drainage of the entire liver is not always assured, this is not important in the absence of infection. In most cases, drainage of 30 percent of the liver parenchyma suffices to relieve the jaundice. If the left lobe of the liver is atrophic or extensively involved with tumor, the anastomsis can be placed in the right liver on the duct of segment 5. This is a more difficult approach as it requires a more important hepatotomy.

The duct of segment 3 is found by opening the umbilical fissure to the left of the round ligament. The fissure is opened for a distance of 3 or 4 cm until the fibrous capsule encasing the portal pedicle of segment 3 is encountered. This capsule contains the bile duct, the portal vein branch, and the branch of the hepatic artery of the segment. The bile duct is the posterosuperior element of the pedicle and is usually 5 mm in diameter owing to the biliary obstruction. To facilitate placement of the jejunal limb in the hepatotomy incision, the mesenteric side of the open end of the jejunum is partially closed by means of several interrupted sutures. The anastomosis is then performed between the end of the jejunum and the side of the opened bile duct; 6–0 monofilament nylon is used for the anastomosis, which is constructed with interrupted sutures. If the anastomosis is satisfactory, a small silastic drain is placed through it to control any leakage that might develop. If there are no problems, the drain is removed in 2 weeks. If the anastomosis is very small a larger drain is placed for calibration which is then removed two months postoperatively.

Early in our experience, hepaticojejunostomy was performed in this setting; the jejunal loop was attached directly to the sectioned hepatic parenchyma without ductal anastomsis. The need for prolonged intubation to maintain biliary drainage as well as complications of bile leakage and fluid collections led us to abandon this technique.

Patients who have advanced disease at surgery can be treated with dilation and transtumoral intubation, using either simple T-tube or U-tube drainage. Most patients who require intubation can be selected preoperatively and spared the surgical exploration.

OPERATIVE ULTRASOUND IN THE TREATMENT OF BILIARY TUMORS

In the past 3 years we have introduced operative ultrasound into our daily practice of hepatobiliary surgery. It provides the following advantages in patients with biliary tumors:

1. The detection of intrahepatic metastases is improved by adequate sonography since detection of small lesions by palpation in enlarged cholestatic livers is difficult. The examination should be performed after decompression of the biliary tree to improve accuracy.
2. Sonography is useful in the detection of dilated intrahepatic bile ducts for the performance of intrahepatic anastomosis (especially helpful in the right liver).
3. It improves the technique of intubation in hilar tumors since the dilated duct can be punctured transhepatically. By means of a guide wire the stent can be advanced under direct sonographic guidance to ensure proper placement.

BILE DUCT CANCERS: RESULTS OF THERAPY

Early Results

Both resection and intrahepatic anastomosis can be performed with low morbidity and mortality in properly selected patients. For resection, the operative mortality has been less than 5 percent, slightly higher for intrahepatic anastomosis (6%).

Complications including episodes of biliary sepsis, gastrointestinal hemorrhage, and biliary fistulas have occurred in 10 percent of the patients. Patients who undergo surgical intubation have a higher mortality (16%) and morbidity, reflecting the more advanced disease in these patients.

Late Results

Patients with bile duct tumors who undergo resection have a 2-year survival rate of 50 percent and good relief of symptoms. We have several long-term survivors, but these patients are rare. In assessing the result of palliative procedures, the quality of life produced after treatment is the principal consideration. A prolonged survival without relief of the symptoms, compounded by complications of the treatment, is of little benefit to the patient. We have evaluated our results by comparing the symptom-free period after treatment with the total survival of the patient. This relationship can be expressed as a percentage, the "comfort index," 100 percent representing a completely symptom-free existence after surgery.

In our experience, both resection and intrahepatic anastomosis have produced survivals that are 75 percent symptom-free. For patients who undergo surgical intuba- tion, the comfort index is less than 50 percent. Patients undergoing nonsurgical intubations tend to have extremely short survival (15% at 6 months).

ANTIBIOTIC SELECTION IN BILIARY TRACT SURGERY

ROBB H. RUTLEDGE, M.D.

The incidence of septic complications in biliary tract surgery has been reported as high as 15 to 20 percent. Combined with good surgical technique, proper antibiotic therapy should decrease this to less than 5 percent. This report considers the bacteriology involved, the antibiotics available, and the author's current practice.

BILIARY BACTERIOLOGY

The importance of bactibilia in septic complications of biliary surgery has been pointed out by numerous authors. Both wound and systemic infectious complica- tions are increased in patients with positive bile cultures at surgery. Further, the bacteria isolated from the wound or blood stream are usually the same as those grown from the bile. One investigator has reported that 65 percent of wound infections and 90 percent of the episodes of septicemia were caused by organisms that had been isolated from the bile. Recently, however, it has been reported that a lower correlation exists between the bacteria in positive bile cultures and postoperative infective complications in patients in community hospitals having elective biliary operations.

Incidence of Bactibilia

Normally the bile is sterile, but the likelihood of bactibilia increases with the complexity of the biliary tract disease. Across the board, about 25 to 35 percent of patients having biliary surgery have positive bile cultures. This breaks down to about 10 percent positive cultures in young elective patients with normal bile ducts, 30 to 50 percent in older patients with previous acute attacks, 50 percent in patients with acute cholecystitis, 75 percent in patients with common duct disease, and up to 100 percent in patients with biliary strictures, biliary-enteric anastomoses, and indwelling biliary drainage tubes. The incidence of positive bile cultures is increased in old age and in patients with nonfunctioning gallbladders by cholecystography.

Since the incidence of septic complications increases with the likelihood of bactibilia, it is important to identify patients with positive bile cultures for appropriate anti- biotic therapy. Some surgeons have favored their identifi- cation by preoperative duodenal drainage and others by intraoperative biliary Gram's stains. Both methods can be cumbersome and unreliable.

Several authors have developed a more practical list of factors that identify the patient who is likely to have a positive bile culture and to be at high risk for post- operative infection (Table 1). These factors include age over 70, recent or current acute cholecystitis or cholangitis, emergency surgery, obstructive jaundice, choledocholithiasis, and previous biliary surgery. The infection rate in this high-risk group is 20 to 30 percent without antibiotic therapy. Numerous studies have shown that this complication rate can be lowered to 5 percent or less with appropriate antibiotics.

Types of Bacteria in Bactibilia

The bacteria in positive bile cultures are the same bacteria that appear normally in the gastrointestinal tract. Whether their biliary arrival is by a transmural, hema- togenous, or ascending route is not totally clear. The three most commonly isolated organisms are *Escherichia coli,* *Klebsiella pneumoniae,* and *Enterococcus.* These results have been repeated consistently in many laboratories throughout the world whether the culture was done from the gallbladder bile, common duct bile, or the gallbladder wall (Table 2).

Gram-negative aerobes are present in about 65 percent of positive cultures, *E. coli* being present in about 50 percent. *Klebsiella penumoniae* is the next most common gram-negative aerobe followed by *Enterobacter sp., Proteus sp.* and *Pseudomonas sp.* The gram-negative aerobes are the most significant target for antibiotic therapy.

TABLE 1 High-Risk Factors for Bactibilia

Age > 70
Acute cholangitis—recent or current
Acute cholecystitis—recent or current
Emergency surgery
Obstructive jaundice
Choledocholithiasis
Previous biliary surgery

TABLE 2 Bacteria in Bactibilia

Organism	Positive Bile Cultures
Aerobes	
Gram-negative	65% - 70%
E. coli*	
K. pneumoniae*	
Enterobacter	
Proteus	
Pseudomonas	
Gram-positive	30%
Enterococcus*	
Streptococcus viridans	
Staphylococcus aureus	
Anaerobes	25% - 35%
Gram-negative	
Bacteroides fragilis*	
Gram-positive	
Clostridia perfringens	

* Four most common organisms

The gram-positive aerobes that are most common in bile cultures are the *Enterococcus* (30%), *Streptococcus viridans*, and *Staphylococcus* species. The importance of the *Enterococcus* is questioned by many authorities. In routine cases, its pathogenicity is low, but in more complicated biliary infections, it may have an important synergistic effect. Superinfections with *Enterococcus* can occur if it is not covered by the antibiotic therapy in critically ill patients.

Several early researchers have shown the importance of anaerobes in bile cultures. The most common isolates are *Bacteroides fragilis* and *Clostridium perfringens*. With the development of good anaerobic culture media and transport methods, the incidence of positive anaerobic cultures is about 25 to 35 percent. The anaerobes are usually in a mixed culture with aerobes, but occasionally are a pure isolate. The incidence of positive anaerobic cultures, especially *B. fragilis* is increased in the elderly and in patients with cholangitis and complicated biliary problems. A positive anaerobic culture does not require antibiotic coverage in elective straightforward cases, but should receive appropriate coverage if the patient is elderly or acutely ill.

Recently, some authors have noticed a change in the bacteria involved in patients with acute cholangitis. They have reported an increased incidence of *Pseudomonas* and *Serratia*. Both of these reports are from referral centers in which many complicated biliary operations are performed and do not represent the findings in a community hospital.

ANTIBIOTICS

There are many effective antibiotics available for biliary surgery. The surgeon must consider the antibiotic's spectrum, pharmacokinetic properties, toxicity, and cost (Table 3).

Antibiotic Spectrum

Gram-negative aerobes are the most important bacteria in the bile, *E. coli* and *K. pneumoniae* being the most prevalent. An aminoglycoside, gentamicin or tobramycin, is the drug of first choice. Amikacin should be reserved for resistant strains. First-generation cephalosporins (cefazolin and cephalothin) are sometimes effective against *E. coli, K. pneumoniae*, and *Proteus*. Second-generation cephalosporins (cefoxitin, cefonicid, and cefamandole) have more activity against many gram-negative aerobes. Third-generation cephalosporins (cefotaxime, moxalactam, and cefoperazone) have even greater gram-negative activity, but development of resistant strains may limit their usefulness. The newer penicillins (azlocillin, mezlocillin, piperacillin, and ticarcillin) are also effective against many gram-negative bacteria. Of these penicillins, piperacillin has the most activity aginst *Pseudomonas* and *Klebsiella*, but does not give complete gram-negative coverage.

Enterococcus, the most common gram-positive organism in bile cultures, is best covered by ampicillin or penicillin G in combination with an aminoglycoside. Piperacillin is also effective, and vancomycin can be substituted in allergic patients. First-generation cephalosporins such as cefazolin are not effective against *Enterococcus*, but are active against *Streptococcus viridans* and the non-penicillinase-producing staphylococci that grow in bile. The second- and third-generation cephalosporins have less gram-positive activity.

The two most common anaerobes in bile are *B. fragilis* and *C. perfringens*. *B. fragilis* is covered best by clindamycin or metronidazole. Cefoxitin, cefoperazone, chloramphenicol, and the newer penicillins are also effective. Except for cefoxitin and cefoperazone, all of these drugs are effective alternatives to penicillin G for treatment of *C. perfringens*. Metronidazole is the single currently available antibiotic with the most complete coverage against nearly all anaerobic bacteria.

The presence of a bacterial strain in a bile culture does not mean it requires antibiotic coverage. In prophylactic situations, only the likely gram-negative aerobes need be covered. In critically ill patients, more complete protection is important. The combination of ampicillin, an aminoglycoside, and metronidazole or clindamycin gives essentially total coverage. Newer penicillins such as piperacillin cover a wide range of biliary pathogens, but at present cannot be recommended as the sole agent in severe biliary sepsis. Similarly, the newer third-generation cephalosporins may be able to replace the more toxic aminoglycosides, but cannot be recommended yet for use alone.

Pharmacokinetic Properties

Distribution. Although not so significant as the antibiotics's spectrum, its distribution in bile, liver, serum, and the subcutaneous tissues is important. Antibiotics with the highest biliary excretion include piperacillin, cefo-

TABLE 3   Antibiotic Therapy in Bactibilia

Antibiotic	Spectrum			Bile Levels	Half-life (Hours)	Average Dose	Cost/Day* To Patient
	Gram-Neg. Aerobes	Enterococcus	B. Fragilis				
Ampicillin	+	+ +	0	High	2	1.0 g q6h	$140
Cefamandole	+	0	0	Very high	1	1.0 g q6h	$130
Cefazolin	+	0	0	High	1½	1.0 g q8h	$ 95
Cefonicid	+	0	0	High	5	1.0 g q24h	$ 40
Cefoperazone	+	0	+	Very high	2	2.0 g q6h	$200
Cefoxitin	+	0	+	High	1	1.0 g q6h	$145
Chloramphenicol	+	0	+	Low	1	1.0 g q6h	$120
Clindamycin	0	0	+ +	High	3	600 mg q6h	$160
Gentamicin	+ +	0	0	Low	2	80 mg q8h	$ 80
Metronidazole	0	0	+ +	Moderate	8	500 mg q6h	$105
Piperacillin	+	+	+	Very high	1	3.0 g q4h	$225
Ticarcillin	+	0	+	Moderate	1	3.0 g q4h	$210
Tobramycin	+ +	0	0	Low	2	80 mg q8h	$ 90

* Piggy-back technique typical community hospital

perazone, and cefamandole. Ampicillin, most of the cephalosporins, clindamycin, and tetracyclines have a high biliary excretion. The older penicillins, aminoglycosides, metronidazole, and chloramphenicol have a lower biliary excretion.

If the bile duct is obstructed, all biliary antibiotic levels are decreased, but the antibiotic's serum, liver, and subcutaneous tissue levels still are important factors. Cefazolin is superior here to cephalothin. Aminoglycosides and chloramphenicol have good serum and tissue levels, although their biliary excretion is low. Nevertheless, biliary excretion is an important consideration, prophylactic or therapeutic, in a patient with an open bile duct.

Half-Life.   Serum half-life is another property to consider in antibiotic selection. Drugs with a longer half-life require fewer injections per day. This saves time and should decrease errors and expense.

Antibiotics with a short half-life are not so effective for prophylaxis. The preoperative injection may already have passed its effective serum level before the operative contamination occurs. Drugs with a half-life of 2 hours or less have a better prophylactic effect if they are repeated at 2-hour intervals during prolonged surgery.

Of the first-generation cephalosporins, cefazolin is preferred because of its longer half-life. Cefonicid, a new second-generation cephalosporin, has a half-life of about 5 hours with therapeutic serum levels detectable at 12 hours. This is much longer than the half-life of cefoxitin or cefamandole. Ceftriaxone, a third generation cephalosporin yet to be released, has an even longer half-life of 6 to 8 hours.

Toxicity

The medication free of risk has yet to be developed. Some medications present more problems with toxicity than others. Penicillin allergies have been fairly frequent. Cephalosporin allergies, in general, have been less common, but do occur. Metronidazole has been reported to be carcinogenic in animals. Chloramphenicol has caused fatal blood dyscrasias. Clindamycin has been associated with severe colitis.

Serious bleeding problems and superinfections have been reported with some of the third-generation cephalosporins. Many of these patients already have hypoprothrombinemia and platelet dysfunction as a result of their biliary disease. Moxalactam, especially, has been associated with these occasionally fatal bleeding disorders. Superinfections with enterococci or other bacteria have also been reported during therapy with third-generation cephalosporins. Both the bleeding and the superinfection problems have been less common with the newer penicillins than with the cephalosporins.

One of the most significant concerns about antibiotic toxicity in biliary surgery is the potential nephrotoxicity of the aminoglycosides. Patients with jaundice, acute cholangitis, or other complex biliary problems are prone to develop renal failure and must be monitored carefully during aminoglycoside therapy. Some authors have pointed out that prolonged aminoglycoside use has contributed to increased morbidity and longer hospital stays in these patients. They advise that the aminoglycosides be reserved for critically ill patients and be discontinued when the bile duct obstruction is relieved and the temperature is no longer elevated.

Cost

Many antibiotics are now available for use in biliary surgery and cost has become a factor. Usually single-drug therapy is less expensive than combination-drug therapy. Drugs with a longer half-life require fewer injections and therefore have a lower cost.

Hospital charges vary, but aminoglycosides are among the least expensive antibiotic drugs used today. First-generation cephalosporins cost less than second-generation ones. Ampicillin, chloramphenicol, and metronidazole are usually more expensive than cefazolin, but are less expensive than cefoxitin. Clindamycin tends to be in the same price range as the second-generation cephalosporins. Third-generation cephalosporins and the newer penicillins are even more expensive. A combination therapy of ampicillin, gentamicin, and clindamycin would be more expensive than a single drug like cefoxitin or even a third-generation cephalosporin or a newer penicillin.

Antibiotic costs are only a small part of the picture of the cost of infection, and a short course of appropriate prophylactic antibiotic therapy is a good financial investment. Several authors have emphasized the financial consequences of infectious complications. The average hospital stay is prolonged by 3 days if a wound infection develops, and the hospital cost is increased by about $3,000. This does not include the added inconvenience or risk to the patient or his extra loss of income because of prolonged disability.

AUTHOR'S CURRENT PRACTICE

There is no uniformity in antibiotic usage in biliary surgery. I am presenting here my current preferences and a discussion of available alternatives (Table 4).

Elective Cases

The majority of authors use prophylactic antibiotics only on high-risk cases likely to have a positive bile culture. However, I have used prophylactic antibiotics on

TABLE 4 Current Practice

Clinical Situation	Antibiotic
Elective cases	
Routine	Cefazolin
Elderly or jaundiced	Cefoxitin
Biliary reconstruction	Aminoglycoside, clindamycin or metronidazole, and ampicillin
Acute cholecystitis	
Routine	Cefazolin
Elderly or jaundiced	Cefoxitin
Critically ill	Aminoglycoside, clindamycin or metronidazole and ampicillin
Emphysematous	Aminoglycoside and a penicillin or metronidazole
Acute cholangitis	
Mild	Cefoxitin
Severe	Aminoglycoside, clindamycin or metronidazole, and ampicillin
Cholangiograms	
Routine T-tube	None
Poor risk or biliary reconstruction	Aminoglycoside and clindamycin or metronidazole

essentially all elective biliary cases. Since I cannot predict before operation which patients will require a bile duct exploration or a biliary drainage procedure, I believe it is better to protect all patients routinely. Further, I frequently do an incidental appendectomy in the younger biliary patients. Unless prophylactic antibiotics are used, it has been shown that wound complications increase if appendectomy is added. The cost of the prophylactic antibiotics is small compared to the cost of a postoperative infection. To date there is no report of the development of resistant bacterial strains to short perioperative antibiotic therapy. Some investigators believe that topical antibiotics such as bacitracin and polymixin are an acceptable alternative if an intraoperative need for antibiotics becomes apparent in a patient who has not received preoperative antibiotics.

It is my usual practice to give 1.0 g cefazolin IM or IV 1 to 2 hours preoperatively. The dose is repeated in 2 hours and then at 8-hour intervals. Treatment is discontinued 24 hours postoperatively unless there is some reason to continue.

Although there are other antibiotics available, none has any significant advantage over cefazolin for routine prophylactic use. It gives good coverage for most gram-negative aerobes and *Staphylococcus aureus*, a frequent cause of wound infections in elective biliary surgery. It does not protect against *B. fragilis* or *Enterococcus*, but this is unnecessary in routine prophylaxis. Cefazolin has good bile, serum, and tissue levels and causes few allergic reactions. Its half-life is 1½ hours, and a second injection should be given 2 hours after the first to ensure high serum levels during closure if the surgery is prolonged. Cefonicid, a new second-generation cephalosporin, has the advantage of a 4- to 5-hour half-life and consequently requires only one or two injections for prophylaxis. Its spectrum is similar to that of cefamandole, but it is not so effective against *Staphylococcus aureus*. Third-generation cephalosporins give less gram-positive coverage, are more expensive, and should not be used at this time for routine prophylaxis.

In elderly jaundiced or recently jaundiced patients, the likelihood of *B. fragilis* involvement is high, and I give cefoxitin instead of cefazolin. If the patient is having a complicated biliary reconstruction or has existing drainage tubes, specific bacteria can be identified preoperatively and exact therapy can be given. Patients of the latter type are more likely to have *Pseudomonas*, *Proteus*, and *Serratia* infections, and more complete antibiotic coverage is needed.

If the patient is allergic to cephalosporins, gentamicin or tobramycin is used for 24-hour prophylaxis because of its good coverge against gram-negative aerobes and *Staphylococcus aureus*. If *B. fragilis* is suspected, metronidazole or clindamycin could be added.

Regardless of the drug chosen, it is essential to start treatment with the antibiotic 1 to 2 hours preoperatively and to stop it in 24 hours. Starting earlier or continuing longer only increases the expense and the likelihood of the development of resistant bacterial strains. It has been shown that even shorter courses of therapy may be equally effective.

Although recommended by many, I do not obtain bile cultures on all elective cases. Instead, I culture only high-risk patients and those having a bile duct exploration. These are the patients who have a correlation between bacteria in the bile and in the wound. The low-risk patients are more likely to have sterile bile and a wound infection due to *Staphylococcus aureus*. The cost of an aerobic and anaerobic culture is equal to the cost of a 24-hour course of gentamicin therapy.

Acute Cholecystitis

At least 50 percent of patients with acute cholecystitis have a positive bile culture. Intravenous antibiotics are started when the diagnosis is made, and surgery is usually performed within 24 hours. Intraoperative bile cultures are taken, but stat Gram's stains are not routinely requested.

Cefazolin is the antibiotic most often used in the typical patient. Cefoxitin is chosen if the patient is elderly or jaundiced because of its *B. fragilis* coverge. If the patient is more critically ill, a combination of an aminoglycoside, ampicillin, and metronidazole or clindamycin might be used instead to give even wider coverage.

Most patients with acute cholecystitis have an unobstructed bile duct. Piperacillin and cefoperazone, with their high biliary excretion and wide gram-negative spectrum, may prove to be useful alternatives to triple antibiotic coverage.

After the gallbladder is removed, antibiotics are continued for 3 or 4 days, depending on the patient's course. When culture reports become available, I may omit an aminoglycoside if it no longer seems necessary or may add a specific antibiotic if the patient needs more intensive coverage.

In the rare case of acute emphysematous cholecystitis, surgical removal is essential. The diagnosis can be made preoperatively by demonstration of air in the gallbladder wall or lumen on the abdominal film. The organisms most commonly cultured from the bile are *Clostridia perfringens* and *E. coli*. Antibiotic coverage should include a penicillin or metronidazole for the *Clostridia*. Piperacillin as a single agent would probably be effective coverage, but is more expensive than a combination of gentamicin and metronidazole.

Acute Cholangitis

Most cases of acute cholangitis are due to choledo-cholithiasis. More recently, cholangitis also has been seen in patients with recurrent strictures, malignant obstruction, and nonoperative interventional procedures. The responsible bacterial flora has widened to include *Pseudomonas, Proteus*, and *Serratia* in these latter complicated cases.

Both bactibilia and biliary obstruction are necessary to produce acute cholangitis. The clinical picture usually appears in the elderly debilitated patient. The bile duct is blocked so that biliary levels of any antibiotic will be low.

Occasional milder cases are treated with cefoxitin for both gram-negative aerobic and *B. fragilis* coverage. However, many of these patients are critically ill, and I often elect to cover the complete spectrum of bactibilia: gram-negative aerobes, *Enterococcus*, and *B. fragilis*. In these patients I have usually used ampicillin, gentamicin, or tobramycin, and metronidazole or clindamycin. The aminoglycoside must be carefully monitored with serum creatinine and antibiotic levels because these patients are prone to develop renal failure. This triple antibiotic coverage has proved to be effective, but is costly and potentially dangerous if the aminoglycoside is continued longer than 5 days. Consequently, the less nephrotoxic newer penicillins may be useful here. Piperacillin is effective against *Enterococcus* as well as the gram-negative aerobes and *B. fragilis*. A third-generation cephalosporin such as cefoperazone, combined with ampicillin for the *Enterococcus*, should also be effective. Controlled studies are not yet available to show that the newer penicillins and third-generation cephalosporins are as reliable as the triple antibiotic program.

Most patients with acute cholangitis respond to antibiotic therapy within 24 to 48 hours. Then an exact diagnosis can be made and appropriate surgery performed promptly. Some patients do not respond to the antibiotic treatment and require an emergency decompression of the bile duct. Then accurate cultures can be made. After the bile duct is decompressed and the patient improves, consideration should be given to stopping any aminoglycoside and changing to a less toxic agent. Antibiotic therapy is usually continued for 4 or 5 days postoperatively.

Cholangiograms

Radiologists and gastroenterologists routinely give a short course of prophylactic antibiotics during their invasive biliary procedures. Less has been written about antibiotics and cholangiograms.

Because I use prophylactic preoperative antibiotics in all cases of biliary surgery, the patient is protected from bacteremia during the operative cholangiogram that is performed routinely after the abdomen is opened. Since the antibiotic is repeated in 2 hours, the patient is also protected during any subsequent cholangiograms performed later in the operation.

Many surgeons routinely give a short course of prophylactic antibiotics to cover postoperative T-tube cholangiograms. Bile cultures are positive in nearly 100 percent of the postoperative patients with tubes. In addition to the usual biliary flora, postoperative bile cultures grow hospital environmental organisms. It has been shown by some investigators that about 10 percent of patients having postoperative cholangiograms develop a bacteremia that is usually well tolerated. Besides emphasizing the importance of keeping the injection pressure below 15 cm water during the study, these investigators recommend antibiotics only for those who would tolerate a bacteremia poorly.

Ordinarily, I do not give antibiotics to cover the routine postoperative T-tube cholangiogram. However, I do give them to the poor-risk patient or the patient with a complicated biliary reconstruction. Frequently, specific antibiotics can be given based on previous cultures. If not, I occasionally use an aminoglycoside with ampicillin and metronidazole. The goal is to prevent bacteremia, not sterilize the bile, and so the medication should be given 1 hour before the cholangiogram and not repeated unless clinically indicated.

THE PANCREAS

ACUTE PANCREATITIS

ANDREW L. WARSHAW, M.D.

Acute pancreatitis is probably a group of diseases whose final common effect is pancreatic inflammation. Each possible inciting factor, be it passage of a gallstone, alcohol, viral infection, ischemia, or metabolic derangements, may initiate the process in a more-or-less unique fashion, but the convergence of enzyme activation, architectural disruption, and ischemic necrosis combine to produce the disease. Endogenous control mechanisms, as yet incompletely understood, exist to combat the process, including antiproteases and a protease-scavenging system utilizing macromolecular complexes and the reticuloendothelial system. The severity and progression of acute pancreatitis is a function of the balance of these various contributing factors. Treatment, including surgical treatment, is designed to affect the balance and to respond to the consequences of the injury.

The clinical course of acute pancreatitis can be separated into three phases, each with its own characteristics and appropriate treatment. The early phase is one of inflammation and vascular instability, generally lasting one to several days. The phenomena during this period may be life-threateningly severe, but are nonetheless reversible. It is during the middle phase, beginning about the fourth day and lasting from one to several weeks, that tissue destruction becomes recognizable. Phlegmon or swelling of the pancreas, recognizable on CT scan in up to 50 percent of patients, may also harbor areas of necrosis of pancreatic and peripancreatic tissues. Thrombosis and erosion of local blood vessels may produce further visceral infarction, fistulas, and hemorrhage. In the late phase, beginning about 2 weeks after onset, the necrotic tissue can become infected, the start of a pancreatic abscess.

EARLY PHASE

In the first few days of the attack, the most prominent and dangerous derangements of function involve the circulation. There is both increased capillary endothelial permeability with consequent loss of plasma volume and reduced peripheral vascular tone leading to peripheral pooling. The resulting hypotension may not respond to replacement of intravascular fluid, even if pursued vigorously. Renal failure and respiratory failure are common. Fortunately, the combination of endogenous control mechanisms and simple medical measures works for 90 percent or more of these patients, regardless of the cause of the pancreatitis. Table 1 lists features of general management that are of proven value, as well as those of more dubious importance.

There are several potential roles for surgical intervention during the early phase: (1) to certify the diagnosis, (2) to counteract the functional derangements, (3) to halt the progression of the pancreatitis, and (4) to excise the disease.

Surgery for Diagnosis

Even today, the diagnosis of acute pancreatitis is often uncertain. All current laboratory and radiologic tests give both false-positive and false-negative results, and the clinical picture may overlap with a number of other diseases, most notably perforated ulcers, acute cholecystitis, intestinal ischemia, closed loop obstruction, or perforation. The serum amylase in particular may increase in any of these entities. When in doubt, especially if a patient has impressive signs of peritoneal irritation, it is safer to perform an exploratory operation than to miss a potentially lethal but surgically correctible lesion. It should not be an embarrassment to find ''only pancreatitis'' in these circumstances, nor should a simple

TABLE 1 Medical Management of Acute Pancreatitis

Effective	Volume replacement with monitoring of urine output, CVP, and left atrial pressure; ventilatory support with monitoring of arterial blood gases
Of value	Antacid therapy, nasogastric suction
Unproven	Antibiotics
Unnecessary	Insulin (except in an established diabetic), calcium supplements
Ineffective	Antiproteases (Trasylol), glucagon
Proposed	Somatostatin, protease scavengers, O_2-derived free radical scavengers, low-molecular-weight dextran, prostaglandins

exploration cause harm or aggravate the pancreatitis. There is no indication to place any drains or tubes in viscera under these circumstances unless there is abundant toxic ascites (to be discussed) or reason to believe that the patient needs biliary decompression for cholangitis.

Surgery for Organ Dysfunction

As noted, circulatory, renal, and pulmonary function are commonly profoundly impaired early in pancreatitis and may not respond to vigorous volume replacement and other supportive therapy. There is evidence that the body-wide effects on function of many organs may be mediated by toxic and vasoactive substances that are absorbed from the brownish peritoneal exudate (toxic ascites) that is present in fulminant cases. Removal of the ascitic fluid should therefore be beneficial. Many surgeons, including myself, have been impressed that peritoneal lavage is effective, but a definitive study has not been performed. The best and most recent one showed no benefit to lavage in severe pancreatitis, but did not address specifically those patients with circulatory dysfunction (shock).

For the present, I will continue to use peritoneal lavage in patients who show signs of shock, tachycardia (>130), ongoing major volume requirements, and progressive renal or pulmonary failure despite 24 hours of vigorous medical treatment. Whether the finding of brown ascites by paracentesis should be a strong index for lavage, as has been suggested, remains to be seen. There is no evidence that lavage benefits any other category of patient and is not indicated, for example, for treatment of pain or purely on the basis of Ranson's signs of severity.

Catheters for peritoneal lavage may be placed percutaneously or surgically. The percutaneous technique suffices in most cases. Under local anesthesia, a Tenchoff catheter, as used for renal dialysis, is placed under direct vision through a short midline subumbilical incision. Standard peritoneal dialysis fluids, containing 500 units of heparin and a broad-spectrum antibiotic with enteric coverage, suffice in most cases. Because of the glucose in the dialysis solution, care should be taken to monitor blood sugar. It is advisable to use only one liter per lavage in order to reduce the risk of precipitating ventilatory compromise, which would necessitate intubation for assisted ventilation. The lavage fluid need not equilibrate in the peritoneal cavity, but can be introduced and drained continuously. If the lavage is working, its effects are apparent almost immediately. Within a few hours, the heart rate falls dramatically toward 100, the blood pressure rises, and the volume requirements fall. The lavage need not be continued for more than a day or two once the improvement has occurred.

If the percutaneous lavage is ineffective after a trial of several hours, laparotomy is recommended to ascertain the diagnosis and to place the lavage catheters directly into the lesser sac. On occasion the toxic ascites is loculated there and has not been effectively removed by the percutaneous catheter in the greater peritoneal cavity.

Of course, some cases of overwhelming pancreatitis do not respond to any treatment.

Surgery to Excise the Disease

Major pancreatic resection and even total pancreatectomy during the early phase of pancreatitis has its advocates, particularly in France. However, there are no objective criteria either for selecting patients for excision or for deciding how much pancreas to remove. Much recoverable pancreas is wasted, and the end-results in preventing death or abscess are no better than the more conservative approach being outlined here. Early pancreatic resection is not recommended.

Surgery to Prevent Progression of Pancreatitis

Gallstone pancreatitis is caused by passage through, or lodging of, a stone at the ampulla of Vater. A common duct stone can be demonstrated in about 70 percent of patients during the first 24 hours of gallstone pancreatitis. This has led some to advocate early common duct exploration (within 48 hours) to remove that stone, with the claim that the progression from edematous to necrotizing pancreatitis will be aborted. The idea has several weaknesses and limitations:

1. The differentiation of gallstone pancreatitis from other forms is often difficult. Biochemical criteria such as an elevated SGOT are helpful, but direct cholangiography (transhepatic or endoscopic) is needed to be sure.
2. Many of the cases studied have undoubtedly had only chemical hyperamylasemia (pseudo-pancreatitis) induced by the obstructing stone, not true pancreatic inflammation.
3. Other investigators have found higher complication and mortality rates among patients subjected to early biliary surgery. Because in 95 percent of cases gallstone pancreatitis subsides on medical management without progression to a fulminant form and 95 percent of the responsible common duct stones pass spontaneously in the first week, surgical intervention to remove stones within 48 hours does not seem justifiable. Cholecystectomy and, if still necessary, common duct exploration can be safely and effectively delayed until the pancreatitis subsides. It is my practice to perform the operative procedure at a later quiescent time during the same admission.

Endoscopic techniques using ERCP and sphincterotomy to remove the common duct stone early in gallstone pancreatitis are also receiving trials. Several preliminary reports suggest that sphincterotomy and clearing of stones can be accomplished safely. Many of the aforementioned limitations are applicable to this approach as well. There is also the concern about aggravating the pancreatitis if contrast is injected into the pancreatic duct during ERCP.

Final judgment about the place of this technique awaits greater experience.

MIDDLE PHASE

The middle phase of pancreatitis, beginning toward the end of the first week, is characterized by inflammatory swelling or phlegmon of the pancreas and peripancreatic tissues. Within the phlegmon, areas of ischemic and enzymatic necrosis may develop, occupying small patches or large confluent areas of the pancreas and surrounding tissues. If the necrotic areas are small, natural repair processes may be successful in healing them. Dead tissue that cannot be cleared sooner or later manifests itself by signs of inflammation and still later by superinfection. The treatment needs during this period stem from the compressing effects of the mass upon adjacent structures, the necessity of debriding necrotic tissues and draining peripancreatic fluid collections, and local vascular injury leading to hemorrhage or visceral vessel thrombosis.

Phlegmon

The pancreatic inflammatory mass, demonstrable by palpation, ultrasound, or CT scan, is treated in the same fashion as the initial phase of the attack, by withholding feedings and giving parenteral fluids. There is evidence that premature feeding may promote progression to tissue necrosis and abscess, and therefore oral feedings should not be started until pain, fever, hyperamylasemia, and leukocytosis have subsided. The phlegmon should be followed by weekly CT scan, if available, to document resolution or to detect the appearance of liquefaction necrosis. Intravenous hyperalimentation (TPN) is of great value in meeting the extraordinary caloric needs of this period. Prevention of stress ulcers by antacid therapy and H_2-blocking agents (cimetidine and raniditine) should be routine. Gastric outlet obstruction by the phlegmon may persist for weeks and, on occasion, has necessitated a gastrojejunostomy. Compression and partial obstruction of the intrapancreatic portion of the common bile duct is common, but always resolves and virtually never requires tube drainage unless there are also gallstones and cholangitis.

Necrosis

Large areas of necrosis of pancreatic and peripancreatic tissue may advertise their presence by signs of inflammation, pain and tenderness, but often remain clinically silent. CT scans are the best available means of demonstrating the lucent, liquefying regional necrosis. Large areas of necrosis should be operated upon for prophylactic debridement before infection can get established. Smaller areas can be followed unless signs of inflammation appear. When in doubt, needle aspiration under CT or ultrasound guidance can be helpful to search for evidence of infection.

Acute Pseudocyst

Fluid collections around the pancreas and in the lesser sac at this stage often represent pancreatic secretions that have leaked from the damaged gland. They are frequently associated with ongoing necrotizing pancreatitis, hemorrhage, visceral injury, and eventually abscess, and are therefore associated with a high mortality (on the order of 20%). On the other hand, acute pseudocysts also have the potential to resolve spontaneously or to evolve by encapsulation into mature pseudocysts. If the patient is stable and not exceedingly ill, it may be safe to watch acute pseudocysts in the hope of spontaneous resolution. If there are any signs of deterioration (increased tenderness, fever, tachycardia, fluid requirements, or leukocytosis), it becomes safer to operate for external drainage of the collection and debridement of necrotic tissues. The presence of semisolid necrotic tissues generally means that attempted percutaneous drainage of the fluid collection will be inadequate.

Hemorrhage

Erosion of major arterial vessels by proteolytic enzymes may produce exsanguinating hemorrhage. I have used arteriography to locate the site and to control the bleeding by embolization with considerable success in a small series of patients. Whereas my previous attempts to control this type of bleeding by surgical means alone had almost always failed, initial angiographic occlusion followed by surgical debridement succeeded in 6 of 8 patients. The angiographic control may in some cases be only partial or temporary, but it appears to provide the benefits of time and reduced blood loss that allow a more orderly and effective operation.

Thrombosis

Vessels (particularly the colic branches of the superior mesenteric artery, the splenic artery, and the gastroduodenal artery) that are exposed directly to the inflammatory process are at risk of thrombosis, perhaps because of the same enzymatic injury that causes bleeding if the vessel wall is penetrated. The resulting ischemia of bowel segments served by these arteries, most often the transverse colon and duodenum, can be manifested by gastrointestinal bleeding from sloughed mucosa, full-thickness bowel infarction, enteric fistulas, or later strictures. The value of arteriography in the detection of thrombosed visceral vessels in such a patient is not established. If bowel infarction occurs, the involved segment must be resected. It is safer under these circumstances to bring out both ends of the remaining bowel as stomas rather than to risk breakdown of an anastomosis. When the duodenum perforates, a pancreaticoduodenectomy rarely is necessary, but limited resection of the compromised duodenal wall and reconstruction with intraluminal decompression by tube is preferable when possible.

LATE PHASE

The transition from sterile necrosis, to infected necrosis, to abscess is often blurred. Infection of the necrotic tissues of the middle phase can be detected as early as the second week after onset; however, it is unusual for clinical signs heralding a pancreatic abscess to be apparent before the third week. The treatment of pancreatic abscess by antibiotics and drainage is discussed elsewhere.

PERSISTING PANCREATITIS

An occasional patient continues to have low-grade signs of pancreatic inflammation for many weeks or even several months, without focal collections or areas of necrosis demonstrable by CT scan to target for debridement or drainage. ERCP may identify irreversible injury to the pancreatic duct or underlying anomalies that do not allow the pancreatitis to subside. In other cases, there may be microabscesses or unrecognized duodenal wall injury.

Resection of the pertinent area, even if it requires pancreaticoduodenectomy, however radical that may seem, may be the only option left. Distal pancreatectomy is indicated when the pancreatic duct becomes obstructed by the necrotizing process and its healing by scar. I have resorted to pancreaticoduodenectomy for removing the head of the gland for persistent acute pancreatitis four times in the last 4 years. The operation was performed 7 to 12 weeks after the onset of the attack in these patients, and all four left the hospital within 2 to 4 weeks.

AFTER THE ATTACK

Once the patient has recovered, it is time to look with ultrasound and ERCP for remediable causes in order to prevent recurrence. Surgically treatable factors include gallstones, pancreatic cancer, ampullary stenosis, accessory papilla stenosis associated with pancreas divisum, and anomalies of the pancreaticobiliary systems (e.g., enteric duplication cysts, choledochal cysts, duodenal diverticula).

PANCREATIC ABSCESS

EDWARD L. BRADLEY III, M.D.

Pancreatic abscess has remained a clinical problem ever since its modern description in 1887. Despite significant advances in perioperative care, morbidity and mortality have not changed significantly over the intervening years.

PATHOGENESIS

Pancreatic abscess has been described in association with trauma, surgery, and miscellaneous diseases and metabolic disorders. However, the vast majority of cases are recognized as being associated with an attack of necrotizing pancreatitis. Several workers have estimated the frequency of development to be 5 percent of all patients with acute pancreatitis. However, it is clear that the risk of abscess formation increases with the severity of the underlying pancreatitis. Because of this relative infrequency, it has been difficult to acquire extensive individual experience or to conduct definitive therapeutic trials.

Although not conclusively demonstrated, it is presumed that the pathogenesis of pancreatic abscess begins with pancreatic and/or peripancreatic necrosis, and not as a primary pancreatic infection. According to this theory, in patients with more virulent forms of pancreatitis, blood flow in the pancreatic microcirculation is severely diminished. This results in parenchymal ischemia and eventual necrosis. In this view, infection is an opportunistic secondary process.

As three quarters of the organisms recovered from pancreatic abscesses are gram-negative, it is likely that transmigration of coliform bacteria serves as the source of the secondary infection. Such transmigration could occur as a result of the release of inflammatory peptides and other vasoactive materials from the contiguous necrotic pancreas. The role of anaerobic bacteria in pancreatic abscess has been controversial. Although I have found significant anaerobic involvement in seven of 22 recent patients, in the past it was not believed that these organisms played any role in pathogenesis. As more reliable methods for recovery of anaerobic bacteria become widely available, this question may be resolved.

PATHOLOGY

In contrast to an infected pseudocyst with its thick walls, a pancreatic abscess without demonstrable walls is often poorly localized and is characterized by its extensive invasive nature. Pancreatic abscesses frequently track far from their peripancreatic origin. Most notable in this regard are the frequent extensions to the colic flexures and down the right and left retrocolic gutters. Furthermore, pancreatic abscesses are multiple in approximately 30 percent of cases. These observations must be taken into account when selecting the type and scope of drainage. Another distinction separating pancreatic abscess from an infected pseudocyst is the nature of the associated fluid. In an infected pseudocyst, there are large amounts of fluid that is often purulent. In a pancreatic abscess, however, the fluid is scant and usually grey and turbid (''dishwater''). Finally, as opposed to an infected pseudocyst, there is a great deal of necrotic tissue present in a pancreatic abscess. Since the tissue is necrotic, it is often difficult to state with certainty at exploration whether the tissue represents pancreas or peripancreatic fat. Occasionally, it is possible to make this distinction bu observing preserved reticulin fibers in the case of necrotic pancreas. In such cases the necrotic pancreas is grey and of a putty-like consistency, interlaced with fine black reticulin fibers resembling hairs. This appearance has been likened to the material recovered from shower drains (''hair ball'').

It is important to make this distinction between an infected pseudocyst and a pancreatic abscess because of the nature of the drainage required. Infected pseudocysts respond to simple external drainage, and death rarely results. Pancreatic abscesses, on the other hand, do not respond well to such simple measures (to be discussed). This therapeutic distinction has not received adequate emphasis in the past and probably accounts for conflicting published data regarding therapy.

Parenthetically, it is likely that pancreatic ''abscess'' is a misnomer in the classic sense. However, as long as clinical decisions are not based on finding a classic abscess in these patients, there seems to be little harm in retaining the term.

CLINICAL PRESENTATION

Pancreatic abscess commonly presents in one of two fashions: early and delayed. In the early type (10% to 15% of cases), the patient presents with fulminant pancreatitis, and pancreatic abscess is suspected on the basis of the extreme prostration, tachycardia in spite of adequate volume replacement as determined by pulmonary artery pressures, and high spiking fevers. In this type, a full-blown abscess may be present by the end of the first week of illness. This presentation is less common than the delayed type, but, because of the fulminant nature of the underlying pancreatitis, carries a higher mortality rate.

In the delayed type, the patient is classically admitted with severe pancreatitis, but responds initially to resuscitative measures. Often the patient appears to improve only to a certain level, and then 2 to 3 weeks after onset, begins to show evidence of sepsis. Tachycardia in the face of adequate volume replacement and pronounced leukocytosis are early predictors of abscess formation in this setting. However, any patient with acute pancreatitis who fails to recover within one week should be suspected of having pancreatic abscess.

DIAGNOSIS

Although clinical suspicion is a prerequisite for initiating a diagnostic program, operative therapy is best founded upon an objective demonstration of the pancreatic abscess. Prior to the widespread employment of computerized abdominal tomography, exploratory surgery was undertaken, in many cases, on the basis of a combination of clinical suspicion and such indirect signs as displacement of the barium-filled stomach. As a consequence, many patients with pancreatic phlegmon underwent unnecessary exploration. Indirect radiographic findings, such as renal displacement on intravenous pyelography and extraintestinal retroperitoneal gas formation (''soap bubble sign''), have limited roles in current diagnosis. Ultrasonography, although highly accurate in the diagnosis of pseudocysts, has not achieved a similar accuracy in discriminiating pancreatic abscesses. It is likely that the demonstrated deficiency is due to the specific gravity of the tissue of interest, i.e., the specific gravity of pseudocyst fluid is sufficiently different from the surrounding tissues to permit discrimination, whereas the necrotic tissue in a pancreatic abscess is not. In any case, as many as 30 percent of cases will not be diagnosed by sonography, and therefore ultrasonography should not be considered definitive.

Computerized abdominal tomograpy has become the primary method for this objective demonstration of pancreatic abscess. It is highly effective in distinguishing between pancreatic phlegmon, abscess, and pseudocyst (greater than 90% accuracy). Recently, additional encouraging data have appeared which suggest that contrast-enhanced computerized tomography can depict pancreatic necrosis with an even higher degree of accuracy (greater than 95%). With this technique, failure to visualize a segment of pancreatic tissue when intravenous contrast has been given is presumptive evidence of interruption of the pancreatic microcirculation and necrosis. At the time of this writing, I have had experience with two cases in which contrast-enhanced tomography was helpful. Further work is needed in this area.

Mention should also be made of the serial monitoring of serum ribonuclease as a marker of pancreatic necrosis. Clinical trials await the development of a rapid assay for ribonuclease and demonstration of specificity for pancreatic necrosis in humans.

Despite some recommendations to the contrary, the diagnosis and treatment of pancreatic abscess should not be withheld until a positive blood culture is obtained. In a careful review of reported cases, only half the surgically demonstrated cases had a positive blood culture prior to surgery. Accordingly, the blood culture should be primarily used to adjust antibiotic therapy.

Finally, considerable current attention is being focused on Gram stains of peripancreatic fluid obtained by guided transcutaneous needle aspiration. This procedure has been advocated to distinguish between pancreatic abscess and phlegmon, in that a pancreatic phlegmon represents a noninfected inflammatory mass. However, despite early impressive reports of accuracy, the intrinsic risks of potentially converting a phlegmon into an abscess by colonic perforation have not been established. Accordingly, it is my feeling that this procedure should be reserved for those 10 percent of cases that will not be identified by computed tomography. In the clinical setting, this situation would arise when the clinical suspicion for pancreatic abscess remains high despite a negative CT scan.

PREVENTION

Some evidence exists to suggest that premature institution of oral feeding in patients with severe pancreatitis may increase the likelihood of abscess formation. Proscribing any oral intake until all signs of inflammation have disappeared may therefore be the key to prevention.

The role of antibiotics in the prevention of pancreatic abscess has been controversial. Although three randomized studies have not shown that prophylactic antibiotics administered to patients with acute pancreatitis altered the incidence of abscess formtion, the conclusion is subject to question because (1) only a small number of patients were present in each study, and for a condition that is present in only 5 percent of such patients, many more patients would be required for meaningful analysis; (2) each of the three studies dealt only with mild or moderate alcoholic pancreatitis, whereas we need information in patients with severe pancreatitis, those more likely to develop pancreatic abscess, and in patients with nonalcoholic pancreatitis; and (3) most importantly, each of the studies used ampicillin, an agent that has subsequently been shown not to enter either pancreatic parenchyma or pancreatic juice.

Primarily because of the suspected pathogenesis of pancreatic abscess and in the absence of evidence to the contrary, I continue to advocate prophylactic antibiotics for patients with severe pancreatitis (three or more Ranson signs). Currently, I use tobramycin, 3 mg per kilogram per day, since it has been demonstrated in the pancreas, and clindamycin, 2.4 g per day, since I have demonstrated anaerobes in one-third of my recent cases. Further studies will address the wisdom of these recommendations.

A short comment is appropriate here regarding the importance of adequate fluid resuscitation in patients with severe pancreatitis. As much as one-third of the circulating plasma volume may be "third-spaced" by circulating inflammatory agents. Systemic hypovolemia leads to splanchnic vasoconstriction with resultant inadequate microcirculatory flow and pancreatic ischemia. Adequate fluid replacement, as determined by pulmonary artery pressure, may well be the single most important measure for the prevention of pancreatic abscess.

Since stress ulceration, respiratory insufficiency, and renal failure are common causes of death in severe acute pancreatitis, their appearance should be anticipated and steps taken to prevent their development. Gastric pH should be kept greater than 4 by a combination of ranitidine and antacids in an effort to prevent stress ulceration. The combination of these agents has proved to be more effective than either alone. Serial monitoring of blood gases exposes insidious hypoxia and determines the need for ventilatory support. Volume replacement is the key to the prevention of renal failure and should be

monitored by pulmonary artery pressures in these severly ill patients. Three to four thousand calories a day are required for maintenance in these patients. In order to avoid pancreatic stimulation, calories are best supplied by intravenous hyperalimentation until all signs of inflammation have disappeared.

TREATMENT

For the past several decades, debridement and closed drainage have been accepted as the optimum form of surgical therapy. What little discussion has arisen seems to have surrounded the specific type of drain employed. However, three large retrospective studies independently concluded that the specific type of drain employed was not a determinant of results. Furthermore, operative mortality has continued to be excessive, ranging from 30 to 60 percent in centers specializing in pancreatic disease regardless of the type of drain. Since surgical drainage is highly effective in relieving other forms of localized sepsis, it is apparent that some features of pancreatic abscess differ from those of other infections. Careful analysis of published case reports support three factors as being primarily responsible for the unacceptably high surgical mortality rates: (1) the diagnosis of pancreatic abscess is frequently delayed and the process is often advanced when first recognized, (2) recurrence or persistence of sepsis after standard debridement and closed drainage occurs in 40 to 50 percent of cases, and is accountable for 80 percent of deaths, and (3) life-threatening complications, such as hemorrhage or intestinal fistulization, are frequent. With such considerations in mind, it seems prudent to examine alternative approaches to standard drainage, in an attempt to improve these unsatisfactory results.

Open Drainage

In 22 patients with pancreatic abscess, identified with impressive accuracy by serial abdominal tomography, the necrotic retroperitoneum was exposed by a transabdominal approach through the gastrocolic omentum. Necrotic tissue was removed by finger dissection (sequestrectomy) and cultured for aerobes and anaerobes. Because of the widespread nature of pancreatic abscess, exposure of the retropancreatic region and both colic flexures was routine. Nonadherent adaptic gauze was placed over the stomach, colon, and any exposed vessels. Dry lap pads were introduced into the depths of the wound. Loosely approximated stay sutures over the lap pads prevented evisceration until intestinal adherence developed. Packing was changed under light general anesthesia every 2 to 3 days. The amount of additional necrotic material encountered during these serial dressing changes was striking. After three or four such dressing changes, the process was carried out under intravenous analgesia on the ward. Wounds were left open to heal by secondary intention. Nutrition was provided by intravenous hyperalimentation. The average length of hospitalization was 76 days.

Nineteen of the 22 patients treated by open packing survived (86%). The mortality rate from this method of management compares favorably with that from closed drainage. No patient experienced persistent or recurrent sepsis.

There were 44 complications in these 22 patients, attesting to the underlying severity of the pancreatitis (average number of Ranson signs, 5.6). In addition to the general complications, there were procedure-specific complications. Two of the three deaths in this series were related to alimentation. One patient died from air embolism from a disrupted subclavian catheter. Another patient expired from the complications of aspiration when oral feedings were begun. The third death occurred in an 85-year-old woman with autopsy-proven myocardial infarction.

Somewhat surprisingly, only 6 of 19 survivors have required a subsequent incisional herniorrhaphy. Other procedure-specific complications included a small bowel fistula secondary to pressure erosion from Marlex following an ill-advised attempt, early in our experience, to hasten wound closure. Another patient experienced massive venous bleeding from an exposed superior mesenteric vein and this was controlled with great difficulty. A pancreatic fistula was present in 10 of the 22 cases. Spontaneous closure of the fistula occurred in all 10 patients.

The marked improvement in these results compared to the results of conventional closed drainage can be attributed to several factors: (1) earlier diagnosis and exploration as a result of serial tomography, (2) elimination of sepsis and prevention of recurrence by open drainage and mandatory packing changes, and (3) anticipation and prevention of frequently associated complications. Of some interest is the observation that seven of the 22 patients had positive cultures for anaerobes in addition to gram-negative bacteria. It is uncertain what role agents effective against anaerobes might have played in addition to eliminating or reducing anaerobic conditions by open drainage. As is the practice in the treatment of other abscesses with systemic sepsis, antibiotics should be discontinued when local wound control is obtained.

The potential seriousness of specific complications of open drainage, such as massive hemorrhage from exposed vessels, should limit the use of this procedure to abscesses of extensive nature. Should a small localized abscess be found, conventional closed drainage may be appropriate. In the event of massive hemorrhage, angiographic embolization may represent a valuable option if local control proves difficult.

Transcutaneous drainage of pancreatic abscesses via guided techniques is mentioned only to discourage its use as primary therapy. Pancreatic abscess differs from other abscesses in the formation of particulate necrotic debris. Such debris, even for 12 to 14 F catheters, is difficult to remove from the abdomen. As expected, results of transcutaneous drainage of pancreatic abscesses via radiologic techniques have been poor. These techniques are best employed in elderly or poor-risk patients.

PANCREATIC PSEUDOCYST

DAVID L. BOUWMAN, M.D., F.A.C.S.

The term "pancreatic pseudocyst" was coined in Germany in the nineteenth century to complete the taxonomic classification of cysts of the pancreas. It initially addressed the phenomenon of fluid collections in the lesser peritoneal sac following blunt trauma to the pancreas. At present the term is applied to organized collections of pancreatic exocrine secretions, lying in or adjacent to the pancreas, with walls consisting of fibrous tissue and with a connection to the pancreatic duct. The cause of a pancreatic pseudocyst is ductal disruption as the result of pancreatitis, either acute, with autodigestion of the gland including the duct wall, or chronic, with proximal stricture and distal blowout of the duct. Less commonly, trauma injuring the duct is the cause.

Pancreatic pseudocysts may be acute or chronic. Alternatively, pseudocysts may be classified as asymptomatic or symptomatic. Each method of classification has significance for therapeutic choices.

ACUTE PSEUDOCYSTS

Acute pseudocysts appear in conjunction with episodes of acute pancreatitis, whereas chronic pseudocysts occur in an isolated fashion in patients with no identifiable acute pancreatitis. The incidence of cystic masses occurring in or near the pancreas in conjunction with pancreatitis is rising as routine ultrasound examination of patients with acute pancreatitis reveals large numbers of previously unrecognized pancreatic and peripancreatic collections. Several important questions may be asked.

First, how many of these newly observed collections are actually acute pseudocysts? These collections might alternatively represent simple tissue edema of the peripancreatic retroperitoneal structures, edematous pancreatic tissue (the so called pancreatic phlegmon), pancreatic abscess, or necrotic pancreas. On occasion the question may be resolved by use of the older clinical criteria indicative of the presence of a pseudocyst: unresolving pancreatitis, continued hyperamylasemia, abdominal mass on palpation, or anterior displacement of the stomach on barium studies. The collections, which are abscesses or necrotic sequestrations, become self evident; however, the identity of many of these collections remains unknown as most of them are seen to have resolved on serial ultrasonographic studies.

Since we know that young or early pseudocysts, less than 6 weeks old, are associated with a high incidence of spontaneous resolution, it is possible that many of these ultrasonographically defined collections that resolve are even younger acute pseudocysts. We do not understand the pressure, secretion, absorption, and ductal resistance parameters that initiate or maintain pseudocyst formation. Many cysts are demonstrated by ERCP to be in free connection with pancreatic ducts that appear to empty easily into the duodenum, and yet the cyst space persists as a result of preferential secretion into it via the ductal connection. It appears that the dynamics that induce an acute pseudocyst initially fluctuate. Only when conditions persistently maintain appropriate fluxes of secretion do pseudocysts persist and mature.

What should be our therapeutic approach toward the collection that might be an acute pseudocyst? It is prudent to observe all pseudocysts for 6 weeks before surgical intervention because a minimum of 40 percent of these cysts do resolve. Duration is associated with persistence; after 6 weeks, pseudocyst resorption becomes rare. Procrastination beyond 6 weeks is dangerous because the incidence of complications rises sharply after this period if no therapeutic intervention is undertaken.

Size is also associated with persistence and progression. Five centimeters have been observed to be the significant size above which cysts persist and are likely to become symptomatic or to develop complications. Persistent ultrasonographic evidence of a peripancreatic collection following resolution of all symptoms in a patient who has suffered acute pancreatitis does not warrant inpatient observation for 6 weeks. Rather, outpatient follow-up with ultrasound surveillance of collection size is indicated at 2-week intervals for as long as the patient is asymptomatic. Development of symptoms, progression of size, or attainment of 6 weeks of age indicates a need for intervention. Persistence of collections 5 cm or less in diameter is an indication for continued follow-up even past 6 weeks as these cysts are expected to resolve.

In patients presenting with acute pancreatitis in whom an acute pseudocyst is suspected, ultrasound is the standard mode of diagnosis. CT scanning should be reserved for patients with equivocal findings or for cases in which even repeat ultrasonographic examination proves to be a technically inadequate study. ERCP is not warranted as a primary diagnostic modality, but should be used for diagnosis when continued symptoms that suggest a pseudocyst exist despite an inability of ultrasound or CT scanning to delineate a cyst.

CHRONIC PSEUDOCYSTS

The majority of chronic pseudocysts, discovered in patients who have no identifiable acute pancreatitis, come to attention because they have become symptomatic. Symptoms include abdominal pain, abdominal swelling, and weight loss. The initial symptoms may also be due to the onset of complications and include peritonitis, obstructive jaundice, gastrointestinal bleeding, or signs of high bowel obstruction. Prolonged observation should not be undertaken to ensure cyst wall maturity. Risks of complications in symptomatic pseudocysts are high enough to warrant immediate intervention. A more leisurely intervention is indicated in incidentally discovered asymptomatic chronic pseudocysts.

Because of the potential difficulty in locating cysts and the possibility of multiple cysts, preoperative ERCP in patients undergoing elective intervention is a valuable guide when available. In the hands of expert, persistent endoscopists, more than 80 percent of pseudocysts can be directly visualized by introduction of contrast medium through communicating ducts. The detailed anatomic road map allows the surgeon additional information in planning his procedure. Use of antibiotics and apropriate technique limits the incidence of infection. ERCP should be performed within 48 hours of the planned surgical procedure.

OPERATIVE THERAPY: INTERNAL VERSUS EXTERNAL DRAINAGE

Internal drainage appears to be the procedure of choice in the operative management of pseudocysts. Functionally, drainage, whether internal or external, tips the dynamics of the situation in favor of cyst resolution by promoting cyst emptying. Since the pseudocyst has no epithelial lining, early obliteration of the cyst by adherence of its walls is the rule after drainage. External drainage has the disadvantage of being temporary, whether accomplished by open operative drainage or by closed percutaneous drainage by CT-guided percutaneous insertion of catheters; as a result, recurrence is common after cessation of external drainage as underlying dynamics reassert themselves. Permanent resolution of cysts following external drainage does not occur with the predictability with which it is achieved after internal drainage, implying that drainage tracts persist after internal drainage procedures.

Internal Drainage

Internal drainage is achieved by the most propitious route at the time of laparotomy. It requires a mature fibrous capsule. The 6 weeks of observation of pseudocysts in the acute situation is also an adequate interval for assuring a mature capsule. It is critical at the time of the operation that the cyst be accurately localized by needle aspiration before incision of its suspected wall, regardless of which procedure is being performed. Under no circumstances should the needle be removed after successful aspiration of the cyst; deflation of small cysts and removal of the needle before incision has resulted in an inability to re-enter the cyst on more than one occasion.

Cystgastrostomy. Because many pseudocysts occur in the lesser sac with incorporation of the posterior wall of the stomach into the organizing anterior wall of the cyst, transgastric incision of the posterior wall of the stomach is a convenient drainage mechanism. Tight adherence of pseudocyst to the stomach must be present, and the cystgastrostomy must be of adequate size. Positioning the opening as low as possible on the shared wall prevents a pocketing effect. Hemostasis of the cut surfaces must be absolute and is best accomplished by a running suture of an absorbable noncatgut suture, such as 3–0 Vicryl.

Cystduodenostomy. A less common analogous situation may occur when a pseudocyst in the head of the pancreas shares a wall with the duodenum. In this situation, a transduodenal cystduodenostomy may be performed. Special care must be taken to avoid interference with the intrapancreatic bile duct. Avoidance of the pancreaticoduodenal arterial arcades is also required. Again, complete hemostasis must be achieved along with an adequate opening between cyst and duodenal lumens. Both cystgastrostomy and cystduodenostomy have the advantage that no potentially leaky anastomosis to the cyst wall is performed.

Cystjejunostomy. When neither cystogastrostomy nor cystduodenostomy is possible, construction of a Roux-en-Y jejunal limb with cystjejunostomy to the jejunal limb by a careful two-layer interrupted anastomosis is the treatment of choice. I prefer a running 3–0 Vicryl inner layer with interrupted 3–0 silk for the outer layer.

External Drainage

The contraindications to internal drainage are the main indications for external drainage. When an immature cyst wall inadequate for a secure anastomosis is discovered at the time of operation for acute or, more rarely, chronic pseudocysts, external drainage is required. Drainage should be carried out via large-bore catheters to afford low resistance; catheters should remain in place as long as drainage occurs. Occasionally marsupialization of a cyst is possible, but the required mature wall also makes these pseudocysts excellent candidates for internal drainage if they are not infected.

Attempts to internally drain infected pseudocysts have resulted in sepsis, anastomotic breakdown, and death. Infected pseudocysts should always be externally drained. If an infected pseudocyst or pancreatic abscess is suspected preoperatively, a trial of percutaneous CT-guided catheter drainage is indicated. Percutaneous CT-guided catheter drainage is also indicated for patients with symptomatic pseudocysts who are prohibitive operative risks. Pseudocysts that do not communicate with the duct on ERCP and amylase-poor pseudocysts are probably also suited for a trial of transcutaneous drainage as they represent inactive cysts that may well be permanently resolved by the temporary drainage afforded by such a maneuver. At this time, data are accumulating that may establish a more central role for percutaneous drainage, but the high recurrence rates reported at present must first be overcome. Unavailability or failure of response following establishment of percutaneous drainage of an infected pseudocyst indicates a need for open external drainage.

RESECTION

Resection of pseudocysts has been advocated but is seldom indicated. Cysts that have burrowed into the omentum, transverse mesocolon, and the colon itself with large inflammatory masses may require resection, and occasionally a well-circumscribed pseudocyst in the distal pancreas invites resection. In most reported series, morbidity and mortality are higher for patients who undergo resection. Although this may be the result of selection of higher-risk patients in whom more advanced disease permitted no alternative, the recognized technical difficulties in dealing with the inflamed tissues of the cyst wall and adjacent pancreas makes it likely that resection itself is the source of the added morbidity. There is no question that successful resection is associated with the lowest recurrence rate of pseudocysts when comparing operative measures.

COMPLICATIONS

Complications of pseudocysts with significant morbidity and mortality include rupture, infection, bleeding, and obstruction of hollow organs. Rupture of a pseudocyst into the free peritoneal cavity results in acute peritonitis with cardiovascular collapse. Immediate resuscitation and operative intervention are required for any hope of salvage. Cystjejunostomy at the point of rupture may be possible in stable cases treated early, but patients in whom treatment was delayed or patients with shock and organ failure should undergo external drainage. Slow leaks result in pancreatic ascites and are addressed in chapter 62. Spontaneous resolution of pseudocysts has been reported via rupture into a viscus. When the stomach is involved, all may go well. Involvement of the colon has been reported with complications. In all instances, bleeding and sepsis from incomplete drainage and bacterial contamination are to be suspected.

Bleeding may take the form of a contained pseudoaneurysm or may present as upper gastrointestinal hemorrhage of occult origin as blood periodically issues from the ampulla of Vater. In patients with pseudocysts who are bleeding, preoperative arteriography is invaluable to establish the site of bleeding, to define vascular anatomy, and to aid in selecting the best intervention. Approaches to the bleeding vessel may include ligature external to the pseudocyst at both sides, ligature of the vessel through the opened cyst, or resection if no alternative exists to achieve hemostasis.

If obstructive jaundice occurs in the setting of a pseudocyst, distorting the head of the pancreas, drainage of the pseudocyst should precede any decision to drain the duct. Intraoperative cholangiography to demonstrate free flow of bile into the duodenum after decompression of the cyst may avoid the need for choledochoenterostomy. On the other hand, continued fibrotic stricture of the intrapancreatic duct secondary to chronic pancreatitis may result in continued obstruction, in which case ductal decompression is indicated.

Failure to recognize and drain all pseudocysts present in a patient with multiple cysts is a recognized cause of inadequate results. Adequate drainage may require multiple cystenterostomies or cystocystostomies between adjacent pseudocysts to create confluent cavities that may be drained by a single cystenterostomy.

PANCREATIC ASCITES AND PANCREATIC PLEURAL EFFUSIONS

ALEXANDER J. WALT, M.B., Ch.B., F.R.C.S.(Eng.), F.R.C.S.(C), F.A.C.S.

By convention, pancreatic ascites is defined as the presence in the peritoneal cavity of a substantial volume of fluid characterized by a serum protein level greater than 2.5 g per deciliter and an abnormally raised amylase content often measuring tens of thousands of units per deciliter. Transient peripancreatic collections of fluid in the early weeks of acute pancreatitis and the fluid associated with pancreatic malignant tumors do not qualify under this definition. The rare clinical picture of acute abdominal pain associated with a sudden rupture of a pseudocyst, in which the patient may present in shock, is also not customarily included under the rubric of pancreatic ascites.

Similarly, pancreatic pleural effusion (PPE) is the presence in one or both pleural cavities of fluid with a protein level greater than 2.5 per deciliter and abnormally high levels of amylase. This pancreatic pleural effusion associated with a leak of pancreatic juice from the pancreas should be distinguished from the sympathetic pleural effusion so often associated with acute pancreatitis. The leakage can be demonstrated to originate from a pancreatic pseudocyst in about 80 percent of patients and from the main pancreatic duct in about 10 percent, but the source is indeterminate in the remaining 10 percent. When the leakage occurs anteriorly into the lesser sac and thence into the peritoneal cavity, pancreatic ascites results. In contrast, when the leak is posterior, the fluid may track cephalad through the aortic or esophageal openings of the

FOLLOW-UP

Even adequate internal drainage of a pseudocyst addresses only the peculiar circumstances that caused that particular cyst. Underlying pancreatic disease is likely to reproduce the same dynamics that created the first pseudocyst and to result in the occurrence of additional cysts. Prolonged follow-up, with attention to symptoms and restudy of the pancreas as necessary, is advisable.

diaphragm into the mediastinum, from which the fluid may break through into one or both pleural cavities. A chronic fistula may then form which perpetuates the lesion of pancreatic pleural effusion (PPE). Rarely, a pancreatic pseudocyst may rupture directly through the diaphragm into a pleural cavity.

Alcoholic pancreatitis is the forerunner of the pancreatic leak in 95 percent of patients by virtue of the ductal changes that it causes and consequent loss of integrity of the ductal wall. In many patients, stenoses of the main duct also may be present as well as concomitant multiple pancreatic pseudocysts. These pseudocysts may not be obvious even on a good pancreatogram owing to the presence of proximal blockage or to rapid dilution of the escaping contrast material. Consequently, a thorough exposure of the entire pancreatic region is essential at the time of laparotomy. In less than 5 percent of patients, and always in children with pancreatic ascites, trauma is responsible for the leak. Many weeks may elapse between the time of injury and the clinical appearance of abdominal fluid.

The presence of intraperitoneal pancreatic juice may have a marked effect on the peritoneum even though the pancreatic enzymes are not activated and no obvious infection is present. The net result, however, is the production of a large volume of fluid rich in protein and, in many cases, a carpeting of the peritoneum with layers of thick fibrin. The color and consistency of the fluid varies. The fluid may be yellowish, brownish, or even bloody, thin or thick, clear or turbid.

CLINICAL FEATURES

In a series of 256 pseudocysts of the pancreas treated at the Wayne State University affiliated hospitals, 42 patients (16.4%) had pancreatic ascites and/or pancreatic pleural effusion. The mean age was 46 years (range 22 to 55), all were alcoholics, and most had been previously hospitalized for pancreatitis. In many, however, years may have elapsed since the last overt attack of pancreatitis. Although about 10 percent of the patients had associated cholelithiasis, calculous pancreatitis does not cause pancreatic ascites. A significant number of patients developed recurrent attacks of acute pancreatitis following successful surgical treatment of their pancreatic ascites.

Almost invariably, these patients present with marked abdominal fluid distention (Table 1). Volumes as large as 16 liters have been measured at operation. Acute pain is not a feature, but 36 of our 42 patients complained of substantial discomfort characterized by a sense of pressure and, in some, a low-grade pain in the back. Tachypnea due to the raised diaphragm and a decreased tidal volume was common. Nausea and vomiting was noted in almost 50 percent. Considerable weight loss, to the point of cachexia in a few patients, occurs in about 30 percent of cases, even in the presence of excessive fluid collection. This loss of lean body mass should not be underestimated.

In patients with PPE, the pulmonary symptoms dominate. Although these patients are also alcoholic, on occasion absolutely no history of previous pancreatitis may be obtainable. Shortness of breath, cough, and chest pain due to the often large effusion are frequently the primary complaints. Following an ostensibly complete thoracentesis, rapid reaccumulation usually occurs. Unless the fluid is measured for protein and amylase, the effusion may be incorrectly attributed to pneumonia, tuberculosis, or other pulmonary disease. The pancreatic effusion is unilateral in about 50 percent and bilateral in the other half. The side of the effusion may not correspond to the side of the pancreas on which the pancreatic pseudocyst or ductal leakage is situated. Seventeen of our 42 patients (40.5%) with pancreatic ascites had concomitant pancreatic pleural effusions. In the Johns Hopkins series, isolated pancreatic pleural effusion was more commonly encountered.

DIAGNOSIS

Awareness of the entities of pancreatic ascites and PPE (the possibility should be considered in all alcoholics) leads to rapid diagnosis by the simple expedient of requesting protein and amylase measurements on both

TABLE 1   Clinical Presentation of Pancreatic Ascites

	No. Patients	%
Abdominal distention and ascites	42	100
Abdominal discomfort/pain	36	86
Anorexia, nausea, vomiting	30	71
Back pain	19	45
Weight loss (>4 kg)	18	43
Fever	7	17
Diarrhea	5	12

ascitic and pleural fluid. In contrast to the low levels of amylase and protein in the ascites associated with cirrhosis (the most common diagnosis causing confusion), the albumin is greater than 2.5 g per deciliter and the amylase is abnormally, and often markedly, raised. These simple measurements provide a conclusive diagnosis. In addition, in most but not in all patients, the serum amylase is raised. This elevation is due to absorption of the enzyme rather than a reflection of any underlying pancreatitis. In fact, reversion of serum amylase levels toward normal may be regarded as indirect evidence of regression of any pancreatic ascites and serves as indirect clinical evidence of successful medical treatment. Furthermore, since the peritoneal and pleural cavities serve as incubators for the leaking amylase, the presence of pancreatic isoenzymes (''old amylase'') are striking in both the serum and the peritoneal and pleural fluid. Measurement of ascitic lipase has also been advocated as a diagnostic index, but lipase measurement is more difficult, expensive, slower, less reliable, and unnecessary.

Upper gastrointestinal series, ultrasonography, and CT scans are of little value because of the small size of any causative pseudocyst and the presence of the large quantity of fluid.

PANCREATIC ASCITES

In the early years after pancreatic ascites was first described in 1952 and pancreatic pleural effusion in 1972, controversy existed about the timing and details of medical as opposed to surgical treatment of these patients. As the natural history and basic pathologic and anatomic nature of the lesion became understood, a reasonably standardized approach has evolved.

Initial Nonoperative Management

In 25 to 45 percent of patients, the pancreatic ascites and/or PPE regress spontaneously on conservative treatment. Medical management consists of (1) reduction of pancreatic secretion, (2) removal of ascites or pleural effusion by repeated paracentesis or thoracentesis, (3) replacement of protein and restoration of lean body mass by total parenteral nutrition (TPN). Pancreatic secretion is reduced by nasogastric suction and avoidance of oral feeding. Although Diamox, atropine, and glucagon have been advocated as agents for inhibiting pancreatic secretion, there are no hard clinical data to support their use in pancreatic ascites. The mortality rate for medical treatment has been about 20 percent in most series, but has fallen since the introduction of TPN and better metabolic care. Most patients who are going to respond to repeated paracentesis by spontaneously sealing the leak show reduction in the reaccumulation of fluid within 7 to 10 days. Paracentesis may be necessary every day or two initially, and great care must be exercised to avoid the introduction of infection. Few patients who have not sealed after 3 weeks can be expected to benefit from the costly, tedious, and increasingly hazardous medical therapy associated with continuing TPN and potential sepsis (Table 2).

If ascites persists after 3 weeks, I favor surgical intervention. By this time, negative nitrogen balance is substantially improved. Operation is routinely preceded by endoscopic retrograde pancreatography (ERP). Thorough paracentesis to make the patient more comfortable in the radiology suite and to improve the quality of the ductal imaging is performed. ERP is done within 24 hours of the projected time of operation. With gentamicin given systemically and also added to the contrast material, no sepsis has occurred in the 17 patients with pancreatic ascites who have undergone ERP in our series. Morbidity and mortality of operation has been greatly reduced since these ductal road maps have become available, and the recurrence of postoperative pancreatic ascites has fallen from a pre-1975 level of 50 percent to 0 percent since pancreatography was introduced as a routine. It needs to be re-emphasized that the pancreatogram may be deceptive in pancreatic ascites as the fluid may dissipate through the site of the leak so rapidly that a pancreatic pseudocyst may not be visualized. Nevertheless, ERP is invaluable as it usually pinpoints the site of the lesion, shortens operative time, makes operation safer, obviates the need to open the duodenum for an intraoperative pancreatogram, and ultimately results in less extensive exploration and a more logical and definitive operative procedure.

Operation

Fortunately, the site of leakage is often found to be situated disproportionately in the tail and left side of the body of the pancreas. In the 80 percent of patients in whom a pancreatic pseudocyst is present, the cyst is small, having decompressed itself into the peritoneal or pleural cavity. Increasingly, I have elected to treat pancreatic ascites definitively by resection of the distal pancreas, incorporating the leaking site of ductal leakage or leaking pseudocyst. If pancreatography has shown evidence of any stricture in the proximal pancreatic duct, a Roux-en-Y loop is placed over the transected end of the pancreas. If the proximal duct is not strictured, the pancreatic duct is suture-ligated and the transected pancreas is closed in a fishmouth manner with a series of nonabsorbable mattress sutures. Some surgeons have advocated the use of staples when the pancreas is sufficiently pliable.

If for any reason the foregoing approach is not desirable or is not feasible, as is the case when the leak is situated in the head of the pancreas, making resection obviously unjustifiable, a Roux-en-Y loop is tacked around the site of leakage. Previous reaction to the leaking fluid produces sufficient fibrosis to give good purchase to the intestinal sutures. Cystogastrostomy is not favored as most pseudocysts are small, and I, as well as others, have observed an unacceptable number of complications with this procedure when it is used to treat pancreatic ascites.

In a small minority of patients, the site of leakage may not be known or may not be visible at the time of laparotomy. The administration of intraoperative secretin may be helpful in determining the source. In a series of 13 patients in whom a laparotomy was done without any definitive treatment being carried out or in whom only external drainage was performed, four patients had no further difficulties, five reaccumulated fluid (one with an associated pancreatic pseudocyst), and four developed pancreatic pseudocysts without ascites.

Miscellaneous Approaches

Irradiation to the pancreas (500 to 600 rads) has been reported as successful in sealing the duct and eliminating the ascites. Irradiation has long been known to inhibit pancreatic secretion temporarily, but its efficacy in pancreatic ascites is difficult to assess as the few patients treated in this manner have also had concomitant TPN. Although transient diarrhea may be a side effect, irradiation bears consideration in patients unresponsive to medical treatment for whom surgery is contraindicated.

The use of a peritoneovenous (LeVeen) shunt has also been reported. In the single patient whom we have treated in this manner after he refused operation, the ascites had not reaccumulated at the time of death from unrelated causes one year later.

PANCREATIC PLEURAL EFFUSION

Nonoperative Management

As the pleural effusion originates from a pancreatic source, the general principles underlying management are similar to those for pancreatic ascites. A nasogastric tube is placed and pancreatic secretion diminished by TPN.

TABLE 2   Management of Patients with Pancreatic Ascites and Pancreatic Pleural Effusions*

Nonoperative Management
  Intravenous hyperalimentation
  NPO
  Nasogastric suction
  Diamox, atropine, glucagon (optional)
  Paracenteses
  Thoracentesis or chest tube

Operative Management
  Direct duct leak
    Roux-en-Y drainage of duct leak
    Pancreatic resection if duct leak is distal
    Roux-en-Y drainage of remnant if proximal duct disease
      is present
  Pseudocyst
    Roux-en-Y drainage of pseudocyst leak
    Cytogastrostomy if Roux-en-Y not possible
    Resect cyst if small and distal
    Roux-en-Y drainage of remnant if proximal duct disease
      is present

* Courtesy of John L. Cameron, M.D.

The pleural fluid is drained by a thoracostomy tube carefully placed and cared for to avoid infection. With expansion of the lung and presumably occlusion of the peritoneopleural fistula by fibrin or inflammatory products, spontaneous disappearance of the effusion occurs in 25 to 40 percent of patients. In those in whom this does not occur within 2 to 3 weeks, a laparotomy preceded by ERP is advisable, followed by a direct attack on the pancreatic lesion within 24 hours. Although the instillation of contrast material directly into the pleural cavity may delineate the fistulous track through and below the diaphragm, ERP is more reliable.

Operative Management

Success in eliminating the PPE surgically lies in the identification and excision or internal drainage of the responsible leaking pancreatic duct. In the absence of a pseudocyst, an isolated fistulous track may be difficult to identify, and one is dependent on pancreatography and local inflammatory changes as guides to the site of leakage.

RESULTS OF TREATMENT

Two of the largest series reported are those of the Johns Hopkins Hospital and the Wayne State University affiliated hospitals (Tables 3 and 4). The observations and results of these mirror each other closely. In our series, the mortality rate was 5 of 26 (19.2%) prior to 1975 and 3 of 16 (18.7%) since. Most deaths were due to aspiration, pneumonia, myocardial infarction, and, in one of our operative cases, sepsis following cyst jejunostomy of an infected pancreatic pseudocyst without previous pancreatography. Although TPN has become a cornerstone of medical management, its potential for initiating infection must be noted and guarded against. While medical treatment is effective in 25 to 40 percent of

patients and should consequently be given a chance, a significant mortality rate, about 10 to 20 percent, continues to be associated with this regimen, in part because some patients are malnourished to the point of cachexia. However, intercurrent complications are substantially less frequent today than in the past.

In patients who do not respond to medical treatment, operation is highly successful when the site of leakage has been identified by pancreatography. Recurrences are rare (none in our series) and recent reported operative mortality ranges from zero to 12.5 percent. Most surgical deaths are due to infection or perioperative myocardial infarction or pulmonary emboli. Low-dose heparin in the perioperative period is probably indicated.

Fortunately, as previously noted, persistence of ascites occurs in only half of those in whom the site of leakage is not definitively dealt with at operation. Irradiation and/or later reoperation may be unavoidable in these. In 30 percent of this special group, pancreatic pseudocysts may be later identified, with or without ascites.

In summary, in a small but significant minority of

TABLE 3 Results of Treatment (Johns Hopkins Hospital)*

Management	Pancreatic Ascites	Pancreatic Pleural Effusions	Both
Nonoperative			
Success	7	2	3
Failure	6	1	2
Death	4	0	0
Total patients	17	3	5
Operative			
Success	8	4	2
Failure	0	1	0
Death	0	0	0
Total patients	8	5	2

* Courtesy of John L. Cameron, M.D.

TABLE 4 Treatment and Outcome (48 Episodes in 42 Patients) at Wayne State University Affiliated Hospitals

	No. of Episodes		Mortality		Recurrence	
	1958-75	1976-81	1958-75	1976-81	1958-75	1976-81
Pancreatic resection	4	7	0	0	0	0
Cyst jejunostomy Roux-en-Y	2	3	0	1	0	0
Cyst gastrostomy	6	1	1	0	1	0
External drainage	7	2	2	0	2	2
Lateral pancreaticojejunostomy		1		0		0
Cyst duodenostomy	1		0		0	
Medical management	4	1	2	1	1	0
LeVeen shunt		1		0		0
Laparotomy only	7		0		6	
Died on OR table		1				
	31	17	6	2	10	2

patients, medical treatment may be successful in the treatment of pancreatic ascites with or without pancreatic pleural effusion. In those in whom medical treatment fails, surgical treatment is effective in achieving cure.

CHRONIC PANCREATITIS

ROGER G. KEITH, M.D., F.R.C.S.(C),
F.R.C.S.(ENG.), F.A.C.S.

Chronic pancreatitis is a disease that usually results from long-term alcohol consumption. The resultant derangements of endocrine and exocrine tissue produce pancreatic insufficiency and diabetes mellitus. Although some forms of chronic pancreatitis are painless, the majority of patients have intractable pain of moderate severity. The mechanism of pain production is not well understood. I have recently identified perineural infiltrates with high eosinophil composition within the interlobular tissue planes in the pancreas. Severity of pain correlates with the eosinophilic perineural infiltrate. Pancreatic duct dilation and elevated intraductal pressure have also been suggested as factors causing pain.

Less frequently, chronic pancreatitis may develop from untreated biliary calculi, lipid disorders, or congenital pancreatic duct anomalies such as pancreas divisium. Distinction between chronic pancreatitis and carcinoma of the pancreas may be difficult in the non-alcoholic patient with chronic pancreatic pain and weight loss.

Pseudocysts are uncommonly associated with chronic pancreatitis. True pancreatic cysts are usually neoplastic; however, significant dilation of the pancreatic ducts does occur with chronic pancreatitis, producing large retention cysts which may be confused with pseudocyst or neoplasm.

The main role of surgical therapy for chronic pancreatitis is relief of pain. Therapy for the majority of such patients is complex. Selection of the candidate for treatment involves assessment of pain-related disability, pancreatic function, and accurate evaluation of alcoholic status. Operative procedures should be specific to the individual anatomic derangements identified by radiologic and biochemical investigation. Success of surgical therapy depends on low operative complication rates, treatment of pancreatic insufficiency and diabetes, and successful support and rehabilitation of the alcoholic patient.

INDICATIONS FOR OPERATION

Pain relief is the primary indication for surgery in chronic pancreatitis (Table 1). The constant pain syndrome is disabling; associated with weight loss and malnutrition, through food-related aggravation; accompanied by analgesic dependency or even addictions. Documentation of daily analgesic requirements from the patient's history, hospital notes, and pharmaceutical records indicates the severity of the pain, and forms a basis for assessing the effectiveness of surgical therapy.

Jaundice from bile duct obstruction in chronic pancreatitis occurs in less than 25 percent of patients. It is universally accompanied by pain, weight loss, and frequently diabetes. Half the patients with chronic pancreatitis show stricturing of the distal common bile duct without complete obstruction, and have an associated elevation of alkaline phosphatase but normal bilirubin. Complete obstruction of the biliary tree or cholangitis requires urgent biliary decompression alone or in combination with definitive pancreatic surgery for treatment of painful chronic pancreatitis.

Duodenal obstruction occurs from progression of peripancreatic fibrosis. Clinical evidence of upper gastrointestinal obstruction can be verified by endoscopy or radiography. Operations for painful pancreatitis with duodenal obstruction must consider gastrointestinal decompression as a component of the procedure.

Pancreatic cysts alone may be responsible for pain. Retention cysts associated with chronic pancreatitis should be treated by decompression, which allows adequate drainage of the in-continuity duct system. Differentiation from neoplasm, either cystic or solid, can only be established by operative biopsy. Operative pancreatography and cholangiography may enhance interpretation of the biopsy reporting "pancreatitis."

SELECTION OF PATIENTS FOR SURGERY

In assessing the patient (Table 2), pain severity must be judged as so disabling that pain relief will allow

TABLE 1 Indications for Surgery

Pain relief
Biliary obstruction
Gastrointestinal obstruction
Pancreatic cysts
Differentiation from carcinoma

rehabilitation, restoration of nutritional deficiencies and withdrawal of analgesic dependency. It must be determined that the pain is of pancreatic origin and not that of biliary tract disease, peptic ulcer disease, or intestinal disorders. In cases of alcoholic pancreatitis, I select only patients who have abstained from alcohol consumption for 12 months or who have maintained sustained abstinence in an established rehabilitation program for a minimum of 6 months. Recurrent alcoholism in a postsurgical patient correlates with recurrent pain and poor long-term results. The evaluation for rehabilitation potential should involve the patient, family, and social service support programs as well as the surgeon and medical colleagues.

Exocrine function is impaired in the majority of patients presenting for surgery. It should be recognized that surgical therapy does not improve pancreatic enzyme secretion. Replacement therapy must be considered for all patients undergoing operation.

Diabetes may not follow decompressive procedures, but does occur following total and near-total pancreatectomy. Insulin-dependent diabetes may not be adversely affected by resective procedures. Recurrent alcoholism creates significant problems in diabetic control following resections for chronic pancreatitis. Each patient's potential for diabetes, and management capabilities, must be evaluated prior to operative treatment.

As most patients have had long-term inadequate nutrition, correction of deficiencies prior to operation must be considered. Severely debilitated patients should be considered for preoperative parenteral alimentation.

SELECTION OF OPERATION FOR CHRONIC PANCREATITIS

There is no single operation that can be recommended for all patients with chronic pancreatitis. Pathologic derangements in chronic pancreatitis are variable, and individual patients require selective operations. The appropriate procedure is determined by preoperative roentgenographic evaluation combined with intraoperative findings.

TABLE 2 Assessment of Patients for Operation

Social evaluation
  Analgesic requirements
  Alcohol abstinence
  Rehabilitation potential

Pancreatic function
  Exocrine function (secretin test)
  Endocrine function (serum glucose)
  Nutritional status

Pancreatic pathology
  Pancreatic duct status (ERCP)
  Parenchymal mass or cysts (ultrasound/CT scan)
  Biliary tract status (ERCP, PTC)
  Gastrointestinal tract status (endoscopy,
    contrast GI roentgenography)

Endoscopic retrograde pancreatography is diagnostic in over 85 percent of cases. Nonvisualization of the pancreatic duct may occur with complete strictures in the head of the gland. The pancreatogram defines the anatomy of the main pancreatic duct and secondary ductules. The presence of intraductal calculi is demonstrated. Segmental strictures and retention cysts also may be seen. Fibrotic pancreatitis with stenosis or dilation less than 1 cm in diameter contraindicates decompressive procedures such as pancreaticojejunostomy. Dilation of the main pancreatic duct beyond 1.0 cm or in-continuity retention cysts may be treated by operative decompression.

Ultrasonic scanning of the pancreas is of particular value in assessing thin patients with pancreatic disease or those in whom cysts may be present. Computerized tomography better demonstrates mass lesions or disease in obese patients. A combination of endoscopic retrograde pancreatography and scanning techniques should be considered in all patients prior to operation, in order to maximally determine pancreatic disease and select the appropriate operative procedure.

Endoscopic retrograde cholangiography identifies strictures of the intrapancreatic portion of the common bile duct in both anicteric and jaundiced patients. Percutaneous transhepatic cholangiography should be reserved for jaundiced patients in whom the endoscopic technique was unsuccessful.

Biliary or gastrointestinal obstruction combined with painful pancreatitis requires selection of a combined operative procedure involving separate pancreatic, biliary, and gastrointestinal decompressions; or an operation combining resection and decompression such as the Whipple procedure. The decision for decompression or resection in these cases should be determined by the status of the pancreatic duct. I prefer to use resective procedures when the duct is stenosed through most of its length. In-continuity gastrointestinal bypass and biliary intestinal bypass can be combined with pancreaticojejunostomy when the duct is dilated.

NONOPERATIVE TREATMENT

Nonoperative procedures include endoscopic stenting and endoscopic ductal obliteration by injection technique. Percutaneous nerve blocks have been used for pain control.

Current experience with endoscopic stenting for chronic pancreatitis with duct dilation does not indicate satisfactory long-term pain relief. Although pancreatic secretion is eliminated by obliterative injection therapy, sustained pain relief is not obtained in most cases. Endocrine function is not altered by either technique.

Percutaneous injection of 50% alcohol or 10% phenol has been used to destroy the celiac ganglion. I have found this technique useful in eliminating pain in selected patients who have contraindications to operative treatment. The duration of pain relief is about one year. Repeat blocks have been ineffective in eliminating recurrent pain. Patients must be informed of the risks accompanying loss of sensation of pain related to other upper abdominal diseases, following successful nerve blocks. The early side effects of postural hypotension and diarrhea are transient, lasting up to 6 weeks.

OPERATIVE MANAGEMENT

The operative procedures used in the treatment of chronic pancreatitis are listed in Table 3.

Pancreaticojejunostomy

Chronic pancreatitis with a diffusely dilated pancreatic duct, uncomplicated by gastrointestinal or biliary tract obstruction, should be treated by an anterior longitudinal pancreaticojejunostomy. Currently, an anterior anastomosis without mobilization of the gland is preferable to the classic operation. The entire anterior surface of the pancreas is exposed by dividing the gastrocolic ligament and mobilizing the hepatic flexure and proximal transverse colon inferiorly. The duodenum and head of pancreas should be fully kocherized. Palpation of the anterior surface of the pancreas should identify the dilated duct as a groove running the length of the body and tail of the gland, less readily appreciated in the head. I confirm the location of the duct by direct fine-needle aspiration of pancreatic secretions. Subsequent dilatation with lacrimal duct probes permits placement of a small cannula for operative pancreatography, if preoperative endoscopic techniques were not successful. Otherwise, a grooved director is passed into the lumen of the duct through the puncture site and the overlying parenchyma incised to open the duct system. I excise a strip of pancreatic parenchyma and anterior duct equal in width to the diameter of the duct itself. This excision is extended a length of 10 cm from the tail of the gland to the neck of the pancreas. Caution must be taken to avoid the anterior pancreaticoduodenal vessels, leaving an adequate margin to anastomose the jejunum to the head of the gland without causing bleeding from this arcade. A Roux-en-Y limb of jejunum is then passed to the anterior surface of the pancreas in a retrocolic position. A side-to-side anastomosis is made in two layers. Nonabsorable suture transfixes the seromuscular coat of the jejunum to the fibrotic capsule of the pancreas below the unroofed duct; then a

TABLE 3 Operative Procedures for Chronic Pancreatitis

Decompression of dilated ducts
  Anterior longitudinal pancreaticojejunostomy

Pancreatic resection
  Distal pancreatectomy
  75% Pancreatectomy
  95% Pancreatectomy
  Whipple procedure
  Total pancreatectomy

Operative nerve block
  Celiac ganglion block

continuous absorbable suture is used to anastomose the mucosa to the margin of the duct epithelium in a continuous manner inferiorly and superiorly. The anastomosis is completed by suturing the jejunum to pancreas superiorly. Any intraductal calculi encountered on unroofing the duct should be removed, particularly those in the neck of the gland, which may obstruct the pancreatic duct in the deeper course through the head. Care must be taken to ensure that the enteroenterostomy lies well below the defect created in the transverse mesocolon, in order to avoid obstruction. Defects in the mesentry should be closed to prevent internal herniation.

Most patients with dilated duct systems have minimal peripancreatic fibrosis and biliary or gastrointestinal obstruction is unusual in such cases. However, if biliary obstruction is associated with ductal dilation, I prefer to combine the pancreaticojejunostomy with a choledochoduodenostomy.

When a retention cyst is encountered in chronic pancreatitis with duct dilation, drainage of the cyst into a Roux limb should be undertaken in a fashion similar to that described for the pancreaticojejunostomy. If the cyst is isolated from the dilated duct system by intervening areas of stenosis, the cyst should be unroofed to its margins with pancreatic parenchyma, the areas of stenosis excised, and a formal pancreaticojejunostomy fashioned, including the cyst bed in the anastomosis to jejunum.

Pancreatic Resections

Resection of pancreatic parenchyma for control of severe pain should be reserved for those selected patients in whom the entire duct system is stenosed by fibrosing pancreatitis. In these cases, evaluation of endocrine function and potential for diabetes is mandatory prior to embarking on resections, which may further compromise islet cell function.

The simplest resection with lowest morbidity is a distal pancreatectomy, removing the tail and body of pancreas up to the left side of the portal vein. In my experience, this procedure has produced minimal disturbance in glucose metabolism. However, pain relief is unsatisfactory and reoperation is frequently necessary.

Subtotal pancreatic resections extending the transection line further to the right of the portal vein have been variously described as 75 percent, 80 percent, and 95 percent pancreatectomy. Understandably, the greater the parenchmal mass resected, the higher the incidence of endocrine insufficiency.

As the initial resective procedure for pain relief in chronic pancreatitis with nondilated ducts, I choose a subtotal resection which I describe as a 75 percent pancreatectomy. This resection preserves one-third of the head of the pancreas from the border of the retroduodenal common bile duct extending obliquely to the confluence of the superior mesenteric vessels overlying the third part of the duodenum, preserving the inferior pancreaticoduodenal vessels and the entire uncinate process. The pancreatic duct at the transection line is examined by fine catheters. If the duct is patent through to the duodenum, it is closed with nonabsorbable sutures. The margin of the transected pancreas is closed with inverting nonabsorbable sutures. If the pancreatic duct is not patent to the duodenum and the transection margin cannot be adequately closed, a limb of jejunum is anastomosed to the cut surface of the gland.

In most patients with obliterative parenchymal disease, peripancreatic fibrosis is extensive. I have not been able to preserve the splenic vessels in this situation. In fact, commonly the splenic vein has been thrombosed. Therefore, splenectomy is usually necessary.

In the 95 percent pancreatectomy the 75 percent pancreatectomy is extended to include removal of the inferior portion of the head of the pancreas including the uncinate process. This operation preserves bile duct continuity, but leaves minimal endocrine tissue. It may be considered for patients with established insulin-dependent diabetes prior to surgery.

The Whipple procedure, pancreaticoduodenal resection with preservation of the body and tail of the pancreas, may be considered for obliterative pancreatitis with maximal involvement of the head. I prefer to reserve this operation for obliterative pancreatitis with bile duct obstruction and compromise of the duodenum producing the gastroduodenal obstruction. This procedure preserves substantial parenchyma, preventing endocrine insufficiency in most cases. However, pain relief is inadequate because of the similar mass of diseased gland left in situ. I prefer to include the antrum of the stomach in the resected specimen and add a truncal vagotomy to ensure hypochlorhydria, which improves efficiency of pancreatic enzyme supplements. I reconstruct with a closed limb of jejunum initially anastomosed in an end-to-side fashion with the bile duct, then similarly to the pancreas over a fine perforated stent, and lastly to the stomach. In my experience, exocrine secretion from the remaining pancreas is inadequate to sustain normal digestion.

Total pancreatectomy is usually reserved for reoperative surgery for pain relief after previous subtotal resections. It may be initially considered in rare cases in which the fibrosis and calcification produce bile duct obstruction, causing the extensive distal disease that is responsible for severe pancreatic pain. Gastroduodenal resection is as for the Whipple procedure, and my reconstruction involves two end-to-side anastomoses with the jejununal limb in a retrocolic position. Only the total pancreatectomy ensures complete freedom from pancreatic pain on a long-term basis.

Operative Nerve Blocks

In spite of a preoperative evaluation that indicates a potentially successful operation, I occasionally find the indicated procedure impossible because of unexpected subacute inflammation or dense peripancreatic fibrosis. In such cases, I use an intraoperative celiac block for control of pain. Fifty percent alcohol is injected into the celiac ganglion and para-aortic splanchnic nerves.

COMPLICATIONS OF SURGERY

Operative Complications

Following pancreaticojejunostomy, a short-term leak of pancreatic secretions may occur. Adequate postoperative drainage prevents the subsquent complications of pseudocyst formation or peripancreatic abscess formation. Prolonged drainage may require nutritional support by means of total parental nutrition, which also minimizes secretory stimulation.

Accumulation of blood and pancreatic secretion at the transection line is more likely to follow subtotal pancreatectomy. Sump drainage of these fluids reduces the incidence of abscess formation. Delayed intra-abdominal bleeding may occur during the second postoperative week, from necrotizing inflammation at the transection line or from portal tributaries.

Early gastrointestinal hemorrhage has frequently been reported following the Whipple procedure. Achieving complete achlorhydria and fashioning a hemostatic gastrointestinal anastomosis should reduce the incidence of this complication. Uncontrolled bleeding usually does not respond to systemic infusion of H_2 receptor blockers and requires reoperation for control of bleeding.

Metabolic Complications

Early postoperative onset of diabetes requires insulin infusion for prompt early control. I find that late insulin requirements are reduced from those required earlier. Late problems with control of insulin dosage should suggest recurrent alcoholism.

Exocrine insufficiency occurs universally following operative treatment of chronic pancreatitis. Oral supplementation with pancreatic enzymes is required for all patients. Following a preliminary 6-month phase of reduced fat intake, I adjust the diet to normal with increasing enzyme supplementation. During the early postoperative course, parenteral alimentation, once initiated, should be continued for at least 2 weeks until adequate oral nutrition is established. Postoperative complications demand long-term support by total parenteral nutrition.

RESULTS OF SURGICAL THERAPY

Sustained total relief of pancreatic pain can only be achieved by total pancreatectomy. Varying relief of pain can be obtained by subtotal pancreatectomy. Residual pancreatic mass determines the degree of residual pain. The greater the denervation of the celiac ganglia from the residual pancreatic mass, the less severe is the residual pain. Recurrence of pain is increased directly by recurrent alcohol ingestion.

Following pancreaticojejunostomy, I have noted a

TABLE 4 Results Following Surgery

Procedure	Pain Relief	Diabetes	Steatorrhea	Weight Gain
Pancreaticojejunostomy	75%	No	Yes	25%
Distal pancreatectomy	40%	No	Yes	15%
Whipple procedure	25%	No	Yes	None
75% Pancreatectomy	75%	Early-No	Yes	25%
		Late-Yes		
Total pancreatectomy	100%	Yes	Yes	25%

decrease in sustained analgesic requirements by 75 percent. Similar pain reduction follows 75 percent pancreatectomy. Following the Whipple procedure, analgesic requirements are only reduced by 25 to 30 percent. Distal pancreatectomy achieves inadequate pain reduction.

Diabetes mellitus is not a consequence of pancreaticojejunostomy in patients undergoing surgery with a normal glucose tolerance. Similarly, distal pancreatectomy and Whipple resections have not altered glucose metabolism adversely. Following total pancreatectomy and 95 percent pancreatectomy, diabetes has been evident from the time of operation. In my experience, 75 percent pancreatectomy has preserved islet cell function in all patients. However, one year after surgery, 25 percent of patients have had chemical diabetes, controlled by diet. At 5 years, 45 percent of patients have developed diabetes; the majority are insulin-dependent.

Nutritional improvement has occurred progressively in all patients in the first year following surgery. A 25 to 30 percent gain over admission weight was noted following all procedures except the Whipple procedure.

In our patients who are selected for operation, the incidence of recurrent alcoholism at one year is 20 percent. Continued regular supportive therapy is required to maintain abstinence and reduce the complications of pancreatic insufficiency rendered through surgical treatment.

The overall results of surgical treatment of chronic pancreatitis are favorable when critical assessment of candidates is undertaken and the appropriate operation selected for each patient (Table 4). Total surgical therapy implies devotion to long-term postoperative support and rehabilitation of patients by the surgical team.

PERIAMPULLARY CANCER

FREDERIC E. ECKHAUSER, M.D.
RICHARD A. POMERANTZ, M.D.
JEREMIAH G. TURCOTTE, M.D.

Carcinoma of the pancreas is now the fourth most common cause of cancer-related deaths in the United States and has surpassed stomach cancer as the second most common gastrointestinal cancer. Statistics generated by the American Cancer Society estimate that there will be approximately 24,000 new cases of pancreatic cancer and a similar number of pancreatic cancer-related deaths in this country in the mid-1980s.

In general, the incidence of pancreatic cancer is greater in males than in females and more common in individuals past 45 years of age. Although the effect of race on the incidence of carcinoma of the pancreas is complicated partly because of racial differences in diet and age distribution, the incidence of pancreatic cancer appears to be higher in blacks than in whites. Many of the proposed etiologic factors are largely speculative; however, clear-cut correlations exist between the incidence of pancreatic cancer and a variety of environmental and dietary factors such as a high intake of fat and animal protein, coffee consumption, and occupational exposure to specific carcinogens such as nitrosamines and beta-naphthylamine.

Despite intensive research aided in part by the National Pancreatic Cancer Project, the prognosis for this disease remains poor, and most patients die of the disease within 6 to 12 months of the diagnosis. Early diagnosis remains elusive, partly because the retroperitoneal location of the gland makes it difficult to examine and investigate. Furthermore, the biological behavior of these tumors results in metastatic spread early in the course of the disease. The term "periampullary cancer" should not be used interchangeably with "pancreatic cancer." Many different cancers occur in the pancreaticoduodenal region, and although all of these tumors may present in an identical manner, each has its own inherent biological behavior. Every effort should be made to distinguish tumors arising in the ampulla of Vater, the intrapancreatic portion of the common bile duct, and the duodenum surrounding the papilla of Vater from carcinomas arising in the head of the pancreas. Periampullary tumors are in general much more amenable to successful operative resection and are associated with a more favorable long-term prognosis.

CLINICAL PRESENTATION

The symptoms produced by cancer of the pancreas depend largely on the extent and size of the tumor. Cancers arising in the head of the pancreas comprise some 60 to 80 percent of all pancreatic cancers and produce pain, jaundice, and weight loss, which are also manifestations of periampullary cancers.

Pain occurs as a presenting symptom in about two-thirds of patients, and most patients develop pain at some time in the course of the disease. The pain associated with pancreatic cancer is frequently characterized as variable in location and severity, steadily progressive, and often aggravated by food ingestion or postural changes. However, the presence of pain per se appears to be of no value in predicting the site of the tumor. Pain localized to the epigastrium and right upper quadrant is fairly characteristic of carcinomas arising in the head of the pancreas, whereas lesions arising in the body and tail of the gland are often associated with left-sided abdominal pain and pain referred to the back, usually in the lumbar region.

Jaundice is a frequent symptom of periampullary carcinoma and invariably occurs at some time in the course of the disease. The jaundice associated with these lesions is usually progressive, but spontaneous fluctuations in the degree of jaundice occur in 10 to 20 percent of patients. The incidence of jaundice is highest in patients with carcinoma arising in the head of the pancreas and in the periampullary region, but may occur late in up to one-third of patients with carcinoma originating in the body and tail of the pancreas. In this setting, jaundice is often caused by secondary spread of the tumor to the liver and to lymph nodes surrounding the common bile duct.

Weight loss is probably the most common symptom of carcinoma of the pancreas and usually precedes other symptoms. The weight loss observed in these patients is usually rapidly progressive and independent of the site of the tumor when considering carcinoma of the pancreas. Likewise, the magnitude of the weight loss does not directly correlate with the extent of the tumor as severe weight loss is occasionally observed in patients with resectable tumors. While anorexia and maldigestion caused by pancreatic exocrine insufficiency may be contributory factors, they alone do not fully explain the extent of weight loss seen in patients with carcinoma of the pancreas.

The most common signs associated with periampullary carcinoma include jaundice, a palpable enlarged liver, and abdominal tenderness. Hepatomegaly is more frequent in patients with periampullary tumors and cancers arising in the head of the pancreas, but also occurs in patients with widely disseminated cancer arising in the body and tail of the pancreas. The gallbladder can be palpated in 15 to 35 percent of patients, and thrombophlebitis, usually migratory, occurs in up to 10 percent of patients.

The development of diabetes or sudden difficulties arising with the control of established diabetes have been observed in patients with carcinoma of the pancreas and may occur before other signs or symptoms appear. Therefore, the sudden appearance of diabetes in a middle-aged or older patient with no family history of the disease, particularly if associated with weight loss and other vague abdominal complaints, should raise one's suspicion about the possible presence of pancreatic malignant disease and serve as an indication for further evaluation.

PREOPERATIVE DIAGNOSIS AND STAGING

Pancreatic Secretory Studies

Pancreatic function studies are highly regarded by a number of investigators, but require duodenal intubation and aspiration of duodenal contents for the purpose of confirming the diagnosis of periampullary or pancreatic cancer. Although the pancreatic secretory response to hormonal stimulation with secretin and/or CCK-PZ may be abnormal in patients with pancreatic cancer, the response to stimulation may be indistinguishable from that observed in patients with chronic pancreatitis. Furthermore, these studies are time-consuming and generally associated with poor patient acceptance.

Secretory studies combined with cytologic examination of the duodenal aspirate can improve our ability to detect the presence of pancreatic cancer. Although the yield from these studies has been variable, confirmatory evidence of periampullary or pancreatic cancer has been observed by some investigators in up to 75 percent of cases. Equivocal results are not helpful and require direct biopsy by one of several alternative techniques.

Conventional Radiographic and Imaging Techniques

Standard barium contrast studies of the upper gastrointestinal tract have little value in demonstrating carcinoma of the head of the pancreas. However, hypotonic duodenography may be useful in evaluating lesions arising in the ampulla of Vater or in the duodenum, and diagnostic accuracies of up to 80 percent for lesions in this region have been reported.

Ultrasonography and CT scanning are useful noninvasive means for visualizing the head of the pancreas, bile ducts, and liver. As a screening examination, ultrasonography is preferable because of its high degree of accuracy, good patient acceptance, low cost, and availability even in smaller institutions. CT scanning may be more useful for identifying metastases or demonstrating invasion of contiguous structures. Furthermore,

CT may be useful to localize pancreatic or peripancreatic masses for transcutaneous aspiration biopsy. The most significant problem associated with CT diagnosis in patients with suspected pancreatic cancer is the high rate of false-positive results. As CT technology improves, machines may be developed that can differentiate the density of cancer from that of normal pancreas. As radiologists develop increasing experience with this evolving technology, we can expect the false-positive rate to decrease significantly.

Angiography

The efficacy of panvisceral angiography in patients with suspected periampullary tumors is somewhat controversial. Selective cannulation of branches of the celiac artery supplying the pancreas, often with pharmacologic enhancement of pancreatic blood flow, have been useful to detect tumors as small as 1.5 cm in diameter in some studies. In this context, selective angiography may be useful in detecting carcinomas of the body and tail of the pancreas when the results of pancreatic secretory studies have been equivocal. Angiography may demonstrate encasement, tortuousity, or amputation of pancreatic arteries and thus may influence preoperative decisions concerning the resectability of such tumors. In addition, angiography may provide invaluable information concerning regional arterial anatomy, which is highly variable in up to 50 percent of cases. Finally, angiography can be useful for detecting metastatic spread to the liver and often distinguishes the neovascularity of pancreatic cystadenocarcinomas and islet cell neoplasms from cancers of ductal origin. Since the biological behavior of these histologically different cancers varies substantially, angiographic information may dictate a more or less aggressive surgical approach. Selective angiography is complex, expensive, and time-consuming, and requires substantial interpretation skills on the part of the radiologist. Consequently, we do not advocate its routine use in all patients with suspected periampullary tumors. However, the benefits delineated previously make it a valuable adjunctive study when other less invasive procedures have confirmed the presence of a pancreatic mass, but have failed either to distinguish between benign and malignant disease or to determine resectability.

Tumor Markers

Sophisticated diagnostic studies are employed only when symptoms suggestive of pancreatic disease are present. Unfortunately, by the time symptoms develop, it is already too late for curative resection in the majority of patients. One means of improving early diagnosis in asymptomatic patients is to develop sensitive markers of neoplasia in the serum, bile, and/or pancreatic juice. Tumor-associated antigens such as carcinoembryonic antigen, alpha-fetoprotein, and pancreatic oncofetal antigen in serum lack sufficient specificity to be reliable markers of early pancreatic cancer. Blood levels of CEA are elevated in the majority of patients with carcinoma of the pancreas, but false-positive and false-negative results are frequently observed and serum levels are often elevated in patients with extrapancreatic carcinoma and benign pancreatic disease. Currently, elevated CEA levels in bile obtained by percutaneous transhepatic drainage have been demonstrated in a small group of patients with proven pancreatic carcinoma. Combining biliary CEA measurements with cytologic examination of the bile and possibly with cholangiography may further improve the diagnostic yield and reduce the number of false-positive or false-negative results. The utility of another and apparently more specific antigen associated with carcinoma of the pancreas (oncofetal antigen) remains to be proved, but preliminary studies indicate that false-positive tests are also found in other diseases. Other serum immunologic studies such as the leukocyte-adherence-inhibition test, a measure of cell-mediated immunity, have thus far not proved to be sensitive markers of pancreatic carcinoma. Other markers such as galactosyl transferase isozyme II and serum RNase have so far not been helpful because of problems related to sensitivity and specificity.

Endoscopic Retrograde Cholangiopancreatography and Percutaneous Transhepatic Cholangiography

Endoscopic retrograde cholangiopancreatography (ERCP) is a useful tool in evaluating patients with suspected pancreatic disease. This modality provides the best way to visualize the pancreatic duct short of intraoperative pancreatography. Duodenoscopy with a side-viewing endoscope allows visualization and biopsy of periampullary tumors arising in the duodenum or the ampulla of Vater. Retrograde injection of dye into the pancreatic ductal system frequently identifies radiologic abnormalities such as strictures of the pancreatic duct, obstruction of the main pancreatic duct, and pancreatic field defects that may aid in confirming the diagnosis of pancreatic cancer. In addition, retrograde cannulation of the pancreatic duct facilitates collection of pancreatic juice for measurement of biochemical and immunologic markers as well as for cytologic analysis. Combining cytology with retrograde cholangiopancreatography increases the diagnostic accuracy to about 90 percent. Angiography and ERCP provide complementary data and should be used together to offer the greatest likelihood of early cancer detection. One added advantage of ERCP is the opportunity to place transampullary stents to decompress the biliary tree in preparation for more definitive procedures. This technique is relatively rapid and has an acceptably low morbidity, but can be accompanied by such serious complications as cholangitis, sepsis, and death in a small percentage of patients. Percutaneous transhepatic cholangiography (PTC) can be useful for delineating the site and sometimes the etiology of bile duct obstruction and has the added advantages of obtaining bile for cytologic analysis and providing a route for external biliary decompression. Like ERCP, PTC has a high success rate, especially in patients with a dilated extrahepatic biliary system, and is associated with relatively low morbidity; however, neither of these studies provides conclusive evidence regarding resectability.

EXPLORATORY LAPAROTOMY AND INTRAOPERATIVE DECISIONS

The definitive diagnostic study is operative exploration performed by a surgeon who is skilled in assessing resectability and capable of performing a pancreatic resection with a low operative mortality. The choice of operation depends on the intraoperative diagnosis, local anatomic factors, and expectations of postoperative mortality and survival rates. Efforts should be made to establish a histologic diagnosis of malignancy and thus avoid unnecessary resection for chronic pancreatitis. The presence of a pancreatic malignant tumor often can be confirmed preoperatively by means of ultrasound or CT-guided percutaneous fine-needle biopsy of the pancreas. However, intraoperative biopsy may be required in up to 25 percent of cases. Tissue from a pancreatic mass usually can be obtained by scalpel biopsy of superficial lesions, direct fine-needle aspiration of the mass for cytologic examination, or transduodenal biopsy using either a Tru-cut or Vim-Silverman needle. Biopsy of the pancreas is relatively safe, reported morbidity and mortality rates being 5 percent and 1 percent respectively.

Once the abdomen has been entered, a careful search should be made for distant metastases to the liver, regional lymph nodes, or free peritoneal surfaces. Histologic confirmation of widespread metastatic disease should preclude any consideration of resection and direct the surgeon's attention toward palliative decompression of the biliary tract and stomach. Once metastases have been excluded, efforts should be directed toward differentiating a common duct stone or chronic pancreatitis from pancreaticoduodenal cancer. In this context, preoperative endoscopy can be helpful to exclude duodenal and ampullary primaries in the majority of cases. In many cases, preoperative PTC combined with cytologic analysis of the bile can distinguish between choledocolithiasis and cancer. Occasionally, it may not be possible to differentiate between chronic pancreatitis and pancreaticoduodenal cancer. Interpretation of frozen section pancreatic biopsies is often unreliable, and false-negative results occur in up to 20 percent of cases, especially when the tumor is small and surrounded by an extensive area of chronic pancreatitis. Many authors have suggested that histologic confirmation of malignancy is not always necessary for resectable lesions, assuming that the clinical criteria of a mass in the head of the pancreas, a dilated common bile duct, and an enlarged duct of Wirsung are present at operation. In this setting, they reported a clinical diagnostic error rate of only 3 percent. Additional operative criteria have been delineated to help distinguish between malignant and benign conditions. Fat necrosis, which is usually considered to be a diagnostic feature of chronic pancreatitis, may also occur in some cancers of the

pancreas. However, with cancer of the pancreas, the area of fat necrosis is characteristically confined to the capsule. Furthermore, the gland distal to the tumor is usually firm or sclerotic. Dilatation of the duct of Wirsung occurs in 50 to 80 percent of patients with pancreatic cancer and can be best appreciated just beyond the shelving edge of the tumor on the anterior surface of the pancreas at the junction of the upper two-thirds and lower one-third of the gland. Ductal dilatation that is not associated with calcinosis of the gland should be considered an important indicator of pancreatic malignancy. On occasion, one must differentiate pancreatic cancer from calculous disease of the biliary system when conventional radiographic studies are nondiagnostic. Choledochotomy with digital palpation of the distal common bile duct may demonstrate a "puckering" or central tapering of the distal common duct that is rare in cases of benign choledocholithiasis. Passage of a probe or small curette toward the ampulla in this setting may cause brisk bleeding that is suggestive of cancer and may yield tissue which, on histologic examination, establishes the diagnosis of malignancy. Careful evaluation at operation combined with thorough review of the history and physical findings should permit differentiation of a common duct stone or chronic pancreatitis from pancreaticoduodenal cancer in the vast majority of cases.

The next major intraoperative decision regards the question of resectability. Irreversible compromise of vital structures can be avoided if a specific sequence of five steps is followed: *Step 1* involves wide mobilization of the duodenum and the head of the pancreas after dividing the lateral duodenal peritoneum. The retropancreatic space separating the pancreas anteriorly from the vena cava and aorta posteriorly should be explored carefully, taking care to examine the superior mesenteric artery as close to its origin as possible. Extension beyond the pancreas to involve the retropancreatic space and the structures contained within makes the lesion virtually unresectable. *Step 2* involves mobilization of the distal stomach and pylorus and identification of structures in the hepatogastric and hepatoduodenal ligaments. Once the hepatic artery and common bile duct have been dissected free of surrounding structures, careful examination can continue for lymph nodes or evidence of direct tumor extension. The portal vein can be examined directly by inserting a finger under the body of the pancreas and gently separating it from the vein in a caudal direction toward the junction of the splenic and superior mesenteric veins. This maneuver can often be facilitated by ligating and dividing the gastroduodenal artery to allow better visualization of the portal vein. Once it has been ascertained that the gastrohepatic and retropancreatic spaces are free of tumor, *step 3* involves exploration of the base of the transverse mesocolon. By reflecting the colon and omentum superiorly, the root of the mesocolon can be exposed. This area is relatively avascular and should be incised transversely as far as the ligament of Treitz. This maneuver allows the surgeon to evaluate the status of the superior mesenteric artery and vein, as well as the middle colic and inferior pancreaticoduodenal vessels. Tumor invading the root of the mesocolon is a contraindication to resection. At this point, the surgeon's index fingers can be introduced from above and below the pancreas into the space between the pancreas and the ventral aspect of the portal vein. Ensuring mobility in this area establishes that the tumor is likely to be confined to the head of the pancreas.

The final two steps are locally destructive, but do not commit one to completing the resection. In *step 4*, the stomach and the pancreas are divided to expose the portal vein for subsequent mobilization of the uncinate process. The presence of short, friable veins in this area requires meticulous dissection, as inadvertent injury may led to troublesome bleeding. Up to this point, no irreversible steps have been taken. Extension of tumor to involve the dorsal wall of the portal vein from a primary involving the uncinate process or encasement of the superior mesenteric artery precludes resection by conventional pancreaticoduodenectomy. Consideration should be given to extended or regional pancreatic resection (to be discussed). If the decision is made to abort the resection, the spleen and tail of the pancreas can be removed and the stomach reanastomosed. *Step 5*, the final step in a conventional pancreaticoduodenectomy, involves division of the common hepatic duct and jejunum. Once the fully mobilized specimen has been reflected to the right, the common hepatic duct can be divided approximately 1.5 to 2.0 cm below its bifurcation into the right and left hepatic ducts.

Reconstruction of gastrointestinal continuity following conventional pancreaticoduodenectomy involves construction of a pancreaticojejunostomy, a choledocho-jejunostomy, and a gastrojejunostomy. Both the pancreatic and biliary anastomoses are placed above the gastric anastomosis to minimize the likelihood of postoperative marginal ulceration. Two techniques are available for performing the pancreaticojejunal anastomosis: end-to-end pancreaticojejunostomy, whereby the stump of the divided pancreas is invaginated into the open end of the jejunum, or end-to-side pancreaticojejunostomy, whereby a pancreaticoductal anastomosis to jejunal mucosa is performed with interrupted absorbable sutures over a temporary indwelling stent that subsequently passes spontaneously through the gastrointestinal tract. We prefer the latter alternative for pancreaticojejunal reconstruction and feel that the two-layer anastomosis provides additional protection against leaks from the pancreatic stump. The choledochojejunal anastomosis is generally straightforward since the common hepatic duct is markedly dilated in the majority of patients with pancreaticoduodenal cancer. Our preference is to spatulate the common hepatic duct in order to construct a 2- to 3-cm end-to-side hepaticojejunal anastomosis with a single layer of absorbable suture material. In all instances we protect the anastomosis in the early postoperative period with a transanastomotic T-tube or Witzel-type choledochostomy tube inserted through a distal jejunotomy and positioned across the choledochojejunal anastomosis. The gastrojejunostomy can be constructed in a variety of ways, but is best fashioned anterior to the colon. Concomitant truncal

vagotomy is performed to reduce the likelihood of postoperative anastomotic ulceration and subsequent gastrointestinal hemorrhage. Most investigators, including ourselves, recognize the ulcerogenic nature of a pancreaticoduodenectomy. Our own experience with approximately 40 patients undergoing Whipple resection suggests that addition of vagotomy may not significantly influence the frequency or severity of postoperative marginal ulceration or hemorrhage. However, we continue to advocate concomitant vagotomy, especially in patients with a favorable long-term prognosis. Prior to closure of the abdominal wall, two closed suction drains are inserted in proximity to the choledochal and pancreaticoductal anastomoses. These drains are left in place postoperatively for 5 to 7 days.

Determining the Extent of Pancreatic Resection to be Performed

The decision for or against pancreatic resection must be based not only on clinical and operative findings, but also on the surgeon's ability to perform pancreatic resection with acceptably low rates of morbidity and mortality. Since only one-third of all patients with cancer originating in the head of the pancreas have resectable lesions and only one-third of these are curable (one-ninth of the total operated population), a mortality rate exceeding 10 or 11 percent must be judged as unacceptable. Considering the world-wide mortality rate of 22 percent for Whipple operations, it is no wonder that some colleagues question the wisdom of resectional therapy for these tumors.

Advocates of total pancreatectomy cite several convincing arguments for their bias: Removal of the entire pancreas eliminates the pancreaticojejunal anastomosis and problems related to leakage from the pancreatic stump. Total pancreatectomy may theoretically be a better cancer operation as it enables the surgeon to obtain a wider margin of normal tissue. It also eliminates the need to transect the pancreatic duct and avoids spilling cancer cells into the operative site, removes all possible multicentric foci of cancer, and facilitates a better lymphadenectomy. The arguments against total pancreatectomy include postoperative endocrine and exocrine pancreatic insufficiency, and an increased risk of peptic ulcer disease. In order to advocate routine total pancreatectomy for cancer originating in the head of the pancreas, one must demonstrate that operative morbidity and mortality rates do not exceed those of the conventional Whipple resection and must also demonstrate an improved long-term survival rate. To date, retrospectively analyzed data from fewer than 200 patients treated in the past decade or two has identified no short- or long-term advantage of total pancreatectomy. It is also important to bear in mind that approximately 25 percent of patients undergoing total pancreatectomy will develop "brittle" diabetes that may be difficult to manage. We recommend total pancreatectomy only when (1) the pancreatic remnant is sufficiently soft and friable that it might result in a tenuous pancreaticojejunal anastomosis, (2) the cancer is multicentric or cancer is identified at the transection margin of the pancreas, and (3) there is pre-existing severe diabetes mellitus.

In some cases, local extension of the tumor may preclude curative resection by conventional pancreatico-duodenectomy. Some investigators advocate regional or extended pancreatectomy in which portions of the portal and superior mesenteric veins along with segments of the hepatic artery and occasionally the superior mesenteric artery are removed along with a wide margin of peri-pancreatic nodal and adipose tissue. Arterial and venous integrity is restored by either direct reanastomosis of vascular remnants or interposition of autologous vein or prosthetic vascular substitutes. To date, this approach seems unjustifiable since surgical mortality is high and survival is not improved.

Management of Unresectable Lesions

When resection for cure cannot be performed, substantial palliation can be achieved with bypass procedures designed to decompress the bile duct, the stomach, or both. Biliary bypass can usually be achieved with an operative mortality rate of 10 to 20 percent and the expectation of a 6-month mean survival. The presence of extrapancreatic metastases at the time of internal biliary decompression reduces life expectancy from 6 to approximately 3 months. The choice of biliary and enteric bypass is immaterial in patients who are unlikely to survive longer than one or 2 months. External biliary drainage by cholecystostomy or tube choledochostomy should be avoided if internal decompression is possible. Biliary decompression using the gallbladder (cholecysto-jejunostomy with or without a diverting proximal entero-enterostomy) is technically easier to perform than a choledochojejunal anastomosis and affords comparable palliation with a similar mortality rate. However, the variable nature of cystic duct anatomy should be kept in mind. In 10 to 15 percent of cases, the cytic duct enters the common duct low, increasing the possibility of future obstruction by continued growth of the tumor. There is some preliminary evidence that Roux-en-Y hepaticoenter-ostomy may produce slightly longer survival rates, and perhaps this technique should be reserved for cases in which long-term prognosis is favorable. Regardless of the method of biliary decompression, 60 to 85 percent of patients experience relief of pruritus, improvement in liver function, and return of appetite following operation.

Nonoperative biliary decompression with specially designed external drainage catheters can be accomplished using a modification of percutaneous transhepatic cholan-giography. Several investigators have used this technique in patients with unresectable lesions and report successful palliation in 70 to 90 percent of cases. Complications associated with these procedures (bleeding, sepsis, and bile leak) are uncommon, but the presence of an external drainage catheter and collecting system is generally associated with poor patient acceptance. In some instances, the catheter can be advanced through the area of obstruction into the duodenum, allowing internal biliary decompression and avoiding the consequences of inter-rupting the enterohepatic circulation. Successful palliation can be expected in up to two-thirds of patients by means of this technique. In general, our indications for percutan-eous external or internal biliary decompression are limited to elderly or frail patients who cannot tolerate surgery or to patients in whom there is demonstrable evidence of an unresectable lesion with extrapancreatic metastases.

The question of whether to perform a routine gastro-enterostomy continues to be a subject of some controversy. Although dudoenal obstruction is a rare presenting symptom of periampullary or pancreatic cancer, up to 15 percent of patients who do not undergo gastroenterostomy at the initial operation eventually require this procedure for treatment of duodenal obstruc-tion. Classically, gastroenterostomy has been recom-mended in conjunction with biliary decompression only when duodenal obstruction appears imminent. The rationale for this bias assumes that construction of an additional anastomosis prolongs operative time and increases morbidity and mortality rates without prolonging survival. A substantial body of evidence has accumulated showing no increase in operative mortality rate resulting from gastroenterostomy performed as a concomitant pro-cedure with biliary bypass. Problems such as gastric stasis resulting from tumor invasion of autonomic neural plexuses and marginal ulceration secondary to diversion of bile and pancreatic juice away from the gastroenteric anastomosis have proved to be more theoretic than real, especially if the patient's life expectancy is adjudged to be weeks or months.

Severe pain is a frequent and debilitating symptom of advanced periampullary or pancreatic cancer and occurs in approximately three-quarters of patients during the course of their disease. Partial pain relief can be afforded with biliary or gastric bypass, but visceral pain due to tumor invasion of retroperitoneal autonomic nerves requires a different aproach. Surgical neurotomy combined with celiac and superior mesenteric ganglionec-tomy can be accomplished at the time of operation. How-ever, this requires additional expertise and prolongs operating time without affording permanent relief of pain. Intraoperative chemical splanchnicectomy, a technique now popular at our instituion as well as others, employs injection under direct vision of either 50% alcohol or 6% phenol along both sides of the celiac axis. Previous studies from this center showed that more than 80 percent of patients undergoing this procedure achieved pain reflief which, in many cases, was permanent. Furthermore, our study failed to show any increase in morbidity or mortality rates associated with this procedure. Based on our experience with intraoperative chemical splanchnicec-tomy, we feel that this procedure should be performed routinely in all patients with unresectable periampullary or pancreatic cancers, irrespective of other intraoperative decisions regarding biliary or gastric bypass.

PROGNOSIS

Therapeutic outcome in any patient with a periampullary or pancreatic cancer varies with the histologic type of the tumor, the clinical stage of the disease, the accuracy of the clinical diagnosis, and the type of operation undertaken as well as intangible factors of age, sex, and host resistance. The biological behavior of cancers arising in the pancreaticoduodenal region is highly variable and significantly influences both resectability and survival rates. The reported resectability rate for ductal cancer originating in the head of the pancreas is a dismal 10 percent. However, resection rates for periampullary tumors arising in the ampulla, common bile duct, and duodenum vary from 40 to 80 percent. Although adenocarcinoma of the pancreas is the most frequent site of pancreaticoduodenal cancer, cancers other than ductal adenocarcinoma can occur in the periampullary area, and resection for such cancers results in relatively satisfactory survival rates. Perioperative mortality rates are similar regardless of the site of origin of the tumor, but 5-year survival rates following resectional therapy vary from a low of 5 percent reported for adenocarcinoma of the pancreas to a high of 40 to 45 percent reported for lesions arising in the ampulla of Vater or the duodenum. Some investigators have suggested that common bile duct cancer has a poorer prognosis than cancers arising in the ampulla of Vater or duodenum, but this observation is not accepted universally. For the most part, periampullary cancers, excluding adenocarcinoma of the pancreas, can be viewed collectively in terms of long-term prognosis.

One additional important point bears mention. Many investigators advocate bypass without consideration of resection for all suspected adenocarcinomas arising in the head of the pancreas and cite as justification the higher operative mortality rates with no improvement in survival following radical resection. While the morbidity rates following radical resection are higher than for bypass, data showing differences in operative mortality are tentative and inconclusive at best. Without pathologic verification of the diagnosis in patients undergoing bypass, it is difficult to interpret the results of bypass operations for resectable tumors that were considered cancers of the pancreas during exploration. Furthermore, even in centers specializing in this disease, up to 10 percent of periampullary tumors arising in the ampulla, common bile duct, and duodenum have been mistaken for tumors originating in the head of the pancreas. Thus, performing bypass for all presumed pancreatic carcinomas not only deprives the occasional patient with pancreatic cancer of the chance for prolonged survival, but also markedly decreases the chance of cure for patients with more favorable periampullary tumors. Our approach to peri-

ampullary and pancreatic tumors has been aggressive, and resection is undertaken if technically feasible. It is important to bear in mind that the decision to resect should not be viewed as an exercise in technical gymnastics, but should take into account nodal status and tumor differentiation. Analysis of survival rates from several large studies of radical resection for periampullary cancer confirm the poor prognosis associated with the presence of lymph node involvement in resected specimens. Nodal metastases should not be regarded as an absolute contraindication to resectional therapy, but this finding would have to be weighed carefully in light of local anatomic factors and the condition of the patient. We recommend using the Whipple operation as the standard procedure for most patients and feel that extended or regional pancreatectomy is not justified. We reserve total pancreatectomy for the patient with (1) a friable, soft pancreatic remnant that might compromise the integrity of a pancreaticojejunal anastomosis, (2) histologic evidence of persistent tumor at the margin of the transected pancreas, or (3) pre-existing severe diabetes.

Adjunctive therapy using chemotherapy and radiation therapy alone or in combination must be considered in light of the low resectability rates for pancreatic cancer. To date, neither single nor multiple drug regimens have proved effective in patients with unresectable pancreatic cancer. External beam radiation therapy alone has not proved to be cost-effective in the majority of cases. However, combining x-ray therapy with a single dose of fluorouracil as a "radiation sensitizer" has extended the median survival from 23 to 41 weeks in a small number of patients treated with this promising modality. Interstitial implantation of radioactive iodine seeds in patients with unresectable pancreatic cancer has not improved survival or afforded any measure of prolonged relief of pain. Intraoperative radiation is a relatively new technique, and preliminary results in small numbers of patients appear promising. With this procedure, an intraoperative dose of radiation is delivered directly through a port designed to encompass the pancreas and peripancreatic tissues. Compared to external beam radiation, intraoperative radiation therapy may reduce the incidence of radiation injury to major contiguous structures such as colon, small intestine, and liver. Although initial results of intraoperative radiation therapy are encouraging, the small numbers of patients accrued to date makes it difficult to draw any certain conclusions regarding the efficacy of this form of treatment.

UNUSUAL PANCREATIC TUMORS

JEREMIAH G. TURCOTTE, M.D.
FREDERIC E. ECKHAUSER, M.D.
WILLIAM E. STRODEL, M.D.

Patients with pancreatic neoplasms usually present with a solid or cystic mass. Ultrasonography, computerized tomography, and magnetic resonance imaging may demonstrate an unsuspected solid or cystic lesion. Seldom is the histologic diagnosis available preoperatively, and the surgeon must decide whether additional diagnostic studies or an operation is indicated. An awareness of the less common lesions that occur in the pancreas is necessary to render an informed opinion.

Tables 1 and 2 list most of the uncommon cystic and solid tumors of the pancreas. Malignant lesions are sometimes cystic, and benign lesions often present as solid neoplasms. In many cases a history and appropriate diagnostic studies are sufficient to either provide a definitive diagnosis or make the surgeon suspicious that he might not be dealing with a more common adenocarcinoma or inflammatory lesion of the pancreas. For instance, typical symptoms of an endocrinopathy may be present, or the patient may have a confirmed diagnosis of pancreatitis. Patients in the pediatric or adolescent age group are suspect for papillary-cystic epithelial cell tumors or pancreaticoblastomas. In many cases only a working diagnosis can be established, and a definitive decision must be made at the operating table.

DIAGNOSIS

Percutaneous fine-needle aspiration biopsy of the pancreatic mass is useful in establishing the diagnosis of malignancy, but is not so reliable in determining the exact histologic type of malignancy. The classic signs of inoperability or unresectability of typical ductal adenocarcinomas of the pancreas may not apply to some of the more uncommon tumors or cysts. Large, potentially curable, endocrine tumors sometimes obstruct the splenic or portal vein or the common bile duct and are still resectable for cure. Papillary-cystic epithelial tumors become densely adherent to surrounding structures, but this does not preclude resection for cure. Many uncommon pancreatic malignant tumors that arise in the body or tail of the pancreas, unlike the typical ductal adenocarcinoma occurring in these areas, are still potentially curable.

TABLE 1 Uncommon Cystic Tumors of the Pancreas

Benign

Microcystic adenoma
Mucinous cystadenoma
Serous cystadenoma
Solitary cysts

Cystic fibrosis
Polycystic diseases
  Von Hippel-Lindau

Retention cysts
  Pancreatic lithiasis
  Pancreatitis

Parasitic cysts
  Amebic
  Ascaris
  Clonorchis sinensis
  Echinococcus
  Strongyloides

Malignant

Mucinous cystadenocarcinoma*

Neoplastic degeneration
  Adenocarcinoma
  Leiomyosarcoma
  Rhabdomyosarcoma

Endocrine tumors*

Papillary-cystic epithelial cell*

Retention cysts
  From obstructing cancer

* Often curable with resection.

TABLE 2 Uncommon Solid Tumors of the Pancreas

Benign

Acinar cell adenoma
Ductal adenoma or papilloma
Microcystic adenoma

Localized pancreatitis
  Focal nodular sclerosis
  Fibrocalcareous pancreatitis

Connective Tissue
  Hemangioma
  Leiomyoma
  Lipoma
  Lymphangioma
  Neurilemoma

Abscess

Dermoid

Malignant

Acinar cell carcinoma
Osteoclastic giant cell
Pleomorphic giant cell
Signet ring carcinoma
Small cell carcinoma
Squamous or adenosquamous carcinoma

Functioning endocrine cell*
Nonfunctioning endocrine*
  Pancreatic polypeptide

Pancreaticoblastoma*
Papillary-cystic epithelial cell*

Connective Tissue
  Fibrous histiocytoma
  Hemangiopericytoma
  Leiomyosarcoma
  Osteogenic sarcoma
  Rhabdomyosarcoma

Lymphoma
Oncocytic
Plasmacytoma*

* Often curable with resection.

The presence of an uncommon pancreatic tumor should be suspected when (1) symptoms suggestive of an endocrinopathy are present, (2) a bulky tumor is present without weight loss, pain, metastases, or obstruction of the bile duct or viscera, (3) percutaneous needle aspiration biopsy demonstrates only benign cells or cells not typical of an adenocarcinoma, (4) a tumor occurs in individuals under 40 years of age and especially in the adolescent or pediatric age group, (5) a cystic mass is present without a typical history of relapsing or chronic pancreatitis, and (6) angiography demonstrates a vascular tumor blush.

Most patients presenting with one of the aforementioned conditions deserve an exploratory laparotomy and a generous biopsy if a definitive diagnosis cannot be otherwise established. Exploration is also often indicated for unusual cystic masses. A frozen section of the cyst wall and any suspicious papillary projection should be obtained before an internal or external drainage procedure is undertaken. Several of our patients with cystic endocrine tumors, papillary cystic epithelial cell tumors, or mucinous cystadenomas were initially treated with drainage procedures based on the false assumption that these were pseudocysts secondary to pancreatitis.

GROSS APPEARANCE

The appearance of the tumor at operation provides a clue to the histologic diagnosis. Endocrine tumors are reddish-brown or reddish-yellow and have a firm rubbery consistency rather than the stoney hard consistency of a ductal or acinar adenocarcinoma. Mucinous cysts of the pancreas have a velvety red epithelial lining and are often multilocular with complete and partial septa rather than unilocular. True pseudocysts are usually tense and filled with clear yellow serous fluid or thick greenish fluid containing particulate matter secondary to previous hemorrhage into the cyst. Cysts secondary to neoplastic degeneration are almost always totally or partially encapsulated with obvious cancerous tissue.

PAPILLARY-CYSTIC EPITHELIAL CELL NEOPLASMS

Papillary-cystic epithelial cell neoplasms of the pancreas have many of the features characteristic of uncommon pancreatic tumors. Synonyms for this tumor include papillary tumor, papillary epithelial neoplasm, solid and cystic acinar tumor, and papillary-cystic neoplasm. The cell type from which this tumor originates remains uncertain. Over 60 cases have been reported in the literature. The great majority of these are females between 2 and 25 years of age. It is likely that many of these tumors were once misdiagnosed as adenocarcinomas or cystic adenocarcinomas of the pancreas. This neoplasm can be large, densely adherent to adjacent structures, or locally invasive. Distant metastases are rare, and most cases have been cured following a generous resection.

Approximately 3 years ago, we had experience with a 14-year-old white female who presented with a large cystic lesion of the pancreas. This was initially thought to be a pseudocyst of the pancreas and was drained externally. When it became apparent that this was a neoplasm, the patient was referred to our institution. Total resection of the tumor required a distal pancreatectomy, a splenectomy, partial gastrectomy, segmental transverse colectomy, and segmental resection of the distal third and fourth portions of the duodenum. The patient's gastrointestinal tract was reconstructed primarily. Her postoperative course was uneventful except for some intermittent fevers. She remains free of neoplasm 2½ years after resection.

NEUROENDOCRINE NEOPLASMS

Neuroendocrine neoplasms sometimes present as cystic masses. When an endocrine tumor is suspected, a gastrointestinal hormone screen can help to identify the mass. A hormone screen includes assays for gastrin, somatostatin, glucagon, vasoactive intestinal polypeptide, pancreatic polypeptide, and insulin. Up to 15 percent of cystic or solid islet cell tumors are silent clinically, but still may secrete polypeptide hormones. Five cases of cystic endocrine tumors of the pancreas have been reported. In four of these cases, an internal drainage procedure was performed on the mistaken assumption that these were benign pseudocysts. Solid endocrine tumors of the pancreas can also be silent and very large. We have had experience with one patient whose tumor was 10 cm in diameter and excreted large amounts of pancreatic polypeptide. Resection of the tumor required a pancreaticoduodenectomy. The patient is free of tumor 3 years postoperatively.

TECHNICAL CONSIDERATIONS

Certain technical considerations deserve emphasis when approaching these unusual tumors. We seldom see complications from wedge or Trucut needle biopsy of the pancreas provided the needle tract or resection site is carefully closed with nonabsorbable suture. Large tumors of the head of the pancreas may require a pancreaticoduodenectomy. This can be accomplished safely even with large and adherent tumors if the major blood vessels are used as landmarks and skeletonized to guide the dissection. A preoperative arteriogram is helpful in planning the resection. As in the case just described, resection of adherent tumors of the distal pancreas may be difficult. Adjacent organs such as the stomach, splenic flexure of the colon, and middle colic vessels should first be identified and isolated from the pancreas or included in the resection if they are adherent or invaded by tumor. The body of the pancreas and the splenic artery and vein can then be divided. The pancreas and spleen are resected from right to left. Reverse distal pancreatectomy is especially appropriate when the spleen or distal pancreas cannot be mobilized because of adhesions or risk of violating tumor margins. If a lymphoma is encountered, a staging procedure including liver and lymph node biopsies and a splenectomy should be performed at the time of the laparotomy.

When an uncommon tumor of the pancreas is suspected, the case should be discussed in detail with the pathologist. Special studies such as electron microscopy and immunoperoxidase stains may be necessary to establish an accurate histologic diagnosis. No doubt some of the reported long-term cures of an adenocarcinoma of the pancreas actually represent a misdiagnosis of an uncommon pancreatic neoplasm.

PANCREATIC ISLET CELL TUMOR

STEPHEN N. JOFFE, M.B., B.Ch., M.D., F.R.C.S., F.A.C.S.

Amine- and peptide-secreting cells are widely distributed in the body. Pearse (1968) proposed the name *APUD* for these cells, as derived from the initial letters of their common cytochemical characteristics: a high content of *a*mine, a capacity for amine *p*recuror *u*ptake, and the presence of the enzyme *d*ecarboxylase. Endocrine cells are found throughout the alimentary tract including the islets of Langerhans in the pancreas, as well as in the pituitary, pineal, thyroid, and adrenal glands. Tumors or hyperplastic lesions of the APUD cells are known as apudomas and usually secrete peptides and/or amines. These cells also contain the enzyme *neuron-specific enolase* (NSE), and the tumors are now preferentially referred to as neuroendocrine tumors. Apudomas may be classified as orthoendocrine, which implies secretion of normal products of their cells of origin, or paraendocrine, implying secretion of hormones characteristic of other glands or cells, and they may be solitary or form part of the multiple endocrine neoplasia syndrome.

Since the identification and surgical treatment of islet cell tumors of the pancreas causing hypoglycemia in 1926 and the description of the Zollinger-Ellison syndrome in 1955, several other islet cell tumor syndromes related to their hormone production have become recognized. These include insulinomas, Verner-Morrison or watery diarrhea syndrome (vipoma), the glucagonoma syndrome, pancreatic polypeptide-secreting tumors (p-poma) and somatostatin-producing tumors (somatostatinoma). In some cases, several hormones have been found in the same tumor. Less common is the ectopic production of ACTH, calcitonin, parathyroid hormone, or serotonin by the pancreatic apudoma. Islet cell tumors may also be non-functioning, and thus patients present without any symptoms and with no recognized hormone secretion. Symptomatology and morbidity are caused by both the hormone secretion (e.g., hypoglycemia) and the direct effects of the tumor itself and its malignant potential.

Management is multidisciplinary and consists of (1) diagnosis, (2) localization, and (3) treatment (Table 1).

Treatment of choice is surgical. A combination of surgery and chemotherapy may be required when the disease is malignant with metastatic spread. Results of palliative therapy are rewarding in controlling functional symptoms and tumor growth as many of these tumors are slow-growing and responsive to appropriate drug treatment.

Studies to determine whether the islet cell disease is localized and benign (adenoma), diffuse (islet cell hyper-

TABLE 1 Management of Pancreatic Islet Cell Tumors

Measures	Methods
Diagnosis	
Clinical	Related to hormone secretion
Measurement	Biochemical
	Bioassay
	Radioimmunoassay (RIA) and characterization (plasma, tumor)
Microscopy	Light
	Histochemistry
	Electron microscopy
	Immunocytochemistry
Localization	
Preoperative	Ultrasound
	CT scanning
	NMR scanning
	Arteriography
	Percutaneous transhepatic selective splenoportal venous sampling
Treatment	
Preoperative	Diazoxide for insulinoma
	H_2-receptor antagonists for gastrinoma
	Somatostatin
Operative	Biopsy
	Enucleation
	Pancreatectomy (partial, subtotal)
	Radical en-bloc ± hepatectomy
	Debulking
Postoperative	Drugs, e.g., steroids, H_2-receptor antagonists, diazoxide, somatostatin
	Cytotoxics, streptozotocin, 5FU
	Radiotherapy

plasia or nesidioblastosis) throughout the pancreas, or malignant with lymphatic or hepatic metastases are essential in selecting a specific operation or nonoperatve management. Each syndrome will be considered here, with emphasis on management.

INSULINOMA (Periodic Hypoglycemia)

Diagnosis

A firmly established diagnosis of an insulin-secreting lesion of the pancreas is a prerequisite to surgical treatment. Inappropriate secretion of insulin in association with hypoglycemia can currently be determined with confidence and accuracy.

Preoperative Localization

CT scan, ultrasound, endoscopic retrograde pancreatography, and contrast studies are of little value in localization. Most insulinomas are too small (0.5 to 3.0 cm) to be shown by these techniques. Selective pancreatic angiography and percutaneous transhepatic pancreatic vein catheterization with venous insulin sampling are the only available techniques that have proved to be of some use.

Pancreatic arteriography is successful in approximately 60 percent of cases, but neither beta cell hyperplasia nor nesidioblastosis can be identified. Selective pancreatic venous hormone sampling for tumor localization is helpful in patients with angiographically occult tumors and the multiple endocrine neoplasia type I (MEN I) syndrome, in which multiple tumors or hyperplasia is likely.

Operative Management

An upper abdominal transverse incision or bilateral subcostal incision allows good exposure of the entire pancreas and surrounding viscera. The initial exploration includes an evaluation of the liver and peripancreatic lymph nodes for possible metastatic disease. Biopsies of suspicious or enlarged lymph nodes are obtained for frozen section. The entire pancreas is then mobilized after the initial evaluation. The lateral peritoneal reflection of the duodenum is incised and the duodenum and head of the pancreas reflected medially to the level of the aorta. The pancreatic head, the uncinate process, and the medial wall of the duodenum are carefully palpated bimanually for tumors that are not readily visualized. The stomach is retracted away from the pancreas, and the entire distal pancreas is inspected and palpated from the superior mesenteric vessels to the hilus of the spleen.

When a benign-appearing insulinoma is seen or palpated in the head, uncinate process, neck, or body and is near either exposed surface of the gland, *enucleation* is usually possible without injuring the ductal

structures. A tumor in the tail or distal body is usually removed by distal pancreatectomy. Rarely, a large benign lesion in the head involving the duct may require a more extensive procedure. Nearly all benign lesions arising in the head or uncinate process can be enucleated.

Malignant lesions in the head, potentially curable, should be treated by a pancreaticoduodenectomy. Body or tail malignant tumors, with or without metastases, are treated by distal pancreatectomy. An incurable malignant insulinoma, as determined by liver metastases, should be treated aggressively with the intent of removing as much primary and secondary tumor as is feasible and safe. These procedures may significantly palliate the hypoglycemia and decrease the need for drugs and chemotherapy.

When undertaking a surgical exploration, it is best to remember that 80 percent of insulinomas are benign and single, 10 percent are multiple and benign adenomas or hyperplastic (nesidioblastosis), and less than 10 percent are malignant with metastases. Half the benign tumors are in the head and neck and the remaining in the body and tail of the pancreas.

The major problem occurs when no tumor is found in either the pancreas or in ectopic locations. This is occurring more frequently with earlier diagnosis of the disease. I do not favor a "blind" distal pancreatic resection in the hope that a small occult tumor will be found on multiple sectioning. All patients receive a trial course of diazoxide preoperatively to evaluate responsiveness.

At the time of surgery, I use intraoperative ultrasound and rapid insulin assay (RIA) following selective splenoportal venous sampling through a catheter fed into a splenic vein. The RIA results are available in 30 to 40 minutes, and this, together with the preoperative venous sampling, helps to determine the extent of surgery. If all tests indicate localization in the body and/or tail, a distal pancreatectomy is performed. If there is no localization and the patient was preoperatively responsive to diazoxide, I only undertake a diagnostic biopsy of the tail to exclude hyperplasia. In patients unresponsive to diazoxide and with no tumor localization, an 80 percent pancreatectomy is performed, leaving only a small portion of the head and uncinate process. A distal pancreatic resection (50% to 60%) is insufficient to control the hyperinsulinism.

I have not confirmed that intraoperative monitoring of blood glucose nor the hyperglycemic rebound within 30 minutes following removal of an insulinoma is useful. Extracorporeal glucose monitoring with the artificial pancreas detects immediately, and rapidly responds to, changes in blood glucose concentrations from tumor manipulation or excision and maintains euglycemia.

Regardless of the extent of resection for benign disease, about 10 percent of patients develop diabetes mellitus postoperatively. Persistent hyperglycemia occurs with malignant insulinomas that cannot be resected and in a few adults with hyperplasia despite an 80 percent resection. Streptozotocin controls the hyperglycemia in about 60 percent of patients with malignant disease. Other techniques for liver metastases include selective hepatic arterial ligation, embolization, and infusion of strepto-zotocin with 5-fluorouracil.

Patients without hyperplasia or a tumor are placed on diazoxide therapy postoperatively to control the hyperinsulinism and are re-evaluated 1 to 2 years later. It is hoped that by this stage, the tumor will have increased enough in size to be found on both preoperative testing and surgical exploration.

Complications

In a multi-institutional review of over 1,000 cases of insulinoma, Stefanini, in 1974, reported an overall surgical mortality rate of 11 percent. Acute pancreatitis or peritonitis was the leading cause of death, and pancreatic pseudocysts were found only after enucleation. The overall morbidity and morality following surgery of the pancreas has declined over the past several years. Persistence or recurrence of hyperglycemia occurred in 16 percent of patients owing to either a nonresectable carcinoma or hyperplasia (7%) or tumors that were missed at operation (9%). The Mayo Clinic reports an overall cure rate of 89 percent in 47 patients treated for insulinoma from 1965 to 1975, with a 0 percent operative morality during the past 23 years. Long-term follow-up in 41 of these patients shows a high incidence of neuropsychiatric symptoms (28%), diabetes mellitus (28%), and peptic ulcer disease (36%).

THE VERNER-MORRISON SYNDROME

Clinical Features

Verner and Morrison in 1958 reported two patients with a pancreatic non-beta islet cell tumor causing watery diarrhea without peptic ulceration. Subsequently named WDHA syndrome after the initial letters of its main characteristics, namely *w*atery *d*iarrhea, *h*ypokalemia, and hypo- or *a*chlorhydria. The syndrome, also called pancreatic cholera or vipoma, is rare, being about one-tenth as common as the ZES, and is sometimes part of multiple endocrine neoplasia.

A non-beta islet cell tumor of the pancreas is usually present (D_1 cells), and about half these tumors are malignant. Tumors occur elsewhere as bronchial (probably oat cell) carcinoma, retroperitoneal neuroblastoma, or adrenal gland tumor, and secrete vasoactive intestinal polypeptide (VIP), a polypeptide humoral agent normally produced by the gut. In large doses, VIP causes vasodilation with facial flushing, increases intestinal blood flow, induces watery diarrhea, and inhibits gastric secretion that causes the clinical features. The diarrhea is explosive, up to 20 to 30 stools per day, and does not respond to simple measures. This causes a profound hypokalemia, but the associated hypercalcemia is unexplained. Bloom's 62 cases had either a pancreatic tumor (84%) or a neural tumor (16%) and high concentrations of VIP

in the blood (greater than 60 pmol/L) and/or in the tumor. Larsson, failing to find elevated VIP in some patients, suggests that another unknown humoral agent is responsible. Occasionally, patients present with the syndrome and elevated levels of pancreatic polypeptide and prostaglandin (PGE_2). The diagnosis is made by eliminating the common causes of watery diarrhea and hypokalemia. Hypochlorhydria is found on gastric secretion tests and the diagnosis confirmed by measuring elevated blood levels of immunoreactive VIP. The pseudo-Verner-Morrison syndrome refers to patients with watery diarrhea, hypokalemia, and achlorhydria who have normal serum VIP levels and no obvious tumor.

Preoperative Localization

Tumor localization is usually obtained with computerized axial tomography. Most symptomatic tumors are larger than 3 cm in diameter. The retroperitoneum and mediastinum should also be evaluated in patients in whom a pancreatic lesion is not identified. It must be emphasized that 20 percent of those with the watery diarrhea syndrome have diffuse islet cell hyperplasia as the etiology. For pancreatic tumors, a characteristic tumor blush of dilated vessels due to the local action of VIP is found on selective arteriography. This latter is also useful for diagnosing hepatic metastases.

Operative Management

The definitive treatment of the Verner-Morrison syndrome is surgical excision of the tumor whether it be pancreatic, adrenal, or a ganglioneuroma. In addition, when hyperplasia or nesiodioblastosis of the islets is the cause, excision of as much pancreas as is necessary to alleviate symptoms (80% pancreatectomy) is required. Preoperatively, the electrolytes (K^+, Mg^{++}) and dehydration need to be corrected, and if the diarrhea is severe and continuous, steroids or somatostatin may be given. Treatment requires early and aggressive surgery to remove the primary and as much metastatic tumor as possible. The operation is performed through an upper transverse abdominal incision, which allows easy identification of nearly all pancreatic tumors and those in the retroperitoneum. The majority of islet cell tumors in this syndrome have been found in the body or tail of the pancreas. If there is no tumor in the pancreas, a careful exploration of the retroperitoneum, including both adrenals, is carried out. If still no tumor is found, a subtotal pancreatectomy (80%) is performed. Islet cell tumors causing the watery diarrhea syndrome have proved to be malignant in 50 percent of the reported cases.

When a tumor is identified as uncurable because of metastatic spread, palliative resection of as much primary and secondary tumor as is feasible is also indicated. Postoperatively, adrenocortical steroids may be effective in controlling the diarrhea induced by residual tumor.

Prostaglandin inhibitors should be used in patients found to have elevated PGE_2 levels.

If the tumor is found to be benign, total alleviation of all preoperative symptoms and metabolic abnormalities is to be expected. Cure or palliation of the tumor also results in normocalcemia. Chemotherapy with streptozotocin or DTIC may also be useful for the follow-up therapy of metastatic disease in this syndrome. There have been reports of cardiac toxicity and nephrotoxicity associated with hepatic intra-arterial perfusion of streptozotocin. Plasma VIP measurement is a useful screening test for the detection of vipomas and an effective tumor marker to detect occult metastases.

GLUCAGONOMA SYNDROME

Clinical Features

McGavran (1966) reported the first patient with diabetes, skin rash, and a high concentration of plasma and tumor pancreatic glucagon. The characteristic necrolytic migratory erythematous rash led Mallinson, in 1974, to diagnose nine cases. Eight were postmenopausal females with symptoms for more than 1 year, and in two, the symptoms exceeded 10 years. Mild-to-moderate diabetes was present in seven of the patients, and a pancreatic tumor was found in eight patients, of which six were malignant with metastases. Other clinical features of the glucagonoma syndrome include a normochromic normocytic anemia, weight loss, glossitis, hypoaminoacidemia, elevated glucagon levels, and an alpha cell tumor of the pancreas. Most patients are clinically identified as a result of their characteristic skin rash. They are usually severely malnourished; both weight loss and hypoproteinemia are the result of the catabolic effects of glucagon. Adult-onset diabetes can be controlled by diet or low doses of insulin. Ketoacidosis has not been described in patients with this syndrome. Although patients have no recognized coagulopathy, there is a high incidence of venous thrombosis. Therefore, these patients should be well hydrated, ambulated early, given embolic stockings, and treated with low-dose heparin. Because the dermatitis may be associated with significant skin infection, the latter should be treated with antibiotics before pancreatic exploration. Antibiotics and steroids can be given, and hyperalimentation should also be considered to alleviate some of the catabolic effects of chronic hyperglucagonemia.

The pancreatic tumors tend to be more in the body and tail of the pancreas, are 4 to 10 cm in diameter, and contain glucagon. The diagnosis is now easily confirmed by the radioimmunoassay measurements of elevated plasma glucagon levels, and the site of the tumor is confirmed by selective angiography and pancreatic venography. An arginine provocation test has been reported to be of some use in the diagnosis of cases in which plasma glucagon levels are equivocal. A single patient is reported with severe constipation and marked small intestinal mucosa hyperplasia who was found to have a tumor of the kidney producing the enteroglucagon.

Operative Management

Approximately two-thirds of patients with glucagonoma syndrome have malignant tumors with metastases at the time of diagnosis. Nevertheless, aggressive surgical efforts are indicated because tumor reduction may alleviate the debilitating effects of hyperglucagonemia, as well as their dermatologic and systemic manifestations. In contrast to insulinomas, glucagonomas are usually large enough to be identified by CT scanning, which, in conjunction with arteriography, can determine the extent of tumor involvement in both the pancreas and liver. An upper abdominal transverse incision is used for exploration of patients with glucagonomas. A thorough exploration is carried out to determine the extent of the tumor. In tumors involving the body or tail, a distal resection should be carried out even in the presence of lymph node or liver metastases. In addition, large tumor nodules that can be easily wedged from the liver should be removed. When a glucagonoma appears localized in the pancreas, enucleation alone is not indicated because of the high incidence of malignancy.

The majority of glucagonoma patients require chemotherapy postoperatively because of the high incidence of metastatic disease. Streptozotocin and dimethyl triazeno imidazole carboxamide (DTIC) have both been used with some success. In addition, if extensive hepatic metastases are present and cannot be excised surgically, an implantable pump for hepatic artery infusion of chemotherapy may be beneficial. Selective hepatic arterial ligation and embolization have also been used with some success for metastatic glucagonomas. Although streptozotocin may be effective, results are not so good as for malignant insulinomas. Cortisone therapy and zinc may alleviate the skin rash when other drug therapy has been unsuccessful.

SOMATOSTATINOMAS

A number of somatostatin-producing tumors of the pancreas have recently been described. These tumors produce an ill-defined clinical syndrome which includes abdominal pain, anorexia, weight loss, diarrhea, gallbladder disease, and adult-onset diabetes. In patients with other pancreatic endocrine tumors, somatostatin cell hyperplasia is often present in the surrounding pancreatic tissue. The reason is not clear, but it has been suggested that this represents an attempt by the pancreas to decrease tumor hormone production. Diagnosis and treatment are based on the same principles as for other pancreatic apudomas.

PANCREATIC POLYPEPTIDOMA

Plasma polypeptide (PP) levels are elevated in a high percentage of patients with vipomas, insulinomas, gastrinomas, and glucagonomas. Some of these tumors contain PP cells, but in others only PP cell hyperplasia in the remaining pancreas is evident (hyperplasia type II). This suggests that elevated PP levels might serve as biochemical markers for pancreatic endocrine tumors. A number of patients with diarrhea have been noted to have pancreatic endocrine tumors composed of only PP cells (p-poma). Pure pancreatic polypeptide apudomas (p-pomas) are rare, although elevated plasma PP levels are found in one-third of cases of pancreatic apudoma. The initial three patients reported with pure p-pomas had no consistent clinical features. One patient presented with watery diarrhea, hypocalemia, and achlorhydria (WDHA syndrome) and with a normal serum VIP, but grossly elevated PP concentration. Treatment of a p-poma should be surgical excision. An elevated plasma PP concentration that occurs postoperatively in the absence of residual tumor is due to PP cell hyperplasia.

MIXED PANCREATIC ISLET CELL TUMORS

Mixed tumors are of clinical importance as the spectrum of symptoms may change with time and metastases may contain only some of the primary tumor cell types. Since raised plasma concentration of hormones may originate either from the primary or metastatic tumor tissue or from hyperplastic extratumoral cells, immunocytochemical studies are necessary. Ideally, the plasma concentration of as many hormones and polypeptides as possible should be measured in all suspected pancreatic apudomas; tumor tissue should be investigated by immunocytochemistry, and hormones measured postoperatively to confirm removal of all tumor tissue. Apudomas have been described as secreting a combination of several polypeptides, e.g., ACTH, MSH, and gastrin.

MULTIPLE ENDOCRINE NEOPLASIA

This term describes a group of syndromes, often familial, in which two or more endocrine glands undergo hyperplasia or tumor formation in the same individual, either at the same time or consecutively. The hyperfunc-tioning glands secrete their normal major hormones (orthoendocrine syndromes) and/or abnormal hormones (paraendocrine syndromes). There are two main varieties.

Multiple Endocrine Neoplasia Type I (MEN I or MEA I) or Wermer's Syndrome. This manifests from the second decade into old age with an equal sex distribution. The glands involved in order of frequency are parathyroids (88%), pancreatic islets (81%), anterior pituitary (65%), adrenal cortex (38%), and thyroid follicular cells (19%). The parathyroids usually undergo chief cell hyperplasia or, less commonly, multiple adenoma formation. The islet cells may be involved by an adenoma (multiple or single), carcinoma, and, rarely, a generalized hyperplasia. In the pituitary, an adenoma or, rarely, a carcinoma or hyperplasia may involve any of the different cell types. The adrenal cortices usually show bilateral diffuse or nodular hyperplasia, but adenomas have been reported. The changes in the thyroid are variable, and occasionally carcinoid tumors are present in the lungs, the pancreas, or the intestine. Peptic ulceration, especially duodenal, is a common feature in some families and may affect more than half the patients. These may form part of the Zollinger-Ellison syndrome owing to an associated pancreatic gastrinoma or to hyperparathyroidism. Many of these lesions are apudomas, and the syndrome may result from a widespread dysplasia of the APUD cells.

Multiple Endocrine Neoplasia Type II (MEN II or MEA II) or Sipple's Syndrome. This syndrome is usually inherited, affects sexes equally, and may manifest itself from the first decade onward, especially between the ages of 20 and 40 years. Three forms of the syndrome are recognized. The most common is medullary carcinoma of the thyroid with a pheochromocytoma in one or both adrenals. Hyperparathyroidism due to hyperplasia or adenoma may be present and is probably due to hypercalcitoninemia. Another variant is a medullary carcinoma of thyroid and pheochromocytoma with multiple small subcutaneous and submucous neuromas of the eyelids, tongue, and buccal mucosa and a diffuse hypertrophy of the lips. These lesions are present from birth. In the last type, all these features are present together with autonomic ganglioneuromatosis and various other congenital abnormalities.

THE SPLEEN

SPLENECTOMY FOR HEMATOLOGIC DISORDERS

SEYMOUR I. SCHWARTZ, M.D., F.A.C.S.

The hematologic disorders for which splenectomy has proved effective include (1) conditions in which the red blood cell has impaired deformability, and (2) situations in which the surface properties of circulating blood cells are altered in such a way as to predispose the cells to phagocytosis. The former category includes hereditary spherocytosis, thalassemia, sickle cell disease, and pyruvate-kinase deficiency. The second group includes immune hemolytic anemia, and idiopathic thrombocytopenic purpura. There are also other conditions such as thrombotic thrombocytopenic purpura, myeloproliferative disorders, and secondary hypersplenism that are associated with excessive intrasplenic destruction of cells as a consequence of diverse pathologic findings.

CONDITIONS WITH IMPAIRED RED CELL DEFORMABILITY

Hereditary Spherocytosis. Anemia with hemolysis is caused by an inherited disorder of the red cell membrane and consequent reduction of cellular deformability, which in turn causes splenic trapping and destruction of cells. The rarer membrane abnormalities leading to ovalocytosis and stomatocytosis are also in this category. Hereditary spherocytosis is transmitted as an autosomal dominant trait. The clinical manifestations are anemia, jaundice, and splenomegaly. The anemia may be mild, in which case the disease may not be diagnosed until adulthood. Jaundice parallels the extent of anemia. Cholelithiasis is present in 30 to 60 percent of patients, but it is uncommon in children under 10 years of age. Infection can lead to life-threatening aplastic crises, particularly in children, but this is uncommon. Splenectomy is the only appropriate treatment and is usually warranted even in mildly affected cases to reduce the risk of cholelithiasis. It is preferable to delay the operation until the patient is older than 4 years of age to reduce the incidence of overwhelming post-splenectomy sepsis, but this is arbitrary. Concomitant cholecystectomy should be performed if gallstones are present. The results of splenectomy are uniformly favorable if the diagnosis is correct. This also pertains to ovalocytosis, but hereditary stomatocytosis often does not respond to splenectomy.

Thalassemia. Thalassemia is also transmitted as a dominant trait and is characterized by a defect in the hemoglobin molecule that leads to the development of intracellular precipitates (Heinz bodies), contributing to premature red cell destruction. The cells are small, thin, and misshapen. Patients with homozygous thalassemia usually have clinical manifestations in the first year of life. In homozygotes and in some heterozygotes, the spleen may reach a size that creates mechanical problems. The patients may experience intermittent left upper quadrant pain related to splenic infarction. They have an increasing transfusion requirement and a propensity for intercurrent infections. Improvement following splenectomy may be significant in patients in whom transfusion requirements are increased and in whom splenic size and/or infarction is symptomatic. Most studies indicate no difference in the risk of infection before or after splenectomy.

Sickle Cell Disease. Sickle cell anemia, which occurs predominantly in blacks, is characterized by crescent-shaped erythrocytes with compromised deformability that leads to trapping in the splenic cords. Although the trait is present in 9 percent of blacks, sickle cell anemia is observed in 0.3 to 1.3 percent of blacks. In double heterozygotes for hemoglobin S, a series of microinfarcts results in autosplenectomy. Occasionally hypersplenism, including symptomatic thrombocytopenia, may constitute an indication for splenectomy. In rare instances, an operation is mandated by the development of a splenic abscess manifested by splenomegaly, splenic pain, and spiking fever.

Hereditary Hemolytic Anemia with Red Cell Enzyme Deficiency. The most common of these disorders is pyruvate-kinase deficiency, which is associated with decreased red cell deformability. Although splenectomy does not eliminate the hemolytic process, it may reduce or eliminate transfusion requirements. The results are not predictable, and postoperative thrombocytosis leading to hepatic, portal, or caval thrombosis has been reported.

CONDITION WITH ALTERED SURFACE PROPERTIES OF CIRCULATING BLOOD CELLS

Immune Hemolytic Anemia. The disorder may be related to certain medications, infections, or a lymphoproliferative disorder. Immunoglobulins, or complement fixed to the red cell surface, as demonstrated by the Coombs' test, result in reduced red cell survival and hemolysis. Immune hemolytic anemia occurs more commonly in women and after the age of 50. Splenomegaly is present in about half the cases. Splenectomy is rarely beneficial in diseases associated with "cold" antibodies, e.g., paroxysomal cold hemoglobinuria. In the warm antibody anemias, splenectomy is indicated for patients who do not respond to steroid therapy or for patients who cannot tolerate the high-dose steroid regimen. A favorable response to removal of the spleen is to be anticipated in 80 percent of these patients.

Idiopathic Thrombocytopenic Purpura (ITP). This disease, the most common hemtologic indication for splenectomy, is acquired and is characterized by destruction and trapping of platelets exposed to circulating IgG antiplatelet factors. The spleen is the source of IgG specific for platelets, and since 30 percent of circulating platelets are in the spleen at all times, the organ plays an integral role in this regard and is also a major site of platelet trapping.

The clinical manifestations include petechiae and/or ecchymoses, bleeding gums, mild gastrointestinal bleeding, hematuria, and vaginal bleeding. Women are affected three times more frequently than men. The spleen is rarely palpable. The platelet count is generally less than 50,000 per cubic millimeter, and the bleeding time may be prolonged. The bone marrow reveals a normal or increased number of megakaryocytes.

The disease is usually an acute and self-limiting process in children. In adults, ITP is usually more responsive, and a sustained response to steroids or plasmapheresis occurs in less than 20 percent of patients. Between 75 and 85 percent of patients subjected to splenectomy have a permanent response, with a rise in the platelet count to over 100,000 per cubic millimeter by the seventh postoperative day. A positive effect of splenectomy is noted even in patients in whom the platelet count does not return to normal as subsequent episodes of petechiae or bleeding rarely occur.

At present, steroids generally constitute the initial therapy. If the platelet count does not increase above 100,000 per cubic millimeter within 6 to 8 weeks or if thrombocytopenia recurs when the drug is discontinued, splenectomy is indicated. The indications for splenectomy for thrombocytopenia in patients with lupus erythematosus are the same as those for ITP.

CONDITIONS ASSOCIATED WITH EXCESSIVE INTRASPLENIC CELL DESTRUCTION

Thrombotic Thrombocytopenic Purpura (TTP).

This is not truly a hematologic disorder, but rather a microvascular disease with hematologic consequences. Arterioles undergo a diffuse subendothelial hyalinization that results in narrowing of the lumens and profound platelet trapping with resultant thrombocytopenia. The clinical manifestations are highlighted by fever, purpura, hemolytic anemia, neurologic abnormalities, and signs of renal disease. The thrombocytopenia is marked early after the onset of the disease, and it is accompanied by fragmented and distorted red cells. Most patients have a fulminant course, and recovery has been reported for patients treated with anticoagulants, steroids, plasmapheresis, heparin, and dextran. The combination of high doses of steroids and urgent splenectomy has achieved the highest success rate (65%).

Myeloproliferative Disorders. Myeloid metaplasia (myelofibrosis) is characterized by increased connective tissue proliferation of marrow, spleen, liver, and lymph nodes. The laboratory hallmark is a peripheral blood smear that demonstrates fragmented, tear-drop, and immature red cells coupled with immature myeloid cells. Thrombocytopenia is present in one-third of the patients, thrombocytosis in one quarter.

Splenectomy should be considered as a palliative procedure in patients with symptomatic splenomegaly or clinically manifest hypersplenism. There is no evidence that splenectomy will adversely affect the hematologic state by removing a significant source of hematopoiesis. Postoperative thrombosis of the splenic and splanchnic venous circulation occurs more commonly in these patients. Prophylaxis against this complication includes avoiding the operation when the patient is thrombocytopenic and using antiplatelet aggregating drugs perioperatively.

Secondary Hypersplenism. Splenomegaly or splenic congestion, which attends a wide variety of diseases, may result in thrombocytopenia, leukopenia, anemia, or any combination of these abnormalities. In patients with lymphomas or lymphocytic leukemia, splenectomy may be indicated for symptomatic splenomegaly or hypersplenism that is of clinical importance or compromises radiation and chemotherapy. The procedure should be performed when the patient's condition is reasonable and not as a preterminal exercise. Splenectomy usually effectively increases the neutrophil count in neutropenic patients with Felty's syndrome and the cytopenia of Gaucher's disease. In patients with secondary hypersplenism related to cirrhosis, splenectomy alone should not be performed because the cytopenia is rarely symptomatic; removal of the organ does not permanently reduce the portal pressure, and the potential venous conduit of the splenic vein, for a decompressive shunt, will be destroyed.

SPLENECTOMY

It is helpful to have the stomach decompressed during the procedure to facilitate ligation of the short gastric veins. The posterior ligamentous attachments are divided first to permit mobilization. The splenic hilus is the ultimate pedicle, and the artery and vein are ligated individually, taking care to avoid injury to the tail of the pancreas. Routine drainage of the left subphrenic space is not advisable, but it has been our policy to drain this space in patients with myeloproliferative disease in whom a large spleen is removed and there is evidence of portal hypertension, i.e., large collaterals. Accessory spleens, which are present in 18 to 30 percent of patients with hematologic disease, should be sought by performing a thorough exploration of the entire peritoneal cavity.

No therapy other than hydration is indicated for patients with postoperative thrombocytosis. If the platelet count rises above 2,000,000 per cubic millimeter, antiplatelet aggregating drugs such as aspirin or dipyridamole may be used. All patients receive Pneumovax pre-operatively, and children receive daily penicillin until the age of 18. Adults are not routinely given antibiotics. The increased incidence of overwhelming postsplenectomy sepsis is an important factor, but is usually related to disease susceptibility such as thalassemia, and also to radiation or chemotherapy or to the general debility of the patient. Patients should not be denied splenectomy because of the potential for this problem, but rather should be maintained on close postoperative surveillance.

TUMORS, CYSTS, AND ABSCESSES OF THE SPLEEN

DONALD E. FRY, M.D.,F.A.C.S.

SPLENIC TUMORS

Primary neoplasms of the spleen are extraordinarily rare lesions. A brief review of the English literature indicates that perhaps only 300 such primary lesions have been reported if one exludes lymphoid neoplasms. Among malignant neoplasms that are primary to the spleen are (1) vascular lesions, (2) lymphoid tumors, (3) tumors of reticuloendothelial origin, (4) tumors of fibrous tissue elements, (5) smooth muscle neoplasms, (6) tumors arising from nerve tissue, and (7) neoplasms arising from embryologic rests. For each of the seven broad classes of neoplasms, a benign counterpart of similar tissue origin is possible. Primary lymphoma is the most common malignant lesion whereas hemangioma is probably the prevalent benign lesion.

Diagnosis is usually achieved by computerized tomography or by angiography. The variable degree of vascularity of these lesions may compromise the diagnostic accuracy of the conventional splenic scan. The absence of a cystic quality for most masses likewise negates the value of ultrasound. Diagnostic inquiry usually is inspired by vague left upper quadrant pain, abdominal fullness, or the ''''small stomach syndrome'' if the lesion assumes a large size. Once mass lesions are identified, potential extrasplenic primary lesions that may metastasize to the spleen should be considered. Breast, lung, and colon primaries are likely sources.

Splenectomy is the principal treatment for these lesions, whether benign or malignant. Frozen sections of small biopsies of mesenchymal or lymphoid lesions are precarious at best in terms of accuracy. Local extension of the disease should cause consideration for resection of contiguous structures in nonlymphoid neoplasms. Chemotherapy or radiation therapy are of limited value, and so surgical resection remains the patient's best chance. Results of resections of hemangiosarcoma, the most common nonlymphoid malignant tumor, have been generally poor. For patients with apparent lymphoma or lymphosarcoma, liver biopsy and appropriate node biopsies should be undertaken to stage the illness. The role of radiotherapy and chemotherapy in the treatment of malignant tumors of lymphoid origin makes these lesions prognostically more favorable.

SPLENIC CYSTS

Splenic cysts can be divided into those that are nonparasitic and those that are parasitic in origin. Both are extremely rare. Among nonparasitic cysts, lesions may be true cysts with an epithelial lining or they may be actual pseudocysts. True cysts include peritoneal inclusions and dermoid and epidermoid cysts. Hematoma from previous trauma or infarction of splenic tissue may result in pseudocysts with a fibrous lining that may calcify with time. Lymphangiomas and hemangiomas are commonly diagnosed as being cysts. Nonparasitic splenic cysts are usually solitary. The usual symptoms are pain and fullness in the left upper quadrant.

Any discussion of parasitic cysts of the spleen primarily involves hydatid disease. Splenic involvement with echinococcal disease is only seen in about 2 percent of patients. Such cysts are very rare in the United States.

Symptoms may be constitutional from the primary disease. If the splenic cyst achieves a sufficiently large size, symptoms of left upper quadrant pain, fullness, or gastric compression may be identified. Patients commonly have peripheral eosinophilia. Calcification may permit diagnosis on plain roentgenograms of the abdomen. Specific studies of complement fixation may prove diagnostic of the primary disease in 85 to 90 percent of patients.

Definitive diagnosis of the splenic cyst, whether of parasitic or nonparasitic origin, is usually best achieved by CT scanning or ultrasonography. When cysts are large, conventional splenic scans may prove diagnostic. Angiography may only be of benefit in very large lesions.

The treatment for splenic cysts is generally splenectomy. Those small cysts that are likely to be from remote trauma, those not parasitic in origin, and those minimally symptomatic may be managed expectantly. Expectant management consists of accepting an undefined risk of bleeding into the cyst, spontaneous rupture, or secondary infection. Lesions that are not centrally located could be handled by hemisplenectomy. This might be particularly desirable in juvenile and adolescent patients, in whom preservation of splenic reticuloendothelial function is thought to be most useful. On the other hand, lesions that are large enough to be symptomatic may not be amenable to anything other than splenectomy.

Splenectomy for hydatid disease poses some special problems. Such cysts have precariously thin walls and may be ruptured into the peritoneal cavity with dissemination of the scolices and/or anaphylaxis. Evacuation of the cysts by aspiration with formalin instillation into the cavity is frequently desirable prior to splenectomy.

SPLENIC ABSCESS

When compared to splenic tumors and cysts, abscesses of the spleen are relatively common. Patients with endocarditis, intravenous drug abusers, and patients with sickle cell disease are vulnerable to splenic abscess. Calderera demonstrated, in experimental animals in the 1930s, that bacteremia combined with ischemia or infarction of splenic tissue will result in splenic abscess. Recent concerns over postsplenectomy sepsis have resulted in retained hematoma and ischemic tissue when limited operation or nonoperative treatment is employed for the patient with splenic trauma. An intercurrent bacteremia from remote infection sets the stage for splenic abscess.

The clinical presentation of splenic abscess can be extraordinarily occult. Patients have the usual fever and leukocytosis. Bacteremia is usually identified, but may be obscured by empiric antibiotic therapy. It is important that the physician have a keen sense of awareness that splenic abscess is a potential problem in patients with sickle cell disease and in drug addicts. Physical findings on abdominal examination may not be impressive, and masses are only palpable when the abscess has achieved a very large size. The diagnosis is established by the abdominal CT scan, by conventional spleen scan, or by skilled ultrasonography.

The treatment of splenic abscess remains splenectomy. Attempts at splenotomy and external drainage may be complicated by recurrent abscess or major bleeding. Disruption of major arterial or venous branches of the spleen into the abscess cavity with life-threatening hemorrhage has been seen to result from splenotomy. Splenic abscesses are commonly adherent to the diagphragm, left lobe of the liver, splenic flexure of colon, or greater curvature of the stomach. Removal of this portion of the abscess "rind" may be hazardous, and it is probably best left alone. Left upper quadrant drainage that exists at the tip of the twelfth rib with large sump systems are useful for continued management of the retained abscess cavity.

Antibiotic selection should focus on likely organisms. Blood culture data may already be available to guide the choice of an antibiotic. In sickle cell patients, gram-negative organisms are likely to predominate, and amino-

glycosides may be needed. Patients with endocarditis usually have gram-positive organisms, and for most species penicillin is appropriate. In drug addicts, virtually any organism is possible, although my experience with seven patients indicated that staphylococci and enterococci predominated. Because methicillin-resistant *Staphylococcus epidermidis* is becoming more prevalent, initial presumptive therapy may require vancomycin until specific culture data are available. A Gram stain of an intraoperative sample of exudate from the abscess may be particularly useful in reducing possible antibiotic choices. As opposed to other intra-abdominal abscesses, the splenic abscess is usually caused by a solitary organism, and this makes the Gram stain especially significant.

TECHNICAL ASPECTS OF SPLENECTOMY

Preoperative preparation for patients with tumors, cysts, or abscesses is generally similar. Large tumors or abscesses may be associated with major blood loss, and appropriate blood resources should be available to cover this eventuality. Immediate preoperative nasogastric decompression is necessary to minimize the risk of gastric injury during splenectomy. Antibiotics should be administered preoperatively to patients with abscesses to maximize protection of the surgical incision and adjacent soft tissues of the peritoneal cavity, which are likely to be contaminated with the drainage and splenectomy process. Since splenectomy for tumors and cysts are clean operations that do not transgress a colonized viscus, preventive preoperative antibiotics usually are not necessary. If adherence of the stomach or intestine to the splenic tumor is likely, particularly when the lesion is large, preoperative cefazolin for wound prophylaxis may be desirable.

Maximal exposure is achieved with a left subcostal incision. For large lesions, this incision can be extended to the tip of the twelfth rib or across the midline along the right subcostal margin. A bed roll placed under the left side of the patient when positioning the patient prior to skin preparation and draping facilitates exposure in the case of a large lesion in which unusual difficulty is anticipated.

Once the abdomen is entered, the extent of intra-abdominal disease needs to be assessed regardless of the primary diagnosis. In patients with malignant lesions fo the spleen, metastases elsewhere within the abdomen are identified. In cases of lymphoma, a liver biopsy and periaortic nodes are taken. In hydatid disease, extrasplenic extent of the disease should also be explored. Heroin addicts and patients with endocarditis may have other abscess foci within the abdomen.

Ligation of the splenic artery in the lesser sac is desirable for splenectomy involving large masses and abscesses. The gastrocolic omentum is divided, and the splenic artery is ligated at the superior margin of the pancreas. Division of the gastrocolic omentum laterally to the splenic flexure facilitates exposure of the pancreas and its relationship to the spleen. Lateral attachments of the spleen are then sharply divided. Division of each short gastric artery is desirable, but can be extraordinarily difficult in cases of upper pole spleen lesions and any lesion that is especially large. Care must be exercised in avoiding injury or devascularization of the greater curvature of the stomach. Malignant lesions that are adherent to the stomach may require that a portion of the stomach be resected with the spleen. Individual branches of the splenic artery and vein are then divided and ligated. The relationship of the pancreatic tail must be appreciated to avoid an inadvertent injury. Meticulous hemostasis must be achieved since the dead space created in the left upper quadrant following removal of large spleens becomes an invitation for hematoma and subsequent subphrenic abscess. The pancreatic tail and the greater curvature of the stomach are likewise carefully inspected for injury.

The use of drains following splenectomy for any cause remains controversial. My review of splenectomies in cases of trauma and for patients with hematologic malignant disease indicates that postoperative abscess is greater in patients *with* drains than in patients *without* drains. The relatively high frequency of staphylococcal abscesses in patients with drains suggests that external migration of microorganisms into the peritoneal space may be a special problem. However, drains are usually a necessity when splenectomy has been performed for abscess. Only on rare occasion can the abscess be removed in its entirety with the splenectomy. Rather, a large abscess cavity is usually left behind and sump drains are necessary to minimize the risks of recurrent abscess. The surgical wound should have the skin and subcutaneous tissue left open for delayed primary closure in patients who undergo splenectomy for abscess.

There are relatively few special considerations in the postoperative management of these patients. In the case of a particularly difficult dissection along the greater curvature of the stomach, retention of the nasogastric tube for 4 to 5 postoperative days may be desirable. Postoperative amylase determinations may be useful when encroachment of pancreatic parenchyma during splenectomy is a concern. Systemic antibiotics should be continued for abscess patients until clinical resolution occurs. For patients with staphylococcal bacteremia and abscess, parenteral antibiotics for 10 to 14 days is probably desirable to prevent recurrent bacteremia and seeding of heart valves.

Postsplenectomy sepsis has become a major concern during the last decade. This infectious complication is relatively rare, but is particularly devastating because of the fulminant and fatal nature of the illness. Postsplenectomy sepsis usually occurs with the encapsulated organisms—*Pneumococcus, Meningococcus*, and *Hemophilus influenza*. Patients with juvenile, adolescent, and hematologic malignant disease are at special risk. The polyvalent pneumococcal vaccine should be used, even preoperatively if possible, for these patients to provide specific immunity against the 23 most common pneumococcal isolates. Approximately 3 weeks are required before specific immunity is conferred by vaccination. Obviously, these patients remain at risk for infection from other pneumococci as well as other bacterial species. Prophylactic penicillin has been recommended, but problems of patient compliance and an incomplete bacterial spectrum make this practice of questionable value. Patients must be made aware of the nature and significance of a rapidly evolving infection.

HERNIA

GROIN HERNIA

RAYMOND POLLAK, M.B., F.R.C.S. (Edin.)
LLOYD M. NYHUS, M.D., F.A.C.S.

Hernias of the groin have been known since ancient Egyptian times, having been first described in the Ebers papyrus of 1600 B.C. A more lucid description was given by Orelius Cornelius Celcus, a Roman, in the first century A.D. The surgery of hernia repair was revived in Salerno in the twelfth century, and in 1556 Piere Franco published, *Traite Des Hernies* shortly before he died. With the development of modern surgery in the seventeenth, eighteenth, and nineteenth centuries, numerous techniques of hernia repair were described as an appreciation of the anatomy of the region developed. Peter Kemper, Antonio Scarpa, Antonio deGimbernat, Henry O. Marcy, Edwardo Bassini, and William S. Halsted all described differing kinds of hernia repairs.

The modern era of hernia surgery has been characterized by a clearer understanding of hernia anatomy as well as by the understanding of the biology and biochemistry of collagen metabolism. These latter studies have largely been the result of excellent work by McVay, Condon, Reid, and Peacock.

INCIDENCE

The incidence of groin hernias throughout all decades of life is uncertain. However, their highest frequency occurs in infancy. The actual incidence of hernia or hydrocele in a childhood population has been estimated to be between 1 and 4 percent. In premature infants, the incidence may be as high as 30 percent in infants weighing less than 1,000 grams at birth. Only 10 to 15 percent of all inguinal hernias occur in women. In childhood and adolescence, 60 percent of hernias occur on the right side and 20 to 25 percent on the left. In small children, 10 to 15 percent of hernias are bilateral at first presentation. The size of the problem is even further magnified when one realizes that over 500,000 groin hernia operations are performed in the United States annually.

ETIOLOGY AND PATHOGENESIS

The classification of groin hernias has had to be rethought of late because controversy still exists as to the etiologic mechanisms that underlie most hernias. Groin hernias have been divided anatomically into inguinal hernias (hernias above the inguinal ligament) and femoral hernias (hernias that occur below the inguinal ligament and protrude through the femoral canal). The inguinal hernias were further subclassified into indirect hernias and direct hernias, based on the relationship of the hernia sac to the inferior epigastric artery and Hesselbach's triangle. Modern authors have preferred to label these hernias as either congenital (a hernia defect in the lower abdominal wall that has been present since birth) or acquired (a defect that appears only later in life and is unrelated to any congenital developmental anomaly). The presence of a patent *processus vaginalis* has been implicated in the causation of indirect inguinal hernias (or congenital hernias), especially in children and young adolescents. However, the presence of a *processus* in older adults (in the sixth and seventh decades) who have indirect inguinal hernias may not be etiologically related to the causation of the hernia. Elegant studies by Peacock and Reid would suggest that, in later adult life, abnormalities of collagen synthesis and breakdown are largely responsible for the deterioration of the transversalis fascia. This results in replacement of this layer by weak areolar tissue and leads to hernia formation. There is now general agreement that the most important musculo-aponeurotico fascial layer in the groin consists of the transversus abdominis muscle, its aponeurosis and fascial coverings, in continuity with the transversalis fascia onto adjacent areas such as the rectus fascia medially and then inferiorly toward the thigh to form the femoral sheath. The more superificial layers of the anterior abdominal wall appear to play little if any role in the support of the inguinal floor. Thus the objective in any hernia repair should be to return the transversus abdominis layer to normal.

TREATMENT

As a rule, a groin hernia is repaired surgically as soon as the diagnosis is made because of the propensity of these hernias to undergo intestinal entrapment with incarceration, subsequent compromise of the blood supply to the entrapped intestine and strangulation, and finally perforation with sepsis and death. The degree of urgency of repair also is dictated by the age of the patient and underlying medical conditions. Certainly in infants and in older adults with congenital or indirect hernias, repair is required as soon as is feasible because of the high incidence of incarceration and strangulation in these age groups. Similarly, femoral hernias should be repaired early to avoid compromise to the viability of the contained intestines.

In large direct hernias that are acquired in an older individual, repair of the hernia should be delayed until the patient is in a suitable physical state to undergo the repair. However, age and infirmity are no deterrent to successful repair of most groin hernias, as many of these can be repaired under local anesthesia. In infants, a question of bilaterality of hernias might exist. In the case of a right-sided hernia, there is a 15 percent chance that a hernia will develop on the left side. Conversely, when the primary hernia is left-sided, there is a 41 percent chance that a hernia will develop on the right side. Although some surgeons routinely explore both deep inguinal rings in infants at the first presentation of a hernia on either side, contralateral exploration in the infant is becoming less common. In adults with bilateral hernias, we do not repair both at the same operation, but stage the repairs in order to reduce the risk of such potential complications as wound sepsis and recurrence.

The use of a truss to keep a hernia reduced has been a practice since medieval times. However, it is a form of procrastination only and does not protect the patient against the common complications of unrepaired groin hernias. A truss may be difficult to apply and uncomfortable to wear, and often fails to achieve the desired objective of keeping the hernia reduced because of a poor match to the patient's body habitus. It is occasionally useful in an obese older individual whose condition does not permit any kind of surgical repair.

SURGICAL MANAGEMENT

Congenital (Indirect) Inguinal Hernia

A congenital or indirect inguinal hernia is invariably associated with a patent *processus vaginalis*. Thus, in principle, all that is required for the repair of this hernia is resection of the patent *processus* and closure of the deep inguinal ring. An incision is made in the lower quadrant of the abdomen approximately 2 fingerbreadths above the pubic tubercle. This incision is taken down through the subcutaneous tissues to the external oblique fascia. The external oblique fascia is then opened in the line of its fibers while care is taken to protect the underlying ilio-inguinal nerve. By means of hemostats or a self-retaining retractor, the external oblique edges are widely separated to expose the underlying spermatic cord (or round ligament). The spermatic cord (or round ligament) is isolated, and a Penrose drain is placed around either structure. The patent *processus vaginalis* is seen to be lying in an anteromedial fashion in relation to the cord and protruding through the deep inguinal ring. The hernial sac is then freed from the cord by sharp and blunt dissection. Cremasteric muscle fibers are divided to prevent the development of hematomas of the cord in the

postoperative period. The round ligament may be safely divided and secured with a 2–0 Vicryl suture in women. Contained intestine within the sac is then carefully reduced into the abdominal cavity prior to opening or placing any ligatures around the sac in a blind fashion. In adults with large hernias, it usually is necessary to open the sac, reduce the visceral contents, and then place a 3–0 silk purse-string suture from within in order to effect closure of the peritoneal cavity. In infants, a silk ligature may be placed around the base of the sac after reduction of any contained intestine, and the excess sac excised and sent for histological examination. The same can be done for smaller hernial sacs in adults, but when the sac is large and redundant, it is best to incise the sac, open it, and sew the sac with a purse-string suture of 3–0 silk from the inside. The redundant sac is then excised after the ligature has been tied and sent for permanent histologic examination.

At this point of the operation in infants, the procedure is completed. There is rarely a need to place any sutures in the transversalis fascia in order to tighten up the inguinal ring. The deep inguinal ring in infants, at this point of the operation, should admit the tip of a Kelly clamp freely without undue tension. If sutures are thought to be necessary, they should be placed in such a way that the venous outflow from the spermatic cord will not be compromised and thus cause testicular swelling in the postoperative period. In adults, however, it is important, prior to placing the purse-string suture, to examine the strength of the posterior inguinal floor as well as the femoral canal to ascertain the absence of a concomitent direct or femoral hernia. If no weakness exists in the inguinal floor and no femoral hernia is noted, the sac can be closed, as already described. In adults, however, it may be necessary to place one or two sutures of 3–0 silk in the deep inguinal ring to close any large defect in the transversalis fascia that may have arisen as the result of the persistence of the patent *processus vaginalis*. When a repair of the inguinal floor is deemed necessary, the technique is the same as for a direct inguinal hernia repair (to be discussed).

Recurrences, though rare, may occur when there is (1) a missed hernia or a failure to recognize a concomitant direct or femoral hernia, (2) failure to recognize a weak posterior inguinal wall, or (3) poor closure of the abdominal deep inguinal ring in adults. This latter error may result in a protrusion of preperitoneal fat into the inguinal ring and so allow the underlining peritoneal sac once again to invaginate the transversalis fascia and form a new hernia.

Acquired (Direct) Inguinal Hernia

A direct inguinal hernia is due to a weakness in the posterior inguinal floor. It usually presents as a diffuse bulge of the posterior inguinal wall. In the repair of these hernias, there is some controversy as to whether the weak and attenuated posterior wall should be excised, or whether the transversalis fascia at the upper margin should be sutured to the tissues below the defect. As for the congenital hernias, the inguinal floor is exposed, the cord retracted laterally, and a search made at its anteromedial aspect at the deep inguinal ring to ascertain the absence of any indirect hernial sac. The presence of an indirect and a direct hernia has been referred to in the past as a ''pantaloon'' hernia. If an indirect sac is found, it is treated as previously discussed. Attention is then turned to the direct component. The flimsy posterior inguinal floor is excised while attention is given to careful hemostasis. With an Allis clamp, the transversus abdominis muscle and its fascia are elevated, and sutures of 2–0 Proline swaged on to curved Mayo needles are placed in the upper margin of the defect. At the same time, an assessment is made of the inferior margin commonly referred to as the iliopubic tract. The iliopubic tract is an extension of the transversalis fascia onto the femoral vessels to form the femoral sheath. Where this layer is found to be strong and adequate, the Mayo needle is placed through the ilio-pubic tract in a medial to lateral direction in order to effect the closure of the direct hernia defect. Approximately six to eight sutures are required, and the sutures are then tied in a medial to lateral direction. Once again, reconstitution of the deep inguinal ring should ensure that the cord is not held too tightly and that a Kelly clamp can easily be admitted between the reconstituted transversalis fascia and the spermatic cord. Where the iliopubic tract is thought to be unsuitable, it should be dissected away to expose Cooper's ligament inferiorly. The Mayo needle can then be passed through this tough ligamentous structure, which will then form the lower border of the reconstituted posterior inguinal wall. With this latter technique, care should be taken to avoid passing a suture through the femoral vein or artery or their pubic branches and tributary (corona mortis). As one reaches the femoral vein in the deeper Cooper's ligament repair, a transition has to be made to a more superficial layer of iliopubic tract. This suture is known as the transition stitch. Once again sutures are tied from medial to lateral, and attention is given to the snugness of the deep inguinal ring about the spermatic cord.

When the posterior inguinal wall defect is large and it is felt that the repair cannot be achieved without undue tension, prosthetic devices such as Marlex mesh may be used with success, but foreign material should be avoided whenever possible. Invariably, in order to ensure a tension-free repair, a relaxing incision is required. This incision is made in the medial aspect of the rectus sheath and causes the rectus sheath to slide into the position of a new posterior inguinal wall. Hernias through the incision in the rectus sheath have been reported in rare instances. Once adequate hemostasis has been achieved, the spermatic cord is allowed to return to its anatomic position and the external oblique is reapproximated with 3–0 or 4–0 Dexon suture. Doing so results in the reformation of the superficial external ring. The subcutaneous tissues are then closed with Dexon or Vicryl suture, and the skin may be closed with interrupted nylon or subcuticular sutures. Recurrences are rare, being less than 3 percent in our series.

Sliding Hernia

A sliding hernia is simply a variety of an indirect inguinal hernia and is usually found in a large indirect hernia. This does not complicate the repair if one realizes that the hernia in its development has pulled down parietal peritoneum with an attached viscus. After exposure of the hernial sac and its sliding component in the usual way, the viscus is excised from the wall of the hernial sac and is reduced into the abdominal cavity. The peritoneal cavity is then closed by ligature or by suturing the sac from within in order to reconstitute the peritoneal cavity. Redundant and excess hernial sac is excised and sent for permanent histologic examination.

Femoral Hernia

Femoral hernia results from a defect in the trans-versalis fascia surrounding the femoral canal in the lower abdomen. Studies by McVay, Anson, and Savage have demonstrated that there is a considerable normal variation in the transverse diameter of the femoral ring. In most series, the majority of these patients are multiparous women. However, femoral hernias are more common in males than in nulliparous females. This raises the question whether femoral hernias are related to the presence of increased intra-abdominal pressure, since there is no congenital diverticulum of peritoneum protruding into the femoral canal and since preperitoneal fat always precedes the peritoneal sac. However, since the great majority of multiparous women do not develop femoral hernias, there must be some congenital predisposition for its develop-ment, which would be a femoral ring that is congenitally larger than normal.

Once the diagnosis is made, the femoral hernia should be repaired as soon as possible to prevent intestinal entrapment and strangulation. Our approach is to again incise the skin and subcutaneous tissues 2 cm above the pubic tubercle for 4 or 6 cm in a lateral direction. The anterior abdominal wall is encountered, and the rectus sheath as well as the external oblique aponeurosis are incised to reveal the internal oblique muscle. This too is incised, as is the transversalis muscle and transversalis fascia, to expose the preperitoneal fat and the underlying peritoneum. By sharp and blunt dissection and the use of adequate retraction, the posterior inguinal floor and the femoral canal is exposed from their posterior aspect. This is the so-called preperitoneal or posterior approach to the inguinal region. With this approach, the tongue of peri-toneum and preperitoneal fat protruding into the femoral canal can be easily seen and is retracted back into the abdominal cavity. This is accomplished by dividing any adhesions between the sac and the margins of the femoral ring. When the viability of the contained intestine is in question, the peritoneal sac may be opened and the contents examined carefully in order to assess bowel viability. If the integrity of the intestine is seen to be intact, the peritoneum can be closed with a running suture of 4–0 Dexon. Attention is then turned to repair of the femoral ring, and this is done by suturing the iliopubic tract above to the strong layer of Cooper's ligament below, using interrupted sutures of 2–0 Proline swaged on curved Mayo needles. It should be noted that the inguinal and lacunar ligaments play no part in the repair. The closure is usually without tension, and a relaxing incision is rarely necessary. Hemostasis is then carefully obtained, and the preperitoneal sac and peritoneal contents allowed to return to their anatomic position. The anterior abdominal muscular layer is then reapposed using 2–0 Vicryl suture for the muscular layer and 2–0 interrupted Vicryl suture for the anterior rectus sheath and external oblique layer. Skin and subcutaneous tissues are closed in the usual fashion and a dressing applied.

Use of Prosthetic Materials for Recurrent Hernia

We do not recommend the use of prosthetic material in primary hernia repair. In patients with recurrent hernia, we use Marlex mesh to buttress the repair as performed through the posterior approach. It will be years before the results of this modification are known. After applica-tion of the prosthetic buttress, the surgeon experiences a sense of well-being. Our concerns about a potentially increased incidence of infection or rejection of the Marlex mesh have not been warranted to date.

Individualizing the Approach

In 25 years of study of this subject, much has been learned regarding individualization of approach and repair. The posterior approach and iliopubic tract repair are satisfactory for femoral hernias, indirect inguinal and large sliding hernias, and recurrent hernias. Incarcerated or strangulated femoral and indirect hernias are ideally approached posteriorly. Small indirect hernias are best treated from the anterior approach by high ligation of the sac and plastic closure of the transversalis fascia at the internal ring. Large indirect and direct hernias are best treated by the anterior iliopubic tract repair or by the McVay-Cooper's ligament repair from the anterior approach. In both these techniques, the posterior inguinal wall is reconstructed. If a direct hernia is repaired from the posterior approach, relaxing incisions are mandatory.

RECURRENT INGUINAL HERNIA

FRED W. RUSHTON, M.D., F.A.C.S.

The frequency of recurrence after repair of inguinal hernia is generally considered to be about 5 to 10 percent, although some authors believe that with extended follow-up the incidence will prove to be much higher. Recurrence may be minimized by strict attention to technical detail at the time of primary repair, although certain biologic factors are involved that may play a major role.

Seventy-seven percent of recurrent hernias occur following repair of an indirect hernia. Direct hernia repairs account for 16 percent of recurrences; combined direct and indirect hernias, 4 percent; bilateral hernias, 5 percent; sliding hernias, 15 percent; and femoral hernias, 3 percent.

ETIOLOGY

The etiology of recurrent hernia may be divided into the categories of (1) technical errors, (2) mechanical factors, and (3) metabolic abnormalities. Recurrences in the first 6 months following repair of an indirect inguinal hernia are most often due to technical errors including (1) inadequate ligation of the hernial sac, (2) improper closure of the internal inguinal ring, (3) failure to recog-nize an associated hernia, (4) damage to the posterior inguinal floor, and (5) failure to evaluate properly the strength of the inguinal floor. Early failure of direct hernia repair may be due to (1) use of an inadequate structure (e.g., the inguinal ligament) for anchoring the trans-versalis fascia, (2) use of attenuated transversalis fascia for the repair, (3) excessive tension at the suture line, (4) failure to make an adequate relaxing incision when indicated, and (5) failure to recognize an associated indirect or femoral hernial sac.

Mechanical factors include increased intra-abdominal pressure due to chronic cough, bladder outlet obstruction, ascites, lower gastrointestinal tract disease leading to straining during bowel evacuation, and multiple pregnancies.

Metabolic abnormalities may lead to attenuation of the fascia. These include (1) defects in collagen metabo-lism and (2) increased levels of circulating elastolytic activity and decreased alpha-1 antitrypsin inhibition, which has been associated with cigarette smoking.

DIAGNOSIS

The diagnosis of a recurrent hernia in the early post-operative period may be difficult because of the induration and tenderness that often follows the surgical procedure, but the diagnosis usually becomes evident in time. Differential diagnosis includes wound hematoma, lymphadenopathy, and abscess. In many cases, both the surgeon and the patient are reluctant to concede that the hernia has recurred, and the diagnosis may be thus delayed.

SITES OF RECURRENCE

The most common site of recurrence of inguinal hernia is at the internal inguinal ring, with 35 to 50 percent of recurrences taking place at this location. About 25 to 30 percent of hernia recurrence occur at the pubic tubercle, and 25 to 30 percent through the floor of the inguinal canal. When undue tension on the transition suture of a Cooper's ligament repair causes that suture to pull through Cooper's ligament at the femoral ring, the result is a femoral hernia (Table 1).

NONSURGICAL MANAGEMENT

Because of today's safe anesthetic methods, it is the rare patient who requires truss management of any hernia, recurrent or primary. If a truss is used, it should be removed only during bathing, since the risk of incarceration may be increased by intermittent use of a truss.

SURGICAL MANAGEMENT

Preoperative preparation should include a thorough pulmonary evaluation, as well as evaluation of the bladder outlet and of bowel function. Patients with large hernias in whom the abdominal viscera have lost the "right of domain" may benefit from repeated preoperative pneumoperitoneum to enlarge the peritoneal cavity.

The management of recurrent hernia, like that of primary hernia, is generally operative. The safe anesthetics of today have rendered nonsurgical management a choice only in the terminally ill patient. Spinal or general anesthesia is usually necessary, although in thin patients local anesthesia has been adequate. An anterior incision is satisfactory in most instances, although in the case of multiple recurrences, the preperitoneal approach allows dissection in a previously unoperated field.

TABLE 1   Sites of Recurrence and Repair Methods of Choice

Site of Recurrence	Incidence	Method of Repair
Internal ring	35–50%	Cooper's ligament repair
Pubic tubercle	25–30%	Simple closure
Floor of canal	25–30%	Fascia adequate: Cooper's ligament repair
		Fascia inadequate: polypropylene mesh backing
Femoral ring	About 3%	Cooper's ligament repair

Anterior Approach

In the anterior approach, the previous incision is excised in an elliptical fashion and extended for 1 to 2 cm laterally. The dissection is begun laterally, identifying the external oblique aponeurosis. The external oblique is cleaned of areolar tissue and the external inguinal ring, inguinal ligament, and spermatic cord are identified. Ideally, the old operative record is available and the surgeon knows in advance the position of the spermatic cord and ilioinguinal nerve. If the record is not available, it should be temporarily assumed that these structures have been left in the subcutaneous tissue as in the Halsted I repair, and the dissection should begin laterally in unoperated tissue and structures identified in areas where they are easily recognizable.

The external oblique aponeurosis is opened in the direction of its fibers, beginning laterally, exposing the spermatic cord and ilioinguinal nerve if these structures have been left in the anatomic position. The spermatic cord is usually easy to identify, even in a previously operated field, since the external spermatic fascia, cremaster, or internal spermatic fascia have generally been left intact. A meticulous search should be made at this point for an indirect hernial sac. The genitofemoral nerve should be identified and preserved, and avoided at the time of the actual herniorrhaphy so that it is not entrapped by sutures, causing postoperative pain. The hernial sac, whether it be direct or indirect, should be identifiable at this point, and a plan for definitive repair may be formulated.

Recurrence at the Internal Inguinal Ring

Hernia recurrence at the internal inguinal ring may be due to inadequate removal of preperitoneal fat and cremaster muscle from the cord structures at the time of the primary repair. Thus it would seem prudent to skeletonize the cord as completely as possible at the second repair. The internal ring may be closed completely if the cord is resected and orchiectomy done, but this is best done only if there is a second recurrence. Although it is tempting simply to tighten the internal ring around the cord structures, there may be unappreciated loss of integrity of the inguinal floor that will lead to a second recurrence. The Cooper's ligament repair, as described by McVay, has proved in my experience to be satisfactory if the transversalis fascia is not attenuated.

After identification of the hernial sac and all the aforementioned structures, the transversalis fascia is assessed for integrity and strength. The anterior surface of the rectus abdominis sheath is cleaned medially, and a vertical relaxing incision is made with a scalpel or with the electrocautery. The transversalis fascia, or "conjoined tendon" is present, is cleaned from medial to lateral until the internal inguinal ring is precisely defined and the dissection is carried onto the iliopsoas fascia from which the transversalis fasica arises. After the inguinal ligament is dissected along its upper border, the iliopubic tract, a transversalis analogue, is identified posterior to the inguinal ligament. This structure has a distinct reddish color that demarcates it from the inguinal ligament.

Suture material of 1–0 silk is utilized for the repair. The first suture of the repair is placed between the anterior rectus sheath and both the lacunar ligament of Gimbernat and Cooper's ligament at the pubic tubercle. The repair is carried laterally, anchoring transversalis fascia (or "conjoined tendon") to Cooper's ligament as far as the medial border of the femoral sheath. The femoral sheath is a continuation of the transversalis fascia on its anterior side and is included in a transition suture along with the transversalis fascia, Cooper's ligament, and the iliopubic tract. The lateralmost portion of the repair brings transversalis fascia to the iliopubic tract (the inguinal ligament is retracted downward to expose the iliopubic tract) and the femoral sheath. The internal inguinal ring should admit a fingertip along with the spermatic cord or may be closed completely if the cord is sacrificed. The external oblique aponeurosis is closed over the cord in younger patients, but in elderly patients who are past reproductive years, the repair may be strengthened by imbricating the external oblique beneath the cord. The subcutaneous tissue is closed loosely with absorbable (polyglactin) sutures, and the skin edges are approximated, preferably with a subcuticular suture to avoid cutaneous sutures in a relatively contaminated field. Steristrips or adhesive plastic dressings are applied to stabilize the skin closure.

Recurrence at the Pubic Tubercle

The pubic tubercle is the second most common site of recurrence and usually can be managed by simple closure. A polypropylene plug has been described, but in my limited experience with its use, the benefits are questionable. Close attention must be paid to the adequacy of the transversalis fascia in the inguinal floor to ensure that a more extensive repair is not required.

Recurrence as a Femoral Hernia

As the transition suture of a McVay hernia repair tears away from Cooper's ligament, a femoral hernia is often created. In addition, femoral hernias are sometimes missed at the time of repair of an inguinal hernia, and the most common site of recurrence of a Shouldice repair is in the femoral ring. The best method of repair is McVay's operation, as described for internal ring recurrence.

Recurrence Through the Inguinal Floor

Fascial defects in the transversalis fascia in the floor are best managed by the McVay repair (as described for inguinal ring recurrences) in patients whose transversalis fascia above the defect is strong enough to provide an adequate patch. When the transversalis is attenuated, fascial backing is required with prosthetic material such as polypropylene mesh (Marlex), polyglactin mesh, fascia lata, preserved human dura, or other fascial substitute. I prefer polyprophylene mesh (Marlex) because of its availability as well as ease to use.

Prosthetic Repair

The repair is done essentially as described by Usher, the fascia being cleaned as described for the McVay repair. A relaxing incision is made in the rectus sheath, and the transversalis fascia is divided from the internal ring to the pubic tubercle. A Marlex sheet is placed anterior and posterior to the transversalis fascia by folding around the cut edge of the fascia and is anchored in place by means of 1–0 polypropylene mattress sutures. Mattress sutures of 1–0 polypropylene are placed from the Marlex-backed transversalis fascia to Cooper's ligament as in the McVay repair, the lateral portion of the repair including a transition suture, as previously described, and incorporating the femoral sheath. A second suture line is then made between the leading edge of the Marlex-backed transversalis fascia and the inguinal ligament. The internal ring should, again, admit a fingertip alongside the spermatic cord. The cord may be left in the anatomic position and the external oblique closed, as in the McVay repair. Recurrences after Marlex-backed repair usually arise at either end of the Marlex sheet, where it does not adequately cover the attenuated transversalis fascia. This may be avoided by making slits at either end of the Marlex sheet so it can be placed around the fascia beyond that involved in the repair.

Preperitoneal Approach

In the case of multiple recurrences, it may be advisable to approach the hernia from the posterior aspect to avoid the extensive scar tissue otherwise encountered. Surgeons inexperienced in the preperitoneal approach should avoid its use since the appearance of the anatomy may be unfamiliar, introducing considerable potential for technical error and later recurrence. The technique begins with a transverse incision approximately 3 cm above the inguinal ligament. The external oblique, internal oblique, and transversalis layers are incised, exposing the peritoneum. Avoiding entry into the peritoneal cavity, a preperitoneal plane of blunt dissection is begun. If a laparotomy has been done for management of incarceration or strangulation, the preperitoneal plane may be developed from the laparotomy incision. With this plane developed, any hernial sac, whether direct or indirect, should be identifiable. The sac may be divided flush with the peritoneal cavity and oversewn; the distal sac is left in place and not ligated.

TABLE 2   Complications of Repair of Recurrent Hernia

> Wound complications
>> Hematoma
>> Cellulitis
>> Abscess
>
> Nerve injury
>> Ilioinguinal
>> Genitofemoral
>
> Spermatic cord injury
>> Vas deferens
>> Spermatic artery
>> Spermatic vein
>> Pampiniform plexus
>
> Bladder injury
>
> Bowel injury
>
> Postoperative pain
>
> Recurrence

In the case of a direct hernia, the arch of the transversalis fascia may be approximated to the iliopubic tract, as described by Nyhus and Condon, until the internal ring is tightened around the spermatic cord. Cooper's ligament may also be used to anchor the transversalis fascia, particularly if the iliopubic tract is attenuated or in the case of femoral hernia. Marlex mesh may be placed in the preperitoneal space and anchored to the fascia as well as to Cooper's ligament to strengthen both the repair and the original incision.

COMPLICATIONS

The most frequent complications of secondary hernia repair are listed in Table 2. Wound complications such as hematoma, cellulitis, and abscess occur more than twice as often following repair of recurrent hernias as following primary hernia repair. Patients having such wound complications tend to have a higher rate of second recurrence. In addition, there is a higher incidence of ilioinguinal nerve injury as well as injury to spermatic cord structures.

In the case of prosthetic repair, the most dreaded complication is that of prosthetic infection. Marlex mesh is somewhat inert and causes minimal foreign body reaction, and although the process is slow, ultimate healing usually occurs. Occasionally it is necessary to remove the mesh to speed healing.

RESULTS OF SECONDARY REPAIR

The incidence of second recurrence after repair of a recurrent hernia has been reported as approximately 30 to 40 percent. Of these, about one-third occur within 1 year after repair, and about three-fourths occur within 5 years. Marlex backing significantly decreases the incidence of recurrence, but carries the potential for prosthetic infection, and the occasional patient complains of pain in the groin for an inordinately long time following Marlex repair.

EPIGASTRIC, UMBILICAL, AND VENTRAL HERNIAS

HAROLD H. LINDNER, A.B., M.D., F.A.C.S.

An epigastric hernia presents as a protrusion of sublinea-alba structures through the relatively wide midline fascia between the ensiform process of the sternum superiorly and the umbilicus inferiorly. The linea alba is present as a result of the junction in the midline of the upper abdominal wall of both the ventral and dorsal sheaths of the rectus abdominis muscles. In the upper half of the abdomen, above the level of the umbilicus, the linea alba is wide (1.25 to 3 cm in width), but the fascial structure narrows gradually as it approaches the umbilicus. Inferior to umbilical level, it is present as a narrow cord with little or no possibility of a herniation through it. Deep to the linea alba, placed in the following sequence, are the transversalis fascia (which in the upper abdomen is

quite thin), varying amounts of preperitoneal fat, the peritoneum, and the peritoneal cavity. Piercing the linea alba on either side of the midline are multiple small blood vessels and nerves which exit through small openings, normally just large enough to transmit the issuing structures.

The incidence of epigastric hernia is given as 3 to 7 percent of the population, but obviously many asymptomatic hernias are not recognized, and the incidence could easily rise as high as 10 percent. Epigastric hernia is three to four times more common in men than in women, and the condition usually makes itself evident between the ages of 20 and 50, despite the fact that there is strong evidence that the hernias exist on a congenital basis. Protrusions are multiple in 15 to 20 percent of cases, and by far the greater percentage (75%) are noted just to the left of the midline.

Two theories are commonly held regarding the etiology of epigastric hernia. The first theory, the one most commonly held, is that the protrusion passes through an area of congenital weakness in the linea alba, making itself known in the third and fourth decades of life as a result of intra-abdominal pressure continually exerting force against the congenitally weak area. Support is given to this theory by the not too uncommon occurrence of the hernia in infants. The second theory purports that the protrusion develops through one of the paramedian foramina of egress of superficial blood vessels and nerves.

The defect in the fascia of the linea alba varies from 0.5 to 2 cm in diameter, the majority of the defects being less than 1.5 cm in diameter. The usual occupant of the opening is preperitoneal fat, a peritoneal sac being found in about 30 percent of the cases. Intraperitoneal structures are rarely present and, if so, are usually small bowel and/or omentum.

Clinical Findings and Differential Diagnosis

A single mass or, occasionally, multiple subcutaneous masses are palpable in the midline superior to the umbilicus. Most often the masses are not tender and are unsuspected by the patient. They are often found only as the result of a physical examination. The smaller protrusions contain only preperitoneal fat, and are particularly liable to incarcerate and strangulate at which time they usually become quite tender. Clinical manifestations of epigastric hernia vary, ranging from mild epigastric distress to severe upper abdominal distress, which often radiates to the lower abdominal quadrants and to the lumbar region of the back. There may be abdominal distention and nausea and vomiting. Following a heavy meal, the symptoms may increase markedly. Some relief may be obtained if the patient assumes a supine position, as this may allow the hernia to retreat from the fascial opening. The differential diagnosis includes peptic ulcer penetration or perforation, biliary tract disease, pancreatitis, hiatal hernia, and a high small bowel obstruction. The mass must be distinguished from a subcutaneous lipoma, fibroma, or neurofibroma. The diagnosis is difficult if the abdomen is obese. Increasing a patient's intra-abdominal pressure may serve to make the mass more prominent. In some cases, in the absence of demonstrable intra-abdominal disease, the inability to palpate the mass and symptoms suggestive of an epigastric hernia are justification for a surgical exploration of the linea alba.

Treatment

Conservative treatment with a compression bandage is usually reserved for the very young or for adults who either refuse surgery or are in poor physical condition and unable to withstand the operative procedure.

Generally, if the epigastric hernia is giving symptoms or if the fascial opening is 0.5 cm or larger, surgical therapy is indicated. An upper midline incision is made from the xiphoid to the umbilicus. The lengthy incision allows for an exploration of the linea alba along its entire length, so that multiple areas of herniation will not be missed. The herniation is dissected free both from the subcutaneous tissues and from the edges of the hernial ring in the linea alba to which it is often adherent. Once the fascial circumference of the ring has been cleared, the superior and the inferior ring edges are together attached to Allis clamps and the entire ring elevated. This allows the surgeon to inspect the hernia for the presence of a sac and to check the contents of the hernia. Clearing the edges of the hernial ring allows the surgeon to place a finger both superiorly and inferiorly at subfascial level to check for other areas of weakness in the linea alba. If such areas are found, the opening in the linea alba is extended to include these areas in the fascial closure. Herniated preperitoneal fat is amputated, and intraperitoneal contents of the hernia, if found, are reduced. No attempt is made to close a peritoneal sac. If intraperitoneal disease is suspected, the upper abdomen can easily be explored by opening the peritoneum the length of the midline incision. The peritoneal layer is closed with a suture line of interrupted 3–0 silk, and the linea alba is closed via a vertical fascia-to-fascia closure using interrupted 3–0 silk.

The operation should be carried out under general anesthesia, and postoperative nasogastric suction is usually sustained for 24 to 36 hours because paralytic ileus and/or acute gastric dilatation occurs postoperatively on occasion. The recurrence rate is relatively high—7 to 10%—higher than the rate for inguinal and femoral hernia repair.

I mention a transverse incisional repair of the hernia only to condemn it. It does not allow for a complete inspection of the linea alba, it is difficult to extend the incision for an upper abdominal exploration, and in our hands, there has been a higher incidence of postoperative complications and recurrences following use of a transverse incision.

UMBILICAL HERNIA

Umbilical hernias generally can be divided into two major classifications: (1) those that are present in infancy and early childhood and are congenital in origin, and (2) those that present during adulthood and are of the acquired type. Since the indications for operative treatment of the two types and the actual techniques of surgical repair vary markedly, each of the hernias will be discussed separately.

Umbilical Hernia in Infants

Infantile umbilical hernia is present because of failure of the midline abdominal fascia to close properly at umbilical level. The hernia is more common in blacks and in children born prematurely, and is found more frequently in male than in female infants. It is commonly associated with (1) an elevated intra-abdominal pressure secondary to intra-abdominal tumor masses, and (2) an ascites associated with cirrhosis, nephrosis, or a failing heart. Following the return of the midgut loop to the abdominal cavity during the eleventh week of fetal life, the two obliterated umbilical arteries and the urachus attach to the inferior quadrant of the umbilical orifice, while the obliterated umbilical vein attaches singly to the superior quadrant of the orifice immediately after parturition. This results in the superior quadrant being more responsive to intra-abdominal pressure, and consequently, in both infants and adults, the superior quadrant is usually the initial site of the protrusion. The herniation usually contains omentum, and frequently a loop of small bowel also is present. Usually a well-developed peritoneal sac is present. Adhesions usually are present between the sac contents and the deep surface of the umbilical ring, and in many cases the adhesions contain small blood vessels. The hernial ring in the midline fascia varies from 0.25 cm to 2 cm in diameter, the smaller rings most frequently showing the symptoms associated with the rare presence of incarceration and or strangulation. Diagnosis is easily made, a bulge at umbilical level being seen when intra-abdominal pressure is raised. Differentially, the condition must be separated from a low-lying epigastric hernia, gastroschisis, and urachal and vitellointestinal abnormalities. Incarceration and strangulation rarely occur (less than 3% in our series), and evisceration practically never occurs. In 90 to 95 percent of cases, fascial defects less than 1 cm in diameter close spontaneously. If the defect is 1.5 cm or larger in diameter, it rarely closes spontaneously. Surgical repair is indicated when (1) the omentum or bowel becomes incarcerated, or (2) the defect in the fasica is wider than 1 cm in girls older than 2 years and in all children older than 4 years. Conservative treatment consisting of a tight belly band is to be condemned as it has no beneficial effect on the hernia. When the need for surgery arises, the child should be given general anesthesia. If at all possible, the cutaneous covering of the umbilicus should be preserved and carefully dissected free from the underlying herniation. The herniated sac is carefully freed from adhesions to both the deep and superificial surfaces of the fascial ring. The midline fascial areas surrounding the ring are thoroughly cleared of adhesions preparatory to closure of the defect. The defect is closed transversely, the edges being brought together directly via interrupted 3–0 silk sutures after the sac has been opened, the contents reduced, and the excess sac cut away. No attempt is made to close the peritoneum individually. I have not used the transverse "pants over vest" closure or the vertical closure in the past 20 years. The umbilical skin and its scanty subcutaneous tissue is sutured down to the underlying fascia with 3–0 plain catgut sutures. Redundant skin is not removed. A firm pressure dressing is applied over the skin closure. If treated properly, this hernia should not recur.

Umbilical Hernia in Adults

Umbilical hernias in adults are due to a gradual weakening of the scar tissue that normally closes the umbilical fibrous ring. In about 80 percent of cases, the protrusion first appears at the superior arc of the umbilical orifice, the weak area of the ring. Umbilical hernia is 10 times more frequent in women than in men. Factors that predispose to adult umbilical hernia are (1) multiple pregnancies with difficult labor, (2) ascites secondary to cirrhosis of the liver, (3) obesity with considerable intra-abdominal fat, and (4) large, intra-abdominal tumors. Umbilical hernia in an adult does not spontaneously regress, but instead usually steadily increases in size. In hernias of long standing, the covering peritoneal sac is markedly thickened, and in the larger hernias, the tissues covering the hernia are so attenuated that the hernia appears to be subcutaneous in position. The hernial sac is usually multi-lobulated, and the skin over the hernia also tends to appear lobulated. A large omental mass is the most frequent occupant of the hernial sac; however, small and large bowel are also frequently present. Strangulation of the hernial contents is a frequent complication, often necessitating emergency surgery. In many cases the neck of the hernial sac is narrow compared to the girth of the herniated tissues. As a result of the small-sized ring and large amounts of herniated abdominal contents, the patients are often chronically constipated and suffer the cramping and nausea that accompanies a subacute, incomplete bowel obstruction. Large hernias often cause marked lumbar backache. Adult umbilical hernias should be treated surgically as soon as they are discovered in order to avoid the need for emergency surgery called for by incarceration and or strangulation of the contents of the sac. The usual surgical repair calls for a preservation of the umbilical depression if possible (difficult in large hernias), a freeing of the hernial sac from the subcutaneous tissues and the edges of the umbilical ring, an opening of the peritoneal sac and replacement of its contents into the abdomen, trimming of the excess sac, and then a closure of the fascial defect in a transverse direction. The fascia is closed in one layer with 2–0 or 3–0 silk. The umbilical defect seldom invades the compartments of the rectus sheath, the herniation passing through the attenuated linea alba. The aponeurosis is closed transversely since the sheath fibers of the three flat muscles of the lateral abdominal wall run in a transverse direction as they join together to make up the anterior and posterior rectus sheaths, and a transverse closure places the sutures at right angles to the direction of the sheath fibers. Thus a transverse closure places the fibers under less tension postoperatively when the patient increases his intra-abdominal pressure during respiration, defecation, or coughing. The larger of the umbilical hernia defects, those that cannot be closed without undue tension, may be closed by use of an inlay of Marlex mesh. Large hernias, general debility of the patient, and intra-abdominal disease are causes of high complication and morbidity rates after repair. In a healthy individual, the repair should give a good result, with only 2 to 5 percent rate of recurrence.

VENTRAL HERNIA

To the operating surgeon, "ventral hernia," in nearly all cases, denotes a postoperative herniation through a previously carried out abdominal incision. However, a diastasis of the rectus abdominis muscles, either congenital or acquired, and the rare herniation present in the Eagle Barrett syndrome, in which there is a congenital absence of the abdominal musculature with a resultant exstrophy of the bladder, must also be mentioned. However, they will not be discussed in this chapter.

All postoperative ventral hernias are of the acquired type and, in nearly all cases, are of iatrogenic origin. Such herniations comprise an important percentage of all hernias operated on in a larger general hospital, constituting 7 to 12 percent of hernioplasties performed. Despite important advances in surgery—improved suture material, improved methods of pre- and postoperative care, introduction of reinforcing and "bridging" materials, and antibiotic therapy—this type of herniation persists in significant numbers and does not appear to be decreasing in frequency (occurring in 5% to 15% of all patients subjected to transperitoneal abdominal surgery). People are living longer today, and consequently geriatic surgery with its many postoperative complications has become common; this fact is probably responsible in part for the continued untoward incidence of incisional hernia.

The conditions that are most often responsible for a postoperative wound weakness are:

1. *Age of the patient.* Geriatic patients tend to heal more slowly and less completely than younger, more active patients.
2. *General physical condition of the patient.* Patients with cirrhosis and ascites, malignant tumor anemia, chronic malnutrition, and electrolyte imbalance and those receiving prolonged steroid therapy tend to heal poorly.
3. *Obesity.* The presence of large amounts of intra-abdominal fat makes for a more difficult wound closure, and large amounts of abdominal wall fat tend to obscure the fascial planes used for closure.
4. *Postoperative wound infections.*
5. *Improper suture material and use of poor fascial tissues for closure.* Nonabsorbable suture material should be used whenever possible, and fascia should be cleaned of overlying fat before being used for closure.
6. *Type of incision.* We feel that transverse and oblique abdominal wounds tend to heal faster and more solidly than vertically-placed incisions.
7. *Postoperative pulmonary complications.* These complications, particularly those accompanied by a persistent cough, may be secondary to preexisting pulmonary disease, secondary to anesthesia, or secondary to the inertia of the patient on the operating table or in the postoperative bed. The patient should be ambulated early.
8. *Unwise placement of drains or colostomy or ileostomy stomas in the primary operative wound.*

Any or several of the aforementioned predisposing factors can set off the train of events leading to a postoperative incisional hernia. Dehiscence, which may be either partial or complete, results from a breakdown of all layers of the wound closure, causing intraperitoneal contents (most commonly omentum and large or small bowel) to spill into the subcutaneous tissues. If the wound breaks through the skin closure, an evisceration results. All patients with dehiscence, with or without evisceration, who can tolerate further surgery should be taken to the operating room immediately. Here, the wound is cleansed with warm saline, the bowel is replaced, and the wound re-closed, either by a layered closure plus retention sutures or by a simple through-and-through closure of all layers, as the surgeon prefers. If possible, I prefer a layered closure, but must confess that in cases in which I have done a simple through-and-through closure, I have been quite satisfied. In the great majority of cases, a wound dehiscence is preceded by a period of serosanguinous wound drainage, which appears anywhere from a few hours to several days prior to the giving way of the closure. Its appearance must always alert the surgeon to the possibility of an impending dehiscence.

There are a group of wounds that show no immediate postoperative drainage or discomfort, but at a later date either suddenly or gradually exhibit a weakness, either along the entire length of the wound or in a segment of its length. The weakness and the accompanying protrusion are due to a complete or a partial giving way of the peritoneal and/or the fascial layers of closure. Such hernias always slowly increase in size and tend to cause some pain when intra-abdominal pressure is raised. A hernia of this type has a relatively high incidence of incarceration and/or strangulation. Such herniations frequently have a loop of small bowel and or omentum plastered against the wound opening at the peritoneal level.

Some important precautions that can diminish the incidence of postoperative incisional hernia include: (1) the use of transverse and oblique abdominal incisions if practical and anatomically feasible, (2) the use of properly selected nonabsorbable suture material, (3) avoidance of closure under tension, (4) avoidance of dead space in wounds, (5) precise hemostasis, (6) the cessation of smoking prior to surgery, (7) proper fluid, electrolyte, and blood balance both prior to and immediately after surgery, (7) proper skin preparations, protection of wound edges, and the considered use of antibiotic therapy both pre- and postoperatively, (8) early postoperative ambulation, (9) nasogastric suction and catheter drainage of the bladder to prevent postoperative distention, and (10) the use of wire, heavy silk, or Dermalon retention sutures in the elderly, the debilitated, patients with malignant disease, and those with poor peritoneal and fascial tissues. The retention sutures must be separated by one-half to three-fourths inch and should be tied relatively loosely over bolsters.

An incisional hernia should be repaired as soon as the patient's condition permits because such a herniation always increases in size, is unsightly, is frequently painful, and may eventually cause a subacute or acute bowel obstruction. Furthermore, ventral hernias are frequently the cause of chronic constipation, particularly in the elderly.

If the patient is unwilling or unable to undergo a surgical repair, the hernia, if not too large, may be fairly well contained by an elastic abdominal support.

Closure of a small incisional hernia, one with a defect of 2.5 to 6 cm, is easily carried out by a pants-over-vest Mayo repair or by a lateral overlapping fascial closure. I prefer to use silk or fine wire suture material and a through-and-through fascial and peritoneal closure. The excess sac is trimmed after the hernial contents have been freed and replaced into the abdomen.

Closure of the larger incisional hernial defect (8 to 16 cm) is usually a most painstaking and difficult procedure. The repair should be preceded by an attempt at weight loss, and because large hernias often lose their right of intra-abdominal domain, the procedure may follow a series of pneumoperitoneum injections to elevate the diaphragm and increase the intraperitoneal area. A nasogastric tube is always placed prior to surgery, and a retention catheter is placed in the urinary bladder. I find such drainage to be of assistance at the time of closure. Spinal anesthesia, because of its relaxant qualities, is the anesthesia of choice. The stretched excess, scarred, covering skin is carefully dissected, freed from the adjacent tissues, and removed. The thickened sac is then dissected free from the surrounding subcutaneous, fascial, and muscular structures, care being taken to dissect the sac free from the ring of the hernia, both superficially and deeply. I routinely open the sac with great care so as not to injure its contents. The sac contents are then slowly dissected free from the inner surface of the sac and replaced into the abdomen. In the larger hernias this dissection can be tedious, as the sac is frequently loculated, with multiple adhesions present in each locule. The excess sac is then cut away, and if possible, the peritoneum is closed as a separate layer with interrupted 3–0 silk sutures. In many cases, I make no attempt to close the peritoneum. It is of vital importance to thoroughly clean and visualize the fascial layers about the circumference of the hernia so that clean, solid fascia can be brought together in the closure and so that the surgeon can accurately judge the degree of tension that will exist if the closure uses the fascia at hand. Some surgeons prefer to use a layered closure, either with or without additional through-and-through retention sutures. I prefer the single suture closure if tension is not present. I use 2–0 silk, placing the sutures through fascia and peritoneum, about 2 cm apart. Meticulous care is given to absolute hemostasis and the obliteration of dead space. When a large dead space exists, a Hemo-Vac is put in place for 48 to 72 hours. The use of tissue grafts, nonreactive metal inserts, and Marlex mesh is held to a minimum. If absolutely needed, I prefer Marlex mesh, the prosthesis but cut to the proper size and then sutured to the deep surface of the abdominal fascia with horizontally placed mattress sutures. The fascial edges are closed with mattress sutures atop the Marlex. If a very large defect cannot be closed without tension, the closure is better left undone if there are no symptoms present. Following closure, I have my patients wear an elastic abdominal support for 3 to 6 months.

The recurrence rate for incisional hernias usually varies directly with the size of the defect that is closed. Small hernias have a low recurrence rate (2% to 5%), medium-sized hernias have a rate of 5 to 10 percent, and large hernias, which are too often closed under tension, have a recurrence rate as high as 15 to 20 percent.

LUMBAR, OBTURATOR, AND SPIGELIAN HERNIAS

WARD O. GRIFFEN, Jr., M.D., Ph.D.

LUMBAR HERNIA

The lumbar region is an area bounded anteriorly by the border of the external oblique aponeurosis, inferiorly by the crest of the ilium, posteriorly by the paravertebral muscles, and superiorly by the twelfth rib. There are two areas in the lumbar region where hernias may occur. The upper area is the site of the larger herniations; smaller herniations occur in the lower portion of the lumbar region, often immediately superior to the iliac crest.

These hernias are considered to be both congenital and acquired. In the superior lumbar triangle, the twelfth intercostal neurovascular bundle penetrates the fascia right at the tip of the twelfth rib. In this area the transversalis fascia is not covered by the external oblique fascia and may be the point of maximal weakness. In the inferior lumbar area there is a triangle of fascia immediately superior to the iliac crest, which is fairly consistent in the adult, but not in the infant. It is speculated that as growth occurs, attenuation of the fascia at the apex of the triangle leads to weakness where a hernia will develop secondary to increased abdominal pressure. In contrast, the acquired variety of lumbar hernias are almost invariably seen after some form of trauma. This may be direct trauma to the lumbar area, resulting in fascial tearing or disruption, but it is more frequently secondary to surgical violation of the area. This may be in the form of drainage of an abscess (e.g., periphrenic abscess following a flank incision for nephrectomy or lumbar sympathectomy) or, in the case of hernias in the lower lumbar region, removal of the iliac crest.

Lumbar herniation is rare, and most surgeons encounter only a few such cases. The most common symptom is protrusion in the lumbar area. The diagnosis is infrequently a major problem because the hernias are usually large when first seen. There may be some discomfort associated with these hernias at any time during their development, but particularly in the early stages of the lower lumbar hernias. In the obvious differential diagnosis is a tumor or mass lesion, but the lumbar hernia is invariably soft and, in the case of the large upper lumbar hernias, usually reduceable. If a great deal of pain is present, one should consider another diagnosis such as a musculoskeletal disorder or herniation of a vertebral disc.

The smaller hernias, particularly those occurring in the lower portion of the lumbar region, may be repaired with simple fascial approximation. Unfortunately, most lumbar hernias are not subjected to repair until they have attained a rather large size, and this represents the major clinical difficulty. In this instance, attenuation of the fascia is sufficiently severe to make primary approximation of fascia difficult, if not impossible. Under these circumstances, it is necessary to reinforce the closure, either with large fascial flaps, which require extensive operative dissection, or with prosthetic mesh.

The patient is placed on an operating room table in an oblique position with the body at approximately 45 degrees. If the hernia is in the inferior portion of the lumbar region, either the previous incision (for iliac crest removal) can be excised or a transverse or vertical incision may be made immediately over the protrusion. If sufficient fascia is present to allow approximation without tension, this can be accomplished, preferably with monofilament nonabsorbable sutures. If the fascia is severely attenuated, Marlex mesh may be sutured to the periosteum of the ilium inferiorly and the fascial edges above. Such mesh has been used as a single layer in the subcutaneous portion or as a double layer, one layer being sutured to the internal layer of periosteum and to the internal surface of the fascia and the second layer being sutured to the external layer of periosteum and the external surface of the fascia. In the repair of these hernias, extensive dissection is not necessary, and primary closure without suction catheter can usually be accomplished.

For repair of the larger hernias occurring in the upper lumbar region, the technique described by Dowd in 1907 or its various modifications are effective in accomplishing the closure. This method requires the development of a generous flap of fascia and aponeurosis from the gluteus maximus below the iliac crest and a portion of the fascia lata lateral to the iliac crest. This flap is then rotated upward and sutured to the lumbar fascia above, the external

oblique fascia medially, and the fascia of the latissimus dorsi posteriorly. Prior to the development of prosthetic meshes, this technique was used with a high degree of success. However, the use of prosthetic meshes to reinforce the fascial flap closure has gained in popularity as a means of ensuring a low recurrence rate. Because of the extensive dissection, subcutaneous suction catheters are often placed and brought out through a stab incision. The possibility of causing infection by using suction catheters in a procedure in which prosthetic material has been used must be weighed carefully. Preoperative, intraoperative, and a brief course of postoperative antibiotics are essential in the management of patients with large lumbar hernias.

OBTURATOR HERNIA

This hernia is important, not because of its frequency, but because of its propensity to produce bowel obstruction. Although it was first described in the eighteenth century, it was not until 200 years later, in 1926, that the anatomic defect was described by Kamper. This defect is almost invariably situated anteromedial to the neurovascular bundle which traverses the obturator canal. It has a preponderance for females in a ratio of 6:1 and is frequently seen in older women who have had multiple pregnancies. This lends credence to the theory that pregnancies begin the attenuation of the fascia in the obturator region which continues with age.

The obturator opening is only about 1 cm in diameter and surrounded by the pubic ramus superiorly and the tough ligamentous portion of the internal obturator muscle laterally and posteriorly. Therefore, a loop of bowel having protruded into this area frequently becomes incarcerated and, in many cases, strangulated by the time the patient undergoes surgical correction.

Making the diagnosis preoperatively is the major clinical difficulty. The most frequent presenting complaint is abdominal pain and vomiting. There is often distention and obstipation, which leads to the diagnosis of mechanical bowel obstruction, which can be confirmed by appropriate x-ray studies. The cause of the obstruction may be obscured because of the lack of surgical scars or obvious groin hernias. Because of the age group, it is often thought that the patient is suffering from an intra-abdominal malignant tumor. Occasionally the patient complains of pain extending down the medial aspect of the thigh and may have discovered that flexion of the thigh usually relieves the pain. In contrast, extension, abduction, or medial rotation of the thigh increases the pain. This is known as the Howship-Romberg sign, and on careful neurologic examination, sensory deficits of the skin of the medial aspect of the thigh and motor weakness of the abductor group of muscles may be demonstrated. Ultrasound of the pelvis has been used to make the diagnosis.

Before the patient is subjected to operation, resuscitation with fluid and electrolytes must be carried out. Once the patient has a satisfactory circulating blood volume, a stable cardiopulmonary situation, and a good urine output, an operation may be carried out. Three approaches have been described. The perineal and inguinal approaches avoid entrance into the peritoneal cavity, but should only be used when the diagnosis is firm and there is no evidence of incarceration or strangulation of the bowel. Because the diagnosis is often obscure and bowel incarceration so frequent, most surgeons prefer the direct abdominal approach, which can be carried out through a lower midline or transverse abdominal incision. The bowel is carefully removed from the area of the hernia and inspected for viability. If strangulation has occurred, segmental resection with end-to-end anastomosis is required. The sac is then inverted and ligated at the level of the obturator foramen, excising the excess peritoneum. This defect can then be closed with two or three monofilament nonabsorbable sutures and reinforced with fascial flap or prosthetic material as desired. Obviously, if the bowel has been resected, particularly if there has been any degree of spillage of intraluminal contents, prosthetics should not be employed. Probably because of the frequent occurrence of strangulating obstruction and the necessity for bowel resection, as well as the age of the population, the mortality rate following repair of this hernia is reported to be 10 percent, the highest for any abdominal hernia repair.

SPIGELIAN HERNIA

A spigelian hernia is a congenital lateral ventral hernia occurring in the semilunar line, which is the aponeurotic zone of the abdominal wall at the margin of the rectus abdominis muscle. The defect usually appears just at the level of the inferior epigastric vessels at the lateral border of the rectus sheath. It is extremely rare for a spigelian hernia to appear above the umbilicus, although it is an anatomic possibility. Most of the spigelian hernias occur in association with the fascial defect created by the inferior epigastric vessels. A defect inferior to these vessels and lateral to the rectus sheath would occur in Hesselbach's triangle and therefore be difficult to distinguish from a direct inguinal hernia. A defect superior and lateral to these vessels is the true spigelian hernia.

As in the case of the obturator hernia, making the diagnosis represents the major clinical problem. The most common symptom associated with this hernia is pain. It is usually exquisitely localized, often associated with exertion, and occasionally associated with gastrointestinal symptoms, predominantly nausea. Unfortunately, when the defect is small, it cannot be palpated, and only localized tenderness may be elicited. At this point the physician is confronted with a relatively healthy patient, usually female, who has few other symptoms. If the index of suspicion is high, ultrasonographic examination of the abdomen may identify excess fat lateral and deep to the abdominal wall muscles, confirming the diagnosis in the early stages. As the defect enlarges, it may be possible either to palpate a bulge when the patient strains or coughs or to palpate the defect. As more omentum protrudes into the defect, and particularly if it becomes incarcerated, the traction on the omentum frequently causes a great deal of nausea. It is rare for a loop of bowel to become incarcerated or strangulated in such a hernia.

Once the diagnosis is suspected or confirmed, operative repair of the hernia is relatively simple. A transverse incision is made over the palpable bulge or defect, if present, or in the area of the semilunar line. If the patient has had some gastrointestinal complaints and has not had an appendectomy, many surgeons opt to open the peritoneal cavity, even when an obvious spigelian hernia is present, to inspect and palpate the pelvic organs and also the appendix itself. If the patient is young and the appendix has a lumen, an incidental appendectomy can be performed without compromising the results of the hernia repair. The hernia itself can be repaired easily with several interrupted nonabsorbable monofilament sutures to approximate the fascial edges. It is extremely rare for reinforcing mesh or fascial flaps to be necessary. Recurrence is rare, although bilateral spigelian hernias have been described and should be looked for during the repair of the symptomatic unilateral one.

ENDOCRINE GLANDS

ADRENAL CORTEX

DAVID O. MOORE, M.D.
JAMES D. HARDY, M.D.

The adrenal cortex is essential for life and may usefully be considered as three organs in one. These components are (1) the outer zone, the zona glomerulosa, which secretes primarily aldosterone; (2) the middle zone, the zona fasciculata, which secretes primarily glucocorticoids (e.g., hydrocortisone); and (3) the inner zone, the zona reticularis, which secretes primarily estrogens and androgens (Fig. 1). There is some overlap in the function of the three zones, the glucosteroids secreted by the middle zone providing sufficient amounts of the mineralocorti-

coid effects of the outer zone to preserve health in many or most patients.

The normal stimulus for secretion of hydrocortisone by the zona fasciculata is ACTH secreted by the anterior pituitary gland. The rate of release of ACTH into the blood is regulated by the blood level of corticoids (negative feedback mechanism). The secretion of aldosterone by the zona glomerulosa is influenced to some extent by ACTH levels, but to a major extent the secretion of aldosterone is believed to be independent of the pituitary.

Tumors of the adrenal cortex, especially malignant ones, may produce secretions representative of more than one of the three adrenocortical zones.

Anatomically, as the surgeon sees the retroperitoneal adrenal glands from the commonly preferred abdominal

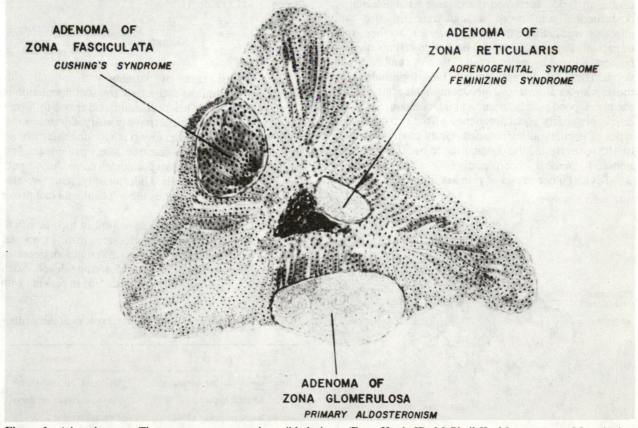

ADENOMA OF ZONA FASCICULATA
CUSHING'S SYNDROME

ADENOMA OF ZONA RETICULARIS
ADRENOGENITAL SYNDROME FEMINIZING SYNDROME

ADENOMA OF ZONA GLOMERULOSA
PRIMARY ALDOSTERONISM

Figure 1 Adrenal cortex. Three separate zones and possible lesions. (From Hardy JD, McPhail JL. Management of functioning tumors of the adrenal cortex. Am J Surg 1960; 99:433.)

approach, the left adrenal, visualized by elevating the pancreas, is bounded by the aorta medially and the left renal vein inferiorly (Fig. 2). The largest vascular structure is the central adrenal vein, which drains into the superior margin of the left renal vein, virtually opposite the ovarian (or the spermatic) vein inferiorly. It is of interest that timed blood samples from these two veins reflect the concentrations and the rates of secretion of steroids, not only 17-hydroxycorticosteroids such as hydrocortisone, but also estrogens and androgens from both the adrenal gland and the ovary or testis.

The right adrenal gland is exposed by dividing the posterior peritoneum beneath the liver, adjacent to the inferior vena cava at a level above the right renal vein, and then following the vena cava (Fig. 3).

The adrenal glands are roughly triangular and a brilliant yellow; each weighs approximately 7 g, with a normal range of perhaps 5 to 10 g. With prolonged and excessive ACTH stimulation, the adrenal cortex becomes hyperplastically enlarged and may in fact exhibit multiple nodules.

PRIMARY ALDOSTERONISM

Primary aldosteronism, a clinical syndrome characterized by hypertension, hypokalemia, and hyporeninemia, results from the excessive production of aldosterone by the adrenal cortex. Conn, who first described this syndrome in 1955, attributed the disease to an adrenal aldosteronoma and noted a high rate of cure with adrenalectomy. Since that time, however, another group of patients have emerged who have aldosteronism due to bilateral adrenal hyperplasia rather than to a unilateral adenoma. These patients are clinically indistinguishable from those with an aldosterone-producing adenoma, but uniformly respond poorly to surgical intervention. Some series report nearly equal frequency of the two pathologic types of primary aldosteronism. Grant et al, in a review of 105 cases, found the distribution to be 60 percent adenoma, 40 percent hyperplasia.

Several other causes of primary aldosteronism exist,

LEFT ADRENALECTOMY

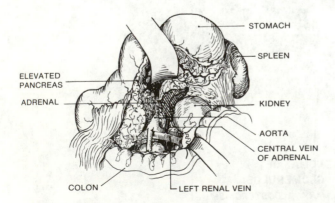

Figure 2 Left adrenalectomy. Surgical approach and exposure of the left adrenal.

RIGHT ADRENALECTOMY

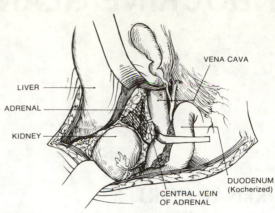

Figure 3 Right adrenalectomy. Surgical approach and exposure of the right adrenal.

all rare but worthy of brief mention. Adrenal cortical carcinoma occasionally has been noted to present as pure hyperaldosteronism.

A very rare familial hyperaldosteronism disorder, first described by Sutherland and associates, may be completely corrected with dexamethasone administration. The inheritance pattern here appears to be autosomal dominant; histologic evaluation of the adrenals of two such patients has revealed bilateral hyperplasia. Ectopic aldosterone-producing tumors have also rarely been described. These tumors may represent elements of adrenal rests (Table 1).

Diagnosis

The identification of patients with primary aldosteronism within the entire hypertensive population is a formidable task. It has been estimated that 2 to 8 percent of hypertensive patients have primary aldosteronism. There is no particular age group at risk and there are no easily discernible clinical features. Many patients are first suspected of having primary aldosteronism due to persistent, severe hypokalemia. Unfortunately, many are also on diuretic therapy, and thus the hypokalemia can prove an unreliable indicator.

Several screening tests are helpful in the identification of patients with primary aldosteronism. In normal subjects, maneuvers that suppress the renin-angiotensin system will lower the serum aldosterone level. Such maneuvers fail to lower serum aldosterone in patients with

TABLE 1 Primary Aldosteronism: Treatment According to Etiology

Etiology	Treatment
Aldosterone-producing adenoma	Unilateral adrenalectomy
Bilateral adrenal hyperplasia	Sprionolactone; no surgery
Glucocorticoid remedial aldosteronism	Dexamethasone
Adrenal cortical carcinoma	Surgical excision

primary aldosteronism because the adrenal is producing aldosterone independent of the renin-angiotensin system.

The saline infusion test is probably the most commonly used initial study. Primary aldosteronism is suspected when serum aldosterone levels fail to fall below 10 ng per deciliter after administration of 2 liters of saline over a 4-hour period. This test is contraindicated in patients with severe hypertension, congestive heart failure, or a recent myocardial infarction. A newer, perhaps safer, test involves the use of captopril. This drug blocks the conversion of angiotensin I to angiotensin II by inhibiting the converting enzyme. Normal subjects and patients with essential hypertension have been shown to have a signficant decrease in serum aldosterone 2 hours following a 25-mg dose of captopril (PO). Lyons et al report a decline in serum aldosterone exceeding 50 percent of the control values in these patients. No such response was noted in those with primary aldosteronism. These patients had higher pre- and post-captopril aldosterone levels when compared to normal subjects and patients with essential hypertension.

Differential Diagnosis and Localization

After completing the screening studies and identifying patients with primary aldosteronism, an effort should be made to localize the lesion and differentiate patients with an adrenal adenoma from those with bilateral adrenal hyperplasia. Recently, it has become possible to evaluate preoperatively a number of patients with both adrenal hyperplasia and adenoma. Patients with adrenal hyperplasia are sensitive to both endogenous and exogenous angiotensin and exhibit increased aldosterone production after assuming the upright position for several hours. The renin-angiotensin system is stimulated by the upright posture, and this slight increase in angiotensin II stimulates hyperplastic cells to produce more aldosterone. Patients with aldosterone-producing adenomas, in contrast, exhibit a fall in serum aldosterone after the patient has maintained the upright position for 4 or more hours. This phenomenon is referred to as anomalous postural decline in plasma aldosterone. One suggested explanation relates to a possible effect of ACTH on the aldosterone-producing adenoma. It has been shown that these lesions, although producing aldosterone autonomously, still manifest some circadian pattern in hormone production, suggesting an influence of ACTH. Whatever the mechanism, this phenomenon has been accepted by many as the best means of differentiating aldosterone-producing adenomas from bilateral adrenal hyperplasia. Grant et al report 93 percent accuracy utilizing this technique.

Localization of the lesion often presents a problem and has led to some controversy. There are many methods, but the most consistently accurate is that of selective adrenal venography. Weinberger et al report 91 percent predictive accuracy using a technique of bilateral adrenal venous sampling during continuous ACTH infusion. Aldosterone and cortisol levels are obtained from the adrenal venous samples and compared to samples taken from the inferior vena cava. This method eliminates the possibility of diurnal variation by provoking constant ACTH stimulation and providing a predictable control in the cortisol assay.

The use of the CT scan in the localization of adrenal cortical lesions is controversial. Grant et al, in the Mayo Clinic series, have embraced the CT scan as the best modality available for the localization of adrenal adenomas. They report 90 percent accuracy using this method. Other investigators, however, have not been as impressed with the CT scan and feel that aldosterone-producing adenomas are easily missed because of their small size and a density similar to that of normal adrenal tissue. Thus, sensitivity of the CT scan is subject to limitations and cannot always be depended on to provide definitive diagnostic information.

The use of ^{131}I-6-β-iodomethyl-19-norcholesterol scans (NP-59) has received recent consideration and may eventually prove particularly helpful when used in conjunction with dexamethasone suppression of the remainder of the adrenal cortex. Functioning adrenal adenomas concentrate the radioactive cholesterol and appear as a "hot spot" on the adrenal scan. In the presence of dexamethasone, the normal adrenal is suppressed, and a decreased uptake of cholesterol is exhibited on the adrenal scan. Patients with bilateral adrenal hyperplasia have also been shown to suppress aldosterone production with administration of dexamethasone, thus providing another means of differentiating adenomas from hyperplasia.

Arteriography has not proved to be sufficiently useful in localizing aldosteronomas. In a review of the recent literature, no investigators reported utilization of this modality in the evaluation of patients with primary aldosteronism.

Treatment

Little controversy exists regarding the treatment of patients with primary aldosteronism. Those with bilateral adrenal hyperplasia have been shown to respond poorly to adrenalectomy and can usually be managed with medical therapy alone. Spironolactone, 100 to 200 mg daily, is commonly required, and the dosage may be increased to as much as 600 mg per day.

Patients with an aldosterone-producing adenoma usually respond favorably to unilateral adrenalectomy. In a large series reported from the Mayo Clinic, 89 percent of patients undergoing unilateral adrenalectomy for an aldosteronoma were normotensive soon after surgery, and 100 percent were improved (Fig. 4). The posterior approach is still favored by many for unilateral adrenalectomy. This incision provides good exposure, is well tolerated, and has few postoperative complications. However, we and others prefer the abdominal approach (see Figs. 2 and 3).

CUSHING'S SYNDROME

Cushing's *syndrome* is the well-described clinical condition resulting from hypercortisolism. Steroids are

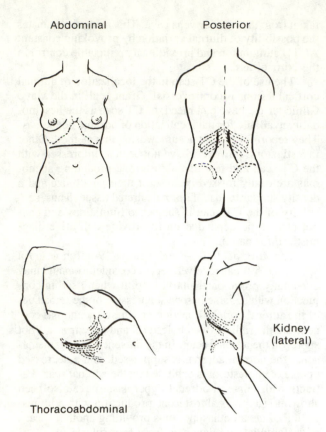

Figure 4 Adrenalectomy. The various incisions to expose the adrenals.

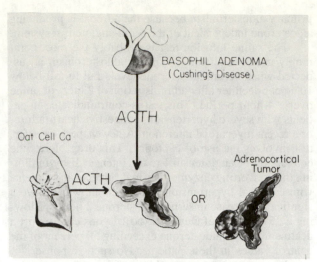

Figure 5 Endogenous hypercortisolism—Cushing's syndrome. The three most common etiologies. (From Hardy JD. Surgical management of Cushing's syndrome with emphasis on adrenal autotransplantation. Ann Surg 1978; 188:290.)

used in the management of a variety of medical problems and often cause an iatrogenic cushingoid state. Exogenous hypercortisolism remains the most common cause of Cushing's syndrome and may be reversed by decreasing steroid dosage.

Cushing's syndrome secondary to endogenous hypercortisolism is a relatively uncommon abnormality, with three major etiologies. All forms of endogenous hypercortisolism have two common features: the loss of the normal diurnal variation in cortisol secretion and a persistently elevated serum cortisol level after a standard low dose of exogenous glucocorticoid (dexamethasone). It is now generally accepted that Cushing's disease is the most common cause of endogenous hypercortisolism. Cushing's *disease* may be defined as hypercortisolism secondary to an ACTH-secreting pituitary adenoma, resulting in bilateral adrenal hyperplasia and hyperfunction. The remaining causes of endogenous hypercortisolism include adrenal neoplasms (adenoma and carcinoma) and ectopic ACTH-producing tumors such as the small cell carcinoma of the lung (Fig. 5).

Diagnosis

When Cushing's syndrome is suspected clinically, there are two relatively simple screening studies to consider. Elevated levels of serum cortisol and urine 17-OHCS with loss of the normal diurnal variation are indicative of Cushing's syndrome. Low-dose dexamethasone suppression is more reliable and should always be done as an initial screening study. One milligram of dexamethasone is given between 10 PM and midnight, and an 8 AM serum cortisol is obtained. This value is compared to the control (pre-dexamethasone) 8 AM cortisol level. Failure to suppress by more than 50 percent and serum values to less than 10 mg per deciliter suggest endogenous hypercortisolism.

Differential Diagnosis

Once the presence of hypercortisolism is established, the various possible etiologies must be considered (Fig. 6). Hypercortisolism due to an adrenal neoplasm differs from that due to the other causes in that the serum ACTH is low. Both ectopic ACTH-producing tumors and Cushing's disease exhibit elevated levels of ACTH and cortisol. These may be differentiated by use of large-dose dexamethasone suppression and metyrapone.

Eighty to ninety percent of patients with Cushing's disease suppress with high-dose dexamethasone, as evidenced by a fall in serum cortisol production. Ectopic ACTH-producing tumors are not suppressed with high-dose dexamethasone. Metyrapone is a pharmacologic agent that blocks the conversion of 11-deoxycortisol to cortisol. This action decreases the serum cortisol level and in turn decreases the negative feedback on the hypothalamus and pituitary, resulting in increased release of CRH (corticotropin-releasing hormone) and ACTH. The final metabolite of both cortisol and 11-deoxycortisol is urinary 17-OH corticosteroids. The pituitary adenoma of Cushing's disease is at least partially governed by the usual negative feedback inhibition of high serum cortisol levels. Metyrapone uncouples this negative feedback inhibition, and the result is increased ACTH production and thus an increase in both 11-deoxycortisol and 17-OHCS.

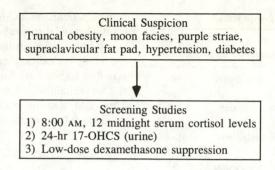

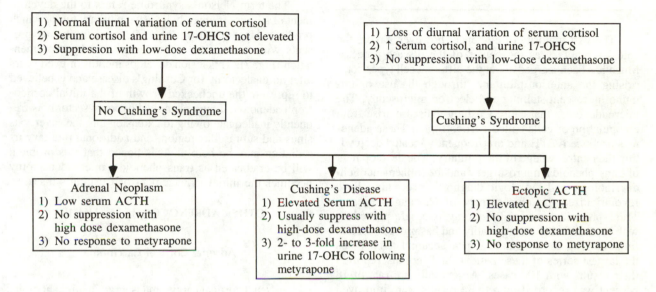

Figure 6 Cushing's syndrome: Diagnostic evaluation.

Patients with ectopic ACTH-producing tumors show no increase in urinary 17-OHCS following metyrapone and can therefore be distinguished from those who have Cushing's disease.

Ectopic ACTH may derive from a variety of neoplasms. APUD tumors, arising from tissues of the neural crest embryologically, possess the potential for hormone production. Small cell carcinoma of the lung is the most frequently observed source of ectopic ACTH. These patients may have the major features of Cushing's syndrome, but frequently manifest their underlying malignant tumor in the form of severe weight loss and lassitude.

ADRENOCORTICAL NEOPLASMS

Approximately 25 percent of patients with Cushing's syndrome have a functioning adrenal neoplasm as the underlying cause of their hypercortisolism. The most common lesion observed is a cortisol-producing, unilateral adenoma which results in increased negative feedback on the hypothalamus and the anterior pituitary, thus inhibiting ACTH release. The serum ACTH level is therefore low in the presence of elevated serum cortisol.

There are several other less common adrenal neoplasms that can cause Cushing's syndrome. These include bilateral adrenal adenomas and microadenomas (Table 2).

Endogenous hypercortisolism, in the presence of low serum ACTH, suggests a functional adrenal neoplasm. The procedures utilized for localization of the lesion include CT scans with thin adrenal sectioning, arteriography, and radioactive iodine-labeled cholesterol scans.

CUSHING'S DISEASE

Cushing's disease is the most common cause of endogenous hypercortisolism. It is almost always caused by excessive secretion of ACTH by a tumor of the anterior pituitary, as proposed by Cushing in 1932. The remarkable advances in radiologic technology have permitted detection of even 1- to 2-mm adenomas by means of arteriography and image intensification. Lateralization of the adenoma has at times been achieved through sampling in the petrosal vein bilaterally. Krieger et al postulate that the abnormality may lie higher, in the hypothalamus, and have reported successful treatment of several patients with cyproheptadine, an antiserotonin drug that presumably inhibits hypothalamic function in producing CRH.

TABLE 2   Adrenal Neoplasms

Pathology	Treatment	% of Total Cases
Unilateral adrenal adenoma Size: 2–6 cm	Unilateral adrenalectomy	90
Bilateral adrenal adenoma Size: 2–6 cm	Bilateral adrenalectomy	2–5
Bilateral microadenomas Size: microscopic	Bilateral adrenalectomy	Rare
Adrenal cortical carcinoma Size: > 6 cm	Unilateral, wide adrenal resection	5

The vast majority of evidence, however, favors the anterior pituitary as the center of the disease process. Much has been learned about the different cell types comprising the anterior pituitary, through the use of immunofluorescent staining and electron microscopy. The microadenomas that cause Cushing's disease arise from a population of cells called corticotrophs. These adenomas produce ACTH and are frequently located deep within the central wedge of the pituitary. The development of transsphenoidal microsurgery and the refinement of endocrinologic and radiologic diagnostic procedures have revolutionized the management of Cushing's disease. Transsphenoidal microadenectomy is a safe procedure with low morbidity and mortality and has proved successful in most cases. Boggan et al have accumulated perhaps the largest series of these patients and recently reported their results with 100 cases. An overall cure rate of 78 percent was recorded, and these results were improved if the tumor was confined to the sella turcica (87% cure). Twenty-five patients proved to have extrasellar extension of tumor at the time of surgery, and the results reflect the inability to remove all the abnormal tissue. Forty-eight percent of these patients were cured, 40 percent failed to respond, and 12 percent developed recurrence.

Management

Prior to the development of transsphenoidal surgery, patients with Cushing's disease were managed in a variety of ways. Total bilateral adrenalectomy was the usual treatment and effected rapid improvement of the cushingoid patient. This approach necessitated permanent steroid replacement, and a significant number of these patients later developed Nelson's syndrome. Hardy et al reported experience with adrenal autotransplantation in an effort to circumvent the aforementioned problems. Adrenal autotransplantation was found to be technically feasible, with all transplants showing at least some degree of viability and function. Indeed, two cases of recurrent Cushing's disease occurred as a result of continued ACTH stimulation of the adrenal transplants. Late follow-up of these autotransplant patients, however, demonstrated no truly significant benefit from adrenal autotransplantation, and there are now few indications for bilateral adrenalectomy in the management of Cushing's disease. Ten to 15 per-

cent of patients with Cushing's disease are not cured with transsphenoidal surgery. Bilateral adrenalectomy can certainly be justified in the management of these patients, especially if medical therapy has been unsuccessful. Other possible indications for bilateral adrenalectomy include the unavailability of neurosurgical expertise in remote areas and also the patient with Cushing's disease who declines intracranial surgery.

NELSON'S SYNDROME

The term Nelson's syndrome refers to the development of a large, frequently invasive pituitary tumor which produces large quantities of ACTH and frequently presents with visual field disturbances and hyperpigmentation (Fig. 7). This lesion develops months or even years after adrenalectomy for Cushing's disease and is believed to represent the unchecked growth of the initial corticotroph adenoma. Transsphenoidal hypophysectomy is frequently inadequate owing to extension into the cavernous sinus and suprasellar region, and additional pituitary irradiation may be helpful. It is hoped that this problem will be eradicated as transsphenoidal microadenectomy becomes the initial management of Cushing's disease.

OTHER ADRENOCORTICAL TUMORS

Adrenal Cortical Carcinoma

Adrenal cortical carcinoma is a rare malignant tumor that accounts for less than 1 percent of all malignant neoplasms. Unfortunately, it has a 75 to 90 percent 5-year mortality rate. In many cases, distant metastasis has already occurred at the time of diagnosis. Owing to the rarity of this disease, few large series of patients exist. Several informative reports have been assembled in recent years which describe the clinical presentation, extent of disease, treatment modalities utilized, and eventual outcome of a number of patients with adrenal cortical carcinoma. King and Lack reviewed 49 cases. The average age at presentation was 28 years for the female patient and 38 years for the males. The most common presenting complaints were abdominal pain and weight loss. A palpable abdominal mass was present in almost half the patients. Clinical findings suggestive of endocrine hyperfunction were present in only 37 percent, with eight of the 49 patients presenting with Cushing's syndrome. Often, the tumors were very large, the average size being 12.4 cm and the average weight 848.6 g. Forty-one of the 49 patients underwent laparotomy, only 24 having resection for possible cure. Thirty-six of the 49 patients died within 9 months following diagnosis. A variety of chemotherapeutic agents were utilized including O,p'-DDD (Mitotane), but no difference was noted in either the length or quality of survival. It should be noted, however, that many of the patients receiving chemotherapy had far-advanced metastatic disease. Some workers have reported beneficial response to O,p'-DDD in a more

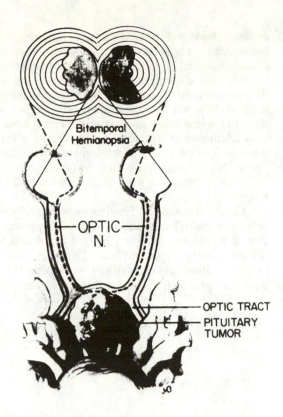

Figure 7 Nelson's syndrome. A large invasive ACTH-producing pituitary tumor occurring after adrenalectomy for Cushing's disease. Patients present with visual field disturbances and/or hyperpigmentation. (From Hardy JD. Surgical management of Cushing's syndrome with emphasis on adrenal autotransplantation. Ann Surg 1978; 188:290.)

salvageable patient population. Radiation therapy was given as both adjuvant and palliative treatment, but there was no evidence that it prolonged survival. The only clinical or pathologic characteristic that correlated with survival was the resectability of the primary tumor. Nine of the 24 patients resected for possible cure were alive 2 or more years following their surgery. Complete surgical excision prior to widespread metastasis remains the only hope for disease-free survival.

Myelolipoma

Myelolipoma of the adrenal is a rare, benign, nonfunctional tumor which should be considered in the differential diagnosis of an adrenal mass. These tumors are composed of both hematopoietic and fatty elements. They occasionally attain large dimensions and may present as a space-occupying mass with symptoms of abdominal compression. In many cases, the presence of this lesion is suggested by its characteristic CT scan and arteriographic findings. Myelolipomas are of low density owing to their high lipid content and are also usually avascular. Adrenal myelolipoma does not appear to be a premalignant lesion, and surgical therapy is therefore limited to unilateral adrenalectomy.

Virilizing Adrenal Tumors

Tumors of the adrenal cortex causing virilization are uncommon and, as one would expect, more easily identified in the female patient. These lesions presenting in childhood cause precocious puberty in the male and clitoral enlargement with development of pubic hair in the female. The clinical findings in adult males are often subtle, and the problem may not be appreciated until the lesion has become large or distant metastasis has occurred. Virilization in the adult female requires a careful evaluation for the possibility of an ovarian neoplasm in addition to adrenal considerations. Virilizing adrenal tumors may be benign or malignant and predominantly secrete large amounts of dehydroandrosterone, which is a major androgen precursor. Dehydroandrosterone may be measured directly in the serum or in urine as 17-ketosteroid. Treatment of this lesion is surgical with unilateral adrenalectomy after appropriate localization of the neoplasm.

Feminizing Adrenal Tumors

Estrogen-producing adrenal tumors are also extremely rare, most of them being discovered in adult males during the second, third, and fourth decades of life. Gynecomastia, testicular atrophy, and impotence are the common presenting complaints. These tumors do occasionally occur in children as well, with precocious puberty being noted in young girls and advanced bone age and gynecomastia seen in boys. Adult females with a feminizing tumor are often difficult to identify and may never be discovered if the lesion is benign. Feminizing neoplasms of the adrenal may be benign or malignant; both are best managed with unilateral adrenalectomy.

ADRENAL INSUFFICIENCY (ADDISON'S DISEASE)

Adrenal insufficiency is a relatively rare problem in the surgical patient, but if unrecognized, it frequently leads to death. A high index of suspicion and early treatment are of great importance in the management of this condition.

In the past, tuberculous involvement of the adrenals was the most common cause of progressive adrenal insufficiency. There has been a steady decline in tuberculosis owing to earlier and better management of that disease, resulting in fewer cases of tuberculous adrenal insufficiency as well. The most common cause of Addison's disease today is idiopathic bilateral adrenal atrophy, which may be an autoimmune phenomenon. Many of these patients have circulating adrenal antibodies, and some of them evidence antibodies to thyroid, parathyroid, and gonadal tissue as well. The adrenal is frequently involved with metastatic disease from a variety of neoplasms including carcinoma of the breast and lung. It is unusual, however, for these metastases to produce sufficient destruction to lead to adrenal insufficiency. The adrenal cortex must be almost completely destroyed before clinical signs of Addison's disease occur. Other infrequent causes of adrenal insufficiency include fungal infections, amyloidosis, and adrenal hemorrhage.

Clinical symptoms of Addison's disease include weakness, bronze skin pigmentation, hypotension, and sometimes nausea, vomiting, and abdominal pain. These patients are frequently mildly hypoglycemic. Other electrolyte abnormalities include hyponatremia and hyperkalemia. The diagnosis can be confirmed by demonstration of reduced urinary corticosteroid excretion and the failure of plasma corticosteroids to increase in response to an infusion of ACTH. The treatment of adrenal insufficiency requires both glucocorticoid and mineralocorticoid replacement and long-term supplementation.

ADRENALECTOMY: PREOPERATIVE AND POSTOPERATIVE MANAGEMENT

Patients undergoing bilateral adrenalectomy need no special preoperative preparation other than the correction of any fluid and electrolyte abnormalities such as hypokalemia or hyperglycemia. However, it is necessary to initiate steroid replacement therapy intraoperatively in order to ensure adequate steroid support for the stress of the operation. Hydrocortisone 100 mg every 6 hours for the first 48 hours as a continuous infusion has worked well. In the immediate postoperative period, intramuscularly administered cortisone is added, 50 mg IM every 6 hours. The intravenous infusion may be discontinued by the third postoperative day, and oral administration of cortisone begun as soon as gastrointestinal function returns.

Chronic maintenance replacement of both glucocorticoid and mineralocorticoid is required. Hydrocortisone, 20 to 30 mg, along with 0.1 mg of 9 α-Fluorohydrocortisone (Florinef) daily usually suffices. The exact dosage must be individualized and manipulated over a period of several weeks in order to arrive at optimal replacement therapy.

PHEOCHROMOCYTOMA

JON A. van HEERDEN, M.B., Ch.B., M.S.(Surg.), F.R.C.S.(C), F.A.C.S.

The term "pheochromocytoma" was initially suggested by Pick in 1912. This name was based on the characteristic chromaffin histologic staining appearance (*pheochromocyte* = a cell that takes on a dusky color; *cytoma* = tumor). This neuroectodermal tumor (apudoma) arises from the chromaffin cells (pheochromocytes) of the adrenergic system. Classically, such tumors originating within the adrenal medulla have been termed pheochromocytomas, whereas those arising in extra-adrenal adrenergic tissue are more appropriately termed paragangliomas; the term "extra-adrenal pheochromocytoma" is thus a misnomer. The extra-adrenal adrenergic tissue is widely distributed, and may conveniently be divided by anatomic site into (1) branchiomeric (carotid body, aortic body, and orbital), (2) intravagal (along the entire course of the vagus nerves), (3) aorticosympathetic (along the course of the para-aortic sympathetic chain, and (4) the visceral-autonomic paraganglia (accounting for tumors occurring in the urinary bladder, duodenum, peripheral blood vessels, and the intra-atrial septum of the heart).

Pheochromocytomas are the cause of high blood pressure in approximately 0.1 to 0.5 percent of patients with hypertension, the incidence among the general population being about one per two hundred thousand. Although these tumors may occur at any age, the peak incidence is in the fourth and fifth decades. Tumors are characteristically extra-adrenal in about 10 percent of patients, multicentric in 10 percent, bilateral in 5 to 10 percent, and familial in 10 percent. Ten percent of tumors occur in the pediatric population, and roughly 10 percent are malignant.

The first successful operative removal of a pheochromocytoma was performed in February of 1926 by Roux in Switzerland. In October of that same year, Dr. Charles Mayo resected a pheochromocytoma in a Roman Catholic nun. She survived for two decades following this procedure.

The majority of pheochromocytomas are sporadic. However, they are associated with multiple endocrine neoplasia (MEN) type II (medullary thyroid carcinoma, pheochromocytoma, primary hyperparathyroidism, mucocutaneous neuromas) in approximately 5 to 10 percent of patients. In rare instances pheochromocytoma may occur in conjunction with neuroectodermal dysplasia, such as von Recklinghausen's disease, von Hippel-Lindau syndrome, tuberous sclerosis, and the Sturge-Weber syndrome. When associated with the multiple endocrine neoplasia type II syndrome, the condition is characteristically bilateral. The pathologic findings in these patients range from early bilateral adrenal medullary hyperplasia to combinations of multicentric bilateral pheochromocytoma, with or without adrenal medullary hyperplasia.

Approximately half of the patient population with pheochromocytoma present with characteristic paroxysmal hypertension episodes (Fig. 1). These episodes were described well by Dr. Mayo in 1927:

''Sudden onset—pain in back—some pain in the occipital region and right side of neck associated with nausea and vomiting. Cold and clammy, rapid respirations, rapid heartbeat.'' ''First noted a slight anxious expression to face. Pupils slightly dilated. Pulse 124, full and pounding, with radial vessels tight and easily rolled. Blood pressure, 300/160 mm Hg after two minutes. Patient felt nauseated. Some vasomotor mottling about mouth and nose. Aorta palpable in episternal notch, neck veins full. Heart sounds pounding. Hands cool and sweaty. No loss of consciousness.'' ''Sudden onset of feeling of suffocation with nausea and vomiting. Blood pressure 260/190 mm Hg. Pulse rate, 144 per minute. Face intensely cyanosed. Respiration labored and rapid—48 per minute.'' In the remaining 40 to 50 percent who present with sustained hypertension, the possibility of a pheochromocytoma should not be excluded.

The catecholamines (dopamine, norepinephrine, and epinephrine) are derived from the essential amino acid tyrosine. Biochemical verification of catecholamine excess can be performed by the measurements of the degradation products of the catecholamines, e.g., urinary metanephrines, vanillylmandelic acid (VMA), and homovanillic acid (HVA), or by direct measurement of dopamine, norepinephrine, and epinephrine in the urine, per se (Fig. 2). In our experience, the least accurate of these modalities has been the measurement of VMA and HVA. The most reliable have been the urinary fractionated catecholamines measured by high-pressure liquid chromatography. The determination of total urinary metanephrines continues to be an excellent screening test with a false-negative rate of about 2 to 4 percent. It bears rememberng that methylglucamine (a component of many iodinated contrast media) may cause metanephrine values to be falsely normal for 72 hours after its administration.

PREOPERATIVE MANAGEMENT

Surgical morbidity and ensuing mortality have been greatly reduced by preoperative surgical preparation with appropriate alpha and beta adrenergic blockade. For more than a decade, I have routinely advocated the use of both dibenzyline (phenoxybenzamine) and the beta blocker Inderal (propranolol). Beta blockade should never precede alpha blockade, since unopposed alpha-adrenergic activity

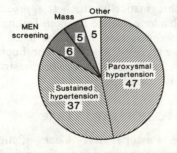

Figure 1 Clinical presentation of pheochromocytoma

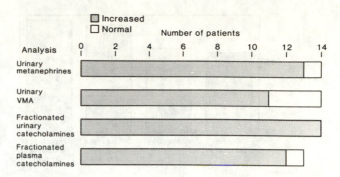

Figure 2 Accuracy of biochemical catecholamine measurements

may result in general vasoconstriction with detrimental cardiac failure. Phenoxybenzamine is usually started at a dose of 20 mg per day with an increase of 10 mg per day until satisfactory control of blood pressure in the erect and supine positions is achieved. A minor side effect of this drug is nasal stuffiness, which is usually well tolerated. This drug should be ''on-board'' for at least 7 to 10 days prior to adrenalectomy. Propranolol is started 48 hours prior to operation at a dose of 30 to 40 mg per day. The dibenzyline is discontinued at midnight on the day preceding operation, and the last dose of propranolol is given with a small sip of water one hour before the induction of anesthesia. Other drugs that are infrequently utilized, and are not our drugs of choice, are the beta$_1$ selective antagonist, metoprolol (Lopressor), and metyrosine (Demser), which is an inhibitor of tyrosine hydroxylase. Metyrosine may reduce the synthesis of norepinephrine by at least 50 percent.

This preoperative preparation is easily managed on an outpatient basis since there is no need for preoperative volume expansion, as was once the practice.

Localization of the Tumor

Selective arteriography, selective venous sampling, retroperitoneal air insufflation, and intravenous pyelography with nephrotomography are of historical interest in the localization of these tumors. All have been replaced by the two modalities of current choice, i.e., computerized tomography and nuclear scintography utilizing ^{131}I-metaiodobenzylguanadine (^{131}I-MIBG). Noninvasive computerized tomography is a highly accurate modality with a resolution capability of 6 to 8 mm, the ability to clearly define a normal adrenal gland, and the ability to document the presence of paragangliomas. The efficacy of this modality has been upward of 96 percent in my experience (Fig. 3). The use of ^{131}I-MIBG, which is an analogue of norepinephrine, is currently showing great promise. This material is selectively concentrated in adrenergic vesicles, and since the normal adrenal medullas are generally too small, they do not ''light-up'' with this technique, which therefore basically concentrates only within abnormal adrenal medullary tissue. This newest modality for localization has been especially help-

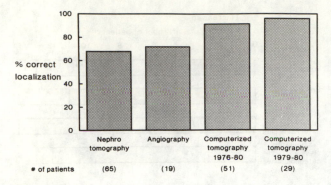

Figure 3 Accuracy of various localizing modalities

ful in the delineation of early adrenal medullary disease in patients with the multiple endocrine neoplasia type II syndrome, in patients with malignant (and metastatic) pheochromocytomas, and in patients with paragangliomas, particularly those that are intrathoracic in origin. The false-negative rate for the MIBG scan is approximately 10 percent.

Anesthesia

Experience in treating patients with pheochromocytomas is essential for both the anesthesiologist and the surgeon, if a successful outcome is to be obtained. The anesthesiologist, in particular, should be aware that adrenergic blockade is rarely complete, and he or she should be comfortable with the management of the rare arrhythmias that may occur intraoperatively and with the episodes of hypertension that are virtually the rule in all patients undergoing resection. I routinely use Valium for preoperative sedation, and the anesthetic agent of choice is enflurane (Ethrane). The relaxants we currently prefer are succinylcholine for intubation and metocurine (Metubine) for postintubation relaxation. Enflurane has been satisfactory and does depress the myocardial irritability that is secondary to catecholamine excess (Fig. 4). Sodium nitroprusside (Nipride) has been the agent of choice for the management of blood pressure fluctuations. A solution is routinely prepared and connected during the early phases of the operation, and the amount administered titrated according to the blood pressure response. Arrhyth-

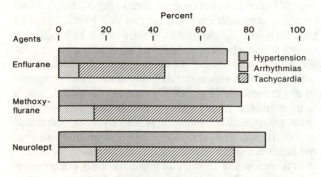

Figure 4 Intraoperative arrythmias and hypertension occurring with various anesthetic agents

mias have been unusual in our experience, and seldom is either propranolol or lidocaine indicated. Contrary to many reports, hypotension has not been a problem following removal of these tumors.

In addition to the placement of an adequate central and peripheral venous line, I have routinely placed a radial artery catheter (after the induction of anesthesia) and have selectively utilized the Swan-Ganz catheter. This catheter, I believe, should be placed in all patients 60 years of age or older and in patients with a history of cardiac disease. In my opinion, routine use is not necessary, although there are those who believe it to be important.

THE OPERATION

The surgical philosophy should be to "steal the tumor away from the patient." This philosophy entails minimal manipulation and pressure on the tumor, with early ligation of the adrenal vein, if possible. Since such a philosophy requires excellent exposure as well as a gentle hand, the posterior approach to pheochromocytomas has not been our practice. The posterior approach requires excessive manipulation and pressure on the adrenal gland, and visualization of the adrenal vein occurs late during the dissection via this approach. Our exposure of choice for pheochromocytomas has been that of an appropriate transverse upper abdominal bilateral subcostal incision. Liberal use of the mechanical third-hand retractor greatly facilitates visualization of both adrenal glands. The right adrenal gland is well exposed by extensive kocherization of the duodenum and downward retraction with the surgeon's left hand on the right kidney. Use of hemoclips has facilitated the occlusion of the single, broad, fragile right adrenal vein, which often enters the posterior aspect of the inferior vena cava. Exposure of the left adrenal gland is achieved by entrance into the lesser sac through the gastrocolic omentum, followed by superior rotation of the pancreas after division of the peritoneum and fibrofatty tissue immediately inferior to the lower border of the pancreas. The single left adrenal vein, which usually enters the left renal vein, is more easily exposed since it is longer than the right, and is less broad. On occasion, the left adrenal vein might enter the left inferior phrenic vein. For larger tumors, especially those suspected of being malignant, a thoracoabdominal incision on either side affords excellent exposure. For paragangliomas located subdiaphragmatically, the best approach is that obtained through a long midline incision. During removal of these tumors, great care should be taken to avoid rupture, which may well lead to tumor implants and recurrent disease, a situation that can be disastrous if the initial lesion was malignant.

POSTOPERATIVE CARE

Immediate Postoperative Care. Patients are admitted to an intensive care unit for the initial 24 hours following resection. Seldom are difficulties encountered in this period. Arrhythmias are extremely uncommon, as are fluctuations in the hemodynamic status, if adequate preoperative blockade has been performed.

Late Postoperative Care.   Prior to the patient's discharge from the hospital, urinary catecholamine levels should be repeated. The patient's blood pressure should be followed carefully, especially if the patient presented with sustained rather than paroxysmal hypertension. If the hypertension was paroxysmal at presentation, 95 percent of these patients should return to a normotensive state. However, if hypertension was sustained at presentation, roughly one-third of this group of patients remain hypertensive and may require additional antihypertensive therapy following resection of the tumor. It has been suggested that a higher percentage of pheochromocytomas and, especially, paragangliomas are malignant, and that long-term follow-up will confirm this fact. It is therefore advisable to perform both a biochemical evaluation of the catecholamine status and a ^{131}I-MIBG scan at yearly intervals following operation.

MULTIPLE ENDOCRINE NEOPLASIA, TYPE II

The disease is characteristically multiple and bilateral in both the type IIA and type IIB syndromes of multiple endocrine neoplasia. For this reason, it has been my philosophy to recommend bilateral total adrenalectomy in all such patients once the presence of excessive circulating catecholamines has been documented. I have been favorably impressed with both the short-term and the long-term results in a series of patients thus treated at our institution. It is evident from the literature that a sizable percentage of patients undergoing unilateral adrenalectomy for this syndrome will subsequently require contralateral adrenalectomy. If this syndrome goes undiagnosed, there is an ever-present danger of unexpected hypertensive crisis during other general surgical procedures. All members of such families should therefore be carefully screened for catecholamine excess, especially if a surgical procedure is contemplated.

MALIGNANT PHEOCHROMOCYTOMAS

Malignant pheochromocytomas are encountered in roughly 8 to 10 percent of patients. The incidence of malignant paragangliomas is much higher—40 percent in our experience. The 5-year survival for all patients with malignant pheochromocytoma is approximately 55 percent. It has been suggested recently that long-term follow-up of patients with seemingly benign, totally resected pheochromocytomas will reveal a higher than heretofore expected rate of malignancy. The histologic diagnosis of malignant pheochromocytoma or paraganglioma is notoriously difficult; unless tumor tissue is demonstrated in ectopic sites such as the liver or lymph nodes, no absolute histologic criteria of malignancy are present.

Patients with metastatic nonresectable disease can be fairly well managed symptomatically with phenoxybenzamine. In addition, catecholamine production may be decreased by the administration of alpha-methylparatyrosin (Demser), a drug that selectively blocks the production of the enzyme tyrosine hydroxylase. Although chemotherapy has not been beneficial, localized radiotherapy has been of value in the symptomatic control of localized bony metastases. I am cautiously optimistic about the possible therapeutic use of ^{131}I-MIBG in the treatment of metastatic pheochromocytoma. Current studies are evaluating the efficacy of this newer modality, which is analogous to the use of radioactive iodine in the treatment of metastatic follicular thyroid carcinoma.

NONTOXIC GOITER

MARIA ALLO, M.D.

Nontoxic goiter refers to thyroid enlargement that is not associated with thyrotoxicosis, hypothyroidism, inflammation, or neoplasm. The usual etiology involves hypersecretion of thyroid-stimulating hormone (TSH) in response to a defect in hormone synthesis within the thyroid gland. In most cases, increase in TSH compensates for the abnormality in hormone biosynthesis, resulting in a patient who is euthyroid but has increased thyroid mass (goiter). In situations in which there is inadequate compensation, hypothyroidism results.

PATHOPHYSIOLOGY

In some parts of the world where there is an iodine deficiency, goiter is endemic. These areas include the Alps, Himalayas, Andes, and the Great Lakes regions in the United States. In the United States and Switzerland, the incidence of goiter has decreased dramatically since the introduction of iodized salt.

Nontoxic goiters occur despite iodine availability in persons who have functional abnormalities of the thyroid related to defective iodination of thyroglobulin. Rarely, ingested agents including antithyroid drugs (PTU, carbinazole, methimazole) or products of plants containing antithyroid drugs (rutabaga, white turnip, casaba meal) have been implicated in goiter.

In the majority of patients, nontoxic goiter produces little problem other than the cosmetically unpleasant appearance of the enlarged thyroid. The majority of patients are euthyroid and asymptomatic women. In fact, approximately eight women develop this syndrome for every man. The longer a goiter has been present, the more it tends to become multinodular. These nodules subsequently may become inactive and involute, degenerate, form cysts, fibrose, or fill with colloid. Longstanding goiters become relatively more autonomous in their function than goiters of more recent onset. This autonomy can be measured by decreased or absent TSH responsiveness to thyroid-releasing hormone (TRH). Some of these patients may show Jod-Basedow phenomenon (hyperthyroidism induced by iodine exposure) or frank thyrotoxicosis from an autonomously functioning thyroid nodule. It is estimated that 25 to 30 percent of persons with goiters in the sixth and seventh decade of life have autonomous function in their goiters. It is unusual for a patient to note any physical abnormalities before an enlargement or asymmetry in the neck is detectable on physical examination. As the goiter grows, however, it may become increasingly associated with symptoms including dysphagia, dyspnea, hoarseness, or tenderness to palpation. Nevertheless, most goiters grow slowly, and the onset of symptoms is insidious and often not recognized immediately. Some large goiters, having occupied the available space in the neck, may grow substernally. These goiters may impinge on the thoracic inlet and produce Pemberton's sign (engorgement of the venous structures in the face and neck secondary to thoracic inlet obstruction, noted when the arms are raised), tracheal compression, esophageal compression with dysphagia, or even a superior vena cava syndrome.

TREATMENT

The treatment of nontoxic goiter is usually directed at eliminating the stimulus for thyroid hyperplasia. One approach is to suppress the hypersecretion of TSH by providing exogenous thyroid hormone. When iodine deficiency is present, treatment should still be directed toward suppressing TSH and providing adequate exogenous thyroid hormone. In these cases, iodine administration should not be employed because it may induce hyperthyroidism. When it does not induce hyperthyroidism, it is frequently ineffective in reducing the size of the goiter. Treatment with 100 to 200 μg of L-thyroxine is usually adequate to suppress the thyroid in the majority of the patients with diffuse relatively recently formed goiters. One can measure the completeness of thyroid suppression by measuring the radioiodine uptake. A RAIU of less than 5 percent is indicative of adequate suppression. In situations in which suppression is not obtained on an apparently adequate dose of L-thyroxine, a thyroid scan performed while the patient is still on L-thyroxine therapy is useful, and may perhaps reveal an area of autonomous hyperfunction which may not be represented by a palpable nodule. Goiters of longer duration are not so responsive

to L-thyroxine and often have areas of mixed function (some nodules that are hypofunctioning and others that are autonomously hyperfunctioning). In patients with large goiters, with longstanding goiters, or with significant cardiovascular disease, in whom some autonomously hyperfunctioning nodules are suspected, a TRH stimulation test is often useful to determine whether or not there is predominant functional autonomy or normal regulatory control. Suppression therapy with L-thyroxine is contraindicated in patients who have lack of response to TRH. It is in these longstanding goiters that thyroidectomy plays an important role. Table 1 lists the indications for thyroidectomy. Enlarged goiters may compress adjacent structures. Esophageal compression may be associated with dysphagia and may sometimes be demonstrated on upper gastrointestinal series as exogenous compression on the esophagus. Tracheal compression may produce dypsnea, cough, stridor, or "nocturnal choking episodes" whereby, because of a change in position while sleeping, the patient obstructs his airway and is awakened from his sleep by air hunger. Substernal or intrathoracic goiters usually extend into the superior mediastinum. These goiters often produce symptoms of compression and may obstruct the thoracic inlet, causing superior vena cava syndrome. Retrograde esophageal varices have been associated with very large substernal goiters. Most substernal goiters can be removed via a cervical approach since the blood supply is retained in the usual position in the neck. Exceptions to this rule are the very rare goiters ($<1\%$) that occupy the posterior mediastinum.

Suspicion of malignancy is an indication for thyroidectomy. Often there is a dominant nodule within a multinodular goiter which may be mistaken for a solitary nodule. Needle aspiration cytology is particularly useful in determining whether these are simple benign colloid nodules or have pathologic changes suspicious for malignancy. In some cases, several cold nodules may be present. The incidence of malignancy in cold nodules within a multinodular goiter is probably 5 to 10 percent. Thus, excision of a goiter to prevent subsequent development of malignancy is not indicated.

It is not uncommon for patients to present with a history of a nodule enlarging overnight. In most cases, this represents hemorrhage into a preexisting degenerating colloid nodule or cyst. Needle aspiration cytology is often useful to define the nature of these rapidly growing nodules. In longstanding goiters with areas of autonomy,

TABLE 1 Indications for Thyroidectomy

Tracheal compression

Esophageal compression

Substernal location

Sudden change in preexisting goiter

Suspicion of malignancy

Thyrotoxicosis

Cosmetic indications

thyrotoxicosis may develop in rare instances. Radioactive iodine is often used to treat these lesions. However, in patients with some contraindication or aversion to radioiodide therapy, surgery may be considered.

Finally, disfigurement can justify surgery, and in patients with large goiters that have not significantly regressed after 6 months to a year of suppression, thyroidectomy is indicated. Plain films of the neck and chest are useful to demonstrate displacement of the trachea or the esophagus. Esophagram is valuable to implicate the goiter as a cause for dysphagia. Thyroid function studies, TBG, and thyroid antibody studies are useful to determine whether the patient is eumetabolic and whether thyroiditis may be the underlying cause of the goiter enlargement. Thyroid scans using technetium-99m or iodine-123 usually demonstrate either heterogeneous uptake or decreased uptake. A needle aspirate showing colloid follicular epithelium and hemosiderin-laden macrophages is consistent with an adenomatous goiter.

In any situation in which surgery is being considered for a large goiter, particularly in patients presenting with hoarseness or stridor, indirect laryngoscopy should be done to assess vocal cord function, and a serum calcium and phosphorus level should be obtained as a baseline. No other specific preoperative preparation is necessary in patients who are euthyroid. However, the anesthesiologist should be alerted to the presence of a large goiter that may be causing some tracheal compression or distortion, making endotracheal intubation difficult and perhaps requiring use of a flexible bronchoscope to facilitate insertion of the endotracheal tube.

OPERATIVE TECHNIQUE

The usual operation performed for a large goiter is subtotal thyroidectomy. The goals of surgery are to eliminate the symptoms of compression, to allow the trachea to resume its normal midline position, and to correct the cosmetic defect associated with the goiter. The patient is usually placed in a semi-Fowler position with the head hyperextended. A Kocher cervical collar incision is used and carried through the subcutaneous layer and the platysma. Superior and inferior flaps are raised, with the thyroid cartilege being the superior landmark and the manubrium of the sternum the inferior one. The strap muscles should be separated and retracted laterally. It is not always necessary to divide the strap muscles, but if they are divided, division should be immediately caudad to their insertion. It is extremely important to carefully and completely separate the sternothyroid muscle from the capsule of the thyroid gland. Critical structures to be identified include the middle thyroid veins, the inferior thyroid artery, the superior thyroid artery, the parathyroid glands, the recurrent laryngeal nerves, and the external branch of the superior laryngeal nerve. Early ligation of the middle thyroid vein permits the thyroid to be rolled anteromedially from the tracheoesophageal groove. In large goiters, particularly those with substernal extension, mobilization of the upper pole may be necessary to allow enough mobilization to deliver the lower part of the thyroid out of the neck. To expose the superior pole of the thyroid, the ligament of Berry should be incised between the medial aspect of the upper pole and the cricothyroideus muscle. The areolar tissue that lies laterally and posteriorly can be bluntly dissected from the upper pole. The three branches of the superior thyroid artery and the associated veins should be individually clamped at the point where they enter the thyroid tissue. After each branch is individually divided, the ends should be ligated carefully. It is injudicious to use cautery or clips that may become dislodged on these vessels since once divided, they may retract cephalad, be very difficult to recover, and be a source of persistent bleeding. Injury to the superior laryngeal nerve can be avoided by dissecting the upper pole vessels laterally to medially on the plane of the thyroid capsule. The nerve generally is medial to the superior thyroid artery and enters the cricothyroideus muscle well above the point at which the superior thyroid vessels enter the capsule of the thyroid gland. The safest method of ligating the inferior thyroid vessels is to do so on the capsule of the thyroid gland by individually clamping these vessels on the vessel without encompassing any thyroid capsule. Vessels may be divided and peeled from the surface of the gland and ligated. The recurrent laryngeal nerve is usually in the avascular area caudad to the lower pole of the thyroid; however, is not uncommon in a large goiter to have the nerve tent along the posterior medial border of the goiter. By approaching the inferior thyroid vessels on the capsule of the gland, injury to the recurrent laryngeal nerve may be minimized. Ligation of the inferior thyroid vessels in the tracheoesophageal sulcus may lead to bleeding and injury to the recurrent laryngeal nerve in an attempt to achieve hemostasis. Posteriorly extending goiters or goiters that displace the trachea may displace the recurrent nerve anteriorly or laterally, and as mentioned earlier, the nerve may stretch over the thyroid capsule. It is critical that the nerve be identified caudad to the lower pole of the thyroid and traced superiorly and that there is awareness of the nerve as the goiter is dislocated medially and anteriorly so as to avoid injury to the nerve.

Parathyroid glands may be identified about 80 percent of the time within the 1-cm circle whose center is the point where the recurrent laryngeal nerve crosses the inferior thyroid artery. Identification of the parathyroids is desirable and care should be taken to avoid injury to the glands themselves and to their blood supply from the inferior thyroid artery.

SUBSTERNAL INTRATHORACIC GOITERS

The vast majority ($>95\%$) of substernal goiters can be removed through a cervical incision. Prior to excision of a substernal goiter, it is desirable to obtain a radioiodine scan to document that thyroid tissue is accounting for the mass in the mediastinum. Lack of uptake does not exclude the diagnosis, nor will it precisely delineate the extent of the goiter. However the presence of uptake is reassuring.

In the approach to a substernal goiter, the upper pole and middle thyroid vein should be divided initially and the isthmus of the gland divided to allow greater mobility of the lobe that has the intrathoracic component. Generally, careful lateral blunt dissection around the intrathoracic component allows it to be delivered from the thoracic inlet. Although morcellation has been advocated by some, we find that approximately 8 percent of patients with substernal goiter have an area of malignancy within the substernal segment. This makes morcellation undesirable, and we rarely find it necessary to free the intrathoracic segment.

Posterior mediastinal goiters are uncommon. They may have a blood supply whose origin is within the mediastinum. In the rare instances in which these are encountered, an enhanced CT scan is helpful to define the relationship of the goiter to the adjacent structures and to determine whether a transcervical or transthoracic approach should be used.

RECURRENT GOITERS

As in any reoperation for thyroid or parathyroid disease, the surgeon performing the second operation should be aware that normal anatomic landmarks may be obscured as a result of previous surgery. A copy of the initial operative note is sometimes helpful to determine what was removed at the time of the first operation and whether the parathyroid glands were identified. A pathology report is often helpful in determining the extent to which the parathyroids may have been disrupted. A lateral approach such as is used for carotid endarterectomy (incision between the sternocleidomastoid muscle and the strap muscles) is sometimes helpful to demonstrate the posterolateral aspect of the thyroid and to identify the recurrent laryngeal nerves and the parathyroid glands, which may be adherent to more anterior structures as a consequence of a previous operation.

DRAINAGE

It is the rule that most thyroidectomy wounds can be closed without drainage. In general, I prefer to leave a drain in patients who have had excision of intrathoracic goiters and prefer to use a small flat closed drainage system with a suction catheter. When large cervical goiters are removed and there is considerable dead space, drainage may be desirable; however, drainage should never be considered a reason for not achieving complete hemostasis.

OPERATIVE AND POSTOPERATIVE COMPLICATIONS

The complications of thyroidectomy for benign goiter are those of other thyroid and parathyroid operations: postoperative hemorrhage, recurrent laryngeal nerve paralysis or neuropraxia, hypoparathyroidism, and, occasionally, laryngeal edema with associated hoarseness and/or stridor. Except in the case of a huge, laterally extending goiter, injury to the cervical sympathetics, phrenic nerve, or thoracic duct should not be a problem. When a goiter with a large substernal component has been removed, one should obtain a postoperative chest film to rule out mediastinal hematoma or pneumothorax. The main problem associated with postoperative hemorrhage is not intrinsic blood loss, but rather bleeding into a closed compartment resulting in tracheal compression. Patients with postoperative respiratory distress—particularly patients in whom the vocal cords were seen to move at the time of extubation and who had a period in the recovery room without stridor, cough, or symptoms of hypoxia—should be examined for bleeding into the incision. The cervical incision should be opened immediately and hematoma evacuated. Postoperative indirect or direct laryngoscopy can indicate whether or not unilateral recurrent nerve paralysis or neuropraxia has occurred. In most cases of unilateral injury, there is either recovery or a compensatory medial movement of the remaining vocal cord with establishment of relatively normal voice. However, even when there is unilateral recurrent nerve paralysis, the presence of laryngeal edema can cause stridor and sometimes obstruction. Elongation and kinking of the trachea secondary to displacement and distortion by a very large goiter can be minimized by suturing the trachea to the strap muscles at the midline. This uncommon occurrence results when a longstanding goiter compresses the trachea, resulting in softening of the tracheal cartilages and deviation of the trachea.

POSTOPERATIVE MANAGEMENT

As mentioned earlier, a chest film should be obtained following removal of any substernal or intrathoracic goiter to rule out mediastinal hematoma or pneumothorax. All patients who have undergone thyroidectomy for adenomatous goiter should be placed on thyroid suppression therapy to prevent recurrent goiter. The patient should be told preoperatively that thyroid hormone treatment will be required for the remainder of his or her life. A dose of 100 to 200 μg of L-thyroxine is generally adequate for suppression.

THYROID CANCER

R. ROBINSON BAKER, M.D.

Malignant tumors of the thyroid gland constitute the most frequent neoplasm of the endocrine system. Slightly more than 10,000 new cases are discovered yearly in the United States, but less than 1,100 patients die annually from this disease.

PATHOLOGY

The various types of thyroid cancers and their incidence are presented in Table 1.

Papillary cancers, with or without follicular elements, are the most common histologic type of tumor. These indolent tumors rarely cause the patient's death. Significant numbers of clinically occult papillary cancers are found incidentally at autopsy. Although papillary hyperplasia is frequently present in an adenomatous goiter and in Graves' disease, a solitary papillary adenoma is relatively rare, and the majority of such lesions are low-grade papillary cancers, frequently with follicular elements. Cervical lymph node metastases are fairly common, but systemic metastases are unusual.

Pure follicular carcinomas are considerably less common. A well-differentiated follicular carcinoma can be extremely difficult to differentiate histologically from a follicular adenoma or a focal area of normal thyroid tissue. A diagnosis of carcinoma is dependent on the histologic demonstration of capsular invasion, vascular invasion, or invasion into the surrounding thyroid tissue. Lymphatic metastasis is uncommon, but systemic metastasis is more common in cases of papillary tumors.

Medullary carcinomas arise from parafollicular C cells in the neural crest. They are composed of solid clumps of cells infiltrated with varying amounts of an amorphous stromal material. An amyloid-like material, which probably represents aggregates of a prohormone of calcitonin, can be detected within this amorphous stroma.

Undifferentiated carcinomas can present with two histologic patterns. A small cell variant, which can resemble a diffuse lymphocytic infiltrate, is slightly more common than the giant cell variant. In contrast to the other thyroid cancers, undifferentiated carcinomas are extremely malignant tumors that frequently invade adjacent structures such as blood vessels, the trachea, and esophagus.

SOLITARY THYROID NODULE

Most patients referred for surgical consultation regarding the thyroid gland have a palpable solitary nodule in the gland and no other abnormality. Certain clinical features in patients with a solitary nodule are associated with a higher incidence of malignancy. Solitary nodules in patients with a history of radiation to the neck have a 50 percent incidence of malignancy. Other clinical findings that increase the chances of malignancy include the recognition of a thyroid mass not previously discernible, a hard or irregular mass when the remainder of the thyroid gland appears unremarkable, fixation of the mass to the strap muscles, and the presence of enlarged cervical lymph nodes. Although many patients with a goiter complain of dysphagia, it is unusual for a patient with a solitary nodule to have any difficulty in swallowing. Hoarseness secondary to invasion of the recurrent laryngeal nerve is unusual in a patient with a solitary nodule due to a malignant tumor. Pain, frequently present in subacute thyroiditis, is rarely associated with a primary malignant tumor of the thyroid gland.

The majority of patients in whom a solitary thyroid nodule is noted on physical examination have no clinical findings suggestive of hyperthyroidism. If such symptoms are present, appropriate thyroid function tests (T_3 and T_4) should be obtained. Diagnostic studies designed to further evaluate the thyroid nodule consist of a thyroid scintiscan and ultrasonography. The scintiscan is obtained for two reasons: (1) to determine whether the palpable lesion is a solitary nodule or simply the only clinical manifestation of a multinodular goiter, and (2) to determine whether the nodule functions or is a "cold nodule" that fails to concentrate the radioactive iodine. Malignant tumors can occur in a multinodular goiter, but the risks of malignancy are considerably less than those of a solitary nodule. If the nodule is solitary, but shows an increased concentration of radioactive material, that is, a hyperfunctioning nodule, there is little likelihood of malignancy. The chances of malignancy are approximately 20 percent in a solid solitary nodule that fails to concentrate radioactive iodine.

Ultrasonographic studies are obtained to determine whether the lesion is sold or cystic; a cystic mass does not exclude malignancy, but does significantly lessen the possibility.

If experienced personnel are available, a percutaneous needle biopsy of the solitary nodule should be performed. A definitive diagnosis can be established in as many a 60 to 70 percent of these biopsies, depending on the adequacy of the biopsy specimen and the experience of the cytologist or pathologist interpreting the material obtained. Percutaneous needle biopsy thus frequently renders unnecessary an exploration of the thyroid gland.

TABLE 1 Classification and Incidence of Thyroid Malignancies

Classification	Incidence
Papillary Carcinoma	70
Pure Follicular Carcinoma	14
Medullary Carcinoma	7
Anaplastic Carcinoma	8
Lymphoma	< 1
Squamous Cell Carcinoma	< 1
Metastatic Carcinoma	< 1

OPERATIVE APPROACH

If a diagnosis cannot be established preoperatively, the initial operative approach for all thyroid nodules is exposure and palpation of both lobes of the thyroid gland. Since it provides maximum exposure of the gland, I prefer a standard Kocher incision. If a solitary nodule is present in one lobe and the contralateral lobe is normal on inspection and palpation, I would proceed with a total lobectomy and excision of the isthmus. A frozen section is obtained, and further management depends on a histologic diagnosis. A benign lesion requires no further treatment. If the pathologist is unable to render a specific diagnosis because of subtle changes in the excised tumor, nothing further is done until a histologic diagnosis has been established. Once a diagnosis of malignancy is established by either frozen section or subsequent permanent section, further surgical management varies with the specific type of thyroid cancer encountered.

PAPILLARY CARCINOMA

As previously noted, papillary carcinoma is the most frequent malignant tumor of the thyroid. This indolent tumor is far more common in young females than in young males. The incidence in males increases with age, and the chances of systemic metastasis appear to increase with age in both males and females.

The treatment of papillary cancer is controversial, and there are no long-term prospective studies evaluating the different operative procedures. Treatment should vary according to the particular clinical situation encountered. If bilateral disease is palpable at operation, there is fairly universal agreement that a total thyroidectomy is indicated. In addition, the neck is explored between the hyoid bone superiorly, the jugular veins bilaterally, and the innominate vein inferiorly. Any suspicious nodes are excised, and specifically, the delphian, subisthmic, tracheoesophageal, and superior mediastinal nodes are removed for histologic study. Postoperatively, the patient receives thyroid replacement therapy (levothyroxine) and is seen at 4-month intervals. If subsequent cervical lymphadenopathy is detected, these nodes are resected; formal radical neck dissections are rarely necessary.

The major source of controversy is the patient under 40 years of age who has a solitary nodule of papillary carcinoma in one lobe of the gland and a normal contralateral lobe. Advocates of a total thyroidectomy cite the following reasons for removing the entire gland: (1) if a lesion is present in one lobe, full-organ histologic sections have demonstrated microscopic foci of tumor either in the parenchyma of the grossly normal contralateral lobe or in the adjacent lymphatics in 85 percent of the cases studied; (2) metastatic lesions cannot be treated with radioactive iodine if any normal thyroid gland is present; and (3) microscopic foci of papillary carcinoma left in place for many years will degenerate into a more malignant tumor. In spite of a high incidence of multicentric origin on histologic section, clinical evidence of subsequent growth of these microscopic tumors is unusual. The clinical recurrence rate in the contralateral lobe after a total lobectomy for papillary carcinoma confined to one lobe is only 5 to 10 percent even after 15 years of followup. Therefore, I do not believe that a routine total thyroidectomy, with the inherent risk of bilateral vocal cord palsy and/or permanent hypoparathyroidism, is indicated on the basis of a high histologic total thyroidectomy completed if recurrence is detected in the contralateral lobe. This approach does not decrease the patients chances of long-term survival.

The second indication for total thyroidectomy is the valid concept that systemic metastases will not take up radioactive iodine if any normal thyroid tissue is present. Although the concept is valid, the incidence of metastatic papillary carcinoma is so low (10%) that it does not seem reasonable to subject the great majority of patients to an operative procedure that will potentially benefit only a few.

The third indication for a total thyroidectomy probably is not valid. There is no convincing evidence that microscopic foci of papillary carcinoma, if left in place for many years, will degenerate into a more malignant tumor.

Although the majority of patients with papillary cancers present with a palpable nodule in the thyroid gland, approximately 10 percent of these patients come to clinical attention with a palpable cervical lymph node and no evidence of a palpable mass in the ipsilateral thyroid gland. The cervical lymph node should be excised through a transverse incision, which can be incorporated into a subsequent larger incision designed to expose the structures in the ipsilateral neck. If the cervical node contains metastatic papillary cancer, the thyroid gland is exposed. In the absence of a palpable nodule, a unilateral lobectomy is performed and the neck explored for other palpable nodes. All suspicious nodes are excised. It is rarely necessary to sacrifice the jugular vein, the sternocleidomastoid muscle, or the spinal accessory nerve.

Postoperatively, the majority of patients with papillary carcinoma of the thyroid gland have been placed on levothyroxine. Papillary carcinomas are responsive to TSH. Replacement therapy with levothyroxine is designed to suppress TSH secretion and therefore remove any hormonal stimulation of microscopic tumor in the remaining lobe, the cervical lymph nodes, or distant metastases in the lungs or liver. Although there is increasing evidence that TSH suppression has no effect on survival of patients with papillary carcinoma of the thyroid gland, patients with papillary carcinoma probably should be maintained on long term levothyroxine therapy until a controlled clinical trial has been completed.

FOLLICULAR CARCINOMA

Follicular carcinomas are encountered considerably less often than papillary tumors. They are usually seen in an older age group and are as common in males as in females. Lymphatic metastases are unusual; systemic metastases to lung and bone are considerably more common than in papillary lesions.

Once a specific diagnosis has been established, either by frozen section or by permanent histologic section, a total thyroidectomy is performed. This procedure is designed to remove the primary tumor as well as all normal thyroid tissue. The central neck is explored for possible lymphatic metastasis. Postoperatively the patients are treated initially with levothyroxine. Two months postoperatively the levothyroxine is discontinued and the patient treated with TSH to stimulate any residual thyroid tissue or functioning metastatic tumor. A whole body scan is performed following an intravenous dose of ^{131}I. If residual thyroid tissue or metastatic disease is demonstrated by the scintiscan, a therapeutic dose of ^{131}I is administered. The patients then return to a maintenance dose of levothyroxine.

MEDULLARY CARCINOMA

Medullary carcinomas that arise from the parafollicular C cells in the neural crest produce a remarkable number of substances with biochemical activity including ACTH, prostaglandins, serotonin, calcitonin, and histaminase. Two of these substances, calcitonin and histaminase, are specific biochemical markers for medullary carcinoma.

Medullary carcinomas can be divided into three general categories: (1) sporadic cases, approximately 50 percent of cases; (2) MEN II$_a$ (medullary thyroid cancer, pheochromocytoma, hyperplasia or adenoma of the parathyroid glands), approximately 40 percent of cases; (3) MEN type II$_b$ (medullary thyroid cancer, pheochromocytoma, hyperplasia or adenomas of the parathyroid glands, and mucosal neuromas involving predominantly the face, lips, and tongue), approximately 10 percent of cases.

The clinical management of the patient with suspected medullary carcinoma includes not only treatment of the thyroid malignant tumor, but also an evaluation of the adrenal glands for a possible pheochromocytoma and the parathyroid glands for a possible adenoma or hyperplasia. When MEN syndrome is discovered, extensive evaluation and testing of siblings is necessary as MEN has been shown to occur in approximately 50 percent of siblings in the involved families. In the absence of symptoms or physical findings suggestive of MEN syndrome, basal calcitonin levels are obtained on all family members. If elevated, a diagnosis is established and a thyroidectomy performed after ruling out the presence of a pheochromocytoma and/or a parathyroid adenoma. Those family members with normal basal calcitonin levels should be screened by provocative testing with intravenous pentagastrin or calcium infusions. If the test is positive, these patients are also candidates for thyroidectomy.

Prognosis varies with the patient's age and mode of presentation. Younger patients with no palpable disease and normal serum calcitonin levels, which are only elevated after stimulation with a calcitonin secretagogue, have an excellent chance of cure if the microscopic foci of tumor are removed. Similarly, patients with elevated basal calcitonin levels also have a good prognosis in comparison to older patients who present with clinical evidence of a thyroid nodule or cervical lymphadenopathy. Patients with disease confined to the thyroid gland, regardless of age or associated syndromes, have a 60 to 70 percent chance of disease-free survival at 5 years. Patients with cervical lymph node metastases, however, have only an approximate 10 percent chance of disease-free survival at 5 years.

Although the disease is more often multicentric in origin and bilateral in patients with MEN compared to sporadic cases, a total thyroidectomy is recommended in all patients with medullary carcinoma. The neck is carefully explored for enlarged lymph nodes, and any suspicious nodes are excised. A formal radical neck dissection is only indicated in the presence of extensive nodal metastasis and/or in the presence of extranodal spread of metastatic tumor. Systemic metastases are not responsive to radiation, and there is little chance of response to systemic chemotherapy.
little chance of response to systemic chemotherapy.

ANAPLASTIC CARCINOMAS

These tumors are unusual and occur predominantly in older patients. They grow extremely rapidly and present as a diffuse goiter extending from the hyoid bone inferiorly to the clavicle. These patients frequently present with tracheal obstruction secondary to either direct invasion by the tumor of the trachea or bilateral recurrent nerve palsies. Dysphagia secondary to esophageal obstruction is also common. Surgical excision is seldom feasible without sacrifice of vital structures in the neck. Occasionally, airway obstruction can be relieved by excision of enough tumor to permit a tracheostomy. Surgical management is otherwise limited to establishing a histologic diagnosis. Chemotherapy and radiation have little if any effect on these tumors, and in contrast to other thyroid tumors, these lesions are not hormonally dependent.

HYPERTHYROIDISM

BROWN M. DOBYNS, M.D., PH.D.

Although there are several types of thyrotoxicosis, the surgeon is primarily concerned with the treatment of Graves' disease (GD) (diffuse toxic goiter) and toxic adenomatous goiter. The surgeon must have a clear understanding of the basic physiology of the thyroid and, in particular, the pathophysiologic difference between Graves' disease and the hyperfunctioning adenoma(s). The surgical technique for the two diseases is decidedly different. A table is prepared to clarify the clinical distinction between the two diseases (Table 1). The details of management will be described in this chapter.

Graves' disease is a peculiar malady characterized by a triad: diffuse hypertrophy of the thyroid, symptoms of hypermetabolism, and exophthalmos, often associated with some degree of emotional instability. Early in the development of this disease, only one or two of the clinical features may have become evident when the patient is first seen. Thus, there may be only exophthalmos or only enlargement of the thyroid, but hypermetabolism may not yet have appeared. The laboratory data may initially be normal, but time will make the diagnosis clear. It is the hypermetabolism accompanied by a goiter that the surgeon should be prepared to treat.

Toxic adenomatous goiter, in which the adenoma(s) is to blame for the thyrotoxicosis, represents merely an autonomous production of thyroid hormone (TH). Clinically it results in a state of hyperthyroxinemia, but not exophthalmos. A mass (or masses) is present which, if single, is easily identified by radioiodine (^{131}I) concentration in the neoplasm with the rapid release of TH, resulting in a partial or complete physiologic shutdown of the remainder of the gland.

The term toxic nodular goiter is a confusing term. The term "nodule" is used by some observers merely to indicate the presence of a "lump" or "lumps" in the gland. If there is hyperthyroidism, the term "nodule" reflects a degree of uncertainty as to whether the lumps are true neoplasms (benign or malignant) or merely lobulations of the gland, and uncertainty whether the "lumps" are to blame for the thyrotoxicosis. The clinical question is whether discrete encapsulated neoplasms are functionally different from the remainder of the gland, and if so, whether they are responsible for the toxicity. It is the nonmalignant neoplasms with autonomous function that produce thyrotoxicosis.

There are several ways hyperthyroidism may be treated: surgery, radioiodine, or antithyroid drugs. The last-mentioned treatment has proved to be of only temporary usefulness. It blocks the synthesis of TH, but frequently, after the drug has been discontinued, the disease recurs. With a recurrence, the clinical features are often modified so that the smoldering persistence of the disease is not recognized. More will be said later of the usefulness of antithyroid drugs.

Radioiodine is taken up by the thyroid and stored in the same way as ordinary iodine. The radiation causes damage or death of thyroid cells that have taken up the isotope. The size of the dose is based on the ^{131}I uptake of a test dose and its retention, the size of the gland, and

TABLE 1 The Clinical Distinction Between Graves' Disease and Toxic Adenomatous Goiter

	Graves' Disease	*Hyperfunctioning Adenoma*
Age group	Younger	10–15 years older
Onset of symptoms	Usually datable	Insidious onset; av. 17 years
General behavior	Restless; useless purposeful movements	Quiet; underestimate the hypermetabolism
Exophthalmos and eye signs	Present in 40% to 80% of cases	Not present
Symptomatic response to iodine	Prompt improvement if no previous iodine	No improvement; may be made worse
Physical features of gland	Diffuse involvement	Lumps to blame - atrophy of extranodular tissue
Thyroid storm	May occur	Does not occur
Iodine therapy, change in gland	Bruit ↓ firmness ↑	No effect
Usual blood pressure pattern	Systolic ↑ diastolic ↓	Systolic ↑ diastolic ↑
Recurrence after surgery	5%	0.1%

the firmness of the gland. The firmness usually represents the degree of infiltration by lymphocytes, interspersed throughout the gland of Graves' disease. Ultimately, most patients become hypothyroid and need medical attention for life.

GENERAL CONSIDERATIONS

Thyroidectomy remains an important method of treating hyperthyroidism when compared to other treatments. When the hyperfunction is diffuse throughout the gland, surgical reduction in the volume of functioning tissue is the objective, leaving a small but appropriate amount of tissue. When the cause of hyperthyroidism is hyperfunctioning adenomatous tissue, thyroidectomy is the treatment of choice for a variety of reasons. Excision of the adenomas is definitive and permanent. Radioiodine in this disease is not uniformly effective. The lesions have nonuniform uptake because spontaneous spotty necrosis is usually found within such lesions. The dose of ^{131}I required is far larger and its effect less predictable. Multiple doses at several-month intervals are often required, prolonging recovery from the disease. The lesions become mummified and usually remain palpable. They are then indistinguishable from other types of neoplasms unless removed. In contrast, the surgical removal is simple. The brief hospitalization is far less costly than multiple ^{131}I treatments. The return to a euthyroid state is immediate, which is much preferred for the cardiac problems that characteristically accompany this chronic disease.

One of the greatest problems in the surgical treatment of hyperthyroidism in recent years has been the availability of surgeons with experience in thyroid surgery and with a knowledge of the pathophysiology of the several forms of hyperthyroidism. The surgical procedures are highly specific for the various situations encountered. Radioiodine became the preferred form of therapy because some surgeons were performing thyroidectomy without this educational preparation. Parathyroid and recurrent laryngeal nerve complications were not only encountered but, in a small percentage of cases, considered by some surgeons to be unavoidable. These particular complications did not occur after ^{131}I therapy. Therefore, opportunities for surgeons to obtain training and experience diminished. However, for those surgeons connected with "thyroid centers," parathyroid and nerve injuries have become very rare and mortality rates have dropped to nearly zero. This complication rate is less than that for cases in which other definitive treatment is prolonged or delayed.

There are clear indications for either thyroidectomy or radioiodine in hyperthyroidism, as shown in Table 2. The advantages and disadvantages are shown in Table 3.

PREPARATION FOR SURGERY

In Graves' disease, hyperthyroidism must be brought under control before surgery is undertaken. The disease is controllable with an antithyroid drug regardless of the severity of the disease, if the patient takes the drug faithfully in divided doses and if the dose is large enough to block incorporation of iodine into the organically bound form in the gland. Propylthiouracil (PTU) is usually the drug of choice. If the patient has had access to large doses of iodine preceding the initiation of PTU, 2 or 3 weeks of effective block may be required before improvement is evident (gland becomes depleted of previously stored TH). Some individuals require larger doses of PTU than others; 400 mg PTU (100 mg every 6 hours) is effective in about 50 percent of patients with Graves' disease, but doses must be taken regularly or iodine in the diet enters the gland and becomes TH, and time is lost. Usually the disease comes under control in 4 to 6 weeks. If there is any question why progressive improvement is not occurring, a small trace dose of ^{131}I will answer the question. If the uptake into the gland is still elevated, either the patient is missing prescribed doses or the dose is not large enough to be effective. In either case, the problem may be promptly clarified. If the uptake in the thyroid remains as high as before the drug therapy was begun, a small dose of potassium perchlorate (or any competitive ion), given 2 or 3 hours following the tracer, will flush the iodide out of the "iodide trap" in the thyroid. A sharp drop in the thyroid uptake curve shows that the tracer is not getting into the organically bound form. Therefore the patient may be expected to soon improve on the dose

TABLE 2 Choice of Therapy in Hyperthyroidism

Radioiodine	Surgery
Older individuals without nodules (age limits variable)	Any individual with discrete mass(es)
	Children and young adults
Individual with reduced life expectancy	Pregnant women (2nd trimester)
	Irresponsible or unintelligent individuals
	Individuals with proven incompetency

TABLE 3 Radioiodine Versus Surgery for Hyperthyroidism

Treatment	Advantages	Disadvantages
Radioiodine	No discomfort No hospitalization Avoid surgical complications Never a recurrence (when treatment is adequate) Minimal effort by physician (except yearly follow-up)	Slow control of disease Slow cell death, no cellular regeneration No pathologic diagnosis available (appropriate if nodules present) Difficulty of sustained follow-up Remote possibility of neoplasms
Thyroidectomy	Majority remain euthyroid (rarely need supplement) Minimal subsequent attention Prompt correction of problem Pathologic diagnosis of any masses	Discomfort of surgery Technical errors, complications Scar

of drug given; otherwise, the amount of antithyroid drug must be increased, sometimes as high as 1,200 mg daily.

When the time for surgery arrives, the decision to proceed is based on clinical judgment. It is hoped that the surgeon may have an opportunity to see the state of the disease before preoperative therapy is begun. He may then be in a better position to judge improvement and decide on the time for thyroidectomy. The thyroxine level in the blood is not a prerequisite to making this decision. All too often serious delays are caused by waiting for this blood level to reach what might be considered normal. Beta blockers are useful in the preoperative preparation of patients with severe thyrotoxicosis because they alleviate many of the symptoms, but it is important to wean the patient off the beta blockers as soon as possible so that the control of the disease can be properly appraised without the masking effect of the blocks.

The criteria upon which judgment is based are several. Disappearance of tremor of outstretched hands, muscle weakness (manifest in the quadriceps), restlessness, and general emotional lability (when the coming operation is discussed) are key considerations. Some of the weight lost should be regained. A decline in pulse rate to 80 to 90 is an excellent basis for judging operability. If there is uncertainty about lability, slight exercise (such as climbing stairs) reveals the cardiac lability according to how high the pulse rate rises and how promptly it returns to the pre-exercise level.

Plans should be made a week or so in advance of the probable date of surgery so that there is no delay when a euthyroid state is approaching. It is most important not to operate on an overtreated patient. Subtle sluggishness often leads to postoperative respiratory problems. A modicum of hyperthyroidism adds no risk and is preferred to overtreatment. With light anesthesia, the patient should awaken promptly as surgery is completed and should be upright in bed within an hour or so and willing to clear mucus freely. Finally, he or she should be taking nourishment within 3 or 4 hours of surgery. This will not occur if the patient is overtreated and particularly if much sedation is used. Although there may be some concern about operating when patients are slightly toxic, true thyroid storm, as it was once known, does not occur in patients treated several weeks with antithyroid drugs even though still mildly toxic. The benefits of an active vigorous patient far outweigh any other risks.

Before the antithyroid drugs came into use, a few drops of saturated solution of potassium iodide (SSKI) a day modified the severity of the disease by partially interfering with the release of TH, so that the risk of insult from surgery was considerably reduced. Many mild cases of hyperthyroidism of the Graves' type were safely treated by thyroidectomy. It has been my policy in cases of mild hyperthyroidism to utilize the effects of SSKI. It has been shown that iodide acts to retard the release of TH even though it is not taken up by the gland, as when blocked by PTU. Thus in mild cases, by giving PTU for several days until the patient is faithfully taking the drug (to establish an effective block to the uptake), SSKI may be introduced additionally. If in a few days the pulse slows

to the 80 to 90 range, and the restlessness and tremor disappear, one may proceed safely with bilateral subtotal thyroidectomy. However, if the mildness of the disease has been misjudged or the modifying effect of SSKI does not take place, no time has been lost. The uptake of iodine has been blocked by PTU (SSKI may or may not be continued) and the PTU is continued until the stored TH in the gland has been depleted and the patient is approaching a euthyroid state.

In recent years there has been less attention directed toward the possibility of untoward reaction to antithyroid drugs. I believe that a baseline white blood count (WBC) is always indicated and that it should be rechecked at intervals of 10 days to 2 weeks; in addition the patient should be warned to report any unexplained high fever, sore throat, or skin rash. Most often the latter signs are not indicative of a drug reaction, but if they are, it is important to know it. The WBC often declines somewhat below the original level, but this decline need not be alarming unless is falls below 3,000. Drug therapy may be continued in spite of some of these signs, but under closer supervision.

The preoperative preparation of the patient with toxic adenomatous goiter (in which the adenomas are to blame for the hyperthyroidism) requires a somewhat different perspective. Most of these patients seek medical attention because of cardiac symptoms, not the signs and symptoms of hyperthyroidism. Usually the patient was aware of the mass for several years. Arrhythmia is the common finding, created by longstanding thyrotoxicosis (see Table 1). The hypermetabolism may be severe, but eye signs are not present, and restlessness and tremor are not commensurate with the hypermetabolism. This is a disease in which true thyroid storm is not encountered unless the diagnosis is incorrect and the problem is Graves' disease with incidental adenomas, mistakenly thought to be the cause of thyrotoxicosis.

Almost all of these patients are in the older age group and so cardiac consultation is important. The adenomatous tissue takes up iodine, but does not store it; rather, it releases the iodine into the circulation rather promptly. We know that only about 25 percent of these patients with hyperfunctioning adenomas (hyperfunctioning when compared to the paranodular tissue) have clinically obvious symptoms of the thyrotoxicosis. We also know that about 95 percent of hyperfunctioning adenomas undergo periodic spontaneous necrosis and subsequent regrowth within the capsule of the neoplasm. This accounts for waxing and waning of symptoms and variations in serum thyroxine levels. Furthermore, the results of ^{131}I uptake may be highly variable. The uptake must be considered in a different frame of reference than that of Graves' disease, i.e., uptakes may be judged to be normal on the basis of what is considered elevated in Graves' disease.

Unless hyperthyroidism is severe with debilitation or unless cardiac problems are a dominant part of the clinical picture, preoperative antithyroid drugs may not be needed or may be given only for a short period. Above all, it is important not to give iodine to these patients, especially if they come from an iodine deficient area or have been on salt restriction. Iodine often makes the condition worse for it provides raw material for making more thyroxine.

PATHOPHYSIOLOGIC PRINCIPLES OF THYROID SURGERY

The surgical procedure for Graves' disease is quite different from the procedure for toxic adenomatous goiter, when the adenomas are to blame for the hyperthyroidism. If there are any palpable masses, it is our policy to give a trace dose of ^{131}I the day before any thyroid operation. This serves a variety of uses during the surgical procedure. It may serve as a basis for interpreting histologic findings in the thyroid tissue being removed. In one case the radioiodine may be concentrated in the masses. In another case it may be primarily in the extranodular tissue. If the adenoma(s) is to blame for the hyperthyroidism, it should be removed, and the nonfunctioning extranodular tissue should be meticulously preserved. A generous bilateral subtotal procedure is not appropriate; otherwise, permanent hypothyroidism will result. If the problem is Graves' disease and the adenomas are incidental, removal of just the adenomas results in persistence of hyperthyroidism. Scanning or imaging clearly demonstrates the single autonomously functioning adenoma that produces thyrotoxicosis. It is well recognized that results of such diagnostic procedures may be easily misinterpreted in the case of multiple masses. It may be that the multiple masses are superimposed in such a way that the interpretation of just where the radioiodine is located may be difficult.

When hyperfunctioning adenomas produce hyperthyroidism, there should be some degree of suppression of the extranodular tissue, but this atrophy is not always grossly obvious at surgery. The answer to these uncertainties during surgery may be simply obtained by placing a few milligrams of each tissue in separate test tubes and measuring the radioactivity in each tube before the definitive surgery is performed. This requires far less time and is much more definitive than interpreting microscopic descriptive anatomy in a frozen section. The use of such an assay makes the diagnosis perfectly clear. In the case of the hyperfunctioning adenomas, they are removed and the paranodular tissue is meticulously preserved. This ensures that the atrophic tissue can subsequently recover its function, and the patient may not need thyroid supplement for the rest of his or her life. If the hyperfunction is in the paranodular tissue, a generous bilateral subtotal thyroidectomy is indicated, including the removal of the incidental adenomas

If the patient has Graves' disease and there are incidental masses lying buried in such a gland, the uptake is scattered through the entire gland. Scanning may be useless or misleading especially if there are multiple masses. The highly functioning paranodular tissue lying in front and behind the mass obscures the fact that that mass may not be taking up much [131]I. Carcinoma may arise in about 2 percent of patients with Graves' disease. Negligible uptake of ^{131}I in an incidental tumor mass can be easily detected by using the assay method already described. Our experience has shown that if a small sample of such a cold neoplasm proves to have less than 0.01 of the ^{131}I in an equal weight of the extranodular tissue, the neoplasm is probably malignant. The finding gives a clue to both the surgeon and the pathologist that special consideration of such a tumor is indicated.

SURGICAL TECHNIQUE

Bilateral subtotal thyroidectomy is a satisfactory method for treating Graves' disease. If a meticulously bloodless field is maintained, the incidence of hypothyroidism is low, the incidence of recurrence is extremely low, and permanent injury to the parathyroids or recurrent laryngeal nerves seldom occurs.

The placement of the thyroid incision is critical to obtaining complete exposure of the thyroid. The thyroid isthmus always bears the same relationship to the larynx, namely, just beneath the cricoid cartilage, which is easily palpable. In some individuals, the larynx lies high in the neck; in those who are heavy-set or older, the larynx has descended until it is partly hidden behind the upper margin of the sternum. Thus, precise identification of the position of the larynx and specifically the cricoid cartilage is a prerequisite to placement of the incision, for it should lie halfway between the superior and inferior poles. This incision should fall in or parallel to a natural skin fold. The incision is made through the platysma muscle to the enveloping fascia. At this level an upper skin flap is raised to the "V" of the thyroid cartilage and the lower skin flap down to the suprasternal notch. The vertical incision in the enveloping fascia permits wide separation of the strap muscles from their origin to their insertion. Thus, even in large goiters, wide exposure is readily available without cutting strap muscle.

In any thyroidectomy, the presence and size of the pyramidal lobe is always noted. Symmetrical enlargement is a manifestation of some form of diffuse hypertrophy, either because the thyroid is biologically inefficient and enlarging to compensate for low hormone production or because it is stimulated to enlarge as a result of Graves' disease. When any thyroid tissue is to be removed, it is imperative that the pyramidal lobe be excised up to the hyoid bone. If allowed to remain, the compensating subsequent hypertrophy may become conspicuous. Furthermore, the thyroglossal duct remnant that is often present, but not obvious until the reaction from surgery causes it to fill with fluid, becomes a postoperative thyroglossal duct cyst or a postoperative draining sinus. Regardless of the procedure contemplated, both lobes of the thyroid should always be completely uncovered because there may be minute masses in one or both lobes. In dealing with thyrotoxicosis, the first objective is to determine whether the thyrotoxicosis is attributable to masses or to the extranodular tissue, as already described.

I prefer to divide the isthmus when bilateral subtotal thyroidectomy is anticipated. The removal of the pyramidal lobe has exposed the posterior plane between the isthmus and trachea. By reflecting the two stumps of the isthmus laterally and freeing the isthmus and anterior part of the respective lobes from the trachea, the lobe may be drawn anteriorly and across the trachea so that the posterior surface of the lobe is exposed.

The objective in Graves' disease is to leave a small single functioning remnant of thyroid tissue on each side of the trachea. There should be adequate tissue removal to control the hyperthyroidism, but sufficient tissue allowed to remain to maintain the patient in a euthyroid state. The remnants of tissue of equal size should lie along each side of the trachea. Ligation of the superior pole vessels should be well above thyroid tissue so that no thyroid tissue remains in that area. Similarly, no tissue should be left at the inferior pole.

Several anatomic features must be clearly identified by any surgeon who performs thyroidectomies. Because the right recurrent laryngeal nerve comes from behind the junction of the innominate and the common carotid artery, it passes in an oblique or transverse direction in the neck and only reaches the tracheoesophageal groove as it approaches the point where it enters the larynx. On the left, the recurrent laryngeal nerve comes from well down in the thorax and therefore lies parallel to the tracheoesophageal groove. I have found it wise to find the nerve first by blunt dissection some distance from the thyroid, because as one proceeds toward the lobe, there are many small vessels that break and bleed easily. When the tissue is spread and windows are made in the connective tissue, the nerve is easily found without bleeding and traced toward its point of entrance into the larynx.

The parathyroids are found by the application of embryologic principles and anatomic relationships. The position of the superior parathyroid is quite consistent while the inferior is variable. The superior is always found near the point where the recurrent nerve enters the larynx. Having already uncovered and clearly identified the cricoid cartilage anteriorly, one has a precise landmark for the point of entrance of the nerve on the lateral aspect of the larynx just above the superior edge of the cricoid. Thus dissection cephalad to this point does not risk injury to the nerve. The superior parathyroid takes its blood supply from an anastomotic vessel between the posterior branch of the superior and the highest branch of the inferior thyroid arteries (Fig. 1). Its vascular attachment to this anastomotic vessel is less than 1 cm from the point of entrance of the nerve. It is quite true that the inferior parathyroid may be found over a wide area in the neck, but it takes its blood supply from the inferior branch of the inferior thyroid artery which accounts for its consistent location.

Contrary to some opinion, the inferior thyroid artery descends as it comes out from under the common carotid and proceeds downward and medially to approximately the midportion of the thyroid lobe, where it divides into an upper and lower branch. The inferior parathyroid derives its blood supply from that lower descending branch, which continues along the posterior surface of the lobe and supplies the superior pole of the thymus, which in most cases lies immediately posterior to the

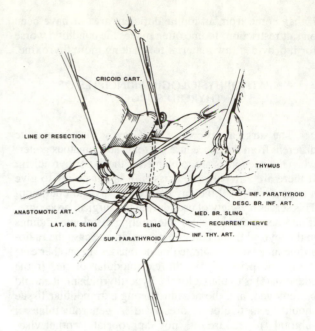

Figure 1 Right lateral view of the thyroid. Shown here is the intimate anatomy at the posterior surface of the thyroid lobe. A knowledge of the relationships in this area is necessary in order to consistently avoid injury to the recurrent laryngeal nerve and parathyroids in subtotal or complete total thyroidectomy. The sling artery that binds the recurrent laryngeal nerve to the posterior surface of the lobe is illustrated. This configuration is a consistent finding on both sides of neck and from individual to individual, regardless of the pathologic distortion of the gland. The principles in the pattern of the blood supply to the parathyroids and the determination of their position is also shown (see text).

inferior pole of the thyroid. If this artery is traced, it is found that the inferior parathyroid derives its blood supply from it, even though that parathyroid is often found down in the thymus. For this reason, anyone performing thyroid surgery must be acquainted with these relationships and, in doing bilateral subtotal thyroidectomy, must see and identify the superior pole of the thymus; otherwise parathyroid injury may occur in a considerable number of cases.

I have called attention to the sling artery, which binds the recurrent nerve tightly to the posterior surface of the thyroid. It lies not far caudad to the point where the nerve enters the larynx and is the usual site at which nerve injury occurs. The ascending branch of the inferior thyroid artery, as it passes upward to join the posterior branch of the superior artery, gives off a medial and a lateral branch, as illustrated in Figure 1. The medial and lateral branches together form a sling through which the nerve passes. The medial branch passes up between the lobe and the trachea and consistently lies in the groove between the lower edge of the cricoid cartilage and the first tracheal ring beneath the upper edge of the isthmus. The lateral branch of the sling artery comes around the lateral margin of the thyroid lobe and breaks up into multiple branches over the lateral surface of the gland. Special attention to this arterial sling avoids injury to the nerve in bilateral subtotal thyroidectomy and permits complete removal of the lobe in total thyroidectomy. When the lateral branch of that sling is carefully clamped and divided, the lobe may be raised and the sling drops down, allowing the nerve to fall away from the lobe (see Figure 1). This does not interfere with the blood supply to the superior parathyroid. In Graves' disease, the remnant of thyroid tissue that is to be preserved lies conveniently over this area. The medial branch of the sling artery is encountered as the isthmus is reflected away from the trachea. Unless it is precisely clamped and tied, bleeding may prompt the surgeon to dissect between the trachea and the lobe to control such bleeding and be inadvertently led to the nerve lying immediately below. This sling formation is uniformly present on both sides of the neck and in approximately the same configuration in all patients. Needless to say, attention to the lateral and medial branches of the sling are vital in controlling the blood supply and in avoiding injury to the nerve. Details of the sling are illustrated in Figure 1. It should be strongly emphasized that ligation of the inferior thyroid artery lateral to the thyroid to control bleeding, as recommended by some, devascularizes not only the remnant of thyroid tissue (a cause of postoperative hypothyroidism), but also both parathyroids that had been so carefully preserved.

In the case of Graves' disease, there is always the question of how much tissue should be allowed to remain. I believe that this is most important in avoiding hypothyroidism. It is a foregone conclusion from the above description that the surgeon will precisely identify the posterior margin of the lobe so that he knows exactly how much tissue is allowed to remain. There are certain general rules that determine the size of the remnants. The regenerative power of the thyroid in young individuals is much greater than it is in adults. Therefore, the remnant in children and adolescents is considerably less than that left in adults. Firmness and pebbly quality of the gland is not only a manifestation of how long the disease has been in progress, but how much lymphocytic thyroiditis has developed in Graves' disease. Thyroiditis is readily recognized by the gross appearance of the gland at surgery. The more gray and crumbly the gland appears, the more extensive will be the thyroiditis. The more extensive the thyroiditis, the greater the probability of future hypothyroidism. Consequently, a smaller remnant is left in the case of a red fleshy gland and a larger one left when considerable thyroiditis has developed. It is scarcely proper to refer to grams of tissue remaining because different operators have a different impression of how much tissue constitutes a gram, but it might be said that in an average case of Graves' disease without thyroiditis and with the blood supply preserved, a remnant of tissue no greater than three-quarters of a centimeter in thickness and no more than 1½ cm in length is left in the tracheoesophageal groove on each side. This is modified by the character of the gland, the age of the patient, and the initial size of the gland. It has been said by some that the resection of the lobe should be wedge-shaped in cross-section. I have found that the remnant of tissue that is to be left is so small that wedging out the center of the lobe to leave a sheet of capsule results in a remnant that is too large and that the preservation of its blood supply is uncertain.

If these general rules regarding the residual remnant are followed, I find from personal experience that hypothyroidism has developed in 12 percent at one year, increasing to 15 percent at the end of 8 years, and that the recurrence rate is about 2 percent, almost all of these recurrences being in young adults and children.

THYROIDITIS

PAUL LoGERFO, M.D.

Thyroiditis occurs in various forms, as identified by laboratory data, clinical presentation, pathologic findings, and prognosis. The major forms are acute thyroiditis, subacute thyroiditis (Quervain's disease), chronic lymphocytic thyroiditis (Hashimoto's thyroiditis), and Riedel's disease. It is not always possible to clearly distinguish some of these forms since some overlap does occur among the various types.

ACUTE THYROIDITIS

This is a relatively rare but often serious illness, and was particularly so before the era of antibiotics. The peak age incidence in the old literature was between 20 and 40 years; the most recent literature indicates that this occurs at the two extremes of age: childhood and old age. The female:male ratio is approximately 5:3. The disease is most often associated with an infection in the neck and occasionally occurs with trauma. The symptoms are usually of sudden onset, the most common symptoms being neck pain, fever, and tachycardia. The pain often radiates to the angle of the mandible or occiput, and the head is held in a flexed position. A rare but serious sign is blood-tinged sputum, which indicates that the infection has extended to the trachea. A typical list of symptoms with their relative frequency is presented in Table 1.

On physical examination the tenderness is usually exquisite and most impressive in one lobe, although occasionally the entire gland is involved. The area involved is usually warm and red. Partial eyelid ptosis from sympathetic nerve involvement occasionally is noted.

TABLE 1 Signs of Acute Thyroiditis

Sign	% Patients Showing Sign
Fever	90
Tachycardia	90
Neck tenderness	95
Neck swelling	50
Erythema	45
Hoarseness	20
Partial ptosis	10
Corneal anesthesia	10
Thyrotoxicosis	Rare
Dysphagia	2–9

Typical laboratory findings are increased white blood cell count, elevated sedimentation rate, normal thyroid function tests, and normal to low ^{131}I uptake. Blood cultures are usually positive, and aspirations of thyroid for culture may be helpful if no clear-cut organism can be identified.

The most common bacterial organisms isolated are *Streptococcus, Staphylococcus*, and *Pneumococcus*. Fungal, parasitic, viral, and tuberculous infections are rare.

The histopathology of acute thyroiditis is the pathology of suppuration. Other conditions such as subacute thyroiditis, thyroglossal duct cyst, and hemorrhage into an adenoma may be confused with acute thyroiditis. In these situations, aspiration biopsy might help to establish a diagnosis.

The current mainstay of treatment centers around identifying an organism and administering the appropriate antibiotic. Abscesses that develop are best treated by some sort of drainage, but lobectomy occasionally becomes necessary. Drainage may be done percutaneously, with large angiocatheters (No. 14 or No. 16) left in place for a 5- to 10-day period. Prognosis with appropriate treatment is excellent, and the problem resolves in 3 to 4 weeks. In the pre-antibiotic era the mortality rate was 25 percent. Lesions that recur are probably cysts that communicate directly with the pyriform sinus or the trachea. These require excision.

SUBACUTE THYROIDITIS

Subacute thyroiditis (de Quervain's disease) is a non-suppurative inflammation of the thyroid gland. It is a self-limited disease which is characterized by neck pain, fever, and other mild systemic symptoms associated with thyroid dysfunctions for several weeks to months followed by complete recovery in most cases.

This disease is much more common than acute thyroiditis and represents 0.5 to 2 percent of all cases of thyroid disease. It is one-fifth to one-tenth as common as Hashimoto's thyroiditis and 10 to 50 times more frequent than Riedel's struma. There is a female predominance (ratio 2:1 to 6:1), which is most common in the third to sixth decade of life.

The cause of this disease remains unknown. Many theories have been proposed over the years, including a viral causation, a genetic predisposition, and auto-immunity. There is some support for each of these theories, but no single theory fits all the clinical and laboratory findings.

The clinical symptoms and laboratory data associated with subacute thyroiditis depend on the stage of the disease. The disease is generally divided into four stages. The first stage usually lasts several months and is characterized by a painful swollen thyroid, mild symptoms, and chemical hyperthyroidism. This hyperthyroidism is secondary to the release of thyroid hormone associated with damage to the thyroid follicles seen histologically. Thyroid scan at this time shows a patchy decreased uptake of radioactive iodine. In the second phase, which lasts 4 to 6 weeks, the gland is firm and large. The primary histologic feature is granulomatous inflammation associated with follicle disruption and depletion of colloid. Radioactive iodine uptake is still depressed, but the patient is clinically and chemically euthyroid. The third phase occurs at 2 to 4 months and is associated with decreased thyroid hormone levels; TSH levels at this time are usually elevated, but thyroid radioactive iodine uptake remains low. Histologically, reparative changes are noted along with granulomatous inflammation. The follicles are beginning to recover. In the fourth phase, thyroid function returns to normal and the gland is reduced to normal size. Thyroid radioactive iodine uptake may be elevated during this recovery phase. The erythrocyte sedimentation rate is usually elevated throughout the first three phases (40 to 70 mm per hour). Anemia with a hemocrit in the range of 32 to 38 percent has been shown to occur in 30 to 40 percent of the cases, but leukocytosis is uncommon. Anti-thyroglobulin and automicrosomal thyroid antibodies are low or absent.

On palpation of the thyroid, there is usually some asymmetry between the lobes, and occasionally, there are firm-to-hard focal areas that suggest thyroid cancer. If these patients are operated on, the findings can be worrisome and often confused with thyroid carcinoma. The best way to make a diagnosis is with a coarse-needle biopsy. Because the firmness of the gland makes it difficult to puncture, biopsy is associated with much more pain than with noninflammatory conditions. Cytology can sometimas be diagnostic (i.e., giant cell), but occasionally the severe inflammatory changes seen can be confused with cancer.

Therapy is directed at treatment of the patient's symptoms, the most bothersome being pain. Mild pain may be treated with anti-inflammatory agents (e.g., aspirin, Indocin). In cases in which the pain is severe, steroids provide rapid relief of symptoms, and the gland may become nontender in 24 to 48 hours. Treatment of the mild hyperthyroidism seen in the first phase of the disease is usually unnecessary, but a short course of Inderal may be helpful in the patient with palpitations. The hypothyroid phase may benefit from some thyroid replacement, but in general there is little support for this therapy. Surgery is unnecessary except to rule out cancer when the diagnosis is in question.

CHRONIC LYMPHOID THYROIDITIS

Chronic lymphoid thyroiditis (Hashimoto's thyroiditis) is an autoimmune disease that is more frequent in women than in men (10:1). The peak incidence is among women 30 to 50 years old, although it has been seen at all ages. Graves' disease and Hashimoto's disease often coexist in the same family and even in the same individual. The reported incidence of the disease has been increasing over the years, and annual estimated incidence is 69 cases per 100,000 people.

There is a strong association between Hashimoto's disease and the HLA-DRW3 locus. Other HLA linkages have been described, but the DRW3 locus is at least twice that seen in the normal population. Most evidence strongly suggests that the immune system is the underlying cause of the disease. Essentially all patients have circulating antibodies against the thyroid at some time in the course of their disease. These antibodies may be directed at thyroglobulin or other thyroid antigens, especially microsomes. The interaction of these antibodies with the TSH receptor produces Graves' disease if the receptor is "turned on" rather than blocked by these antibodies. The antibodies themselves do not produce the disease unless cell-mediated mechanisms of the immune system are activated. The exact method of this interaction is unclear.

Patients with chronic lymphoid thyroiditis generally present with firm, painless thyroid glands weighing 40 to 60 grams (normal 15 to 20 g). The goiter is usually diffuse, but nodularity may be present. In some patients, this nodularity changes considerably from month to month and makes follow-up difficult. Large glands may produce pressure symptoms in the neck and superior vena caval syndrome can be seen, particularly if the major share of the gland is substernal. Exophthalmos is rare, but does occur in the absence of Graves' disease.

Thyroid function tests are variable, depending on the stage of the disease. Overt hypothyroidism increases with the duration of the disease. Hyperthyroidism may be seen early in the disease process (3% to 5%) and is referred to as hashitoxicosis. During this period, ^{131}I scans usually show patchy uptake, which is low. Fluorescent scanning indicates a low iodine pool, and iodine perchlorate discharge is frequently abnormal. Thyroid antibodies (thyroglobulin and microsomal) are usually present, depending on assay technique.

The diagnosis is best made by coarse-needle biopsy since cytology is often misleading, especially if extensive Hürthle cell hyperplasia is present. Laboratory tests may be helpful, but biopsy is still the best diagnostic test. Nodules that grow or are dominant should be examined by biopsy to rule out lymphoma. Glands undergoing extensive change are examined at 6-month intervals, stable glands yearly. Surgical intervention is rarely necessary unless respiratory compromise or dysphagia develops, in which case the treatment is isthmectomy. Occasionally, an enlarged gland presents a cosmetic problem and must be treated surgically if thyroid replacement does not shrink it to a satisfactory size.

Hashimoto's disease usually progresses to hypothyroidism, but occasionally remissions are seen in young women with a mild form of the disease. Treatment generally requires thyroid replacement in the final stages of the disease. This replacement is associated with a decrease in the size of the gland in 75 percent of patients. Since Hashimoto's disease may coexist with a variety of autoimmune disorders (e.g., rheumatoid diseases, pernicious anemia, adrenal insufficiency, myasthenia, idiopathic thrombocytopenic purpura), these may be the main determinants of the patient's clinical course. The most serious complication of the disease itself is the development of lymphoma or myeloproliferative disease. The risk of lymphoma is 67 times as high as would be expected in the normal population.

RIEDEL'S STRUMA

Riedel's struma is a rare entity, and the incidence in thyroidectomy specimens ranges from 0.03 to 0.14 percent. This is really a fibromatosis that involves the thyroid and surrounding structures. The lymphocytic infiltrate and mild vasculitis that are usually present help distinguish this condition from fibrosarcoma, but this distinction is difficult at best. According to the literature, this disease is generally confused with Hashimoto's disease and/or subacute thyroiditis (Table 2).

Riedel's struma is usually seen in the fourth to fifth

TABLE 2 Clinical Features of Forms of Thyroiditis

	Riedel's Disease	Subacute Thyroiditis	Hashimoto's Thyroiditis
Age incidence	30–70 yr (most 50 yr or over)	Any age (most 30–50 yr)	Any age (most 20–50 yr)
Sex incidence (F/M)	2–4/1	~4/1	4–10/1
Symptoms	Pressure, goiter	Pain, tenderness, goiter	± Goiter, may be hyper-eu-, or hypothyroid
Thyroid involvement	Unilateral 30%	Bilateral (one side may be more affected)	Focal or diffuse
Thyroid antibodies	None or very low	±	+
Follow-up	Hypothyroidism rare; may recur following treatment, stabilize or regress	Thyroid function reverts to normal in almost all cases	Usually progresses to hypothyroidism

decade of life, the male:female ratio being 2:1 to 4:1. The usual presenting sign is goiter, and the patient may give a history of slow or rapid growth. The lesion is usually painless, but produces pressure symptoms in the neck. The most common symptom is dyspnea, which mayh progress to a stridor that is out of proportion to the size of the gland. Vocal cord paralysis is rare; mild dysphagia may be present.

On physical examination, the thyroid is stony hard and fixed to surrounding tissues. In about one-third of the cases, the disease is unilateral. Local lymphadenopathy may be present and may suggest the clinical diagnosis of thyroid cancer (anaplastic). Systemic signs are usually absent unless the disease process is representative of a fibromatosis process elsewhere in body (e.g., mediastinum, biliary tree, orbit, or retroperitoneum). The patient is almost always clinically and chemically euthyroid except in cases of massive replacement of the gland. Hypoparathyroidism may be present. The main problem confronting the surgeon is to rule out carcinoma and to decompress the trachea in patients with dyspnea. Extensive experience with needle biopsy is not available, and I have not been able to clearly make the diagnosis using this technique. Operation may be difficult because of the extensive adherence to surrounding structures with loss of tissue planes. Tracheal decompression is not easy when disease is extensive and recurrence rates are 15 to 16 percent. The mortality rate is 6 to 10 percent, and most deaths are secondary to asphyxia due to tracheal compression. Thyroid replacement is necessary if hypothyroidism is present. Steroids may be helpful in decreasing recurrences, but there is little solid evidence for this.

HYPERPARATHYROIDISM

ORLO H. CLARK, M.D.

Primary hyperparathyroidism is a common disorder, affecting approximately one in 700 people. It occurs most commonly in women, especially those over age 45, and is the most common cause of hypercalcemia in unselected patients. The etiology of primary hyperparathyroidism is unknown. Most cases are sporadic and associated with a benign solitary parathyroid adenoma (approximately 85%). Other cases may be caused by primary hyperplasia (10%), multiple adenomas (4%), or parathyroid carcinoma (1%). Hyperparathyroidism may also be familial and associated with multiple endocrine neoplasia (MEN) type I and type II. Patients with MEN are more likely to have hyperplasia or multiple adenomas and are also prone to both recurrent and persistent hyperparathyroidism. Hyperparathyroidism is also more common in persons who have received low-dose therapeutic irradiation.

DIAGNOSIS

Hypercalcemia is the usual clue to the diagnosis of hyperparathyroidism, although some patients have intermittent hypercalcemia and others are normocalcemic. Hypercalcemia has numerous causes, malignant disease being the most common cause among hospitalized patients. Most such patients (85%) have bone metastases. Some, however, have no evidence of bone metastasis, and their tumors appear to secrete hormone-like substances such as parathyroid hormone (ectopic hyperparathyroidism), prostaglandin, vitamin D-like sterols, or other substances. In most patients with malignant tumor-associated hypercalcemia, the duration of the hypercalcemia is short (weeks) and the tumor is apparent on thorough evaluation. The most common tumors associated with ectopic hyperparathyroidism are squamous cell carcinoma of the lung and hypernephroma. In some patients with ectopic hyperparathyroidism, the tumor may not be evident on physical examination, but is detectable by radiologic examination of the lung or kidneys. Multiple myeloma is another cause of malignant tumor-associated hypercalcemia with which tumor may not be apparent on physical examination. These patients usually have abnormal bone roentgenograms, abnormal serum proteins and urinary proteins by electrophoresis, and an abnormal bone marrow. Other causes of hypercalcemia include increased ingestion of vitamin D, vitamin A, milk products, and alkali. Thiazide-containing diuretics and lithium can also cause mild hypercalcemia, although another coexistent cause of hypercalcemia should be considered in these patients since most other patients receiving these medications are not hypercalcemic. It should be noted in the history whether the patient's intake of vitamins and milk products has increased. Granulomatous diseases (e.g., sarcoidosis, tuberculosis, berylliosis), other endocrine disorders (e.g., hyperthyroidism, hypothyroidism, Addison's disease, pheochromocytoma, vipoma), and other disorders (e.g., benign familial hypocalciuric hypercalcemia, immobilization, laboratory error, tight tourniquet) must also be considered.

The clinical manifestations of some of these other conditions, such as hyperthyroidism, are usually apparent, making the diagnosis relatively easy. The duration of the hypercalcemia is significant: if someone has hypercalcemia for 3 or 4 years, malignant disease and most conditions other than hyperparathyroidism are unlikely. If the patient was formerly documented to be normocalcemic, benign familial hypocalciuric hypercalcemia (BFHH) is essentially ruled out. Patients with BFHH can be differentiated from patients with primary hyperparathyroidism because they have a low urinary calcium level (usually less than 200 mg per 24 hours) and a mean ratio of calcium clearance to creatinine clearance of 0.01 or less. These patients also have family members who are hypercalcemic before the age of 10 years. Patients with primary hyperparathyroidism, even when it is familial, rarely develop hypercalcemia before age 10.

The most common laboratory abnormalities in patients with primary hyperparathyroidism include hypercalcemia, hypophosphatemia, an increased ratio of chloride to phosphate (33 or higher), hyperuricemia, and, in about 15 percent of patients, an increased serum alkaline phosphatase level. The serum parathyroid hormone (PTH) level is increased in most patients with primary hyperparathyroidism (if a sensitive PTH assay is available), and one can therefore make the diagnosis of primary hyperparathyroidism by inclusion (i.e., increased serum PTH level and increased serum calcium level) rather than by excluding the aforementioned other causes of hypercalcemia. The most common symptoms in patients with hypercalcemia include a mild increase in fatigue, a lack of enthusiasm for life, increased thirst (polydipsia) or polyuria, nocturia, musculoskeletal aches and pains, and constipation. Associated conditions include hypertension, nephrolithiasis, gout and pseudogout, peptic ulcer disease, and pancreatitis. Some patients are asymptomatic.

SELECTION FOR PARATHYROIDECTOMY

There is general agreement that patients with symptomatic hyperparathyroidism and those with a serum calcium level 1 mg per deciliter above the upper limit of normal should be treated by parathyroidectomy. Symptoms of fatigue, musculoskeletal aches and pains, and such associated conditions as nephrolithiasis or peptic ulcer disease usually improve following successful parathyroidectomy. The abnormal laboratory tests (serum calcium, phosphate, and alkaline phosphatase levels) also return to normal. Urinary calcium levels and renal function improve and serum uric acid levels decrease. The same metabolic benefits that occur in patients with symptomatic hyperparathyroidism, such as improvement in renal function and bone density, also occur in patients with asymptomatic hyperparathyroidism, and the success rate of parathyroidectomy performed by an experienced surgeon is about 95 percent. When 147 patients with minimal hyperparathyroidism were followed at the Mayo Clinic for 10 years, 38 of these patients (26%) developed some complications of concern to the patient or the physician and were treated surgically, 35 patients died, 23 were lost to, or declined, follow-up evaluation, and 13 had indeterminate or questionable hyperparathyroidism. Thus, although only 26 percent of the original patients required surgical treatment, 50 percent of those who could develop problems from or progression of their hyperparathyroidism (that is, those who were alive and available for follow-up examination) were operated on within 10 years because of problems.

It therefore appears that even patients with minimal or asymptomatic hyperparathyroidism should be treated surgically unless there is a strong contraindication to surgery. Medical treatment with oral phosphate to decrease the serum calcium level, furosemide (Lasix) to increase urinary calcium excretion (after salt loading), and, in women, estrogens to decrease the effect of parathyroid hormone on bone is only partially effective. When medical treatment includes phosphate, serum creatinine levels should be carefully monitored because deteriorating renal function sometimes occurs in these patients.

LOCALIZATION PROCEDURES

In the last few years, noninvasive localization procedures including ultrasonography (10 mHz, real time, small parts scanner), computerized tomography (CT) scanning, and scanning with ^{201}Tl chloride and ^{99m}Tc pertechnetate have become much more precise. In the best of circumstances, about 75 percent of the abnormal parathyroid gland(s) will be localized by these procedures. These results approach 90 percent when two or more procedures are used. However, several important facts must be considered:

1. An experienced surgeon, as stated previously, can cure 95 percent of patients. Localization procedures are therefore not essential, but are helpful.
2. All localization studies have a higher failure rate in patients with multiple abnormal glands (hyperplasia or multiple adenomas). Thus, the largest parathyroid gland may be identified, but smaller abnormal parathyroid glands may be missed.
3. Failure to identify parathyroid gland does not negate the diagnosis.
4. As many as 40 percent of patients with hyperparathyroidism may have small thyroid nodules, and many other patients have lymphadenopathy, so that not all lesions seen by these localization studies are parathyroid tumors. Both false-positive (identifying parathyroid glands in the wrong place) and false-negative (not identifying parathyroid glands when they are present) studies occur with all of these localization procedures.
5. The 75 percent success rate occurs when experienced radiologists or physicians are interpreting these studies and "state of the art" equipment is used. Invasive studies such as highly selective venous catheterization for parathyroid hormone (PTH) and digital angiography as well

as fine-needle biopsy to confirm that the suspected lesion is a parathyroid tumor are only recommended for patients who have had previous parathyroid operations. Selective venous catheterization is quite helpful in patients with persistent or recurrent hyperparathyroidism. When used with the noninvasive studies, the precise location of the elusive parathyroid tumor can often be determined. Digital angiography prior to selective venous catheterization sometimes identifies the tumor (approximately 40%), but also demonstrates the venous system and this is helpful for the venous catheterization.

PREPARATION FOR OPERATION

Patients should be prepared for parathyroidectomy just as they are for other operations. If there is any hoarseness or if the patient has had previous neck surgery, indirect laryngoscopy to view the vocal cords is required. All patients should be well hydrated, especially those with mild-to-moderate renal dysfunction. All electrolyte abnormalities such as hypo- or hyperkalemia should be corrected, if possible. The indications for the operation as well as its inherent risks (approximately 1% to 2% incidence of hypoparathyroidism, hoarseness, bleeding, or infection in experienced hands) and benefits should also be discussed with the patient.

SURGICAL TREATMENT

Various surgical approaches have been recommended for treating patients with primary hyperparathyroidism. Each had certain advantages, and the approach used depends on the expertise of the surgeon and the pathologist and the availability of preoperative localization tests. These approaches include (1) unilateral exploration, (2) bilateral exploration with identification of four glands, and thymectomy for patients with primary or secondary hyperparathyroidism due to parathyroid hyperplasia, (3) prophylactic subtotal parathyroidectomy regardless of the operative findings, and (4) total parathyroidectomy with autotransplantation. Most surgeons favor a bilateral exploration with identification of all parathyroid glands and removal of the abnormal parathyroid gland. Some surgeons use the same approach for all patients with primary hyperparathyroidism, whereas others may prefer one approach but use the others in certain circumstances. For example, in an opera singer, one may perform a unilateral exploration knowing that the failure rate may be slightly higher, but the risk of a change in the voice is lower.

A unilateral approach has been advocated by Wang and Tibblin and their colleagues. When an abnormal parathyroid gland is identified preoperatively, this technique saves time. Since only one recurrent nerve and two parathyroid glands are at risk, the complication rate should be lower than when more extensive operative

procedures are performed. However, the failure rate is slightly (3% to 5%) higher. The major problem with this approach is that some patients have multiple adenomas and others have hyperplasia with parathyroid glands that vary in size. The latter group of glands may be erroneously diagnosed as having an adenoma and a normal gland. Some pathologists also have difficulty differentiating between normal and hyperplastic parathyroid tissue by frozen section examination of a small biopsy specimen.

Most surgeons and the author advocate a bilateral neck exploration with removal of the solitary parathyroid adenoma and identification of the three other glands. Biopsy of one normal gland is optional. When there is more than one abnormal parathyroid gland, hyperplasia must be suspected, although double adenomas do occur. In these cases, biopsy of the normal-appearing parathyroid glands should be obtained and the enlarged parathyroid glands removed. All suspected parathyroid tissue in patients with multiple abnormal parathyroid glands should definitely undergo frozen section examination. In patients with hyperplasia, a subtotal parathyroidectomy should be performed. The important point to emphasize here is that all of the glands should be identified first. Then, a biopsy is obtained from the parathyroid gland that is to remain before any of the other parathyroid glands are removed. The smallest and most readily accessible parathyroid gland is the one to leave. If the parathyroid remnant is viable and of proper size, the other parathyroid glands should then be removed. In patients with hyperplasia, I also perform a bilateral thymectomy because at least 15 percent of these patients have a fifth parathyroid gland, and it is usually situated in the thymus. Failure to do this will result in persistent hyperparathyroidism in some patients with hyperplasia.

A prophylactic subtotal parathyroidectomy was formerly recommended by several surgeons. Today, however, no one advocates this approach except perhaps for patients with familial hyperparathyroidism or MEN I. Patients with familial hyperparathyroidism and MEN I are the most difficult to treat successfully because of a high incidence of both persistent and recurrent hyperparathyroidism. Because these patients sometimes develop recurrent hyperparathyroidism even after postparathyroidectomy hypoparathyroidism, Wells and others advocate total parathyroidectomy with parathyroid autotransplantation. With this approach, recurrent hyperparathyroidism that follows total parathyroidectomy and autotransplantation of parathyroid tissue to the forearm can usually be treated by removal of the transplanted hyperplastic parathyroid tissue under local anesthesia. Unfortunately, in some patients the recurrence is due to the growth of residual parathyroid tissue that was not removed from the neck, despite a presumed "total" parathyroidectomy.

Total parathyroidectomy with autotransplantation is not advocated for other patients because it is also associated with about a 5 percent incidence of early and late failure, causing permanent hypoparathyroidism. Total parathyroidectomy with autotransplantation, however, is the treatment of choice for patients with neonatal hyperparathyroidism. This is a life-threatening condition, and operations that fail to recover virtually all of the hyperfunctioning parathyroid tissue often prove disastrous. Cryopreserving parathyroid tissue is recommended for all patients treated by autotransplantation in case the transplanted tissue does not function adequately. It is also recommended for patients who require reoperation when the condition of the remaining parathyroid glands is unknown.

What should be done when no enlarged parathyroid gland is identified during the operative procedure? In general, if three or fewer parathyroid glands are identified in the neck, the remaining parathyroid gland is still approachable via the cervical incision. When four glands are identified in the neck, a fifth gland is usually situated within the mediastinum. When no abnormal parathyroid gland is identified, all normal-appearing parathyroid glands should be subjected to biopsy and frozen section examination to confirm that they are parathryoid glands. The position of each gland and its relationship to the recurrent laryngeal nerve should be documented so that one can determine which gland is missing and where the nerve is situated if reoperation becomes necessary. When only three normal-appearing glands are identified, the thymus should be removed on the side where only one gland has been identified. If no abnormal parathyroid tissue is identified in the thymus, the retroesophageal area should be explored, the carotid sheath opened, and either a thyroid lobectomy or thyroidotomy performed. All extra fibrofatty tissue should be removed between the carotid and the trachea on the side where the parathyroid gland is missing. An undescended parathyroid gland situated at the level of the carotid bulb should also be considered.

At the time of exploration, the surgeon is responsible for making sure that all abnormal parathyroid tissue approachable via a cervical incision has been removed. After a thorough exploration, if no abnormal parathyroid tissue has been identified, the glands previously subjected to biopsy should be marked with clips or with a long nonabsorbable suture. Normal-sized parathyroid glands should *not* be removed. The operation should then be completed, except in patients with serum calcium levels greater than 13 mg per deciliter. In these latter patients a median sternotomy should be performed. Remember that the size of the parathyroid gland generally corresponds with the serum calcium and serum PTH levels. Thus, patients with profound hypercalcemia usually have relatively large parathyroid glands.

PERSISTENT OR RECURRENT HYPERPARATHYROIDISM

Localization studies are helpful in patients with primary hyperparathyroidism who have not had previous operations and are essential for patients requiring reoperation. In the latter group, the diagnosis must be reconfirmed. Patients with benign familial hypocalciuric hypercalcemia, ectopic hyperparathyroidism due to malignant disease, and other conditions can occasionally mimic patients with hyperparathyroidism, and these conditions must be ruled out. The previous operative note(s) and pathology reports must be carefully analyzed to determine whether the patient has adenomatous or hyperplastic disease and where the abnormal remaining parathyroid gland is most likely to be situated. Correlating this information with that of the localization tests is often helpful. Noninvasive localization tests (echography, CT scanning, and thallium-technetium pertechnetate scanning) should be performed and, if equivocal or negative, should be followed by highly selective venous catheterization for PTH. Using this approach, I have been able to identify the abnormal parathyroid tissue in more than 90 percent of patients who have persistent or recurrent hyperparathyroidism, and this in spite of loss of normal tissue planes, scarring, and previous ligation of many of the thyroid and other cervical vessels. The surgical approach for patients who require reoperation is to use the previous cervical incision, but then to use a lateral approach, posterior to the strap muscles and anterior to the sternocleidomastoid muscle. This frequently eliminates the need to dissect through the extensive adhesions and immediately places the dissection in the area behind the thyroid gland, where most parathyroid glands are situated.

PATHOLOGY

It is imperative to confirm by frozen section examination all tissue suspected of being abnormal parathyroid tissue. Occasionally, a thyroid adenoma or other mass may mimic a parathyroid tumor. The pathologist must be able to state whether or not the tissue in question is parathyroid tissue. It is also helpful to know whether the parathyroid tissue is hyperplastic (contains little to no fat either between the cells or within the cytoplasm of the cells). The size of the gland also helps to determine whether it is normal or abnormal (greater than 65 mg). The size and appearance of the other parathyroid glands determines whether the abnormal parathyroid gland is an adenoma (other glands normal) or a hyperplastic parathyroid gland (other glands abnormal). Parathyroid carcinoma should be suspected in patients with profound hypercalcemia when there is invasion into adjacent structures or nodal metastases. Patients with cancer should have the adjacent fibrofatty tissue, lymph nodes, and the ipsilateral thyroid lobe removed. A modified neck dissection should be performed if the nodes are clinically positive.

COMPLICATIONS

The possible complications of parathyroidectomy include injury to one recurrent laryngeal nerve with resultant hoarseness or bilateral injury with immobilization of the vocal cords in the midline and difficulty in breathing. Hypocalcemia may occur owing to "bone hunger" or a devascularization or removal of all of the parathyroid glands. Infection, bleeding, corneal abrasions, or keloid formation are also possible. Overall, the incidence of complications should be less than 2 percent.

Other rare postoperative problems include acute gout or pseudogout, pancreatitis, or acute psychosis. Most patients have benign postoperative courses, are eating within 24 hours, and may be discharged from the hospital within 2 days after surgery.

Postoperative pain is usually not severe, and if nausea occurs, it can be treated with Compazine. Following the operation, the serum calcium and phosphate levels should be determined daily. When both the serum calcium and serum phosphate levels are low, bone hunger is usually the cause. This situation can be anticipated in patients with osteitis fibrosa cystica, who have an increased alkaline phosphatase level preoperatively. A low serum calcium and increased serum phosphate level postoperatively suggest hypoparathyroidism. Regardless of the cause of symptomatic or profound hypocalcemia, patients need to be treated with calcium and sometimes with vitamin D. Oral calcium supplementation with Titralac (400 mg elemental calcium per 5 cc) or Os-Cal (500 mg calcium per tablet) usually controls symptoms of temporary hypocalcemia. This treatment is sometimes necessary for several weeks. Treatment with calcium intravenously (calcium gluconate, 10 to 20 ml injected slowly) may be necessary in more severe cases. It must be remembered, however, that (1) the local infiltration of calcium must be avoided because it may result in extensive local tissue necrosis and full-thickness skin loss, and (2) hyperventilation with resultant alkalosis may cause or aggravate the clinical manifestations of hypocalcemia.

In patients with profound hypocalcemia, treatment with 1,25 dihydroxy vitamin D_3 (Rocaltrol, 0.25 to 1.0 μg/day orally) is sometimes required. If hypoparathyroidism is permanent, the serum phosphate should be kept normal with phosphate binders (Alu-Caps or Basalgel, two or more capsules or tablets with meals), and continued treatment with vitamin D is helpful.

FOLLOW-UP AND RESULTS

The results of parathyroidism are gratifying. Ninety-five percent or more of these patients are successfully treated at the initial operation, and the complications of the operation are infrequent. Postoperatively, the abnormal preoperative laboratory tests (calcium, phosphate, alkaline phosphatase, uric acid) usually return to normal. Symptomatic patients often feel better with more energy, less fatigue, and less constipation. They also have fewer episodes of nephrolithiasis and renal colic, the subperiosteal resorption disappears, and brown tumors become sclerotic. Two-thirds of the patients with peptic ulcer disease also become asymptomatic and renal function may improve.

RECURRENT AND PERSISTENT PRIMARY HYPERPARATHYROIDISM

MARTIN D. JENDRISAK, M.D.
SAMUEL A. WELLS, Jr., M.D.

The first operation for the preoperative diagnosis of primary hyperparathyroidism was performed in Vienna by Mandl in 1925. The patient ultimately expired 6 years later with recurrent hypercalcemia. Captain Charles Martell, a merchant marine, was the first patient to undergo an operation in the United States for this condition. Postoperatively he developed persistent hypercalcemia, and he underwent six unsuccessful operations between 1926 and 1933 before his mediastinal adenoma was finally removed. He expired soon thereafter from renal failure. Recurrent and persistent hyperparathyroidism remain diagnostic and therapeutic challenges for even the most experienced surgeon.

The widespread use of multichannel biochemical serum analysis has resulted in increased recognition of hypercalcemia due to primary hyperparathyroidism. The reported incidence of this disease in the general population ranges from .08 per 1,000 per year to five per 1,000. As hyperparathyroidism is being recognized more frequently, the number of patients in whom the first operation is unsuccessful has also increased.

A clear distinction between persistent and recurrent hyperparathyroidism should be made. Persistent hyperparathyroidism is the more common cause of postoperative hypercalcemia and, by definition, represents a continuation of an elevated serum calcium level through the immediate postoperative period or its development within one month of the operation. This is almost always the result of a missed hyperfunctioning parathyroid gland or inadequate resection of abnormal parathyroid tissue. The much less common recurrent hyperparathyroidism is believed by Clark and colleagues to result from the subsequent development of abnormal hyperfunction of a parathyroid gland or glands previously observed to be normal. According to Muller, recurrence is defined by the following criteria: (1) histologic identification by biopsy and frozen section of all parathyroid glands at the initial operation, (2) complete removal of the enlarged glands, (3) a normocalcemic state for a minimum post-operative period of one year, and (4) the finding of an enlarged parathyroid gland at the site of a previously normal-sized gland.

Persistent hypercalcemia subsequent to an operation for hyperparathyroidism may be due to nonparathyroid diseases such as malignant tumor, sarcoidosis, hyper-vitaminosis A or D, the milk-alkali syndrome, hyper-thyroidism, or immobilization. These possible causes must be excluded prior to consideration of a repeated neck exploration. However, the hypercalcemia may result from an ectopically located hyperfunctioning parathyroid gland or a missed supernumery parathyroid gland. The inex-perienced surgeon may have failed to appreciate a normally positioned enlarged parathyroid, or he may have conducted an incomplete search or failed to resect an adequate mass of hyperfunctioning tissue. The initial operative approach affords the best chance for cure of hyperparathyroidism and should be characterized by a meticulous dissection. A repeated neck exploration is technically more difficult than the first procedure and is attendant with greater risks of recurrent nerve damage, permanent hypoparathyroidism, and even death.

ANATOMY OF THE PARATHYROID GLANDS

A thorough appreciation of normal and abnormal anatomy of the parathyroid glands is essential to the appropriate surgical management of hyperparathyroidism, especially in recurrent and persistent disease. The upper parathyroid glands are normally located close to the posterior surface of the upper portion of the thyroid gland, very near the entry of the recurrent laryngeal nerves into the larynx. During embryologic development, the inferior parathyroid glands descend from the pharynx to the lower thyroid pole, and this accounts for the variability in their location. They are generally associated with the lower pole of the thyroid gland or the thyrothymic ligament adjacent to the inferior thyroid veins. Less often, the inferior para-thyroid glands may be located high in the neck as undescended parathyroid tissue or in the superior mediastinum within the thymus.

With enlargement, the position of the parathyroid glands may change. The upper parathyroid glands normally reside posterior to the recurrent laryngeal nerve and inferior thyroid artery. The enlarged gland may descend inferiorly in the tracheoesophageal groove or into the posterior mediastinum. The lower parathyroid glands may be located adjacent to or within the thymus in the anterior-superior mediastinum. Generally, 80 to 85 percent of single enlarged parathyroid glands are in a relatively normal location adjacent to the thyroid gland. In rare instances, parathyroid glands may be intra-thyroidal, usually within the lower pole of the gland. Although there are usually four parathyroid glands, five or more may be present. It is doubtful whether fewer than four parathyroid glands are ever present, and so the failure to find four usually indicates that one has been overlooked or is located in an ectopic position.

INITIAL PARATHYROID EXPLORATION

The goal at the initial exploration for hyperpara-thyroidism is to identify all four parathyroid glands and to remove those that are enlarged. Hyperfunctioning para-thyroid glands are enlarged and of a dark color, ranging from tan to reddish-brown. The normal parathyroid glands are usually yellow with an abundant blood supply. If one, two, or three parathyroid glands are enlarged, they should be resected, and biopsy obtained from the remaining normal parathyroid gland(s) to ensure identity. The sites of the remaining parathyroid glands should be marked with a silk suture. In the case of "parathyroid hyper-plasia," in which four enlarged parathyroid glands are found, either a 3½ gland parathyroidectomy or a total parathyroidectomy with heterotopic autotransplantation should be performed. In a radical subtotal parathyroidec-tomy, three glands and a portion of the fourth are excised, leaving a well-vascularized remnant of approximately 50 to 70 mg of tissue. When two or three parathyroid glands are enlarged and the others appear normal, the situation probably represents a variant of "hyperplasia" or what is sometimes referred to as multiglandular disease or "multiple adenomas." In this situation, most authors agree that resection of the enlarged glands with biopsy of the normal gland(s) is almost always curative. The remaining parathyroid remnants are marked with non-absorbable suture should future reexploration be required.

In the event that an enlarged parathyroid gland cannot be found at the usual locations during neck exploration, the systematic search for ectopic parathyroid glandular tissue should be carried out. The identified normal para-thyroid glands should be subjected to biopsy to confirm their identity, and then each gland should be marked with a nonabsorbable suture. In the event that only three normal parathyroid glands are found while the fourth gland escapes detection, the surgeon should assess whether the upper or lower parathyroid gland is missing. In the case of a missing lower parathyroid gland, as much of the thymus as possible should be delivered into the neck by firm traction and then resected. An enlarged parathyroid is often found within the thymus. Enlarged superior para-thyroid glands may descend along the esophagus into the posterior-superior mediastinum and are often overlooked because the depth of dissection is not carried to the pre-vertebral fascia. Generally, a finger can be safely inserted behind the inferior thyroid artery posterior to the recurrent laryngeal nerve to palpate an enlarged gland and aid in its deliverance into the field.

If all of these maneuvers are unsuccessful, dissection should be carried in a cephalad direction to the pharynx where occasionally a parathyroid gland may be found. An undescended parathyroid is commonly associated with thymus tissue in the superior neck and has been called "undescended parathymus." The thyroid lobe on the side of the missing gland should be carefully palpated. Occasionally, an intrathyroidal parathyroid tumor may be palpated and excised. More often, however, a superior parathyroid gland may be partially or totally covered by a large nodular thyroid lobe and thereby appear intrathyroidal. Even if no intrathyroidal lump is palpable, total excision of the ipsilateral thyroid lobe should be considered as a nonpalpable parathyroid may be found when the excised tissue is sectioned. Finally, the carotid sheath should be opened and explored since parathyroid tumors have, in rare instances, been found there. If four normal glands are found within the neck, the surgeon should search all of these ectopic sites for a supernumerary gland. One should not remove whole normal parathyroid glands if no tumors are found.

Mediastinal exploration for a missing adenoma should not be a part of the first operation. The rationale for deferring mediastinal exploration includes the possibility that the diagnosis of hyperparathyroidism may be in error. Occasionally, the hypercalcemia may regress or even be eliminated by the first neck exploration owing to inadvertent disruption of the blood supply to the occult gland. In 80 to 90 percent of cases of persistent hyperparathyroidism, the missing parathyroid is located in the neck or is removable through a cervical incision. Deep mediastinal exploration was required in 3 percent of Beazley's 35 patients, in 19 percent of Wang's 110 patients, in 10 percent of Brennan's 30 patients, and in 9 percent of Granberg's 53 patients.

EVALUATION OF THE PATIENT WITH PERSISTENT OR RECURRENT HYPERPARATHYROIDISM

It is important that the severity of the parathyroid disease be carefully assessed in order to justify the increased risk of re-exploration of the neck with possible sternotomy. Billings and Millroy recommend that re-exploration be limited to patients with symptomatic hypercalcemia, deteriorating renal function, enlarging renal calculi, or rising serum calcium. In a totally asymptomatic patient with a serum calcium concentration below 11 mg per deciliter and no evidence of skeletal or renal disease, most authors agree that a nonoperative course should be considered.

If re-exploration is the decided course, the operating surgeon should carefully review the previous operative notes, pathologic findings, and sections of all resected tissues. Although re-exploration of the neck may be safely carried out as early as one week postoperatively without undue difficulty, it is rarely undertaken because most surgeons wish to perform localized tests. Usually several weeks are allowed to pass before reoperation. If generalized parathyroid gland enlargement was documented grossly and either a 3- or a 3½-gland parathyroidectomy with confirmed histology was performed, one may opt to repeat the neck exploration without performing localization procedures. This same course may also be undertaken if the previous neck exploration had been performed by an inexperienced parathyroid surgeon, as the probability of finding the missing adenoma by repeat exploration is high. In other patients who remain hypercalcemic after a failed operation, an attempt should be made to localize the hyperfunctioning parathyroid tissue prior to re-exploration.

TECHNIQUES FOR LOCALIZATION OF ABNORMAL PARATHYROID TISSUE

Noninvasive techniques for localization of hyperfunctioning parathyroid tissue include barium swallow, radionuclide imaging, and computed tomographic (CT) scanning. The presence of an enlarged parathyroid gland may be suggested indirectly by the demonstration of esophageal indentation at barium swallow and cine esophagography or by the identification of a cold area in the thyroid gland by radionuclide imaging. These techniques are rarely helpful. A more direct approach to identify overlooked parathyroid tissue includes CT scans, parathyroid scanning with thallium-201, and high-resolution real time ultrasonography. CT scans are especially helpful in locating mediastinal parathyroid glands. Radionuclide imaging and high-resolution ultrasonography are of value in localizing hyperfunctioning parathyroid glands in approximately 40 to 60 percent of patients who are undergoing repeated neck surgery. Neddle aspiration (with parathormone assay) of an enlarged parathyroid gland is often helpful in identifying a specific mass lesion or parathyroid tissue.

The invasive localization techniques include arteriography and selective venous sampling with assay of plasma for parathormone. Arteriographic demonstration of a parathyroid adenoma was first performed by Seldinger in 1954. Selective injection of thyroid arteries results in successful identification of hyperfunctioning parathyroid tissue in 50 to 70 percent of cases. Initial thyroid scanning is done to assess the amount of thyroid tissue previously resected and to aid in the interpretation of vascular blushes seen on subsequent arteriography. Since arteriography may be associated with morbidity (particularly in the elderly) including transient cortical blindness, cerebrovascular accidents, and transverse myelitis, it should only be performed by an experienced vascular radiologist. By determining plasma levels of PTH from selectively sampled thyroid veins, one is able to identify sites of increased secretion. Actually this technique serves to correctly lateralize rather than localize the side of the neck in which the hyperfunctioning tissue resides, being especially helpful to identify multiple and ectopic tumors. These combined techniques of arterial and venous catheterization can accurately localize hyperfunctioning tissue in 70 to 85 percent of reoperated cases. Most authors would utilize sequentially noninvasive and (if negative) invasive localization studies in patients previously explored by an experienced endocrine surgeon.

STRATEGY FOR REOPERATION

After the data from the previous operations have been reviewed and the appropriate preoperative diagnostic studies have been evaluated, re-exploration of the neck is undertaken. The patient should be prepared for median sternotomy. If an enlarged parathyroid gland has been localized to the deep mediastinum, a median sternotomy may be performed without a lengthy neck exploration,

TABLE 1 Recently Reported Experiences of Reoperation for Hyperparathyroidism

Author and Date	Patients (N)	Number of Patients with Glands Removed		Pathologic Findings			
		Via Neck	Via Chest	Adenoma	Hyperplasia	Carcinoma	Other*
Martin et al (1980)	25	16 (64%)	1 (4%)	7 (28%)	9 (36%)	1 (1%)	7 (28%)
Roslyn et al (1981)	26	20 (77%)	6 (23%)	19 (73%)	--	--	--
McGarity and Goldman (1981)	28	17 (74%)	6 (26%)	--	--	--	--
Granberg et al (1982)	53	42 (79%)	5 (9%)	26 (49%)	20 (38%)	1 (2%)	8 (15%)
Billings and Millroy (1983)	33	24 (73%)	3 (9%)	17 (52%)	9 (27%)	1 (3%)	6 (18%)
Brennan and Norton (1985)	175	--†	--†	105 (60%)	56 (32%)	5 (3%)	9 (5%)

* Includes patients with the diagnosis of sarcoidosis, familial hypercalcemic hypocalciuric hyperparathyroidism (FHHH), and unidentified causes.
† It is reported that 26% of the inferior glands were located in the anterior mediastinum, but the incidence of sternotomy is not given.

especially if the normal complement of parathyroid glands had been previously identified in the neck. Usually, however, an attempt should be made to extract a mediastinal gland through a cervical incision; thus the need for a median sternotomy would be eliminated. If a mediastinal parathyroid is not identified by localization studies, a median sternotomy should be performed only after a thorough cervical re-exploration has been performed. At operation, any suspicious areas indicated by the localization studies should be explored first. Frequently, however, the whole neck must be re-explored superiorly to the angle of the jaw, laterally to and including the carotid sheaths, posteriorly to the vertebral column, and inferiorly to the innominate vein. If not previously done, the thyroid lobe on the side of the missing gland should be resected. Lymph nodes should always be taken for histologic studies to exclude the presence of sarcoidosis. Only after an exhaustive neck exploration should the surgeon consider sternotomy. In 60 percent of 35 patients reported by Beasley and associates and in 49 percent of 51 patients reported by vanVroonhover and Muller, the previously missed parathyroid glands were located in a normal anatomic position. McGarity and Goldman report normal location of hyperfunctioning parathyroid tissue in 9 of 22 cases. The majority of parathyroid glands located ectopically within the mediastinum can be removed through a cervical incision.

The previous transverse neck incision is utilized for repeat neck exploration. The strap muscles are often adherent to the thyroid lobes, in which case it is often easier to dissect the vertical plane between the sternocleidomastoid muscle and the strap muscles. This plane is often unscarred, and by retracting the carotid sheath laterally and the thyroid gland medially, the surgeon exposes a relatively normal area containing the recurrent laryngeal nerve and parathyroid glands. The surgeon should carefully search the entire neck looking for parathyroid glands in their normal and abnormal locations. If no enlarged parathyroid glands are found, one should proceed to mediastinal exploration.

MEDIASTINAL EXPLORATION

The sternum is divided from the sternal notch to the xiphoid and separated with a self-retaining retractor. If a parathyroid gland is not readily visible, the thymus is excised. The resected thymus must be carefully evaluated since a hyperfunctioning parathyroid gland may be present but not readily visible. If the parathyroid is not found within the substance of the thymus, one must search near the great vessels, over the pericardium, and in the retroesophageal area of the posterior mediastinum. This latter area is most difficult to explore through a median sternotomy. When an enlarged parathyroid is found in the neck or chest, it should be removed. If at least one additional normal gland had been left after the first operation and is still intact after repeted surgery, the patient will have normal parathyroid function, which emphasizes the importance of not removing normal parathyroid tissue during an initial unsuccessful operation. If three normal glands have previously been excised from the neck and the fourth parathyroid gland is enlarged and identified in the neck or mediastinum, a portion of the parathyroid should be implanted into the forearm muscle to prevent

TABLE 2 Reoperative Results for Primary Hyperparathyroidism

Author and Year	Number of Patients	% Cured of Hypercalcemia
Hellstrom (1957)	20	70
Clark and Taylor (1972)	11	82
Romanus et al (1973)	11	73
Beazley et al (1975)	35	74
Livesay and Mulder (1976)	20	63
Clark et al (1976)	11	82
Wang (1977)	112	91
Brennan et al (1978)	30	83
Edis et al (1978)	51	84
vanVroonhover and Muller (1978)	51	98
Organ and Albano (1980)	12	100
Roslyn et al (1981)	26	100
Prinz et al (1981)	27	78
Bruining et al (1981)	53	81
McGarity and Goldman (1981)	28	82
Granberg et al (1982)	53	83
Billings and Millroy (1983)	33	88
Brennan and Norton (1985)	175	90

permanent hypocalcemia. If one is unsure of the number of parathyroid glands remaining in the neck, the excised hyperfunctioning parathyroid tissue should be cryo-preserved and the patient observed. If hypocalcemia occurs and the patient cannot be weaned from calcium and vitamin D, the frozen parathyroid tissue can be grafted subsequently under local anesthesia.

PARATHYROID AUTOTRANSPLANTATION

The enlarged parathyroid gland is removed from the neck and frozen section confirmation obtained. The gland is sliced into $1 \times 1 \times 3$ mm slivers and placed either in chilled saline or tissue culture medium. If delayed auto-transplantation is chosen, the technique of cryopreservation can be performed. The parathyroid pieces are frozen in tissue culture media containing 10% dimethylsulfoxide and 10% serum, and stored in liquid nitrogen until used. Tissue viability has been documented for periods up to 18 months. If the patient cannot be weaned from vitamin D and oral calcium (usually after a course of 4 to 6 months), the cryopreserved parathyroid tissue is thawed and autografted into the forearm muscle under local anesthesia. Fifteen to twenty pieces of parathyroid tissue are implanted, each in a separate intramuscular pocket. The fascia overlying the parathyroid is closed with non-absorbable suture to prevent the parathyroid tissue from being extruded and to serve as a marker for location of the imbedded parathyroid tissue should subsequent re-exploration be required for tissue removal. Care must be taken at this time to prevent hemorrhage into the muscle pocket, which would adversely affect tissue viability. Heterotopic autotransplantation to the forearm is ideal because hyperfunctioning tissue can be readily identified and removed under local anesthesia. Utilizing these techniques, permanent hypoparathyroidism is a preventable complication of re-exploration for persistent or recurrent hyperparathyroidism.

RESULTS

Early series reported success rates for recurrent or persistnet hyperparathyroidism in the range of 60 to 70 percent. More recently, however, with several large series reported, the expected success rate approaches 90 percent (Tables 1 and 2). Reoperation for parathyroid disease remains a major challenge for both the patient and the surgeon. Clearly, operative risks increase with each succeeding reexploration, but with careful attention to confirmation of the diagnosis, review of prior operative procedures, appropriate utilization of localization procedures, and thorough intraoperative management, relatively high success rates can be expected.

THE BREAST

FIBROCYSTIC DISEASE OF THE BREAST

ARMANDO E. GIULIANO, M.D.

Fibrocystic disease is the most common diagnosis for breast problems seen in women. Unfortunately, the term is vague and imprecise, referring to a broad spectrum of clinical and microscopic findings, many of which may represent variants of normal histologic changes. The clinical significance of fibrocystic disease, its treatment, and its relationship to malignant disease are confusing and often misunderstood.

CLINICAL SPECTRUM OF FIBROCYSTIC DISEASE

Most women who see their physician with a breast problem complain of a mass or pain and tenderness. Women with fibrocystic disease present with mildly tender, multiple palpable masses in the breast that fluctuate with the menstrual cycle. These are often associated with pain prior to menses. Usually the patient notices these changes while in her twenties, and they generally abate with menopause. It is estimated that at least 50 percent of women between the ages of 25 and 50 have clinical findings compatible with the diagnosis of fibrocystic disease. Breasts are composed of fat, fibrous tissue, and epithelial ducts. Since this tissue is under the influence of circulating hormones, it is not surprising that variations in the breasts occur in response to hormonal fluctuations during the menstrual cycle. Most patients who present with "fibrocystic disease" probably have a variation of the normal end-organ response to physiologic changes in circulating hormone levels. Nodularity and sensitivity of the breasts may be a result of this normal hormonal variation.

MICROSCOPIC APPEARANCE OF FIBROCYSTIC DISEASE

The microscopic findings in biopsies of patients with fibrocystic disease are varied and range from gross fluid-filled cysts to firm fibrous tumors. Macroscopically, one may see blue or yellow cysts of varying sizes. At other times, the transected tissue may be a firm greyish-white mass. The microscopic pattern is notoriously pleomorphic, and usually more than one histologic appearance is seen. In general, there are four dominant features seen in fibrocystic disease: (1) cysts, (2) sclerosing adenosis, (3) duct hyperplasia, and (4) fibrosis.

Cysts probably result from duct dilatation. Usually, the cysts are filled with a serous turbid fluid and lined with a smooth membranous wall of cuboidal or columnar epithelium. An isolated cyst is often an alarming clinical finding since it is a dominant mass and can be confused with carcinoma on physical examination. Fibrosis results from proliferation of the stromal fibrous connective tissue. In isolated fibrosis there is no evidence of epithelial or ductal proliferation. Often this entity is called "mammary fibrosis" rather than fibrocystic disease. Usually, however, there is proliferation of the epithelium of the ductules in addition to proliferation of the fibrous stroma. This pattern with proliferation of both the intralobular fibrous tissue and the small ductules or acini is named "sclerosing adenosis." If only the terminal ductules proliferate, it is generally referred to as "blunt duct adenosis." "Sclerosing adenosis," however, implies both ductal and perilobular connective tissue proliferation. On the other hand, "epithelial hyperplasia" is predominantly a proliferation of the epithelial cells lining the ducts and lobular ductules. This epithelial proliferation may be mainly in the terminal ductules or lobules, in which case it is called "lobular epithelial hyperplasia," but usually it is in the small ducts themselves ("ductal epithelial hyperplasia"). When the epithelium proliferates and projects papillary extensions into the ducts, the pattern is termed "papillomatosis." "Metaplasia" results in transformation of the cuboidal epithelium into a columnar epithelium with epithelial proliferation.

Many of these histologic findings are present on any surgical biopsy specimen. In general, it is of value to know which histologic type predominates, particularly to determine whether the epithelium is hyperplastic. These microscopic findings of fibrocystic disease are so common that most clinical surgeons have not seen a breast biopsy diagnosed as "normal." Indeed, in autopsy studies, 60 to 90 percent of breasts show one or more of these histologic findings. Eighty percent show macroscopic cysts.

RELATIONSHIP OF FIBROCYSTIC DISEASE TO CANCER

Many patients fear that the nodules of fibrocystic disease will become malignant. Although this is probably not true, the relationship between fibrocystic disease and cancer is controversial. Much literature is devoted to demonstrating the increased risk of malignancy with fibrocystic disease. The presence of fibrocystic disease reportedly imparts a two- to five-fold increase in the incidence of breast cancer. Since one in eleven American women will develop breast cancer, and somewhere between 60 and 80 percent of all breasts have fibrocystic disease, the finding of both on a biopsy specimen should not be uncommon. However, a more critical analysis of the literature suggests that fibrocystic disease itself may not be a significant risk factor for the development of cancer.

Although breasts removed for cancer usually have fibrocystic disease in them, the finding of fibrocystic disease in cancerous breasts appears to be no more common than finding fibrocystic disease in normal breasts at autopsy. Actually, some studies show a lower incidence of fibrocystic disease in cancerous breasts than in normal breasts. In addition, prior breast biopsies appear to be no more common in women who develop breast cancer than in those who do not.

Studies examining the histologic findings in breast biopsies of women who ultimately develop breast cancer suggest that patients who have fibrocystic disease manifested by epithelial hyperplasia histologically are at an increased risk of developing breast cancer. Studies by several investigators suggest that women having fibrocystic disease with epithelial hyperplasia have approximately twice the risk of cancer as do women with nonproliferative lesions. If there is epithelial atypia (atypical hyperplasia), the risk of cancer in one recent study was approximately five times more than that for women with nonproliferative breast lesions. Most pathologists believe that the spectrum of premalignant breast disease progresses from epithelial hyperplasia to atypical hyperplasia to carcinoma in situ, and finally to infiltrating carcinoma. Of course this theory cannot be proved, but is is not unreasonable based on our knowledge of malignant disease in other organs.

CLINICAL EVALUATION

Most patients who seek the advice of a physician for a breast problem are concerned that they have a malignant tumor. An essential part of the surgeon's care must be to determine whether the patient does or does not have carcinoma of the breast. The diagnosis of fibrocystic disease is of little clinical value, particularly if an underlying malignant tumor is overlooked. A careful history should be taken, not only with respect to the clinical problem, but also relating to the risk of developing breast cancer. A careful physical examination is then performed. The breasts are inspected for symmetry and appearance of the skin, nipples, and areolae. A clear, watery, colorless, or greenish discharge is not uncommon in fibrocystic disease, and if any discharge is present, is should be noted and tested for blood. Although most bloody discharges are associated with an intraductal papilloma, a bloody discharge requires further investigation since it may indicate malignant tumor. The patient should raise her arms above her head, and the skin should be examined for retraction or dimpling. Similarly, skin dimpling can be elicited by flexing the pectoralis major muscles by having the patient squeeze her hips with one hand on each iliac crest. A methodical bimanual examination is made of each breast in a systematic fashion. Each examiner tends to develop his or her own method of breast examination, but the most important factor is that a complete and careful examination be performed with the examiner palpating the entire breast. Usually the patient complains of a single area or nodule which she has located. The examiner must be certain that this area is identified. On physical examination, most breast nodularity is in the upper outer quadrant.

If the lesion is localized, aspiration of a discrete mass suggestive of a cyst is indicated. The skin and overlying tissues may be anesthetized by infiltration with 1% Xylocaine, but this is not usually necessary. An 18-gauge needle is introduced. If a cyst is present, the typical watery fluid (straw-colored, gray, greenish, brown, or black) is evacuated and the mass disappears. The patient is reexamined at intervals thereafter. If no fluid is obtained, if the fluid is bloody, if a mass persists after aspiration, or if at any time during follow-up a persistent lump is noted, biopsy should be performed.

MANAGEMENT

The overwhelming majority of patients with the clinical findings of fibrocystic disease require no specific treatment. Generally, reassurance and discussion of the problem with the patient suffices to allay her anxiety and fear of cancer. It is often helpful to explain that fibrocystic disease is probably a normal variant of the response to physiologic hormonal fluctuation, and the patient does not have a "disease." However, in light of the high incidence of breast cancer among American women, each patient should be instructed in the technique of breast self-examination and advised to have periodic screening examinations and mammograms. Mammograms are indicated for older women with fibrocystic disease to search for an occult malignant tumor. However, the woman in her twenties or early thirties with clinical fibrocystic disease and no dominant mass is not likely to benefit from mammography. In general, these patients' breasts are extremely dense and mammograms are not helpful. However, a screening mammogram should be obtained at least once even in young patients. Ultrasound may be extremely helpful in distinguishing a cystic from a solid lesion. Since fibrocystic disease may be indistinguishable from carcinoma on the basis of clinical findings, a biopsy is mandatory for every patient with a dominant mass or one who has a cyst that had bloody fluid or recurred after complete aspiration, even if there are no suspicious areas on the mammogram. The pain associated with fibrocystic disease is best treated by avoiding trauma and wearing a supportive brassiere. Mild analgesics may be indicated for the times when the patient has the most pain.

Hormonal therapy is generally not advisable. Tamoxifen, a potent antiestrogen that binds to cytosol receptor sites, has been used to induce regression of fibrocystic breast nodules. Bromocriptine, which inhibits secretion of prolactin, has similarly been effective in relieving symptoms attributed to fibrocystic disease. However, most clinical experience is with the drug danazol. Danazol is an androgen derivative that suppresses pituitary secretion of LH and FSH and interferes with gonadal steroidogenesis. The drug appears to be effective in reducing breast pain and nodularity. However, there is a high incidence of side effects, predominantly menstrual disorders and hot flashes. These render this drug of limited clinical value for the management of fibrocystic disease, except perhaps for the most unusually severe cases.

The role of caffeine consumption in the etiology and treatment of fibrocystic disease is controversial. Minton has shown that elimination of methyl xanthenes from the diet results in dramatic reduction of the clinical symptoms of fibrocystic disease. However, conflicting reports have appeared evaluating the role of caffeine consumption in the etiology and treatment of fibrocystic disease. Since the symptoms of fibrocystic disease frequently fluctuate, it is difficult to determine whether reduction in caffeine intake is related to diminution of symptoms. However, a number of studies suggest that elimination of methyl xanthenes from the diet will improve the symptoms of fibrocystic disease. Whether this improvement of symptoms is related to an etiologic role of caffeine or to a placebo effect is unknown. Most women with fibrocystic disease are unwilling to eliminate coffee from their diet once they understand that fibrocystic disease itself is not a premalignant condition. Interestingly, most patients with breast pain and premenstrual tenderness have decreased their intake of caffeine by the time they see their physician. Similarly, there is little evidence that vitamin E intake alters the course of fibrocystic disease. Most significantly, there is little to suggest that use of vitamin E or elimination of caffeine will alter a hyperplastic epithelium.

Surgical Considerations

In general, operations for fibrocystic disease should be limited to biopsies to excise a dominant mass in order to determine that it is not malignant. Prophylactic subcutaneous mastectomy has been recommended both as treatment for fibrocystic disease and prevention of cancer. In general, prophylactic subcutaneous mastectomies are not indicated. Most patients with fibrocystic disease probably do not have a risk of developing breast cancer significantly higher than other patients. In addition, subcutaneous mastectomy is not a guarantee against the development of breast cancer. The treatment of fibrocystic disease with total mastectomy is rarely indicated. In general, mastectomy (any type) should not be performed for fibrocystic disease.

The patient with fibrocystic disease who has a dominant mass that appears solid on attempted aspiration should undergo biopsy. A common error is to obtain a mammogram that shows no evidence of malignancy and then to defer biopsy. Regardless of the mammographic findings, a dominant mass should undergo biopsy. In general, biopsy can be performed in an outpatient setting under local anesthesia. The mass should be totally excised whenever possible and sent to the pathologist for diagnosis.

BREAST CANCER: STAGE I AND II

RUDOLPH ALMARAZ, M.D., Ph.D.

It is estimated that one out of eleven American women will be diagnosed as having breast cancer. This translates into over 110,000 new cases of breast cancer per year and accounts for approximately 27 percent of all cancers in women. Controversy continues over the management of all stages of breast cancer, but in this chapter only stage I and stage II will be discussed. The staging system shown in Table 1 is the one most widely used and was adopted by both the UICC (International Union Against Cancer) and the AJC (American Joint Commission on Cancer Staging and End Results Reporting). It is based on the TNM system of clinical staging. From a clinical point of view, stage I and stage II breast cancer are also known as "primary operable breast cancer" and therefore are primarily treated surgically.

RISK FACTORS

Unfortunately, the etiology of breast cancer is unknown at present, but certain risk factors have been identified, and they play a significant role in the etiology and pathogenesis of human breast cancer. Perhaps one of the most impressive risk factors is that of genetic predisposition. There are groups of women identified whose risk for breast cancer has been estimated to be approximately 50-fold higher than that experienced by control women. These high-risk women are sisters of breast cancer patients whose mother also had breast cancer. The disease in this family situation usually develops in the premenopausal period and is often bilateral. Another less heritable form is found in patients who have had two affected sisters but unaffected mothers. The risk in these women is at least three-fold higher than that of controls, and this disease process appears to be primarily in the postmenopausal period.

There still exists significant controversy over the risk factors for breast cancer in women with proliferative

TABLE 1 Staging of Breast Cancer

T   Primary tumors
T1   Tumor 2 cm or less in its greatest dimension
    a. No fixation to underlying pectoral fascia or muscle
    b. Fixation to underlying pectoral fascia or muscle
T2   Tumor more than 2 cm but not more than 5 cm in its greatest dimension
T3   Tumor more than 5 cm in its greatest dimension
    a. No fixation to underlying pectoral fascia or muscle
    b. Fixation to underlying pectoral fascia or muscle
T4   Tumor of any size with direct extension to chest wall or skin
    Note: Chest wall includes ribs, intercostal muscles, and serratus anterior muscle, but not pectoral muscle
    a. Fixation to chest wall
    b. Edema (including peau d'orange) ulceration of the skin of the breast, or satellite skin nodules confined to the same breast
    c. Both of above
    d. Inflammatory carcinoma

Dimpling of the skin, nipple retraction, or any other skin changes except those in T4b may occur in T1, T2, or T3 without affecting the classification.

N   Regional lymph nodes
N0   No palpable homolateral axillary nodes
N1   Movable homolateral axillary nodes
    a. Nodes not considered to contain growth
    b. Nodes considered to contain growth
N2   Homolateral axillary nodes containing growth and fixed to one another or to other structures
N3   Homolateral supraclavicular or infraclavicular nodes containing growth or edema of the arm

M   Distant metastasis
M0   No evidence of distant metastasis
M1   Distant metastasis present, including skin involvement beyond the breast area

Clinical Stage-Grouping

Stage I	T1a	N0 or N1a	
	T1b	N0 or N1a	M0
Stage II	T0	N1b	
	T1a	N1b	
	T1b	N1b	M0
	T2a or T2b	N0, N1a, or N1b	
Stage III	T1a or T1b	N2	M0
	T2a or T2b	N2	M0
	T3a or T3b	N0, N1, or N2	M0
Stage IV	T4	any N	any M
	any T	N3	any M
	any T	any N	M1

"benign" fibrocystic disease. Benign fibrocystic disease is diagnosed commonly in American women, and its relationship to breast cancer should be addressed. Recent studies have indicated that nonproliferative lesions of fibrocystic disease do not have an associated significant risk of malignancy. On the other hand, the risk in women with atypical hyperplasia (atypia) has been noted to be about five times higher than in women with nonproliferative lesions. The risk of breast cancer in women with atypia and a family history of breast cancer has also been noted to be about 11 times higher than in women with nonproliferative lesions without a family history of breast cancer. In summary, recent data indicate that the majority of women (approximately 70%) diagnosed as having fibrocystic disease are not at an increased risk of cancer. There is, however, a patient population with atypical hyperplasia and a family history of breast cancer who have a clinically significant elevation of cancer risk. These women should be followed closely with yearly breast examination and yearly mammography.

EARLY DETECTION OF BREAST CANCER

It must be emphasized that women should begin self breast examination at an early age. In order to encourage this, many school systems have started programs that teach adolescent girls the basic principles of self breast examination. It is hoped that such programs will educate women in the necessity of such examinations and thus aid in the early detection of early breast cancer. Self breast examination should be performed on a monthly schedule and should be done approximately one week postmenstrually. Women with a strong familial history of cancer should also be followed with regularly scheduled mammography. Also, women with extensive fibrocystic disease and breasts that are difficult to examine should undergo routine mammography in order to identify early breast cancer. The interval for routine mammography is variable, but the study probably should not be done more often than once a year. In women 40 years of age or older, a combination of careful routine self breast examination, yearly examination by an experienced breast surgeon or gynecologist, and mammography every 18 months is sufficient to follow most women with only minimal-to-moderate risk of developing breast cancer. Women at very high risk should undergo mammography on a yearly basis after the age of 30.

Any abnormal mass that is easily palpated in women who are at high risk should be excised for a definitive diagnosis. In premenopausal women, abnormal masses can often be aspirated in hopes of identifying benign cystic masses. If a mass cannot be aspirated or is suspicious in nature, the mass should be excised in its entirety for definitive diagnosis. Biopsy should not be avoided if the mass is thought to be abnormal, even if a mammogram does not demonstrate any abnormality, since mammography is only approximately 85 percent accurate in diagnosing cancer.

Since mammography has become a part of a routine breast examination by many family physicians and gynecologists, nonpalpable xeromammographic lesions are being discovered more frequently. These lesions are generally represented as microcalcifications or as well-circumscribed lesions showing architectural distortion within the mass. All clearly abnormal xeromammographic abnormalities should be excised. If the abnormality is questionable and a mass cannot be palpated, it is usually acceptable to follow this patient closely, to repeat mammography in 6 months, and to examine the patient at that time for any abnormalities. I have found preoperative localization of nonpalpable xeromammographic lesions by an experienced radiologist to be quite helpful. This localization is done in the mammography suite, percutaneously, and is followed with injection of a dye into the abnormality. Shortly after localization, the patient is taken to the operating room where, under sterile conditions and either general or local anesthesia, the mass is excised in its entirety, sparing normal breast parenchyma. The specimen excised is sent to the mammography suite, and its total excision is confirmed by mammography. The lesion is then sent for histopathologic examination. Unless a lesions is felt to be clearly consistent with carcinoma preoperatively, I usually recommend only an excisional biopsy of the abnormality. In women with clearly palpable or easily diagnosed breast cancer, surgical options are often discussed with the patient before a biopsy is performed so that she can make her choice early enough to permit all required surgery to be performed during one procedure. When significant uncertainty exists as to the possibility of carcinoma, I believe that excision alone is adequate before any definitive decisions are made. The anxiety evoked by the fear of having breast cancer and facing possible mastectomy is often of significant magnitude and should be avoided unless there is strong clinical suspicion of cancer. On the other hand, if the clinician feels strongly that the diagnosis is certain, I feel the patient should be offered the option of proceeding with definitive therapy at the time of her biopsy in order to prevent any further delay in her treatment, and thus minimizing the severe anxiety that may accompany waiting. If the patient wishes to have definitive proof of her lesion before she chooses her surgical options, it is perfectly reasonable to perform only an excisional biopsy and then discuss all of the options subsequently.

Every patient with the diagnosis of breast carcinoma should have recent bilateral mammography in order to fully evaluate both breasts. Mammography is often done preoperatively, but if, for some reason, it has not been done, it should certainly be done before a definitive procedure is performed. Further preoperative evaluation includes the complete history and physical examination, a recent chest film, and blood chemistries in search of abnormalities in liver function or bone metabolism. If a patient gives a history of bone disease, a preoperative bone scan should be obtained, or if there is any abnormality in the liver function tests, a preoperative liver scan should also be obtained. It is important to carefully stage the patient's disease preoperatively to ensure appropriate treatment. In cases of early breast cancer, the likelihood of distant metastasis is minimal, but still possible, and should be investigated.

DETERMINANTS

Among the many factors to be considered in counseling a patient on her options for the treatment of primary operable breast cancer are her age, her general medical condition, the histology of the primary tumor, the size and shape of her breasts, her genetic risk factors, and her own personal desires.

Histologic Type and Multicentricity

It has become apparent from recent data that certain breast cancers do not respond adequately to simple excision followed by adjuvant radiation therapy. Among the types noted to be associated with a high local recurrence rate are preinvasive lesions. Tumors involving more than 50 percent of the intraductal component and demonstrating preinvasive cancer at the margins of resection, significant pleomorphism, and a high mitotic index cannot be adequately treated with adjuvant radiotherapy. Furthermore, if margins of the previous excisional procedure are inadequate the risk of local recurrence is greater, and many radiation therapists are not recommending adjuvant radiation therapy as a conservative option in these patients unless negative margins can be obtained. Patients who present with stage I or stage II breast cancer and have either lobular carcinoma in situ or intraductal carcinoma should also be advised to undergo modified radical mastectomy because (1) there is still no convincing evidence that radiation therapy is as effective as mastectomy, and (2) these two types of in situ lesions, if treated by biopsy alone, have a high risk of developing subsequent carcinoma owing to their multicentricity. With respect to lobular carcinoma in situ, patients who have been observed for 25 years have demonstrated an increasing risk of developing subsequent carcinoma. More than half these patients have been diagnosed more than 15 years after the biopsy. In addition to this risk, the bilateral nature of this histologic type is to be considered, and contralateral breast biopsies should be performed. I do not recommend bilateral mastectomies in this situation; if biopsy of the contralateral breast shows no disease, that breast can be observed carefully by physical examination and routine mammography. According to recent data, 30 to 70 percent of patients with intraductal carcinoma treated by excision alone developed breast cancer in the ipsilateral breast within a 10-year period.

Axillary Lymph Node Staging

Since most institutions are considering adjuvant chemotherapy or hormonal manipulation in both pre- and postmenopausal women with documented axillary lymph node metastases, it is critical to properly stage an individual with primary breast cancer. The importance of adequate staging raises the question of how extensive the axillary lymph node dissection should be to ensure proper staging as well as proper treatment of the axilla. It is a well known fact, that Clinical assessment of axillary lymph nodes is, at best, accurate only in approximately two-thirds of patients. Approximately one-third of clinically negative nodes are histologically positive, and the same fraction of clinically positive nodes are found to be histologically negative. Reports of large series indicate that the pathologic status of axillary lymph nodes is the most important determining factor in the prognosis. Among patients observed for more than 30 years, those who had histopathologically negative nodes have at least an 80 percent survival, whereas those who had histopathologically positive nodes have a survival of 40 percent. In addition, the number of lymph nodes involved is probably also significant. Patients with less than four involved axillary lymph nodes are apt to have a better long-term survival than those with more than four positive nodes.

One of the leading controversies in the management of primary operable breast cancer concerns the role of lymph node dissection as a means of therapy. Physicians who believe that lymph node metastases are a harbinger of systemic disease support the concept that complete axillary dissections are not required because they have no therapeutic benefit and sampling or limited axillary dissections are adequate for staging. Other physicians have compared axillary lymph node biopsies to axillary lymph node sampling by pathologic evaluation of axillary nodes removed after complete axillary dissection, and have demonstrated that axillary node biopsies failed to detect metastases in over 40 percent of patients. Axillary node sampling or partial axillary dissection failed to recognize approximately 25 percent of patients with axillary metastases. Even if no therapeutic benefit is expected from a complete axillary dissection, the procedure is required for adequate staging. I therefore recommend complete axillary dissection for all cases of invasive breast carcinoma. This procedure includes removal of all lymphatic tissue from the axillary tail of the breast up to the axillary vein. The pectoralis major muscle and latissimus dorsi muscle are the medial and lateral boundaries of the dissection. I remove the pectoralis minor muscle in performing the dissection because this permits complete dissection of all level I through level III lymph nodes.

In approximately 12 to 14 percent of patients with inner quadrant lesions and histologically negative axillary lymph nodes, there exist histologically positive internal mammary lymph nodes. It therefore becomes necessary to perform internal mammary lymph node staging in these patients in order to properly stage them and thus provide adequate adjuvant chemotherapy or hormonal therapy.

SURGICAL OPTIONS FOR PRIMARY OPERABLE DISEASE

There are actually three options available in managing primary operable breast cancer. These include a wide excision (partial mastectomy) alone followed by no adjuvant therapy, a wide excision of the primary (partial mastectomy), complete axillary dissection and adjuvant radiation therapy, and a modified radical mastectomy. The first option has been investigated but is associated with an approximately 30 to 35 percent incidence of local recurrence. This is an option which I feel should not be considered in a healthy woman unless there is a medical contraindication to further surgical therapy or to the addition of adjuvant radiation therapy. The two main options available for primary operable breast cancer, are those mainly of modified radical mastectomy, and partial mastectomy, complete axillary dissection and adjuvant radiation therapy postoperatively.

Modified Radical Mastectomy

The preferred modified radical mastectomy for the treatment of infiltrating breast cancer is the Patey type. This procedure involves a total mastectomy, complete axillary dissection, and removal of the pectoralis minor muscle. I tend to preserve both nerves, namely, the long thoracic and the thoracodorsal nerve and vessels, although some prefer to remove the thoracodorsal nerve and vessels along with the specimen. For in situ lobular or intraductal carcinoma, I prefer the modified radical mastectomy described by Auchincloss, which preserves the pectoralis minor muscle. This allows for a total mastectomy and dissection of the low and midaxilla (levels I and II), but does not provide adequate access to dissection of level III nodes, which do not have to be removed in these situations. The radical mastectomy is rarely advocated in the treatment of stage I or stage II breast carcinoma.

Partial Mastectomy, Axillary Dissection, and Radiation Therapy

According to long-term data from Milan and their prospective randomized trial, quadrantectomy (entire quadrant of breast including pectoral fascia), axillary dissection, and postoperative radiation therapy for stage I breast cancer has a survival rate identical to that for radical mastectomy. However, this prospective randomized trial is still of short duration, and the real long-term results of such data are unavailable. Nonetheless, the data available at this time clearly indicate no difference in survival between these options. Other series, however, report a slightly higher incidence of local regional recurrence with partial mastectomy and adjuvant radiation therapy than with modified radical mastectomy, but current data seem to indicate that salvage surgery (i.e., modified radical mastectomy) does provide an acceptable 5-year survival (55%). Patients who have recurrence in the axilla alone or in the axilla and breast have been demonstrated to have only a 30 percent survival after 10 years.

Another therapeutic dilemma is the case of the woman who chooses to have a partial mastectomy, axillary dissection, and adjuvant radiation therapy and is found to have positive lymph nodes. The timing of the administration of adjuvant cytotoxic chemotherapy and adjuvant radiotherapy becomes an issue, although there is evidence in such cases that adjuvant radiation therapy can safely be administered simultaneously with cytotoxic chemotherapy without significant morbidity. Patients in this situation are often advised by surgeons to undergo a complete modified radical mastectomy in order to avoid adjuvant radiation therapy and then to proceed with systemic chemotherapy or hormonal therapy since the patient's main risk at this point is probably systemic disease. Incidental positive nodes found after axillary dissection should not necessarily indicate the need for complete mastectomy.

It is important to point out that all treatment options should be presented to a patient with breast cancer before any definitive procedure is performed. The multidisciplinary approach required for optimal care includes the professional yet sympathetic input from the surgical oncologist, the radiation therapist, and the medical oncologist. It is important that all these individuals have the patient's best interest at heart and are cooperative in their efforts. Such a relationship between these physicians is seen as reassuring and comforting to a woman and her family who find themselves in this distressing situation.

ADJUVANT CHEMOTHERAPY AND HORMONAL THERAPY

Available data clearly indicate the benefits of adjuvant cytotoxic chemotherapy in premenopausal women with documented positive lymph nodes. The agents primarily used include cytoxan, methotrexate, Adriamycin, 5-fluorouracil, and prednisone. Controversy continues over the benefit of these adjuvants in postmenopausal women.

Women with breast cancer who possess positive estrogen and progesterone receptors seem to benefit from the administration of antiestrogen therapy. Encouraging are the evolving data indicating the benefit of oral tamoxifen in postmenopausal women with positive lymph nodes. This agent is safe and has minimal side effects, and thus its use should be encouraged in this clinical situation.

BREAST CANCER: SURGICAL STAGING AND RADIATION THERAPY

JULIAN W. PROCTOR, M.D.
STANLEY E. ORDER, M.D., Sc.D.

The surgeon who is committed to the treatment of breast cancer derives considerable satisfaction from his participation in the preservative management of breast cancer by surgical staging and the radiation therapy that follows. The three major problems of breast cancer—(1) local regional control, (2) dissemination, and (3) the psychological impact of therapy—may be addressed by this more conservative approach to breast cancer management.

This review addresses the indications for this therapy, its important technical aspects, complications, results, and controversies, and its effect on the three major problems of breast cancer.

RECONSTRUCTION AFTER MASTECTOMY

Great strides have been made in the area of plastic surgery involving breast reconstruction. Newer, more natural prostheses are available for postmastectomy patients. The introduction of subpectoral muscle placement of prostheses has also improved the postoperative reconstruction results and provides patients with more natural-feeling prosthetic breasts.

The introduction of autologous muscle flaps for reconstruction has expanded the role of reconstruction after mastectomy, particularly in large-breasted women and in women sustaining significant radiation injury to the anterior chest wall after adjuvant radiation therapy.

In summary, some form of breast reconstruction can be offered to most women contemplating mastectomy. The timing of breast reconstruction is variable, but I personally feel it can be offered to most women at the time of initial mastectomy. The old concept of waiting 6 months is not always necessary or even fair to most women. Women with preinvasive lesions or stage I disease are not at high risk for local regional recurrence, and thus should be offered the opportunity for immediate breast reconstruction. Women who undergo bilateral prophylactic mastectomies because they are at high risk of developing breast cancer should certainly be offered bilateral reconstruction immediately. The ultimate decision regarding the timing of breast reconstruction should be made jointly by the surgical oncologist, the plastic surgeon, and the patient herself.

LOCAL CONTROL

Size of the Lesion

The dose of radiation necessary to control breast cancer increases as the primary lesion increases in size. Therefore, ideal candidates are patients with T1 and T2 lesions. Patients who have such lesions excised and undergo radiation therapy, in our experience, may expect a 95 percent local control rate at 5 years and a 90 percent local control rate at 10 years. T3 lesions are less easily controlled even when excised, and except for special criteria, as enumerated by Hellman when he reported a series from Harvard, most radiation oncologists would not treat patients with 5 cm or larger lesions by the methods described.

Lymph Nodes

Most authorities, regardless of orientation, agree that the number of tumor-positive nodes in the axilla relates

TABLE 1 Recommendations for Surgical Technique

Primary excision discontinuous with axillary dissection

Circumferential incisions for upper quadrants

Radial incisions for lower quadrants

Placement of the scar over the primary site

Measurement of depth of tumor bed or use of metal clips

Level I and II axillary dissection with a clip marking the upper limit of dissection

Inking of resection margins

Modified from Fisher B. National Adjuvant Breast Cancer Program (NASBP)

to prognosis. Although fine distinction may be drawn between one positive node and 3 to 4 or more positive nodes, a variety of adjuvant chemotherapy and/or hormonal management decisions are made on the basis of such data in combination with hormonal status and tumor hormone receptors.

Role of the Surgeon

By providing an adequate description of location and size of the primary lesion, by performing a complete surgical excision of the primary lesion with clean margins in association with an axillary dissection of level I and II lymph nodes, and by submitting 6 to 8 nodes for pathologic examination, the surgeon supplies the guidelines for radiation therapy and/or a combined modality program. In doing so, the surgeon must consider the following:

1. If the primary excision has tumor cells at the margin, either re-excision or a higher dose of radiation is necessary for local control.
2. An adequate level I and II surgical staging of the axilla (6 to 8 lymph nodes) renders axillary radiation unnecessary and therefore reduces the probability of both arm edema and local recurrence.
3. Surgical scars that extend to the posterior axillary lines or around the chest wall, or across the chest anteriorly, require more fields of radiation to cover the operative field, thus increasing radiation risks.
4. A cosmetically unappealing excision has an adverse psychological effect on the patient. The criteria for surgical excision that appear in Table 1 were suggested by Fisher et al.

The knowledge that such conservative treatment (i.e., surgical excision, axillary dissection, breast retention, and definitive radiation) is available encourages patients to carry out self-examination and to see the surgeon earlier. Both retrospective and prospective studies have reported local and regional control (Table 2), good cosmesis, and more acceptable psychologic impact on patients. The surgeon retains his role and his value as an oncologist while displaying a new sophistication in patient management.

IMPORTANT TECHNICAL ASPECTS OF RADIATION THERAPY

In the past, before the era of sophisticated treatment simulation, treatment planning computers, and other treatment modifiers, the quality of cosmesis without major complications was not so easily achieved. In our experience, using Johns Hopkins techniques, 90 percent or more of the patients should have excellent cosmetic results. Obese women are generally not ideal candidates, owing to the need for either greater energy or increased dose to achieve an acceptable tumor minimum dose.

Essentially there are two techniques for breast irradiation. One technique uses tangential breast fields, including the internal mammary chain, with a second and separate supraclavicular field. The second technique uses a field encompassing the supraclavicular fossa and internal mammary chain (the field being called the "hockey stick") and a second set of tangential opposed fields encompassing the breast. These fields are compared in Table 3.

The potential disadvantage of lung irradiation may be resultant pneumonitis or lung fibrosis; however, this is a rare occurrence with modern techniques. The irradiation of the internal mammary chain is of particular importance in inner quadrant lesions, central lesions, and lesions with postoperative axillary nodes, owing to the increased incidence of positive internal mammary nodes. Heart irradiation can be a potential disadvantage if the volume of heart in the field is large and if Adriamycin is to be used. Irradiation of the spine could reduce future radiation palliation for spinal metastasis.

"Matchline fibrosis" is fibrosis that occurs between the supraclavicular and tangential breast fields. The uninitiated surgeon may become concerned over the induration in this region. Several techniques have been worked out. A variety of blocks reducing the irradiation from linear accelerators or the use of cobalt-60 irradiation modifies such problems.

Lung irradiation may be reduced by placement of the patient on an angled breast board that makes the lung parallel to the field of irradiation. Three planes of treatment planning for radiation dose distribution improve the cosmetic results.

TABLE 2 Local Control of Stage I–II Breast Cancer Managed with Excisional Resection and Radiation Therapy (1,893 patients)

	5 Years	10 Years
Yale	92%	---
Institute Curie	94%	89%
Marseilles	94%	88%
Long Island	---	90%
Toronto	91%	82%
Royal Marsden	85%	74%
Villejuif	92%	---
Milan	94%	---
Harvard	91%	---

TABLE 3 Comparison of Radiation Therapy Techniques in Breast Cancer

Field Technique	Advantages	Disadvantages
Tangential breast, supraclavicular	Spares heart and thoracic spine	Potential increase of lung volume; not as secure in coverage of internal mammary chain
Internal mammary chain, supra-clavicular (hockey stick), tangential breast	Secure internal mammary radiation; reduces potential lung irradiation	Irradiates heart and thoracic spine

Finally, fractionated electron radiation of the surgical scar produces less cosmetic deformity of the local region than is produced by radioactive seed implantation techniques.

COMPLICATIONS OF RADIATION THERAPY

In properly managed patients, arm edema has occurred in less than 5 percent of the patients since the axilla is not treated. Breast cosmesis is not satisfactory in 5 percent of patients, and this may be improved by patient selection. Brachial plexopathy may occur in less than 1 percent of patients, pneumonitis in less than 2 percent. The incidence of rib fractures varies from 1 to 5 percent, whereas fibrosis at the matchline occurs in at least 15 to 20 percent of patients, and although it does not cause symptoms, it reduces cosmetic perfection.

RESULTS OF RADIATION THERAPY

The reported local regional control at 5 years should be 90 percent or greater, and at 10 years, 80 to 92 percent (Table 2). Neither surgery nor radiation therapy influences systemic disease.

CONTROVERSIES

Breast cancer remains controversial only because there are no absolute methods of guaranteeing disease-free survival. Radiation oncologists are attempting to reduce fields and doses of radiation to further enhance cosmesis, to reduce complications, and to continue to achieve high local regional control rates. Medical oncologists report adjuvant programs to increase duration of disease-free survival, but "cure" remains elusive.

The patient with an inner quadrant lesion, T1 or T2, and negative axillary nodes, although historically having a good prognosis, is often denied best treatment because internal mammary nodal assessment is not available.

Randomized trials have clearly demonstrated equality between the various radical surgical procedures and the modified procedures and radiation therapy. Yet some surgeons cannot accept change and privately carry out excision and axillary dissection without radiation therapy; they do not share with their patients the information regarding the 25 percent or greater incidence of local regional failure. A randomized study should be designed to address such a question.

Those surgeons, radiation oncologists, and medical oncologists who are patient advocates realize the advantages and disadvantages of all of the procedures and remain committed to the multimodality approach and to patients, not to techniques or specialty.

MAJOR PROBLEMS OF BREAST CANCER

In early-stage breast cancer (T1-T2), excisional resection and axillary dissection allow for cosmetic preservation of the breast with excellent local regional control greater than 90 percent at 5 years. However, the modified masectomy does not require 5 weeks of committed time and, in appropriate patients who are unconcerned about cosmesis, remains an appropriate technique of management.

Excisional resection and axillary dissection without radiation therapy, if not part of a formal scientific study, is not a standard of the oncologic community. Initial consultation with the surgeon and the radiation and medical oncologists remains the best management plan.

Disseminated Disease

Although discussion continues regarding premenopausal and postmenopausal status and estrogen and progesterone receptor positivity, "best opinion" may only be achieved after adequate surgical staging, at which time it is decided whether research or standard care should be applied.

Psychologic Impact

The breast remains one of the more revered organs of artistic expression and a symbol of femininity. Why should a woman remove her breast without cause or advantage? At the minimum, a woman should be told the truth, as far as it is known, and whatever appropriate treatment she chooses should be supported by all physicians concerned.

Procedures available for the treatment of breast cancer include (1) radical mastectomy (Halsted), (2) modified radical mastectomy, (3) simple mastectomy and postoperative radiation (McWhirter), (4) modified radical mastectomy with postoperative radiation (Einhorn), (5) extended mastectomy (Urban), (6) simple resection (Crile), (7) excisional resection and/or axillary dissection with radiation therapy (Peters, Montague, Hellman, and others), (8) quadrantectomy with postoperative radiation (Veronesi), and (9) excision and staging with varied postoperative radiation(Fisher, Lichter).

Radiation therapy remains a method of increasing local regional control and preserving breast cosmesis.

UNUSUAL FORMS OF BREAST CANCER

ARTHUR J. DONOVAN, M.D.

Malignant tumor of the breast may arise from epithelium of the ducts within the breast, from the cells within the breast lobule, and in rare instances, from stromal elements. The majority of infiltrating carcinomas of the breast are of duct cell origin. The pattern in over three-quarters of cases is that of a scirrhous growth with considerable fibrotic reaction in the area about the tumor. The tumor infiltrates and extends its tentacles into the surrounding tissue.

PATHOLOGIC VARIANTS

There are a number of pathologic variants of adenocarcinoma of duct cell origin which have a somewhat more favorable prognosis than does the scirrhous form. These pathologic variants include ductal carcinomas with a pushing rather than an infiltrating border, medullary carcinoma, comedocarcinoma, papillary carcinoma, colloid carcinoma, and tubular carcinoma.

Medullary carcinoma tends to be bulky and contains areas of hemorrhage and cyst formation. There are sheets of cells with scant stoma that is infiltrated with lymphocytes. In comedocarcinoma, the ducts are blocked with cellular debris, and on cut surface the debris projects from the ducts in a manner resembling "blackheads" (comedones). Papillary carcinoma is an infiltrating lesion which on occasion can be difficult to distinguish from a duct papilloma. The papillomatous process extends through the duct wall into the surrounding tissue. Colloid carcinoma is soft and ill-defined; it can be bulky and contains large mucinous lakes. Tubular carcinoma is well differentiated with an orderly pattern of growth. All of the aforementioned tumors are associated with a lower incidence of lymph node metastasis and a less aggressive biological behavior.

Cancer may develop from the mammary lobules (see chapter on *Lobular Carcinoma in Situ*). Infiltrating lobular carcinoma is an uncommon lesion and has a propensity for bilaterality. With lobular carcinoma, either in situ or infiltrating, tumor is present in the other breast in at least 50 percent of patients. As with the variants of infiltrating duct carcinoma just described, infiltrating lobular carcinoma also has a somewhat more favorable prognosis.

With a good technologic approach, the results are excellent in achieving the desired goals. However, its success is determined in part by the judgment and skill of the surgeon in achieving local regional control and improving the quality of life for his patient.

The treatment of these pathologic variants of breast cancer is that of invasive cancer. The behavior of the individual tumor cannot be predicted, and the usual treatment of breast cancer should be pursued. A discussion of the current controversy as to acceptable therapy of breast cancer is beyond the scope of this chapter. Suffice it to say that my choice for surgery is a modified radical mastectomy. The combination of segmental mastectomy, axillary dissection, and radiation therapy to the breast is acceptable as therapy for selected patients such as those with clinical stage I cancer (tumor <2 cm; clinically negative nodes). If pathologic examination reveals tumor in lymph nodes, adjuvant chemotherapy is recommended.

CLINICAL VARIANTS

In addition to the aforementioned variants of infiltrating breast cancer that are identifiable on histologic examination, several unique clinical forms of breast cancer deserve special consideration. They may or may not have specific pathologic features and include Paget's disease of the nipple, inflammatory breast cancer, cancer occurring during pregnancy, bilateral breast cancer, breast cancer in the male, and malignant cystosarcoma phylloides.

Paget's Disease

Paget's disease of the breast is an adenocarcinoma of the breast that arises in the main excretory ducts beneath the nipple. The tumor grows out through the ducts onto the nipple and produces an eczema-like lesion. This may initially appear to be innocuous and its significance may not be recognized. Diagnosis may be delayed. The breast cancer is palpable in less than half the cases. Biopsy of the nipple establishes the diagnosis based on typical histology. Paget cells are large cells with clear cytoplasm and small dark nuclei. When these cells are seen in a nipple biopsy one may be assured that there is an underlying breast carcinoma, whether or not it is palpable. The prognosis is better in those cases in which there is not a palpable underlying cancer. The conventional therapy for Paget's disease of the nipple has been modified radical mastectomy. In the absence of palpable nodes and of a palpable mass in the breast, radiation therapy might be considered. Results have not been reported that establish its efficacy in treatment of this form of breast cancer. Conventional surgical therapy with adjuvant chemotherapy based on nodal status remains the therapeutic choice.

Inflammatory Breast Cancer

Inflammatory breast cancer is a specific clinical and pathologic type of tumor. The skin of the breast is red and inflamed. There may be a rather sharp edge to the area of redness which closely represents streptococcal cellulitis or erysipelas. Dermal edema and peau d'orange are noted. The patient complains of a burning pain in the breast. There is an underlying mass of infiltrating carcinoma. Histologic study of a biopsy of the skin shows that the dermal lymphatics are plugged with tumor cells. Inflammatory breast cancer must be distinguished from a breast cancer that has invaded the skin and in which there is a localized area of redness, with or without ulceration, and from the rare case of carcinoma with duct obstruction and an associated bacterial cellulitis. If the diagnosis is suspected, a skin biopsy should be performed for confirmation.

In the past, the course for inflammatory breast cancer has been one of rapid progression without long-term survival. A direct surgical approach with resection fosters rapid local extension of the tumor and is contraindicated. There has been recent experience with multimodality therapy for inflammatory breast carcinoma. In several trials, chemotherapy, radiation therapy, and surgery have been used in various combinations. Conceptually, the approach is one of initial attempt to control local disease with either chemotherapy or radiation therapy. If there is a favorable regression of the breast disease in response to this initial therapy, surgery is performed as a secondary procedure. Most of these protocols consist of three to five courses of induction chemotherapy. Multiple drug combinations are used, such as the Cooper's regimen of cytoxan, methotrexate, 5-fluorouracil, vincristine, and prednisone. Adriamycin has been selected by some because of the high sensitivity of breast cancer to this particular agent. When the response to chemotherapy has been one of regression of the evidence of inflammatory skin involvement, a modified radical mastectomy may be performed. Postoperatively, the patient usually receives radiation therapy to the chest wall and lymphatic drainage areas. Maintenance chemotherapy is administered for at least 18 months. Five-year survival rates in the range of 25 percent have been reported with this aggressive therapeutic approach. This is a major advance over an essentially zero 5-year survival reported for surgery alone or radiation therapy alone. Because of current interest in multimodality therapy of inflammatory breast cancer, new information is evolving rapidly. The patient with inflammatory breast cancer should no longer be assumed to be incurable.

Breast Cancer and Pregnancy

The diagnosis of breast cancer that develops during pregnancy is often delayed. Because profound changes occur in the structure of the breast during pregnancy, mass lesion may be overlooked. Any solid lesion of the breast identified during pregnancy must promptly undergo biopsy to establish its pathologic nature. The prognosis of breast cancer that develops during pregnancy was formerly thought to be dismal. This is not necessarily true. Numerous studies have documented that for a given stage, the prognosis for breast cancer developing during pregnancy does not differ significantly from that in the non-pregnant female. A much higher percentage of patients with breast cancer diagnosed during pregnancy do have a more advanced stage of the disease with positive lymph nodes and overt dissemination. In cases with disseminated disease, the hormonal environment during pregnancy may foster more aggressive growth of tumor. This stimulation may also extend into the period of lactation.

The treatment of breast cancer that occurs during pregnancy should be that of any breast cancer, and the priority should be the treatment of the breast cancer, not the management of the pregnancy. If disease is limited to the breast and ipsilateral axilla, modified radical mastectomy is indicated. The risk of precipitating an abortion is greatest in the first trimester. During the second trimester of pregnancy, patients tolerate the surgical treatment of breast cancer well. Individual judgment is necessary regarding the patient in the third trimester, in whom surgery can induce premature labor. With disseminated disease, it may be preferable to terminate the pregnancy by cesarean section as soon as it is believed that the fetus is viable and then to proceed with therapy of the cancer. Lactation should be suppressed in any patient with breast cancer that is diagnosed during pregnancy. If lymph nodes are involved, administration of chemotherapy would be contraindicated because of possible fetal effects and should be delayed. Radiation therapy is contraindicated during pregnancy. Patients who have had breast cancer are generally advised not to become pregnant until at least 5 years following treatment and then if they are free of the disease.

Bilateral Breast Cancer

A clinical diagnosis of bilateral breast cancer is made in approximately 7 percent of patients at the time of initial diagnosis and in at least another 7 to 10 percent of patients during their subsequent lifetime. The incidences just cited are significantly lower than the incidence of bilateral breast cancer that would be detected if one were to do routine biopsies or serial histologic sections of the opposite breast in a search for covert cancer. Many of the cancers detected by detailed scrutiny for covert cancer might well be so-called pathologist's cancer, which would never achieve clinical significance. The incidence of bilaterality is higher with medullary carcinoma and with lobular carcinoma. Mammography should be performed on the opposite breast prior to treatment of carcinoma of the breast to detect occult carcinoma that may be already present in the opposite breast. Urban has recommended, in women with proven cancer of one breast, a routine biopsy of the upper outer quadrant of the opposite breast as well as of the mirror image of the site of the cancer. The latter biopsy is performed if the initial cancer is not in the upper outer quadrant. This recommendation has not been widely adopted, other than for medullary and lobular carcinomas. The greatest risk factor for development of breast cancer is a prior cancer of the breast. Therefore, patients who have been treated for breast cancer should have an annual mammogram of the remaining breast.

When a patient has a carcinoma in the other breast, synchronous or dysynchronous, the question arises whether it is a second primary or a metastatic lesion. Although the pathologist may be able to provide some guidance in this regard, it has been customary to assume that it is a second primary and to treat the lesion accordingly.

Breast Cancer in the Male

Less than 1 percent of breast cancer occurs in males. The lesion may be confused with senescent gynecomastia, and the diagnosis is often late. Breast cancer in the male tends to infiltrate locally, and pectoral involvement is somewhat more likely than in the female, probably because of the lesser mass of breast tissue and the close proximity of breast tissue to the muscle. There is a higher incidence of lymph node metastasis than in the female, as well as a higher incidence of hormone dependence, as reflected in estrogen binding. Cancer of the breast in males should be treated by modified radical mastectomy, at which time a segment of the underlying pectoral muscle is generally excised. Chemotherapy should be employed as would be indicated in the case of breast cancer in the female. If one considers the prognosis by stage of disease, the prognosis is similar to that in the female. Overall, survival is poorer because of the higher incidence of axillary lymph node involvement.

Cystosarcoma Phylloides

Cystosarcoma phylloides of the breast is a tumor that is usually benign but of which there is a malignant variant. The tumor consists of proliferation of both stromal and glandular elements. The lesions vary in size from 1 or 2 cm to more than 25 cm. The tumor has a specific histologic pattern with a very cellular stoma and is distinct from a fibroadenoma, irrespective of size of the lesion. If more than five mitoses are seen in a high-power field, the lesion may be classified as malignant, but the malignant nature of a cystosarcoma is best documented by gross invasion of surrounding tissues or by metastases. Metastases are blood-borne and predominantly pulmonary. Lymph node metastases of stromal elements are extremely rare. Metastasis of epithelial elements may be due to an associated adenocarcinoma rather than the epithelial elements of the cystosarcoma phylloides. This tumor has a propensity for local recurrence. It is not particularly sensitive to radiation therapy or chemotherapy.

LOBULAR CARCINOMA IN SITU

LOREN J. HUMPHREY, M.D., Ph.D.

Management of carcinoma of the breast should be based on a solid data base. Projected recurrence or survival data, small numbers of cases, or minority reports have little place in standard treatment. The patient deserves the best regimen based on sound biologic considerations and mature data critically reviewed. This presentation on lobular carcinoma in situ will focus on the natural history of this pathologic lesion of the breast. Rhetoric regarding hypothesis or reference to divergent opinions will be left to appropriate forums. However, data on which differing conclusions or opinions are proffered will be scrutinized. Not withstanding exigencies for judgment, this approach should lead to a treatment plan that is based on today's data and is optimum in survival and quality of life for the patient.

PATHOLOGIC DATA

Since the classic description in 1941 of lobular carcinoma in situ, pathologists have agreed on criteria for its diagnosis. Critical to this agreement as well as management is the consideration of this lesion when it occurs alone. Hence, in contrast to invasive carcinoma and ductal carcinoma in situ, no mass is present, precluding the gross identification of lobular carcinoma in situ. As in ductal carcinoma in situ, the lesion involves epithelial lining. However, in lobular carcinoma in situ, the acini and small ductules emerging from the lobules exhibit characteristic changes. Epithelial cells lining these ducts generally appear uniform in size and shape, but are markedly increased in size and number. As these changes progress, the lumina are not recognizable.

Differential diagnosis is not difficult for the experienced pathologist. Ductal carcinoma extending into the lobule, as well as well-differentiated ductal carcinomas, are separated by their characteristic ductal features. Previously, clinicians thought it of great importance to differentiate ductal carcinoma in situ from lobular carcinoma in situ because of alleged marked differences in biologic behavior. Recent data from the Breast Cancer Detection Demonstration Projects (BCDDP) show that ductal carcinoma in situ also has a significant incidence of multicentricity, as much as 32 percent.

CLINICAL DATA

Incidence. The true incidence of lobular carcinoma in situ is unknown, and older figures are undergoing scrutiny owing to the current detection of more minimal breast cancers. Since lobular carcinoma in situ is not a palpable lesion, incidence in occult lesions might give a better appreciation of its incidence under clinical circumstances. In a study of some 550 cases of occult lesions detected by mammography, 14 (2.5%) were lobular carcinoma in situ. However, of the 550 biopsies, only 175 were malignant (either invasive or in-situ cancer), and hence 8 percent of occult cancers were lobular carcinoma in situ. These figures are pertinent to the physician who is managing the occult lesion. The imprecise incidence data for lobular carcinoma in situ have little meaning for the clinician. As noted above, the data do not pertain for lobular carcinoma found concomitant with other cancer forms since under those circumstances it seems to have a different biologic behavior.

Age. Patients with lobular carcinoma in situ are premenopausal. An occasional patient is menopausal, although the mean age for the patient with lobular carcinoma in situ is some 5 years younger than that of the patient with invasive carcinoma.

MULTICENTRICITY VERSUS BILATERALITY

From collected data of six studies, lobular carcinoma in situ was multifocal in 120 of 172 patients (69%). The range varied from 56 to 86 percent. At the same time, 20 to 45 percent have synchronous or develop metachronous contralateral lobular carcinoma in situ. Pertinent to our deliberations regarding optimal treatment of these lesions rests the query regarding the biologic behavior of this lesion. For example, data support the view that multicentricity and bilaterality are manifestations of similar factors involved in the transformation leading to invasive breast cancer. Along with this, one must focus on lobular carcinoma in situ occurring as an entity by itself in order to form a picture of the natural history of lobular carcinoma in situ. Therefore, such entities, a signet-ring carcinoma of the breast, invasive lobular carcinoma with associated lobular carcinoma in situ, or other forms of synchronous invasive carcinoma should be treated as mandated by those forms.

THE CONTINUUM

Most germane to building a logical plan for optimal treatment is the subsequent behavior of lobular carcinoma in situ. Only in the past few years has confidence in the natural history of fibrocystic disease or gross cystic disease of the breast emerged. This so-called disease is a spectrum of histologic changes, most being hormone dependent. The fact that severe ductal epithelial hyperplasia is associated with an increased risk for the development of ductal carcinoma raises the speculation of a continuum. Most experts have concluded that this lesion, severe ductal epithelial hyperplasia, when associated with atypia, will proceed to ductal carcinoma in situ in 50 to 80 percent of cases.

Similarly, data show that the patient with lobular carcinoma in situ has around a 30 percent chance of developing invasive cancer. Numbers are smaller for lobular carcinoma in situ than for ductal carcinoma in situ, and invasive cancer following biopsy may take 20 to 25 years to develop. As an approximation from retrospective studies, risk for developing invasive cancer by 15 years is about 30 percent for the patient with lobular carcinoma in situ. Hence, the clinician has no data on which to judge whether a specific patient is in the continuum, as with florid, atypical epihelial hyperplasia.

OPTIMAL THERAPY

Given the foregoing information, the clinician must approach the patient with the objective of prolonging her life while attempting to maintain quality of life as near normal as possible for her. The reason the expert surgeon has always given options is based on the fact that patients weigh quality of life against prolongation of life differently. Seldom does the surgeon know his patient well enough to balance these facets of his objective. Nevertheless, he must assist the patient by giving the nature of his data based on small numbers, frequently from nonrandomized and at times noncritical retrospective studies. Hence, informed with general information about bilaterality, multicentricity, and synchronous and metachronous invasive cancers, he must reflect for the patient his understanding of the continuum for her specific lesion. One way to assess this for the patient is as follows:

Affected Breast. Following biopsy that shows lobular carcinoma in situ, there is about a 69 percent chance of having other areas of lobular carcinoma in situ and about a 5 percent chance of having, at that moment, an invasive cancer. Over the next 15 years there is about a 15 percent chance of developing invasive cancer and about a 30 percent chance by 20 to 25 years. Considering the average age of 45 years for lobular carcinoma in situ, one-third of such patients will have invasive carcinoma by 65 or 70 years of age.

The options for treatment are (1) no further therapy or (2) total mastectomy. Subcutaneous mastectomy is not an option because this procedure does not prevent the development of cancer in the residual breast tissue. Thus the patient, with her doctor's assistance, weighs the worry of harboring a cancer at that time (5%) or of developing a cancer at any time over the next 20 to 25 years (30%).

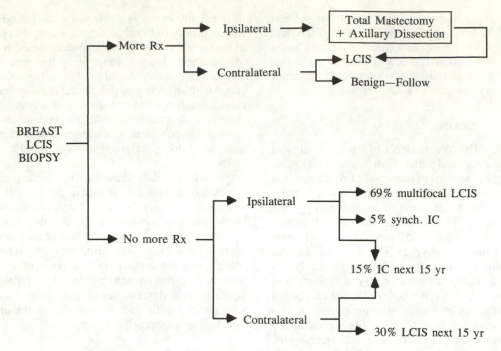

Figure 1 Management of lobular carcinoma in situ. IC = Invasive cancer; synch. = synchronous; Rx = treatment.

She should appreciate that survival is less when treated expectantly compared to total mastectomy soon after biopsy, but this apparently is not as great a difference, as is now realized in invasive cancer treated by biopsy (wedge) versus mastectomy.

Axillary Lymph Nodes. Discussion of this as part of the total mastectomy is precluded if the patient decides to have no further therapy after biopsy. However, if the patient elects total mastectomy, either low axillary lymph node removal or axillary dissection should be carried out. Since the morbidity and mortality are the same, the latter is recommended. With a 5 percent chance of a concomitant invasive cancer and since even minimal or occult cancers have a 15 to 35 percent incidence of lymph node metastases, I strongly urge this procedure. Axillary dissection is not necessary for lobular carcinoma in situ, which rarely has metastases, but for the 5 percent chance, this extra 20 minutes saves the patient another trip to the operating room.

Contralateral Breast. With over 30 percent of the women having lobular carcinoma in situ on contralateral biopsy at the time of discovery of their first lesion, contralateral biopsy of upper outer quadrant and mirrored image biopsy, if pertinent, is recommended (Fig. 1). Given the information that breast biopsy for a palpable mass has a

1 in 8 chance of being cancer and a biopsy for a suspicious mammographic shadow has a 1 in 5 or 6 chance of being cancer, most patients readily accept this. On the other hand if the patient has opted to have no further therapy on the original side after biopsy, biopsy of the contralateral side with a 30 percent chance of lobular carcinoma in situ makes little sense since the original breast harbors a 60 percent chance or more of lobular carcinoma in situ and 5 percent chance of invasive cancer.

In conclusion, data strongly suggest that following a breast biopsy with the diagnosis of lobular carcinoma in situ only, ipsilateral total mastectomy and axillary dissection with contralateral upper outer quadrant and mirrored image biopsy is the optimum form of therapy. With today's excellent reconstruction, the women over 40 years can expect a very acceptable end result as part of this treatment. Nevertheless, for women whose quality of life is much more dependent on keeping their own breasts, they should be reassured that their alternate course of action is not one fraught with certain death, but one with a definite chance of having or developing invasive cancer and consequently some risk of decreasing chances of survival. Certainly, for women of both persuasions, continued follow-up is necessary.

DISSEMINATED BREAST CANCER

MARTIN D. ABELOFF, M.D

Despite vigorous efforts at early detection and adjuvant therapy, metastatic breast cancer remains a major problem in the United States where over 38,000 deaths are estimated for 1985. Thus, virtually all practicing surgeons face the challenge of participating in the management of patients with disseminated breast cancer.

Before discussing more specific aspects of patient management, several general principles are worthy of emphasis. Unlike certain lymphomas and germ cell tumors, once metastases occur in a patient with breast cancer, cure is usually not achievable. However, in contrast with many other solid tumors, breast cancer is responsive to a variety of chemotherapeutic and endocrine regimens. Skillful use of these therapies can result in improvement in the quality of life as well as prolongation of life for the patient with disseminated breast cancer. The selection of these therapies can be based not only on clinical criteria, but also on the results of the estrogen and progesterone receptor assay.

SYSTEMIC THERAPIES

There are a variety of chemotherapeutic and endocrine regimens that can be successfully utilized in the treatment of advanced breast cancer. As noted in Table 1, there are some general characteristics of endocrine therapy and combination chemotherapy that aid in the decision-making process. Endocrine therapy results in an overall response rate of approximately 30 percent in an unselected population of patients with metastatic breast cancer. This response is generally achieved with relatively mild toxicity, and the median duration of response often exceeds 1½ years. However, the rate of response to endocrine therapy can be quite slow and it may take many weeks or months to achieve a complete or partial regression of tumor. In addition, endocrine therapy generally is not very effective against extensive visceral metastases or rapidly growing disease. In contrast, combination chemotherapy achieves an overall response rate of approximately 55 percent, and responses usually begin within 2 months of initiating chemotherapy. The median duration of response averages somewhat less than one year, and the toxicity is generally moderate and sometimes severe. However, combination chemotherapy can frequently achieve dramatic regression of even far-advanced visceral metastases.

Endocrine Therapy

Ablative Therapy

The earliest form of systemic therapy for advanced breast cancer was bilateral oophorectomy, which was introduced by Sir George Beatson in 1896. Following the availability of replacement hormone therapy, adrenalectomy and hypophysectomy also became part of the therapeutic armamentarium. Adrenalectomy and hypophysectomy, however, have now largely been replaced by "medical adrenalectomy" with aminoglutethimide.

Bilateral oophorectomy does remain an effective form of therapy for selected premenopausal patients with metastatic breast cancer. For the patient in generally good medical condition, surgical oophorectomy offers a significant opportunity for tumor regression with no subsequent drug administration. In the appropriate patient population, the surgical mortality is approximately 2 percent, and the morbidity is also limited. Castration can also be accomplished by radiation, but this approach should generally be limited to patients in whom surgery is contraindicated. Remissions take a longer time to achieve after radiation castration because the estrogen secretion by the ovaries generally declines over a period of several months to reach levels comparable to those achieved by oophorectomy.

Additive Hormonal Therapy

Hormones useful in the treatment of metastatic breast cancer include the antiestrogens, aromatase inhibitors, estrogens, androgens, progestational agents, and corticosteroids. Significant experience has been accumulated in the use of these agents, either as single agents or in combination, and therefore suggestions can be made as to appropriate sequence of administration.

One of the most important recent advances in the therapy of breast cancer has been the development of nonsteroidal antiestrogens such as nafoxidine and tamoxifen. Nafoxidine and other antiestrogens have not been clinicaly useful because of a low incidence of severe adverse reactions such as photosensitivity. Tamoxifen has remarkably few serious side effects. In general, the side effects of tamoxifen are confined to exacerbation of menopausal symptoms, mild nausea or vomiting, transient and often clinically insignificant thrombocytopenia, and mild hypercalcemia. Increased tumor pain or an inflammatory flare can be seen in a small percentage of patients.

Because of the low degree of side effects and a level of therapeutic effectiveness that is comparable to other endocrine therapy, tamoxifen has become the first-line

TABLE 1 Characteristics of Major Therapeutic Modalities for Disseminated Breast Cancer

	Endocrine Therapy	Combination Chemotherapy
Time to response	8–12 weeks	4–6 weeks
Overall response rate	25%–35%	50%–60%
Mean duration of response	16–20 months	10–12 months
Toxicity	Generally mild	Moderate to severe

endocrine therapy for postmenopausal women and is either first- or second-line therapy for premenopausal patients.

Since 1944, when Alexander Haddow reported the therapeutic efficacy of estrogens in postmenopausal patients with breast cancer, additive estrogen therapy had a time-honored role in the management of metastatic breast carcinoma. However, additive estrogens have a significant incidence of insidious and potentially serious side effects including fluid retention, anorexia, nausea and vomiting, and induction of life-threatening hypercalcemia. Although estrogens are still used in the treatment of postmenopausal patients, they generally have been relegated to a later position in the therapeutic schema.

In recent years, however, increasing attention has been given to aminoglutethimide. This drug was originally developed as an anticonvulsant agent, but was found to cause adrenal insufficiency by inhibiting the enzymatic conversion of cholesterol to Δ-5-pregnenolone. It was thus originally thought that aminoglutethimide caused an objective antitumor response in patients with breast cancer by performing a "medical adrenalectomy." More recently, aminoglutethimide has been shown to be an aromatase inhibitor, i.e., it inhibits the enzymes necessary for the conversion of steroid precursors to estrogens in body tissues such as adipose tissue and liver.

The proposed different mechanisms of action for aminoglutethimide have clinical relevance. When given in conjunction with hydrocortisone in doses sufficient to achieve a "medical adrenalectomy," aminoglutethimide has significant side effects including transient lethargy and nausea, transient rash often accompanied by fever, and neurologic symptoms. Recent data suggest that aromatase inhibition can be achieved at significantly lower doses than that required to achieve a "medical adrenalectomy." It remains to be seen whether these low doses will have the same antitumor effect and whether the side effects can be significantly ameliorated. The toxicities of aminoglutethimide are in general more acceptable than the morbidity and mortality related to adrenalectomy and hypophysectomy. Oncologists who are experienced with the use of aminogluthethimide report response rates comparable to those for other hormonal treatments with acceptable morbidity. However, in general, aminoglutethimide does not appear to be as well tolerated as tamoxifen.

Like the other forms of endocrine therapy, synthetic analogues of progesterone have been found to result in an effective response rate of approximately 20 to 30 percent in patients with advanced disease. Megestrol acetate is frequently used at a dose of 40 mg four times a day and is currently being compared with tamoxifen as first-line hormonal therapy for patients with advanced breast cancer. Progestational agents, in general, can cause significant fluid retention and other steroidal side effects, but the adverse effects are usually modest.

Androgens and corticosteroids also have low-order effectiveness in patients with metastatic breast cancer. The objective response rates appear to be in the range of 10 to 20 percent. However, the masculinizing effects of androgen therapy are often unacceptable for patients with metastatic breast cancer. Likewise, the multitude of signi-

ficant side effects that can be caused by systemic corticosteroids militate against the prolonged use of this agent in patients with metastatic cancer.

Systemic Combination Chemotherapy

Metastatic breast cancer is responsive to a variety of cytotoxic chemotherapeutic agents. Doxorubicin (Adriamycin) is probably the most effective single agent. As is the case with many other human malignant tumors, combination chemotherapeutic regimens consisting of multiple drugs that are individually active against breast cancer is generally more effective than single-agent therapy in the management of metastatic breast carcinoma. However, there is not any single regimen that is definitively best in this disease.

The commonly used combination chemotherapeutic regimens are cyclophosphamide, methotrexate, and 5-fluorouracil (CMF) often given in conjunction with prednisone and/or tamoxifen (CMFPT); cyclophosphamide, doxorubicin, and 5-fluorouracil (CAF); thiotepa, doxorubicin, vinblastine, tamoxifen, and halotestin (TAVTH); and mitomycin-C plus vinblastine (MV).

As noted in Table 1, these regimens all have an objective response rate of approximately 50 to 60 percent in patients who previously have recieved no prior chemotherapy for their metastatic breast cancer. The time to response is generally short, and the duration of response averages one year. These regimens generally have more toxicity than endocrine regimens, but within recent years there has been considerable progress in the amelioration of side effects secondary to cytotoxic chemotherapy. The use of steroids as an antiemetic has greatly decreased the morbidity of chemotherapeutic regimens. In addition, much has been learned about the pathophysiology of nausea and vomiting syndromes. For example, it has been documented that a significant number of women with breast cancer develop an anticipatory syndrome of nausea and vomiting, and this often can be at least partially treated with behavioral modification therapy. There has been some reduction in the incidence of alopecia with the use of ice caps, and in general, supportive care has significantly improved.

Combined Hormonal and Chemotherapy

In an attempt to produce more meaningful responses and accordingly prolong survival, considerable interest has been focused on combining endocrine treatment and chemotherapy. Recent reviews of these combined modalities indicate that simply combining endocrine therapy and chemotherapy may produce more complete responses, but does not increase overall survival in patients with advanced disease. There is ongoing research to evaluate effectiveness of using one form of therapy to stimulate or prime the tumor for an enhanced response to another form of treatment. These synchronization regimens have resulted in some encouraging results in patients with locally advanced breast cancer, but it is too early to tell whether this will result in better survival. Since cure is seldom achieved for patients with metastatic breast cancer, one must guard against using all therapies simultaneously and thereby eliminating options at the time of inevitable relapse. Combined chemotherapy and hormonal therapy should at this time be considered largely investigational.

Guidelines for Systemic Therapy

A number of clinical and laboratory findings influence the selection of therapy for an individual patient with metastatic breast cancer (Table 2). However, the estrogen and progesterone receptors are the single most useful determinants of therapy in metastatic breast cancer.

Estrogen and progesterone receptors should be quantitatively measured on all primary breast cancers and in virtually all cases in which biopsy is obtained from metastatic tumor tissue. Patients with positive estrogen receptors (i.e., greater than 10 femtomoles per milligram of protein) generally have a 60 percent likelihood of responding to endocrine maneuvers. The quantitative statement of the estrogen receptor protein is important in that the higher the ER protein content, the greater the chance of response to hormonal manipulation. Likewise, the presence of positive progesterone receptors in addition to positive estrogen receptors enhances the probability of response to a hormonal therapy.

It is essential that the tumor tissue be handled properly so that the receptor assays are accurate. False-positive results are most unusual, but false-negative results can occur owing to mishandling of the tumor specimens.

If a patient's tumor is negative for these receptors, the chance of responding to a hormonal maneuver is less than 5 percent. On the other hand, if the receptors are positive, the chance of responding to endocrine therapy is in the range of 50 percent or better. Whenever possible, endocrine therapy is utilized since the morbidity of the therapy is less than that of combination chemotherapy. However, other clinical factors (as noted in Table 2) have impact on this decision.

A patient who has extensive visceral metastases and/or rapid rate of progression of the disease may not have adequate time for hormones to exert a therapeutic effect. For these patients, combination chemotherapy is recommended. Likewise, patients who have a short disease-free interval, i.e., less than 18 months from the time of diagnosis of breast cancer to the first evidence of relapse, may initially require systemic chemotherapy for control of their metastatic cancer.

Menopausal status per se does not dictate the choice between endocrine and chemotherapy. Neither does age, and in general, therapy should be based on physiologic considerations and not arbitrary age cutoffs. However, menopausal status does affect the choice of hormonal therapies. Women who are premenopausal at the time of the development of their metastases are generally considered candidates for oophorectomy or tamoxifen whereas postmenopausal patients are usually considered candidates for tamoxifen, and oophorectomy is not recommended in these circumstances. Estrogen therapy is not given to premenopausal women with metastatic breast carcinoma.

If a patient responds to an additive hormonal therapy and then relapses, a trial of hormone withdrawal can result in another response. A brief waiting period is justified after hormone withdrawal to see whether this "rebound response" occurs. One response to hormonal treatment generally justifies trying another hormonal therapy at the time of relapse, provided the disease has not become rapidly progressive in visceral areas.

A very important factor, which is not mentioned in Table 2 and should be considered in making these management decisions, is the patient's individual needs. As previously mentioned, the treatment of metastatic breast cancer rarely results in cure of the disease. None of the therapies are completely without side effects, and as we move down the therapeutic flow to second- and third-line therapies, the duration of responses and the improvement in the quality of life generally diminishes. At every step in this process, the patient should be informed of the therapeutic options available, but also should have the opportunity to know the limitation of such therapy and the associated morbidity.

LOCAL TREATMENT AND SUPPORTIVE CARE

Although the emphasis in this chapter has been on the systemic therapies of metastatic breast cancer, it is worth making note of the significant palliation that can be achieved by the adroit use of local radiotherapy and various forms of supportive care. Local radiation therapy can be used to effectively manage local and regional recurrences and painful bone lesions. In fact, the management of bone metastases in metastatic breast cancer poses many challenging problems. Lytic lesions in weight-bearing areas must be approached vigorously with radiation therapy, and on occasion, prophylactic orthopedic pinning is helpful to the patient. In addition, spinal cord compression due to bony and/or extradural lesions is a major cause of morbidity in patients with metastatic breast cancer. Thorough diagnostic work-ups to rule out spinal cord compression should be done in patients with metastatic breast cancer and persistent back pain. This involves

---

TABLE 2   Characteristics Useful in Selecting Systemic Therapy

Estrogen and progesterone receptors

Disease-free interval

Sites of metastases

Rate of progression

Menopausal status, age

the use of myelography in conjunction with CT scan technology.

The management of malignant effusions, the skillful management of pain with systemic analgesics as well as neurosurgical pain relief procedures, the management of metabolic complications including hypercalcemia are all important in the overall treatment of the patient with metastatic breast cancer. Last, but certainly not least,

considerable time should be spent with the patient and the family so that appropriate psychological support can be made available to women with this illness. The thoughtful use of these supportive measures in conjunction with the available systemic therapies can certainly lead to meaningful prolongation of survival for many patients with metastatic breast cancer.

CHEST WALL

THORACIC WALL TRAUMA

FREDERICK W. WALKER, M.D.

Thoracic injuries are the cause of approximately 25 percent of all trauma deaths in the United States. Many of these deaths could be prevented with prompt diagnosis and treatment. Fortunately, few of these injuries require major surgical intervention. Approximately 80 percent can be managed by simple procedures that do not require the abilities of a trained thoracic surgeon. It is incumbent on the general surgeon, and on other physicians treating the injured patient, to be familiar with thoracic trauma as an integral aspect of overall management.

This chapter will have an audience of physicians with a wide variety of experience levels. While its primary purpose is to provide an overview of thoracic wall trauma for the relatively inexperienced, it will address several misconceptions that have been handed down over the years and which may, therefore, still be held by those with considerable expertise.

GENERAL FEATURES

In the American College of Surgeons' approach to the trauma victim entitled "Advanced Trauma Life Support," the ABCs of resuscitation refer to airway, breathing, and circulation. Frequently, chest trauma affects all three of these functions with life-threatening or potentially life-threatening injuries. The chest wall is the first line of defense against almost all thoracic injuries, both blunt and penetrating. Penetrating injuries, in general, deliver the most serious damage to the intrathoracic contents. These will not be addressed in this article. Injuries that are limited to the thoracic wall usually fall within the sphere of blunt trauma.

In some respects, the thoracic wall can be thought of as a "barometer" of the amount of energy transferred from the "environment" to the victim. This estimation governs the overall approach to the traumatized patient. The relationship between energy transmitted and damage observed is not linear. The isolated but unprotected fall by the inebriate may fracture multiple ribs, although there is a small energy transfer. On the other hand, considerable damage can be done to intrathoracic and intra-abdominal organs from decelerative injuries with huge energy

transfers, and yet the thoracic wall remains unscathed. Certain locations of chest wall trauma, such as sternal, first rib, and left lower rib fractures, have strong correlations with associated internal injuries. It is often the hidden injuries that are most devastating, rather than those that are the most obvious.

The general rules of resuscitation, which include maintenance of the airway, adequate ventilation, and restoration of circulation, prevail here as well. The chest wall is inspected rapidly during the primary survey, but it is essential that a detailed and complete examination be performed again, as part of the secondary survey. Missed penetrating wounds, such as those on the back or in the axilla, are not uncommon. Blunt injuries that appear trivial on first inspection may become more demonstrable with the passage of time.

PENETRATING WOUNDS

As already mentioned, penetrating injuries to the intrathoracic organs will not be covered here. It is important to note that wounds that affect only the chest wall do occur. Patients who are reported, from the field, to have been shot or stabbed in the chest may prove, on closer examination, to have wounds limited to the chest wall. These wounds can cause hematomas and infections, and patients can bleed extensively from lacerations to the intercostal or internal mammary arteries.

One of our patients, who attempted to commit suicide by driving a sharpened pencil (to the depth of its eraser) into his left chest wall, managed to miss his heart, penetrate his diaphragm, and miss all intra-abdominal organs in the pencil's path. This same patient was 2 weeks postoperative from a self-inflicted knife wound to the left chest wall which had penetrated the pericardium but not the heart. Both times, his major injury was chest wall trauma.

BLUNT TRAUMA

Blunt trauma to the chest wall may result in rib and sternal fractures, including flail chest. Many of these injuries are associated with pulmonary or myocardial contusions, hemo- or pneumothorax, tracheobronchial disruption, ruptured diaphragm, and aortic disruption. It is important to keep in mind that some of these victims of blunt trauma may have aspirated foreign bodies at the time of the accident. These may include teeth, partial or fragmented dental plates, chewing gum, pieces of regurgitated food, and other foreign bodies. What are felt to be "pure" pulmonary contusions may, in fact, be the result of aspiration. Initial chest films should be examined carefully for the presence of any possible foreign objects. The examiner's index of suspicion should be particularly high when the patient has suffered any intraoral trauma with broken or missing teeth or lacerations of the tongue or gums. Many of these patients require bronchoscopy to relieve obstruction of the pulmonary segment and reinflate the affected lobe.

CHEST TUBE INSERTION

Many patients who have trauma to the chest wall require the insertion of an intercostal catheter. The sudden, and sometimes irreversible, decompensation of the patient with a thoracic injury such as a tension pneumothorax makes it appropriate to treat "suspected" rather than "proven" injuries. In retrospect, significant intrathoracic lesions may be ruled out, but cautious judgment is always the preferred approach.

The insertion of chest tubes is a skill that is generally passed down from house officer to house officer. While there are undoubtedly many satisfactory techniques, and considerable experience evolves into appropriate individuality, there are some commonly misconstrued concepts that I will attempt to rectify here. Three valid concepts are frequently joined to produce one invalid technique.

First, chest catheters placed intraoperatively are usually "tunneled" through the chest wall to the outside. This is done from the inside out, under direct vision, with access to the catheter from both the inside and the outside, and with muscle relaxation. This same concept, when carried over into the trauma situation, has merit, but must be tempered with certain modifications.

Second, inexperienced chest tube inserters are frequently hesitant in the use of the scalpel, and are taught to make the incision directly over a rib so that over-enthusiastic division of tissue will not lead to premature chest entry. This, too, is certainly acceptable.

Third, one is taught to enter the chest just over a rib (as in thorocentesis) to avoid the neurovascular bundle. When these three tenets are combined, however, the result is often unsatisfactory. If the tract is created from the skin incision to the space immediately above, the tunnel is "too short." If the tract is made to the second space above, still going perpendicularly to the ribs, the long distance makes for a painful insertion and frequently leads to an anterior tube placement. Muscle splinting by the patient further hinders correct placement.

The proper direction of the tunnel is toward the posterior chest, and pleural passage need only be a few fingerbreadths from the skin incision. The skin may still be incised over a rib, but a shorter tunnel should lead to the space immediately above that rib and 3 to 4 cm posterior to the skin opening. This type of tunnel leads to a proper posterior placement, is far less painful, utilizes either a trocar or a Kelly clamp, and allows the surgeon to place a finger into the chest to make sure that the lung is not adhered to the parietal pleura. It makes a potentially difficult assignment into one that is carried out with ease.

RIB FRACTURES

Rib fractures are extremely common injuries. They may result from motor vehicle accidents, industrial and home mishaps, sports injuries, and personal assaults. If the "environment" that has caused the fracture is small in area, the rib fractures occur at the point of impact. Examples of this are a baseball bat, bicycle handlebars, or the patient's arm (as in the aforementioned fall). If the area is large, like a fall onto a flat surface, the ribs fracture at distant sites as the force is transmitted along the rib to a point of relative weakness. Commonly, the anterior fracture site is at the costochondral junction. These fractures may not show up on the x-ray film. The posterior site is often the posterior axillary line or at the "neck" of the rib, close to the spine.

Patients complain of shortness of breath and chest pain following an accident that may have occurred many hours prior to presentation. Sometimes the nagging pain interferes with sleep and necessitates a 2 AM visit to the emergency room (ER). Unless there are complications such as hemo- or pneumothorax, the physical examination may show only decreased ventilatory volume and muscle splinting. Tenderness may occur in a wide area, but in many cases excellent point tenderness can be elicited. On occasion, gentle anteroposterior compression of the chest produces pain at the distant site of a rib fracture.

Radiographs may prove to be more "documentary" than "therapy-directing." The presence of a roentgenographically demonstrable fracture is not so significant as the physical findings. The major complication of an otherwise uncomplicated rib fracture is atelectasis and pneumonia secondary to splinting. This can occur as a result of contusion as well as fracture, and the patient, not the roentgen findings must be treated.

The initial chest roentgenograms should be a PA and lateral, with the lateral being done on the side of the injury. The standard left lateral view is done because of interest in the heart. The trauma surgeon must individualize the lateral film to better visualize structures that were on the same side as the accident. The roentgenogram is examined carefully for hemo- and pneumothorax as well as for early signs of pulmonary contusion. Looking for a foreign body is also important. Rib detail films can be obtained to further clarify those areas that are not well seen on the standard films.

The treatment of simple rib fractures, which includes one or possibly two ribs, is centered on the relief of pain so that the patient can breathe deeply and cough. Methods of restricting chest wall movement, such as taping, are perhaps useful on the football field in the final game of the season, but have no use once the patient is being seen by a physician. Frequently, adequate oral analgesia is all that is needed. Low-dose narcotics may provide more significant pain relief than will the nonsteroidal anti-inflammatory drugs, since the source of the pain is direct nerve irritation by the fracture fragment and not the result of inflammatory swelling.

Intercostal nerve blocks are a frequently utilized therapeutic modality. These are performed, using a 30-gauge needle, with either bupivacaine hydrochloride, 0.25%, or a mixture of bupivacaine and lidocaine, 0.5%. When mixing the two drugs, use strengths of 0.5% and 1% respectively, so that the final concentrations are as indicated above. The maximum recommended dose of lidocaine alone is 400 mg (80 cc of a 0.5% solution), and of bupivacaine alone is 200 mg (80 cc of a 0.25% solution). When mixed, a total volume of 40 cc should be sufficient to perform an adequate rib block. If one finds a need to use more, an alternative therapy is indicated. Usually, one space above the highest fracture and one space below the lowest are blocked. A maximum of 4 to 5 spaces should be blocked.

The intercostal nerves exit the spinal column midway between two ribs. At a point just lateral to the articulation of the transverse process, the rib broadens and a groove forms on the inferior surface of the rib for the neuro-vascular bundle. The nerve joins the rib at this point and lies in this groove for the remainder of its course. Nerve blocks are consistently more effective if placed at a point where the nerve is just diving deep to the lower rib border. One should not block the nerves too close to the spinal cord because of the risk of creating a total spinal block. In addition, the nerve's location is more inconsistent, and the chances of a successful block are less. Three to 5 ml of anesthetic at each nerve is usually sufficient to obtain an adequate block.

As with all other peripheral nerve blocks, the first step is to anesthetize the skin, thereby allowing the pain-less insertion of a ''booster'' dose should the first prove ineffective. No surgeon achieves a 100 percent success rate on every injection, but patients are quite satisfied if the second attempt is made painlessly. The block should provide pain relief for 18 to 24 hours. This is often enough to break the ''pain cycle,'' and additional blocking is not needed. Repeat blocking can be performed when neces-sary. Usually no more than one re-block is attempted.

Most patients with rib fractures can be treated on an outpatient basis. Obviously those with significant other injuries, with pulmonary or cardiac disease, or with fractures in locations highly suggestive of additional injury should be admitted to the hospital. Close observation and vigorous pulmonary care and pain relief can then be simul-taneously carried out.

Several reports have suggested that fractures of the first rib are associated with a higher severity of injury. This is because a greater amount of energy is theoretically required in order to break such a short and stout structure. Many articles advise both esophageal swallows and aortic arteriography for all patients sustaining such injuries. More recent reports indicate that the association may not

be high enough to warrant this additional risk. However, a period of observation is clearly mandated in all of these patients. Arteriography should be utilized whenever upper rib fractures are associated with any neurovascular symptoms or findings.

FLAIL CHEST

By definition, a flail chest occurs when more than one adjacent rib is fractured in more than one place. As was noted previously, the anterior fracture site may be at the costochondral junction and therefore be unobserved on roentgenogram. The examining physician should be able to pick up a significant flail segment on physical examination despite this lack of roentgenographic confirmation. In truth, it is the significance of the flail and the extent of underlying pulmonary contusion that determine the outcome for the patient, not the roentgeno-graphic location of the fracture sites. If a flail segment is so small as to be inapparent on clinical examination, it may likewise prove to be insignificant in its contribution to the patient's overall condition.

Partially because the etiology and evolution of pulmonary contusion has been misunderstood in the past, it was felt that all flail chests deserve maximum interven-tion. In earlier years, this included either the use of gauze pads or sandbags taped to the chest to keep the flail segment inverted or the use of wires or towel clips placed around the ribs and put on traction to maintain eversion of the segment. Attempts of early wiring of flail segments of ribs have been undertaken with suboptimal results. All of these methods introduce risks that are unacceptably high to justify their use in all flail chests. In addition, more efficient methods of internal stabilization have been perfected for use in selected cases.

The era of ''internal pneumatic stabilization'' was brought about by the introduction of the volume ventilator and the ability to maintain positive end-expiratory pressure (PEEP) throughout the ventilation cycle. By raising the functional residual capacity (FRC) of the lungs, pul-monary volumes were maintained at a higher level. This was thought to keep the segment from moving so great a distance and, thereby, reduce pain; it was frequently referred to as ''internal splinting.'' Since the true value of utilizing PEEP to increase FRC is that a greater percent-age of the alveoli remain open throughout the respiratory cycle (above ''critical closing volume''), it may have been this early treatment of pulmonary contusion that led to more satisfactory results using this method. Long-term mechanical ventilation was frequently utilized in the flail chest patients. It was maintained until the ribs had healed or at least stabilized wth a soft callous. This led to many complications. The most significant of these is the need for long-term intubation, which led to tracheostomy and its associated complications. The use of the low-pressure cuff has rendered early tracheostomy unnecessary in most patients, and the ability to closely monitor the patient's cardiac output and pulmonary status has allowed us to utilize ventilatory support only for patients who truly require it.

An early film of the chest wall injury frequently does not show evidence of pulmonary contusion. An axiom is that the x-ray findings lag behind the condition of the lungs, both in its evolution and its resolution. Many patients with chest injuries have other associated injuries which create accompanying degrees of shock. Resuscitation of the patient's shock has frequently led to deleterious effects in the lungs, particularly when the resuscitation is performed with large amounts of crystalloid solution. The use of colloid solution has been advocated by some as a means of eliminating this complication, but most physicians doubt its effectiveness. In almost all resuscitations, the crystalloid volume should be limited to 2 liters, after which whole blood or reconstituted packed red blood cells should be the infusion of choice.

Arterial blood gases should be performed on arrival to the Emergency Room and frequent redeterminations utilized to pick up early evidence of shunting. This may require arterial line insertion and clearly is an indication for observation in an intensive care setting. Frequently, patients who can be monitored more closely can have intubation and ventilation deferred until later in the course because they can be instituted rapidly when needed. Patients who cannot be treated at the resuscitating hospital are better managed by intubation for airway protection, ventilation, and oxygenation prior to transfer to another facility.

In the Intensive Care Unit, if a flail chest is treated with mechanical ventilation, treatment of the pulmonary contusion is instituted utilizing fluid restriction and steroids. Close monitoring of the patient's respiratory flora and careful pulmonary toilet by experienced individuals are mandatory to prevent further complications. Supplemental oxygen with humidification is used in all patients. It is not necessary to delay weaning the patient until the ribs are stabilized. The ability to monitor the degree of shunting and the use of intermittent mandatory ventilation (IMV) techniques make weaning a patient much easier and more effecitve than it was in the early days of the use of volume ventilators. As mentioned before, the input and output status of the patient should be watched closely. Kidney function should be monitored on an ongoing basis.

The treatment of flail chest has undergone some degree of evolution since its early descriptions and the individualized approach is clearly the standard of care at this point in time.

STERNAL FRACTURES

Fractures of the sternum are relatively uncommon. Most occur as deceleration injuries, usually from falls. They can occur in patients who are not wearing appropriate restraints when involved in motor vehicle accidents. The use of shoulder and lap belt restraints can significantly reduce the incidence of sternal fracture and its associated complication, myocardial contusion. The reduction in the legal speed limit from 70 to 55 has also created a reduction in the incidence of this injury.

The contused or fractured sternum is extremely tender. The diagnosis can usually be confirmed by lateral chest film, but is occasionally difficult to pick up. In most instances, a stable fracture needs no additional treatment. If, by palpation, one is able to move the fractured segments easily, consideration should be given to internal fixation to prevent the development of a pseudoarthrosis and chronic pain. General anesthesia is used, a small vertical incision is made, and the fractured segments are stabilized by means of wires such as are used following median sternotomy for cardiac surgery. A small drill should be used to make the holes through the sternum, and the wires are generally placed in a vertical direction.

The major injury associated with sternal fracture is myocardial contusion. A complete EKG should be obtained upon arrival at the hospital, and continuous monitoring for 24 hours should be utilized to detect arrhythmias early. The most common arrhythmia following myocardial contusion is atrial fibrillation, but occasionally ventricular dysrhythmias are also elicited. Determination of CPK isoenzymes can be performed over the next several days. It is uncommon, but possible, for papillary muscle dysfunction to occur following blunt trauma to the chest. Auscultation of the patient's heart is required immediately following the injury and at the 24 and 48 hour points to detect new murmurs.

TUMOR OF THE CHEST WALL

WILLIAM A. GAY, Jr., M.D.

Although adenocarcinoma of the female breast is by far the most common of chest wall tumors, discussion of this entity is beyond the scope of this chapter. In addition, this chapter will not consider either those tumors arising from mesothelial cells on the pleural surface or those arising from ganglia or nerve roots in the posterior mediastinum. It will focus instead on primary tumors of the supporting structures of the chest wall.

Although primary tumors of the chest wall are uncommon, the fact that more than half are malignant underscores the importance of the appropriate diagnosis and management of these patients. Additionally, about half the tumors, either benign or malignant, arise in cartilaginous tissue. Bones of the chest wall are also among the more common sites for metastatic involvement. In particular, malignant tumors of the breast, lung, kidney, and thyroid seem to have a predilection to metastasize to the chest wall. Malignant tumors of the chest wall, whether primary or metastatic, have a poor prognosis, possibly due to a long delay between discovery and treatment. Early recognition and prompt treatment of these highly lethal tumors is therefore of paramount importance.

Most patients with tumors of the chest wall present with either pain or a mass or both. Pain, although more common in malignant tumors, is also present in as many as one-third of patients with benign tumors. Sometimes local trauma may have focused the patient's attention on the tumor, but except perhaps for fibrous dysplasia, trauma probably has little role in the etiology of these masses.

Size and location of tumors may sometimes by helpful in determining the likelihood of malignancy. For example, tumors of the sternum and tumors exceeding 4 cm in diameter, regardless of location, are virtually always malignant. Just as in tumors of other types, fixation to or involvement of the overlying skin is highly suggestive of malignancy.

Certain laboratory examinations may be helpful. An elevated alkaline phosphatase level suggests metastatic disease. Similarly, acid phosphatase levels may be elevated in metastatic involvement of the bones from a prostatic primary. Sometimes the sedimentation rate (ESR) is elevated in Ewing's sarcoma. The presence of immature blood cells in the peripheral smear may suggest a myeloproliferative disorder. Similarly, the electrophoresis of serum proteins may uncover proteins specific for myeloma.

The most important accessory information, however, is obtained by the roentgenographic evaluation of the chest wall. Some abnormality is almost always detectable. PA and lateral views of the chest are routinely obtained, and occasionally oblique views are necessary. CT is usually advisable to delineate the tumor and the extent of local involvement. Benign tumors characteristically are sharply delineated with intact cortical margins. Poor delineation and cortical disruption are characteristic of malignant tumors.

Unless there is a strong suspicion of myeloma or metastatic disease, needle biopsy is not recommended as a method of choice for obtaining tissue. The treatment of choice for most tumors of the chest wall is surgical excision. Therefore, tumors less than 2 cm in size should be carefully excised with good margins. This procedure usually proves curative. Tumors larger than 2 cm require a carefully planned open biopsy, obtaining tissue adequate for a diagnosis and avoiding techniques that may compromise a future definitive resection. Obviously, the myeloproliferative tumors are exceptions to this as are most metastatic lesions.

BENIGN TUMORS

Chondroma

Chondromas are typically located at the costochondral junctions and are often seen in patients in their teens and 20s, usually presenting as a painless mass. X-ray examination typically shows a medullary mass that thins, but does not penetrate, the overlying cortex. Most chondromas occur in the ribs (30% or more), but they may occur in any site in the body where cartilage is found. Left untreated, they can grow to very large size.

The skin and muscle tissue overlying the tumor is nearly always freely movable, and the tumor usually is not tender. Proper treatment consists of excision of the involved costal cartilage along with a short segment of the accompanying rib.

Fibrous Dysplasia

This tumor, approximately equal in incidence with chondroma, usually presents as a slow-growing painless mass in the posterior rib area in young individuals. Characteristically, its growth may cease at puberty. Chest films reveal the cortex to be thinned overlying a fusiform osteolytic lesion in which trabeculations may be visible. Excision of the involved rib segment with a reasonable margin on either end is usually curative.

Osteochondroma

This tumor, which is much less common than chrondromas or fibrous dysplasia, is usually seen in young patients. The characteristic roentgenogram shows an excrescence of cartilage with a calcified cap projecting out of the rib itself. Tumor growth usually stops at the time of closure of the nearest bony epiphysis. Malignant degeneration of this tumor is rare when the lesions are solitary, but may be as high as 20 percent in the hereditary form of multiple exostoses. Surgical excision usually results in cure. However, one should be careful to excise the cartilaginous growth center. If doubt exists, a segment of the rib itself should be excised.

Desmoid Tumors

Desmoid tumors of the chest wall are rare, but are locally aggressive in their growth. These tumors, unlike others of the chest wall, occur twice as frequently in women as in men. The preferred site of origin seems to be the intercostal musculature. Occasionaly the tumors arise in areas of previous surgery or trauma. Because of its locally invasive nature, complete resection is indicated.

MALIGNANT TUMORS

Chondrosarcoma

Chondrosarcoma, the most common of the primary malignant tumors of the chest wall, is usually located at the costochondral junction. However, it may occur anywhere along the course of the rib and may also occur in the sternum. The tumor is usually slow-growing, but is frequently painful and may involve adjacent ribs, pleura, and muscle, or even extend into the underlying lung. Usually larger than 4 cm at the time of discovery, these tumors are easily palpable and may be tender and fixed to the surrounding tissues. X-ray examination usually shows a large lobulated mass with evidence of soft tissue involvement and bony destruction with scattered mottled calcification.

Thorough surgical excision is the treatment of choice. These tumors rarely metastasize; therefore, the poor 5-year survival statistics (25% to 30%) attest to late discovery and inadequate excision in most instances.

Osteogenic Sarcoma

This tumor, a rapidly growing malignant tumor, occurs most frequently in patients in their teens and early 20s. Although rare on the chest wall, the poor prognosis associated with osteogenic sarcoma should arouse suspicion whenever a chest wall tumor presents in a young person. These tumors tend to metastasize early, the usual site of metastatic involvement being the lung. The tumor usually presents as a painful, rapidly expanding mass originating on a bony structure of the chest wall. The characteristic "sunburst" appearance of the tumor on the x-ray film is virtually diagnostic. Careful inspection of the lungs for metastatic disease should precede surgical therapy. Wide local excision to include adjacent bones and soft tissue is the procedure of choice. Ipsilateral pulmonary metastases may be removed by wedge resection. However, contralateral disease should be removed at a separate operation. Recent therapeutic trials with chemotherapy show considerable promise, and a combined multidisciplinary approach for control of these tumors may be on the horizon. At this time, however, the prognosis in primary osteogenic sarcomas of the chest wall is poor, with an overall 5-year survival of less than 10 percent.

Ewing's Sarcoma

Ewing's sarcoma characteristically occurs in the long bones of the body, but may also be seen in the bony structure of the thorax. The tumor is most common in the adolescent age group and characterized roentgenographically by the typical "onionskin" calcification produced by the periosteal elevation over the tumor. Generalized malaise and fever may accompany the finding of a tender chest wall mass. An elevated sedimentation rate (ESR) may arouse suspicion of this particular tumor. Open surgical biopsy is necessary for histologic diagnosis. A combination of surgery, radiation, and chemotherapy is most likely to yield optimal results in this aggressive tumor, but the overall prognosis is poor.

Myeloma

The incidence of myeloma (plasmacytoma) occurring in the chest wall may actually be higher than reported since this tumor represents a systemic disease and many cases are diagnosed by needle biopsy and are not reported as primary chest wall tumors. Although the roentgenographic features of myeloma in the skull are characteristic, the tumor is not so readily recognizable in the ribs or sternum. Generalized symptoms, such as fever and malaise, may be present. Additionally, the myeloma protein may be present in the serum of the patient. If the suspicion of myeloma is strong, needle biopsy is preferable to open surgical biopsy. Systemic chemotherapy is usually the treatment of choice.

Other Tumors

Other types of soft tissue sarcomas such as fibrosarcoma, angiosarcoma, neurosarcoma, and liposarcoma have been reported to occur on the chest wall. Additionally, occasional cases of Hodgkin's disease and other forms of lymphosarcoma arising in the sternum have been reported. The solitary form of histiocytosis, eosinophilic granuloma, may occasionally present as a painful lytic lesion in a rib, and with the fever and leukocytosis that may accompany, it can result in the mistaken diagnosis of osteomyelitis.

SURGICAL TECHNIQUES

Whereas most benign chest wall tumors lend themselves to simple excision, careful preoperative planning of the required reconstruction should be done before undertaking the surgical resection of a malignant mass. Wide surgical incision, however, is just what its name implies, and no compromise should be made in removing the primary tumor in its entirety. Previous biopsy sites should be included in the resection of all malignant tumors. Full-thickness resection of the chest wall is recommended for all sarcomas, including entry into the pleural space at least one normal interspace beyond the tumor.

The physiologic effects of a chest wall defect should be taken into consideration preoperatively. For example, a large chest wall defect underlying the scapula posteriorly would be much better tolerated than a similar-sized defect anteriorly or laterally. Hence, most posterior defects do not require extensive stabilization or reconstruction. Conversely, large defects in the anterior and lateral aspects of the chest wall may require imaginative reconstructive techniques. Occasionally, adjacent ribs may be excised and split to form free rib grafts to bridge a significant gap. In addition, the use of prosthetics such as Marlex mesh for this purpose has become common.

Skin closure is usually possible; however, when there is involvement of the skin with tumor or prior damage from radiation, the surgeon must be prepared to provide for an airtight integumentary cover for the resulting defect. Local flaps including breast, deltopectoral cutaneous, latissimus myocutaneous, and thoracoabdominal cutaneous tissues have been used. Omental pedicles have also been used in combination with large split-thickness skin.

Sternal excisions usually require minimum reconstruction and infrequently lead to the requirement for prolonged ventilatory support. Sometimes the sternum is only partially involved with a tumor, allowing preservation of the uninvolved end for midline stability.

PNEUMOTHORAX

H. PAT EWING, M.D.

INCIDENCE AND ETIOLOGY

Pneumothorax may be defined as a collection of air or gas within the pleural space. It may occur either spontaneously (idiopathic) or as a result of some kind of trauma including iatrogenic trauma. In the era of fast-moving automobiles, ubiquitous firearms, and other weapons of assault, traumatic pneumothorax has become the most common form. Of increasing importance are the iatrogenically induced pneumothoraces occurring as a result of such procedures as subclavian vein catheterization, percutaneous and transbronchial lung biopsies, balloon dilation of esophageal strictures, and positive pressure ventilation, sometimes with high levels of positive end-expiratory pressure (PEEP). As may be imagined, traumatic pneumothorax presents in association with a wide range of precipitating causes and underlying problems, and the significance of the finding as well as the management vary depending on the circumstances. In contrast to traumatic pneumothorax, idiopathic or spontaneous pneumothorax occurs without external interference. Typically, it occurs in the young male patient 20 to 40 years of age. It is therefore frequently seen around college campuses and in the military; but it may occur at any age and in women. It has been associated with a wide range of diseases including bronchogenic and metastatic pulmonary carcinoma, endometriosis, (catamenial pneumothorax), scleroderma, Marfan's syndrome, cystic fibrosis, most pneumoconioses, and tuberculosis, which was once thought to be the primary cause. It is now well recognized that in the otherwise healthy patient, spontaneous pneumothorax almost always occurs as a result of rupture of subpleural blebs, which are most commonly located over the apeces of the lungs or on the superior segments of the lower lobes. The reason for the development of these subpleural blebs is uncertain, but biochemical changes in the protein content of the involved lungs would suggest a complex problem of tissue degeneration rather than a purely mechanical bronchiolar obstruction. The relationship to smoking is uncertain, but cigarette smoking is a common practice in the patient population most susceptible to the condition. In patients over 40 years of age, idiopathic pneumothorax is frequently seen in association with chronic obstructive pulmonary disease and bullous emphysema. Management under this circumstance may need to be modified because of the underlying pulmonary disease.

CLINICAL PRESENTATION

The clinical picture of pneumothorax varies depending on the size of the pneumothorax and the associated disease. Spontaneous pneumothorax may be asymptomatic if it remains small. However, the typical picture is that of sudden onset of sharp chest or shoulder pain, which may be mild or severe and abates over several hours. It is characteristically associated with the onset of dyspnea, tachypnea, and tachycardia. There may be a nonproductive cough. With the development of a tension pneumothorax or of a hemopneumothorax secondary to tearing of pleural adhesions, the patient may become hypotensive and show signs of cardiovascular compromise. This is reported to varying degrees in 15 to 30 percent of the patients. Bilateral simultaneous spontaneous pneumothorax is reported to occur in approximately 2 percent of patients with spontaneous pneumothorax.

Pneumothorax is associated with varying degrees of respiratory distress. On physical examination, there are usually decreased breath sounds on the involved side and there is a hyperresonance to percussion. With a large pneumothorax and some element of tension, the trachea may be shifted toward the uninvolved side. The diagnosis is confirmed roentgenographically, and in the clear-cut case, it is easily recognized by the faint line representing the visceral pleura as outlined by radiolucent air on both sides, but lung markings are absent peripherally. However, the diagnosis may be obscured if the film is taken with inappropriate exposure or with the patient supine, or during inspiration rather than expiration. Particular care must be taken when giant emphysematous bullae are present since these may mimic the picture of pneumothorax.

TREATMENT

Observation

As with the clinical picture of pneumothorax, the management varies with the size and associated findings.

A very small asymptomatic and uncomplicated pneumothorax may be safely managed with expectant observation. Serial chest films confirm the stability and slow resolution of the pneumothorax. Needle aspiration of the small (10% to 20%), asymptomatic pneumothorax is not necessary and may potentially complicate the problem owing to the danger of laceration of the lung or intercostal vessels with subsequent hemorrhage. In a patient with severe chronic obstructive pulmonary disease and emphysematous changes or bullous disease of the lung, even a small pneumothorax may be symptomatic, and these patients are best managed by insertion of an intercostal tube once the diagnosis is established. A small, asymptomatic traumatic pneumothorax may also be treated conservatively with observation in some instances. This may include the small iatrogenic pneumothorax produced as a result of inadvertent puncture of the lung during subclavian vein catheterization or following needle biopsy or transbronchial biopsy of the lung. However, close observation is required since many of these patients subsequently require invasive intervention. Furthermore, the usual traumatic pneumothorax seen in the emergency room is associated with multiple other injuries and varying degrees of pulmonary hemorrhage and contusion. These patients should be managed with early intercostal tube drainage. Many of them require endotracheal intubation for anesthesia or pulmonary support; intercostal tube drainage, in this circumstance, is always indicated to prevent the rapid development of life-threatening tension pneumothorax.

Needle Aspiration

Most authors agree that an uncomplicated spontaneous pneumothorax does not require evacuation unless it occupies an estimated 20 percent of the hemithorax in expiration. The large pneumothorax with complete or nearly complete atelectasis of the involved lung, or those associated with underlying emphysematous disease, pleural effusion, or hemothorax, certainly require intercostal tube insertion for adequate drainage and reexpansion of the lung. However, management of the moderate-sized uncomplicated spontaneous pneumothorax remains somewhat controversial. These pneumothoraces sometimes are managed by a single aspiration or repeated aspirations of the pleural space by means of a plastic intravenous 16-gauge catheter, which is inserted through the appropriate intercostal space. The air is expelled under water using a three-way stopcock and a large syringe. Aspiration is continued until resistance is felt or until it becomes apparent that reexpansion will not be accomplished (usually after 2 to 4 liters have been aspirated.) In selected patients, the procedure has been reported as being 70 percent successful, and it has the advantage of avoiding unnecessary intercostal tube drainage in the patients. On the other hand, attempted aspiration carries with it the disadvantage of being frequently unsuccessful and requiring repeated procedures. The lung is seldom completely reexpanded, and the added danger of further injury to the lung with laceration, infection, and hemorrhage is introduced. It requires close observation and repeated chest films, and a significant number of patients subsequently require intercostal tube drainage, which has been unnecessarily postponed. Consequently, intercostal tube drainage is the treatment of choice of many thoracic surgeons when faced with an uncomplicated moderate-to-large spontaneous pneumothorax.

Closed-Tube Thoracostomy

Intercostal tube drainage or closed tube thoracostomy is therefore indicated in most instances of pneumothorax except for the small, uncomplicated spontaneous pneumothorax, which may be successfully managed with observation. In experienced hands, the intercostal tube may be inserted under local anesthesia with minimal discomfort to the patient, and it need not be a particularly painful or traumatic experience. Although techniques may vary, the following description makes mention of the salient points that have proved important in our experience.

First, the area of insertion is carefully prepared and is draped in a sterile fashion. A small amount of local anesthetic is infiltrated into the skin to allow a 2-cm incision over the rib beneath the intercostal space which is to be entered. Using a longer needle, a more generous dose is then necessary to anesthetize sequentially the appropriate intercostal nerve and the periosteum of the ribs above and below the intercostal space, as well as to infiltrate the intercostal muscle and pleura that are to be penetrated. Although toxic doses of the local anesthetic must be known and avoided, a liberal dose permits a practically pain-free insertion.

Proper positioning of the tube is of critical importance if one is to avoid problems with inadequate drainage. In the final analysis, the tube should be inserted into the appropriate area as determined by the chest film. Usually, for the treatment of pneumothorax, placement through the second intercostal space in the midclavicular line or through the fifth or sixth intercostal space in the midaxillary line is appropriate. In the acutely traumatized patient, the midaxillary approach is usually preferred. Under such circumstances, insertion of the drainage tube is often performed under less than ideal conditions, and it must frequently be accomplished under some duress. Complications are more likely to be avoided and adequate drainage more likely to be achieved if a large-bore (28 to 32 F) tube with multiple side holes is used and is inserted high on the chest wall. It is usually directed posteriorly at the time of insertion because of the frequent concomitant hemothorax, which is poorly drained by an anterior tube. Furthermore, the exact position of the hemidiaphragm is not always known in the acutely traumatized patient, and a chest film of the supine patient with hemopneumothorax is seldom helpful. Consequently, in the true emergency, it is probably better to err on the side of placing the tube too high on the chest wall. The fifth intercostal space in the midaxillary line is usually appropriate, and at this level, subdiaphragmatic insertion can be avoided.

One of the disadvantages of using the lateral fifth or sixth interspace for tube insertion is that the major fissure is located in this area. Tubes positioned within the major fissure often drain poorly and have to be repositioned. This problem sometimes can be avoided by directing the tube posteriorly and superiorly rather than centrally at the time of insertion. A simple pneumothorax uncomplicated by pleural effusion or hemothorax may be effectively treated by using a smaller tube (20 to 24 F), which is placed either anteriorly or laterally, but is directed anteriorly and to the apex to more effectively drain the pneumothorax.

After the skin incision has been made, blunt dissection with a hemostat is continued through the subcutaneous tissue, over the top of the rib, and through the external intercostal muscle layer. The pleural space may then be entered gently, either bluntly with a hemostat or with a trocar. Although some surgeons use a trocar almost routinely, in general it seems safer to use a trocar only when a large free pleural space has been documented. The trocar technique has the advantage of allowing a more rapid insertion and makes the procedure considerably less difficult, particularly in the obese patient. However, it also increases the risk of lung injury if pleural adhesions are present. Proper technique must be used to prevent too deep a penetration of the trocar. If a large free pleural space has not been demonstrated, the pleural space should be gently entered with a hemostat and then explored with the index finger. If there is no free pleural space, a different insertion site should be used. In the case of chronic pleural disease, care must be taken to be certain that the true pleural space is entered since a thick, tough parietal pleura may be bluntly dissected off the rib cage and the tube may be positioned extrapleurally. If the drainage site is low on the chest wall, the exploring finger should feel for the liver or spleen since the tube may easily be inserted beneath the diaphragm. With the acutely traumatized patient requiring emergency tube thoracostomy, the use of the trocar should probably be avoided since it seems to increase the risk of complications.

The tubes most commonly used include the 28 to 36 F red rubber or latex tubes with multiple side holes or the clear plastic intercostal catheter with a radiopaque marker added to aid roentgenographic visualization and determination of the position of the most proximal side hole. Some surgeons still effectively use a Foley catheter, but the clear plastic catheter seems to be preferred by most. Some prefer the latex tube because the more irritative quality of this material is more likely to produce pleural adhesions. However, this must be a localized effect and seems to be of doubtful clinical value.

Following insertion, the tube is sutured to the skin and connected to some system that allows controlled negative pressure with high volume capabilities in the event of a large air leak. The standard 2- or 3-bottle underwater seal system continues to work well, but disposable plastic units accomplishing the same ends of underwater seal drainage with controlled suction are now frequently used because of their convenience and ease of transportation. Such innovations as the Emmerson suction device allow easy control of the amount of negative pressure. Controlled negative pressure of 10 to 20 cm H_2O is usually all that is needed. However, it may be necessary to increase negative pressure to as much as 60 cm H_2O to adequately handle a large air leak and allow complete lung reexpansion.

Management of the chest tube usually is not difficult, but it requires persistent and tedious care if good drainage is to be maintained and complications avoided. The dressing around the chest tube should be changed as often as is necessary to keep the area clean and to avoid infection. Care should always be taken to carefully secure the tube with adhesive tape since continued traction may tend to displace the most proximal side hole to a position outside the thoracic space. This is a particular problem in the obese patient and is a common cause of continued development of subcutaneous emphysema after chest tube insertion. In the presence of pleural blood or effusion, the chest tube may need to be frequently stripped to prevent obstruction with clot or fibrin debris. A section of soft latex tubing may need to be connected to the chest tube to facilitate this. The level of fluid in both the underwater seal container and the suction bottle must be checked and adjusted daily. In the past, it has been frequently recommended that the chest tube be clamped whenever transportation of the patient is necessary to avoid problems with reflux of fluid back into the pleural space or loss of the underwater seal. However, clamping of a chest tube tends to cause more problems than it solves, particularly if there is a continued air leak. It may then result in recurrent pneumothorax or extensive subcutaneous emphysema. It seems more advisable to recommend that the chest tube not be clamped, but that more attention be paid to proper care and positioning of the chest bottle device during any necessary transportation. The chest tube is usually left in place until after the air leak has stopped and the lung remains completely expanded for 1 to 2 days.

Thoracotomy, Bleb Resection, and Pleural Abrasion

The indications for thoracotomy for management of a pneumothorax are (1) a persistent air leak after 10 to 14 days of adequate chest tube drainage, (2) a large air leak that cannot be adequately handled by the chest tube, (3) a recurrent ipsilateral spontaneous pneumothorax or bilateral simultaneous pneumothoraces, or (4) a hemopneumothorax with evacuation of more than 1,000 cc of blood.

Indications for surgery following a traumatic pneumothorax include excessive hemorrhage, massive air leak, massive chest wall injury, and the possibility of diaphragmatic, esophageal, or cardiac injury. Description of the surgical approaches in these instances is beyond the scope of this paper.

In the case of spontaneous pneumothorax, the necessity for thoracotomy is variously reported as 10 to 40 percent. The incidence of a recurrent spontaneous pneumothorax following treatment with closed-tube thoracostomy is reported to be around 20 percent. Surgical technique varies. The standard posterior lateral thoracotomy incision through the fourth intercostal space offers the best exposure. A median sternotomy incision has been advocated because it gives access to both lungs and therefore allows bilateral bleb resection and pleural abrasion to be done at the same time when indicated. It has also been argued that this incision results in less morbidity in the patient with severe chronic obstructive lung disease. On the other hand, it offers relatively poor exposure of the superior segments of the lower lobes, particularly on the left, which are common sites for bleb formation and may need to be resected or stapled at the time of surgery. Furthermore, in the event of a persistent air leak following surgery, a median sternotomy incision predisposes the patient to the development of extensive subcutaneous emphysema if the mediastinal pleura has not been carefully closed at the time of surgery. Regardless of the approach, appropriate surgical management usually entails ligation, plication, or surgical stapling of the apical blebs or bullous disease. In addition, some form of pleural abrasion is required to promote pleural symphysis and prevent a recurrent pneumothorax. In the experience of many, vigorous abrasion of the entire parietal pleural surface with dry gauze is adequate and efficacious. In the past, some have advocated resection or cauterization of the parietal pleura. This is effective, but in our experience it has not been necessary. Vigorous abrasion of the entire pleural surface with a dry gauze is all that is needed. Recurrence of pneumothorax following bleb resection is rare.

Closed chemical pleurodesis using such irritants as tetracycline, talc, silver nitrate, or nitrogen mustard has been advocated for treatment of recurrent pneumothorax. However, one may expect this method of management to be uncomfortable for the patient, and it has little advantage over thoracotomy in this regard. In addition, it is frequently ineffective. Consequently, it is generally reserved for patients who, because of advanced age or severe pulmonary disease, have a prohibitive expected surgical mortality.

CLINICAL PROBLEMS AND COMPLICATIONS

Tension Pneumothorax

A common concern regarding the patient with pneumothorax is the development of tension pneumothorax. This potentially catastrophic complication may occur in any patient, but it is more common in (1) the patient on positive pressure ventilation, particularly the neonate, (2) patients with massive trauma, and (3) patients with severe chronic obstructive pulmonary disease. Tension pneumothorax is relatively rare in the young patient with idiopathic pneumothorax, although it may occur.

The tension component is produced as a result of the development of a valve mechanism, which allows air to be trapped in the pleural space during the period of negative pleural pressure required for inspiration, but prevents its expulsion during expiration. Clinically, it is associated with severe respiratory distress and subsequent cardiovascular collapse. Although it has been suggested that cardiovascular collapse in tension pneumothorax is caused by decreased venous return and a mediastinal shift with "kinking" of the vena cava, experimental evidence seems to discount this. Cardiac output and arterial pressure are partially protected because of a reflex tachycardia as well as incomplete transmission of pleural pressure to the mediastinum and increased thoracic pressure fluctuations as the patient struggles to breath. However, there is a rapid and progressive development of a severe respiratory restrictive defect with subsequent hypoxemia and hypercarbia and secondary cardiovascular decompensation. The condition may be fatal if not recognized promptly and appropriately managed. The traumatic tension pneumothorax is most commonly seen in the patient with major bronchial disruption. Its presence should alert the surgeon to the possibility of the need for emergency thoracotomy. In the presence of tension pneumothorax or in patients at high risk, conservative management should not be attempted. The condition may be temporarily relieved by insertion of a large-bore needle into the thoracic space, but closed-tube thoracostomy should be undertaken on an urgent basis.

Hemorrhage

Hemorrhage is common with a traumatic pneumothorax, but may also occur with a spontaneous pneumothorax if pleural adhesions result in a parenchymal pulmonary tear. Development of a hemothorax following insertion of an intercostal tube is usually the result of injury to the intercostal vessels or to the lung itself. These injuries may be avoided with proper technique and are rarely a problem to the experienced surgeon. The presence of a significant hemothorax is an indication for closed-tube thoracostomy to avoid subsequent problems such as development of a pleural rind and lung entrapment. These tubes must be positioned posteriorly in the pleural space to allow adequate drainage. In the event of continued hemorrhage, thoracotomy is usually undertaken when blood loss is 1,000 cc or greater.

Reexpansion Pulmonary Edema

Reexpansion pulmonary edema is an unusual problem; nevertheless, it should be remembered because of the potentially lethal results. It was first described by Carlson et al in 1954. The clinical picture is characterized by the progressive development of cough, dyspnea, hypoxemia, cyanosis, and production of the frothy pink sputum of fulminant pulmonary edema following chest tube insertion and lung reexpansion. The chest film shows characteristic changes of pulmonary edema limited to the treated lung. The reason for the derangement is uncertain, but associated factors include prolonged atelectasis of the lung, rapid reexpansion of the lung frequently with rather high negative pressure, and, probably, some partial bronchial obstruction tending to prevent lung reexpansion. The hypoxemia may be severe, and supplemental oxygen and positive pressure ventilation may be necessary to prevent death. Fortunately, gradual clearing of the lung may be expected over 2 to 12 days.

Pneumothorax in Pilots and Air Travelers

Finally, a not uncommon problem for the contemporary physician concerns appropriate recommendations for management of the pneumothorax in a patient who will be flying at high altitudes as in a commercial airliner. Owing to Boyle's law, one may expect the size of a pneumothorax to vary directly with atmospheric pressure. Consequently, at high altitudes, a previously small pneumothorax may double or triple in size. Flying in

pressurized cabins limits but does not remove the problem since the cabin is usually pressurized to a differential of 8.6 psi. Consequently, if a patient with pneumothorax is transported by air, it is essential that the pneumothorax be treated with a chest tube and that the tube be connected either to a source of continuous negative pressure or to some type of flutter valve such as the Heimlich valve to prevent a potentially dangerous increase in the size of the pneumothorax. Once pneumothorax has been treated, however, the danger of flying is not great. A patient who had a spontaneous pneumothorax which resolved without treatment is permitted by the Federal Aviation Administration to return to flying within 6 to 12 months provided the pneumothorax has completely resolved and the patient does not have reason to expect a likely recurrence. Following a repeat pneumothorax, the patient must have surgical correction, but he is permitted to return to duty 3 months following the surgery. Most pilots may be returned to unrestricted flying.

HEMOTHORAX

KEVIN TURLEY, M.D.

Hemothorax is defined as the presence of blood in the pleural space. The modes of accumulation may be either traumatic or spontaneous. The former is the more common, with blood entering the pleural cavity directly from the chest wall, lung, mediastinum, or great vessels. The latter has multiple etiologies, and distinction between hemothorax and bloody pleural effusion is often unclear.

Since spontaneous etiologies are more varied and less common, I shall first direct attention to them and then discuss the incidence, diagnosis, and management of blunt and penetrating trauma subsequently. The pathophysiology of both and the clinical course in each, however, reflect a common natural history. As blood enters the pleural cavity, coagulation occurs that is precipitated by foreign material or inflammation. A bloody pleural effusion free of such contamination is rapidly absorbed.

Occasionally, fibrin is deposited, and fibrothorax with entrapment of the lungs may develop. Fibrothorax is more common in the presence of bacterial contamination or the presence of a foreign body within the pleural space. Adequate pleural drainage eliminates such problems regardless of the etiology. However, when pleural drainage is not possible, a fibrin sac develops, producing a pseudomembrane that becomes thick and nonpenetrable (a fibrin peel). When bacteria or bile is involved in the

production of this peel, a dense entrapment of the lung may develop, resulting in loss of pulmonary function if removal is not attempted. It should be noted that spontaneous resorption is possible in more than 80 percent of trauma patients and occurs through the pleural surface. Spontaneous resorption likewise occurs in those with spontaneous hemothorax in whom no continued source of hemorrhage is present.

SPONTANEOUS HEMOTHORAX

Multiple etiologies of spontaneous hemothorax have been identified. Spontaneous pneumothorax secondary to tearing of pleural adhesions is the most common etiology and usually afflicts young males in the third decade of life. The second most common etiology is pulmonary arteriovenous malformation with rupture into the pleural space, and this also occurs in young males in the third decade of life. Other pulmonary sources include bullous emphysema, necrotizing infections, pulmonary embolus with infarction, and tuberculosis, as well as hereditary hemorrhagic telangiectasia, primary pulmonary neoplasm, and metastases of all types including melanoma and trophoblastic tumors. Pleural sources include primary neoplasms of the pleura and endometriosis. Blood dyscrasias including thrombocytopenia, hemophilia, and complications of systemic anticoagulation, as well as von Willebrand's disease, have been implicated. Finally, abdominal and cardiovascular pathology in the form of pancreatic pseudocysts, splenic artery aneurysms, hemoperitoneum from multiple causes, as well as rupture of thoracic aortic aneurysms and aortic dissections, may produce hemothoraces; the onset of bleeding may be sudden or insidious and has no relationship to the activity of the patient. The patient experiences dyspnea with or without pleural pain; other systemic symptoms reflect the rate of hemorrhage and the pain pattern reflects the adjacent structures involved.

TRAUMATIC HEMOTHORAX

Traumatic hemothorax can result from either nonpenetrating or penetrating injuries. In nonpenetrating chest trauma, 25 to 75 percent of the patients present with hemothorax, which is bilateral in 5 to 20 percent of cases. In penetrating chest trauma, as many as 80 percent present with hemothorax, which is commonly associated with a pneumothorax. Again, the signs and symptoms are related to the rate and amount of intrathoracic bleeding, the patient's remaining pulmonary reserve, and associated injuries.

Patients with an accumulation of less than 500 cc of blood and without a major associated pneumothorax rarely present with significant hemodynamic or respiratory compromise, whereas those with an accumulation of more than 2,000 cc of blood or with a rapid accumulation may present with signs of hypovolemic shock and severe respiratory compromise. Patients who had a pre-injury decrease in pulmonary reserve demonstrate signs of respiratory compromise with even minimal injury. Severe cardiovascular compromise results from mediastinal shift, obstruction of caval return, and inflow occlusion, producing severe hypotension.

TREATMENT

In the majority of patients, as many as 85 percent in reported series, tube thoracostomy is adequate therapy. A large-bore, 36 F or greater, chest catheter in the fifth interspace at the anterior axillary line is the preferred drainage system. The tube should be placed through a skin incision, with blunt dissection of the chest wall structures and entry into the pleural space. The use of a sharp trocar should be avoided, as secondary injury from this method is common. After placement of the chest tube, repeat chest roentgenograms should be obtained to assess the adequacy of evacuation of the hemothorax. Residual pneumothorax in the apical region can be evacuated through a second chest tube in the second intercostal space anteriorly.

The goal of therapy is prompt evacuation of the pleural space and expansion of the lung, which allows apposition of the pleural surfaces. Frequently, this local hemostatic mechanism controls the hemorrhage and no further therapy is required. The more efficiently this goal is achieved, the less chance there is of a chronic fluid collection. If continued chest tube drainage at a rate greater than 200 cc per hour or more than 1,500 cc total is noted, emergency thoracotomy and surgical control of the bleeding site is necessary.

In patients with penetrating trauma who require thoracotomy for continued intrathoracic bleeding, the source of hemorrhage is usually an injured systemic artery: an intercostal artery, the internal mammary artery, an esophageal branch of the aorta, the subclavian artery, or the thoracic aorta. Occasionally, the source of hemorrhage is the pulmonary parenchyma or a hilar pulmonary vessel. Systemic arterial hemorrhage is usually controlled by direct suture ligation, although occasionally vascular reconstruction of the subclavian artery, innominate artery, or descending aorta may be required.

Injury to the pulmonary parenchyma that cannot be readily controlled by direct suture ligation may require pulmonary resection for control of hemorrhage. In general, pulmonary resection should be limited to the least amount of pulmonary tissue that will allow control of the hemorrhage and maximize parenchymal salvage. Wedge or segmental resection is the procedure of choice; however, lobectomy or even pneumonectomy may occasionally be required, particularly if injury to the hilar vessels is the source of the hemorrhage. In patients with exsanguinating hemorrhage from injury to the hilum of the lung, immediate division of the inferior pulmonary ligament and clamping of the pulmonary hilum with a vascular clamp may be lifesaving. This is particularly true when the rate of intrathoracic bleeding and inability to resuscitate the patient leads to emergency thoracotomy in the emergency room. If this is necessary, definitive surgical control of the hemorrhage should be delayed until the patient has been resuscitated and transferred to the operating room, where optimal conditions for surgical therapy are present.

Delayed thoracotomy may be necessary for persistent bronchopleural fistula following a hemopneumothorax or for persistent hemothorax. In the former case, a bronchopleural fistula that is present more than a week after injury is usually an indication for investigation of the source of the fistula and consideration for surgical correction. In patients with residual clotted hemothorax, conservative management usually allows resolution of the hemothorax without long-term sequelae. Resolution frequently requires as long as 6 weeks to occur. During this period, needle aspiration is rarely indicated and, in fact, is probably contraindicated. Needle aspiration is the source of contamination of the hemothorax and on occasion may be the etiology of recurrent intrathoracic hemorrhage. Development of empyema has been shown to be related to shock on admission, pleural contamination, pneumonia, and prolonged catheter drainage. In the absence of these conditions, adequate chest tube drainage usually is sufficient for resorption of traumatic hemothoraces, with fewer than 15 percent requiring subsequent thoracotomy for decortication. This plan of management has frequently returned patients to full activity 6 months after traumatic injury without detectable sequelae from the traumatic hemothorax.

THE TRACHEA

TRACHEAL STENOSIS

GORDON F. MURRAY, M.D.

Important factors in the surgical management of tracheal stenoses are the age of the patient, the etiology and chronicity of the stenosis, and the extent of the lesion. An understanding of these features of the stenosis is required to facilitate the choice of operation which is at once the safest and most effective for the patient. Perhaps most critical to a successful therapeutic conclusion is a careful assessment of the pathologic anatomy of the tracheal narrowing (Table 1). Tracheal narrowing may be due to functional stenosis of the airway secondary to compression or to intrinsic disese of the trachea itself (tracheomalacia). My experience has been primarily in the pediatric age group, and operative intervention is directed at relief of compression (usually vascular) or restitution of tracheal luminal integrity (tracheopexy). Intraluminal disease with maintenance of the external diameter of the trachea invites the application of exciting new methods of endoscopic therapy, chief among which is the carbon dioxide laser. When there is transmural injury and loss of full-thickness dimensions of the trachea, resection and primary anastomosis remains the desired surgical approach. In the unsuitable patient, treatment of tracheal stenosis by stenting with a silicone T-tube is a useful adjunct in management.

The goal of operative treatment of tracheal stenosis is the restoration of a normally functioning trachea. A tracheal lumen of at least one-half the diameter of a healthy trachea is essential for complete recovery of the patient.

TABLE 1 Pathologic Anatomy of Tracheal Stenosis

Functional stenoses (stenoses without mucosal defects)
  Compression
  Tracheomalacia

Mucosal stenoses (luminal cicatricial stenoses with
  maintenance of external diameter)
  Granulation tissue
  Mucosal ulceration and scarring

Structural stenoses (mural cicatricial stenoses with
  loss of substance and external diameter)
  Stomal defect
  Cuff injury

The method used should be as rapid as possible, but also completely safe. With rare exceptions, definitive operation is not required for the urgent or even long-term management of tracheal stenosis. The emergency treatment of obstruction may require nothing more than reassurance, humidification, sedation, and adequate treatment of endotracheal infection by appropriate antibiotic therapy. In many cases, dilation can be performed under general anesthesia and under direct vision with rigid bronchoscopes. A crucial factor in the outcome of dilation is the time elapsed since the tracheal trauma: the more recent the injury, the greater the chance of success of conservative therapy. If the patient cannot ventilate satisfactorily and his medical condition contraindicates early repair, a tracheostomy can be established. The latter alternative must be carefully planned and is more often required in the patient with panmural cicatricial stenosis. If the area of stenosis is accessible with a cervical exposure, the tracheostomy should be made directly through the area of already damaged trachea. The establishment of the tracheostomy at any distance from the diseased area is decried, since it lengthens the extent of the future resection. If the stenosis is mediastinal, the tracheostomy may be accomplished several centimeters away from the damaged segment to permit reconstruction in healthy trachea. I particularly emphasize that the definitive reconstruction is an elective procedure, and the surgeon must be confident that the operation can be performed safely and with excellent opportunity for a permanent solution to the airway problem.

FUNCTIONAL STENOSIS

Nearly all of my experience with tracheal stenosis that does not involve a mucosal defect (compression, tracheomalacia) has been in the pediatric age group. Anomalies of the great vessels, especially the innominate artery and aorta, are the most common causes of extrinsic compression of the trachea. The diagnosis requires roentgenograms of the chest and an esophagogram. There may be vascular compression of the trachea alone or compression of both the trachea and the esophagus by a vascular "ring". Arteriography is often advised prior to thoracotomy, especially if interruption of vascular structures is required to relieve the compression. Owing to improved clinical acumen and diagnostic facilities, the

345

significance of vascular anomalies as a cause of tracheal stenosis has recently become better appreciated. The more common types of congenital vascular anomalies which produce partial or complete encirclement of the trachea are listed in Table 2.

Innominate Artery Compression

I have become increasingly aware that compression of the trachea by the innominate artery is the most common stenotic airway problem in infants and young children. It is also apparent that the majority of innominate artery compressions occur when the origin of the artery is situated normally with respect to the trachea. (Occasionally, the origin of the vessel is truly aberrant and arises farther to the left than usual.) Clinical significance is related to the severity of symptoms: inability to clear the airway of secretions results in cough, respiratory distress, inflammation, and further secretions and obstruction. Recurrent tracheobronchitis and pneumonia may prompt consideration of operative intervention. However, history of reflex apnea is the most dangerous symptom, as death can be sudden and unexpected. The term *reflex apnea* is used to describe 2- to 3-minute episodes of apnea and cyanosis which may terminate in loss of consciousness. Mouth-to-mouth resuscitation by the physician or parent may be required during an episode. I would emphasize that the presence of reflex apnea is an absolute indication for investigation and surgical treatment when tracheal compression is proved.

Diagnostic Investigation

The initial specific examination of the child with reflex apnea and suspected tracheal compression is a lateral chest roentgenogram. Radiologic evidence of anterior tracheal compression should be regarded with suspicion, and a contrast esophageal study should then be performed. The latter study not only can identify associated esophageal pathology such as severe gastroesophageal reflux, but also gives information about the presence of an aortic arch anomaly. Bilateral indentation of the esophagus implies the presence of a vascular ring (e.g., double aortic arch) which will require arteriography for definition. Posterior compression of the esophagus suggests an anomalous subclavian artery passing behind

the esophagus, and this also requires delineation by aortography. Recognition of the existence of a vascular ring is obviously important, since suspension of the innominate artery is precluded. Fortunately, the presence of an associated vascular anomaly is reliably excluded by the finding of a normal esophagogram, and the surgeon can proceed to endoscopic examination. I utilize a rigid bronchoscope with fiberoptic illumination and a telescopic attachment. The classic bronchoscopic appearance is that of a pulsatile, anterior compression of the trachea immediately above the carina. Luminal narrowing is more severe on the right, resulting in a tear-drop configuration of the obstruction. Interestingly, the right radial pulse is easily obliterated by levering the bronchoscope forward. A complete tracheobronchial examination can usually be carried out, and appropriate cultures obtained. Careful attention to the airway in the operating room for a half hour following diagnostic bronchoscopy usually renders intubation unnecessary, and I have never had to proceed with emergency arterial suspension.

Surgical Management

General anesthesia is maintained through an endotracheal tube placed under direct vision with the aid of a pediatric flexible bronchoscope. Often ventilation is enhanced by passing the tube beyond the area of compression. The patient is placed in the supine position with the right chest slightly elevated. An anterior 3- to 4-cm incision is made in the right second intercostal space. An extrapleural thoracotomy is usually possible, but has minimal advantages. The thymus must always be mobilized, and I do not hesitate to excise a portion of the gland to ensure an empty anterior mediastinum for the suspension. The innominate vein is retracted superiorly and the vena cava to the right. The pericardium is regularly entered to expose the proximal innominate artery and the summit of the aortic arch. It is important that no effort be made to identify the limits of the trachea. *The connective tissue between the innominate artery and the trachea must be left intact* to provide for a suspension mechanism of the anterior tracheal cartilages when the artery is itself suspended. Elevation of the innominate artery is accomplished with three horizontal mattress sutures of 4–0 Polydec with pledgets. The first suture is placed in the anterior surface of the aortic arch in line with the origin of the innominate artery, the second in the artery at its origin from the arch, and the third in the proximal first centimeter of the innominate vessel. The mattress sutures are first passed through the body of the sternum, and all anchor points on the artery are evenly advanced to the undersurface of the sternum. Dramatic relief of the compression is often achieved and can be appreciated by anyone who views the results through the bronchoscope. Less often, the pulsatile component of the compression is removed, but residual narrowing persists. In any case, all infants have enjoyed a marked improvement in ventilatory function and are free of apneic episodes. I am convinced that there are clear indications

TABLE 2 Vascular Ring Anatomy

Double aortic arch
Right aortic arch and left ligamentum arteriosum
Anomalous left subclavian artery
Pulmonary artery sling
Anomalous innominate artery
Innominate artery compression

for the operation of innominate artery suspension in infants with severe symptoms characterized by cyanosis, stridor, extreme difficulty in clearing secretions, and, above all, reflex apnea. Not only are the anxieties of the parents and the attending physician immediately relieved, but a life-threatening lesion is eliminated and the infant is restored to a normal life expectancy. I have not applied this technique (tracheopexy) to infants who are symptomatic with tracheomalacia following tracheoesophageal fistula repair, and I note that others report less gratifying results in this circumstance.

MUCOSAL STENOSIS

With lesser degrees of injury to the tracheal wall, bronchoscopic removal of granulation tissue or destruction of scar tissue may suffice to restore a satisfactory airway. In this particular circumstance, the surgeon is dealing with a partial-thickness lesion and compromise of the tracheal lumen but maintenance of normal external diameter. A wide variety of endoscopic methods have been applied to these obstructing lesions including biopsy forceps, coagulation, cryotherapy, and forceful dilation. It must be appreciated that all of these techniques may jeopardize the perilous position of the patient with tracheal obstruction. Even gentle manipulation of an inflammatory lesion may be followed by bleeding or edema and may precipitate a complete tracheal occlusion. I have, in one child, elected to approach a particularly formidable endotracheal obstruction by formal surgical tracheotomy and excision of the scar. The intraoperative dilemma of identification of the level of the disease (the external diameter and appearance of the trachea is normal) is effectively pinpointed in this instance by bronchoscopic observation of the insertion of a 25-gauge needle through the anterior wall of the trachea. The tracheotomy can then be made precisely at the level of the offending lesion and the patency of the airway quickly restored.

Treatment by Laser Resection

The technologic development of transbronchoscopic use of the carbon dioxide surgical laser has added a powerful tool to the management of intraluminal cicatricial stenoses (Table 3). The carbon dioxide laser beam is an invisible light near the infrared spectrum which can be focused and delivered to the obstructing lesion by mirrors.

TABLE 3 Characteristics of the Carbon Dioxide Laser

Wavelength (nm)	10,600
Transmission system	Mirrors
Absorption in tissues	High
Coagulation	Low
Penetration	Shallow
Cutting effects	High

(Since the beam travels in a straight line, lesions in the tracheobronchial tree must be visible with a rigid bronchoscope.) The laser beam energy is released when it is absorbed in tissues containing water. (The field must be clear of secretions, since the beam will be adversely affected by them.) The interaction of the laser beam with tissue results in almost instantaneous elevation of the intracellular and extracellular fluid to 100 °C, producing destruction of the cellular elements. The depth of penetration is shallow, which allows progressive destruction of lesions without fear of perforating the trachea. The laser has a hemostatic effect with sealing of both lymphatic and vascular channels, and there is no observable postoperative edema due to the rapid thermal drop-off from the edge of the beam. Importantly, treatments can be carried out repeatedly without a cumulative deleterious effect.

Carbon dioxide laser therapy is indicated in the presence of a symptomatic obstructing tracheal lesion in which the external diameter of the trachea is maintained. The anatomic definition of such a lesion can usually be assured by roentgenograms, computerized tomography, and bronchoscopy. Treatment is initiated by passage of a rigid bronchoscope under general anesthesia. Following inspection of the lesion, the carbon dioxide laser beam assembly is attached to the bronchoscope. Ventilation is maintained by a Sanders attachment. (Risk of fire or explosion must be avoided by the use of compressed air rather than oxygen during the time of laser application.) The *eyes of the patient, operator, and all personnel must be protected* from possible incident reflections of the laser beams. Experience with the carbon dioxide laser indicates that it will be an effective and satisfactory method of treating symptomatic obstructing tracheobronchial lesions. Among the inflammatory lesions successfully treated, granulation tissue has occurred commonly, with most remaining patients having membranous cicatrix.

STRUCTURAL STENOSIS

Resection is the only definitive treatment possible when there is extensive injury to the cartilages over a distance. Alternative measures are unlikely to succeed in the patient with full-thickness destruction of the tracheal wall and are not without significant risk. The operative techniques of segmental resection and primary anastomosis described by Grillo in the first edition of *Current Surgical Therapy* most consistently achieve a good result. Several principles for successful primary reconstruction can be emphasized (Table 4). Since the operative approach usually requires only a cervical incision or, at most, an upper mediastinal division of the sternum, the physiologic stress is minimal. When the operation is done with extreme precision, anesthesia is given properly, and first-quality postoperative care is provided, even patients with extremely poor respiratory reserve can undergo primary repair. Contraindications to surgical segmental resection are therefore few (Table 5).

TABLE 4 Principles for Primary Anastomosis

Accurate definition of the precise level and length of the lesion

Full evaluation of the functional state of the larynx

Resection through healthy trachea

Preservation of tracheal circulation

Avoidance of injury to the recurrent laryngeal nerves

Avoidance of tension at the anastomosis

TABLE 5 Contraindications to Primary Anastomosis

Systemic contraindications
  Diseases or circumstances that would require respirator
    support postoperatively
  Disease process certain to require early repeat
    tracheostomy
  Quadriplegic patients who should not be subjected to
    tracheal reconstruction (unable to raise secretions)
  High-dose steroid therapy

Local contraindications
  Uncorrected laryngeal disease
  Recently or markedly inflamed tracheostomy
  Presence of florid granulation tissue and inflammation
    at the site of the stenosis

Silicone Tracheal T-Tube

I continue to see patients for whom surgical reconstruction is unfeasible or inappropriate. In this circumstance, the Montgomery silicone T-tube is a useful adjunct to the surgical management of complex tracheal lesions. Rarely, structural stenosis of the trachea which is not circumferential may respond to long-term use of the silicone T-tube alone. Tracheal narrowing in only one projection of the chest roentgenogram may suggest the potential for this therapeutic selection. When the T-tube is used as the definitive treatment to stent an abnormal area of the trachea, it should remain in place for 9 months or longer. More often, the silicone T-tube is utilized as (1) a temporary airway prior to definitive resection, (2) an adjunct to segmental subglottic resection, and (3) rescue following uncertain or unsuccessful tracheal resection.

The Montgomery T-tube is soft and pliable, has a polished nonabrasive surface, and is commercially available in a variety of diameters and lengths. The T-tube preserves the voice and results in normal physiologic mechanisms for humidification of the airway. Tracheal-bronchial secretions do not tend to accumulate on the smooth inner silicone surface, and my experience indicates that these tubes may be left in place for periods as long as a year. Cooper has found them to be particularly useful in selected patients with complex reconstructions following resection of high subglottic strictures. In this situation, the proximal limb of the stent lies just above the level of the vocal cords. With the tube in this position, most patients maintain adequate voice and are not troubled by problems of aspiration.

A vertical tracheostomy stoma is utilized for insertion of the T-tube. The tube selected should have the largest diameter accommodated by the trachea. General anesthesia is used for the insertion, and a technique permitting spontaneous respiration simplifies the procedure. The insertion is facilitated by initial placement of a long umbilical tape through the tracheostoma and out the mouth. To accomplish this, a rigid bronchoscope is passed through the larynx and a forceps is used to bring the tape cephalad through the scope. The lower end of the umbilical tape is passed through the upper limb of the T-tube and out the horizontal limb. Both ends of the tape are carefully grasped to prevent inadvertent withdrawal. Insertion is completed by advancing the lower limb of the tube through the stoma directly toward the carina. The entire T-tube, including most of the horizontal limb, is advanced until the upper limb enters the trachea. Forceful traction on the upper end of the umbilical tape straightens out the upper limb of the T-tube and places the tube in its intended position. The bronchoscope is used to confirm the proper position of the T-tube. Alternative techniques for insertion of the flexible silicone tube have been described, but I have found that use of the umbilical tape, as just described, is reliable and simplifies insertion.

VASCULAR SYSTEM

ABDOMINAL AORTIC ANEURYSM

JAMES F. BURDICK, M.D.

PRESENTATION AND EVALUATION

The patient with an abdominal aortic aneurysm (AAA) is commonly asymptomatic, and the diagnosis made as an incidental finding. The major indication for elective repair is the high risk of fatal rupture, which can occur even in relatively small aneurysms. Other complications of abdominal aortic aneurysm that may occasionally represent indications for repair include distal embolization (usually of the microembolic variety to end arterioles in the feet), aortovenous fistula to the inferior vena cava or iliac vein, and aortoenteric or aortoureteric fistula (both rare). Finally, in a patient with a known AAA, any pain between the diaphragm and the groins, regardless of its character or exact location, represents a potential leak and is an indication for urgent intervention.

Even patients with stable but severe medical risks are rather likely to die of their AAA rather than other causes. It is generally accepted that risk of rupture increases with size of the aneurysm. Therefore, if the aneurysm is approximately 5 cm or greater in transverse diameter, repair is indicated in almost all cases. In relative order of importance for the decision to proceed to elective repair, the following factors must be considered (Table 1): size, severity of patient's other medical problems (which increase the operative risk and limit the life expectancy), whether the visceral vessels are involved in the proximal portion (which would necessitate a higher-risk procedure), and inclination of the patient. It is

Table 1 Considerations in Elective Repair of Abdominal Aortic Aneurysm

Size (>5 cm)

Severity of other medical problems

Anatomy of the aneurysm

(Patient inclination)

important to note that the surgeon should approach the patient with a clear recommendation for surgery (or observation) based on the criteria just mentioned since the patient may find it difficult to resolve the various probabilities that must be factored into the decision.

Evaluation of the aneurysm itself (Table 2) is most expeditiously done with sonography, although CT scanning also provides an accurate picture of an aneurysm and may help to detect visceral artery involvement or dissection into the wall. During noninvasive assessment, it is important to investigate other suspiciously widened femoral or popliteal pulses since patients with AAA have a higher incidence of other such peripheral aneurysms. It is our routine to perform preoperative angiography, although an intravenous pyelogram may be substituted for this. The position of the aneurysm neck, with its relationship to the renal arteries, should be assessed, and the angiogram usually helps to decide what run-off vessels will be employed. Although concomitant iliac occlusive disease is uncommon, this should be assessed. Finally, one of the most important advantages of preoperative angiography is to allow the surgeon to plan in advance the best revascularization for the lower colon. The incidence of colonic ischemia after aortic surgery is far lower than in the past, apparently owing to the present realization that appropriate flow through internal iliac and/or inferior mesenteric arteries will be necessary at the end of the procedure.

The medical work-up should pay particular attention to the possibility of atherosclerotic involvement of the coronary or carotid arteries. If there is evidence of hemodynamically severe occlusive disease in either of these distributions, further evaluation with even the possibility of coronary artery bypass or carotid endarterectomy should be undertaken, prior to repairing the aneurysm. Whether to elect such preaneurysmectomy coronary or cerebral revascularization, in patients without other indications for the procedures, is controversial. At any rate, this would only be done in cases with hemodynamically severe lesions, since only these represent a particular threat during anesthesia or blood-loss-related hypotension. In addition, the patient's pulmonary status should be assessed since chronic obstructive pulmonary disease is common in these individuals. It is best to work up and treat obstructive uropathy in advance of elective AAA repair. Age, at least below 85 to 90 years, is not a major consideration, since a fit individual with a large

TABLE 2 Work—up of a Patient with Abdominal Aortic Aneurysm

Sonography:	The "gold standard"
CT scan:	For more detailed anatomy or question of dissection
Angiography:	Not for diagnosis Note status of renal, iliac, and inferior mesenteric arteries Ensure hydration, and an observation interval after the angiogram

aneurysm is likely to survive elective repair and the aneurysm represents by far the greatest specific threat to such a patient.

PROCEDURE

Conventionally, the approach is through a midline abdominal incision. A useful alternative to consider is the extended retroperitoneal approach. This allows easy exposure and clamping in the region of the visceral aorta, and produces much less postoperative pulmonary and gastrointestinal morbidity, so that is is preferable for older patients or those with chronic lung disease. The major contraindications to its use are a large right iliac aneurysm, which is difficult to control from this approach, or a right renal artery stenosis, which is difficult to approach directly from the left extended retroperitoneal approach. The groins must always be draped into the field, although this is generally an unnecessary precaution. Regardless of choice of incision, the arteries may be dissected carefully around three quarters of their circumference, but the older technique of placing a clamp and a tape directly around the entire artery is unnecessary since it is possible merely to clamp the artery (or the aortic neck) with some undissected material remaining opposite the operator. Great care should be taken with dissection and clamping in the region of the distal aorta and iliac arteries, since these are often densely adherent to the vena cava and iliac veins. However, proximally, near the neck, there is a large amount of tissue between the aorta and vena cava, and the only venous structures at risk are crossing lumbar veins from the left renal hilum to the left lumbar region, or underneath the aorta on the vertebral column. Ureters are occasionally encased in the wall of aortic or iliac artery aneurysms and must be diligently sought and protected. A fearsome disaster, which is fortunately rare, is the development of massive visceral and distal embolization due to disruption of material within the lumen of the diseased aorta. Dissection should always be done carefully to avoid this. However if the patient has had a definite history of such embolization in the months prior to the operation, an extreme degree of caution, involving early heparinization and clamping of the iliac vessels, is advisable since it is the general experience that these patients are at the greatest risk for this complication of extensive microembolization.

Prior to cross-clamping, unheparinized blood should be withdrawn for preclotting the graft if the usual knitted prosthesis is to be employed, and then heparin is administered at a usual dose of 5,000 to 8,000 units. Careful attention to hemodynamics, with communication between the anesthesia team and the surgeon, is required during cross-clamping. As soon as the aneurysm is opened, heavy stitches should be available for immediate suturing of any bleeding lumbar orifices, in order to minimize blood loss. If clamping has, for instance been above the renal arteries, there may be some back flow from these vessels. This bleeding may be controlled by placement of a Fogarty catheter balloon in the orifice held inflated with a three-way stop cock. The dissection at the region of the neck should be done with care to ensure an adequate margin of aorta below the clamp for anastomosis. It is generally expeditious and safer to employ the Creech technique of sewing the posterior portion of the graft within the aortic wall at the region of the neck rather than dissect around and divide the aorta completely, although this varies from case to case. A running suture of 3–0 Prolene is used for the proximal anastomosis. After testing the anastomosis and the graft preclot, the graft is clamped just below the anastomosis, using protective rubber shod clamps, and the initial limb is reimplanted if an aortoiliac graft is elected. It is my present policy to employ a sleeve graft whenever the aortic bifurcation and iliac arteries are in reasonably good condition, although others feel that the bifurcation graft is almost always better.

During the completion of the first outflow anastomosis, communication between the surgeon and anesthesia team is important, so that preparation for unclamping is made. This will always include the administration of additional intravascular volume and bicarbonate, and perhaps tapering of vasodilating agents. It is important to carefully flush first the inflow, and then back out the outflow, to ensure that no debris is present in the graft or the anastomotic region. Following this, the stitch is tied down. Then the flow is restored to the limb with great care, while the blood pressure is monitored so that this process goes smoothly with no period of hypotension. The surgeon may need to spend several minutes holding the graft limb and partially releasing it, preferably while actually watching the arterial pulse tracing, to ensure that the blood pressure will remain adequate with the flow restored. Similar care is necessary for the second side of a bifurcation graft.

After the graft has been completely sewn in, the femoral pulses should be palpated, and the clamp sites on the iliac artery should be inspected to ascertain that the outflow is good bilaterally. If cross-clamping was done near the renal vessels, these should be assessed, and if necessary Gerota's capsule should be opened and the renal parenchyma itself palpated and visualized to ensure that it is firm and of a healthy, purple-pink color. If there was any question on the preoperative arteriogram about revascularization of the lower colon and pelvic region, the inferior mesenteric artery should be dissected free and divided at the region of the aneurysm temporarily, to determine whether there is excellent backbleeding indicating a good head of pressure in the anastomoses to the lower colon. If IMA pressure or backbleeding is poor, it is advisable to revascularize it by anastomosis to the side of a graft limb.

OPERATIVE PROBLEMS

With experience, major venous hemorrhage is generally avoidable. The vena cava is separated nicely from the aorta proximally, but the vena cava and iliac venis can become densely adherent to the lower aorta and common iliac arteries. In this area dissection must be done cautiously with this in mind. Proximally, the large left renal vein-lumbar collateral, which travels on the left side of the aorta, must be avoided, and venous bleeding from crossing lumbar vessels underneath the aorta can occur. A series of Allis clamps applied with care, perhaps twisted or pushed in appropriate directions, can usually gain temporary occlusion of a large venous rent, allowing careful fine suturing which will not tear and cause larger holes. The use of a Teflon felt strip to totally reinforce the anastomosis on the aorta is rarely necessary in the abdomen, but additional sutures placed to stop this or other arterial bleeding should be based on Teflon felt pledgets to protect the arterial side of the suture from tearing through the artery.

The femoral pulses and pedal pulses, as well as the general appearance of the feet, should be determined before the patient leaves the operating room. If absence of the femoral pulse is discovered prior to closure, the condition can be corrected by opening the graft limb and performing either thrombectomy or an extension of the graft down to the groin. If this is determined after closure, it may be more expeditious to explore the femoral artery and, if Fogarty thrombectomy is successful, not to reopen the abdomen.

POSTOPERATIVE COMPLICATIONS

Cerebrovascular disease is common in these patients, and this may complicate the postoperative course. For this reason, many centers recommend prophylactic carotid endarterectomy for lesions that are hemodynamically significant prior to performing a major procedure such as aneurysm repair. Similarly, myocardial infarction is not uncommon in spite of the best efforts of surgeon and anesthetist to protect the heart by maintaining a good filling pressure and low peripheral vascular resistent throughout the patient's course. Patients with critical coronary artery disease should probably have this repaired at a separate procedure prior to aneurysm repair, unless the aneurysm is leaking or otherwise symtomatic.

Pulmonary status should be assessed in patients prior to aneurysm repair. If there is significant chronic obstructive pulmonary disease, the retroperitoneal approach is preferable. This allows avoidance of a large midline incision and entry into the peritoneal cavity, and the repiratory function of these patients is much less compromised by the procedure postoperatively. Renal failure may occur due to preoperative angiogram dye, intraoperative embolizaiton of the renal arteries or renal parenchyma, intraoperative or postoperative hypotension, or direct anatomic compromise of arteries or ureters. It is important to perform angiography at least 48 hours prior to aneurysm repair, to ensure that good hydration and urine output remain present during this interval and any major decrement in renal function is identified prior to proceeding with the repair. The other possible causes for renal failure must be avoided by appropriate care insofar as possible during the procedure.

Finally, in spite of the best efforts of the surgeon to revascularize the extremities successfully, there is in rare instances an ischemic event that results in loss of a foot or leg. This slight risk must be clear to the patient prior to proceeding with the procedure. If the patient is in stable condition, additional procedures to restore circulation if acute complications of this sort occur are appropriate and relatively safe. The most devastating example of this is the rare occurrence of multiple small emboli from the atherosclerotic debris lining the aorta which can occur during dissection of the aorta. It is remarkable how uncommon this is, but it may cause such severe occlusion of end vessels in the extremities, or even in the gastrointestinal tract or kidneys, that these are not salvageable. In the absence of more proximal vascular occlusion, which is surgically accessible, there is little to do except manage these patients with heparin or dextran and vasodilating agents.

Blood loss is a significant problem during many aneurysm repairs. Several maneuvers can help to mitigate morbidity from this. In the first place, it may be possible to obtain as many as three or four units of the patient's own blood by a multiple "piggy-backing" preoperative donation technique. These will then be available, before becoming outdated, at the time of surgery. In the second place, it is appropriate to allow some degree of hemodilution to occur during the procedure which can spare some need for transfusion. Some thought to the points at which blood loss commonly occurs, such as inadvertent venous damage, bleeding during opening of the aneurysm and ligation of lumbar and middle sacral arteries, and during testing of anastomoses and flushing, will allow conservation of erythrocytes to some degree. All of these may be of assistance, but hemologous blood transfusion is still commonly required. Patients should understand that this does not represent a noticeable risk of acquired immunodeficiency syndrome. The transfer of hepatitis or occurrence of a transfusion reaction are the greatest dangers, although the probability of even these complications is remarkably small for each individual unit of blood transfused.

Overall, the expectation is a 10 to 15 percent morbidity in patients undergoing elective AAA repair. Recent series, even of patients over 65 years of age, indicate a 0 to 9 percent mortality rate.

RUPTURED ABDOMINAL AORTIC ANEURYSM

E. STANLEY CRAWFORD, M.D.
HUGH GATELY, M.D.

Rupture of an abdominal aortic aneurysm continues to be an important treatable cause of death. Aneurysms of the infrarenal abdominal aorta may be traumatic, syphilitic, congenital, infected, or anastomotic, but more than 95 percent are due to arteriosclerosis. Although abdominal aortic aneurysms can thrombose, embolize, form enteric or caval fistulas, or become infected, the threat of rupture is such a frequent and lethal complication that it completely dominates the indications for operative treatment. A ruptured abdominal aortic aneurysm is considered to be an aneurysm with a defect in its wall that allows the escape of blood into the retroperitoneal tissues or the free abdominal cavity. This definition does not include expanding aneurysms with intact walls, aneurysms with evidence of edema or inflammation within the wall, dissecting aneurysms, or aneurysms in which there is evidence of old, well-circumscribed false aneurysm formation. Primary aortoenteric and aortocaval fistulas represent separate entitites and are discussed elsewhere in this monograph.

It is estimated that about 28,000 abdominal aortic aneurysms are seen every year in the United States, and that 5,000 patients present with rupture. That aneurysms of the abdominal aorta are potentially lethal was shown by Estes in his classic description of the natural history of abdominal aortic aneurysms based on his experience with 102 patients. Survival in this group of patients followed without operation was only 18.9 percent at 5 years, 63.3 percent of the deaths being due to rupture of the aneurysm. Szilagyi and Ottinger, in separate studies, have confirmed that rupture is a potential danger of abdominal aortic aneurysms. Gliedman, in a study of patients with symptomatic abdominal aortic aneurysms, discovered that 30 percent were dead within 1 month and 74 percent within 6 months of the onset of symptoms.

The first successful resection of an abdominal aortic aneurysm was on March 29, 1951 by Dubost, who restored aortic continuity with a homograft after excising the lesion. On November 6, 1952 DeBakey and his associates in Houston were the first in the United States to replace an abdominal aortic aneurysm. The first operations on ruptured abdominal aortic aneurysms were performed in 1953 and reported the following year by Bahnson, by Cooley, and by DeBakey.

Over the last three decades, the risk of elective aneurysmectomy has fallen from 12 to 15 percent down to 2 to 5 percent. Crawford and associates examined a 25-year experience with infrarenal abdominal aortic aneurysms and the factors influencing survival. Over this period, the mortality rate dropped from 19.2 percent to 1.9 percent in spite of a tenfold increase in the number of high-risk patients subjected to operation. In surgical series, the incidence of ruptured aneurysm ranges from 4 percent to 37 percent of all aneurysms treated surgically. In the senior author's experience, rupture has occurred in 6 percent. The chance of survival once rupture has occurred varies between 17 and 66 percent, averaging 45 percent. Approximately 30 percent of patients with ruptured abdominal aortic aneurysms are those known to have aneurysms who have been followed nonoperatively. Conversely, the majority of patients present with no prior history of abdominal aortic aneurysm, making the diagnosis difficult at times.

Although most aneurysms that rupture are large (6 cm), it is important to note that smaller aneurysms do rupture. In various studies, 9 to 39 percent of abdominal aortic aneurysms smaller than 6 cm ruptured during follow-up. Szilagyi, in a large study with careful follow-up and analysis of data, showed that small aneurysms (6 cm) had a 15 to 20 percent risk of rupture, and 5-year survival with resection was approximately 65 to 70 percent and without resection approximately 48 percent, in comparable groups of good-risk patients. The greatest cause of death in the nonsurgical group was a ruptured aneurysm, accounting for 34.6 percent of deaths. Bernstein has shown that the rate of expansion of small abdominal aortic aneurysms is variable, with rupture occurring in spite of close follow-up. Therefore, we believe that an aneurysm two times the size of the native vessel proximal to the lesion should be considered for operation, even if it is 3 to 4 cm in diameter.

Age has been related to survival by several authors, whereas others have shown no relation. Results of these previous studies of patients undergoing emergency operation for ruptured abdominal aortic aneurysms have suggested that age should be more accurately based on a physiologic rather than on a chronologic basis. Lawrie et al have reported that 60 percent of patients older than 80 years survived operation. In the senior author's series, 80 percent of octogenarians have survived operation.

PRESENTATION

The classic clinical presentation of a ruptured abdominal aortic aneurysm is easily recognized: severe abdominal and/or back pain followed by hypotension and shock with a palpable, pulsatile abdominal mass. Pain is the most common and constant feature; it may radiate to the groin or back and is often excruciating. Severe hypotension or shock (systolic blood pressure 90 mm Hg) is present in approximately 30 to 40 percent of patients. Shock may occur suddenly; therefore, the presence of a normal blood pressure does not justify delay in transporting the patient to the operating room. Flank ecchymoses may present in a small percentage of patients. Not all symptomatic abdominal aortic aneurysms show evidence of rupture. Expansion of abdominal aortic aneurysms or inflammatory aneurysms may produce symptoms without rupture. Hypotension is rare in these conditions; nevertheless, symptomatic aneurysms should also be considered an urgent indication for surgery in order to prevent problems associated with frank rupture.

PREOPERATIVE EVALUATION

All patients with a suspected diagnosis of ruptured abdominal aortic aneurysm with hypotension should be taken immediately from the emergency center to the operating room after blood is drawn for typing and saline and routine crossmatching of 10 units of packed red blood cells, 10 units of platelets, and 10 units of fresh frozen plasma. In a small percentage of symptomatic patients without hypotension and without known or palpable abdominal aortic aneurysm, CT scanning, ultrasound, or aortography may be employed to establish the presence of an aortic aneurysm. Abdominal CT and ultrasound are highly sensitive in identifying the location and size of the aneurysm. Aortography, although not always accurate in confirming the diagnosis of abdominal aortic aneurysm, is helpful in identifying associated aneurysms, occlusive disease, and renal artery anatomy. For the majority of patients, however, these tests are unnecessary and may cause a fatal delay.

Placement of lines for monitoring and infusion should be performed in the operating room and should not delay surgery in the moribund patient. If the patient is in severe shock or suffers cardiac arrest preoperatively, the abdomen is rapidly entered without regard to blood availability via a long midline incision without prepping the patient, and with only oxygen administered by the anesthesiologist while aortic control is obtained at the diaphragmatic hiatus with a hand. Resuscitation then proceeds with placement of several large-bore intravenous lines by cut-down technique or percutaneously while the patient is intubated and anesthesia induced. When hypotension is less severe, a radial artery line, central venous line, Foley catheter and nasogastric tube may be placed prior to induction of anesthesia. Two grams of a second-generation cephalosporin are given intravenously before the skin incision is made. Vasopressors and excess IV fluid are avoided to prevent extravasation of more blood prior to surgery.

SURGICAL TECHNIQUE

The operative field is prepared and draped in all patients before induction of general anesthesia and intubation. With blood infusing through blood warmers, a midline incision from xiphoid process to symphysis pubis is performed. If rapid control is necessary, this is accomplished without dissection at the diaphragmatic hiatus with an assistant's hand or an external compression device while avoiding trauma to adjacent organs. We believe that left thoracotomy is contraindicated for proximal control because of operative delay and postoperative morbidity. If the patient is hemodynamically stable, but the aneurysm has ruptured freely intraperitoneally or there is a large retroperitoneal hematoma, proximal control is again accomplished at the diaphragm. The left lobe of the liver is retracted laterally and superiorly, the stomach retracted inferiorly, the gastrohepatic omentum incised, the right crus of the diaphragm incised in the direction of its muscle

fibers, and the aorta bluntly freed with finger dissection and then vertically cross-clamped. Heparin is not used. The transverse colon is then laid superiorly on the abdominal wall and the small bowel eviscerated to the patient's right. The retroperitoneal hematoma may cause marked displacement of the left renal vein, duodenum, and inferior vena cava. Therefore, the duodenum is identified and the center of the aneurysm is entered using electrocautery, and care is taken to avoid injuring the duodenum or the descending colon mesenteric vessels. The aortic wound edges are retracted with No. 2 silk stay sutures, atheromatous material is removed, and blood is aspirated with the Baylor cell saver. The uninvolved proximal aortic neck and renal artery origins are identified from within the aneurysm. Distal back bleeding from the iliac arteries is controlled in the majority of patients by packing with a lap sponge to prevent stasis distally. Peripheral vascular clamps or balloon catheters are used when vigorous back bleeding is encountered. One end of a woven Dacron tube graft is sutured to the proximal uninvolved aorta from within the aneurysm using a running 3–0 Prolene suture. It is important that the aortic suture bites be large to prevent anastomotic leaks. The proximal aorta and graft are flushed by temporary removal of the proximal clamp to check for hemostasis. With the graft filled with blood, the graft is clamped distal to the anastomosis and the proximal clamp removed, restoring blood flow into the visceral and renal arteries.

Tube grafts were used in 70 percent of our series to simplify operation. Indications for bifurcation grafts included (1) severe iliac occlusive disease and (2) aneurysmal involvement. Woven Dacron is the graft material of choice because of its low porosity and because there is no need for preclotting. Sodium bicarbonate and mannitol solution are given, and the distal anastomosis performed. If anastomoses to the common iliac arteries are required, they are accomplished end-to-end with continuous 4–0 Prolene.

Prior to completion of the distal anastomosis, proximal flushing is performed and distal back bleeding assessed by clamp removal if previously applied. If distal backbleeding is poor or absent, Fogarty balloon catheters are passed distally to remove thrombus. Once the anastomosis is complete, the anesthetist is notified so that appropriate adjustments can be made in volume replacement and vasopressors. The clamp is removed slowly, and distal circulation is restored. The adequacy of femoral pulses is assessed as well as perfusion of the feet and left colon. The aneurysmal wall is then sutured around the graft with a running 2–0 Prolene suture after covering the graft with one gram of Mandol powder. Coagulopathies are prevented and treated as indicated by using fresh frozen plasma, platelets, and cryoprecipitate.

Aneurysmal dilatation may involve the renal arteries. In this event, proximal control is required at the diaphragm. Juxtarenal aortic aneurysms were present in 9.3 percent of cases in our series, the survival rate being 85.7 percent.

Patients with aortocaval fistulas present with an abdominal bruit, widened pulse, venous hypertension, peripheral edema, arterial insufficiency of the lower extremities, and congestive heart failure. Operative management must avoid embolization of thrombus either distally to the legs or through the vena cava to the lungs. The vena caval defect is closed through the aneurysmal sac.

Patients with primary aortoenteric fistulas present most commonly with massive upper gastrointestinal bleeding, although melena and hematochezia may occur. The anatomic proximity of the duodenum to the aneurysm makes this the most common site of the fistula. Rupture into the jejunum or colon is rare. The etiology of the primary fistula is different from that of a secondary fistula following graft placement and probably reflects adherence of the bowel to an inflammatory reaction around the aneurysm rather than an active infection. The initial procedure on abdominal exploration is proximal control of the aorta at the diaphragm. A careful search is then made for the enteric fistula. If the surrounding tissue is clearly viable, a primary enteric closure is performed. If the surrounding tissue is ischemic, the bowel must be locally resected and anastomosed. Abdominal aortic aneurysm resection and graft replacement is performed, as previously described, and the patient is maintained on antibiotics. Local excision, aortic closure, and extra-anatomic bypass are not necessary.

RESULTS

The results of operation for ruptured abdominal aortic aneurysms vary considerably in the recent literature. Mortality rates vary from 15 to 68 percent and depend on the condition of the patient at the time of operation. In most series, patients with preoperative hypotension have a mortality rate at least twice that of normotensive patients. Factors that have influenced mortality in other series include age of the patient, preoperative hypotension, length of cross-clamp time, number of blood transfusions required, amount of blood loss, length of operation, and postoperative complications.

Seventy-five patients underwent operation for ruptured abdominal aortic aneurysms over a 28-year period in our series. Intraoperative and overall mortality rates were 2.6 percent and 24 percent respectively. Increased mortality rates were associated with preoperative hypotension, BUN levels higher than 25 mg per deciliter, creatinine levels higher than 1.8 mg per deciliter, and a hematocrit less than 30 vol per deciliter. Increased mortality rates were associated with lengthy operative times—more than 130 minutes, estimated blood loss greater than 2,200 ml, and blood transfusion of more than 7 units.

The mortality rate for patients older than 70 years was 26 percent, and 8 of 10 patients in their ninth decade of life survived. The difference in the mean age of the survivors was 68.1 years, and that of the 18 nonsurvivors, 70.4 years. This was not significant. Death occurred in 12 of 28 patients (42.9%) with preoperative shock and in three of four patients (75%) who required cardiopulmonary resuscitation prior to induction of anesthesia.

COMPLICATIONS

Complications following operation for ruptured abdominal aortic aneurysm are not uncommon. Postoperative complications influence hospital morbidity and mortality, as reported in several studies. The most serious sequelae of ruptured aneurysms are renal failure and myocardial infarction. Renal failure carries a mortality greater than 90 percent in patients with ruptured aneurysms. The incidence of renal failure after elective abdominal aortic aneurysm resection averages approximately 3 percent, with a mortality rate of 45 percent. The incidence of acute renal failure after operation for ruptured aneurysms averages approximately 30 percent, with a mortality rate of 75 percent. Multiple factors contributing to the occurrence of acute renal failure include prolonged hypotension, blood loss, and suprarenal aortic clamping. Renal insufficiency requiring hemodialysis occurred in 9.3 percent of the senior author's series, with a mortality rate of 57 percent. Ischemic colitis after surgery for ruptured aneurysms is more frequent than after elective operation and represents a major cause of postoperative morbidity and mortality. Other possible complications include distal thrombosis, coagulopathy, and paraplegia.

PREVENTION

The opportunity of improving results in this group of patients lies in treatment before rupture. Certain basic concepts require emphasis.

1. Untreated aneurysmal disease terminates with rupture and 100 percent mortality.
2. Elective operation offers 98 percent survival, and an average of 48 percent die if treatment is delayed until after rupture.
3. Rupture does not correlate accurately with size, and consequently, this criterion should be abandoned as a contraindication to surgery. An aneurysm twice the size of the native vessel proximal to the lesion should be considered for operation.
4. Since approximately 70 percent of patients present with ruptured abdominal aortic aneurysms without prior history, screening should be performed with ultrasonography on an annual basis for those older than 55 years and especially for obese patients.

FEMORAL AND POPLITEAL ANEURYSMS

JAMES S. T. YAO, M.D., Ph.D.

Of all peripheral aneurysms, the popliteal aneurysm is most common. When it is present, it is frequently associated with an abdominal aortic aneurysm (35%) or with common femoral and superficial femoral artery aneurysms (30%). In contrast, an isolated femoral aneurysm is uncommon. It occurs with only one-third the incidence of popliteal aneurysm. For some unknown reason, popliteal aneurysm is more common in males and is rarely found in females. Most aneurysms are atherosclerotic in origin. Therefore, associated atherosclerotic lesions causing cerebral ischemia, hypertension, and coronary artery insufficiency are not an uncommon finding in these patients.

The natural history of an aneurysm is progressive expansion to rupture, thrombosis, or distal embolization. Of these, thrombosis, either acute or chronic, is most common. Unlike aortic aneurysms, rupture of a peripheral aneurysm is rather uncommon and occurs in only 7 percent of reported series. Another common clinical manifestation is atheromatous embolization, and a popliteal or femoral aneurysm serving as the source of embolization must be suspected in a patient who presents with the so-called "blue toe" or "purple toe" syndrome.

SYMPTOMS

Symptoms may be due to ischemic events or compression of surrounding structures. Major ischemic events are thrombosis or embolization. Thrombosis may occur acutely, simulating acute embolism, or it may occur insidiously, with presenting symptoms of intermittent claudication. Embolization is manifested by the blue or purple toe syndrome or by a petechia-like lesion of the foot. Compression of surrounding structures, such as a vein or nerve, by the aneurysm is a distinct, though uncommon, clinical feature. Symptoms may include limb swelling or referred pain along the path of the femoral or posterior tibial nerve. Although rupture of the aneurysm is relatively rare, when it occurs, a pulsatile hematoma with extreme pain is a common finding.

DIAGNOSIS

By virtue of its characteristics, a popliteal or femoral aneurysm can be diagnosed by careful palpation of the femoral triangle or popliteal fossa. Because of bilaterality (50%) of popliteal aneurysms and the high frequency of associated aortic aneurysm, a search for other aneurysms must be made. Acute thrombosis of a popliteal aneurysm may cause acute ischemic symptoms simulating arterial embolism, and misdiagnosis may subject the patient to unnecessary embolectomy. Therefore, the finding of a contralateral popliteal aneurysm helps to establish the diagnosis of acute thrombosed aneurysm. Other helpful diagnostic signs to establish the presence of an aneurysm are loss of pedal pulses, gangrene of the digits, atheromatous embolization, and swelling and numbness along the distribution of the femoral or posterior tibial nerve.

When the diagnosis is suspected, both B-mode ultrasound scan and computed tomography (CT) help to confirm the diagnosis. Arteriography is important for preoperative evaluation, but may not be diagnostic because of a laminar thrombus, which obscures the true size of the aneurysm. However, preoperative arteriography is necessary to the planning of the surgical approach. Information provided by the arteriogram includes (1) the extent of aneurysmal degeneration of the superficial femoral artery; aneurysm of the popliteal artery may be a manifestation of aneurysmosis, and arteriography outlines these changes; (2) multiplicity of aneurysms; (3) the outflow or runoff below the popliteal trifurcation; (4) the collateral status; and (5) the extent of involvement of a femoral aneurysm in relation to the profunda femoris artery. Not infrequently, distal embolization to the foot vessels is seen despite the presence of pedal pulses. Once again, because of the multiple nature of these aneurysms, routine CT scanning of the abdominal aorta and iliac artery should be done in all patients with femoral or popliteal aneurysms. The CT scan is also helpful to establish the diagnosis of a thrombosed popliteal aneurysm.

MANAGEMENT

A popliteal aneurysm is the harbinger of disaster, and its presence is an indication for surgical intervention. Unless there is an absolute contraindication, surgery must be done regardless of the size of the aneurysm and the age of the patient.

Preparation for surgery is similar to that for femoropopliteal or distal bypass. A preoperative antibiotic is indicated if the use of prosthetic material is contemplated. Careful examination of the saphenous vein system will determine whether a prosthetic graft is needed. The lower half of the abdomen, including the groin, and the distal part of the leg must be included in the preparation of the surgical field. For femoral aneurysm, the contralateral groin must be prepared in case there is a need for alternative inflow reconstruction.

Popliteal Aneurysm

The modern surgical technique is femoropopliteal or femorodistal bypass with exclusion of the popliteal aneurysm by proximal and distal ligation of the aneurysm. Prior to the reconstruction, special attention must be paid to the arteriographic findings in the superficial femoral artery as well as arteries distal to the popliteal. The latter determine the site of distal anastomosis.

In acute thrombosis, preoperative arteriography may fail to demonstrate any arteries distal to the popliteal trifurcation, especially if the arteriogram is done by the translumbar route. Even in the presence of a pulsatile aneurysm, turbulent flow within the aneurysm may cause delayed filling of distal arteries with the contrast medium. Nonvisualization by preoperative arteriography is not an inoperable situation, however, and the use of a prebypass on-table arteriogram helps to determine operability.

The technique of prebypass arteriography consists of exposure of the common femoral artery through a standard groin incision under general anesthesia, just as one would proceed with a femoropopliteal bypass. A 20- by 24-inch x-ray cassette in a disposable sterile cover is positioned obliquely (corner to corner) under the leg and foot. A 16-gauge intravenous cannula is introduced into the common femoral artery, and the artery is cross-clamped proximally. Approximately 50 cc of contrast medium (Renografin 60) is injected manually. The clamp across the common femoral artery is then released, and after a delay of 10 seconds, the single exposure is made. In my experience, 95 percent of cases with nonvisualization of the distal vessels by preoperative arteriography have a bypassable tibial or peroneal artery identified for distal anastomosis.

Once operability is established, the bypass technique is similar to the standard femoral-infrapopliteal bypass. First, the saphenous vein is identified in the groin wound, traced along its path, and harvested by making a separate skin incision in the thigh. If the superficial femoral artery appears normal on the arteriogram, the proximal anastomosis may be placed on the superficial femoral artery in the adductor canal, or on the popliteal artery above the knee. When there is degenerative change or aneurysmal dilatation of the superficial femoral artery, the proximal anastomosis must be placed on the common femoral artery. If this is the case, the common femoral artery is exposed with careful attention to preservation of lymphatic tissue between the femoral artery and the saphenous vein.

Placement of the distal anastomosis of the vein graft depends on arteriographic findings. In most instances, it is possible to place the anastomosis below the aneurysm, on the below-knee popliteal artery or the tibioperoneal trunk, which can be exposed by the standard medial approach. The gracilis and semitendinosus muscles may be divided to facilitate the exposure. By incising the deep or soleal fascia along the tibia, one exposes the posterior tibial artery. If bypass to the peroneal artery is needed, the deeper fascia may be opened to facilitate exposure of the peroneal artery along the fibula. For exposure of the anterior tibial artery, a separate incision is made over the anterior compartment. The anterior tibial artery is situated between the heads of the anterior tibial muscle and the extensor digitorum longus muscle.

Once exposure of the proximal and distal arteries is complete, a tunnel is made through the popliteal fossa between the heads of the gastrocnemius muscle. The harvested saphenous vein is then passed through the tunnel, and the proximal and distal anastomoses are constructed end-to-side with running 6–0 Prolene suture. At the completion of the bypass, the popliteal aneurysm is excluded from the circulation by ligation of the artery proximal and distal to the aneurysm. If heavily calcified plaque makes ligation difficult, the artery proximal to the aneurysm must be transected and closed with running sutures. In most instances, there is no need to tamper with the aneurysm, and excision of the aneurysm seldom is necessary. Large aneurysms, especially in patients with compression symptoms, may need to be decompressed after ligation. Failure to do so may result in persistent compression to the surrounding structures because of the size of the aneurysm.

In my practice, a prosthetic graft is used only when the saphenous vein is unavailable, and I prefer to use a polytetrafluoroethylene (PTFE) graft. A completion arteriogram is routinely made by injecting contrast medium through the vein graft. The completion arteriogram is helpful to determine the integrity of the distal anastomosis and to obtain information on the foot vessel anatomy.

Femoral Aneurysm

A standard vertical groin incision is used to expose the femoral aneurysm. If the aneurysm is very large, the inguinal ligament may be divided to facilitate exposure of the common femoral artery. In a very large aneurysm, a separate transverse oblique incision placed above the inguinal ligament with retroperitoneal exposure of the external iliac artery may facilitate proximal control. The superficial femoral and profunda femoris arteries must be identified and closely inspected to determine the involvement of the profunda femoris artery.

A prosthetic graft, preferably a polytetrafluoroethylene (PTFE) graft, is anastomosed end-to-end. Once proximal and distal control is complete, the aneurysmal sac is opened and the graft is sutured circumferentially within the lumen of the aneurysm. If the profunda femoris artery is involved in the aneurysmal sac, it must be reimplanted onto the PTFE graft. Depending on the size of the artery, a short segment of PTFE (8 mm or 10 mm) is used for the replacement.

FALSE ANEURYSM AND ARTERIOVENOUS FISTULA

ALBERT E. YELLIN, M.D., F.A.C.S.

Traumatic false aneurysm (FA) and arteriovenous fistula (AVF) are seen with increasing frequency in civilian vascular surgery practice. Mechanisms of injury include gunshot wounds, stab wounds, and blunt trauma with and without related skeletal fractures. Many are iatrogenic, caused by angiographic or cardiac catheterization procedures, multiple arterial punctures, intra-arterial balloon pump, orthopedic screws, nails, external fixators, and various surgical procedures, most notoriously lumbar disc surgery.

False aneurysms result from an injury through all layers of the arterial wall, with the subsequent hemorrhage contained by the adjacent tissues as a perivascular hematoma. The clot may tamponade the hole in the artery or blood may continue to flow into a cavity within the clot. The major arterial flow continues across the site of vessel injury. Most such lesions occur with a partial circumferential tear that prevents retraction and thrombosis of the vessel ends. Occasionally, a false aneurysm occurs around a circumferentially transected vessel, in which blood flow traverses a channel through the surrounding clot. Hematoma size does not correlate with the size of the arterial injury. Following blunt trauma and disruption of the intima and media, the clot may be contained by a thin adventitial sheath. Since this layer of the arterial wall is intact, some refer to this lesion as a true aneurysm. It might be more appropriate to lump all of these together as "traumatic aneurysms."

Owing to the proximity of the associated veins, many wounding agents result in a simultaneous puncture or laceration of both adjacent artery and vein. High-pressure arterial blood may readily follow the path of least resistance into the low pressure venous circulation, resulting in a traumatic AVF. On occasion, a false aneurysm or mycotic aneurysm might erode and rupture into an adjacent vein.

With rare exceptions, FA and AVF should be definitively treated when diagnosed. Untreated, they occasionally close spontaneously; however, most persist, enlarge, and cause increasing symptoms. Untreated, a false aneurysm may suddenly rupture with exsanguinating hemorrhage or thrombose and cause distal ischemia. Occasionally, the clot may fragment, embolize distally, and result in multiple distal occlusions. With time, a chronic FA develops. The original clot might slowly liquefy and organize. The adjacent inflammatory reaction surrounds the area with a fibrous saccular capsule, and this capsule may mimic an aneurysm wall. Under the continued head of arterial pressure, these gradually enlarge and may impinge on adjacent veins, nerves, or other viscera. Eventually, an untreated AVF enlarges and shunts an increasing amount of arterial blood into the venous circulation. The distal arterial walls thin and become attenuated. The proximal artery thickens and becomes aneurysmal. The venous outflow bed becomes thick-walled and "arterialized." As more of the proximal arterial blood flows through the fistula, and particularly if there is a "steal" or reversal of flow in the distal artery, ischemia might develop, and the hemodynamic systemic effects of a high cardiac output shunt may evolve. AVF in the distal extremities rarely cause congestive heart failure (CHF), whereas those involving the aorta, vena cava, and their major branches can lead to high-output CHF.

DIAGNOSIS

Any patient with trauma or a skeletal fracture in proximity to a major blood vessel may have a false aneurysm despite the absence of any abnormal physical findings. A patient with a history of trauma and a pulsatile mass is likely to have a false aneurysm. There may be an overlying systolic murmur or thrill and diminished distal pulses. Rarely, and more often in chronic situations, there may be evidence of distal embolization. The size and locations of the mass may produce symptoms related to compression of adjacent structures. An infected, mycotic FA may have clinical manifestations of an abscess, but if pulsatile, its true nature should be evident. *It should not be incised and drained*! Post-traumatic AVF are often initially asymptomatic, but may gradually develop the characteristic overlying machinery type murmur, evidence of venous hypertension, dilated veins, diminished distal arterial pulses, and tachycardia, the latter usually disappearing if the fistula is temporarily occluded.

If either lesion is suspected and if time and the condition of the patient permits, the precise location and extent of the lesion is best delineated by an appropriate arteriogram. Ultrasound or CT scans can be used to locate lesions within the head, thorax, or abdomen, but arteriography is still required to delineate the magnitude of the lesion, whether single or multiple (particularly in shotgun wounds), and to help plan the vascular reconstruction. The question of whether all patients with penetrating injuries in proximity to a major vessel, but without abnormal physical signs, should have an arteriogram in an attempt to identify occult injuries remains controversial. Although I use diagnostic angiography liberally, I do not use it routinely on *all* such patients! Major life- or limb-threatening injuries usually have some abnormal physical findings. Small or occult injuries, if initially missed, can invariably be treated successfully when identified at a later date. Patients with close-range shotgun injuries with deep tissue penetration should undergo arteriography. Frequently, numerous small FA and AVF are identified, scattered over the pattern made by the pellets. It is essential that all the lesions be identified prior to surgery.

NONSURGICAL MANAGEMENT: ARTERIOGRAPHIC EMBOLIZATION

Traditionally, vascular injuries including FA have been treated by direct repair of major blood vessels or by ligation of noncritical vessels. Similarly, the preferred treatment for traumatic AVF consists of surgical division of the fistula with reconstruction of involved critical vessels, or quadruple ligation of noncritical afferent and efferent vessels. Occasionally, the anatomic location of the injury makes a direct surgical approach technically difficult or hazardous, or the condition of the patient may preclude surgery, in which case an alternate treatment must be sought.

In recent years, angiographic transcatheter embolization techniques have been used to treat a wide variety of traumatic lesions. They are an ideal alternative when surgery might be hazardous or unwarranted. Success and safety depend on close communication between surgeon and radiologist in terms of patient selection and techniques. When a patient with a possible vascular injury is sent for diagnostic angiography, the surgeon should alert the angiographer to the possibility of therapeutic embolization if the vessels involved are noncritical, if there is little likelihood of subsequent tissue ischemia, and if there is minimal possibility that the embolic material will migrate distally or through an AVF into the right heart. If such a lesion is identified, the surgeon should, while the patient is still in the angiographic suite, view the films, assess the risks of a failed embolization attempt, and decide whether surgery or embolization is most appropriate. A wide variety of embolic materials are available for use, including steel balls, stainless steel pellets, metal filings, acrylic, methylmethacrylate, Silastic, silicone, and polystyrene spheres. These can be inserted through large catheters into large vessels. The smaller catheters used in highly selective catheterization of small vessels require microspheres or fine biodegradable material such as autologous clot or gelatin sponge. Particle size should be selected for the size of the vessel. Ultrafine particulate material can embolize distally, occlude terminal arterioles, and cause ischemic tissue necrosis. Some materials have unique characteristics, lending themselves to certain applications.

1. *Polyvinyl alcohol foam.* This can be extruded from a small catheter, and when it contacts blood, it rapidly expands to 10 to 15 times its original volume. It is well suited for occlusion of medium to large vessels.
2. *Isobutyl-2-cyanocrylate.* This is a liquid tissue adhesive that rapidly polymerizes when in contact with normal saline, blood, or blood vessel intima. It adheres firmly to the vessel wall and is ideal for occluding medium or large vessels.
3. *Detachable silicone balloons.* A silicone rubber balloon that can be inflated or deflated via a valve is attached to the catheter. It is filled with radiopaque dye, positioned at the site to be occluded, and then inflated. The catheter is detached, leaving the balloon in place. Various-sized balloons are available and can be used to occlude large AVF.
4. *Stainless steel coils.* Dacron-tufted stainless steel coils, appropriately sized, are introduced through a 5 F or 7 F catheter and extruded at the site to

be occluded. The coils, once in the blood vessel, spring into their coiled position and lodge at the site. The tufted Dacron promotes thrombosis. These coils are useful in occluding various-sized vessels and AVF. Frequently gelatin sponge, autologous clot, or other materials are used in conjunction with coils to more rapidly achieve total occlusion.

Following embolization, a completion angiogram is obtained to ensure that the desired result has been achieved without displacement or migration of embolic material. If necessary, additional embolic material can be introduced until the desired result is attained. Nonabsorbable material that emoblizes to the heart or lungs may require catheter extraction.

Applications of these techniques are limited only by the skills of the radiologic team and careful understanding of the risk-benefit ratio by surgeon and radiologist. Several examples include:

1. *Noncritical vessel.* FA or AVF of the distal profunda femoris artery, hypogastric artery, or similar medium-sized arteries leading to the muscle groups can be occluded without tissue loss. Therefore, these are ideally suited to embolization.
2. *Difficult location.* Lesions involving distal branches of the external carotid artery are often difficult to approach surgically without risk of major nerve injury or considerable disfiguring dissection. These vessels are noncritical and can readily be embolized.
3. *Hazardous conditions.* The vertebral artery, as it passes through the bony intervertebral foramina, is anatomically difficult to approach. The surrounding bony structures make it difficult to approach the vessel for proximal and distal control. Massive hemorrhage frequently occurs when the surgeon chisels through the bone and enters into the FA or AVF. If arteriography demonstrates cross-filling of the posterior circulation by collaterals, the affected vertebral artery can safely be embolized. Similarly, FA or AVF involving hypogastric vessels consequent to blunt trauma or penetrating trauma poses a major surgical challenge. Exposure is difficult and hemorrhage usually massive when the lesion is entered. Frequently, pelvic AVF are not apparent until months or years after the original injury, when massive arteriolized venous collaterals fill the pelvis. Owing to the noncritical nature of the branches of the hypogastric artery, these lesions are best embolized. Embolization may be used to reduce the volume of flow prior to a surgical procedure.

Embolization is a procedure associated with low risk and a high success rate. It is reasonable to consider its use in all cases in which arteriography is used to identify a vascular injury. Numerous unnecessary surgical procedures might then be avoided. The careful selection of patients minimizes complications and results in a high success rate.

SURGICAL MANAGEMENT

Almost all FA or AVF involving a major vessel require vascular repair. A small 1- to 2-mm FA caused by a low-velocity shotgun pellet or an instrument like an ice pick can be treated nonoperatively. These are similar in nature to the FA that often occur following arteriographic procedures and invariably close. Careful follow-up is required to ensure that the lesion does not enlarge. Surgery should be planned in such a fashion as to avoid entering the pulsatile hematoma or fistula until after control of the appropriate vessels has been obtained proximally and distally. For lesions on the distal extremities, excellent vascular control can be achieved by using a proximally placed pneumatic tourniquet.

The size of the lesion will determine the choice of incision. The incision must be designed to enable the surgeon to rapidly expose all necessary vessels. Small incisions, particularly when confined by adjacent bones, limit exposure and can result in massive hemorrhage. Lesions of the ascending aorta and its arch vessels are best approached through a median sternotomy; however, proper exposure of the left subclavian artery is achieved via a trap-door incision or anterolateral thoracotomy in the third intercostal space (ICS). The descending mid-thoracic aorta is best exposed by a posterolateral thoracotomy removing the fifth rib subperiostally and a portion of the fourth rib posteriorly. Exposure of the distal thoracic aorta requires an incision of the seventh intercostal space and division of the diaphragm. Exposure of the intrathoracic aorta is facilitated by use of a Carlens double-lumen endotracheal tube, which maintains ventilation of the right hemithorax, but permits the collapse of the left lung. The proximal abdominal aorta above the superior mesenteric artery is difficult to expose. A thoracoabdominal incision, division of the diaphragm, and mobilization of the spleen, tail, and body of the pancreas toward the midline provide excellent exposure for the proximal abdominal aorta and its major visceral branches. The distal aorta and the remainder of the peripheral vessels are exposed in the usual fashion.

Once the vessels have been isolated above and below the injury, they should be encircled with vascular tapes and/or vascular clamps. At this point, a decision should be made regarding systemic anticoagulation. Many vascular surgeons do not employ systemic heparin in trauma cases, owing to the minimal likelihood of distal thrombosis in relatively normal nonatherosclerotic vessels. Moreover, the presence of major soft tissue injury or associated intra-abdominal or intracranial injury might preclude systemic heparinization. Regional heparinization can be employed during the arterial reconstruction if deemed necessary. Once vascular control is achieved, the FA or pulsatile hematoma is entered and clot rapidly evacuated. Hemorrhage is controlled by the pneumatic

tourniquet, tapes, or clamps, and the site of injury, usually a small side-wall hole, is identified. If the hematoma is entered before control is achieved, direct pressure with a finger is used to control hemorrhage. Careful dissection adjacent to the injury exposes sufficient vessel to encircle with tapes or clamps. Blindly placing clamps in an effort to control hemorrhage invariably lacerates adjacent veins and increases bleeding, or possibly injures accompanying nerves. Bleeding coming from collaterals can be controlled by intraluminal vascular balloon catheters, and Foley bladder catheters can be used to occlude the lumen of large vessels.

Once control is achieved and prior to beginning the vascular repair, consideration is given to the warm ischemia time distal to the point of occlusion. Carotid artery repair should be performed with the protection afforded by a temporary shunt, unless the repair involves a few rapidly placed sutures. The protection afforded by a shunt minimizes the need for undue haste. If there is major loss of artery, necessitating a graft, the shunt should be placed through the graft and then inserted into the proximal and distal carotid. Shunts may also be beneficial in surgery on the innominate artery. Occasionally, popliteal artery FA may be associated with distal thrombosis and ischemia. A carotid shunt can be inserted in the popliteal artery if the operative period and vascular occlusion time will be extensive. Prolonged renal artery repairs can produce ischemia. Continuous irrigation of the kidney with iced saline, lactated Ringer's, or Collins' solution through a catheter in the renal artery will reduce small vessel thrombosis and extend the safe ischemia time. Packing the kidney with slush, ice, or iced sponges prolongs ischemia time. Spinal cord ischemia with paraplegia is a disastrous complication which can occur after clamping the thoracic aorta. Attempts to avoid this include the use of partial bypass (femorofemoral), left heart bypass, or a heparin-bonded external shunt. Pump bypass is complex and time-consuming, requires systemic heparinization, is unfamiliar to many surgeons, and does not eliminate the danger of paraplegia. Therefore I have abandoned bypass or shunts and rely on rapid repair of the aortic injury. Maximum intercostal collateral flow can be maintained by placing the occluding clamps as close to the site of injury as possible.

Acute FA or AVF may be due to similar types of trauma, and the nature of the injury to the blood vessel may have the same characteristics. They are repaired in the same manner as other acute vascular injuries. Non-critical vessels can be ligated. Definitive treatment of an AVF involving noncritical vessels requires that all afferent and efferent vessels be ligated and the fistula divided. Devitalized soft tissue is debrided. The artery is best repaired by lateral arteriorrhaphy if the injury is small and the edges of the vessel are clean. Larger side-wall holes may require a patch graft of vein or synthetic material in order to avoid a critical stenosis. If the vessel is transected, retraction may pull the ends apart. The vessel should be mobilized proximally and distally for sufficient length to permit fashioning of an end-to-end anastomosis without tension. This may necessitate dividing several noncritical branches. Gunshot injuries (particularly high-velocity wounds) and blunt trauma may cause considerable arterial injury. All damaged vessels must be debrided, invariably leaving a gap that cannot be bridged by direct end-to-end anastomosis. In such instances an interposition graft should be used, preferably of autologous vein. Synthetic material such as Dacron should be avoided in a contaminated or infected field. Expanded polytetrafluoroethylene grafts have been placed in areas of contamination with some success. Occasionally, autologous artery has been removed from another site and used for a critical repair in a contaminated field. The clean donor site can be bridged by a synthetic graft.

The intima of the thoracic aorta frequently retracts when the aorta is torn by blunt trauma. It is tempting to attempt direct suture repair of lacerations that are partially circumferential; however, the sutures frequently pull through the attenuated adventitia. Such injuries are best repaired by interposing a short segment of synthetic graft.

Venous injuries involving major veins should be repaired if the patient's condition is stable. Venous repairs must be meticulously performed to help reduce the chance of thrombosis. Lateral repair, venous patch graft, and venous interposition grafts (saphenous vein, internal jugular vein) can be used. Compartment pressure measurements, dermotomy, and fasciotomy should be employed on extremity injuries if there has been significant venous injury, soft tissue injury, hematoma formation, or edema to avoid the disastrous consequences of an unrecognized compartment syndrome.

A completion arteriogram should be obtained following all repairs of medium or small vessels to ensure that there is no technical error which might lead to thrombosis or narrowing of the repair. A satisfactory pulse distal to the repair does not guarantee a good result or render an arteriogram unnecessary. An unsatisfactory arteriogram should prompt immediate correction. If distally propagated thrombus is demonstrated, an arteriotomy should be made and a thrombectomy performed.

EXTRACRANIAL OCCLUSIVE CEREBRAL VASCULAR DISEASE

JOHN A. MANNICK, M.D.
ANTHONY D. WHITTEMORE, M.D.
NATHAN P. COUCH, M.D.

Important symptoms of extracranial arterial occlusive disease can be caused by arteriosclerotic lesions of the great vessels arising from the aortic arch and lesions of the vertebral and internal carotid arteries. Of these, lesions involving the first portion of the internal carotid artery are by a considerable margin more common and more likely to produce symptoms of cerebral ischemia.

INDICATIONS FOR ENDARTERECTOMY

The indications for carotid endarterectomy listed in Table 1 include those about which there is considerable controversy at present as well as those that are widely accepted in the medical community. There is widespread agreement that transient ischemic attacks (TIAs) of ipsilateral monocular blindness or of contralateral paresis or paresthesias in a patient with a significant arteriosclerotic stenosis of the origin of the internal carotid artery are an indication for carotid endarterectomy, the goal being relief of symptoms and prevention of stroke. It seems clear that the majority of transient ischemic attacks occur on the basis of embolization from the surface of

arteriosclerotic lesions. However, attacks can undoubtedly be produced by simple hypoperfusion, though this probably occurs in a minority of individuals with such symptoms. Direct evidence for microembolization can often be seen in the retinal arteries of patients with transient ischemic attacks, where cholesterol emboli are visible as bright Hollenhorst plaques. While there is no good prospective study comparing carotid endarterectomy with nonoperative therapy with antiplatelet agents in patients with TIAs, reports from surgical groups experienced in carotid endarterectomy continue to report long-term results superior to those reported for treatment with antiplatelet drugs. There is also general agreement that protracted TIAs, which are termed reversible ischemic neurologic deficits, or RINDs, should be treated by carotid endarterectomy.

There is less agreement about the role of carotid

TABLE 1 Deciding for Carotid Endarterectomy

Indications
  Transient ischemic attacks or reversible ischemic neurologic deficits
  Nonhemispheric ischemic symptoms
  Fixed neurologic deficits
  Strokes in progress
  Asymptomatic stenosis

Contraindications
  Acute profound stroke
  Internal carotid occlusion
  Severe intracranial disease

endarterectomy in patients with significant carotid stenoses and so-called nonhemispheric symptoms. These patients present with symptoms of bilateral motor or sensory deficits, unsteadiness, and cortical visual disturbances suggestive of vertebral basilar ischemia. In our experience it is not unusual to find bilateral hemodynamically significant internal carotid stenoses in such patients, and carotid endarterectomy has brought prompt symptomatic relief in the majority of such individuals. This has also been the experience of a number of other surgeons.

There is also a growing consensus that patients with small fixed neurologic deficits or those who have experienced more severe deficits with full recovery of function of the affected parts may benefit from endarterectomy of lesions in the internal carotid arteries supplying the affected hemisphere in order to prevent further infarction. Because of the disastrous results obtained with early attempts at emergency carotid endarterectomy for frank completed strokes, it has been recommended for many years that patients with fixed neurologic deficits should not be operated on for 4 to 6 weeks following the occurrence of the stroke. Because this policy has the disadvantage of placing the patient at risk for further embolization from the offending internal carotid plaque during the recommended waiting period, we have recently begun to offer prompt carotid endarterectomy to patients who present with minor fixed deficits in the territory supplied by a stenotic internal carotid. Experience with 28 such individuals has indicated that prompt surgery has not resulted in new deficits or an increase in the deficits already present.

Perhaps the most controversial indication for carotid endarterectomy at present is the patient with an asymptomatic carotid bruit. The term "asymptomatic bruit" is probably a misnomer since a bruit in the neck may or may not be caused by an internal carotid stenosis, and it is a stenotic lesion rather than a bruit that is a possible indication for surgery. There is little evidence to suggest that an asymptomatic internal carotid stenosis of a degree insufficient to interfere with flow is hazardous to the patient. Even asymptomatic lesions that narrow the carotid lumen by as much as 50 percent may remain stable for years. However, there is now evidence from prospective studies that high-grade stenoses that are preocclusive, i.e., stenoses that narrow the carotid lumen by 75 percent or more, are associated with a real risk of stroke because of the propensity of such lesions to thrombose. This risk is probably as high as 30 percent over the first 2 years following detection of the lesion. It seems logical, therefore, to study asymptomatic patients with neck bruits by noninvasive means, in order to determine the presence or absence of a high-grade internal carotid lesion. Ultrasonic imaging techniques have now improved to the point that they are very nearly competitive with angiography in their ability to assess accurately the degree of internal carotid narrowing caused by an arteriosclerotic plaque. It is our policy at present to perform angiography on asymptomatic patients with high-grade internal carotid stenoses revealed by ultrasonic imaging and to offer such individuals prophylactic endarterectomy if the angio-

graphic findings confirm the noninvasive studies. Many other vascular surgical groups follow a similar policy.

DIAGNOSTIC STUDIES

Investigation of all patients with neck bruits by angiography was at one time felt to be hazardous as well as costly since conventional angiography performed by the retrograde Seldinger technique, with studies of the origins of the great vessels in the aortic arch and selective injection of the carotid arteries, carried a small but appreciable risk of stroke, particularly in patients with cerebrovascular disease. However, in the last 2 years, the quality of intravenous digital angiography has improved in many medical centers. We now use this technique as the preferential one for delineating carotid artery lesions. It is more comfortable for the patient than conventional angiography and is associated with essentially no risk of stroke. It has the disadvantage of requiring the injection of a large volume of contrast medium, and it does not give a clear delineation of the small intracerebral vasculature. However, a detailed knowledge of the fine vascular architecture within the brain is seldom necessary to make a decision for or against carotid endarterectomy. The intravenous digital angiogram, in most instances, gives a satisfactory veiw of the entire internal carotid artery, including its intracerebral portion, so that carotid siphon lesions are clearly revealed. If the intravenous digital angiograms in a given instance are unsatisfactory, we proceed immediately to an intra-arterial digital examination, which requires a very small additional amount of angiographic contrast medium. The intra-arterial digital technique, although not so safe as an intravenous digital angiogram is probably safer than a conventional angiogram with respect to the complication of stroke.

Although the safety of the intravenous digital angiogram makes it an attractive means for screening patients with asymptomatic bruits or cerebral symptoms not clearly suggestive of TIAs, it is clearly more costly, more time-consuming, and less acceptable to the patient than ultrasonic carotid imaging, which we prefer as a screening test combined with occuloplethysmography to confirm the hemodynamic significance of any lesions observed with the direct imaging technique.

EMERGENCY ENDARTERECTOMY

The majority of carotid endarterectomies for the indications discussed above can be performed as elective or semi-elective procedures. However, emergency carotid endarterectomy is occasionally necessary. We perform such emergency procedures for patients who have crescendo TIAs, that is, TIAs of increasing frequency or severity over a span of a few hours. We also perform emergency carotid endarterectomies in patients with so-called stuttering strokes, or strokes in progress, if the fixed deficit is small and there is the waxing and waning of a more profound temporary deficit. Some surgeons regard a stroke in progress as a contraindication to carotid endarterectomy because they are afraid of inducing a more profound permanent deficit. However, several reports from other surgical groups and our own experience suggest that many individuals with stuttering strokes or strokes in progress can have their progressive symptoms arrested by prompt carotid endarterectomy and are left with only a minor fixed deficit.

In an occasional patient, usually one who already has been admitted to the hospital for work-up of a symptomatic carotid stenosis, the neck bruit suddenly disappears coincident with the onset of a profound stroke in the ipsilateral hemisphere. Emergency carotid endarterectomy, if it can be performed within an hour of the onset of symptoms, may sometimes result in complete relief of the patient's symptoms. However, this is not invariably the case, and a profound fixed neurologic deficit is ordinarily a contraindication to carotid endarterectomy.

In concert with most vascular surgeons, we believe that patients who have suffered complete internal carotid occlusions benefit from ipsilateral carotid endarterectomy seldom enough to rule out such operations on a routine basis. However, certain patients with complete internal carotid occlusion and stenosis of the ipsilateral external carotid artery may benefit from external carotid endarterectomy to increase collateral circulation to the affected hemisphere.

TECHNIQUE OF CAROTID ENDARTERECTOMY

Controversy concerning the technique of carotid endarterectomy currently centers on the choice of anesthesia, the extent of exposure of the internal carotid artery necessary to perform the endarterectomy, and the use of an internal shunt to maintain arterial blood supply to the ipsilateral cerebral hemisphere while the carotid endarterectomy is performed (Table 2).

Anesthesia

A number of experienced vascular surgeons prefer local anesthesia for carotid endarterectomy and selective shunting based on the tolerance of the awake patient to carotid clamping. This technique clearly has its virtues; however, after experience with this method in more than 125 patients, we prefer general anesthesia for carotid endarterectomy because it is usually more acceptable to the patient and the surgeon and, in our hands, permits a more precise and controlled operation.

TABLE 2 Established Methods of Cerebral Protection During Carotid Endarterectomy

Local anesthesia with selective shunting

General anesthesia with routine shunting

General anesthesia with selective shunting
    Stump pressure
    EEG monitoring

Shunt

Although there are still advocates of carotid endarterectomy under general anesthesia without the use of shunts under any circumstances, the evidence seems overwhelming that some patients suffer permanent ischemic damage to the ipsilateral hemisphere during the performance of a careful endarterectomy if a shunt is not used. Surgeons experienced with routine use of a shunt report excellent results. However, there is also little doubt that the use of a shunt can occasionally cause an embolus or intimal damage, which can result in a permanent neurologic deficit. Selective shunting under general anesthesia requires some objective means of assessing the quality of the collateral circulation to the affected hemisphere. Some surgeons prefer to use the back pressure in the internal carotid artery as a gauge of the state of the collateral circulation. This so-called "stump pressure" is measured after application of clamps to the external and common carotid arteries, and if it is below 50 mm Hg, for example, many surgeons decide to use an internal shunt. We believe, along with a number of other groups, that continual EEG monitoring during carotid endarterectomy under general anesthesia offers an accurate indication of the need for an internal shunt and also offers the advantage of assuring the surgeon that the shunt is working by the return of normal electrical activity to the affected parts of the brain after the shunt is inserted.

Exposure

We believe strongly that the exposure of at least half an inch of clearly normal internal carotid artery above the plaque in the first portion of this vessel is necessary for the performance of a safe endarterectomy. This exposure ordinarily involves dissection in a plane posterior to the twelfth cranial nerve, which arches over the first portion of the internal carotid artery. Division of a small arterial branch to the sternocleidomastoid muscle permits entry to this plane. Detachment of the ansa hypoglossi is also a helpful maneuver. Division of the posterior belly of the digastric muscle may be necessary for adequate exposure in some individuals. We have not found it necessary to dislocate the jaw in order to permit adequate exposure for a carotid endarterectomy.

The endarterectomy ordinarily ends cleanly in the internal carotid, at a point where intima of normal thickness and consistency is reached. It is important to be able to inspect the distal intimal edge to ensure that there are no loose tags of intima left protruding into the lumen at that point and that the edge is firmly adherent circumferentially so that it will not be dissected by restoration of blood flow and form an obstructing intimal flap. It is also important to carefully irrigate and debride the area of endarterectomy to remove all loose or partially attached pieces of residual intima. We find that the use of loops of 2½ power magnification is of considerable aid in this regard. We ordinarily close the arteriotomy primarily using a running suture of 6–0 polypropylene. We do not routinely use patch grafts and feel that they have the disadvantage of creating an unnatural widening of the artery with associated turbulence. However, an autogenous venous patch is occasionally necessary to permit adequate closure of a small or friable internal carotid.

COMPLETION ANGIOGRAPHY

On completion of the endarterectomy, we routinely perform completion angiography by injecting 10 ml of contrast medium into the common carotid proximal to the endarterectomized segment. It is important to know at the completion of the procedure that there are no technical errors or distal clamp injuries that might result in thrombosis of the endarterectomized segment.

MORBIDITY AND MORTALITY

The chief cause of operative mortality following carotid endarterectomy is myocardial infarction, and the next most common cause is stroke. However, with modern anesthetic management and careful surgical technique, the operative mortality for carotid endarterectomy should be under 1 percent. Utilizing general anesthesia and selective shunting based on EEG monitoring, the operative mortality for the last 450 patients undergoing endarterectomy on our service has been 0.5 percent.

The most distressing complication of carotid endarterectomy is clearly perioperative stroke (Table 3). The vast majority of such strokes are undoubtedly caused by emboli dislodged at the time of the carotid surgery. Obviously, great care must be exercised to avoid manipulating the area of the plaque prior to application of the occluding clamps. A second cause of stroke is thrombosis of the endarterectomized segment in the early postoperative period, which almost invariably is the result of technical error and usually can be avoided by the routine use of intraoperative angiography on completion of the procedure. Ischemia resulting from failure to use a shunt is a less common, but important, cause of postoperative neurologic deficit. The incidence of permanent neurologic deficit associated with carotid endarterectomy should be

TABLE 3 Complications of Carotid Endarterectomy

Stroke or transient deficit caused by
  Embolus at time of surgery
  Ischemia during carotid clamping
  Thrombosis of the endarterectomized area
  Intracerebral hemorrhage or edema

Wound related problems
  Cranial nerve palsies: IX, X, XII, and mandibular branch
    of VII
  Hematoma
  Tracheal obstruction

Cardiac problems
  Arrhythmia
  Myocardial infarction

1 percent or slightly less in experienced hands, and an additional 1 or 2 percent of patients experience transient neurologic deficits in the postoperative period. The incidence of late strokes in patients who undergo carotid endarterectomy is approximately 1 percent per year. Other postoperative complications include injury to the ninth, tenth, and twelfth cranial nerves, the superior laryngeal nerve, and the mandibular branch of the facial nerve. Cranial nerve palsies have invariably been temporary in our experience.

CORONARY BYPASS

The performance of carotid endarterectomy in association with other surgical procedures, particularly coronary artery bypass grafting, is a subject about which there is no clear consensus at present. Some surgeons find that the complications of carotid endarterectomy performed in association with coronary artery surgery are excessive, and others have found the reverse. In our experience, carotid endarterectomy for preocclusive asymptomatic or symptomatic carotid lesions performed concomitantly with coronary artery bypass grafting in patients with severe symptomatic coronary disease has resulted in no increased risk of mortality or stroke beyond that associated with the coronary artery operation alone. We therefore continue to recommend this combined procedure in selected patients.

Symptomatic arteriosclerotic lesions of the great vessels rising from the aortic arch or of the vertebral arteries are less commonly encountered than symptomatic lesions of the carotid bifurcation. However, the former lesions clearly require surgical repair in some patients. Some patients with symptoms suggestive of vertebral-basilar insufficiency are found to have lesions of the vertebral artery origins and of the carotid bifurcations. In many such cases, symptoms are relieved by carotid endarterectomy, and this procedure should certainly be tried first. However, there remains a small group of patients who have clear-cut vertebral-basilar symptoms and high-grade lesions of the origins of both vertebral arteries in the absence of carotid disease. Such patients may be relieved by surgical repair of the stenotic origin of one of the two vertebral arteries. Two procedures—endarterectomy of the vertebral orifice from an arteriotomy in the subclavian artery and reimplantation of the first portion of the vertebral artery into the common carotid artery—have yielded satisfactory long-term results in our experience. A lesion at the origin of one vertebral artery is almost never the cause of symptoms because of the confluence of the two arteries in the skull to form the basilar system.

SUBCLAVIAN STEAL SYNDROME

The subclavian steal syndrome, which results from reversal of flow in the ipsilateral vertebral artery caused by occlusion or high-grade stenosis of the origin of the subclavian artery proximal to the vertebral take-off, was once considered an important source of cerebral ischemia and stroke. However, it is now clear that this lesion seldom produces symptoms and almost never produces stroke. Surgical correction is probably best accomplished in the rare symptomatic patient by carotid to subclavian bypass in the neck. However, lesions at the origin of the left common carotid or innominate artery may cause cerebral symptoms either by embolization or by hypoperfusion. About ten years ago there was a consensus that such lesions could be more safely managed by crossover bypass grafts in the neck. More recently, however, there

has been a trend toward a direct approach to these lesions in the mediastinum. The latter approach seems particularly appropriate for lesions that appear to be the source of emboli to the brain since more distal bypasses run the risk of permitting continued embolization from the offending plaque. Endarterectomy of the origin of the innominate artery or bypass grafts originating in the ascending aorta to repair left common carotid or innominate lesions can now be performed with low mortality by surgeons experienced with these techniques.

AORTOILIAC OCCLUSIVE DISEASE

G. MELVILLE WILLIAMS, M.D.

At the outset I will be foolhardy and state my belief that all patients with atherosclerotic disease of the aorta and iliac vessels can and should be treated aggressively because of the high rate of success of therapy. This statement is made possible because of innovations in invasive angiography and also because the retroperitoneal approach to the aorta has been used extensively with minimal mortality and morbidity.

DIAGNOSIS

The diagnosis is made on the basis of history and physical examination. Patients complain of pain, numbness, or tingling in the legs, thighs, or buttocks when walking and of sexual impotency. The femoral pulses are missing or significantly reduced. Rarely, some patients complain of calf pain only, but on close questioning these individuals never walk up stairs so that the principal muscles used are those in the calf and the others are not truly tested. The diagnosis is confirmed by tests routinely available in vascular laboratories. The Doppler flow signals are significantly dampened in the femoral arteries, and thigh and ankle pressures are generally diminished. An occasional patient complains of significant claudication and has relatively normal ankle pressures. In these, an exercise test should be carried out. A fall of 30 mm Hg or greater in the calf pressure indicates the existence of significant occlusive disease. Thus, prior to entrance into the hospital and certainly prior to angiography, the diagnosis is established, and the only decisions to be made are those pertaining to the type of therapy.

THERAPY

Because the results of balloon dilation are so good, I believe that all patients with diminished femoral pulses and ischemic symptoms should be admitted for angiographic examination. Admission is necessary because the transaxillary or translumbar approach is commonly required to identify accurately the extent of the disease. Furthermore, the majority of these patients undergo some therapeutic procedure that requires hospitalization.

Given a proper lesion, balloon dilation should be the procedure of choice. In my experience with treating 141 vessels, the 3-year patency rate is 89 percent. Complications, most of them minor, were observed in only 10 percent of the patients. Two patients developed distal embolization, and in each case the embolic plaque was removed successfully under local anesthesia. Blue toe syndrome developed in a third, who subsequently underwent bypass with normalization of distal circulation.

Balloon dilation is now advocated for patients who have only minimal symptoms of claudication and ankle/arm indices greater than 0.7. Such individuals are commonly athletically inclined and are grateful to be able to play ''singles'' again. Should such individuals have diffuse disease or, more commonly, plaque formation of the aorta, no therapy is recommended. These patients are given Trental, and about one-third stay on the medication. Surgery is recommended only if the claudication becomes intractable, the resting ankle/arm index falls below 0.5, or symptoms of rest pain, ulceration, or gangrene develop.

Patients are candidates for femorofemoral bypass if they have the aforementioned symptoms or findings and if one iliac system is normal or can be made normal without a pressure gradient (after intra-arterial Priscoline) by means of balloon dilation. Femorofemoral bypass is 100 percent successful at 30 days. Furthermore, I have never had to convert a femorofemoral bypass to an aortofemoral bypass because of progressive occlusive disease of the iliac system serving both limbs.

Over a 4-year period (1980 to 1984), I performed 57 aorto-bifemoral bypasses employing the retroperitoneal route. There was one early death in a patient who had had the thoracic aorta replaced for aneurysm disease previously. This patient developed paraplegia together with disseminated intravascular coagulation. There have been no deaths since 1980. During this period, I abandoned axillary-bifemoral bypass except for patients who had infected grafts. The management of patients with aortoiliac occlusive disease is summarized in Table 1. The 3-year actuarial limb patency rate is 92 percent.

Technical Considerations

I have had equally good results with balloon dilation irrespective of whether the stenosis is dilated antigrade or retrograde. Under circumstances of acute iliac occlusion, thrombolytic therapy has been successful in restoring iliac artery flow, and in several of these cases, balloon dilation of stenotic segments has sustained the patency of the vessel, justifying a 6-hour infusion followed by repeat arteriography in such patients.

Excellent descriptions of femorofemoral bypass can be found in the literature, and I have no innovations to add to the standard approach. After experience with both 8-mm Gore-tex and Dacron, I prefer the latter. As time passes, the Dacron remains more pliant, allowing palpation of the pulse more readily. The graft material is less expensive, and the patency rates are equal.

In performing 200 aortic reconstructions by employing the retroperitoneal approach, I have learned some lessons. The approach is associated with greater blood loss than the standard and is inappropriate for patients with bleeding disorders or those who refuse blood transfusions. It is also inappropriate if a major indication for the procedure is vascular impotence. The left internal iliac is readily exposed and treated, but the right is exceedingly difficult to approach, and endarterectomy should not be performed through the left flank incision. Finally, coexisting disease of the gastrointestinal system or stenotic lesions in the middle of the right renal artery cannot be treated as well, and midline laparotomy provides better exposure for the correction of these problems.

The retroperitoneal approach is the one I favor for all other patients. The most important single principle is to develop the plane of aortic exposure well posteriorly.

TABLE 1 Management of Patients with Aortoiliac Occlusive Disease

Angiographic Finding	Treatment
Unilateral iliac artery disease	
Localized stenosis	Balloon dilation
Diffuse disease	Femorofemoral bypass
Bilateral diffuse iliac and/or Aortic occlusive disease	Aorto-bifemoral bypass

The second most important point is to limit the aortic dissection to the area immediately inferior to the left renal artery. There is no point in performing a "low" aortofemoral bypass. The further from the renal arteries, the more extensive the atheromatous disease and the greater the difficulty in achieving aortic exposure and control.

Thus, the standard procedure consists of making a left flank incision in the eleventh interspace and extending the incision posteriorly to the erector spinae muscles. The anterior extent of the incision stops well short of the rectus muscle, and in most instances the incision is no more than 6 inches long. The retroperitoneal space is developed as for sympathectomy. The left renal artery is identified by palpation or inspection, and the proximal portion of the left renal artery is dissected to its junction with the aorta. The lumbar branch(es) of the left renal vein are ligated and divided. This maneuver develops the aortic plane, and the lymphatic and areolar tissue along the lateral wall of the aorta is ligated and divided simply and safely. The surgeon can now pass a finger over the anterior and posterior surfaces of the aorta which is all the dissection needed for applying the occluding clamp later. The table is now rotated to make the pelvis as flat as possible, and the groins are exposed in standard fashion. The tunnel to the right groin must be developed carefully, following the course of the iliac vessels. If the plane does not develop easily, a counter-incision in the right lower quadrant should be made.

I drain the retroperitoneal space for 24 hours following surgery and make the stab wound for the drain early. The clamp to control backbleeding from the aorta is placed through the stab wound. This keeps the handle out of the surgeon's working space. The proximal clamp is applied immediately below the left renal artery. End-to-end anastomosis is performed in all cases of distal aortic and common iliac disease. End-to-side anastomosis is the procedure of choice in patients who have bilateral external iliac disease and patent internal iliac and inferior mesenteric arteries. The end-to-end anastomosis is made obliquely to prevent stenosis at this suture line. Whenever an endarterectomy of the proximal aorta is required, a strip of Teflon felt is used to buttress the aortic side of the anastomosis.

An end-to-side anastomosis requires that control of the aorta be as great as or greater than that required for the end-to-end. The arteriotomy is made on the left lateral wall of the aorta, and the graft is positioned to lie in the gutter rather than anteriorly. This is not only simpler, but it lessens the possibility of erosion of the graft into the gastrointestinal tract.

The importance of the profunda femoral artery in aortofemoral bypass cannot be overemphasized. I believe that all patients who have stenosis of the profunda in conjunction with aortoiliac occlusive disease should undergo femoral profundaplasty. This entails division of a branch of the femoral vein that crosses the proximal portion of the profunda femoral artery. Once this vessel is divided, excellent exposure of the profunda down to its first branching points is achieved. In most cases, the vessel becomes normal at this point. When the superficial femoral artery is occluded or significantly diseased, the femoral arteriotomy should be extended across the origin of the profunda femoral artery. Following removal of the plaque, the limb of the graft is sutured in place creating a patch over the orifice of the profunda.

Simultaneous Aortofemoral and Femoropopliteal Bypass Grafting

The only indication for a simultaneous aortofemoral and femoropopliteal bypass is the existence of gangrene or significant nonhealing ulceration in patients with diffuse and *moderate* aortoiliac occlusive disease. These patients require restoration of blood flow to the greatest possible degree in order to achieve limb salvage. Furthermore, if the femoral pulses are present and the resting thigh pressure is systemic, aortofemoral bypass alone will not salvage the extremity. The surgeon does not have time to wait and see the effectiveness of the preliminary aorto-bifemoral bypass.

On the other hand, patients who have total aortic occlusion or absent pulsations in the groin, even those lacking perfusion of the superficial femoral artery, are likely to be improved enough by this procedure alone to make femoral popliteal bypass superfluous. Of course, this rule, like all others, must be tempered by the findings at surgery. Should there be acute thrombus material in the aorta coupled with the existence of a small profunda vessel, the surgeon must infer that the thrombosis was caused by poor runoff. To achieve limb salvage, the simultaneous performance of aortofemoral graft and femoropopliteal bypass is required.

EVOLUTION OF TREATMENT

In a very short time, reconstruction of the aorta and iliac arterial systems has progressed from reliance on aortofemoral bypass (which worked) or axillary femoral bypass (which did not) to a three-tiered approach, benefiting greatly by advances in less stressful means of accomplishing the same ends. We are not quite at the stage of advocating balloon angioplasty of the iliacs to prevent the development of more extensive iliac disease. The 5- and 10-year results of balloon dilation have to be assessed for this to be true. Nonetheless, its application to all patients with claudication seems justified by the short-term results currently available. Furthermore, the patient with bilateral symptoms can undergo dilation on one side, enabling the surgeon to perform a femorofemoral bypass, which is much less morbid than aortofemoral bypass and provides almost equally good results. Finally, the retroperitoneal approach affords the surgeon an exposure equivalent to that achieved with midline laparotomy while sparing the patient a major intraperitoneal procedure.

FEMOROPOPLITEAL OCCLUSIVE DISEASE

JOHN J. BERGAN, M.D.

Treatment of femoropopliteal arterial occlusive disease is important in vascular surgery. The decision must be made whether to initiate surgical care, recognizing that nonoperative techniques can do little to relieve ischemic symptoms. If decision for intervention is made, the method of therapy must be selected. It is the objective of this section to identify the causes of femoropopliteal arterial occlusive disease, to explain the hierarchy of ischemia, and to describe the choices of surgical management. Finally, a discussion of ancillary measures that may or may not be applied following surgery will conclude the section. Reconstruction distal to the popliteal artery will not be considered.

CAUSES OF FEMOROPOPLITEAL ARTERIAL OCCLUSIVE DISEASE

The causes of arterial occlusion in the femoropopliteal segment are the same as in other arteries in the body. Of primary importance is atherosclerosis, and of secondary importance is thrombosis of aneurysms of the popliteal, superficial femoral, or common femoral artery. A less frequent but important cause of arterial occlusion is trauma. In particular, anterior or posterior knee dislocation can cause arterial wall and/or intimal injury with consequent thrombosis. Least frequent causes of femoropopliteal occlusion are popliteal entrapment and adventitial cystic disease of the popliteal artery.

Statistically, one-half of all arterial occlusions distal to the inguinal ligament are located at the junction of the superficial femoral and the popliteal artery, at the level of the adductor magnus tendon. One-half of the remaining arterial occlusions are in the popliteal segment, and the rest are scattered throughout the peroneal and tibial vessels. This implies that arterial reconstructions should originate proximal to the most common arterial occlusions and extend distally to bypass the majority of occlusions in the popliteal artery.

SEVERITY OF ISCHEMIA

It is generally appreciated that single arterial occlusions cause physiologic derangements distal to the femoropopliteal axis. A single arterial occlusion at the adductor hiatus can cause claudication in the calf. This symptom can be confirmed by history-taking, and physical examination should reveal absent popliteal and ankle pulses. Doppler-derived segmental limb pressures show an ankle/brachial ratio of about 0.5, but such ratios may be as high as 0.8 or as low as 0.3.

When multiple levels of arterial occlusion occur, such as occlusion of the superficial femoral artery and the popliteal artery and/or one or more tibial arteries, a greater degree of ischemia is produced. Physical findings with regard to pulse taking may be identical to those with single-segment occlusions, with absent ankle pulses, but segmental limb pressures show an ankle/brachial ratio of 0.3 or below.

This information indicates that claudication occurs with an ankle/brachial ratio of about 0.5, and rest pain begins with an ankle/brachial ratio of 0.3 or lower. The single most important exception to this rule is sudden arterial occlusion. When this occurs, whether due to thrombosis of a popliteal aneurysm or trauma, the ankle pulses are absent by Doppler examination. Therefore, the ankle/brachial ratio is reduced to 0.0. Some hours after the occlusion, arterial perfusion may resume, Doppler signals may become evident, and the ankle and brachial pressures may allow calculation of a ratio.

The precise regularity of ischemic symptoms allows a great deal of information to be obtained from history-taking and physical examination. This can be applied to the differential diagnosis of limb pain, which must include acquired spinal stenosis, radiculopathy, primary diabetic neuropathy, and inflammatory disease of joints, muscles, and tendons.

SURGICAL THERAPY

Methods of relieving limb ischemia due to femoro-popliteal arterial occlusions include bypass grafting with autogenous vein or prosthetic tubes, as well as percutaneous transluminal angioplasty. Of lesser importance are profundaplasties and lumbar sympathectomy alone or combined with any of these procedures.

Vein or Prosthetic Bypass

As is true of all surgery, autogenous tissue has been found to be the best resource in revascularization of the femoropopliteal axis. In the femoropopliteal arborization, the operation that has stood the longest test of time is the reversed autogenous saphenous vein bypass, although cephalic vein can be used and the in situ technique has been championed by some. The usual indication for the procedure is disabling claudication. In some situations of severe acral ischemia, however, it may be chosen to do a femoropopliteal bypass and ignore more distal arterial occlusions that are contributing to the ischemia. Gradually, over a period of time, surgeons have extended femoropopliteal reconstructions to the below-knee level, and at present, most operations are done to this level

unless some situation arises in which the bypass can be placed to the above-knee popliteal artery.

The anesthetic of choice is general endotracheal anesthesia, although continuous epidural anesthetic has been used by some. After suitable preparation and draping, the thigh and leg are externally rotated and the knee flexed.

The first incision is linear, over the common femoral artery and its bifurcation. This incision extends one-third above and two-thirds below the inguinal ligament crease and is made in such a way that the saphenous vein at its termination is exposed. Careful preservation of lymph nodes and lymphatics in this area requires that a separate incision be made after the saphenous vein is removed to expose the common femoral artery. The skin incision is common, but the two deep incisions preserve lymphatic tissue between the artery and vein.

The second incision is placed in the anteromedial thigh where the anterior border of the sartorius lies. The midportion of the saphenous vein is approached from its deep side, thus preserving the blood supply to the medial skin flap. If desired, the deep fascia can be incised, the sartorius retracted laterally, and the superficial femoral artery-popliteal junction identified.

The third incision is made in the anteromedial calf, parallel to the tibia and extending nearly to the knee joint. Within this incision, the saphenous vein can be removed from the medial flap, taking extraordinary care to preserve the blood supply to the flap. After the deep fascia is incised, the semimembranosus and semitendinosus tendons can be cut, and there is no need to repair them.

After the saphenous vein is removed, it can be gently distended, tributaries ligated, and bleeding points suture-ligated with 6–0 polypropylene suture. There is no conclusive proof that any particular irrigating solution produces better long-term patency rates than any other. Our choice is room-temperature saline or lactated Ringer's solution.

Tunneling is accomplished using submuscular planes, and the reversed saphenous vein can be pulled from above downward by means of long, semicurved aortic clamps. Similarly, prosthetic material can be passed in the same fashion, with care being taken to avoid twisting of the vein or prosthesis. With regard to prosthetic grafts, polytetrafluoroethylene (PTFE) is favored, simply because aneurysmal degeneration of umbilical vein grafts has been noted frequently in patent bypasses beyond the third year. It is not determined whether externally reinforced PTFE grafts function better or less well than nonreinforced grafts, but is is accepted that thin-walled PTFE grafts are not disadvantaged and are easier to work with than earlier models of PTFE with a thicker wall. Woven or knitted Dacron grafts have been used in the past as femoropopliteal bypasses and have functioned fairly well, but they are no longer favored.

Prior to arterial clamping, the patient is systemically heparinized with 5,000 units of heparin, and the anastomoses are performed end-to-side, with care being taken to align the anastomosis as nearly parallel to the artery as possible. In no instance should the graft take off from the parent artery at a right angle. The introduction of polypropylene suture has changed anastomotic techniques. The suture, being monofilament and frictionless, allows careful placement of each suture in the artery wall and vein wall so that there is no compromise of the suture line. The 6–0 suture is used for the common femoral and popliteal anastomoses; 7–0 and smaller sutures are used for tibial anastomoses. The heparin anticoagulation need not be reversed, but meticulous attention must be paid to hemostasis.

In all arterial reconstructions below the inguinal ligament, an intraoperative arteriogram should be done to demonstrate the distal anastomosis and outflow. Although technical abnormalities are not usually seen, an assessment of the outflow of the tibial vessels, and especially the arborization in the foot, determines prognosis for the limb and indicates whether a subsequent arterial exploration might be advantageous if the reconstruction fails. Poor tibial outflow into the foot and absence of pedal arches constitute a grave prognostic sign which would indicate that, when the graft fails remotely after operation, perhaps the limb should be abandoned rather than subject the patient to multiple arterial reconstructions.

In our prospective, randomized study, patency of grafts at 48 months was as follows: saphenous vein, 68 percent; PTFE, 38 percent; above-knee saphenous vein, 61 percent; above-knee PTFE, 38 percent; below-knee saphenous vein, 76 percent; below-knee PTFE, 54 percent. This shows the wisdom of taking grafts to the below-knee position when possible.

Percutaneous Transluminal Angioplasty

Percutaneous transluminal angioplasty (PTA) has been advocated in the treatment of femoropopliteal arterial occlusions. However, its use should be restricted to short-segment stenoses of the femoral or popliteal vessels. It may be possible to disobliterate total occlusions, whether they are short or long, but the prognosis for such disobliterations is poor.

Profundaplasty

Profundaplasty has been advocated as a means of revascularizing the calf and foot without the hazards of bypass grafting. However, profundaplasty alone has proved to be disappointing. It seems to have its greatest effect when combined with inflow arterial reconstructions, such as aortofemoral bypass. In such instances, the profundaplasty achieved by anastomosing the graft to the profunda femoris artery has greatest effect.

Lumbar Sympathectomy

The subject of lumbar sympathectomy comes up in any discussion of treatment of femoropopliteal occlusions because it was introduced as the first form of treatment for such occlusions prior to the advent of arterial reconstruction. There is no conclusive proof that lumbar sympathectomy, alone or in combination with arterial reconstructive procedures, can do more than temporarily relieve coldness of the foot. Neither in the situation of rest pain nor in superficial skin necrosis has it been shown conclusively that lumbar sympathectomy has any beneficial effect. Although some patients have objectively demonstrable increases in arterial perfusion and ankle pressure, no method has been devised to predict reliably which patients will do so. Our group does not use lumbar sympathectomy in the treatment of severe ischemia.

POSTOPERATIVE CARE

The truism of postoperative care beginning in the operating room is nowhere more important than in femoropopliteal arterial reconstruction. Postoperative hematomas can be avoided by meticulous hemostasis, and care should be taken to achieve such hemostasis by electrocautery or irrigation with hemostatic solutions. Following closure of the wounds with continuous braided absorbable suture, the skin edges are approximated with intradermal 3–0 suture. The knots are carefully buried. Such attention to details of wound closure decreases postoperative morbidity. Initially, the limb is wrapped in sterile gauze, but 24 hours postoperatively, this and all other bandages are removed.

Monitoring in the recovery room and intensive care unit should be carried out by trained personnel who are capable of detecting Doppler signals at the ankle and assessing ankle pressure. In all cases, the ankle pressure should exceed the preoperative level. It is to be expected that the initial ankle pressure will be the highest to be obtained. Frequently after autogenous vein bypass grafting to the popliteal level, the pressure decreases 4 to 8 hours postoperatively, and then increases to a higher level so that by 24 hours, the maximum level has been achieved. If the ankle pressure decreases to the preoperative level or below, failure of the bypass is to be expected and the patient should be returned to the operating room.

Similarly, if a tense hematoma is encountered in any of the wounds, the patient must be returned to the operating room for evacuation of the hematoma. Such hematomas act as a compartment syndrome and compromise arterial blood flow and nerve function.

There is no proof that anticoagulant therapy improves the patency rate of femoropopliteal grafts. They are used by our group only in cases of multiple previous graft failures. Similarly, antiplatelet therapy has not been proved to improve graft patency. However, coagulation abnormalities have been encountered in patients undergoing femoropopliteal bypass, and when abnormal platelet function is seen, antiplatelet therapy should be given to reverse this tendency.

It is critically important to prevent edema of revascularization. Such edema is of lymphatic origin and is not due to venous obstruction. It should be treated by leg elevation and elastic bandaging.

Finally, in situations of severe ischemia relieved by bypass grafting, one expects the ischemic neuropathy existing before the operation to be manifest as an increased level of neuropathic pain following the procedure. This decreases gradually in a pattern much like that of removing a stocking. The patient should be reassured that such neuropathic pain indicates function of the bypass.

Monitoring of the reconstruction should be done at 6-month intervals using objective criteria, such as pulse-taking by an experienced physician or ankle pressures derived by the Doppler technique. Any decrease in objective indicators of bypass function calls for arteriography and correction of the abnormality before total occlusion of the graft occurs.

TIBIOPERONEAL ARTERIAL OCCLUSIVE DISEASE

JOHN J. RICOTTA, M.D.

Over the last decade, improvements in surgical technique and perioperative care have allowed vascular surgeons to extend arterial reconstruction to the level of the tibial and peroneal arteries. Patients with symptomatic atherosclerotic disease in these vessels represent perhaps the greatest challenge to modern vascular surgery. Life expectancy in this patient population is significantly less than in patients with more proximal arterial disease. In general, these patients are older than those with femoro-popliteal occlusive disease, and the incidence of diabetes in this population may exceed 50 percent. Both of these factors increase the operative risk. In addition, many of these patients have multisegmental occlusions of aorto-iliac, femoropopliteal, and infragenicular arteries. Patency rates of arterial reconstruction are lower than in patients with proximal disease, and this becomes especially true if autogenous graft material is not available.

As a result of these factors, meticulous preoperative evaluation, strict selection criteria for operation, and optimal perioperative patient support are essential. With proper management, however, several investigators have shown that adequate patency rates and excellent palliation may be achieved in these patients.

SELECTION OF PATIENTS

Only patients with profound ischemia of the lower extremity, as manifested by unremitting ischemic rest pain, nonhealing lesions of the foot, or ischemic gangrene of the forefoot, should be considered for tibioperoneal reconstruction. Patients whose only complaint is claudication are generally managed nonoperatively. This position is taken because of the limited patency rate reported for bypass grafts to the tibial vessels. In general, these patency rates, at best, approach 60 percent at 2 years and 40 to 50 percent at 5 years when saphenous vein is used. Experience has shown that when prosthetic material is required for bypass, the majority of grafts become occluded in 3 years. Graft occlusion is usually accompanied by a recurrence of limb-threatening ischemia. These factors, more than any others, serve as a rationale for limiting tibioperoneal revascularization to patients in whom major amputation would be the only alternative.

When patients present with nonhealing lesions or gangrene of the lower extremity, the extent of ischemia in the surrounding tissues must be determined. Gangrenous areas that extend beyond the forefoot generally are indications for below-knee amputation and preclude attempts at arterial revascularization. Many patients present with necrotizing infection and/or plantar space abscesses. Recognition of infection with radical debridement and/or drainage should be instituted prior to any decision on arterial bypass.

Occasionally patients present with distal lesions of the toes that have resulted from proximal arterial emboli, small-vessel thrombosis, or vasculitis. In these instances, the remainder of the forefoot and lower extremity is usually well perfused. A careful search for underlying atheroembolic disease in the proximal arterial tree is important in these patients. In general, surgical attention should be directed toward the more proximal disease. The gangrenous distal lesions often heal with local wound care and may be managed conservatively. If patients have persistent lesions or continue to complain of ischemic pain, a lumbar sympathectomy may be beneficial.

Some patients present with rapid onset of rest pain resulting from acute arterial occlusion. This may be due to proximal arterial thrombosis, arterial embolism, or thrombosis of a preexisting graft. If limb viability is not threatened, urgent tibial revascularization is generally avoided, and this acute occlusion is treated by thrombo-embolectomy or anticoagulation. The role of thrombolytic therapy in this group of patients remains to be defined.

PHYSICAL EVALUATION

Preoperative evaluation should focus on (1) precise anatomic localization of the occlusive process, and (2) accurate assessment of blood flow to the foot, and (3) evaluation of the extent of any tissue necrosis present. A thorough physical examination of the lower extremities is imperative. This includes palpation and auscultation of the aorta and the iliac, femoral, popliteal, and pedal vessels. Objective data are obtained by the use of segmental blood pressures and plethysmography, supplemented by Doppler femoral wave forms. Doppler interrogation of the tibial and peroneal vessels at the ankle as well as evaluation of the pedal arch is an essential part of the preoperative physical evaluation. This technique allows the clinician to determine the dominant vessel supplying the pedal arch in most cases. Confirmation of the presence of a pedal arch and identification of the major vessels supplying the arch provide invaluable information in the planning of arterial reconstruction.

Physical examination of the foot is extremely important. Patients with advanced arterial ischemia may show signs of skin and muscle atrophy in the forefoot and loss of hair in the lower leg. Even more important is the presence of dependent rubor and the "elevation-dependency" test. In this test, the patient is examined in the supine position. The legs are elevated at a 45-degree angle for a 60-second period, after which they are brought back to the horizontal position. In the presence of significant inflow disease, pallor should be noted within 60 seconds of elevation, and capillary and venous filling should be delayed for at least 30 seconds after the legs have been brought back to the horizontal position. This test is helpful in distinguishing the symptoms of diabetic neuropathy from those of rest pain.

ANGIOGRAPHIC EVALUATION

A thorough angiographic evaluation is of utmost importance in patients who are being considered for arterial reconstruction. Such an evaluation involves complete angiography of the aortoiliac, femoropopliteal, and infragenicular vessels. Standard intra-arterial angiography with muliplanar views is essential in these patients. Digital techniques may also play a role in evaluation. The angiographic approach should be guided by the results of physical examination and noninvasive laboratory evaluation. It is important to identify significant lesions in the aortofemoral system, and this can be done by the use of oblique views and femoral artery pressures in selected cases. When there is evidence of a proximal pressure-reducing lesion, this can sometimes be improved by balloon angioplasty carried out either in the angiography suite or at the time of arterial revascularization. Although the detection of inflow disease is important in most cases, treatment of inflow lesions alone will not usually relieve symptoms in patients with multiple occlusions in the lower extremity. Angioplasty or extra-anatomic bypass such as a femoral-femoral graft is most important as a means of providing adequate inflow to sustain the more distal arterial reconstruction.

In addition to evaluation of proximal arterial disease, it is important to accurately delineate the state of the distal vessels. The long-term patency of femorotibial reconstructions has been related to the status of the "runoff" vessels

and the presence of a pedal arch. Every attempt should be made to visualize the tibial vessels down to the level of the foot. Although reactive hyperemia has been used in our center to enhance visualization, this procedure is often uncomfortable to the patient. A good alternative is the use of intra-arterial vasodilators such as Priscoline with delayed filming. Intra-arterial digital techniques may enhance visualization of these vessels. Even with these techniques, approximately 10 to 15 percent of arteriograms in patients with advanced distal ischemia do not show a runoff vessel supplying the pedal arch. In these cases, intraoperative femoral arteriography using 30 cc of contrast medium with proximal femoral artery occlusion is an extremely helpful technique.

The complications of arteriography must be remembered. As stated previously, many of these patients are diabetic and may have compromised renal function. Adequate pre-angiographic hydration is essential. In patients with creatinine levels greater than 2 mg per deciliter, limited arterial studies may be indicated. In this case, unilateral femoral angiography may provide adequate information for operation. Alternatively, use of digital subtraction angiography with intra-arterial injection has allowed us to limit dye load in uremic patients, although the quality of the studies has not equalled that of a standard arterial injection.

PREOPERATIVE PREPARATION

Prior to a vascular reconstruction, a thorough evaluation of the patient's operative risks is required. As previously stated, these patients are usually elderly and have a significant incidence of hypertension, diabetes, compromised renal function, and atherosclerotic heart disease. Many of these patients are also heavy smokers. Preoperative evaluation focuses on control of hypertension and diabetes and assessment of pulmonary function and myocardial reserve. A careful cardiac history is taken, with emphasis on past history of myocardial infarction and the presence and extent of any current angina. Symptoms of congestive heart failure are also important. Resting EKG is taken, and if necessary, echocardiography or radioisotope cardiac scans are performed. Pulmonary function tests are performed as clinically indicated, and renal function tests including creatinine and, if indicated, creatinine clearance are performed. Although many of these patients have multiple medical problems, it is unusual to deny a patient arterial bypass because of excessive operative risk. Lower limb reconstruction rarely involves excessive blood loss or fluid shifts, and appropriate preoperative preparation combined with regional anesthesia can be applied with success even in high-risk patients. Epidural anesthesia is particularly useful in this regard. Occasionally, however, if a patient is moribund or has a limited life expectancy, an expeditious amputation is often the best treatment.

Local control of infection is extremely important in this group of patients. Debridement of necrotic tissue and drainage of any localized focus of infection should be performed before arterial bypass is undertaken. Adequate cultures should be obtained prior to institution of antibiotic coverage. Initial antibiotic coverage should be broad and include both gram-positive and gram-negative organisms. Coverage is later adjusted on the basis of the bacteriologic data. Paients with evidence of gross infection should be treated preoperatively for at least 24 hours, or until there is evidence of control of any infectious process. It is not always possible to delay revascularization until infection has completely subsided; however, there should be good evidence that the infectious process is responding to systemic antibiotics and local wound care. When revascularization is undertaken in the presence of an open wound or infection, prosthetic material should be avoided whenever possible.

OPERATIVE TECHNIQUE

A variety of operative techniques are applicable to femorotibial reconstruction. All of these approaches share several common goals. These include establishment of adequate inflow proximally and outflow distally, avoidance of prosthetic graft material whenever possible, and limiting the length of prosthetic material used. The different operative options will be discussed separately.

Standard Femorotibial Bypass

This procedure is employed with the common femoral artery as inflow source and one of the infrageniculate arteries (anterior tibial, posterior tibial or peroneal) as the outflow source. The common femoral artery should have a normal or near normal pressure whenever possible. As previously mentioned, hemodynamicially significant proximal disease should be corrected by angioplasty or extra-anatomic bypass. In general, I try to avoid aortofemoral bypass in patients who will need a subsequent tibial reconstruction for limb salvage since this increases the operative risk. I have not hesitated to perform a tibial reconstruction for limb salvage in patients with a clinically adequate femoral pulse even in the presence of angiographic evidence of inflow disease. The outflow vessel is selected through a combination of Doppler examination and angiography. Ideally, the vessel should communicate with the plantar arch. Careful examination of the posterior tibial, lateral malleolar, and dorsalis pedis arteries with compression maneuvers at the ankle will serve to identify these vessels. Although some authors have avoided the use of the peroneal artery, I do not hesitate to use this as an outflow vessel, if there is evidence that it supplies the plantar arch. In general, the site of distal anastomosis should be beyond any major vessel occlusion. At times, this may require that the bypass be carried down to the level of the ankle, or even onto the pedal arch. In my experience, intraoperative pre-bypass angiography has been helpful in this regard, and I have rarely found bypass to the dorsalis pedis artery necessary.

The tibial peroneal trunk, posterior artery, and proximal peroneal artery are approached through a medial incision. The anterior tibial artery and lower half of the peroneal artery are exposed through a lateral approach. Exposure of the lower portion of the peroneal artery requires resection of the fibula. When using the lateral approach, I have tunneled the graft through the interosseous membrane and have avoided extra-anatomic tunneling along the lateral portion of the leg. Proximal and distal vascular control may be obtained by the use of fine neurosurgical clips or intraluminal vessel occluders. Some authors have reported success using a proximal thigh tourniquet, but I have had no experience with this approach. I have abandoned the use of vessel loops because they may be associated with significant arterial damage or spasm and they distort the vessel anatomy.

When reversed saphenous vein is used, this may be harvested through single or multiple skin incisions. Precise placement of the incisions prevents development of skin flaps and tissue necrosis. The vein should be harvested atraumatically. Periadventitial injection of a dilute papaverine solution helps to reduce venospasm. For reverse vein bypass, the saphenous vein should be 3.5 to 4 mm in minimal inner diameter and free of areas of fibrosis or large varicosities.

When performing a standard femorotibial bypass, using either vein or prosthetic material, one performs the distal anastomosis first. A long arteriotomy, at least 15 to 20 mm, is used. This provides a hemodynamically better flow through the anastomosis and, I believe, retards the development of neointimal hyperplasia. Anastomoses are performed using fine monofilament suture and loop magnification. On occasion, interrupted sutures may be used at the "heel and toe" of the anastomosis, but I have not found it necessary to use an interrupted technique for the entire anastomosis when saphenous vein is employed. Once the distal anastomosis is performed, the vein graft is distended with a solution containing heparinized saline and papaverine and passed proximally in an anatomic position. The proximal anastomosis is then performed to the common femoral artery at its bifurcation. This anastomosis is completed with a continuous fine monofilament suture. The arteriotomy in the common femoral artery is made in such a way that the orifice of the profunda femoris artery can be visualized. If necessary, profundaplasty may be carried out at the time of tibial bypass. Whenever possible, endarterectomy of the common femoral artery is avoided. After completion of the bypass graft, intraoperative angiography is mandatory and is performed by injecting 30 cc of Renografin into the bypass graft, which is occuded proximal to the injection site. The graft is checked for position, kinking, and status of the distal anastomosis. At this time, it is also possible to assess the quality of the recipient tibial vessel and the status of the pedal arch.

In Situ Saphenous Vein Bypass

Interest in the in situ saphenous vein bypass technique is increasing. This technique, which has been in use for about 20 years, recently has been modified and publicized. Results of this technique suggest that veins as small as 2.5 mm in internal diameter may be used for bypass without compromising long-term patency, thus increasing the availability of autogenous vein for bypass. This technique has the additional advantage of avoiding excessive size discrepancy between vein and artery, which often is seen when the reverse bypass technique is used in tibial vessel reconstruction. These advantages explain the increasing popularity of in situ saphenous vein bypass in distal vessel reconstruction.

The in situ technique requires a reliable and relatively atraumatic method for incising venous valves. In general, the proximal venous valve in the greater saphenous vein is excised under direct vision. The remainder of the valves are serially excised using specially designed instruments such as the valve cutter or valvulotome. In this technique, the saphenous vein is left in its bed, and excessive dissection of the vein is purposely avoided. Access to the vein for valve disruption is via side branches. After the proximal venous valves have been excised, the proximal anastomosis to the common femoral artery is performed. This is in contrast to the sequence of anastomosis when the reversed saphenous vein is used. After the proximal anastomosis is performed, the vein is allowed to distend with the patient's own blood to demonstrate the site of more distal valves, which are then disrupted by means of the techniques already described. After all the valves have been disrupted, the distal anastomosis is then performed as described for the reverse vein. Any remaining venous collaterals are then ligated to diminish the incidence of postoperative arterial venous fistulas. An angiographic study of the entire graft, as well as the runoff vessel, is required. Special attention is directed toward persistence of any venous valves or the presence of any arterial venous fistula.

Femorotibial Bypass Using Prosthetic Material

On occasion, bypass to the tibial vessels is undertaken with prosthetic material. Every attempt is made to avoid this because of the marked decrease in patency rate as compared to bypasses with autogenous vein. Nevertheless, approximately 5 to 10 percent of patients require a prosthetic femorotibial bypass. These patients must be carefully evaluated since it is well known that the majority of these bypasses will occlude within 2 to 3 years. Despite this, patients with limb-threatening ischemia should not be denied attempts at revascularization simply because of the unavailability of autogenous vein. These patients often have a limited life expectancy and may die before their arterial bypass occludes. In addition, a patent prosthetic bypass may allow healing of a traumatic ulcer or a minor amputation. This may result in limb salvage even if the graft becomes occluded at a later date. These considerations suggest that even when prosthetic bypass is required, effective palliation can be achieved in properly selected patients.

A variety of materials are available for prosthetic bypass, the most commonly used being polytetrafluoroethylene (PTFE) and human umbilical vein. The technique of bypass is similar to that described for reversed autogenous saphenous vein. It is particularly important in these patients, however, that a long arteriotomy be performed in the distal vessel since intimal hyperplasia is more common when prosthetic materials are used. The relative merits of these two types of prosthetic will not be debated here. However, when PTFE is used, it is important that the graft be distended with heparinized saline and that blood be kept out of the lumen of the graft until arterial flow is reestablished. Use of umbilical vein requires some technical adaptation, and interrupted suture technique generally is required for at least part of the anastomosis to avoid fragmentation of the intimal lining of the graft.

Adjunctive distal arterial fistula has been advocated to maintain graft patency when prosthetic grafts are used to vessels with limited runoff. My experience with this technique has been limited, and at present I believe it is of unproven value.

Sequential Bypass

Sequential arterial bypass has been advocated in patients with multisegmental disease as a means of improving runoff. Such bypasses may consist of femoropopliteotibial bypasses or femorotibiotibial bypasses. The latter may be indicated when there are two tibial arteries supplying the lower leg which are not clearly connected by collaterals. In this situation, it may not be clear which of the two tibial arteries are dominant, and a sequential bypass may decrease the outflow resistance and therefore increase the flow through the bypass graft. Femoropopliteotibial bypasses are indicated when there is a suitable isolated popliteal segment present which gives rise to significant geniculate collaterals. It should be noted that such a sequential bypass to the popliteal artery cannot be easily performed using the in situ to saphenous vein technique.

Finally, sequential bypasses have become popular when only a limited amount of saphenous vein is available for bypass. In these situations, a femoropopliteal bypass is constructed with prosthetic material, and this bypass is used as an inflow source (in a "hitchhike" or "piggyback" fashion) for a tibial bypass for which autogenous vein is used. If such a composite sequential bypass is employed, the distal prosthetic anastomosis should be kept above the knee whenever possible.

Short-Segment Bypass Grafts

A variety of short-segment grafts have been proposed which use arteries distal to the common femoral artery as inflow sources. Thse bypass grafts are especially useful when the amount of saphenous vein present for bypass is limited. The superficial femoral artery and even the popliteal artery may serve as adequate inflow sources under appropriate conditions. For these arteries to be considered as adequate inflow sources, they must be free of any angiographic stenosis greater than 20 percent and should have a systolic pressure within 10 mm Hg of radial artery pressure. These conditions are noted most often in diabetics whose disease is limited to the infrageniculate arteries. Although this situation is unusual, good results have been reported with the short-segment bypasses and my experience supports this. Either reversed or in situ technique may be applicable here.

POSTOPERATIVE CARE

Postoperatively, the status of the distal arterial tree is monitored by the sequential determinations of ankle blood pressure and calculation of ankle-to-brachial index. A significant drop in ankle-brachial index (greater than 15%) or a return to preoperative values is a prognostic sign and may, in some cases, dictate the need for repeat angiography and/or reoperation. Failure of an angiographically proved patent graft to raise the ankle/arm index more than 15 percent over baseline values may indicate that an inappropriate recipient artery has been selected. It should be noted, however, that ankle blood pressure may continue to rise for a week or more after revascularization if graft is anatomically patent.

In the immediate postoperative period, attention is turned to the maintenance of adequate hemodynamics of fluid balance in the patient. Avoidance of vasospasm and vasoconstriction is important. Maintenance of adequate urine output in these patients is important, and monitoring is facilitated by use of an indwelling Foley catheter for several days. Postoperative heparinization is rarely indicated, although dextran sometimes is employed. However, I feel that antiplatelet agents must be administered following revascularization, and in fact, there is evidence to suggest that at least one dose should be given prior to bypass. Currently, I give my patients aspirin, 325 mg twice a day, and Persantine, 50 mg three times a day, beginning the day before surgery. A knee immobilizer should be used while the patient is in bed and should be worn for the first 2 or 3 months postoperatively while the patient is sleeping. Many patients have some swelling of the lower extremity following revascularization. This is usually of limited significance and can be treated with mild compression stockings or ace bandages.

Antibiotics should be continued in these patients until all invasive monitoring equipment such as central venous lines, arterial lines, and Foley catheters have been removed or until there is evidence that soft tissue infection has been controlled.

CAUSES OF GRAFT FAILURE

As previously mentioned, graft failure is more common following femorotibial reconstruction than following femoropopliteal reconstruction. Causes of graft failure are similar to those seen in more proximal arterial reconstructions, i.e., technical error, neointimal fibrous hyperplasia, and progression of atherosclerotic disease. Technical problems usually result in thrombosis within 30 days of bypass. Neointimal hyperplasia results in graft failure 6 to 24 months postoperatively, whereas progression of disease is usually seen later than 18 months after surgery if patients are properly selected. Technical error generally can be avoided by the use of intraoperative completion angiography. Neointimal hyperplasia cannot be avoided, but I believe its effects can be minimized by the use of antiplatelet agents and long distal arteriotomy. Progression of atherosclerotic disease, at present, is an unsolvable problem. Proper selection of the distal anastomosis is important to minimize distal vascular resistance. Use of a sequential bypass may be of help in this regard. The limitation of the distal vascular bed and progression of tibial artery disease represent major causes of later graft occlusion and are likely to be the greatest reasons for differences between results of femorotibial reconstruction and those of femoropopliteal reconstruction.

OCCLUSIVE DISEASE OF THE UPPER EXTREMITY

TERENCE QUIGLEY, M.D.
JERRY GOLDSTONE, M.D.

Ischemic symptoms in the arm or hand may result from a great variety of causes including atherosclerosis, arterial spastic disorders, inflammatory arteriopathies, and trauma. Although the final common pathway producing symptoms must necessarily be a lack of blood flow, the exact etiology is often difficult to ascertain. Thus, the entire spectrum of diseases must be considered in patients with symptoms indicating an obstructive arterial lesion of the upper extremity (Table 1). It is extremely important that a thorough history and physical examination be performed on every patient complaining of pain, coolness, discoloration, or dysesthesia in the hand. The physician must use all available clinical and laboratory tools in order to make a precise diagnosis. In patients who require surgical treatment to correct ischemic symptoms, the operative procedures may be difficult and the results occasionally unrewarding. Thus, the selection of patients for surgery and the choice of procedure can tax the judgment of even the most experienced surgeon.

DIAGNOSIS

The History

In addition to the usual demographic data, a detailed history of the patient's activities at work and in the home provides valuable information as to the chronicity of the problem and the potential cause. The patient may only come to realize the pattern of his or her disease during this questioning. Thoracic outlet syndrome, cervical disc disease, and other nerve compression syndromes may mimic arterial occlusive disease, and the history could make differentiation possible. It is important to keep in mind that the thoracic outlet syndrome and arterial occlusive disease may coexist. Specific questioning concerning the patient's past medical history and any remote traumatic injuries may provide valuable clues to the diagnosis. A medication history is extremely valuable

TABLE 1 Etiology of Upper Extremity Ischemia

Primary arterial
  Atherosclerosis
  Aneurysm
  Embolism
  Congenital defects
Trauma
  Injury (blunt or penetrating)
  Occupational (vibratory)
  Iatrogenic
    Catheter injury
    Angiography
    Dialysis shunting procedures
    Radiation
  Frostbite
Arteritis/Immune disorders
  Raynaud's disease
  Connective tissue disorders
    Systemic lupus erythematosus
    Polyarteritis
    Scleroderma
    Takayasu's arteritis
    Buerger's disease
  Allergic arteritis
Musculoskeletal
  Thoracic outlet syndrome
  Carpal tunnel syndrome
  Compartment syndrome
    Postinjury
    Venous occlusion
Drugs
  Ergot poisoning
  Abuse
  Iatrogenic (dopamine, levophed)
Hematologic
  Blood dyscrasias
  Polycythemia
  Sickle Cell Anemia

information, being diagnostic in the case of ergotism and suggestive if the patient is a drug abuser. Questions about systemic and musculoskeletal symptoms may point to inflammatory arteritis or collagen vascular disease.

Physical Examination

Both upper extremities should be examined together so that comparisons are easily made since many of the systemic causes of upper extremity ischemia tend to by symmetrical. Visual inspection should include any evidence of muscle atrophy, posturing, or obvious deformity as well as any color or skin changes in the fingers. Temperature changes should also be noted. The blood vessels from the neck to the wrist should be individually palpated for evidence of aneurysm and to record the quality of the pulses. An Allen test should be performed at the wrist to assess the patency of the radial and ulnar arteries and the adequacy of the palmar arch. Auscultation of the neck and axillary area can detect the presence of bruits. A complete neurologic examination, including thorough sensory and motor evaluation, is necessary. An Adson maneuver (assessment of the radial pulse during hyperabduction and external rotation of the arm) and an elevated arm stress test (rapid opening and closing of the fists while the arms are held over the head) should be performed to assess the status of the thoracic outlet.

Testing Procedures

Blood should be drawn for a complete blood count, erythrocyte sedimentation rate, and, if indicated, serologic testing that may uncover a systemic metabolic disorder responsible for arm and hand ischemia. Scleroderma, systemic lupus erythematosus, and other connective tissue disorders can be diagnosed by such tests as an antinuclear antibody, cryoglobulin, rheumatoid factor, and serum complement levels.

Noninvasive vascular testing can be useful in determining the presence of segmental vascular occlusion or the patency of the arteries of the wrist and digits. Blood pressure should be obtained in both arms, and if necessary, Doppler arterial pressure and wave form recordings should be obtained in the upper arm, just distal to the antecubital fossa and at the wrist. The Doppler instrument is sensitive in detecting blood flow, and the pressure measurements and wave forms are objective data that can be followed over time.

X-ray studies may well provide the definitive data necessary to establish a diagnosis. Angiography should probably be performed prior to any surgical procedure on the ischemic upper extremity. It is important to include the aortic arch and the innominate and subclavian arteries in every evaluation, especially if an embolus (micro or macro) is suspected. If a musculoskeletal cause of arm ischemia is suspected, such as the thoracic outlet syndrome, hyperabduction maneuvers should be performed during the angiogram. Additionally, neck films should be obtained to rule out a cervical rib. If a vasospastic disorder is suspected, intra-arterial nitroglycerine during the angiogram may provide diagnostic and therapeutic information. It is important to alert the radiologist concerning the clinical suspicions so that maximal data can be obtained from the examination.

THERAPY

The therapeutic approach to the patient depends largely on the etiology of the ischemic problem and the extent of the injury (Table 2). For the patient with arteritis or a metabolic disorder, the treatment is primarily nonsurgical. Steroid preparations, vasodilators, rheologic agents, and platelet inhibitors all have a role in the management of these patients. Cervical sympathectomy and/or amputation may be indicated when severe ischemia or necrosis is present. Arterial reconstruction is rarely indicated or possible for ischemia of this type.

Cervical Sympathectomy

Our current indications for cervical sympathectomy include causalgia, vasospastic disorders not responsive to oral vasodilating agents, and advanced digital ischemia not amenable to arterial reconstruction. We prefer the anterior, supraclavicular approach to the cervical sympathetic chain. The anterior scalene muscle is divided, and the subclavian artery is followed proximally to the vertebral artery origin. Sibson's fascia is incised at this point, and the sympathetic chain is palpated against the vertebral body posterior to the vertebral artery. The distal half of the stellate ganglion, the T2 and T3 ganglions, are removed. A transient Horner's syndrome is occasionally noted, but the procedure is otherwise well tolerated by the patients. Unfortunately, the long-term results of cervical sympathectomy are unpredictable and often disappointing.

Scalenectomy and First Rib Resection

The thoracic outlet syndrome is best treated by surgical decompression of the thoracic outlet. Cervical ribs, if present, are removed through an anterior supra-

TABLE 2   Treatment of Upper Extremity Ischemia

    Medical
        Vasodilators
        Steroids
        Antiplatelet agents
        Rheologic agents (antimetabolites)
    Surgical
        Arterial reconstruction
        Cervical sympathectomy
        Amputation
        Fasciotomy

clavicular approach with concomitant removal of the anterior scalene muscle. Anterior scalenectomy and/or first rib excision is indicated for symptoms relative to nerve or vessel compression by these structures. Our approach to the first rib is transaxillary. If an anterior scalenectomy is indicated by the nerve pain distribution, a separate supraclavicular incision provides the exposure necessary to remove this muscle and identify any of the other anatomic anomalies that may be implicated in the thoracic outlet compression syndrome as described by Roos. Occasionally, the musculoskeletal compression may be so severe that the subclavian artery may have an area of poststenotic dilatation. We would consider surgical reconstruction only if distal embolization has occurred or thrombus is present and, in our opinion, represents a serious risk for embolization. In that case the artery would be approached directly and replaced with an arterial autograft, Dacron, or PTFE through a supraclavicular incision. Saphenous veins are generally inadequate for subclavian replacement. If distal exposure of the axillary artery is necessary, we use an infraclavicular incision with division of the fibers of the pectoralis minor and major muscle.

Direct Arterial Reconstruction

Primary arterial disease and traumatic injuries of the upper extremity require direct arterial reconstruction. Our approach and method of repair vary with the clinical situation, which can be classified as either acute or chronic.

Acute ischemia of the arm and hand is usually the result of trauma or an embolus. Rarely, an atherosclerotic stenosis progresses to the point of occlusion, causing limb-threatening ischemia. Traumatic injury usually is obvious, and an angiogram provides the information necessary to plan an operative approach. In the injured extremity, priority should be given to providing arterial inflow. Orthopaedic stabilization can precede arterial repair if (1) the patient is seen early, within 1 to 2 hours, (2) the arm and hand are clearly viable, or (3) a subsequent orthopaedic procedure is likely to disrupt the arterial repair.

The patient is placed supine on the operating table with the arm resting on an arm board. We do not use a tourniquet, preferring direct pressure if necessary. (One leg is prepared for harvesting the saphenous vein in *all* procedures involving arterial repair of the arm.) A longitudinal incision is placed over the site of injury unless it will cross the antecubital crease, in which case a transverse "step" incision is made. Once proximal arterial control is obtained, heparin is administered (50 to 100 units per kilogram) intravenously. Direct repair of the artery is attempted, or a saphenous vein graft is interposed. In our experience, prosthetic grafts below the antecubital crease have a dismal patency rate. We also feel that prosthetic material is contraindicated in open traumatic wounds, the Houston experience with PTFE notwithstanding.

For all arterial reconstructions below the axilla, we recommend the use of magnification in performing the anastomosis or repair. Vessel occlusion is performed iwth double-looped Silastic slings to minimize trauma. A 6–0 or 7–0 polypropylene interrupted suture is used. We routinely pass a 2 F or 3 F balloon thrombectomy catheter distally to ensure patency of the vessels at least to the level of the palmar arch. A completion angiogram is performed to examine the repair and to assess the status of the distal arm vessels and digital arteries. We use a 21-gauge plastic catheter placed proximal to the repair and occlude the inflow during the angiogram. Seven to 10 cc of contrast medium is sufficient to detail the hand anatomy. We routinely inject 30 to 45 mg of papaverine prior to the contrast injection to enhance visualization of the distal vessels. If there is thrombus in the digital arteries, heparin administration is continued in the postoperative period to maintain the PTT at twice the control value. The decision to place the patient on Coumadin depends on the status of the hand after 4 or 5 days. Distal arterial spasm may be significant in the immediate postoperative period, confusing the clinical picture.

Perhaps the most common cause of upper extremity ischemia is catheter manipulation. Thrombosis of the brachial artery should be treated by immediate thrombectomy through a transverse arteriotomy according to the principles already outlined. If the catheter has caused significant trauma to the brachial artery, we do not hesitate to transect, debride, and perform a primary anastomosis. Heparin is continued for 24 hours if the thrombosis is extensive. In the infant or child, we would be cautiously optimistic in the presence of a viable hand and avoid operative intervention. Brachial thrombectomy in children less than 10 years old may be very difficult and result in further ischemia.

Compartment syndromes of the forearm are treated aggressively with fasciotomy as indicated. Venous thrombosis of the upper extremity may also cause increased pressures in the forearm compartments and should be treated in a similar manner if indicated.

Chronic occlusions of the upper extremity *causing*

symptoms can be treated electively. Atherosclerosis of the branches of the aortic arch is common. There is no indication to revascularize the upper extremity in the asymptomatic patient. The decision to approach these lesions surgically should be made individually. Generally, only limb-threatening ischemia is an indication for arterial reconstruction in this situation, although incapacitating effort-related symptoms may require surgical treatment. We prefer endarterectomy of these vessels in almost all cases. The technique is easily learned, it is well tolerated even in the elderly patient, and the results are durable.

Our approach to the innominate and proximal right subclavian arteries is via a median sternotomy, with or without a supraclavicular incision. The distal subclavian and axillary arteries may be approached through a supraclavicular or infraclavicular incision, as indicated by the location of the disease. On the left, the proximal subclavian is approached via a third-interspace posterolateral thoracotomy. We use these incisions for both elective and traumatic cases.

Surgically correctable atherosclerosis of the arm arteries distal to the subclavian is unusual. Diabetic patients may have advanced arterial disease into the hand, but the vessels are generally patent, and the involvement of the digital arteries is not amenable to reconstruction. Reconstruction may be indicated, however, in patients who suffer a complication of a dialysis shunting procedure. Using the principles already outlined, aggressively provide inflow to the hand by means of autogenous grafts in this subset of patients.

The postoperative care of these patients is directed toward the maintenance of the desired result. Pulses are monitored by palpation or with the Doppler instrument. Anticoagulation may be indicated, as already discussed. If immobilizaton is necessary, the arm and hand should be maintained in the "position of function."

Supported in part by the Pacific Vascular Research Foundation

DEAD FOOT

CHARLES S. O'MARA, M.D.

The most common cause of foot gangrene is chronic atherosclerotic occlusive disease (Table 1). The high prevalence of atherosclerosis in our culture, combined with a steady growth in the number of elderly patients, has resulted in an increased frequency of lower extremity gangrene. Despite our better understanding of the pathophysiology of limb ischemia as well as improved diagnostic and surgical techniques, proper treatment of the patient with gangrene of the foot remains a challenging problem. The principal objectives of treating a patient

with a dead foot include removal of all necrotic tissue, relief of pain, and primary healing of the amputation site. Patient salvage, which was the main goal of treatment in past decades when amputations for gangrene usually were done at a level above the knee, is not enough. In addition, the surgeon must strive for successful amputation at the most distal possible level to afford maximal patient rehabilitation.

PRIMARY AMPUTATION VERSUS REVASCULARIZATION PLUS AMPUTATION

Several factors must be considered in resolving the crucial issue of whether a patient should either have

TABLE 1 Common Causes of Foot Gangrene

Chronic atherosclerotic occlusive disease

Peripheral arterial embolism

Trauma

Massive venous thrombosis

Vasospastic disorders

Frostbite

primary amputation alone or undergo arterial reconstruction combined with amputation (Table 2). As a general rule, I favor an aggressive approach with lower limb revascularization when necessary to ensure successful amputation at the lowest possible level and therefore to allow optimal rehabilitation of the patient. Standard vascular surgical procedures, such as aortofemoral, femoropopliteal, and femorotibial bypass, can be done with a high expectation of hemodynamic improvement when applied prudently and when done by an experienced surgical team. In addition, in selected situations percutaneous transluminal balloon dilation of arterial stenoses can significantly augment limb blood flow without risk of general anesthesia. The concern that failure of an arterial bypass procedure may compromise the chance of salvaging a successful below-knee amputation is unjustified when proper attention is given to operative technique and wound care.

The initial decision about whether to perform primary amputation or to combine arterial reconstruction with amputation involves evaluation of both the extent of the gangrenous process and the prediction of amputation healing potential. The extent of gangrene should be categorized as either (1) limited gangrene of the toes and/or distal foot or (2) extensive gangrene of the entire foot or a major portion of the forefoot. Provided the blood supply to the amputation site is sufficient for healing, limited gangrene is ideally treated with toe, ray, or transmetatarsal amputation to allow continued prosthesis-free ambulation. Extensive foot gangrene is best managed by below-knee amputation. The importance of preserving the knee joint, especially in elderly patients, cannot be overemphasized. Over 80 percent of elderly patients retain bipedal gait after a successful below-knee amputation, whereas less than half that number walk again after an above-knee amputation. Furthermore, the time for rehabilitation is roughly doubled in the above-knee amputation group when compared to that for below-knee amputees. In addition, atherosclerosis is a symmetric disease, and it is recognized that one-half of unilateral

amputees who survive 3 years or longer eventually lose the other limb. The likelihood of the bilateral amputee's ever walking again is greatly improved by preservation of at least one knee joint.

Several clinical guidelines are useful in assessing amputation healing potential. For example, digital and transmetatarsal amputations usually heal in the presence of a palpable pedal pulse. Likewise, blood supply is usually satisfactory to allow healing of a below-knee amputation when the popliteal pulse is palpable. The absence of a palpable pulse does not preclude amputation healing. The presence of necrosis, dependent rubor, or cellulitis at the intended level of skin transection is a contraindication to performing amputation at any level.

Information from one or more objective tests can provide additional help in the preoperative prediction of healing (Table 3). In my experience, the Doppler instrument and the photoplethysmograph have proved to be both practical and reasonably accurate tools for predicting amputation healing. Digital and transmetatarsal amputations are likely to heal if Doppler pressure at the ankle is greater than 50 mm Hg or if pulsatile flow is present at the metatarsal level as determined by photoplethysmography. A proximal calf pressure greater than 70 mm Hg has a high correlation with sufficient blood supply to heal a below-knee amputation. A calf pressure lower than 70 mm Hg is less likely to heal. However, despite their objectivity, these tests are not infallible. Some patients with low segmental Doppler pressures heal an amputation without problem, and the converse of this statement is also true. Moreover, segmental Doppler pressure determinations may be spuriously elevated because of arterial mural calcification, which not uncommonly occurs in diabetic patients. In this situation, assessment of the quality of Doppler pulse velocity waveforms may be helpful. Despite such limitations, I believe that lower extremity amputation should not be performed without some type of preoperative objective testing to ensure healing of the most distal amputation possible.

When clinical judgment and objective tests indicate that limited foot gangrene can be satisfactorily treated by toe, ray, or transmetatarsal amputation or when extensive foot gangrene can be managed successfully with primary below-knee amputation, further consideration of vascular reconstructive surgery is not necessary; the patient should undergo primary amputation. In contrast, when satisfactory healing of the most distal amputation site is unlikely, the surgeon should consider additional factors with the objective of possibly performing arterial reconstructive surgery to improve blood supply at the optimal

TABLE 2 Considerations in Deciding to Revascularize

Extent of gangrene

Prediction of amputation healing

Operative risk

Age and life expectancy

Rehabilitation potential

Arteriographic findings

TABLE 3 Objective Means of Predicting Amputation Healing

Segmental Doppler pressure measurements

Photoplethysmography

Segmental pulse volume recordings

Xenon-133 skin clearance

Skin fluorescence measurement

Laser Doppler perfusion monitoring

level of amputation. These other factors include operative risk, age of the patient, and rehabilitation potential. An accurate assessment of the patient's ability to safely tolerate arteriography, anesthesia, and surgery is obtained by carefully evaluating the patient's medical condition, especially cardiac, pulmonary, and renal function. In the elderly patient with multiple medical problems and a limited life expectancy, an aggressive approach including arterial reconstruction is not justified. Likewise, in a debilitated patient with poor rehabilitation potential, obtaining the lowest possible amputation level becomes must less important. For example, it would be unwarranted to perform arterial reconstructive surgery to permit healing of a transmetatarsal amputation in a patient who was bedridden prior to the onset of limited foot gangrene. Furthermore, bypass surgery to preserve the knee joint is unwarranted in patients who have significant ipsilateral neurologic deficit following cerebrovascular accident or in patients who have a severe knee or hip flexion contracture, which precludes satisfactory use of a below-knee prosthesis.

When augmentation of blood supply is necessary to heal an amputation at the lowest possible level, arteriography is done unless the operative risk of bypass surgery is inordinately high, the patient's age is far advanced with a very short life expectancy, or his rehabilitation potential is extremely limited. Proper hydration prior to arteriography is essential to prevent development of renal failure induced by contrast media. This complication is more common in diabetic patients and in patients with a contracted intravascular volume caused by chronic diuretic therapy. When the patient's renal function is impaired, use of intra-arterial digital subtraction angiography should be considered to minimize the amount of contrast material and therefore to decrease the risk of exacerbating renal dysfunction.

If arteriographic findings suggest that arterial reconstruction is technically feasible and is likely to restore satisfactory blood supply at the optimal amputation level, vascular surgery is recommended. Bypass to the distal popliteal artery or to a tibial or peroneal artery may be required for salvage of a transmetatarsal amputation. Or, bypass to the proximal popliteal artery may be essential to ensure success of a below-knee amputation. Providing pulsatile flow to the femoral artery or performing profundaplasty may be necessary to allow healing of an amputation at below-knee or distal thigh level.

INFECTED GANGRENE

The gangrenous foot complicated by infection represents a special management problem. The goal of treatment is eradication or control of the local infection prior to definitive amputation. In addition to the risk of systemic sepsis, the local infection may cause surrounding ischemic but viable tissues to become necrotic, thus extending the gangrenous process. A Gram stain should be performed initially and antibiotics started according to results of the stain. Mixed organisms are usually present, and a cephalosporin and an aminoglycoside are appropriate. Antibiotics are subsequently adjusted, based on culture results. If infection responds to the antibiotics, they should be continued for 5 to 7 days, after which definitive amputation may be carried out. Lack of response to antibiotics within 12 hours, as manifested by persistent fever, rising leukocyte count, local spread of erythema, or signs of systemic toxicity, requires immediate open surgical drainage under regional or local anesthesia.

In the diabetic patient, if the local infection is advanced on initial presentation, as indicated by plantar tenderness, fluctuance, or evidence of spread along tendon sheaths, a drainage procedure should be performed immediately. Similarly, the nondiabetic with obvious abscess formation should undergo early drainage.

The type of drainage procedure required is dictated by physical findings. If sepsis is limited to the forefoot, open transmetatarsal amputation involving one, several, or all five toes may be adequate; the crucial requirement is the establishment of adequate drainage. Over the next several days the wound is treated with povidone-iodine-soaked dressings; intravenous antibiotics are continued; and appropriate noninvasive and arteriographic studies are performed to assess the possibility of healing at the transmetatarsal level as well as the feasibility of vascular reconstruction if needed. If it is apparent 5 to 7 days after a transmetatarsal drainage procedure that healing at this level is not likely and arterial reconstruction is not feasible, higher definitive amputation should be performed. If, on the other hand, a bypass procedure is technically possible and would re-establish satisfactory blood flow to the transmetatarsal level, and the patient's condition is favorable, arterial reconstructive surgery is performed after this 5- to 7-day interval. The open transmetatarsal amputation, once revascularized and adequately debrided, may be closed. When sepsis encompasses the foot proximal to the transmetatarsal level, the most efficacious drainage procedure is a guillotine amputation at the supramalleolar level. The incision may be made through cellulitic skin, although it should be proximal to discrete pockets of purulence. Definitive amputation may be performed about 5 days later.

ACUTE GANGRENE

There are two clinical situations that can tax even the most experienced surgeon's judgment. The first is represented by the patient who has impending gangrene of the foot secondary to an acute arterial occlusion that is unreconstructable. The second is typified by the patient who presents with an acute occlusion that has been allowed to progress to frank tissue necrosis, even though the occlusive process may have been reconstructable early in the course of ischemic changes. In each of these situations, the surgeon must balance the objectives of patient salvage with the desire to preserve as much viable tissue as possible. Recruitment of collateral flow can be expected to occur following an acute arterial occlusion, even though some of the tissues may have become frankly necrotic.

If amputation can be delayed long enough, sufficient collateral flow may develop to allow amputation at a lower level than that predicted on initial evaluation. I treat patients who present in this setting of acute ischemia with an intravenous bolus of 5,000 to 10,000 units of heparin followed by a continuous intravenous heparin infusion adjusted to maintain the partial thromboplastin time at about two times control value. The rationale of heparinization is to prevent thrombus propagation in the arterial system, as well as to prevent venous thrombosis that might further compromise capillary perfusion. In the patient with a contraindication to heparinization, an infusion of low-molecular-weight dextran at 20 cc per hour may be used.

The crucial factor determining need for emergent amputation in the patient with acute ischemia is the amount of ischemic or necrotic tissue present. When only a portion of the foot is involved, a conservative approach is in order as long as pain is not severe and there is no supervening infection. These patients should be kept at bed rest on full anticoagulant therapy for as long as 1 to 2 weeks until adequate tissue demarcation has occurred. Susceptibility of ischemic tissue to secondary infection is justification for the use of prophylactic broad-spectrum antibiotics, usually a cephalosporin. This delay in amputation increases the likelihood that a more distal limited amputation will heal.

When the ischemic or gangrenous process extends proximal to the foot, the risks are greater because of the potential complication of calf muscle necrosis. This condition is manifested by significant swelling, rigidity, and pain in the calf as well as skin discoloration and decreased sensation in the leg. With progressive myonecrosis, the life-threatening complications of systemic acidosis, hyperkalemia, and myoglobinuria may result. The presence of systemic toxicity, significant changes on physical examination, myoglobinuria, or cardiovascular instability is indication for immediate amputation, almost always at the above-knee level. In the absence of these specific indications, one may continue to closely observe the extremity. If observation is elected, it is important to maintain a brisk diuresis (75 to 100 cc per hour) with liberal volumes of intravenous fluid and use of mannitol. Since myoglobin precipitates in renal tubules at an acid pH, the urine should be prophylactically alkalinized with a slow infusion of sodium bicarbonate. Observation may be continued as long as there is further improvement in collateral blood supply and there are no signs of systemic or renal toxicity. Amputation at the lowest possible level is performed once satisfactory demarcation between healthy and ischemic tissues has occurred.

AMPUTATION LEVELS

Certain details of the commonly performed amputations for ischemia deserve mention. For each amputation level, attention must be given to complete hemostasis and atraumatic deep tissue and skin closure.

Meticulous operative technique is equally as important as adequate blood supply in ensuring healing at the amputation level. A brief course of prophylactic antibiotics is routinely used perioperatively. Because these patients are at increased risk of venous thromboembolism, subcutaneous minidose heparin is frequently employed.

Toe Amputation

Amputation of a single toe is done by transection through the proximal phalanx, leaving a small segment of bone to protect the metatarsal head. Amputation by disarticulation should not be done because it leaves avascular cartilage, which predisposes to supervening infection and failure to heal. Skin flaps may be of any design provided an adequate base is left to allow closure without tension. The most commonly used incision is circular.

The presence of dry gangrene of a toe without infection or significant pain allows a choice to be made between surgical intervention and autoamputation of the toe. During the autoamputation process, epithelialization occurs beneath the gangrenous eschar. When epithelialization is complete, the toe falls off and leaves a cleanly healed stump. With autoamputation, the most distal site of healing occurs naturally; in addition, a surgical procedure and the subsequent healing process are avoided altogether. However, the process of autoamputation often requires several months to occur.

Ray Amputation

When gangrenous or ischemic skin of a necrotic toe approaches the metatarsal-phalangeal crease and precludes healing of a simple toe amputation, a conservative amputation can still be performed by extending the toe amputation to include the distal metatarsal head. The incision for a ray amputation begins vertically on the dorsum of the foot, extends medially and laterally to encircle the toe, and meets on the plantar aspect of the foot. The distal metatarsal shaft is divided at its neck, soft tissues are removed by sharp dissection, and care is taken to avoid injury to adjacent digital arteries. The surgical specimen consists of toe, metatarsophalangeal joint, and distal metatarsal shaft and head. Involvement of multiple toes and gangrene of only the great toe are relative contraindications to ray amputation. For these specific circumstances, more stable weight-bearing and less difficulty with ambulation are usually afforded by transmetatarsal amputation.

Transmetatarsal Amputation

Gangrene that involves several toes and/or the great toe is best treated by transmetatarsal amputation. This amputation may also be used if the gangrenous process extends a short distance onto the dorsal skin past the metatarsophalangeal crease, but it is important that the plantar skin be uncompromised. I prefer a total plantar flap designed by use of a dorsal incision at the level of the mid-metatarsal shafts and a plantar incision across the metatarsophalangeal crease. It is important to place the dorsal skin incision 0.5 to 1 cm distal to the anticipated line of bone transection. Once the specimen is removed, tissues of the plantar flap are thinned sharply, removing exposed tendons and leaving the underlying musculature attached to the skin flap, which is rotated dorsally for closure. Weight-bearing on the foot is not allowed until 2 to 3 weeks after surgery, when the stump is well healed.

Transmetatarsal amputation provides an excellent functional result compared to more proximal amputations. Disability is minimal, and prosthetic requirements are relatively simple. Shoe modification incorporating either a steel shank in the sole or custom molding with a roller-shaped sole allows normal toe-off during ambulation. Foam padding is used to fill the toe portion of the shoe. It is essential that the shoe fit properly and be well constructed to avoid stump ulceration and breakdown.

Below-Knee Amputation

Below-knee amputation is the most common amputation used for foot gangrene when foot necrosis precludes more distal amputations. When the amputation level is selected objectively, primary healing can be expected in more that 95 percent of below-knee amputations. Moreover, the vast majority of patients with unilateral below-knee amputations are able to ambulate with a prosthesis.

I prefer to use a long posterior flap and no anterior flap in performing a below-knee amputation. The tibia is transected 8 to 10 cm below the tibial tuberosity and beveled anteriorly. The fibula is cut 2 cm shorter than the tibia. The skin incisions should be about 1 cm distal to the intended point of bone division. The tibial and peroneal vessels are transected and suture-ligated. The posterior tibial nerve is sharply transected as high as possible after ligation with absorbable suture to minimize neuroma formation. The posterior calf musculature is transected, leaving gastrocnemius muscle as part of the posterior skin flap. The bony edges of the tibia and the fibula are made smooth. No instruments are used on the skin. With appropriate attention to hemostasis, use of a drain is unnecessary. The stump is wrapped in a fluffy dressing, and a posterior plaster splint is padded and applied with an Ace wrap to prevent development of a flexion contracture of the knee. The splint is removed after 7 days, at which time range of motion exercises are begun if the stump appears healthy. At 3 to 4 weeks, sutures are removed and the patient begins to wear a temporary prosthesis.

TABLE 4   Pain Syndromes After Below-Knee Amputation

Ischemia
Infection
Phantom limb
Neuroma
Causalgia

Pain, the most common postoperative complication, may occur secondary to several etiologies of varying significance (Table 4). Severe pain in the stump during the first few postoperative days is an ominous sign of infection or nonhealing due to ischemia, or both. Such pain is an indication for careful daily examination of the stump. Phantom limb pain is almost universal. The pain initially occurs during the first week and can persist for months or longer, but the severity generally diminishes with time. Development of a tender point in the stump, weeks to months following surgery, is suggestive of a neuroma. Relief of this pain by local anesthetic injection is confirmatory evidence of the presence of a neuroma and is an indication for local exploration and excision. Causalgia, a burning pain in the stump, has been described in rare instances and, in some patients, has responded to sympathectomy.

Above-Knee Amputation

Amputation at the above-knee level is performed if blood flow is inadequate to heal at a more distal level, if a patient is disabled and not expected to walk again, if there is profound life-threatening infection with questionable viability of the lower extremity, and/or if extensive infection or gangrene precludes a below-knee amputation.

Several points are important in performing a successful above-knee amputation. As much femur length as possible should be preserved to prevent hip contracture. Equal anterior and posterior flaps—the fish-mouth incision—are recommended since the anterior and posterior flaps are equally vascularized in the thigh. The femur should be sectioned about 4 to 5 cm higher than the distal extent of the skin incisions. The muscle groups should be sutured to prevent the lateral migration of the femur that tends to occur after this procedure. Drains usually are not used. Bed rest is continued for one week after operation.

The primary advantage of above-knee amputation is the high likelihood of primary healing. However, prosthetic rehabilitation is difficult. Only 40 to 50 percent of unilateral above-knee amputees can be expected to ambulate, and less than 10 percent of bilateral lower extremity amputees, when one side is an above-knee amputation, will successfully ambulate.

PERIPHERAL ARTERIAL EMBOLUS

GAIL E. BESNER, M.D.
NICHOLAS L. TILNEY, M.D., F.A.C.S., F.R.C.S

Peripheral arterial emboli still carry a significant morbidity and mortality, although options for appropriate treatment are increasing. The majority of emboli originate in the heart, arising in a fibrillating atrium (70%), from mural thrombi developing after myocardial infarction (20%), from cardiac valves or valve prostheses, or secondary to myocarditis or endocarditis. A few are tumor emboli from the heart chambers, particularly myxomas. Emboli also arise from ulcerating plaques on the atheromatous aorta, from aneurysms of the aorta or of the iliac, femoral, or popliteal arteries, or they may be paradoxical emboli or foreign bodies. They can complicate cardioversion, arteriography, or the use of the intra-aortic balloon pump. The source of 10 percent is unknown.

Emboli may lodge in many peripheral arterial sites which, in descending frequency, include the common femoral arteries, superficial femoral arteries, popliteal/tibial system, iliac vessels, aortic bifurcation (saddle embolus), axial/brachial system, and visceral arteries.

An acute embolus can produce a broad spectrum of signs and symptoms. Most acute occlusions present early, with the patient complaining of pain and numbness in the involved extremity. Peripheral nerves and muscles are most sensitive to the ischemic insult, which causes loss of sensation followed by muscle paralysis. Unless blood flow is promptly restored, tissue necrosis is usually inevitable. The greater the extent of ischemia, the more severe are the systemic effects following revascularization, particularly if delayed; in the most advanced stages, muscle swelling and necrosis is marked, with accompanying acidosis, hyperkalemia, and myoglobinuria. Once flow is restored, complications may include cardiac arrhythmias, renal failure, and respiratory distress. Revasularization of the acutely ischemic leg carries a mortality rate as high as 25 percent, particularly as many of the patients are older and have generalized cardiovascular disease.

EVALUATION OF THE LIMB

Accurate assessment of the cause of acute limb ischemia is necessary in determining urgency of surgical intervention, prognosis, and surgical approach. Acute arterial emboli may be confused with acute arterial thrombosis, aortic dissection, or phlegmasia cerulia dolens. The patient with arterial thrombosis may have a sudden onset of symptoms similar to those of an individual with an embolus, but may give a history of claudication or other symptoms of chronic peripheral vascular disease. Advanced venous thrombosis may also present as a painful pulseless extremity, but massive swelling and cyanosis usually differentiate this condition from the cold, pale, and pulseless extremity of the patient with an embolus. Arteriography is critical in differentiating embolism from thrombosis. The patient who has suffered an embolism usually has normal vessels with a sharp cut-off and obvious meniscus at the proximal end of the clot. The patient with a thrombosed vessel may have obvious arteriosclertoic involvement of other vessels, with atheroma in the involved artery tapering toward a point of obstruction.

Regardless of etiology, the most reliable predicator of limb salvage is the viability of the extremity on presentation rather than the actual ischemic time. Nevertheless, prompt revascularization results in the greatest limb salvage, whereas longer periods of occlusion may lead to increased ischemia and increased risk of limb loss.

INITIAL PATIENT MANAGEMENT

Once the diagnosis of arterial embolism is made, the patient should be given heparin systemically. Volume resuscitation should be carried out intravenously as needed. In patients with myoglobinuria, mannitol can be given to produce osmotic diuresis to flush pigment from the tubules and prevent acute renal failure. Hyperkalemia should be corrected with Kayexalate, intravenous insulin and glucose, or dialysis if necessary. Acidosis, produced by metabolic products such as lactates and pyruvates, can be controlled with sodium bicarbonate.

The therapeutic options are usually clear-cut, depending on physical findings and extent and duration of ischemia (Fig. 1). Amputation must be performed in individuals with far-advanced ischemia and evidence of irreversible muscle damage or obvious nonviability of the lower extremity. This procedure should not be delayed, as extensive venous thrombosis, sepsis, or pulmonary emboli may intervene. In contrast, significant sensory or motor changes in a viable limb may be reversed by prompt embolectomy. In individuals with a viable extremity presenting before sensory or motor changes have occurred, a choice between embolectomy and thrombolysis can be made.

Heparinization

Systemic heparinization in those with acute emboli prevents propagation of thrombus in the occluded arterial segment. A loading dose is given intravenously, 5,000 to 7,500 units depending on the size and weight of the patient, followed by a constant heparin infusion via an IVAC pump, usually 1,000 units per hour and titrated to prolong the partial thromboplastin time to twice normal. Surgical embolectomy should be performed immediately if systemic anticoagulation is contraindicated.

Nonoperative treatment with high-dose heparin as the sole therapy may be appropriate for relatively localized arterial thrombosis in some high-risk patients, but has little role as the only treatment of acute arterial embolus, which should be treated with either embolectomy or thrombolytic agents.

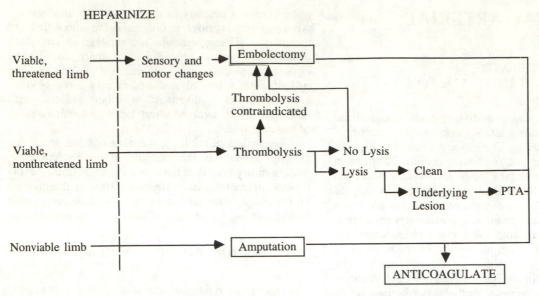

Figure 1 Therapeutic options available for patients with peripheral arterial emboli (PTA = percutaneous transluminal dilatation).

Thrombolytic Therapy

Thrombolysis is appropriate in the patient with an embolism who has a viable extremity in which the ischemia is not severe enough to cause motor or sensory signs. If motor weakness or sensory changes are greater than hypesthesias alone, however, embolectomy should be carried out as an emergency surgical procedure. Thrombolysis may also be useful when surgery may be hazardous or in patients in whom the embolus is relatively inaccessible, particularly in the small vessels of the lower leg. Patients with focal areas of cyanosis such as the toe, where occlusion of digital arteries has occurred, may also be considered for thrombolytic treatment; this should always be carried out under close supervision of the vascular surgeons.

Urokinase is the best agent available for thrombolysis. Developed in 1947 by MacFarland and Pilling, it is a proteolytic enzyme derived from human kidney tissue cultures. A nonantigenic protein, it does not induce drug resistance or adverse reactions, and acts directly to convert plasminogen to plasmin, the active enzyme that depolymerizes fibrin within the clot. Thus, urokinase + plasminogen → plasmin and plasmin + fibrin → fibrin split products. Use of urokinase is contraindicated in persons with active bleeding, a cerebrovascular accident or craniotomy in the preceeding 2 months, coagulopathy, recent surgery or invasive procedures at inaccessible sites, pregnancy or recent delivery, or uncontrolled hypertension.

The agent is administered via an infusion catheter placed through the femoral artery. A flexible, heparin-coated guide wire is inserted into the arterial lumen and advanced into the occlusion. The catheter is then passed over the guidewire with the tip in the proximal aspect of the clot. Urokinase is then infused directly into the clot, using an initial high-dose regimen of 4,000 IU per minute for 2 hours. If distal clot persists on repeat arteriogram, the guidewire and catheter are advanced. The high-dose infusion is continued and the procedure repeated until complete recannulization has occurred. The catheter is then withdrawn to a more proximal position and the infusion decreased to a rate of 1,000 IU per minute and continued if repeat arteriograms show progressive clot lysis; the mean perfusion time is approximately 18 hours. If an underlying arterial stenosis is found following clot lysis, percutaneous transluminal angioplasty can be performed as necessary. In addition to urokinase administration, heparin is infused intravenously to prevent thrombus formation on the catheter. Once successful thrombolysis is achieved, full anticoagulation is resumed 12 hours later.

Responses to urokinase infusion include (1) complete thrombolysis without residual lesions; (2) partial lysis with clinical improvement resulting in relief of symptoms or allowing healing of a distal amputation site; (3) partial lysis revealing a distal vascular occlusion, which may be inoperable; (4) failure due to inability to lyse clot, usually represented by old organized thrombus, atherosclerotic obstructing lesions within the clot, or inability to reach distal clot.

In some series, complete clot lysis has been obtained in as many as 73 percent of patients, with clinical improvement rendering surgery unnecessary in 80 percent of these. The best predictor of the success of this technique is the ability to recannulize the clot within the first 2 hours of enzyme infusion. If this occurs, the likelihood of complete clot lysis is excellent, whereas failure to create a channel through the clot within this time period should alert one to consider surgical embolectomy. Prompt recannulization is a better predictor of success than clot age, size, duration, location, or origin. Indeed, thromblysis is usually more effective in lysing thrombotic than embolic occlusions, probably because many emboli, though acute in nature, actually represent organized clots that may have been present at the site of origin for prolonged periods.

Complications of enzyme infusion include bleeding, usually occurring at the catheter entry site in the groin, migration of small pieces of clot into the distal vasculature, and reperfusion injury. Compared to streptokinase, urokinase has a higher incidence of successful lysis, a shorter infusion time (18 versus 41 hours mean), and a lower incidence of bleeding. In addition, since no antibodies are made against urokinase, it can be used repeatedly. Although in general, early postoperative thromboses and emboli are best removed surgically, urokinase has occasionally been successful as early as 3 days postoperatively.

EMBOLECTOMY

Surgical embolectomy should be performed absolutely in patients with a viable but severely ischemic leg with sensory and motor deficits. As proximal emboli are more easily removed by means of the Fogarty catheter, patients presenting with such lesions should be operated on immediately; adjunctive thrombolysis should be reserved for distal emboli that cannot be extracted with the catheter.

The Fogarty embolectomy catheter was first described in 1963. Prior to this time, several methods of embolectomy were employed, including direct removal by opening the vessel over the embolus, use of a corkscrew device that was passed down the vessel and pulled back in hopes that the clot would adhere to it, and use of arteriotomies proximal and distal to the clot, flushing or squeezing the leg in a retrograde fashion. The mortality rates associated with these methods were high; emboli associated with arteriosclerotic heart disease, for instance, carry a mortality rate as high as 74 percent, and those lodging in aorta or iliac systems have a mortality rate over 90 percent. Since use of the Fogarty catheter has been common, the morality rate for emboli associated with arteriosclerotic heart disease has decreased to less than 25 percent, as many of these previously formidable procedures now can be performed relatively easily under local anesthesia.

The Fogarty catheter is hollow and flexible, and a soft balloon covering its tip can be inflated with a syringe at its proximal end. Either saline or air can be used, air used commonly for the smaller catheters and saline for the larger ones, as this is thought to give better control of balloon size. Embolectomy of the lower extremities can be performed following isolation of one or both femoral arteries, the latter approach being used for aortic saddle emboli. Such a procedure can be undertaken under local anesthesia. Control of common femoral, superficial, femoral, and profunda femoris arteries is obtained. The patient is then given heparin systemically and the vessels are clamped. A transverse arteriotomy is made at the femoral bifurcation, and the embolectomy catheter inserted and passed distally through the embolus. The balloon is then inflated by the surgeon, who gently withdraws the catheter along with the clot. Balloon size is controlled with the syringe and adjusted so as to merely coapt the arterial wall. The femoral and popliteal systems can usually be explored with a 3 or 4 F catheter; a 5 F catheter is inserted proximally to remove obstructive material in the distal aorta or iliac system.

At the completion of the procedure, an operative arteriogram should be performed. Palpable pedal pulses without obvious clinical improvement may suggest residual embolic material in distal vessels or arterial spasm that may clear in time. Occasional failure of femoral embolectomy may also be explained anatomically, based on cadaver studies. The popliteal artery continues distally as the peroneal artery, with the anterior and posterior tibial arteries branching off acutely from the main trunk. Thus, when the embolectomy catheter is passed distally down the popliteal artery, it usually enters the peroneal artery selectively. Its passage down the tibial arteries can be expedited by exposure of the popliteal artery and its bifurcations and guidance of the catheter tip directly down the appropriate branch. Other maneuvers to advance the catheter distally into tibial branches via the femoral arteriotomy include rotating the catheter, introducing more than one catheter, or bending the knee. Gently inflating the balloon at the site of obstruction, then deflating it as the catheter is advanced, may also guide the tip into the center of the lumen and allow distal advancement.

Reperfusion Injuries

Reperfusing a seriously ischemic extremity following embolectomy can produce serious sequelae. Upon reestablishment of arterial flow, metabolic breakdown products that have accumulated in the injured muscle are washed out into the systemic circulation. These include lactic and pyruvic acid, potassium, and myoglobin. As noted, a sudden rush of acidotic hyperkalemic blood can produce cardiac arrhythmias and hypotension, while myoglobin precipitating in the renal glomeruli may cause acute renal failure. Buffering agents and antiarrhythmic drugs can be used, and dialysis can be instituted if necessary. If signficant edema of a reperfused, previously severely ischemic extremity develops, fasciotomy should be performed immediately to prevent the development of a compartment syndrome. Such a maneuver can save otherwise threatened limbs.

Amputation

Embolectomy is not indicated when there is obviously irreversible muscle damage and myonecrosis; patients with irreversible ischemia who have undergone embolectomy have a high mortality rate and negative limb salvage. The cardiac status of the borderline patient can be used as a reasonable criterion for proceeding, or not, with

TABLE 1 Summary of Embolectomy Reviews

Author	Year	No. of Patients	Amputation (%)	Mean	Mortality (%)	Mean
1937–1963						
Haimovici	1950	228	48		50	
Warren	1954	200	14	22%	29	34%
Edwards	1966	82	17		42	
Darling	1967	260	9		32	
1963–1979						
Fogarty	1967	91	4		15	
Cranley	1970	246	5		24	
Levy	1970	125	14	12%	26	22%
Thompson	1970	163	17		14	
Green	1973	110	12		19	
MacGowan	1973	174	13		27	
Hight	1974	124	22		30	
1980–1985						
Silvers	1980	106	13		22	
Lorentzen	1980	130	23		14	
Carvana	1981	61	25		11	
Kendrick	1981	90	29	19%	18	19%
Abbott	1982	313	14		25	
Sheiner	1982	134	13		20	
Dale	1983	65	27		11	
Connett	1984	111	5		14	

embolectomy. If an individual has poor cardiac function, this treatment modality should probably be avoided as his already diseased heart may not withstand the additional stress related to revascularization. Once the decision for amputation has been made, it should be instituted without delay.

Postoperative Treatment

Recurrent embolization may occur in the post-operative period; thus, systemic heparinization should be continued. Peripheral pulses and warmth of the extremity should be assessed frequently. If reocclusion occurs, reoperation usually is indicated, and a careful search for the source of embolus is continued. As many as one-third of patients develop recurrent emboli, which carry a significantly higher morbidity and mortality than the initial embolic event. Compared to a limb rate of 10 percent after the first embolic episode, the amputation rates after second and third emboli are 20 percent and 50 percent, respectively. Although some studies have shown that there is no statistically significant effect of Coumadin in preventing recurrent emboli, many patients are still given Coumadin postoperatively, depending on the initial source

of the embolus. It is obviously critical to detect the sources of the embolus and correct the problem as soon as possible.

Results

The leading causes of death in patients with acute arterial emboli in most series are myocardial infarction (40%), congestive heart failure (33%), pulmonary embolus (16%), cerebrovascular accident (8%), and renal failure (3%). The amputation rates and patient mortality in several major series of embolectomies, both prior to and subsequent to the introduction of the Fogarty catheter in 1963, are reviewed in Table 1. It is clear that the mortality rate has declined since use of the embolectomy catheter began, although it is equally clear that even in the 1980s, it still approaches 20 percent, which indicates the potential severity of the condition. This persistently high mortality rate reflects the fact that arterial emboli represent a small part of the spectrum of overall atherosclerotic heart disease and that these patients often die of the underlying coronary artery disease that may have precipitated the formation of the embolus.

BUERGER'S DISEASE

BRUCE A. PERLER, M.D.

Since the initial description of this syndrome by Leo Buerger in 1908, the existence of Buerger's disease, or thromboangiitis obliterans, as a distinct clinical entity has been repeatedly questioned. Much of the confusion recently has resulted from incorrectly diagnosing young men with arterial ischemia as having Buerger's disease, when in fact they were suffering premature arteriosclerosis. Buerger's disease is a real entity, clinically and pathologically distinct from arteriosclerosis obliterans and other causes of arterial insufficiency (Table 1). The disease occurs almost exclusively in young men, and all are smokers. When these patients present with claudication, it almost always involves the instep of the foot. The patient's initial complaint, however, may be severe rest pain involving the distal foot. The pain frequently has a "burning" quality and may appear out of proportion to the appearance of the foot. The involved area is often tender to palpation. Skin ulceration and secondary infection frequently occur, and gangrene of the toes and forefoot is common. Arterial occlusion frequently occurs in the upper extremity as well, resulting in pain and ulceration of the fingers. Buerger's disease also may involve the mesenteric and cerebral vasculature, although much less frequently. As many as 40 percent of patients with Buerger's disease experience migratory superficial thrombophlebitis. Patients with Buerger's disease, as opposed to those with premature arteriosclerosis, experience normal longevity.

Pathologically, the disease is a segmental inflammatory panangiitis involving all layers of the wall of small and medium-sized arteries and veins. Large numbers of lymphocytes and fibroblasts and an occasional giant cell are seen within the vessel wall, although the normal structure of the vessel is preserved, in contradistinction to arteriosclerosis. The end result is an inflammatory thrombosis of the vessel.

AGGRESSIVE DIAGNOSTIC EVALUATION

A number of pathologic conditions may present as extremity or distal ischemia in the young patient and be confused with Buerger's disease. Since most of these conditions are more precisely and effectively treatable than

TABLE 1 Clinical Profile

Male
Young (less than 40)
Smoker
Foot claudication
Rest pain
Migratory superficial thrombophlebitis
Normal life expectancy

Buerger's disease, an aggressive diagnostic work-up should be the intial step in the management of these patients (Table 2). I believe every patient presenting with digital ischemia should undergo a diagnostic arteriogram to rule out arteriosclerosis as the cause. Thrombosis in situ of small and medium-sized vessels previously involved with arteriosclerosis may present with symptoms suggestive of Buerger's disease, particularly in the young diabetic patient. Recognition of the arteriosclerotic process is essential in formulating appropriate long-term medical management, although the options for surgical revascularization in this setting are usually limited. Distal atheroor microemboli from proximal arteriosclerotic lesions such as ulcerated plaques or true or false aneurysms may be detected arteriographically and should be surgically corrected. A complete hematologic profile should be obtained including platelet and red cell counts to rule out polycythemia vera as a cause of digital vessel thrombosis. An erythrocyte sedimentation rate should be performed as a screening test for collagen vascular disease, and if the rate is high, antinuclear antibody, rheumatoid factor, and L-E prep must be obtained. Mercury strain-gauge plethysmography in the vascular laboratory should be performed to rule out a vasospastic disorder such as Raynaud's disease. Total serum protein and serum protein electrophoresis should be measured to rule out cryoglobulinemia, macroglobulinemia, and other serum protein disorders.

MEDICAL MANAGEMENT

The treatment of Buerger's disease must be aimed at the primary disease process as well as its ischemic complications. Although the precise cause of the disease is unknown, and most smokers do not develop Buerger's disease, smoking is the sine qua non for its existence. Total, uncompromising, and permanent abstinence from tobacco is an absolute necessity and the mainstay of its medical management. As opposed to arteriosclerotic complications of tobacco abuse, pipe and cigar smoking may be as harmful as cigarette smoking in Buerger's patients. There is some evidence that even environmental exposure to the smoke of others may exacerbate the disease process. Most patients who achieve complete abstinence from smoking experience a remission, which is often permanent as long as they remain nonsmokers. However, it may take several weeks or months after the patient has stopped smoking for the remission to occur.

PHARMACOLOGIC MANAGEMENT

Potent analgesic agents are almost always required to control the pain experienced by patients during acute exacerbations of Buerger's disease. In many cases the severe distal rest pain responds only to narcotics. Unfortunately, the young patient with Buerger's disease may easily become addicted to these drugs, particularly while attempting to break his smoking habit, and the physician must be cognizant of this potential complication.

If the patient appears to be entering a cycle of increasing analgesic requirement, inpatient admission and management is advisable to try to break the cycle, even before tissue loss has occurred. The mainstay of treatment, of course, is complete withdrawal from tobacco. All other measures are supportive and will be unsuccessful if the patient continues to smoke.

The severe pain experienced in the toes and forefoot is ischemic in etiology, and therefore supportive measures are designed to promote perfusion through the microcirculation. Strict bed rest with the patient in the reverse Trendelenburg position is often helpful in this regard. Since small-vessel thrombosis is a fundamental pathologic process in Buerger's disease, a 5- to 7-day course of heparin (1 mg per kilogram), administered as a continuous intravenous drip, may be beneficial in the acute setting. A reasonable alternative is a continuous infusion of low-molecular-weight dextran at 20 cc per hour. Dextran appears to impair platelet adhesiveness and the stability of thrombus by altering factor VIII function. Prolonged use of dextran, an osmotic expander, has been associated with the development of congestive heart failure, but this should not occur in these young patients. A combined infusion of heparin and dextran is not unreasonable as long as coagulation is closely monitored.

Recently, certain prostaglandins have been used in the treatment of Buerger's disease of the lower extremity. Prostaglandin E_1 is a potent vasodilator that also inhibits platelet adhesiveness. The drug usually is administered as a continuous drip (0.1 to 0.2 mg per kilogram per minute) through a femoral artery catheter placed either percutaneously or by surgical cutdown. The drug may also be administered through a central venous catheter. Sporadic reports have cited relief of the intense pain and healing of toe ulcers with infusions of this drug. The best results have been achieved in those patients with the most distal arterial occlusions. Infusions have been carried out from 48 hours to as long as 30 days in some centers. Prostaglandin E_1 rarely lowers systemic blood pressure since the decrease in peripheral resistance that occurs is compensated by an increase in cardiac output. Complications reported with the intra-arterial route of administration include catheter sepsis, mycotic aneurysm formation, and local hemorrhage.

I would strongly discourage the administration of steroids to patients with Buerger's disease. Their use has been entirely empiric and of no proven benefit. Furthermore, steroids may adversely influence healing in areas of tissue breakdown and may impair the patient's ability to eradicate infection occurring in these ischemic tissues. Similarly, I see no role for the use of traditional oral vasodilators in Buerger's patients.

SURGICAL MANAGEMENT

Wound Care

The surgeon is often initially asked to see the Buerger's patient after he has reached a true limb-threatening state, that is, when actual skin ulceration has occurred. Early recognition and aggressive therapy are mandatory to minimize tissue loss. I believe that an open foot lesion in the Buerger's patient is an absolute indication for in-hospital management. The ischemic foot is particularly susceptible to septic complications, and infection of an ischemic ulcer can quickly deteriorate to gangrene. In addition to the aforementioned principles of management, swabs of the ulcer should be taken for Gram stain and culture. Fungal infections are particularly common in the patient with Buerger's disease, and fungi may be noted on histologic stains. Unless something unusual is noted, I favor treating these patients initially with a broad-spectrum intravenous antibiotic, such as a cephalosporin, until culture results are available. Limited local debridement may be required to promote adequate drainage. I favor Betadine wet-to-dry dressings to these ulcers to continue the debriding process. If sepsis is suspected under the nail bed, partial or total nail removal should be performed early. Plain films of the bone underlying a skin ulcer should be obtained to rule out osteomyelitis. Roentgenographic signs of bone involvement include periosteal elevation, bone rarefaction, and new bone formation.

Meticulous foot care is essential to prevent the spread of necrosis during these acute exacerbations of Buerger's disease. Soft gauze heel pads are used to prevent pressure necrosis while at bed rest. In the ischemic foot, pressure and rubbing between adjacent toes may result in the development of so-called "kissing ulcers," and this complication can be prevented by the judicious placement of lamb's wool between adjacent digits. Dressings should be secured to the foot with gauze bandages, thus avoiding the potential injury that may result from tape applied directly to ischemic skin.

Vascular noninvasive laboratory testing should be performed early to objectively assess the patient's arterial disease. I use the Doppler ultrasound flow probe to measure segmental limb pressures to quantitate the overall severity of the ischemia, localize the anatomic level of arterial obstruction, and predict the likelihood of ulcer healing (Table 3). Analysis of the pulse waveform using mercury strain-gauge plethysmography at the transmetatarsal and proximal phalangeal levels provides further evidence in this regard. In the patient who appears to have inadequate perfusion to heal based on these criteria or who is clinically deteriorating despite maximal medical management, arteriography should be performed to define the potential for successful surgical reconstruction. Since Buerger's disease typically involves the most distal arteries and since opacification of the pedal vessels is crucial in

TABLE 2   Diagnostic Work-up

Arteriography
Hematologic profile
Erythrocyte sedimentation rate
ANA; rheumatoid factor; L–E prep
Mercury strain-gauge plethysmography

TABLE 3 Likelihood of Foot Ulcer Healing (normotensive patient)

| | Doppler Ankle Pressure (mm Hg) | | |
	Likely	Probable	Unlikely
Nondiabetic	>65	55–65	<55
Diabetic	>90	80–90	<80

order to assess the potential for surgical treatment, I believe intra-arterial digital subtraction angiography is the optimal method for adequately assessing the distal arterial anatomy.

Bypass Grafts

When Doppler studies suggest inadequate perfusion to heal foot lesions, or when there is minimal evidence of healing despite optimal medical care, I favor an attempt at distal bypass grafting if the arteriogram demonstrates a patent posterior tibial or dorsalis pedis artery. Autogenous saphenous vein is the only acceptable bypass conduit in my opinion because of the markedly inferior patency rates noted with prosthetic grafts to the tibial or pedal vessels. The Buerger's patient with distal arterial occlusive disease is an excellent candidate for the non-reversed, in situ saphenous vein graft, although excellent results may be obtained with the standard reversed vein graft in these patients. Since recurrent superficial thrombophlebitis is such a common finding in Buerger's disease, I would recommend performing a saphenous venogram prior to surgery to make certain that the vein is patent and usable. In this way one would avoid creation of a large surgical wound in an ischemic limb in the patient who turns out to have an unusable saphenous vein. I have no reservations about using the distal superficial femoral or popliteal artery as the site for the proximal anastomosis if these vessels are disease-free and only a short segment of adequate vein is available.

Sympathectomy

Unfortunately, owing to involvement of the pedal arteries and/or the saphenous vein in the patient with Buerger's disease, most patients are unable to undergo a distal bypass graft in this setting. I would seriously consider performing a lumbar sympathectomy as a limb-salvage procedure in the patient with nonhealing foot ulcers and/or infection if direct vascular reconstruction is not feasible. Although there is no scientific evidence that sympathectomy is associated with a better long-term prognosis in the patient with Buerger's disease, there is clinical evidence that the procedure may benefit some patients in the acute setting. Sympathectomy appears to improve arterial perfusion at the skin level, and although the effect occurs unpredictably and appears to last no more than a few weeks to months, in some Buerger's patients this may provide enough of an incremental increase in flow to tip the balance in favor of ulcer healing. The best

results are obtained when the procedure has been performed early, before gangrenous changes have occurred. There is absolutely no evidence that sympathectomy retards the progression of the disease, and therefore I see no role for performing a "prophylactic" sympathectomy on the contralateral side.

I prefer to perform lumbar sympathectomy under general anesthesia with the patient supine. A roll is placed under the patient on the appropriate side above the iliac crest to elevate that side about 30 degrees. A transverse incision is carried out from the lateral border of the rectus muscle at the umbilicus to the tip of the twelfth rib. The external oblique fascia is incised, and the internal oblique and transversalis muscles are bluntly separated. The intercostal neurovascular bundle should be identified and carefully protected since inadvertent trauma to it may cause bothersome postoperative pain symptoms. The peritoneal sac is identified and mobilized medially in blunt fashion, beginning the mobilization in the lateral portion of the wound to minimize the chance for entering the peritoneal cavity. Once the retroperitoneum has been identified and entered, the key to identifying the lumbar sympathetic chain is maintenance of a bloodless field and careful palpation. The chain should feel like a taut thin cord adjacent to the spine. Once it is identified by palpation, I elevate it with a nerve hook, divide it between hemaclips, and sharply dissect proximally and distally, clipping and dividing overlying vessels and branching rami. The ilioinguinal and genitofemoral nerves are located posterolaterally and should be protected. The ureter should have been mobilized with the peritoneum to minimize the chance of inadvertent injury. Other potential complications are injury to the inferior vena cava and its branches on the right, and lumbar branches from the aorta on the left. I close the wound in layers over a suction drain, which is usually removed in 24 hours. A mild ileus is not unusual for a day or so.

Amputations

Amputation is frequently required in the patient with Buerger's disease who has nonhealing ulcers, gangrene, or osteomyelitis. The surgeon should amputate at the most distal level at which healing has a reasonable change to occur, based on general clinical criteria (Table 4). A button-toe amputation has a reasonable chance of healing if Doppler analysis demonstrates a pulsatile waveform at the proximal phalangeal level or toe pressure is greater than 30 mm Hg in the normotensive patient. Meticulous surgical technique is equally important. I create medial

TABLE 4 Clinical Criteria for Amputation Healing

Active infection controlled

Healthy skin at site of incision

No dependent rubor proximal to amputation site

Venous filling time <20 seconds

No pain proximal to amputation level

and lateral flaps in a single toe amputation, being careful not to bevel or undermine the skin. The joint space must not be entered in transsecting the bone. The wound is closed with widely spaced, simple 4–0 nylon sutures; strict bed rest is maintained for 5 to 7 days; and broad-sprectrum antibiotics, usually a cephalosporin, are continued for 5 days.

When skin necrosis extends proximal to the meta-tarsophalangeal joint, a transmetatarsal amputation (TMA) of one or several toes is required. A strongly pulsatile forefoot Doppler or mercury strain-gauge waveform is the best predictor of healing of a TMA in adition to the general clinical criteria noted in Table 4. The plantar incision, begun 1 cm proximal to the web space, should be perpendicular to the skin and carried in a single cut through tendon directly down to bone. Inadvertent dissection of tissue planes may compromise the small arterial vessels that lie with the tendons. The dorsal incision is placed at the mid-tarsal level to allow for a total plantar flap. I close the wound in a single layer with widely spaced 4–0 nylon simple sutures to minimize skin trauma and allow for possible serous drainage between the sutures. Forceps are *never* used on the skin! (If deep infection is unexpectedly encountered, the wound may be left open on betadine wet-to-dry dressings and allowed to heal by second intention. A loosely applied bulky dressing should be left intact for 48 to 72 hours unless severe pain (suggestive of ischemia) or signs of infection develop. Bed rest is maintained for 10 to 21 days, depending on my assessment of the degree of arterial insufficiency in the foot prior to the amputation. Prophylactic antibiotics, usually a cephalosporin, are continued for 5 days unless operative cultures dictate a change in the regimen.

In a minority of patients with Buerger's disease, when gangrenous changes extend to the metatarsal level or a TMA fails, a below knee amputation (BKA) may be required. I utilize a long, posterior myocutaneous flap. The tibia is beveled anteriorly and the fibula transected 2 cm shorter than the tibia in order to prevent pressure necrosis on the BKA stump. The tibial nerve is transected at as high a level as possible and ligated with a nonabsorbable suture to minimize the chance of painful neuroma formation. The fascia is closed with nonabsorbable interrupted sutures, and the skin with interrupted 4–0 nylon. A posterior plaster splint is applied and maintained for 7 days to prevent the development of flexion contracture. Broad-spectrum antibiotics are maintained for 5 days and bed rest for 7. Range of motion exercises are begun at one week and crutch walking at 10 days.

IMMUNOLOGIC CONSIDERATIONS

Recent studies have demonstrated the association of Buerger's disease and certain HLA antigens, suggesting that the disease is a specific immunogenetic entity. Cellular sensitivity to human type I or type III collagen has been detected in peripheral lymphocytes in a number of patients with this disease. It is intriguing to consider that, in the future, immunologic tests may be available to identify smokers at particular risk for the development of Buerger's disease before it is clinically apparent, as well as to allow the development of specific immunologic therapy for this devastating arteriopathy. For the present, however, the mainstay of therapy remains complete abstinence from tobacco, compulsive preventive foot care, aggressive in-hospital management of the acutely ischemic limb, surgical reconstruction when technically feasible, and amputation to control gangrene and infection.

INTRA-ARTERIAL INJECTIONS AND INFUSIONS

ROBERT W. HOBSON II, M.D.
CREIGHTON B. WRIGHT, M.D.

Intra-arterial injections or infusions may be used therapeutically or may result in acute and chronic arterial insufficiency in drug abuse cases by either systemic or inadvertent intra-arterial administration. This chapter will review therapeutic use of intra-arterial thrombolytic therapy as well as vascular insufficiency caused by drugs of abuse.

THROMBOLYTIC THERAPY

Systemic thrombolytic therapy with streptokinase or urokinase has been proposed for acute and chronic arterial thrombi or emboli. Other indications have included treatment of deep venous thrombosis, pulmonary embolus, and acute coronary arterial thrombosis. Efficacy and indications for streptokinase and urokinase have been essentially equivalent; however, streptokinase has been employed more widely in this country because of its lower cost. Intravenous administration of the drug in a high-dose protocol has been associated with an increased incidence of complications, resulting in recommendations for intra-arterial infusions employing low-dose regimens. Streptokinase has been particularly effective in native arterial occlusions of femoropopliteal and tibial arteries, particularly in poor-risk surgical patients, in cases in which thrombi are diffuse and less amenable to catheter thrombectomy, and in other circumstances in which avoidance of operation is desirable. Its effectiveness in acute arterial thrombosis occurring as a result of percutaneous transluminal angioplasty also has been reported; however, thrombolytic therapy has been less effective in cases of prosthetic graft occlusions. In a further attempt to reduce associated hemorrhagic complications, fluoroscopic placement of the infusion catheter near or within the proximal thrombus for intra-arterial administration of a low-dose regimen has been used successfully. Streptokinase is administered at a dose of 5,000 to 10,000 units per hour, generally for 48 to 72 hours, followed by intravenous heparinization. Pre-infusion and postinfusion coagulation studies are performed including serial hematocrit, platelet count, prothrombin time (PT), partial thromboplastin time (PTT), thrombin time (TT), fibrinogen, and fibrin split products. Since streptokinase activates the body's normal plasminogen-plasmin system, monitoring of these various parameters will be useful in therapy. We also have relied on reductions in fibrinogen to indicate activation of the fibrinolytic system, noting increased clinical effectiveness under those circumstances.

Documented major complications with thrombolytic therapy may occur in 35 to 40 percent of patients. Severe local and distant hemorrhage, migration of proximal thrombus distally with worsening ischemia, local catheter bleeding, and pseudoaneurysm formation have been reported. Recognizing these complications, contraindications to intra-arterial streptokinase include operation within the previous 10 days, history of recent previous gastrointestinal bleeding, blood dyscrasias, severe hypertension, subacute bacterial endocarditis, and prior allergic reactions to the drug.

Recent clinical trials with intra-arterial recombinant human tissue plasminogen activator (t-PA), a DNA-synthesized thrombolytic agent, have demonstrated its affinity for fibrin-bound plasminogen without producing generalized fibrinolysis. Reduction in hemorrhagic complications should increase interest and use of this drug in preference to streptokinase. Preliminary data presented from the Cleveland Clinic confirmed the selective fibrinolytic potential of t-PA while preserving systemic fibrinogen and plasminogen. No significant changes occurred in PT, PTT, or TT, and fibrinogen levels were maintained at about 50 percent in most patients treated. Further reports will be necessary to establish the drug's efficacy; however, this initial series may allow wider application of fibrinolytic therapy without the higher incidence of hemorrhagic complications.

Our current recommendation (Table 1) is to utilize intra-arterial streptokinase in native arterial occlusions in high-risk surgical patients in whom avoidance of operation is desirable. The drug has no use in clinical situations in which acute arterial occlusion is accompanied by progressive ischemia, as reflected in increasing neurologic deficits or paralysis. Prompt operation in these cases is

TABLE 1 Protocol For Use of Intra-Arterial Streptokinase (SK)

Native arterial occlusions preferred
Less effective with prosthetic occlusions
Local catheter delivery of SK
Dose: 5–10,000 U/hour
Monitor for hemorrhagic complications
Evaluate lysis of thrombus with follow-up arteriography
Convert to systemic heparinization after SK therapy

mandatory, but is associated with significant mortality and limb loss. Therefore, thrombolytic therapy is recommended for patients who do not have such severe ischemia, in whom excellent results can be achieved.

INTRA-ARTERIAL DRUGS OF ABUSE

In the nontherapeutic situation of drug abuse, capacity for identification of arteries, veins, and false aneurysms is low and the skill of the injector variable. Addicts inject arteries in the upper and lower extremities and inject directly into false aneurysms when driven to seek progressively deeper routes of intravascular access. The description of acute, inadvertent, intra-arterial injection and its associated symptoms of burning discomfort, severe pain, and transient vascular obstruction or vasospasm has been characterized as a "hand trip." Gangrene has been reported following intravascular injection of such drugs as heroin, Demerol, Seconal, Pentothal, Nembutal, Sparine, Darvon, Talwin, Vistaril, Atarax, Thorazine, Dexedrine, and quinine. Complications from repeated intra-arterial injections of excipients may also contribute to syndromes of acute and chronic arterial occlusion. Some common "street drug" excipients are caffiene, lactose, magnesium stearate, quinine, starch, stearic acid, and talcum powder.

In addition to these problems caused by the drug, the excipient, and the route of administration, the drug abuser may become stuporous or comatose and leave in place a tourniquet, or other obstructive device on the injected extremity. Unusual posturing, either with an arm over the back of a chair, lying on the arm, or some other position, may allow compression of the arterial and venous circulations independent of the drug or route of injection. In contrast, improper pressure over the site of vascular injection, in the hospital setting or otherwise, may lead to superficial hematomas, pulsatile hematomas (pseudoaneurysms), or extravasation of the injected agent with varying degrees of local and systemic toxicity.

Although infrequent with in-hospital sterile preparations and techniques, localized or systemic infections can occur, but they have been much more prevalent among addicts. Arteriovenous fistula is generally associated with perivascular trauma of a penetrating nature, usually following use of larger needles, but such fistulas have been known to follow cardiac catheterization, use of arterial monitoring catheters, and apparently atraumatic intravenous punctures with smaller needles.

TABLE 2 Management of Drug-Induced Vascular Injury

Prevent thrombosis or thrombic extension
    Anticoagulants (heparin)
    Low-molecular-weight dextran
Improve flow
    Nerve blocks
        Brachial plexus
        Stellate ganglion
        Sympathectomy
    Vasodilators (papaverine)
Thrombolytic agents
    Streptokinase
    Urokinase
Arteriography and direct intervention
    Thrombectomy
    Direct arterial repair as indicated
    Fasciotomy
    Debridement
    Amputation

Another clinical feature of the addict is the ''puffy hand'' syndrome. The etiology is not entirely clear. It probably relates to a combination of superficial and deep phlebothrombosis, extravascular drug administration, cellulitis, and/or acute or chronic lymphangitis with obstruction. As noted in cases of acute venous obstruction in the lower extremity and in cases of limb replantation, obstruction in major venous outflow, particularly when combined with lymphatic obstruction, can lead to gangrene even in the presence of patent arteries or arterial anastomoses.

Physical examination may bring to light the entire spectrum of vascular insufficiency from vasospasm, congestion, and cyanosis to established gangrene. Careful palpation and recording of all pulses in both the affected and unaffected extremity or extremities is mandatory. All puncture sites and ecchymoses should be noted and correlated with clinical records.

Use of a portable Doppler device (BF4A-Medsonics Inc.) is extremely valuable as the next step. Arterial pressure gradients can be measured with blood pressure cuffs. In the upper extremity, Doppler auscultation of the palmar arch and digital arteries, with assessment of the major inflow, whether radial or ulnar, can be performed by temporary arterial compression of each artery at the wrist as described in Allen's test. The Doppler may also identify high-flow signals characteristic of arteriovenous fistula and, with local compression, can localize these abnormalities. B-mode ultrasonography also may be useful for transcutaneous visualization of arterial obstruction and as a technique for sizing true or false aneurysms.

Based on the clinical history, physical examination, and Doppler studies, arteriography may be useful early in the management of these patients. Identification of mechanical injury to arteries as well as documentation of distal emboli and thrombi will guide further treatment. Toxicologic studies may also be necessary to identify specific overdoses and allow definitive therapy for systemic drug toxicity, while surgical intervention for the specific ischemia is under way. General features of therapy are outlined in Table 2.

RENOVASCULAR HYPERTENSION

RAYMOND ENGLUND, M.D.
RICHARD H. DEAN, M.D.

A causal relationship between renal artery occlusive disease and hypertension was demonstrated over fifty years ago. Controversy still remains, however, regarding its frequency, clinical characteristics, diagnostic evaluation, and management. Since renovascular hypertension (RVH) probably accounts for less than 5 percent of the entire hypertensive population, there is little enthusiasm for population-wide screening for its presence. However, the probability that RVH is present increases with the severity of hypertension. Although it is rare in the large group of mildly hypertensive patients, it is a common cause in severely hypertensive patients (40%).

Three age groups are particularly prone to this type of hypertension. Hypertension in the pediatric age group has a high probability of being secondary to RVH. Similarly, young adult females with recent onset of hypertension have a high incidence of RVH secondary to fibromuscular dysplasia of the renal arteries. In the third group, the older atherosclerotic age group, hypertension may be accelerated and difficult to control. In these circumstances the development of atherosclerotic renal artery stenosis and secondary RVH is a common circumstance. Regardless of age, however, patients with either recent-onset severe hypertension or accelerated hypertension should be evaluated for RVH.

Certain physical diagnostic signs also increase the possibility of RVH. These include the finding of an epigastric or flank bruit and intravenous pyelographic findings of decreased size of one kidney, unilateral delay in the nephrogram phase, or late hyperconcentration. Absence of these or other positive screening data should not persuade one against pursuing diagnostic evaluation in search for RVH, for all such screening tests may be falsely normal.

Notwithstanding newer digital subtraction angiographic techniques, standard aortography and renal arteriography are required to definitively evaluate the renal vasculature and either confirm or exclude the presence of renovascular disease. However, identification of such a renovascular lesion does not establish the diagnosis of RVH. Instead, proof of the functional significance is desirable through the use of renal vein renin assays. In patients with unilateral lesions, renal vein renin assays should be positive with a ratio of at least 1.5:1.0 between the involved and uninvolved sides before presumptive proof of the diagnosis is established. Since a positive test depends on lateralization to an involved side, the renal vain renin assay is less accurate when bilateral disease is present. In such patients with equally severe bilateral disease and nonlateralizing renal vein renin assays, we proceed to interventional therapy only when hypertension is severe and control with medications is difficult.

DRUG THERAPY

Through the development of increasingly specific and powerful antihypertensive medications, blood pressure control can be achieved in most patients regardless of the severity or underlying cause. Drug compliance is often difficult, however, due to the frequent and commonly severe side effects of such multidrug regimens. Similarly, when hypertension develops early in life, drug therapy of potentially correctable hypertension has the additional disadvantage of obligating the patient to decades of treatment with its accumulative attendant economic impact on the patient. Finally, drug management only attenuates the secondary blood pressure manifestations of the underlying disease and does nothing to alter the progressive nature of the renovascular lesion with its adverse effects on excretory renal function. For these reasons, drug therapy should play a supportive role in the management of RVH, and greatest emphasis should be placed on identification and correction of the underlying renovascular disease.

PERCUTANEOUS TRANSLUMINAL ANGIOPLASTY (PTA)

Introduced by Gruntzig less than a decade ago, this new interventional modality gained widespread publicity and use prior to identification of its success or durability in the respective types of renovascular occlusive lesions. Reports now appearing demonstrate wide discrepancies in its value among the various types of disease. Medial fibroplasia of the ''string of beads'' variety appears to be amenable to dilation yet the probability of cure is less than that promised by operative management. Similarly, atherosclerotic lesions situated distal to the renal artery ostium appear to respond favorably to PTA. However, dilatation of unifocal fibrodysplastic lesions and ostial and bilateral atherosclerotic lesions appear to be associated with either a high incidence of unsuccessful dilation or rapid recurrence of the lesion and hypertension. Notwithstanding these limitations, it is of value for use in the patient at increased risk for operative treatment and in patients with a relatively short expected survival time. Nevertheless, such interventions should always be undertaken in a collaborative effort with the vascular surgeon in the event of technical misadventure. Although uncommon in experienced hands, PTA may produce acute occlusion, rupture, or dissection of the renal artery, and the surgical team should be prepared for management of such complication.

OPERATIVE THERAPY

A variety of operative techniques have been used to correct renal artery stenoses. From a practical standpoint, however, two basic operations have been most frequently employed: aortorenal bypass and thromboendarterectomy. Thromboendarterectomy is limited to atherosclerotic lesions and is preferably employed when severe bilateral orofacial lesions are to be corrected. Although Wylie popularized the transaortic technique for performance of this procedure, it requires postendarterectomy assessment to prove the presence of complete endarterectomy and absence of residual intimal defects. This can be performed either by completion intraoperative angioplasty or by the direct visualization afforded by angioscopy. For these reasons, we prefer a transverse aortotomy that is carried out each renal artery to a point beyond the lesion. By doing this, the entire procedure can be performed under direct vision and success assured without the necessity of angiography.

In our experience, aortorenal bypass has been the most versatile method of renal revascularization. Three types of grafts are usually available: autogenous saphenous vein, autogenous hypogastric artery, and a synthetic prosthesis. We prefer to use saphenous veins in adults who require bypass. If it is small, less than 4 mm in diameter, we employ an expanded polytetraflouroethylene prosthesis. In children, however, the saphenous vein appears to be more susceptible to aneurysmal dilatation, and we prefer to use the autogenous hypogastric artery. It is important to note, however, that the hypogastric artery may be involved with an arteriopathy similar to the renal artery lesion and is thus susceptible to degenerative changes as well.

Long-term angiographic studies have shown that the vast majority (90%) of grafts that are initially patent without abnormalities remain durable over long-term follow-up. Sequential follow-up angiography is important in children because of the risk of aneurysmal degeneration of any autogenous graft. Similarly, a low incidence of late false aneurysm formation at the suture lines of synthetic grafts has been noted. This argues for repeat long-term angiography or scanning to exclude the presence of this formation in patients with such grafts.

Results of Operative Treatment

In assessing the value of the surgical management of renovascular hypertension, one must consider mortality rate, efficacy in controlling blood pressure, technical success rate, durability of the procedure, and maintenance of renal function. According to a recent assessment of the results of operation in 182 patients with at least 6 months follow-up in our center, one patient died as a result of renal revascularization alone (mortality rate 0.5%). Technical success as judged by routine postoperative angiography was present in 97 percent of these patients. Four patients from this group developed graft occlusions or stenosis. Although complete cure was achieved in 31 percent of the atherosclerotic group and 77 percent of the fibromuscular dysplasia group, a beneficial blood pressure response was achieved in 94 percent of patients. This discrepancy in cure rates is due to pre-existing mild essential hypertension in many of the patients within the atherosclerotic group. Since the risk of morbid cardio-vascular events secondary to hypertension is severity-related, such reduction in severity of hypertension in the majority of atherosclerotic patients is almost as beneficial as cure. Similarly, the durability of the initial result is important. A recent report of late results in a group of patients managed from 15 to 23 years previously in our center demonstrated that overall benefit from operation persisted. Although there was a decrease in the percentage of patients who sustained a cure in both the fibromuscular dysplasia and atherosclerotic group, the percentage who had a beneficial response (cured and improved) remained unchanged over long-term follow-up.

In summary, many questions remain unanswered in the field of renovascular surgery. Drug therapy is still preferred in some institutions. Percutaneous transluminal angioplasty is being used inappropriately in other centers without definitive diagnostic evaluation. Current results with the operative management of RVH are predictable in centers experienced with its use, and the theoretic advantages of potential cure of hypertension and retrieval of renal function by operation are obvious. Nevertheless, long-term comparative studies are necessary to delineate the respective merits of operative management, PTA, and drug therapy.

RAYNAUD'S SYNDROME

BRUCE J. PARDY, B.Med.Sc., Ch.M., F.R.C.S. F.R.A.C.S.

Raynaud's syndrome is characterized by cold sensitivity of the hands and, less often, of the feet, together with episodic digital ischemia secondary to digital artery vasospasm precipitated by cold and emotion. While all patients have vasospasm, a proportion also have organic arterial occlusive disease. This principally affects the digital arteries, but the superficial palmar arch and the ulnar artery at the wrist are also frequently involved. Raynaud's syndrome is benign in those with vasospasm alone, but may cause severe disability when organic occlusive disease is present. The complications of chronic digital ischemia comprise recurrent or persistent nail-related infections, abscess, finger ulceration, and focal necrosis.

TREATMENT

Reassurance

Most patients are seeking reassurance because they have heard that the fingers sometimes become gangrenous and that amputation may be required. The strongest reassurance is given to those patients without evidence of organic digital arterial disease (Table 1). Even patients with the most severe forms of Raynaud's syndrome are informed that finger gangrene of any consequence is

TABLE 1 Raynaud's Syndrome: Vasospasm Only Versus Vasospasm Plus Organic Arterial Disease

Vasospasm Only	Organic Arterial Disease
Female	Female or male
Onset in teens	Onset in adult life
Both hands involved	One or both hands involved
Family history of cold sensitivity	No family history
No history of severe persistent or recurrent finger sepsis, ulceration, or finger necrosis	This history present
No evidence of underlying disorder	Evidence of connective tissue disease, hematologic disease, Buerger's disease, atheroma, or malignancy
No evidence of proximal arterial occlusion or aneurysm	Subclavian bruit, subclavian aneurysm, cervical rib, reduced brachial pressure
No evidence of distal arterial disease; hand blood flow not radial artery dependent	Absent ulnar pulse, reduced ulnar pressure; hand blood flow radial artery dependent
Fingernails and pulps healthy	Thickened or curved finger-nails, pitted pulps, atrophied pulps
Hand films normal	Subcutaneous calcinosis, acroosteolysis, finger pulp atrophy

extremely rare, and that with the proper therapy, finger amputation need almost never be performed.

Removal of Etiologic Agent

Careful enquiry is made to elicit any relevant drug or occupational factor. Drugs that can precipitate or aggravate Raynaud's syndrome include ergotamine preparations and beta-blockers; the role of oral contraceptives is currently uncertain. Beta-blockers often aggravate cold sensitivity of the toes of middle-aged hypertensive females in winter. Strong advice is given against the use of tobacco. Occupational factors that may require modification include working with vibrating tools, contact with vinyl chloride, working in a cold environment, and the handling of frozen foods.

Maintenance of Body and Extremity Warmth

In cold weather, the trunk should be overdressed to the extent that the patient at all times feels warm, and the hands and feet should be protected against the cold. Charcoal hand warmers give comfort during prolonged periods of cold exposure, and electric gloves are helpful in the home and while driving short distances (e.g., to and from work). Electric socks are also available.

General Care of Ischemic Parts

Digital skin nutrition is impaired, and the tissues adjacent to the fingernails are particularly prone to inflammation and infection. Care should be taken to protect the fingers against injury, and particularly against prolonged contact with dishwater. Protective gloves should be worn as often as possible, and footwear should be comfortable and warm (e.g., down boots).

Treatment of Underlying Condition

The possiblity of an underlying connective tissue disease, hematologic disease, proximal arterial disease, or malignant disease must be considered and, if present, managed appropriately.

Oral Drug Therapy to Increase Extremity Blood Flow

I believe that the urge to treat patients with oral drugs should be resisted. Certain drugs have been shown to improve hand blood flow, but it is difficult to evaluate their effects on finger blood flow. No drug has been convincingly shown to be of long-term clinical benefit. Not only are drugs expensive, but many have unpleasant side effects. I never use oral therapy to improve finger blood flow. Drugs favored by some physicians include nifedipine, pentoxifylline, guanethidine, and stanozolol.

Antibiotics

Finger infection in patients with Raynaud's syndrome is almost exclusively caused by *Staphlyococcus aureus*. The treatment is floxacillin, 500 mg four times daily, and I give a 3-week course. Toe infection is much less common, but is difficult to eliminate because the ischemia tends to be more severe. Any fungal infection must be dealt with, and antibiotic therapy must cover a mixed bacterial population that usually includes coliforms.

Intravenous Prostaglandin E$_1$

For the treatment of patients with persistent finger pain secondary to a visible lesion (i.e., not vasospasm alone), I prefer intravenous prostaglandin E$_1$, with or without local surgery. The drug is given as a continuous central intravenous infusion, and this increases blood flow in the distal phalanx of even the most severely affected fingers. This increase in blood flow is probably effected both by direct vasodilation and by a centrally induced vasodilation secondary to increased body heat production. Prostaglandin E$_1$ is also an inflammatory agent, and this action may promote healing.

Because of its potency, prostaglandin E$_1$ is best administered by means of a syringe pump. I dilute the drug in 0.9% saline solution and use a dose rate of 0.8 mg per 24 hours in females and 1.2 mg per 24 hours in males, and a volume rate of 0.5 ml per hour. The patient is warned of possible side effects, which include influenza-like symptoms with anorexia, fever, headache, and general body ache; hand and foot swelling secondary to increased blood flow; and occasional joint inflammation. Rings are removed from the fingers because of drug-induced swelling, and the patient is instructed not to get out of bed unattended because of the possiblity of postural hypotension. The maximal enhancement of finger blood flow appears to be achieved after infusion for 48 hours, and blood flow may be increased for several months.

In practice, prostaglandin E$_1$ infusion for 84 hours is employed to encourage persistent large ulcers to heal, but complete healing may take several months. It is emphasized that prostaglandin E$_1$ has been of no value in patients who have pain from vasospasm alone, and this calls into question the use of vasodilators in this condition.

Intra-arterial Prostaglandin E$_1$

Occasionally, great disability may be caused by necrosis and sepsis of a toe. If intravenous prostaglandin E$_1$ is ineffective, the drug is administered via a cannula in the superficial femoral artery. An epidural cannula, with an outer diameter of 1.1 mm, is inserted at the groin for a distance of 20 cm into the surgically exposed artery. The drug is diluted in 0.9% saline and given with heparin. The initial dose rate of prostaglandin E$_1$ is 0.01 mg per 24 hours and that of heparin is 5,000 IU per 24 hours. The subsequent prostaglandin E$_1$ dose rate is adjusted according to the degree of induced leg swelling and knee pain. The duration of therapy may be as long as 3 weeks.

Sympathectomy

I believe that there is today almost no place for upper limb sympathectomy in the management of Raynaud's syndrome. Patients without organic arterial disease are rarely sufficiently incapacitated to warrant sympathectomy, and the procedure does not confer long-term benefit in patients with severe disease. In contrast, the occasional patient with severe foot cold sensitivity may obtain relief for many years after chemical or surgical lumbar sympathectomy.

Digital Amputation

Many patients referred to me have previously had one or more fingers partially amputated, and careful questioning usually reveals that the indication for amputation was not gangrene, but persistent severe finger pain unresponsive to therapy. As described later, persistent severe pain with localized tenderness is diagnostic of closed sepsis, and this should be managed by surgical drainage, not amputation. Finger amputation is to be avoided because not only is this disfiguring, and damaging to morale, but there may be persistent phantom pain, severe stump cold sensitivity, and hyperesthesia.

Local Surgery Under Prostaglandin E₁ Cover

In the past, the surgical principles of debridement of necrotic and septic tissue, drainage of pus, removal of a "foreign body" (fingernail) from infected tissue, and removal of bone underlying a pressure ulcer have not to any extent been applied to the fingers of patients with Raynaud's syndrome. The reason for avoiding finger surgery has been the fear of producing nonhealing wounds and of precipitating gangrene. However, it is my experience that local surgery in even the most ischemic fingers is safe when carried out under prostaglandin E_1 cover. The indications for local surgery are:

1. *Necrotic and septic tissue.* The removal of eschars and of necrotic and septic tissue relieves pain and promotes healing.
2. *Recurrent, severe, nail-related sepsis.* The presence of the fingernail encourages established infection to persist and makes recurrent infection more likely, the situation being somewhat analogous to the ingrowing toenail. Removal of the nail terminates established sepsis, and removal of the nail bed prevents recurrence of nail-related sepsis. Treatment consists of removal of the nail and nail bed. Oblique incisions are made on each side of the dorsum of the terminal phalanx, extending from the nail fold to just short of the distal interphalangeal joint. One proximal

and two lateral skin flaps are raised, and the nail and nail bed are removed. All tissue down to bone is removed, from the level of the nail fold distally to just short of the joint proximally. The nail fold flaps are replaced, but not sutured. The cosmetic defect of nail bed removal is surprisingly slight and is acceptable to patients.
3. *Apical pressure ulcer.* This is one of the most common indications for surgery. The diagnosis of apical pressure ulcer is based on such findings as an apical ulcer that is usually covered by a small eschar, blanching of the finger pulp on finger extension, pulp atrophy both clinically and radiologically, and the presence of bone in the base of the ulcer at operation. A transverse incision is made over the ulcer, and the soft tissues gently freed from the distal 0.5 cm of the terminal phalanx, which is excised. This allows the soft tissues to fall in over the shortened bone.
4. *Drainage of abscess.* The classic signs of abscess are usually absent because the finger is incapable of hyperemia. The diagnosis is often made because of persistent severe pain associated with tenderness over the site of a small eschar, although occasionally, a collection of pus may be present without any pain. At operation, the overlying eschar is removed, and this reveals a collection of pus extending down to bone. The area is debrided.
5. *Severe disruption of the dorsal tissues of the terminal phalanx.* Rarely, severe necrosis and sepsis of the dorsal tissues of the terminal phalanx necessitate filleting of the terminal phalangeal shaft and tuft and removal of the nail and nail bed. A transverse incision down to bone is made on the dorsum of the finger just distal to the distal interphalangeal joint. Lateral extensions are then made, passing just ventral to the nail and meeting on the pulp. All dorsal tissue is removed, and the distal phalanx is excised as far as its base. The skin is closed with three dorsal sutures. Although it is radical, this procedure preserves all the pulp skin and is not attended by the previously mentioned problems associated with amputation.
6. *Ulcerating subcutaneous calcium.* Ulcerating calcium can usually be lifted out with a needle in the awake patient. However, if there is any difficulty, this may be performed under general anesthesia. No attempt should be made to remove nonulcerating calcium from the subcutaneous tissues. Despite the roentgenographic appearance, the calcium is diffusely spread and cannot be removed. Attempts to do so result in acute sterile inflammation and seem to promote further calcium formation. Surgery is performed only after intravenous infusion of prostaglandin E_1 for at least 48 hours, and after operation the infusion is continued for a further period of not less than 48 hours. If infection is present or suspected,

floxacillin is given for 3 weeks. Surgery is performed under general anesthesia and usually requires two assistants.

Wound Management

All surgical wounds are covered with partial-thickness skin, which is taken from the thigh before the finger procedure. The skin is laid over the whole finger wound. A strip of nonadhesive dressing 1 cm wide is passed from the dorsum of the finger, across the pulp to the ventral aspect of the finger, and held with an overlying strip of adhesive tape.

The finger is then covered with stockinette, which is held by adhesive tape passing to the dorsum of the hand. The dressing is removed by the patient on the third day after operation. Thereafter, the wound is left exposed by day and is dressed at night, as described, by the patient. Fluid collections under the skin dressing may require needle aspiration, and the patient leaves the hospital on the fourth postoperative day.

The partial-thickness skin does not take as a graft; it merely acts as a dressing, and becomes mummified within about 10 days. Fortunately, infection does not prevent use of the skin dressing. The patient is advised that the skin will turn black and that it will not separate until healing of the underlying tissues is complete. This may take several weeks when the finger blood supply is moderate, but up to 6 months when blood flow is severely impaired. During this time the finger is useful and free of pain. Advice is also given to keep the fingers as dry as possible and to avoid soaking.

THORACIC OUTLET SYNDROME

DAVID B. ROOS, M.D.

The numerous variations and combinations of neurovascular symptoms that constitute the thoracic outlet syndromes (TOS) often make definite diagnosis and effective management difficult. Ancillary tests commonly used in other neurovascular problems, such as EMG, nerve conduction times, arteriograms, and noninvasive vascular laboratory studies, rarely offer information significant enough to clarify the diagnosis of thoracic outlet syndrome. The physician must rely on his clinical suspicion, experience, and diagnostic acumen to evaluate patients with neurovascular complaints of the upper extremities adequately. By carefully categorizing the

RESULTS OF TREATMENT

The importance of reassurance cannot be understated. I usually take patients off their oral drug therapy at their first visit, and there has been no reported exacerbation of symptoms. All complicated finger ulcers, no matter how large, have healed with intravenous prostaglandin E_1.

The results of local surgery have been highly satisfactory, and in my experience of operating on over 140 fingers, the need for formal digital amputation has been totally eliminated. Typically, a patient who has been in severe pain for several months is free of pain and is healing within one week of entering the hospital. Permanent removal of the fingernail has been successful in preventing recurrent terminal phalangeal sepsis, and shortening of the phalangeal bone tuft allows apical ulcers to heal and prevents recurrence. It is not always possible to remove the nail bed completely in patients with scleroderma because the tissue planes are poorly defined, and when small spikes of nail reappear, the patient is advised to keep these well filed.

It is my general impression that over a period of several years, the fingers of patients with severe Raynaud's phenomenon, particularly those with scleroderma, seem to improve. The need for prostaglandin E_1 therapy becomes less frequent, and the hands more mobile and useful. The benefits of prostaglandin E_1 and local surgery seem to be limited mainly to the terminal phalanx, and recurrent ulceration of the middle phalanx has occasionally been noted shortly after prostaglandin E_1 therapy. Finally, prostaglandin E_1 therapy and local surgery have been entirely safe; although drug side effects are numerous, there have been no complications.

symptoms, one often finds the protean complaints of the patient to conform to definite patterns seen in many other patients with these syndromes.

Of the three major categories of TOS—neurologic, venous, and arterial—the neurologic type, caused by compression or irritation of the nerves of the brachial plexus, is by far the most common, comprising about 97 percent of all cases of TOS. According to the symptom patterns, this type may be further divided into *upper* brachial plexus involvement (Table 1), in which the C5, C6, and C7 nerves are primarily affected, and *lower* plexus involvement (Table 2), in which C8 and T1 nerves are affected. The upper plexus type is caused by abnormal formation of the scalene muscles in relation to the upper three nerves of the plexus, usually combined with acute or chronic muscle contraction or spasm of the cervical muscles. This causes pain in the anterior aspect of the neck over the brachial plexus just behind the ster-

TABLE 1 Symptom Pattern of Upper Plexus Involvement

Pain
  Side of neck behind sternocleidomastoid muscle
  Side of head, sometimes in ear or jaw
  Upper anterior chest area (infraclavicular)
  Rhomboid and suprascapular areas
  Outer shoulder and arm to dorsum of hand

Aggravated by
  Turning or tilting head
  Lifting and straining

Weakness
  Abducting arm
  Biceps muscle
  Triceps muscle

TABLE 2 Symptom Pattern of Lower Plexus Involvement

Pain
  Back of neck and head
  Suprascapular and back of shoulder
  Back of shoulder joint radiating down back of
    arm through inner elbow and forearm

Aggravated by
  Arm elevation
  Reaching
  Lifting

Weakness
  Grasp
  Finger abduction-adduction
  Fingertip extension

Paresthesias
  Axilla, inner or entire arm, intermittent
  Small and ring fingers
  May spread to entire hand and arm at night
  Arm feels heavy, tired, cold

nocleidomastoid muscle. The pain radiates anteriorly from the ear down through the neck and over the clavicle into the upper chest, posteriorly into the rhomboid and scapular areas, and laterally across the suprascapular and trapezius muscle areas and down the *outer* arm in a typical C5-C6 distribution. The lower plexus type of TOS is distinctly different, with abnormal muscle compression or irritation of the C8 and T1 nerves causing pain in the supraclavicular fossa radiating to the back of the shoulder, to the infraclavicular area, into the axilla, and down the *inner* arm through the ulnar nerve distribution to the ring and small fingers.

The second category of TOS results from compression of the subclavian vein as it passes between the clavicle and first rib. The anatomic structures causing abnormal compression of this vein are usually soft tissue anomalies of the subclavius muscle and tendon passing over and anterior to the subclavian vein, abnormal insertion of the anterior scalene muscle under the vein, a congenital fibromuscular band from the anterior scalene muscle passing directly under the vein and attaching to the sternum, bone anomalies such as exostosis of the first rib under the vein, or a fractured clavicle callous compressing the vein against the first rib. The symptoms of external compression of the subclavian vein are intermittent swelling, cyanosis, heaviness, and aching of the arm that comes on with exertion or, paradoxically, with elevation and clears with rest and dependency. If the symptoms are constant, if collateral veins develop across the anterior shoulder and pectoral areas, and if symptoms worsen with dependency, the subclavian vein has probably thrombosed as a result of abnormal external compression mechanisms.

Arterial symptoms comprise the third major type of TOS and are the result of anatomic anomalies affecting the subclavian artery as it passes through the outlet from the mediastinum to the axilla. The most common of these anomalies is a long cervical rib, and rarely, soft tissue abnormalities not appreciated on x-ray films. Poststenotic dilatation from the cervical rib may cause aneurysmal dilatation, emboli to the fingers, or, rarely, acute thrombosis of the artery resulting in severe ischemia of the entire extremity. Although this type is the least common, comprising only about 1 percent of all TOS cases, it is the most devastating to the patient and most difficult to manage.

DIAGNOSIS

The diagnosis of TOS depends on a high index of suspicion, familiarity with the various syndromes, a detailed history, and careful physical examination of the neck, shoulder, arm, and hand. Careful differentiation of TOS from other nerve compression syndromes, i.e., ruptured cervical disc, cubital tunnel syndrome, and carpal tunnel syndrome, must be made before effective treatment can be advised (Tables 3, 4).

The Adson test with the hand in the lap and the head turned and extended to the ipsilateral side has been found to be useless for this diagnosis. Radial pulse variations with the arms elevated or shoulders braced also have little or no bearing on the diagnosis of TOS as pulse changes in those positions are variations of normal found in 60 to 90 percent of the general population without symptoms. Electromyograms and nerve conduction studies seldom give useful information and usually are not worth the considerable expense and patient discomfort they entail.

Routine arteriograms are useless and merely confirm,

TABLE 3 Differential Diagnoses for Thoracic Outlet Syndrome

Cervical disc syndrome

Carpal tunnel syndrome

Cubital tunnel syndrome at elbow

Cervical arthritis (spondylitis)

Brachial plexitis

Inflammatory shoulder problems
  Bursitis
  Tendinitis
  Capsulitis

Angina pectoris

Central nervous system tumor

Pancoast tumor of the lung

Multiple sclerosis

TABLE 4 Thoracic Outlet Syndrome Versus Cervical Disc and Carpal Tunnel Syndrome

	Thoracic Outlet	Cervical Disc	Carpal Tunnel
Symptoms			
Pain	Intermittent: neck, shoulder, arm (chest)	Constant: neck, rhomboid, suprascapular	Intermittent: volar wrist. forearm, 1st, 2nd, and 3rd fingers
Numbness	Intermittent: ulnar nerve area, 4th and 5th fingers, or entire hand and arm	Constant: radial nerve distribution, forearm, 1st and 2nd fingers	Intermittent: median nerve distribution, palm, 1st, 2nd, and 3rd fingers
Weakness	Grasp, 4th and 5th fingers adduction and extension	Biceps, triceps, deltoid, wrist extension	Grasp, pinch, thenar muscles
Swelling	None or intermittent or constant in fingers, hand, or arm	None	Occasional, intermittent
Aggravation	Arm elevation, lifting, reaching, turning head	Turning neck, lifting, coughing, straining	Sustained grasp, pinch, wrist flexion
Signs			
Percussion	Tender brachial plexus	Tender midline and paracervical	+ Tinel test volar wrist
Compression	Tender brachial plexus	Neck pain with cervical compression	Wrist compression causes median nerve symptoms
Symptoms reproduced by	3 minute elevated arm stress test (EAST); brachial plexus compression	Turning and tilting head; cranial compression	Flexing wrist 1 minute (Phalen test)
EMG and nerve conduction	Usually normal, seldom indicated	Usually normal	Often normal, may show delay at wrist
X-ray findings	Usually normal; may show cervical rib, long C7 transverse process; venogram, arteriogram occasionally required	Degenerative arthritis, narrowed discs, myelogram + 85%	Usually normal; may show arthritis in hand
Treatment			
Conservative	Avoid arm elevation; hunch shoulders, heat, massage, muscle relaxants, analgesics	Cervical collar, home traction, analgesics	Minimize grasp and pinch; wrist splint; ? steroid injection; anti-inflammatory drugs
Indications for surgery	Severe pain; impaired hand function; atrophy; treatment failure	Severe pain, increasing weakness; treatment failure	Severe pain, hand dysfunction, thenar atrophy, treatment failure
Operation	Resect first rib and anomalous bands for C8-T1 symptoms; total anterior scalenectomy for C5,6,7 symptoms	Discectomy (fusion)	Resect transverse carpal ligament

in a very expensive way, the insignificant information that can be more easily obtained by feeling the pulse and listening for bruits with a stethoscope. Arteriograms are indicated only in unusual and specific cases in which one suspects, from the history and examination, that the patient may have an aneurysm or arterial occlusion, or is forming clots and emboli. However, venograms are required to clarify the diagnosis of subclavian vein compression or thrombosis as various conditions may cause swelling and discomfort in the arm. When indicated, venograms should be performed with the arm dependent and then elevated above shoulder level to demonstrate external compression mechanisms and collateral vein formation, which are required for the diagnosis of subclavian vein thrombosis.

CONSERVATIVE TREATMENT

Once the patient's symptoms are clarified by a careful history and examination, the diagnosis usually becomes apparent, and decisions regarding management fall reasonably into place. For the mild type of neurologic symptoms, avoiding unusually strenuous arm activities (i.e., weightlifting, frequent use, or sleeping with the arms above shoulder level) and using hot showers and local heat applications to the neck and shoulder muscles to ease muscle tension affecting the nerves of the brachial plexus often afford adequate relief. For more severe symptoms that may interrupt sleep and affect job performance, a trial of physical therapy with either hot or cold packs for muscle pain and spasm, massage, ultrasound, muscle stretching, and posture correcting exercises is indicated. The more vigorous type of "thoracic outlet syndrome exercises" often prescribed by physical therapy departments usually increase muscle spasm, pain, and TOS symptoms, and patients with moderate-to-severe syndromes cannot tolerate them. Muscle relaxant medications, frequent hot showers at home, and analgesics may be indicated. If the patient can control the symptoms, maintain adequate job performance, get reasonable sleep, and continue normal activities with his family, conservative treatment should be continued. If these measures do not control the symptoms, and the patient requires strong medication, job performance suffers, personality changes of depression and frustration from the unresponding severe symptoms increase, prolonged conservative management will not suffice. The most effective means of relieving the more severe cases of TOS of any type requires surgical decompression of the brachial plexus and the subclavian vessels.

SURGICAL TREATMENT

Various operations have been used to try to alleviate the distressing symptoms of the severe thoracic outlet syndromes. Supraclavicular resection of the first and cervical rib was the original operation for TOS, first performed in 1910. Dividing the anterior scalene muscle and removing a short segment became popular after Adson's report in 1928. Scalenotomy was generally abandoned later owing to poor results, and removal of the first rib again became the basic operation, through the posterior parascapular approach in 1962, and then through the transaxillary approach after 1966. The latter operation offers much greater and safer exposure of the T1 nerve of the plexus and the subclavian artery and vein. The entire first rib can be resected along with the various anomalous fibromuscular bands that are always present in severe cases in order to decompress the thoracic outlet completely. These essential objectives cannot be achieved through the supraclavicular, infraclavicular, or posterior approaches.

Other associated procedures sometimes required in TOS cases can also be performed simultaneously through the transaxillary approach. These include complete removal of the various anomalies compressing the subclavian vein, even performing a thrombectomy in carefully selected cases; removal of a cervical rib; performing an extrapleural thoracic sympathectomy for causalgia or sympathetic dystrophy; and sectioning the pectoralis minor muscle in rare cases in which it seems to compress the neurovascular structures in the axilla.

In patients presenting with severe symptoms of upper brachial plexus involvement caused by anomalous scalene muscle formation, the obsolete scalenotomy, or removal of the first rib alone, using any approach, usually proves ineffective. The divided scalene muscle will reattach itself by heavy scar formation, to the first rib or Sibson's fascia,

and symptoms will recur because the underlying anomalies remain. Reoperation to remove the entire anterior scalene muscle then becomes much more difficult and hazardous owing to extensive scar involvement of all five nerves of the brachial plexus and the phrenic nerve. It is much easier, safer, and more effective to perform a total anterior scalenectomy during the first operation.

Many patients may be found to have severe symptoms from involvement of both the upper and lower nerves of the plexus. In these cases, complete decompression of all five nerves is required for optimal relief. In such patients, I prefer to decompress the lower nerves and the thoracic outlet first through the transaxillary approach with the patient in the 80-degree lateral thoracotomy position, and then turn him on his back and perform a supraclavicular total anterior scalenectomy.

An occasional patient has multiple nerve entrapments with definite carpal tunnel syndrome in addition to TOS. In these cases, decompression of the median nerve in the carpal tunnel should be performed immediately after completing the procedures indicated for the outlet syndromes.

All of the operations mentioned in this chapter have been thoroughly described in the literature. The surgeon faced with operating on patients with these syndromes should carefully review the various techniques that may be required and the detailed anatomy involved before undertaking these potentially difficult and hazardous procedures. In all of these syndromes, significant anatomic anomalies play a major role in causing the neurovascular symptoms. Therefore, the surgeon must be mentally prepared to recognize and deal with anatomic abnormalities he may encounter that are not depicted in the standard anatomy textbooks if he is to achieve optimal results with the least complications or scar tissue recurrences.

Dealing with TOS patients requires familiarity with the various symptom complexes that may be encountered and great patience with people suffering unpleasant, sometimes incapacitating and frightening, symptoms. This often requires considerable time and communication to understand these patients thoroughly. However, if an accurate diagnosis is made, if surgical candidates are chosen with care, if the appropriate operations are performed with meticulous technique, and if postoperative care is appropriate and compassionate, significant, if not total, relief may be achieved in 85 to 95 percent of cases, even after all attempts at conservative treatment have failed. These patients may be some of the most challenging, yet gratifying and appreciative people seen in surgical practice.

MESENTERIC ISCHEMIA

FRANK J. VEITH, M.D.
SCOTT J. BOLEY, M.D.

ANATOMY AND PHYSIOLOGY

The mesenteric circulation can be defined as that portion of the splanchnic circulation supplying the small and large intestines. The major arteries contributing to this intestinal vascular bed are the superior mesenteric artery (SMA), the inferior mesenteric artery (IMA), branches of the celiac axis (CA), and the middle and inferior hemorrhoidal branches of the internal iliac artery.

The intestines are protected from ischemia to a great extent by their abundant collateral circulation. Communications between the celiac and the superior and inferior mesenteric beds are numerous, and as a general rule, at least two of these vessels must be compromised to produce symptomatic intestinal ischemia. Moreover, occlusion of two of the vessels occurs frequently without evidence of ischemia, and total occlusion of all three vessels has been observed without symptoms.

The major collateral circulation from the celiac axis is through the superior pancreaticoduodenal artery into the inferior pancreaticoduodenal artery, which is the first branch of the superior mesenteric artery. Collateral blood flow from the inferior mesenteric artery comes primarily through the arch of Riolan ("meandering mesenteric artery"), which connects the left colic and middle colic arteries. The inferior mesenteric artery in turn may receive collateral circulation from the internal iliac artery through the inferior hemorrhoidal to superior hemorrhoidal arterial connections.

Collateral pathways around occlusions of smaller mesenteric arterial branches are provided by the primary, secondary, and tertiary arcades in the mesentery of the small bowel and by the marginal arterial complex of Drummond in the mesocolon. Within the bowel wall itself there is a network of communicating submucosal vessels that can maintain the viability of short segments of the intestine whose extramural arterial supply has been lost.

In the resting state the mesenteric circulation receives up to 25 percent of the cardiac output. This percentage may increase after eating or decrease during exercise. Motor control of the mesenteric circulation is mediated primarily through the sympathetic nervous system. Although beta adrenergic receptors are present, alpha adrenergic receptors predominate. Thus increased sympathetic activity produces vasoconstriction, which increases resistance and decreases blood flow.

In response to the fall in arterial pressure distal to an obstruction, collateral pathways open immediately when a major vessel is occluded. Increased blood flow through this collateral circulation continues as long as the pressure in the vascular bed distal to the obstruction remains below the systemic pressure. If vasoconstriction develops in this distal bed, the arterial pressure there rises and causes diminution of collateral flow. Similarly, if normal blood flow is reconstituted, flow through collateral channels ceases.

The degree of reduction in blood flow that the bowel can tolerate without damage is remarkable. Reduction of mesenteric arterial flow of 75 percent or greater for up to 12 hours can be tolerated without morphologic changes in the bowel.

Intestinal ischemia may result from a reduction in blood flow, from redistribution of blood flow, or from a combination of both. A reduction in blood flow to the intestine may reflect generalized poor perfusion, as in shock or with a failing heart, or it may result from either local morphologic or functional changes. With hypotension there is both decreased splanchnic blood flow, as a result of vasoconstriction, and redistribution of flow away from the mucosa because of arteriovenous shunting within the bowel wall. Narrowings of the major mesenteric vessels, emboli, vasculitis as part of a systemic disease, or mesenteric vasoconstriction all can lead to inadequate circulation. However, whatever the cause, intestinal ischemia has the same end results: a spectrum ranging from completely reversible functional alterations to total hemorrhagic necrosis of portions or all of the bowel. Two situations that can dramatically produce or sustain diminished intestinal blood flow in the absence of vascular occlusion are bowel distention and systemic conditions producing lowered cardiac output and transient fall in mesenteric arterial blood flow.

ACUTE MESENTERIC ISCHEMIA

The earliest report of a patient with acute mesenteric ischemia (AMI) was that of Tiedermann, who described the first clinical case of superior mesenteric artery occlusion in 1843. The first successful bowel resection for intestinal infarction was reported by Elliott in 1895. Further progress in the management of these catastrophes did not occur until the 1950s. Klass, in 1950, attempted the first superior mesenteric artery embolectomy, and one year later Stewart performed the first successful operation of this type. Successful operative approaches to acute superior mesenteric artery thrombosis, as well as chronic mesenteric ischemia, were reported in that decade. Ende, in 1958, first described nonocclusive mesenteric ischemia, and during the 1960s various attempts to treat this latter condition using local and regional anesthetic blocks as well as systemic and intra-arterial vasodilators were reported.

Incidence

The exact incidence of AMI is difficult to ascertain. In one large metropolitan medical center, the incidence in the late 1970s was 1 per 1,000 admissions. Recently, there appears to have been a real increase in the occurrence of AMI as well as in its recognition, and with this increased incidence there has been a change in the distribution of cases attributed to each of the different causes. Whereas, in the past, mesenteric venous and arterial thrombosis were most common, in recent series arterial emboli and nonocclusive mesenteric ischemia were responsible in 70 to 80 percent of patients.

Etiology

Superior Mesenteric Artery Embolus (SMAE). Today, emboli are responsible for 40 to 50 percent of episodes of AMI and usually originate from a mural or atrial thrombus. Formerly, such thrombi were most often due to rheumatic vascular disease, but arteriosclerotic heart disease is now the most common cause. Many patients have a previous history of peripheral arterial embolism, and approximately 20 percent have synchronous emboli in other arteries.

Arterial emboli tend to lodge at points of normal anatomic narrowings, usually just distal to the origin of a major branch, such as the inferior pancreaticoduodenal or middle colic artery.

The artery may be completely occluded, but more often the embolus only partially obstructs blood flow. Mild-to-marked vasoconstriction is often present in arteries both proximal and distal to the embolus.

Acute Superior Mesenteric Artery Thrombosis (SMAT). Acute thrombosis of the SMA almost always is superimposed on severe atherosclerotic narrowing, most commonly at its origin. Thirty to fifty percent of patients with SMAT give a history of abdominal pain during the preceding weeks or months. When total occlusion of the SMA is demonstrated by angiography in a patient with abdominal pain, but there are no abdominal findings, it is important to differentiate an acute occlusion from a longstanding one, as the latter may be coincidental to the present illness. The presence of prominent collaterals between the superior mesenteric and celiac or inferior mesenteric circulation in such a patient suggests a chronic occlusion; the absence of collaterals indicates an acute occlusion.

Nonocclusive Mesenteric Ischemia (NOMI). Since Ende's first description in 1958, the proportion of mesenteric vascular accidents resulting from NOMI has risen from 12 percent to over 50 percent in some recently reported series. The pathogenesis of the entity is believed to be splanchnic vasoconstriction occurring in response to a decrease in cardiac output, hypovolemia, dehydration, vasopressor agents, or hypotension. This vasoconstriction may persist even after the initiating cause has been corrected. Predisposing conditions include myocardial infarction, congestive heart failure, aortic insufficiency, renal and hepatic disease, or major abdominal or cardiac operations. Digitalis and diuretic therapy have also been implicated. In addition, a more immediate precipitating cause such as pulmonary edema, cardiac arrhythmias, or shock is usually present, although the intestinal ischemic episode may not become manifest until hours or days later.

Acute Mesenteric Venous Thrombosis (MVT). This entity was cited as the most frequent cause of intestinal infarction 50 years ago, but is uncommon today. MVT can be primary (agnogenic) or secondary to a variety of conditions, including hematologic disorders,

hypercoagulable states, intra-abdominal sepsis, local venous stasis, and abdominal trauma. Recently there has been a spate of reports of minor and major mesenteric venous thromboses in patients taking oral contraceptives.

Diagnosis

Clinical Presentation. Early identification of AMI depends on recognition of those patients who are at risk: (1) patients over 50 years of age with heart disease and longstanding congestive heart failure, cardiac arrhythmias, or recent myocardial infarction, or (2) patients with hypovolemia or hypotension, such as in burns, pancreatitis, or hemorrhage. The development of abdominal pain in a patient with one of those conditions should raise the suspicion of AMI. Previous or simultaneous arterial emboli increase the possibility of the ischemia being due to an SMA embolus.

Abdominal pain is present in 75 to 98 percent of patients with intestinal ischemia, but it varies in severity, nature, and location. A history of postprandial abdominal pain for several weeks or months preceding the acute episode is common in patients with SMA thrombosis. A characteristic early clinical feature is a disparity between the severity of the pain and the paucity of significant abdominal findings on physical examination. Sudden severe pain accompanied by forceful intestinal emptying is strongly suggestive of an acute arterial occlusion, especially when there are minimal or no abdominal findings.

Unexplained abdominal distention or gastrointestinal bleeding may be the only indication of acute intestinal ischemia, since pain may be absent in up to 25 percent of patients. Distention, though usually absent early, may be the first sign of impending intestinal infarction. Gastrointestinal bleeding may precede any other symptom of mesenteric ischemia, and stools are positive for occult blood in up to 75 percent of patients.

Early in the course of an ischemic episode there are no abdominal findings. However, as infarction develops, increasing tenderness, rebound tenderness, and muscle guarding reflect the progressing intestinal changes. Significant abdominal findings are strong evidence for the presence of nonviable bowel. Nausea, vomiting, fever, rectal bleeding, hematemesis, intestinal obstruction, back pain, shock, and increasing abdominal distention are other late signs.

Laboratory Values. Leukocytosis above 15,000 cells per cubic millimeter occurs in approximately 75 percent of patients with AMI, and metabolic acidosis with increased base deficit is present in about 50 percent. Elevations in other serum and peritoneal fluid values have been reported, but the consistency and specificity of these findings have not been established.

Ancillary Techniques. Several diagnostic radioisotopic techniques have been developed in experimental animals, but have not been evaluated clinically. Laparoscopy has been used to identify transmural infarction, but is not reliable in the earlier stages of intestinal ischemia.

Roentgenologic Studies. Signs of intestinal ischemia on plain film studies occur late and usually indicate bowel infarction. Ideally, all patients should be studied before the signs of ischemia develop. In series of cases in which a significant portion of the patients have had such signs, the mortality has been dismaying.

Angiography. Angiography can establish AMI in most cases, identifying both the cause of the ischemia and the site of an SMA occlusion if one is present. Moreover, it provides the surgeon with a road map to accomplish adequate revascularization when it is indicated. Angiographic signs of mesenteric vasoconstriction in patients who clinically are suspected of having AMI, and who are not hypotensive or receiving vasopressors, are presumptive evidence of nonocclusive mesenteric ischemia. The angiographic catheter provides an access for the administration of vasodilators into the SMA as part of a management plan.

Management Plan

Although the diagnosis of AMI has been made with increasing frequency during the past 20 years, until recently the mortality rate for this catastrophe remained at 70 to 90 percent. This poor outlook could be attributed mainly to three factors: inability to make the diagnosis before intestinal gangrene developed, progression of the bowel infarction after the primary initiating vascular or systemic cause has been corrected, and the increasing frequency of NOMI, with its reported mortality rate of over 90 percent. Improved survival of patients with AMI has been achieved with an aggressive approach directed at these factors. The new features in this approach are (1) the earlier and more extensive use of angiography to diagnose mesenteric ischemia and determine its cause before intestinal infarction occurs and (2) the intra-arterial infusion of papaverine to interrupt the splanchnic vasoconstriction that is the direct cause of NOMI and a major factor in occlusive forms of AMI, and that persists after successful management of the underlying local or systemic cardiovascular cause. These concepts are incorporated into a comprehensive roentgenologic survey and a therapeutic plan.

General Management. When AMI is suspected, initial treatment is directed toward correction of predisposing or precipitating causes of the mesenteric ischemia. Relief of acute congestive heart failure, correction of cardiac arrhythmias, and replacement of blood volume precede any diagnostic studies. In general, efforts at increasing intestinal blood flow will be futile if low cardiac output, hypotension, or hypovolemia persists. Plain roentgenographic studies of the abdomen are then obtained, and subsequent abdominal angiography is routinely performed unless some other intra-abdominal condition is diagnosed on the plain film examination. Based on the angiographic findings and the presence or absence of signs of peritoneal irritation on physical examination, the individual patient is then treated according to the schema outlined in Figures 1 to 3.

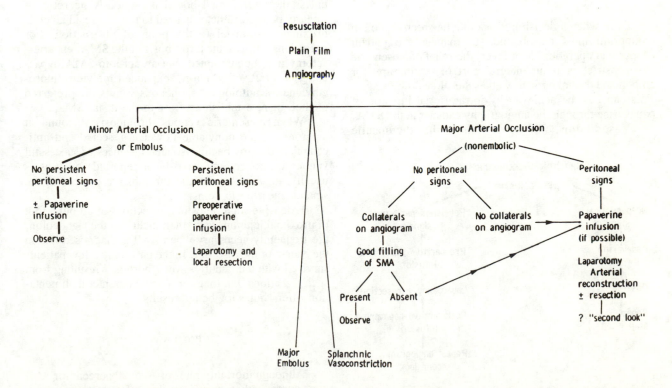

Figure 1 Schema of plan of management for minor superior mesenteric artery occlusions (in branches of the SMA distal to the ileocolic artery) and acute thrombosis of the SMA at or proximal to the origin of the ileocolic artery.

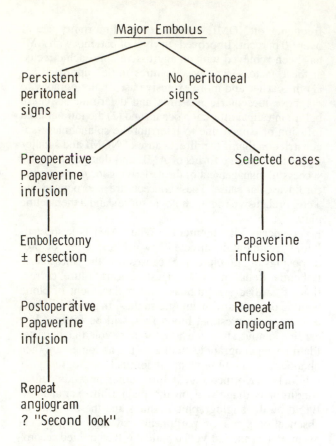

Figure 2 Schema of plan of management for emboli in the SMA at or proximal to the origin of the ileocolic artery.

Even when a decision to operate has been made, an angiogram must be obtained to manage the patient properly at operation. Moreover, the relief of mesenteric vasoconstriction is an integral part of the therapy for emboli and thromboses, as well as the "low flow" stages. This can best be achieved by intra-arterial infusion of papaverine through the angiography catheter in the SMA.

Vasodilator Therapy. When the therapeutic

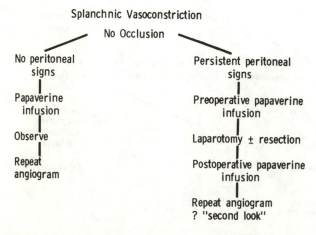

Figure 3 Schema of plan of management for nonocclusive mesenteric ischemia (angiography revealing splanchnic vasoconstriction).

regimen includes the use of papaverine, the drug is infused at a constant rate of 30 to 60 mg per hour using an infusion pump. Systemic arterial pressure and cardiac rate and rhythm are continuously monitored as these amounts of papaverine theoretically could have systemic effects. The duration of the papaverine infusion varies with both the purpose for its use and the clinical and angiographic response of the patient.

Surgical Principles. Laparotomy is indicated during the course of AMI either to restore intestinal arterial flow, such as after an embolus or thrombosis, or to resect irreparably damaged bowel. Revascularization should precede any evaluation of intestinal viability since bowel that initially appears infarcted may show surprising recovery after restoration of blood flow.

After revascularization, if short segments of bowel are nonviable or questionably viable, these are resected. If extensive segments of bowel are involved, only the frankly necrotic bowel is resected and a planned re-exploration or "second look" is performed within 12 to 24 hours.

A decision to perform a "second look" operation is made at the initial laparotomy if there is questionable viability of either a major portion or multiple segments of intestine. The purpose of the "second look," as proposed by Shaw, is "not just to allow a clear definition between dead and live bowel to take place, but also to allow time for the institution of supportive measures, which may render more of the bowel viable."

Embolectomy is indicated for all emboli impacted in the main SMA at or above the origin of the ileocolic artery unless the entire small bowel is obviously necrotic. A Fogarty balloon catheter is used to remove residual clots proximal and distal to the point of obstruction. For occlusions due to acute thrombosis of the SMA, endarterectomy may be attempted, but an aorta-to-SMA bypass using a graft of Dacron, expanded polytetrafluoroethylene, or autologous saphenous vein is the preferred method of re-establishing flow to the distal SMA.

When mesenteric venous thrombosis is found at laparotomy, the nonviable bowel is resected and anticoagulant therapy begun. Isolated instances of successful venous thrombectomy have been reported, but this is usually not possible, as the thrombi are present in the smaller mesenteric veins.

Extensive small intestinal resections of all but a foot of proximal jejunum, and often including the right colon, are frequently necessary when AMI is diagnosed late in the course of the disorder. In the past, only a few patients survived with the "short bowel syndrome" resulting from such resections, but long-term home parenteral alimentation offers hope for better results.

Prognosis

Although mortality rates of 70 to 90 percent for AMI were consistently reported for almost 50 years, an aggressive approach to management has lowered the mortality to under 50 percent. Although many patients with AMI are elderly and suffer from severe cardiovascular disease, they can survive the acute intestinal ischemic episode if diagnosed early and managed properly. A recent review of experience with 47 patients with SMA emboli showed that if the "doctor delay" was less than 12 hours, and the patient was managed as described above, 2 out of 3 patients survived.

FOCAL INTESTINAL ISCHEMIA

Ischemia insults localized to short segments of the small bowel produce a broad spectrum of clinical features without the life-threatening systemic complications associated with ischemia of more extensive portions of the gut.

Etiology

The most frequent causes are atheromatous emboli, strangulated hernias, collagen diseases, blunt abdominal trauma, segmental venous thrombosis, and, especially during the 1960s, enteric-coated thiazide-potassium chloride preparations. Lesions associated with systemic diseases may occur late in the course of the illness or may be the heralding event of the generalized disorder.

Pathogenesis

With focal ischemia there is usually adequate collateral circulation to prevent transluminal hemorrhagic infarction. Hence, the most common lesions are infected infarcts resulting from partial necrosis of the bowel wall and secondary invasion by the intestinal bacterial flora. Limited tissue necrosis may result in complete healing, a chronic enteritis simulating Crohn's disease, or a stricture with partial or complete intestinal obstruction. When the local insult is severe enough to produce transmural necrosis, perforation or a localized peritonitis may ensue.

Clinical Presentation

Patients with short segment ischemia present in one of three clinical patterns, depending upon the severity of the infarct.

In the acute presentation, seen with transmural necrosis, there is a sudden onset of abdominal pain that often simulates an attack of acute appendicitis.

Another group of patients present with signs and symptoms of chronic enteritis, crampy abdominal pain, diarrhea, occasional fever, and weight loss. The clinical picture may be indistinguishable from that of Crohn's disease of the small bowel.

The most common presentation is that of chronic small bowel obstruction, with or without a history of some antecedent episode of trauma, pain, or hernia incarcera-

tion. Intermittent abdominal pain, distention, and vomiting are direct results of the obstruction; and bacterial overgrowth in the dilated loop proximal to the obstruction may lead to the metabolic and clinical derangements usually associated with the "blind loop syndrome," this is, anemia, diarrhea, and steatorrhea.

A preoperative diagnosis of focal ischemia is difficult to make. A previous episode of transient pain or trauma, or a known systemic illness can suggest the correct diagnosis.

Treatment

The treatment of acute focal ischemia is usually surgical, but some patients without signs of peritonitis can be managed expectantly. In those instances the diagnosis is based on the roentgenographic findings of "thumbprints" indicative of acute ischemia; serial studies should reveal a changing pattern. Both clinical and roentgenographic findings must resolve or the nonsurgical approach should be abandoned.

Patients who present with chronic enteritis or obstruction should be operated on immediately after proper preparation. Awareness of these lesions produced by segmental ischemia is essential because a limited resection is the operation of choice both for obstructing lesions and for focal enteritis.

CHRONIC INTESTINAL ISCHEMIA

Etiology

In this entity, also known as abdominal angina, intestinal angina, or recurrent mesenteric ischemia, there is inadequate intestinal blood flow to satisfy the demands of the increased motility, secretion, and absorption that develop after meals. Thus patients with chronic intestinal ischemia are actually experiencing recurrent acute episodes of insufficient blood flow during periods of maximal intestinal work load. The ischemia is manifest either by visceral pain or abnormalities in gastrointestinal absorption or motility. Therefore, the pain is similar to that arising in the myocardium with angina pectoris or in the calf muscles with intermittent claudication. Atherosclerotic involvement of the mesenteric vessels is almost always the cause of this form of intestinal ischemia. Although partial or complete occlusion of the SMA, CA, and IMA is fairly common, few patients have documented chronic intestinal ischemia. Moreover, there are many patients with occlusion of two or even all three of these vessels who remain asymptomatic. The various small vessel diseases such as thromboangiitis obliterans (Buerger's disease) or periarteritis nodosa may also produce chronic intestinal ischemia and even lead to segmental intestinal gangrene.

Clinical Presentation

The one consistent clinical feature of chronic mesenteric ischemia is abdominal discomfort or pain. Most commonly this occurs 10 to 15 minutes after eating, gradually increases in severity, reaches a plateau, and then slowly abates in 1 to 3 hours. The pain pattern is so intimately related to the ingestion of food that the patient reduces the size of his meals, becomes reluctant and afraid to eat, and has massive weight loss. Bloating, flatulence, and derangements in motility with constipation or diarrhea are also seen.

Diagnosis

There is no specific reliable diagnostic test for abdominal angina. The diagnosis must be based on the clinical symptoms, the arteriographic demonstration of an occlusive process of the splanchnic arteries, and, to a great measure, on the exclusion of other gastrointestinal disease. Angiographic evaluation includes flush aortography in frontal and lateral views and selective injections of the SMA, CA, and, if possible, the IMA. The degree of occlusive involvement of the three major arteries can be best assessed on the lateral projections, and the collateral circulation and pattern of flow are best seen on the frontal views. The presence of prominent collateral vessels indicates a significant stenosis of a major vessel, but also connotes a chronic process. Angiographic demonstration of stenoses or occlusions of one, two, or all the major vessels does not by itself establish the diagnosis of arterial insufficiency.

In the past a major indication given for early operative intervention for chronic intestinal ischemia was the prevention of acute intestinal infarction. However, over 75 percent of cases of AMI are due to embolus or non-occlusive disease, and in neither condition are prodromal symptoms present. Neither has the incidence of intestinal infarction in patients with occlusive disease of the splanchnic vessels ever been determined. Hence the fear of impending intestinal infarction is not an indication for operation if other criteria do not warrant it. There is one special situation in which reconstruction or bypass of obstructed splanchnic arteries is indicated in the absence of abdominal complaints. This indication arises in a patient who is undergoing an aortic operation for aneurysm or peripheral vascular disease and in whom aortography has demonstrated occlusive involvement of the SMA or CA and the presence of a large "meandering artery."

Surgical Approach

Although several procedures have been advocated for restoring normal flows and pressures distal to an occlusion in the CA or SMA, the present preferred operation is a bypass from the infrarenal aorta to the SMA alone. However, some surgeons believe that in the presence of CA and SMA occlusion, adequate surgical management must include restoration of normal flow and pressure to both vessels and their branches. Knitted Dacron (6 mm), polytetrafluoroethylene, or an autologous saphenous vein (reversed and at least 5 mm in diameter) are all acceptable graft materials.

Patency rates with such bypass grafts to the SMA or CA have generally been good, and symptomatic relief in properly selected patients has been excellent. However, Stoney and his associates have recently reported poor results with retrograde bypasses. They attribute this to an unusual and rapidly progressive form of atherosclerosis that involves the subdiaphragmatic aorta and occurs more commonly in females and in relatively young subjects. On the basis of their extensive experience with this entity, they advocate either a thoracoabdominal retroperitoneal approach, with antegrade prosthetic grafts originating from the uninvolved distal thoracic aorta, or a "trapdoor" transaortic endarterectomy supplemented with venous patch grafts when indicated.

CELIAC AXIS COMPRESSION SYNDROME (CACS)

This controversial syndrome is discussed here, although we and others do not consider it to be a manifestation of gastrointestinal ischemia. One of the major difficulties in assessing the validity of the CACS is that different criteria are used by various authors to define it. Postprandial abdominal pain, weight loss, diarrhea, an abdominal bruit, and angiographic demonstration of extrinsic compression of the CA constitute the findings on which the diagnosis should be based. This compression is due to the crural fibers of the diaphragm, the celiac ganglion, or both, which produce a smooth asymmetric narrowing of the superior aspect of the CA. The surprisingly high frequency of CA narrowing among asymptomatic individuals and the lack of close correlation between the severity of symptoms and the degree of narrowing in symptomatic patients indicate the need for considerable caution in attributing a patient's symptoms to the arterial stenosis.

The most difficult aspect of the treatment of the CACS is the selection of patients for surgical relief of the compressed artery. Results of surgical procedures have varied from series to series, and no specific criteria can be well correlated with a successful outcome. In view of the continuing lack of objective evidence that stenosis of the CA produces any pathologic changes in the viscera supplied by that artery, we believe that only patients fulfilling strict criteria should be operated on. These criteria are abdominal pain, preferably related to eating; significant weight loss; an abdominal bruit; and angiographic demonstration of the typical narrowed celiac axis. In a large medical center with special interests in vascular surgery and vascular disorders of the gastrointestinal tract, we have not encountered a single patient with these findings during the past 10 years.

The surgical approach to CACS varies with the surgeon's beliefs concerning the cause of the pain. Those who believe it is ischemic emphasize the necessity for re-establishing CA blood flow. Those who believe that the pain is neurogenic emphasize the division or resection of the celiac ganglion. A practical approach includes incision of the median arcuate ligament and local resection of the periarterial portion of the celiac ganglion as an initial step. In a few cases in which a significant aorta-to-celiac axis

pressure gradient remains, dilation or arterial reconstruction may be warranted.

This work was supported in part by grants from the Manning Foundation and the Anna S. Brown Foundation.

DIABETIC FOOT

BRUCE A. PERLER, M.D.

Diabetic foot problems are enormously important in terms of both patient morbidity and the national health care dollar. At least one in five diabetic hospital admissions is for treatment of foot complications; in fact, diabetic foot infections are responsible for more days of hospitalization than any other of the known complications of diabetes mellitus. In 1980 it was estimated that more than two hundred million dollars of direct hospital costs were incurred in the management of diabetic foot infections. The diabetic patient is 17 times more likely to develop gangrene of the foot than the nondiabetic, and more than three-fourths of nontraumatic limb amputations are performed in diabetics. About 50 percent of diabetics who undergo amputation of one leg eventually require amputation of the contralateral extremity.

Several factors contribute to the development of diabetic foot complications, including peripheral sensory neuropathy, arteriosclerotic occlusive disease of both large and small arteries, and an unusual susceptibility to infection. In my opinion, the great tragedy in diabetic foot disease is that much of this tissue and limb loss could be avoided with compulsive preventive medicine and aggressive management of early foot lesions.

OUTPATIENT MANAGEMENT

Preventive Medicine

Patient education is an essential component of the overall management of the diabetic foot and is the responsibility of the general surgeon as much as the internist and podiatrist (Table 1).

TABLE 1 Principles of Routine Diabetic Foot Care

Daily inspection
Daily washing
Skin care: moisturizing/drying
Proper toe and toenail care
Proper footwear

The feet should be examined daily for abrasions, blisters, ingrown toenails, and cracked skin. Areas most susceptible to skin breakdown include the plantar aspect of the foot over the metatarsal heads, the heel, the inner surfaces of the toes, the interdigital web spaces, and other areas of abnormal bony prominence. The feet should be washed daily with a mild soap in lukewarm water since hot water may scald the neuropathic foot and go unnoticed. Prolonged soaking should be avoided since it will cause skin maceration and predispose to infection. The foot should be thoroughly dried following washing since excessive moisture, particularly between the toes, predisposes to fungal infection.

The minor skin fissures and cracks that serve as the portal of entry for infection result from excessively dry skin; daily application of a skin moisturizer reduces the likelihood of this complication. A number of lanolin-base products, such as Nivea, Lanolin, Alpha-Keri, Eucerin, and Vasoline Intensive Care lotion, are recommended. Many of the perfumed lotions contain alcohol, which may harm the skin, and therefore should be avoided. Antifungal powders such as Desinex should be used in the diabetic patient with excessive foot perspiration, especially in the interdigital spaces.

In my experience, more diabetic foot morbidity results from improper toenail care than any other cause. For this reason, I strongly urge my patients to have their nails trimmed by an experienced podiatrist. The nail should not be cut shorter than the edge of the toe, and should be cut straight across and shaped according to the contour of the toe and adjacent nails. Lamb's wool or soft gauze should be placed between adjacent toes to prevent the development of so called "kissing ulcers" on adjacent toe surfaces. Diabetics should avoid wearing sandels or other open-end footwear and should never go barefoot. New shoes should be broken in gradually to prevent excessive foot trauma. Many diabetic patients develop anatomic foot deformities secondary to chronic neuropathy and require specially designed footwear. I rely heavily on my podiatric colleagues for their expertise in this regard.

Treatment of Early Lesions

Hyperkeratosis is a normal protective response of the foot to intermittent pressure and occurs in an exaggerated fashion in the diabetic, resulting in corn and callous formation. Once a corn forms it serves as a secondary focus of trauma on the deeper tissues and may result in an underlying hematoma, tissue breakdown, and eventual deep infection. The corn should be sharply trimmed with a scalpel, and the debridement should be limited to the nonvascular hyperkeratotic tissue. Once it is trimmed, U-shaped pads should be applied to minimize the pressure forces responsible for the development of the corn. The anatomic deformities that occur in the diabetic foot from longstanding neuropathy predispose to callous formation over the metatarsal heads. Although the pain caused by these callouses will lead the nondiabetic patient to seek medical attention early, in the neuropathic diabetic foot the lesion may go essentially unnoticed, leading to sub-keratotic hematoma formation, ulceration, the development of a sinus tract, and potentially limb-threatening infection. Therefore, these callouses should be aggressively trimmed down to the level of viable skin and podiatric consultation obtained to help design footwear to minimize trauma to the metatarsal heads. Usually the application of a metatarsal bar to the shoe and/or a molded fitted insole will prevent recurrence of these callouses. In the foot with severe structural deformities such as hammertoes, orthopedic surgical consultation may be necessary.

Incurved or ingrown toenails usually result from improper nail trimming and may lead to serious invasive infection in the diabetic foot. An inwardly curving lateral nail edge causes irritation and inflammation in the underlying toe with the repeated trauma of walking. In this situation cotton should be placed beneath the nail edge after gently removing the underlying debris. If the nail edge is sharp, it may actually penetrate the lateral nail groove leading to a localized cellulitis or purulent collection. The nail edge must be excised. The patient should be treated with a broad-spectrum oral antibiotic (Keflex, 500 mg four times a day) and povidone-iodine soaks, and followed closely until resolution.

Toe and foot ulcers that are small (less than 2 cm in diameter), superficial (no exposed bone), uninfected, and occurring in a nonischemic foot may be managed on an outpatient basis, at least initially. In addition to the general principles of foot care discussed previously, obviously necrotic tissue should be sharply debrided after sterile prep. I treat clean ulcers with a Neosporin or Bacitracin ointment and dry sterile dressing changed three times daily. If superficial crusting is present, normal saline wet-to-dry dressings are applied four times a day. These patients should be instructed to look for signs of infection or progression of tissue breakdown and should be seen in the office at least on a weekly basis. A thorough arterial examination with Doppler pressure measurements is mandatory, and if arterial perfusion is compromised, inpatient management is advised (to be discussed).

Heel ulcers are an exception. The subcutaneous fat tissue deep to the skin of the heel provides almost no barrier to the spread of infection or the extension of necrosis. Once the deep tissues are violated, the necrotic process quickly extends to the calcaneous. Therefore, unless signs of deep infection are present, I avoid debriding the eschar over a heel ulcer. With adequate perfusion and proper heel padding, these lesions slowly heal without requiring aggressive surgical debridement.

INPATIENT MANAGEMENT

Superficial ulcers that are not improving with outpatient management, ulcers occurring in the foot with arterial compromise, and invasive infection are absolute indications for hospitalization of the diabetic patient.

Ischemic Foot Ulcers

The diabetic patient with a nonhealing foot ulcer should be placed on strict bed rest in the reverse Trendelenburg position unless there is superimposed infection. The foot should be protected from further pressure-induced injury by using a soft gauze heel pad and lamb's wool between the toes. The ulcer should be debrided and any drainage sent for Gram stain and culture. I favor povidone-iodine wet-to-dry dressings to continue the debriding process. Foot roentgenograms are recommended to look for evidence of osteomyelitis. Radiologic signs of bone involvement include periosteal elevation, bone rarefaction, and new bone formation. I treat these patients with minidose heparin, 5,000 units subcutaneously every 12 hours, to prevent the development of venous thromboembolic disease. Noninvasive vascular laboratory testing should be performed at presentation to objectively assess the patient's arterial perfusion. I use the Doppler ultrasound flow probe to measure segmental limb pressures, quantitate the overall severity of the ischemia, localize the anatomic level of arterial obstruction, and predict the likelihood of ulcer healing (Table 2). In general, the diabetic patient requires a somewhat higher level of Doppler ankle pressure to attain healing than the nondiabetic owing to the presence of small vessel arterial occlusive disease and/or because ankle pressures may be artifactually elevated in diabetics as a result of tibial vessel calcification.

If arterial perfusion appears inadequate to promote healing, or when no clinical improvement is noted after a 7- to 10-day hospital course, I recommend proceeding with diagnostic arteriography. Diabetics are especially prone to the development of contrast-induced renal failure, and intravenous hydration prior to the arteriogram is the single most important factor in preventing this serious complication. In a patient with pre-existent renal dysfunction, the use of intra-arterial digital subtraction angio-

TABLE 2 Likelihood of Foot Ulcer Healing (normotensive patient)

	Likely	Probable	Unlikely
Doppler ankle pressure (mm Hg)	>90	80–90	<80

graphy is an excellent method for obtaining high quality studies with a minimal dye load. The nonhealing foot ulcer in the ischemic diabetic foot is a truly limb-threatening lesion, and I recommend early aggressive surgical revascularization in this setting in order to effect healing, or at least to lower the ultimate amputation level.

Neuropathic Ulcer (Mal Perforans)

Deep ulceration on the plantar aspect of the foot at the level of one or several metatarsal heads, the mal perforans ulcer, is a characteristic lesion in the diabetic foot. Although small-vessel disease may play a minor contributory role, usually these patients have easily palpable pedal pulses, and unless osteomyelitis is already established, these ulcers should heal with proper wound care. The exuberant callous and necrotic ulcer edges are sharply debrided just to viable tissue. The ulcers are cultured and treated with povidone-iodine wet-to-dry dressings, changed three times daily. I keep these patients on strict bed rest for several days, until evidence of ulcer healing is noted. Once signs of healing are evident, the patient may become ambulatory and be discharged to his home. It is of crucial importance, however, to make certain that the patient's footwear has been examined by a podiatrist and proper insole support constructed to eliminate the cause of this callous and ulcer formation.

When bone or joint space is exposed at the base of the ulcer, osteomyelitis is very likely. Bone involvement is more likely when neuropathic ulcers present with complicating cellulitis or frank abscess formation. Plain films of the foot are obtained to look for signs of osteomyelitis, although these films may be negative when bone involvement is early. A bone scan is a much more sensitive indicator of early osteomyelitis than is the plain x-ray film.

Unfortunately, many of the radiographic changes seen on both plain film and bone scan in osteomyelitis are similar to the bony abnormalities that occur in the chronically neuropathic foot. Therefore, osteomyelitis as a complication of a neuropathic ulcer is frequently a clinical diagnosis. If an ulcer sinus tract persists in a foot with normal arterial perfusion despite maximal supportive therapy or, as is more commonly the case, the ulcer heals only to recur several weeks later, the overwhelming odds are that the metatarsal head is infected. In rare cases the surgeon may effect a cure by performing a local currettage of the exposed bone. However, when this approach fails to effect permanent healing, resection of the involved toe and metatarsal head will be necessary (to be discussed). I have seen little success with long-term (4 to 6 weeks) intravenous antibiotic treatment of metatarsal osteomyelitis in the diabetic foot, which is advocated by some authors.

Infection

Cellulitis in the diabetic foot is an urgent indication for hospital admission. The foot must be carefully examined for signs of undrained infection and plain films obtained to look for pockets of air suggestive of deep sepsis. Ulcers should be sharply unroofed, ingrown toenails excised, and Gram stain and cultures obtained. The patient should be placed at strict bed rest with the affected foot elevated unless there is also an element of arterial ischemia, which can be documented with Doppler examination. Since infection may spread rapidly in the diabetic foot, I recommend initial treatment with intravenous antibiotics. In the absence of abscess formation or signs of lymphangitis, I use a cephalosporin. Improvement, documented by reduced pain, swelling, and erythema and by a falling white blood cell count, should be noted in 24 to 48 hours. If there is no significant improvement, I usually add an aminoglycoside (checking creatinine and blood urea nitrogen levels every other day). Failure of cellulitis in the diabetic foot to respond to this regimen is indicative of loculated infection that must be identified and drained. If the patient responds to this initial regimen, I continue the intravenous antibiotics for 5 days and then switch to an oral agent such as Keflex and begin ambulation. If there is no exacerbation of the cellulitic process with ambulation, the patient may be discharged to his home to complete an additional 5 days of oral antibiotic therapy.

Plantar Abscess

Abscess formation in the diabetic foot, manifested by fluctuance, plantar tenderness, and evidence of spread along the tendon sheaths, is a true surgical emergency requiring immediate drainage and debridement in the operating room. A common misconception is that diabetic foot infections should be drained through limited incisions since healing potential is limited. I strongly disagree. Undrained or inadequately drained infection in the diabetic foot rapidly spreads along the tendon sheaths and deep plantar spaces, resulting in necrosis and a high likelihood of eventual limb loss. The involved area should be widely opened along its entire extent by means of a longitudinal incision since transverse incisions tend to devitalize more tissue. Probing along the exposed tendon sheaths with a blunt instrument helps to define the extent of infection. The incision must be so designed as to promote dependent drainage with the patient at bed rest in the supine position.

Following the drainage procedure, I manage these patients with povidone-iodine wet-to-dry dressings changed four times daily to continue the debriding process. Frequent wound checks and repetitive sharp debridements may be necessary. The adequacy of arterial perfusion should be documented with Doppler study and arteriography performed if perfusion is felt to be inadequate to effect healing. I prefer to wait 5 to 7 days, if possible, before proceeding with revascularization in this setting. If the circulation is not compromised at presentation, or following revascularization, the wound may be closed with a split-thickness skin graft or allowed to heal secondarily.

When diabetic foot infection is complicated by frank

gangrene at the time of presentation, the goal should be eradication of infection before definitive amputation is performed, since local infection may cause surrounding ischemic but viable tissue to become necrotic, thus extending the gangrenous process. If gangrene involves one or several toes or the distal forefoot, open transmetatarsal amputation (TMA) may be required as part of the initial drainage procedure. Once the sepsis is controlled, usually after 5 to 7 days of dressing changes and intravenous antibiotics, vascular reconstruction may be performed, if necessary, to effect healing at the transmetatarsal level. When gangrene and sepsis extend proximal to the metatarsal level at presentation, a guillotine amputation at the supramalleolar level is the most efficacious method of drainage in preparation for definitive below-knee amputation.

At the time of the initial drainage procedure, deep aerobic and anaerobic cultures should be obtained. Mixed bacteriologic species are usually responsible for the diabetic foot abscess. *Staphylococcus aureus*, enterococci, *Proteus* species, *Escherichia coli*, *Pseudomonas aeroginosa*, *Bacteroides* species, and other anaerobic gram-positive cocci are most frequently identified from these wounds. I favor "triple antibiotic therapy" in the initial management of a diabetic plantar abscess, usually penicillin, an aminoglycoside, and clindamycin. Later changes in antibiotic coverage are dictated by the deep culture results and the response to therapy. Antibiotics are usually continued for a full 7-day course.

Amputation

Transmetatarsal amputation of one, several, or all five toes was initially introduced and continues to be most useful for the management of the diabetic patient with neuropathic metatarsal head ulceration or toe gangrene extending proximal to the proximal phalynx. Extension of skin necrosis, dependent rubor, or cellulitis to the intended level of skin incision makes healing of a TMA unlikely. In my opinion, the presence of pulsatile flow at the metatarsal level, as determined by the pulse volume recorder, by the mercury strain-gauge system, or by photoplethysmography, is the most objective evidence to predict healing at this level. Segmental pressure determinations are much less reliable, particularly in the diabetic in whom arterial medial calcinosis may yield spuriously high ankle pressure measurements.

Meticulous surgical technique is just as important as arterial blood supply in ensuring healing of a TMA. When the first or fifth toe is to be removed, I use a racquet-type incision at the base of the toe, being careful not to violate the adjacent joint space. The incision is extended proximally with a longer plantar flap so as to create a dorsal incision that will not be on the weight-bearing surface. The bone is cleared of surrounding tissue, transected well proximally, and rongeured smooth so as to avoid pressure on the skin flaps. The wound is closed with interrupted 4–0 nylon sutures, and I rarely use a drain. The same approach may be used for adjacent two-toe TMAs.

In performing a full five-toe TMA, the plantar incision is performed 1 cm proximal to the web space, perpendicular to the skin, and carried down directly to bone. Care must be taken to avoid undermining the skin. The dorsal incision is made at the mid-tarsal level to create a total plantar flap. A neurotrophic plantar skin ulcer may be excised with a proximal wedge-shaped extension of the plantar incision. A single layer closure with widely spaced 4–0 nylon sutures minimizes skin trauma and allows for serous drainage between the sutures. Forceps are never used on the skin! A bulky dressing is loosely applied and not removed for 48 to 72 hours unless severe pain (suggestive of ischemia) or signs of sepsis develop. Postoperatively, the patient is kept on strict bed rest for up to 21 days to ensure healing, and sutures remain in place for 4 weeks.

When a TMA is not feasible, fails to heal, or following a guillotine amputation of the foot for sepsis, a below-knee amputation is strongly recommended to maximize the chance of successfully rehabilitating the diabetic patient. I utilize a long posterior myocutaneous flap. The tibia is divided and carefully bevelled anteriorly, and the fibula divided 2 cm higher than the tibia to prevent pressure on the subcutaneous blood flow after wound closure. The tibial nerve should be sharply divided as far proximally as possible after ligating with an absorbable suture to minimize the likelihood of painful neuroma formation. Hemostasis is obtained with absorbable suture material and must be meticulous. The musculofascial layer is closed with interrupted absorbable sutures and the skin with interrupted 4–0 nylon stitches. No instruments should be used on the skin. With appropriate attention to hemostasis, a drain is not necessary. The stump is wrapped in a fluffy dressing and a posterior plaster splint carefully applied and secured with an Ace-wrap to prevent the development of a flexion contracture during the early postoperative course.

The primary dressing is left intact for 5 days unless signs of sepsis such as fever, elevation of the leukocyte count, or severe pain suggestive of ischemia are noted. During the first week, quadriceps strengthening exercises are encouraged. The splint is removed at 7 days, after which range-of-motion exercises may begin if the stump appears healthy. Bed rest is maintained for the first week and minidose heparin employed for venous thrombosis prophylaxis. At 10 days the patient begins crutch walking. At 4 weeks the sutures are removed and thereafter a temporary prosthesis is fashioned.

LOWER EXTREMITY VARICOSITIES

SESHADRI RAJU, M.D.

"Varicosities" are among the oldest diseases known to man, having been described prior to biblical times. By common usage, the term has come to signify a broad variety of pathologic conditions that present with dilated veins on the skin surface. Even some cutaneous nevi with dilated venular components are referred to as "varicosities" by some patients. For purposes of this discussion, a broad definition will be used to cover chronic insufficiency of the deep, as well as superficial, venous systems of the lower extremity. It should be noted that not all patients with chronic venous insufficiency present primarily with varicosities (Table 1), even though varices may be present on close examination.

CLASSIFICATION

By longstanding convention, varicosities of the lower limb are classified as primary or secondary. Primary varicosities were thought to represent a dysfunction of the superficial venous system, often from genetic predisposition, with anatomically and functionally intact deep veins. In contrast, secondary varicosities were thought to arise from abnormalities in the deep venous system, usually obstruction or reflux, due to previous phlebitic episodes in the deep veins. It has been well documented by several authors that only a minority of patients with deep venous reflux give a history consistent with previous phlebitis. Even though many of these patients might have been victims of silent deep venous thrombosis, it is likely that deep valve reflux of a developmental nature is a significant etiologic factor not sufficiently appreciated previously. The etiology of "primary" superficial varicosities had been explained on the basis of sapheno-femoral valve incompetence of congenital nature (Trendelenburg school) or due to incompetence of the perforator valves (Linton school), allowing the high venous pressure in the deep system during calf systole to be transmitted to the superficial veins. Cockett later helped to further popularize the latter concept. Since there is no morphologic difference between the sapheno-femoral and perforator valves on the one hand, and other venous valves in both varicose and normal extremities, such theories based on selective insufficiency of a single or small group of valves located at specific anatomic sites had always sounded somewhat implausible. With modern laboratory and phlebographic techniques, it can now be shown that even though reflux dysfunction of specific valves at specific sites may be more prominent than that of others, reflux in the all-important deep venous valves occurs to a greater or lesser extent in the overwhelming majority of patients with venous insufficiency. Thus, the distinction between "superficial" and "deep" venous insufficiency and again between "primary" and "secondary" varicosities is not so clear-cut as previously thought.

VENOUS HEMODYNAMICS

Patients presenting with venous insufficiency should undergo a detailed history and examination to document symptomatology, work restriction, and the distribution and extent of the varicosities. A Trendelenburg test and a three-tourniquet test to localize perforator incompetence, when present, may be carried out; however, it is my practice to omit these maneuvers when a laboratory venous profile is ordered, since it provides the information sought in a more detailed fashion. The astute examiner should be wary of unusual causes of lower limb varicosities, such as arteriovenous fistula, Klippel-Trenaunay syndrome, and abdominal tumor compressing or invading the vena cava. Antithrombin-III deficiency can also produce varicosities from thrombosis and obstruction of major veins at an early age. Failure of varicosities to empty on leg elevation in the supine patient is usually a clue to the presence of an unusual etiology. Pregnancy produces exacerbation of varicosities, sometimes to a florid degree. Regression is seldom complete postpartum, however. Little can be done during the pregnant state except for reassurance and supportive measures, such as elevation and elastic stockings.

Many different techniques to assess venous hemodynamics have been described recently. The techniques used in my laboratory are listed in Table 2. Irrespective of the combination of techniques used, it should be emphasized that a thorough laboratory examination is a vital part of managing a patient with venous insufficiency or lower limb varicosities. Even patients with "familial" varicosities may have surprisingly severe dysfunction of the deep venous system when subjected to appropriate laboratory scrutiny. A well-executed Doppler venous examination can detect obstruction as well as reflux in the venous system with a fair degree of accuracy. It is particularly important to compare the findings with those in the opposite limb to appreciate subtle variations that are frequently the only indication of underlying disease. Additional embellishments of technique, such as compression maneuvers, can further help to identify reflux as well as obstruction. The photoplethysmograph (PPG) may be used interchangeably with ambulatory venous pressure measurement to provide a measure of reflux at the distal

TABLE 1 Presenting Symptoms in 147 Patients Tested for Suspected Venous Insufficiency

Primary Symptoms	Incidence (%)
Pain	10
Swelling	21
Ulcer	53
Discoloration	2
Varicosities	14

From Raju S. Venous insufficiency of the lower limb and stasis ulceration. Ann Surg 1983; 197:689.

TABLE 2 Techniques Used in the Laboratory for Venous Assessment

Doppler venous examination

Photoplethysmography (PPG)

or

Ambulatory venous pressure measurement

Valsalva foot venous pressure elevation*

Arm/foot venous pressure differential*

Reactive hyperemia-induced foot venous pressure measurement*

* Technique is carried out in the supine patient with the same venipuncture in the dorsum of the foot.

portions of the lower limb. I have found that the relatively simple technique of measuring elevation of foot venous pressure in the supine position during Valsalva provides a good indication of reflux for following patients undergoing surgery (normal less than 4 mm Hg elevation; reflux greater than 4 mm Hg). In my laboratory, measurement of arm and foot venous pressure at rest and with reactive hyperemia is utilized to detect overt as well as compensated venous obstruction.

With the foregoing laboratory examination, an objective measure of venous hemodynamics is available so that the severity of symptoms can be correlated with laboratory data. Clinicians attending patients with venous insufficiency problems would attest to the frequent overlay of functional symptoms in this patient group. Some patients facing socioeconomic pressures are looking for disability declarations on the basis of minimal underlying venous disease. The venous laboratory, if nothing else, helps to sort out these difficult clinical situations.

SELECTION OF PATIENTS

Phlebography is usually not necessary in patients for whom surgery is not contemplated. Patients with only mild derangement of venous hemodynamics, as determined in the laboratory, should be treated by conservative measures. Similarly, patients of advanced age who have lived with their venous dysfunction for years are not candidates for surgery. A limb is seldom lost due to stasis ulceration, but antitetanus prophylaxis should be prescribed for all such patients with ulceration treated conservatively. Patients with numerous and differing complaints of pain, even though severe in description, should not be treated surgically, especially when the objective hemodynamic data do not correspond with the symptomatology. The motivation of the patient in terms of rehabilitation and return to work should be carefully probed before surgery is offered when pain is a major presenting complaint. Patients with stasis dermatitis or ulceration are usually good candidates for surgery, as a successful outcome can be established per resolution and cure of the presenting condition. In my experience, swelling alone, without pain or ulceration, is an unsatisfactory indication for surgery, as swelling frequently exacerbates in the postoperative period. Patients do not generally appear to be bothered by the postoperative swelling when the relief of accompanying pain or stasis ulceration is achieved by surgical intervention. Except in young patients with obviously prominent varicosities, cosmetic considerations should not generally govern decisions for surgical intervention. Middle-aged women who focus their anxiety of gathering years on cutaneous nevi or other skin blemishes may be referred to a dermatologist specializing in laser therapy, as acceptable results are obtained with this technique.

SAPHENOUS VEIN STRIPPING

Subcutaneous varicosities, such as short and long saphenous varicose veins, seldom cause symptoms by themselves. The presence of pain, stasis skin changes, or swelling usually denotes accompanying deep venous insufficiency. Saphenous vein stripping is a logical surgical procedure when the presence of varicosities is a presenting complaint and venous testing shows only mild or moderate deep venous abnormalities. Since only a few patients fall into this category (see Table 1) in my practice, isolated saphenous vein stripping has become a relatively rare surgical procedure in our institution. When performed, the stripper should be passed up from the ankle and the vein stripped down from above. This sequence of maneuvers avoids injury to the saphenous nerve and prevents inadvertent stripping of the femoral artery.

For most patients with symptoms denoting deep venous dysfunction, even when varicosities are part of the symptom complex, it is our view that a valve reconstruction procedure is appropriate therapy, especially when objective laboratory data support moderate-to-severe deep-valve reflux. These patients should undergo ascending and descending phlebography. Ascending phlebography defines deep venous anatomy and reveals such pathologic conditions as obstruction and recanalization. Perforator incompetence can also be identified with appropriate modifications of technique. Descending venography delineates valve structure and demonstrates reflux when present. Reflux through the valve during Valsalva is particularly significant, as a normal valve is made completely competent by the Valsalva maneuver. Attention is especially focused on the uppermost valve in the superficial femoral vein, which is the easiest valve to repair.

TECHNIQUE OF SUPERFICIAL FEMORAL VEIN VALVULOPLASTY

Through a groin incision, the common femoral, superficial femoral, and deep femoral veins are carefully dissected out, freeing the tri-junction of smaller branches. The saphenofemoral junction should also be dissected out and ligated in continuity. In many patients, the veins and the adjacent tissue planes are clearly free of previous inflammatory process, providing further support to the belief that many of these patients have a congenital basis for their reflux. The uppermost valve in the superficial femoral vein is usually clearly identified on external inspection by the characteristic bulge. After systemic heparinization (10,000 units in adults), an atraumatic bulldog clamp is applied to the superficial femoral vein some distance below this valve, and the intervening vein segment is manually emptied by gentle stripping. The venous segment promptly fills by reflux from above, confirming the preoperative descending venographic finding. Further bulldog clamps are applied to the common femoral and deep femoral veins, and a transverse venotomy is placed some distance above the valve bulge, usually opposite the entrance of the profunda femoral vein. As the valve commissures are surprisingly higher than would be expected by external inspection, one should favor placing this incision in a more cephalad direction rather than risk inadvertent transection of the commissure. With the aid of good magnification and lighting and frequent irrigation of the field with ice-cold Ringer's lactate solution, the valve cusps can usually be identified without difficulty. Retraction of the cut edge with strategically placed 5–0 Prolene stay sutures, which can be later utilized for closing the venotomy, is mandatory for good exposure. Since the valve cusps are transparent and sometimes adhere to the periphery, diligent search with a blunt probe should be carried out to identify the valve cusps and define the anatomy. The most frequent anatomy is a redundant bicuspid valve, presenting with pleats and folds at the free edge. In most instances, no evidence of previous phlebitis can be discerned. Number 7–0 polyproplene sutures with the finest needle available are utilized to place commissural sutures. A double-needle suture is used, each needle utilized for gathering up the free edge of the valve cusp on either side of the commissure. The needles exit to the outside at the commissural attachment and the suture is tied on the outside vein wall. Enough valve cusp should be gathered by each suture, so that when both commissural sutures are tied, the opposing edges of the valve cusps will present as a sharp crescent. Usually, a fifth of the valve cusp edge at each commissure has to be gathered to achieve a satisfactory result. The valve cusps are surprisingly tough and take sutures well. With practice, a satisfactory result can be achieved with only one suture at each commissural end. Hand irrigation with ice-cold solution usually provides a reasonable picture of the opposing characteristics of the repaired valve cusp. The venotomy is next closed with the previously placed Prolene stay sutures in an interrupted fashion. A vital part of the procedure is the retesting of the competency of the valve by manual stripping, as described previously. *The valve should now be demonstrated to be competent by this technique*. If not, the valve should be re-explored and the repair improved. After completion of the procedure, the heparin is reversed with protamine, meticulous hemostasis is secured, and the wound is closed without drainage. The foot of the bed is elevated in the postoperative period, but the patient is ambulated the next day. Postoperative venous thrombosis, either at the site of venotomy or distally in the calf, is surprisingly rare, only three instances having been identified in my experience with over 75 valve reconstructive procedures. It was found that long-term postoperative anticoagulation of a mild degree (2.5 mg Coumadin per day) prevented postoperative episodes of acute limb edema previously seen without such anticoagulation. Pain relief after a successful procedure is dramatic, and stasis ulcerations usually heal spontaneously within a few weeks after surgery. In approximately 70 percent of operated patients, excellent to good results have been achieved, with a follow-up period ranging from 1 to 7 years. Follow-up should include periodic laboratory venous testing. Even though excellent symptomatic relief and resolution of stasis features are obtained, ambulatory venous pressure measurements are seldom completely normalized even though a 10- to 15-mm Hg improvement in postexercise ambulatory pressure is frequently obtained in most patients. Apparently, this degree of reduction is adequate for significant symptom relief in most patients. I have recently demonstrated that by employing the Valsalva technique for foot venous pressure measurement as an index of reflux, normalization of the high preoperative values can be obtained with valve reconstruction.

AXILLARY VEIN VALVE TRANSPLANT

In approximately 20 percent of the patients coming to surgery, a primary valvuloplasty procedure would be unsuitable, as the valve structure itself has been destroyed by previous phlebitis and recanalization. Many of these cases are evident preoperatively, and the ascending venogram gives the picture of recanalization with irregular channel size and contrast density. Descending venography usually reveals a reflux pattern without an identifiable valve apparatus in the superficial femoral vein region. Where there is no hemodynamic obstruction on venous testing, as evidenced by a normal arm/foot venous pressure differential (less than 4 mm Hg) and absence of significant foot venous pressure elevation on reactive hyperemia (less than 6 mm Hg), these patients can be considered for an axillary vein valve transplant. The technique has been described previously by me and by others. When the axillary segment is transposed in the superficial femoral vein, there is seldom a major size disparity problem. Owing to retraction of the divided superficial femoral vein, only one-half inch of this vein must be sacrificed to be replaced by one inch of valve-bearing axillary vein segment. Of course, the axillary vein valve should have been demonstrated to be competent in situ before excision and transfer. As I have previously reported, this valve sometimes is found to be incompetent, an indication of the global and developmental nature of the valve deformity. The transferred axillary vein valve should be enclosed in a snug 8- or 10-mm Dacron sleeve jacket to prevent late dilatation. Infection of the jacket has not occurred in our experience, even in instances in which re-exploration was carried out to evacuate a serum or lymph collection. I have also utilized the jacket principle in a few instances to enclose an in situ superficial femoral vein valve. Preoperative investigations had revealed reflux, but at surgical exploration the valve became competent when the superficial femoral vein contracted with manipulation. In such instances, a snug-fitting Dacron sleeve was applied without a formal valve repair, resulting in a successful outcome. I use a modified Linton procedure in the relatively rare instance in which the superficial femoral vein valve is competent, but symptoms can be ascribed to incompetent popliteal valve and perforators. It is also used as a fall-back procedure when valvuloplasty or other types of reconstruction have subsequently failed. In terms of surgical trauma inflicted and postoperative complications and morbidity, the modified Linton procedure is clearly inferior to primary valve reconstruction; hence, the reluctance to use it more often, as some have advocated, in place of valvuloplasty.

DALE PROCEDURE

The results of treatment for hemodynamic venous obstruction in the lower extremity are unsatisfactory. In the relatively rare patient in whom tumor or trauma has resulted in segmental venous obstruction, good results may be obtained by employing the Dale procedure, which utilizes the saphenous vein to perform a femorofemoral vein bypass to reroute blood flow around a venous obstruction. In my experience, symptomatic relief is less satisfactory in patients with postphlebitic obstruction, even though acceptable patency rates can be obtained with this technique. Several centers, including ours, are currently engaged in evaluating stented PTFE grafts to bypass obstruction in the venous system. Adequate follow-up data have not yet been generated to recommend this new prosthetic device for wider use.

VENOUS THROMBOSIS

ROBERT W. BARNES, M.D.

Venous thrombosis ("thrombophlebitis" is a misnomer except in superficial venous thrombosis) may result in five clinical syndromes, and these require accurate diagnosis to permit appropriate therapy. *Acute deep vein thrombosis* (DVT) refers to the initial clinical episode of thrombosis of the deep veins of the upper and lower extremities or the vena cavae. *Recurrent deep vein thrombosis* refers to repeated episodes of venous thrombosis in a patient with a past history of clinical DVT. *Superficial thrombophlebitis* refers to venous thrombosis involving the superficial veins of the upper or lower extremities or the torso. The *post-thrombotic syndrome* ("postphlebitic" syndrome, venous stasis, chronic venous insufficiency) refers to the late sequelae of prior deep vein thrombosis with leg pain, swelling, brownish discoloration, and dermatitis with or without ulceration. *Pulmonary embolism* is the major complication of venous thrombosis and may be acute or recurrent with resultant chronic pulmonary hypertension.

These clinical syndromes are frequently misdiagnosed and mismanaged. Unfortunately, the bedside diagnosis of the venous thrombosis syndromes is notoriously inaccurate, seldom exceeding a sensitivity or specificity of 50 percent. For this reason, the clinician must employ objective diagnostic techniques. Invasive radiologic procedures including venography and pulmonary angiography remain the diagnostic standard. However, several noninvasive diagnostic techniques have been developed over the past 20 years to improve the clinician's diagnostic accuracy and to increase his awareness of the patho-physiology of acute and chronic venous disease. It is the purpose of this chapter to review some of these diagnostic advances and to provide my algorithms for the use of these techniques in planning therapeutic strategy.

PATHOPHYSIOLOGY

Venous thrombosis results in two major pathophysiologic sequelae: venous outflow obstruction and venous valvular incompetence. Venous obstruction results in the usual clinical manifestations of acute deep vein thrombosis, superficial thrombophlebitis, and pulmonary embolism. Venous valvular incompetence, with or without concomitant venous outflow obstruction, accounts for the symptoms of the post-thrombotic syndrome. Patients with recurrent deep vein thrombosis may suffer the recurrent effects of venous outflow obstruction if repeated attacks of venous thrombosis actually occur, but such patients often have symptoms due to chronic venous insufficiency associated with valvular incompetence.

Venous outflow obstruction results in distal venous hypertension in the extremity. Such venous hypertension results in the clinical manifestations of pain, edema, prominent superficial veins, and cyanotic discoloration of the skin. The symptoms are intensified by ambulation, and leg pain of venous origin may result in so-called venous claudication.

Venous valvular incompetence of the deep and communicating (perforating) veins leads to superficial venous hypertension during ambulation. Normally ambulation, with contraction of the calf muscles, results in decompression of the superficial veins, so-called ambulatory venous hypotension. In the presence of deep and communicating venous insufficiency, with or without venous outflow obstruction, superficial venous pressures may change little during ambulation, so-called ambulatory venous hypertension. The resultant increased venous pressures are transmitted to the capillary bed where extravasation of the red blood cells may lead to hemosiderin deposition in the skin, the so-called venous stasis hyperpigmentation in the post-thrombotic syndrome. Eventual tissue edema, hypoxia during ambulation, and superficial trauma may result in a chronic venous stasis ulcer.

DIAGNOSTIC TECHNIQUES

Doppler Ultrasound

A continuous-wave portable Doppler ultrasonic velocity detector, operating at 5 mHz, is useful to detect venous obstruction as well as valvular incompetence of the deep, communicating, and superficial veins of the upper and lower extremities. The technique depends on sound pattern recognition of normal and abnormal venous velocity signals. In experienced hands, an accuracy exceeding 95 percent may be achieved. The technique is the least expensive and the most versatile of the various noninvasive techniques. However, the accuracy is highly dependent on the skill and experience of the technologist or physician performing the test. An advantage of Doppler ultrasound is the fact that specific sites of the venous system may be studied to document the presence of venous obstruction and/or venous valvular incompetence. In addition, anatomic discrimination of superficial, communicating, and deep veins is possible with this device.

Ultrasonic Real-Time Imaging

High-resolution B-mode ultrasonic imaging of the venous system has recently been possible to permit visualization of venous thrombi and the integrity of venous valves. The technique is expensive and requires considerable experience on the part of the technologist to achieve adequate visualization of major deep and superficial veins. Combined technologies of B-mode imaging and Doppler ultrasound, so-called duplex scanning, permit both imaging and Doppler flow assessment of venous thrombosis and valvular insufficiency.

Venous Volume Plethysmography

The phleborheograph (PRG) permits recording of venous volumetric changes in the lower extremity using multiple pneumatic cuffs applied to the limb. Normal fluctuations in leg volume are attenuated in the presence of venous thrombosis. Furthermore, pneumatic compression of the distal limb results in acute increases in proximal limb volume in the presence of venous outflow obstruction. This plethysmographic device records objectively those changes noted on a routine venous Doppler examination. In experienced hands, the technique is the most accurate noninvasive method to detect venous thrombosis, with an accuracy exceeding 95 percent in some reported series.

Venous Outflow Plethysmography

Calf volumetric changes after deflation of a proximal veno-occlusive thigh pneumatic cuff may be recorded with a variety of transducers, including a strain gauge (SPG), impedance electrodes (IPG), or pneumatic cuff (PVR). Proximal venous thrombosis of the popliteal, femoral, iliac, or caval venous system may result in attenuation of venous outflow recorded by one of these methods. In experienced hands, the sensitivity of venous outflow plethysmography is greater than 90 percent. The techniques are limited by their insensitivity to isolated calf vein thrombosis.

Venous Reflux Plethysmography

Noninvasive assessment of altered venous hemodynamics in patients with chronic venous insufficiency may be recorded with strain-gauge plethysmographic (SPG) or photoplethysmographic (PPG) techniques. Normally the calf venous volume decreases approximately 2 percent in response to erect leg muscle exercise. In the presence of chronic venous insufficiency, such volumetric changes are attenuated, and the recovery time to baseline is accelerated. The photoplethysmograph is particularly useful to record altered skin blood content changes in the presence of chronic venous insufficiency. Using in vivo calibration techniques, the PPG may permit noninvasive indirect assessment of ambulatory venous pressures in patients with the post-thrombotic syndrome.

125I Fibrinogen Uptake Test

Human 125I-labeled fibrinogen may be injected intravenously to detect sites of active venous thrombosis by means of external scintillation counting techniques. The fibrinogen uptake test is extremely sensitive to active calf vein thrombosis or thrombosis in the distal thigh. The technique is useful to screen patients for suspected recurrent deep vein thrombosis. Because of the expense and time required for the test, the technique is not suitable for routine diagnosis for patients presenting with acute deep vein thrombosis. The technique is also limited by its insensitivity to venous thrombosis other than the active stage of the disease. Finally the technique does not detect proximal thigh or iliac venous thrombi.

Radionuclide Phlebography

The major deep veins of the lower extremities from the popliteal veins upward may be rapidly imaged using technetium-99m injected intravenously in a superficial vein of the foot or ankle. The isotope may be visualized as it ascends the venous system using a gamma camera. The isotope, if labeled on human albumin, may be subsequently used to obtain a perfusion lung scan. Radionuclide phlebography has the advantages of being painles on injection and providing excellent imaging of the iliac veins and vena cava. The technique is not suitable for discriminating isolated calf vein thrombi.

Contrast Phlebography

Contrast phlebography (venography) remains the diagnostic standard to evaluate venous thrombosis. The technique provides excellent visualization of the calf veins provided appropriate techniques are used. The femoropopliteal venous system is usually well visualized. However, the iliac veins and inferior vena cava may not be adequately visualized with peripheral injections unless digital subtraction techniques are used. Separate femoral venous injections may be required to adequately visualize the central venous system. The technique suffers the limitations of expense, irritation of conventional contrast media, and nonportability.

Table 1 summarizes the attributes of various venous diagnostic techniques.

THERAPEUTIC OPTIONS

Anticoagulation

Intravenous heparin therapy remains the treatment of choice for most patients with acute or proven recurrent deep vein thrombosis as well as patients suffering pulmonary embolism. Continuous intravenous administration is preferred with an initial bolus of 5,000 U followed by continuous infusion of 1,000 to 1,500 U per hour to achieve prolongation of the activated partial thromboplastin time to approximately twice the control value. Patients with active deep vein thrombosis or pulmonary embolism may require larger amounts of heparin, up to 3,000 U per hour, to achieve therapeutic prolongation of the partial thromboplastin time. After several days, the heparin dosage usually must be reduced as the thrombotic process is controlled. Heparin should be maintained for at least 7 to 10 days. During the final 4 or 5 days of heparin therapy, concomitant administration of oral sodium warfarin (Coumadin) may be instituted.

Fibrinolysis

Patients with recent onset of proven acute deep vein thrombosis of less than 5 days duration may be treated with fibrinolytic agents, provided there is no surgical or medical contraindication to such therapy. In my own experience, most patients with venous thrombosis either have had clinical evidence of disease for more than 5 days or have some recent surgical or medical problem that contraindicates therapeutic fibrinolysis.

Anti-inflammatory Agents

Anti-inflammatory agents have no role in the treatment of acute or recurrent deep vein thrombosis. However, superficial thrombophlebitis is preferentially treated with nonsteroidal inflammatory agents such as ibuprofen or indomethacin. Heparin therapy does not seem to alter the inflammatory course of superficial thrombophlebitis, but is indicated if concomitant deep vein thrombosis is present.

Surgical Therapy

Venous thrombectomy is rarely performed because of the frequent recurrence of venous thrombosis after this procedure. An exception to this is the patient with impending venous gangrene (phlegmasia cerulea dolens) in whom venous thrombectomy may provide temporary venous decompression of the lower limb to prevent tissue loss or amputation.

An inferior vena cava filter (Greenfield) is recommended for patients who have proven acute or recurrent

TABLE 1   Characteristics of Diagnostic Techniques in Venous Disease

Technique	Simplicity	Portability	Objectivity	Inexpensiveness	Sensitivity Proximal	Calf	Specificity
Doppler	+	+	0	+	+	±	±
B-mode imaging	0	±	+	0	+	±	+
Volume plethysmography	0	±	+	0	+	±	±
Outflow plethysmography	±	±	+	±	+	0	±
Reflux plethysmography	±	±	+	±	+	+	+
^{125}I fibrinogen	±	+	+	±	±	+	±
Isotope venography	±	0	+	0	+	0	±
Contrast venography	0	0	+	0	+	+	+

+ = good   ± = fair   0 = poor

deep vein thrombosis or pulmonary embolism in whom anticoagulants are contraindicated or are associated with hemorrhagic complications during the course of therapy. The preferred route of insertion is via the right internal jugular vein, and the filter is discharged just caudad to the renal veins. In selected instances, the filter may be placed above the renal veins in patients with renal vein thrombosis and associated pulmonary embolism or in whom a thrombotic complication of a previous intracaval device has occurred. The advantage of the Greenfield filter is that the device is associated with a low incidence of caval thrombosis (less than 5%). Furthermore, if an embolus is trapped by the filter, continued blood flow around the thrombus is possible because of the conical configuration of the device. Such trapped thrombi may be lysed if caval thrombosis does not occur.

Pulmonary embolectomy is reserved for patients who have life-threatening massive pulmonary emboli that do not respond to vigorous medical management including fibrinolytic therapy. Such patients may undergo transvenous suction pulmonary embolectomy with a catheter developed by Greenfield and may require concomitant partial circulatory support. If the patient requires partial cardiopulmonary bypass, an open pulmonary embolectomy is recommended.

Prophylaxis

Primary prophylaxis to prevent deep vein thrombosis in high-risk patients is controversial. I recommend low-dose subcutaneous heparin therapy, 5,000 U every 8 to 12 hours, for patients with previous proven deep vein thrombosis who are undergoing major operative procedures. For orthopaedic patients, I recommend intravenous low-molecular-weight dextran, 1,000 cc during the course of the operation and then 1,000 cc for the 2 successive postoperative days. Alternatively, sequential pneumatic compression of the lower extremities is recommended for patients undergoing hip or knee joint replacement.

Secondary prophylaxis of patients treated with heparin therapy for acute or recurrent deep vein thrombosis involves oral warfarin (Coumadin) for 3 to 6 months after the onset of thrombosis. Oral anticoagulants are administered in a dosage to prolong the prothrombin time approximately 1.3 times control values. This lower-dosage regimen has been shown to be as effective as the previous higher-dose therapy and is associated with a reduced risk of bleeding complications.

CLINICAL SYNDROMES

I use diagnostic and therapeutic algorithms for patients with venous thrombosis syndromes. The following section reviews the application of these algorithms for the management of patients with venous disease.

Acute Deep Vein Thrombosis

Figure 1 shows the diagnostic algorithm for patients with suspected acute deep vein thrombosis. Unless contraindicated, intravenous heparin therapy is started while the diagnostic work-up proceeds. If available, noninvasive studies should be performed to screen for the presence or absence of venous obstruction. I rely on Doppler venous evaluation by an experienced technologist. Alternatively, venous outflow plethysmography, phleborheography, or radionuclide phlebography could be used for such screening. If the noninvasive study is unequivocally normal, the heparin is discontinued and the patient is evaluated for another cause of symptoms mimicking venous thrombosis. However, if isolated calf vein thrombi are suspected on the basis of clinical manifestations, a venogram is recommended because of the fallibility of noninvasive techniques in detecting isolated calf clots. If the noninvasive study is abnormal, the patient may be treated for deep vein thrombosis unless a concomitant clinical condition is present that may lead to a false-positive noninvasive study. Such conditions as malignant tumor, trauma, or a possible ruptured Baker's cyst should prompt the clinician to order a venogram to prove whether the noninvasive study was falsely positive. If the noninvasive study is equivocal, a venogram is recommended to clarify the diagnosis.

Figure 2 depicts the therapeutic approach to a patient with proven acute deep vein thrombosis. If the patient has threatened venous gangrene (phlegmasia cerulea dolens), venous thrombectomy is performed to decompress the venous circulation. A concomitant inferior vena cava filter is inserted, and anticoagulant therapy is then instituted. If the limb is not threatened with gangrene, thrombolysis may be considered if the thrombosis is of recent (<5 days) onset and there are no contraindications to fibrinolytic therapy. In my own experience, thrombolysis is seldom practical. Unless contraindicated, intravenous heparin therapy is instituted, as already outlined. Heparin is continued for 7 to 10 days and overlapped with warfarin therapy during the final 5 days of treatment. Once the prothrombin time has been prolonged to 1.3 times control, heparin is discontinued and warfarin is maintained for 6 weeks to 6 months, depending on the predisposing factors to recurrent venous thrombosis. If complications occur while the patient is on heparin therapy, such as bleeding or a pulmonary embolus despite adequate heparin therapy, a Greenfield inferior vena caval filter is inserted. If heparin therapy is contraindicated and proximal deep vein thrombosis involving the popliteal veins or higher is present, an inferior vena caval filter is inserted. If isolated calf vein thrombi are present, the patient is observed with repeated Doppler examinations, and a Greenfield filter is inserted only if the thrombosis extends into the popliteal veins or higher.

Recurrent Deep Vein Thrombosis

Figure 3 depicts the diagnostic and therapeutic algorithm for managing patients with clinically suspected

SUSPECT ACUTE DEEP VEIN THROMBOSIS

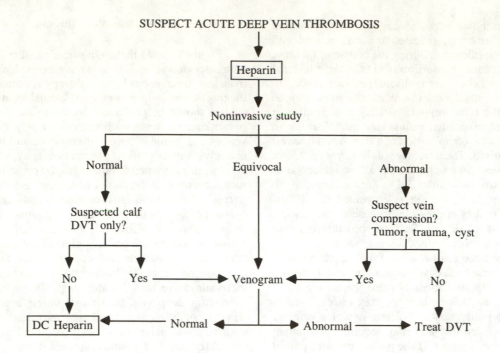

Figure 1 Algorithm for diagnostic evaluation of patients with suspected acute deep vein thrombosis.

recurrent deep vein thrombosis. A noninvasive study is initially performed to confirm the presence of venous disease and the relative contribution of obstruction and venous incompetence. If the noninvasive study is normal, another diagnosis should be suspected and appropriately evaluated. Most patients with suspected recurrent venous thrombosis have patent but incompetent deep veins, suggesting old venous thrombosis with recannalization and valvular destruction. Such patients may be treated for the post-thrombotic syndrome with leg elevation, elastic support, and other measures to control chronic venous insufficiency. I do not recommend anticoagulation for such patients. If venous obstruction is documented, the diagnosis is ambiguous because the clinician must know whether the obstruction represents recent active thrombosis or old venous occlusion due to previous thrombosis. If available, a radioactive iodine fibrinogen uptake test may be used to clarify the diagnosis. If this test is not available, a venogram is recommended to identify fresh clot outlined by contrast material, which is the hallmark of recurrent active venous thrombosis. Patients with such evidence of recent venous thrombosis are given anticoagulant therapy with heparin, followed by secondary prophylaxis with sodium warfarin. If no evidence of recent thrombosis is seen, and the obstruction appears to be chronic, the patient is treated for the post-thrombotic syndrome without anticoagulants.

Superficial Thrombophlebitis

The patient presenting with symptoms and signs of superficial thrombophlebitis presents a diagnostic dilemma because such symptoms may be confused with those of lymphangitis or cellulitis (Fig. 4). If a predisposing varicosity is obviously thrombosed, the diagnosis is not in question. However, if the patient only manifests redness, inflammation, and tenderness along the course of a superficial vein, lymphangitis may be present which mimics superficial thrombophlebitis. For such patients, a venous Doppler study is the most definitive method to clarify the diagnosis. If normal venous flow signals are established in the inflamed area, lymphangitis or cellulitis is the most probable diagnosis, and the patient is treated with antibiotics, usually penicillin. However, if venous thrombosis is indicated by Doppler examination, the diagnosis of superficial thrombophlebitis is confirmed. If the process extends near the saphenofemoral junction, the Doppler examination should clarify the status of the deep veins. If the deep veins are also thrombosed, the patient should be treated for deep vein thrombosis with anticoagulation. However, if the deep veins are patent, I recommend ligation of the saphenofemoral junction under local anesthesia to prevent the thrombosis from extending into the deep veins. If the superficial thrombophlebitis does not approach the saphenofemoral junction, I recommend nonsteroidal anti-inflammatory agents to treat superficial thrombophlebitis.

Postthrombotic Syndrome

Figure 5 shows the diagnostic and therapeutic algorithm for patients with suspected postthrombotic syndrome. A noninvasive study is recommended to evaluate the relative contribution of obstruction or

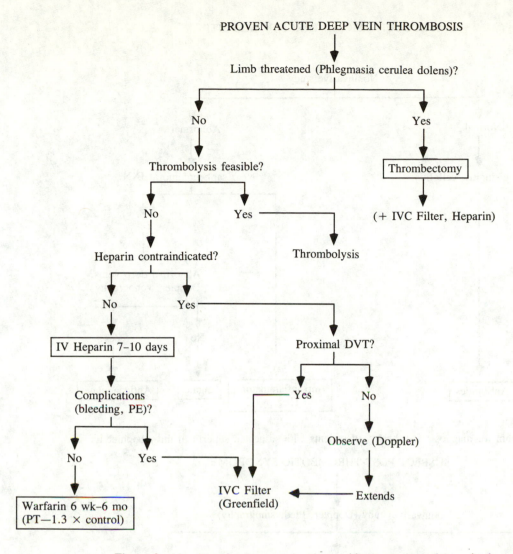

PROVEN ACUTE DEEP VEIN THROMBOSIS

Figure 2 Algorithm for therapy of patients with proven acute deep vein thrombosis.

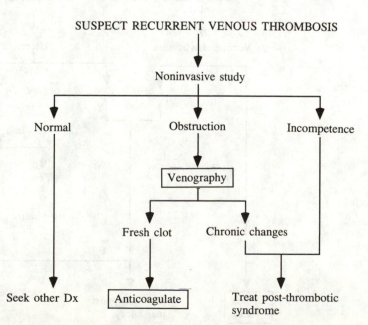

SUSPECT RECURRENT VENOUS THROMBOSIS

Figure 3 Algorithm for diagnosis and therapy of patients with suspected recurrent deep vein thrombosis.

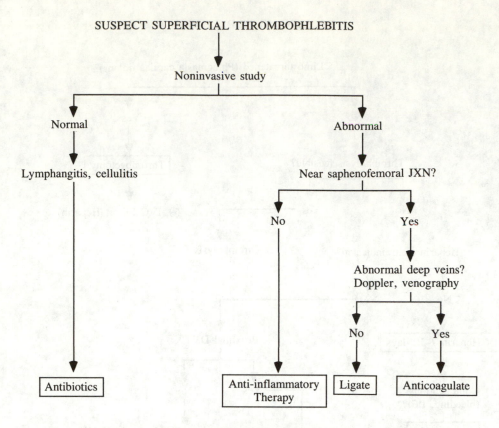

Figure 4   Algorithm for diagnosis and therapy of patients with suspected superficial thrombophlebitis.

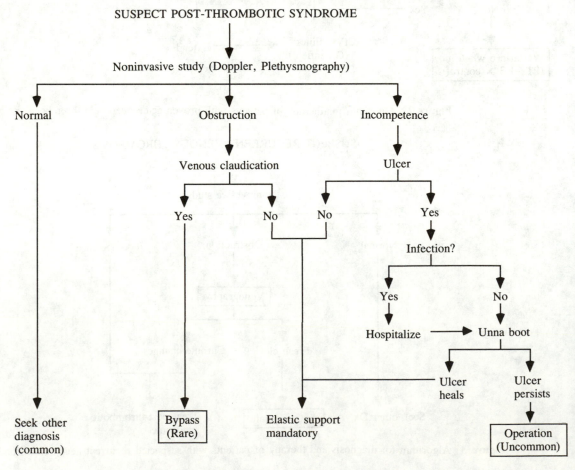

Figure 5   Algorithm for diagnosis and therapy of patients with suspected post-thrombotic syndrome.

incompetence in patients with venous disease. Occasionally the noninvasive study is normal, and the clinical manifestations of leg pain, swelling, and pigmentation may reflect a condition mimicking venous insufficiency, such as contact dermatitis, chronic congestive heart failure, vasculitis, or collagen vascular disease. If the patient manifests primary deep venous obstruction, venous claudication usually can be managed by conventional measures. If venous claudication becomes a limitation to the patient, venous bypass procedures occasionally may be performed, although these remain of limited efficacy.

For primary valvular incompetence in the absence of venous stasis ulceration, elastic support therapy usually suffices to control symptoms. The patient with a grossly infected ulcer may have to be hospitalized with leg elevation and antibiotic therapy. Once the ulcer is relatively clean and uninfected, ambulatory therapy with a medicated bandage (Unna boot) may be instituted. This support bandage usually permits healing of the ulceration. If it persists, excision and grafting or ligation of incompetent communicating (perforating) veins may be recommended. Surgical reconstruction of venous valves or transposition of valve-bearing segments into the venous system remains an experimental approach for the control of chronic venous insufficiency.

Pulmonary Embolism

Figure 6 depicts the diagnostic algorithm for evaluating a patient with suspected pulmonary embolism. The patient is initially given anticoagulant therapy with heparin, and a ventilation-perfusion lung scan is obtained. Because of the high sensitivity of lung scanning, a normal study virtually rules out a pulmonary embolus, and heparin therapy may be discontinued in such patients. If the ventilation-perfusion lung scan is abnormal, the diagnosis of pulmonary embolism may still be in question because of the poor specificity of lung scans. I recommend a noninvasive venous study to define a potential source of pulmonary embolism in the extremities. If the noninvasive study is abnormal, the patient may be appropriately treated for pulmonary embolus. However, if the noninvasive study is normal, a pulmonary arteriogram is recommended to clarify the diagnosis.

Figure 7 depicts the therapeutic algorithm for management of patients with proven pulmonary embolism. If the patient has class IV embolus with persistent shock despite intensive medical management for massive embolism, an embolectomy using a Greenfield suction catheter or open pulmonary embolectomy is recommended. Such patients should have concomitant

SUSPECT PULMONARY EMBOLISM

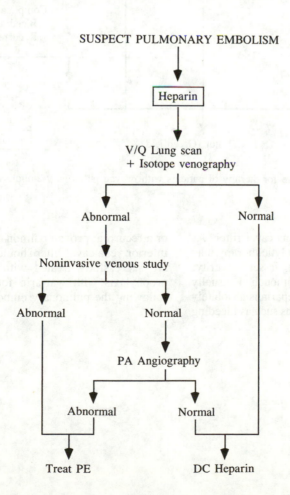

Figure 6 Algorithm for diagnostic evaluation of patients with suspected pulmonary embolism.

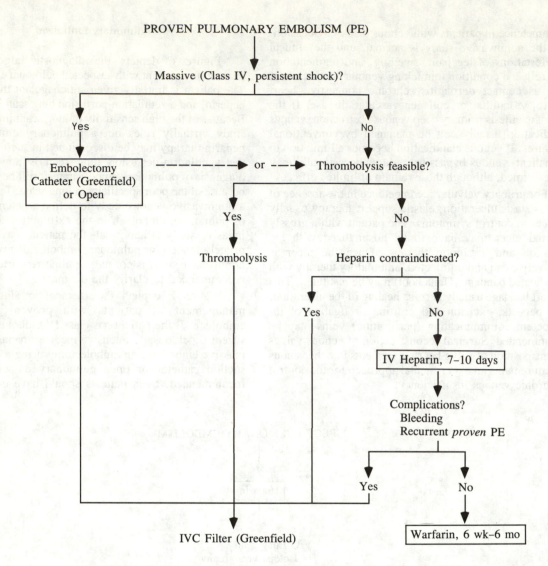

PROVEN PULMONARY EMBOLISM (PE)

Massive (Class IV, persistent shock)?

Yes — Embolectomy Catheter (Greenfield) or Open

or → Thrombolysis feasible?

No — Heparin contraindicated?

Yes — Thrombolysis

No — IV Heparin, 7–10 days

Complications?
Bleeding
Recurrent *proven* PE

Yes — IVC Filter (Greenfield)

No — Warfarin, 6 wk–6 mo

Figure 7 Algorithm for therapy of patients with proven pulmonary embolism.

placement of a Greenfield inferior vena caval filter. As an alternative to embolectomy, fibrinolytic therapy may be instituted. For an embolus of lesser severity, thrombolysis may be employed, although I usually recommend heparin therapy. When heparin is absolutely contraindicated or causes complications such as bleeding or a recurrent proven pulmonary embolus, a Greenfield inferior vena caval filter should be placed. Patients who are successfully treated with heparin are then given prophylaxis with warfarin for 6 weeks to 6 months following the pulmonary embolus.

PULMONARY THROMBOEMBOLISM

WALTER G. WOLFE, M.D.
VITO MANTESE, M.D.

Pulmonary embolism remains a frequent and often fatal disorder in spite of the improved understanding of its pathogenesis, diagnosis, and management. From a clinical standpoint, suspicion and early diagnosis are the hallmark of successful therapy of this disease. The incidence in the United States is approximately 650,000 cases a year with a mortality approaching 250,000. Interestingly, in almost 400,000 patients the diagnosis is not initially made, and of these, approximately 140,000 die of the disease.

CLINICAL PRESENTATION

As indicated, one of the difficulties in establishing the clinical diagnosis of pulmonary embolism is the similarity of a number of other cardiorespiratory disorders that mimic this disease. The signs and symptoms include dyspnea, chest pain, and hypotension. It is also clear that many of the patients who suffer pulmonary embolism have underlying cardiac disease, and therefore dyspnea and tachypnea may be among the most common clinical findings. Accentuation of the pulmonary second sound may be common, whereas more commonly associated signs such as hemoptysis, friction rub, cyanosis, and chest splinting are present in an even small number of patients. Finally, only one-third of the patients manifest signs and symptoms of venous thrombosis. In patients with pulmonary embolism, approximately 33 percent have the disease originating from calf veins and 67 percent have disease in the iliofemoral venous system. Although pulmonary thromboembolism usually originates from the deep venous system, it has been described as originating from the right atrium, from septic thrombi in the pelvis, and from tumor emboli as is seen with hypernephroma. Therefore, a high index of suspicion for this disease is extremely important so that (1) the physician thinks of pulmonary thromboembolism as a clinical possibility, and (2) appropriate diagnostic studies are performed to rule the diagnosis in or out.

The chest film is always of benefit in establishing the diagnosis of pulmonary thromboembolism. The findings on chest film must be correlated with those on the scan and perhaps the arteriogram. At times diminished pulmonary vascular markings may be seen on the plain chest film (Westermark's sign). Most often, however, evidence for chronic obstructive disease, atelectasis, and at times a pulmonary infiltrate are commonly seen. In addition to the Westermark's sign, engorgement of the pulmonary artery may be present in the hilum in some patients. All of these signs are nonspecific, but are useful when correlated with the perfusion and ventilation scan. In general, a normal six-view ventilation-perfusion scan is consistent with the diagnosis of *no pulmonary embolism*. Currently, the use of probability statements in interpreting V/Q scans is being used by radiologists, and these interpretations may be misleading and dangerous. In our opinion, if clinical suspicion is great, even patients with low or intermediate probability scans should be studied with arteriography. The high probability scan, if there is no contraindication to anticoagulation, is most likely to make the diagnosis of pulmonary embolism. If there is concern over the use of anticoagulation, the arteriogram should be used to establish an objective clinical diagnosis of pulmonary embolism. In general, a normal angiogram means that there is no pulmonary embolism, if the angiogram is done in two views and selective injections are made in both pulmonary arteries. One must remember that perfusion defect alone does not necessarily indicate pulmonary emboli.

DIAGNOSIS OF DEEP VENOUS THROMBOSIS

Just as pulmonary angiography is the optimal study for diagnosing pulmonary embolism, venogram is the study that establishes the diagnosis of venous thrombosis. Venograms, which can be done as outpatient studies, are safe, the incidence of resulting thrombophlebitis being less than 1 percent. In patients in whom venous thrombosis is suspected, the angiogram should be done before anticoagulation is considered.

PROBLEMS OF DIAGNOSING PULMONARY EMBOLISM AND DEEP VENOUS THROMBOSIS

The diagnosis of pulmonary embolism and/or deep venous thrombosis changes the patient's life style for the rest of his or her life. From the time of diagnosis and even after successful therapy is discontinued, each pulmonary episode raises the suspicion of recurrent thromboembolism. Similarly, with deep vein thrombosis, the morbidity caused by edema and pain may be significant. The objective diagnosis is also extremely important because *long-term anticoagulation remains one of the most dangerous therapies in use today*. The foregoing points dictate that definitive diagnosis be made before therapy is instituted.

Once the diagnosis is established, intravenous heparin is clearly still the best form of treatment. Heparin is given intravenously, either continuously or intermittently, *but not subcutaneously*, for the treatment of acute pulmonary thromboembolism. Continuous intravenous therapy is our preference. In fact, some studies have indicated that continuous intravenous therapy is safer with regard to maintenance of clotting time. In general, the patients are given either 5,000 or 10,000 units as a loading dose, after which the continuous intravenous heparin is administered and the activated partial thromboplastin time (APTT) monitored. This is taken up to approximately two times normal. If clotting time is used, this should be taken to approximately three times normal. In general, 800 or

1,000 units per hour are needed for maintenance; we try not to exceed 1,000 units per hour, depending on the effect on the APTT. Platelet count also must be carefully monitored. The main complication of this therapy is bleeding, although bleeding is much less common with the use of continuous intravenous heparin as the range in PTT is kept tighter. The therapy is continued for 7 to 10 days, during which time repeat perfusion scans usually demonstrate improvement in resolution of thrombi. Once the patient is clinically asymptomatic, the therapy is slowly tapered while Coumadin is started. The patient is then maintained on Coumadin for 3 to 6 months after which he or she is reevaluated as to whether anticoagulation can be discontinued.

In general, other forms of therapy such as streptokinase and urokinase have been used, but do not demonstrate results, after 7 days, that are significantly different from those of heparin. There are no apparent differences in mortality in large series, though streptokinase does demonstrate an increased activity in lysis of clots early on, and in massive pulmonary embolism, there appears to be less impairment of lung function at one-year follow-up in patients who were treated with streptokinase. With streptokinase, the complication of bleeding is increased by a factor of approximately three as compared to that with heparin therapy. In general, streptokinase therapy is discontinued after 48 to 72 hours, and heparin therapy is then instituted. If streptokinase therapy is used, there should be minimal invasive monitoring during therapy to diminish the problems with bleeding. Obviously, careful coagulation studies are necessary as well as clinical evaluation of blood pressure and pulse rate every 2 hours during streptokinase therapy because of the serious complications of bleeding.

SURGICAL MANAGEMENT

Surgical management is considered in three specific instances. The first is caval interruption for prevention of recurrent emboli from the vena cava and lower extremities. The second is the pulmonary embolectomy for acute pulmonary embolus associated with hypoxemia and hypertension not responsive to oxygen and cardiotonic drugs. The third is pulmonary embolectomy for chronic pulmonary embolism associated with dyspnea, hypoxemia, and pulmonary hypertension in patients who have not resolved their obstruction on heparin therapy.

Caval Interruption

Caval interruption, whether it be ligation of the cava or placement of a filter, should not be undertaken without objective evidence that the patient has deep venous disease involving the cava and iliofemoral systems. It has usually been our position that these patients are best managed with chronic anticoagulation, and we reserve procedures with interruption of the cava for patients who have well-documented recurrent episodes while receiving adequate anticoagulation therapy. This policy is based on the well-

known fact that interruption of the cava alone does not completely prevent subsequent embolism. Furthermore, the use of filters may not prevent recurrent emboli, and in many cases, even when filters are placed anticoagulation therapy is continued. Ligation of the cava in males is usually done through a right flank incision; however, in females we generally use a transabdominal route so that both ovarian veins can be ligated. A significant morbidity rate occurs with ligation, and many of these patients have leg edema. If caval ligation is done, the legs should be elevated immediately, and elastic stockings should be used to help control and prevent leg swelling. The Greenfield filter is used most often, and this is usually placed through the transfemoral or transjugular route, depending on the location of the thrombus in the veins. The most common indication for some form of vena caval interruption is proven recurrent emboli or a contraindication to, or complication from, the use of anticoagulation. We have used the filter in patients who had free floating thrombus in the iliocaval system or in patients who have recurrent embolism while on adequate anticoagulation. Recurrent emboli must be documented, however, before we consider any form of caval interruption.

Pulmonary Embolectomy

Trendelenburg, in 1908, performed the first pulmonary embolectomy. His procedure was associated with an extremely high mortality rate, and it was not until the advent of cardiopulmonary bypass that the mortality rate for removal of acute pulmonary emboli became acceptable. Usually, patients with massive pulmonary emboli survive for a period of several hours, although there are certainly instances of sudden death. Once the diagnosis is made, patients who are unresponsive to medical treatment and who have persistent refractory hypotension and hypoxemia despite maximal resuscitation measures (i.e., immediate heparinization and administration of vasopressors and inotropic agents) are taken to the operating room for pulmonary embolectomy. The sternotomy is performed, cardiopulmonary bypass is instituted, the pulmonary artery opened, and the emboli removed. Both lungs should be adequately explored and irrigated using gentle pressure and compression in an attempt to remove as much embolic material as possible. Cardiopulmonary bypass is then discontinued and the sternotomy closed. The patient may then undergo ligation of the vena cava or placement of a filter, or he or she may be maintained on long-term anticoagulation, depending on the clinical indications. The results are excellent, and the mortality has declined in recent years. Still significant, however, are the many associated clinical problems in these patients, which are most frequently cardiac. The mortality rate is still approximately 25 percent.

Chronic Pulmonary Embolism

Chronic pulmonary embolism is now recognized as an important cause of cor pulmonale. These patients usually present with chronic dyspnea, have high right-sided pressures, and, in most instances, do not respond to heparin therapy and are unable to resolve their emboli by their natural fibrolytic system. Evaluation includes pulmonary angiography, measurement of right-sided pressures, and measurements of blood gases. Most of these patients are class III or class IV and are considered for chronic pulmonary embolectomy. The ideal candidates for pulmonary embolectomy are those who have a proximal main or lobar occlusion. For peripheral chronic emboli, the results are poorer, and it is more difficult to remove these clots. In the evaluation, bronchial arteriography is helpful in demonstrating the patency of the distal pulmonary artery.

The surgical approach may be a median sternotomy, with the patient on cardiopulmonary bypass, or a right or left thoracotomy without cardiopulmonary bypass if only a unilateral embolectomy is necessary. Ideal candidates for this operation are patients who are symptomatic with (1) proximal pulmonary artery occlusion, (2) adequate collateral vessels and filling of the distal pulmonary artery through the bronchials, and (3) high right-sided pressures and hypoxemia, but minimally impaired lung function. It is in this group that the best long-term results are obtained. If the main pulmonary artery is opened to complete the chronic pulmonary embolectomy, it can be closed primarily. However, when either the right or left main pulmonary artery is opened and the embolectomy accomplished, the vessel is almost always patched with either vein or pericardium. In the patients who have survived, long-term results have been excellent with improvement of their NYHA class by at least one and sometimes two positions.

Deep venous thrombosis and pulmonary thromboembolism are a major cause of morbidity and death, and continue to be difficult clinical problems. The *diagnosis is made too often without objective diagnostic tests, but paradoxically also not as frequently as indicated in many autopsy series.* Once the clinical diagnosis of pulmonary thromboembolism is considered, it must be *objectively* established or ruled out. Heparin anticoagulation with conversion to Coumadin is still the treatment of choice in acute pulmonary emboli; in rare instances, caval interruption and pulmonary embolectomy may be necessary.

LYMPHEDEMA OF THE EXTREMITY

ROBERT C. SAVAGE, M.D.

Our knowledge of lymphatic anatomy and physiology has improved appreciably in the last 30 years with the development of lymphangiography and other investigative techniques. However, the pathophysiology of lymphedema remains poorly understood. This lack of fundamental information is reflected in our clinical frustrations. That is, no medical or surgical treatment of lymphedema is curative at present. Most surgical techniques are confounded by at least partial recurrence of edema.

Similar to the varicose ulcer patient, patients with lymphedema are often shunted from physician to physician seeking new solutions. Surgical interest in lymphedema has historically been low because the procedures are frequently tiresome, unexciting, and yield incomplete results. However, renewed interest in lymphatic research and the development of new surgical methods offer promise for patients with lymphedema. Moreover, the tendency away from radical node dissections combined with refined radiotherapy techniques may decrease the incidence of secondary lymphedema in the future.

A coordinated treatment program for the lymphedematous patient, followed over the long term, can yield gratifying results for both physician and patient. The dismal outlook alluded to earlier has been propagated by medical personnel with limited experience or inclination for treating these neglected individuals.

CLASSIFICATION

Lymphedema has been classified as either primary (idiopathic) or secondary (Table 1). A complete discussion of the various types and etiologies is inappropriate for this forum.

TABLE 1 Lymphedema Classification

Primary lymphedema

  Congenital: onset at birth
  Praecox: early age (usually teens or twenties)
  Tarda: after age 35
  Milroy's disease: primary lymphedema that is congenital and familial

Secondary lymphedema

  Postsurgical
  Postradiation
  Infection
  Trauma
  Tumor
  Factitious
  Recurrent phlebitis
  Recurrent lymphangitis
  Rare bites

Primary lymphedema has been further divided according to lymphangiographic findings (Table 2). Lymphedema praecox with hypoplasia in females is the most common variety.

The causes of secondary lymphedema vary widely, depending on the individual physician's geographic location and referral patterns. Worldwide, the most common etiology is filariasis, whereas in the United States lymphedema occurring from tumor, surgery, or radiation is more frequently encountered.

MEDICAL MANAGEMENT

It should be emphasized that most patients with lymphedema are handled well by medical means. Surgery should be reserved for cases that have failed a sincere, aggressive trial of medical therapy. Nonoperative techniques satisfy the great majority of patients.

Two categories of medical therapy exist: mechanical and pharmacologic. Mechanical adjuncts of importance include (1) strict extremity elevation, (2) customized, graded pressure garments, (3) intermittent pneumatic pressure devices, (4) fastidious skin hygiene, and (5) weight control. Pharmacologic techniques of some value are (1) antibiotics for the treatment and prevention of cellulitis and lymphangitis, (2) topical antifungal agents, especially for those with hyperkeratoses of the feet, and (3) diuretics, which may offer temporary improvement, although long-term effects are disappointing and can be hazardous if improperly supervised.

SURGICAL TREATMENT

Relative Indications

Patients with lymphedema who have failed an intensive trial of medical therapy present for surgery for a variety of reasons. Extremity function may be impaired by excessive size and weight or easy fatigability. Pain is not uncommon with severe swelling. In addition, many individuals suffer from repeated bouts of cellulitis and lymphangitis.

Since most patients with primary lymphedema are young females, aesthetic considerations cannot be dis-

TABLE 2 Lymphangiographic Classification of Primary Lymphedema

Classification	Description
Aplasia	No subcutaneous lymphatics (rare)
Hypoplasia	Lymph nodes and/or vessels small and few in number
Hyperplasia	Many large nodes and/or vessels that are sometimes tortuous and varicose

counted. Body contour abnormalities and difficulty in wearing contemporary clothing are important considerations in the maturing adolescent.

Finally, lymphangiosarcoma, a rare but frequently fatal complication, has been described after longstanding primary and secondary lymphedema.

Lymphedema surgery is primarily a "quality of life" undertaking. Therefore, as in any elective procedure, general medical condition and age are important factors in the selection of patients.

Preoperative Management

Once it has been decided that the patient is a surgical candidate, a number of preparatory steps may be helpful. Obviously, any active infection must be controlled with appropriate antibiotics and topical hygiene. In addition, perioperative antibiotic coverage, especially against streptococci and staphylococci, is probably also of value. Any fungal difficulties should be addressed with Tinactin therapy or similar agents.

Strict extremity elevation, pressure stockings, and short-term diuretics are recommended for optimal preoperative swelling reduction. In these days of cost containment, these measures should be started on an outpatient basis. However, incomplete patient compliance frequently necessitates some hospitalization before surgery for optimal results.

Intermittent external compression devices can be useful preoperatively and are becoming more readily available for home care. However, patient satisfaction with this technique varies because of the time necessary for improvement.

If any of the more formidable surgical procedures is planned, blood should be crossmatched in advance. This is done preferably by self-donation, to minimize potential side effects and to maximize conservation of available blood products.

Surgical Approach

Many surgical procedures have been described for the treatment of lymphedema (Table 3). These techniques are of two basic types: physiologic and excisional. Currently no surgical *cure* is available short of amputation, which is obviously contraindicated except in the *most* extreme cases. However, several techniques are available which can yield marked objective improvement and a high degree of patient satisfaction.

Most lymphangioplasty techniques, with the subcutaneous implantation of various materials as "lymphatic wicks," have been abandoned because of transient improvement coupled with high infection and extrusion rates. Better tolerated alloplastic materials (e.g., Teflon) may have some limited role in the relatively poor-risk patient or in those with major concerns about excessive scarring.

Goldsmith's omental flap for the treatment of lymph-

TABLE 3 Surgical Techniques

Excisional
  Charles procedure—radical skin and sub-
    cutaneous excision with subsequent grafting
  Kondoleon procedure—fascial excision
  Staged excision of skin and subcutaneous fat

Physiologic
  Lymphangioplasty—subcutaneous implants,
    e.g., silk, nylon, Teflon, rubber, fascia
  Pedicle skin flaps
  Dermal flaps—e.g., the Thompson procedure
  Axial pattern and musculocutaneous flaps
  Lymphatic anastomosis techniques:
    Lymph node to vein
    Lymph vessel to vein
    Lymphaticolymphatic
  Omental flap
  Intestinal flap

edema also has fallen into disfavor because of excessive morbidity (e.g., pulmonary embolus, intestinal obstruction, hernia, and wound infections). In addition, other investigators have been unable to demonstrate long-term lymphatic connections between the omentum and the involved extremity. Intestinal flaps of ileum and mesentery have not gained widespread acceptance because of the potential complications of laparotomy.

Pedicle skin flaps, although used extensively in the past, are now uncommon because of the requirement of multiple stages, potential flap necrosis, and unsightly donor sites. The recently described axial and musculocutaneous flaps should markedly improve flap survival and donor site appearance. However, much more experimental and clincial experience is necessary before defining their roles in lymphedema therapy.

Various lymphatic anastomosis techniques have been advocated for both primary and secondary lymphedema. To me, their use in the treatment of primary lymphedema makes little physiologic sense. Several reports have shown partial early improvement, in cases of secondary lymphedema, as a result of lymph-node-to-vein or lymph-vessel-to-vein anastomosis. Others have been frustrated by late thromboses and edema recurrence. Many of these trials included concomitant skin and subcutaneous excisions, plus postoperative medical adjuncts, raising serious doubts about what aspects of the treatment contributed to the clinical improvement. Finally, as emphasized by Clodius, in cases with chronic fibrosis, the reconstituting of lymphatic conduits is likely to be an incomplete solution.

The more recently described lymph-vessel-to-lymph-vessel microsurgical repairs may offer more promise for the future in selected cases. However, appropriate proximal and distal lymphatics must be available. Furthermore, these can be long, tedious procedures requiring special surgical expertise as well as a young, healthy patient. Many of these procedures have also been supplemented by surgical excisions, thereby obscuring result analysis. Finally, long-term studies on significant numbers of patients with objective documentation of improvements is not yet available. The ultimate role of this procedure may be in the treatment of early secondary edema or as prophylaxis when done concomitantly with nodal dissection.

Thompson's extensive experience with his buried dermal flap has demonstrated impressive improvements. Other authors have argued that its primary advantage is from its concomitant excision of lymphedematous tissue, rather than from the establishment of superficial-to-deep lymphatic connections. In addition, less experienced surgeons have had a higher incidence of flap necrosis, wound infection, and dehiscence.

The Charles procedure, with radical excision of all involved skin, subcutaneous tissue, and fascia and subsequent graft coverage, although still widely used, should be abandoned except in extreme cases. The postoperative "spindle" appearance is grotesque. Hypertrophic scar formation, contracture, graft loss, sensory deficits, ulceration, exophytic keratoses, and aggravation of distal edema are additional drawbacks.

The staged excision of skin and subcutaneous tissue under skin flaps, I feel, represents a reasonable compromise for most patients seeking surgery for lymphedema. While it is true that all cases have some partial recurrence, objective and subjective improvement is gratifying in the great majority of candidates.

The technique I prefer is similar to that repopularized by Dr. Timothy Miller. This is a two-staged approach, which allows the relatively safe removal of a large amount of lymphedematous tissue.

The first procedure usually is performed on the medial aspect of the leg. A high pneumatic tourniquet is initially placed to limit blood loss. A straight incision is made along the medial thigh and calf, then curved behind the medial malleolus. Skin flaps, approximately 1.5 to 2 cm in thickness, are then raised anteriorly and posteriorly to the midsaggital plane. However, conservative undermining is advisable about the malleolus per se. All underlying fat, fibrous tissue, and fascia is then excised, except a strip of fascia overlying the posterior tibial artery at the ankle. The saphenous vein usually is sacrificed; however, if possible, its preservation is desirable. The sural nerve should be positively identified and maintained. An equal amount of redundant skin is then removed from both the anterior and the posterior flaps, allowing for closure under minimal tension. If the viability of a skin flap is in question, the use of intravenous fluorescein is occasionally helpful for diagnostic purposes. The flaps are then closed over silicone suction drains after hemostasis has been obtained. Closure in two layers allows for early suture removal, at about 1 week, and conversion to Steri-Tapes.

A similar procedure is performed on the lateral aspect of the leg, if necessary, approximately 2 to 4 months later. Special attention should be paid to the preservation of the sural nerve and the peroneal nerve when performing the lateral approach.

With proper attention to atraumatic technique, hemostasis, and avoidance of excessive tension, complications should be minimal. The most common problems have been small areas of skin flap necrosis or dehiscence, and hematoma. Obviously, any sizable hematoma should be drained. Minor flap loss or separation is usually treated with dressings and, on rare occasions, with small split-thickness grafts.

All patients experience some element of decreased sensation, which generally improves over time and is rarely of concern. However, the patient should be appropriately forewarned preoperatively.

Recurrent lymphedema is minimized by the continued use of elevation and customized stockings. If residual edema becomes clinically significant, the procedure can be repeated on the medial aspect of the leg for additional contouring.

TRAUMA AND EMERGENCY CARE

ABDOMINAL TRAUMA

GREGORY LUNA, M.D.
C. JAMES CARRICO, M.D.

Abdominal trauma accounts for about 10 percent of all significant injuries and ranks third behind head and chest injuries as the cause of death following accidents. The importance of abdominal injuries is heightened by the recent observation that they represent the most common cause of preventable deaths following injury. An organized approach to the evaluation and treatment of abdominal injuries can result in a significant reduction in morbidity and mortality, since the majority of these preventable deaths result from delayed diagnosis or incomplete understanding of the anatomic extent of the abdominal viscera.

The external landmarks that encompass the abdomen extend from the nipples to the inguinal ligaments anteriorly, and from the inferior border of the scapula to the ischial tuberosities posteriorly. The importance of these external points of reference lies in the potential for penetrating wounds seemingly removed from the abdominal cavity to injure abdominal viscera. Although the bony structures of the thorax, spine, and pelvis provide protection against blunt injury to roughly 50 percent of the abdominal contents, this protection is at best partial. Considerable energy is required to disrupt the bony structures surrounding the trunk, and part or all of this energy may be transmitted to the underlying tissues. Thus, structures in all parts of the abdomen ("true," thoracic, pelvic, and extraperitoneal) are subject to blunt injury without disruption of the musculoskeletal system.

Recent controversies in management of abdominal trauma can be grouped in three categories: (1) the optimal means to identify visceral injuries, (2) departures from traditional management of specific organ injuries, particularly the spleen and colon, and (3) the distinction between nonproductive and unnecessary laparotomies. Admitting that these areas are interrelated, we will address them sequentially.

DIAGNOSIS: IDENTIFICATION OF VISCERAL INJURIES

The evaluation and treatment of the injured victim begins with the ABCs. Adequate airway, ventilation, tis-

sue oxygenation, and cellular perfusion are always the primary goals. Once these ABCs have been secured, injuries must be prioritized. Early identification of all significant injuries allows the development of an orderly and efficient sequence of resuscitation and treatment. Rarely does even a severe abdominal injury cause a patient's demise as rapidly as a progressing head or thoracic injury.

The principal goal of diagnostic investigations in abdominal trauma is the *identification* rather than *specification* of injury. Emergency laboratory and radiologic evaluations should be performed *only* if the information gained will have a direct bearing on the immediate treatment of the patient. Neurologic and hemodynamic stability must dictate the extent of initial diagnostic investigations.

Initial "laboratory" should include: a blood sample for typing and crossmatching and for hematocrit and amylase determinations and a urine sample for RBC, WBC, and glucose determinations. Unstable or seriously injured patients should have an arterial blood gas determination. This provides vital information about oxygenation, ventilation, and perfusion. Portable anteroposterior chest, cervical spine, and pelvic roentgenograms should be obtained early in the evaluation. Further radiologic studies depend on the patient's stability, location of and mechanism of injury, and presence or absence of existing clear indication for laparotomy. For example, patients with blood at the urethral meatus, severe blunt pelvic or perineal trauma should undergo a retrograde urethrogram prior to insertion of a Foley catheter; excretory urograms and cystograms should be obtained in patients with gross hematuria or injuries in close proximity to the kidneys, ureters, or bladder; contrast and tomographic examinations of the duodenum and pancreas may be of value in victims of blunt trauma with hyperamylasemia and no obvious indication for laparotomy.

Penetrating Abdominal Trauma

For patients with penetrating injuries, the principles of management are straightforward. Unless injuries to the intraperitoneal or retroperitoneal abdominal contents can be definitively ruled out, abdominal exploration is warranted. Consequently, patients with gunshot wounds between the external landmarks previously described should undergo laparotomy. Stab wounds of the abdomen are

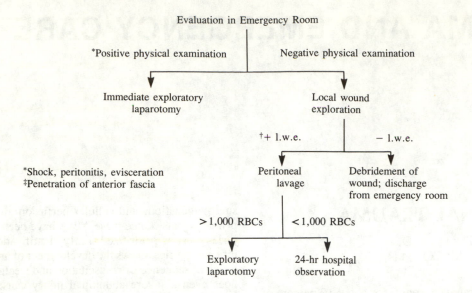

Figure 1 Evaluation of stab wounds of the abdomen.

evaluated as shown in Figure 1. Hypotensive patients and those with peritoneal irritation require laparotomy; in our experience, this comprises approximately one-third of the entire group. The remaining patients should undergo thorough wound exploration under local anesthesia. If the superficial muscle fascia is not violated, the exploration is terminated. (This accounts for half of all local wound explorations and one-third of all anterior stab wounds.) For anterior stab wounds, if the fascia has been penetrated, a peritoneal lavage is carried out and a RBC count obtained. Patients with less than 1,000 RBCs per cubic millimeter can be safely observed. This approach reduces the rate of nonproductive laparotomies to less than 10 percent and *rarely* allows an injury to be missed.

Peritoneal lavage is not as useful in patients with stab wounds to the flank and back (because of the increased probability of retroperitoneal injuries). If local exploration cannot establish a low probability of significant injury in such patients, laparotomy is in order. Currently, even the newer imaging techniques have little to offer in the evaluation of patients with penetrating injuries.

Blunt Trauma

Blunt trauma to the abdomen offers a much greater diagnostic challenge, particularly when evaluating the patient with multiple injuries. In such patients, and even in those with isolated abdominal injuries, physical signs may be more difficult to interpret than in the patient with penetrating trauma. The mechanism of injury, stability at the scene and during transport, and the presence of associated injuries all give vital clues to the probability of visceral injury. High-speed deceleration such as motor vehicle accidents and falls from a level higher than two stories frequently results in visceral injury. Victims of blunt trauma who are hypotensive in the prehospital setting have a 30 to 40 percent chance of having sustained a severe abdominal injury. Fractures of the lower ribs, pelvis, and thoracic and lumbar spine all indicate significant trauma to the trunk, particularly if there is displacement or comminution of the fragments. A Malgaigne pelvic fracture alone is associated with a 40 percent change of intra-abdominal injury.

Patients with clear evidence of abdominal injury (e.g., peritonitis, hypotension) require laparotomy, not further investigations of the source of inflammation or bleeding. In contrast, the optimal means of rapid identification of a visceral injury that is not immediately obvious depends on the personnel and equipment available. Many facilities lack the expertise or immediate availability required to utilize computerized tomography. Peritoneal lavage remains the "gold standard" for diagnosis following blunt injury and can be rapidly performed and interpreted by a surgeon with extremely high sensitivity and essentially no morbidity. Accidental visceral injury and false-negative and false-positive results have been essentially eliminated by the adoption of the open technique, whereby the peritoneum is visualized prior to insertion of the catheter.

Lavage is indicated whenever a patient at significant risk for abdominal injury has equivocal physical findings, when the examination cannot be accurately followed, or when apparent blood loss cannot be accounted for by other injuries. Lavage has proved to be a reliable predictor of visceral injury (sensitivity greater than 95%) when the red blood cell count is greater than 100,000 per cubic millimeter. If one accepts the concept that the primary goal is identification rather than specification of injury, the lack of specificity of peritoneal lavage is outweighed by its sensitivity. Exceptions to this generalization will be discussed subsequently. The other limitation of peritoneal lavage is its lack of sensitivity in identifying retroperitoneal injuries.

INJURIES TO SOLID ORGANS

Treatment of solid organ injuries entails control of hemorrhage, debridement of devitalized or avulsed tissue, and drainage of excretory or secretory products. Specific techniques depend on the severity of injury, stability of the patient, magnitude of associated injuries, and morbidity of organ resection.

Bleeding from parenchymal tears and injuries to major vessels account for the majority of immediate deaths. Rapid intraoperative control of bleeding prior to attempts at definitive repair is critical. Uncertainty regarding the source of bleeding and extent of injuries, make a midline incision from the xiphoid to the subumbilical region optimal. If massive hemoperitoneum is encountered, evisceration of the small bowel, evacuation of blood, and rapid assessment of the abdominal contents are necessary to identify the source of hemorrhage. Direct pressure on the bleeding source allows temporary control while injuries are assessed.

Injuries to organs that perform physiologic functions essential to life, i.e., the liver, pancreas, and kidneys, require particular consideration during surgical repair. Although extensive resections are occasionally necessary to control hemorrhage or to repair major ductal injuries, once hemostasis is achieved, the primary goal of treatment is to remove devitalized tissue and provide egress for extravasated bile, pancreatic juice, or urine.

The Liver

The liver is the most commonly injured solid viscus with an overall mortality rate of 10 to 20 percent, the majority of deaths resulting from uncontrollable hemorrhage. Penetrating wounds carry a more favorable prognosis than blunt injuries unless associated with a major vascular injury or damage to multiple organs. Simple lacerations or cracks through Glisson's capsule with limited parenchymal damage account for the majority of injuries.

Twenty to forty percent of hepatic injuries will have stopped bleeding at the time of exploration. Nonbleeding wounds should be left alone. We continue to use perihepatic closed-suction drains except for the most superficial lacerations. If no significant drainage occurs, these drains are removed 36 to 72 hours postoperatively.

Treatment of active hemorrhage requires a progression of maneuvers to accomplish temporary hemostasis followed by definitive control (Fig. 2):

1. Manual compression of the liver between the surgeon's hands or against the posterior abdominal wall and diaphragm affords excellent temporary control of severe bleeding and is often sufficient for premanent hemostasis with minor bleeding from parenchymal tears. Topical application of hemostatic agents and absorbable sutures placed parallel to the wound are usually effective in controlling bleeding from superficial wounds.

2. Vigorous bleeding following release of manual compression indicates injury to larger vessels. Temporary control by inflow occlusion of the porta hepatis (Pringle maneuver) often allows visualization and direct ligation of the bleeding vessel. Bleeding from deep in the substance of the liver on rare occasion requires exposure by extending the wound in Glisson's capsule and "finger fracture" division of the underlying parenchyma to bring the bleeding point into view. Selective hepatic artery or portal vein ligation has been recommended if direct ligation is not possible or is unsuccessful. Owing to variations in arterial anatomy and the potential for infarction of major segments or even entire lobes, this technique should be reserved *only* for the rare inflow injury not amenable to direct ligation. Omental pedicles are occasionally useful for venous oozing from deep lacerations. Major (formal) resections are rarely necessary, although large segments of devitalized tissue should be debrided. Drainage is indicated with any deep laceration, debridement, or resection.

3. Major bleeding that cannot be controlled by pressure or inflow occlusion indicates hepatic vein or vena caval injury. Repair requires control of the vena cava above and below the liver as well as thorough mobilization of the liver. Extension of the midline incision into a median sternotomy allows access to the suprahepatic vena cava and upper right hepatic vein. Division of the falciform and both triangular ligaments optimizes liver mobility and exposure. Mobilizing the duodenum (Kocher maneuver) completes the access to the infra- and retrohepatic vena cava. Our enthusiasm for atriocaval shunting has waned. It is rarely necessary and should not be used in a hypotensive patient.

4. Massive transfusion and hypothermia often accompany severe hepatic injuries. These factors may result in a coagulopathy rendering hemostasis by surgical maneuvers alone virtually impossible. If this complication cannot be prevented or rapidly corrected, gauze packing and closure to allow warming and correction of the bleeding diathesis may prove lifesaving. Packing should also be considered in cases of diffuse bleeding from the liver surface when major vessels have been controlled and when immediately available resources are limited, necessitating control of bleeding prior to transfer of the patient.

Liver failure following even severe injury is uncommon unless there is underlying acute or chronic hepatocellular disease. Immediate complications result from persistent bleeding, prolonged shock, or massive transfusions. Delayed morbidity specific to the liver injury includes parenchymal and intra-abdominal abscesses, biliary fistulas, and vascular malformations.

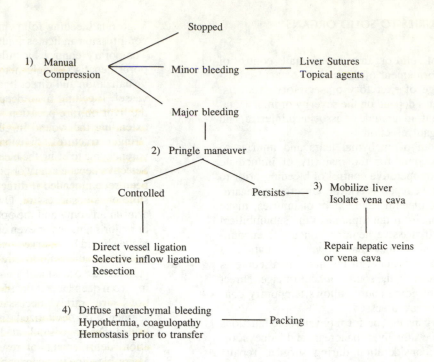

Figure 2 Control of Hepatic Bleeding

The Pancreas

Isolated injuries to the pancreas from either penetrating or blunt trauma are relatively uncommon. Major complications and death result from delayed diagnosis and the high frequency of associated injuries. Overall mortality rates from pancreatic injuries range from 5 to 10 percent. Primary postoperative complications include pseudocyst, fistulas, and abscesses, often related to unrecognized injury or inadequate drainage. Endocrine or exocrine insufficiency following surgery is rare except when a major resection is performed.

Because of the retroperitoneal location of the pancreas, recognition of the presence of a pancreatic injury is the first crucial step. This is relatively straightforward in patients with penetrating trauma since retroperitoneal penetration in the area of the pancreas requires complete inspection of the gland. Mobilization of the right colon and direct entry into the lesser sac affords excellent anterior exposure. Mobilization of the duodenum then permits "bimanual" examination of the pancreatic head.

Delayed recognition usually occurs in patients with blunt trauma who lack initial indications for laparotomy. The lack of sensitivity and specificity of hyperamylasemia militates against exploration based solely on this laboratory test. Computerized tomography, ultrasound, and contrast studies of the duodenum should be used to investigate pancreatic or duodenal injuries suspected on the basis of an elevated serum amylase. Laparotomies performed for blunt trauma require the same anatomic investigation if a pancreatic injury is suspected.

Once the injury is identified, specific management depends on the location and severity of the injury and, particularly, the integrity of the major duct and ampulla. Simple contusions and superficial tears in the capsule (type I) should be managed by drainage alone. Soft closed-suction drains placed into the lesser sac are adequate and should be removed when the effluent amylase concentration returns to normal serum values. Deeper lacerations or extensive contusions (type II) require examination of the major pancreatic duct. We usually begin with a cholecystocholangiogram. If this is not adequate, a contrast examination of the duct can be obtained via a lateral duodenotomy, cannulating the ampulla with a Silastic catheter. Injection of soluble contrast medium under minimal pressure clearly outlines ductal anatomy. Lacerations or fractures that do not involve the major duct generally require only hemostasis and extensive drainage.

Ductal disruptions from blunt injury most often occur over the spine, to the left of the portal vein. Transections of the body of the gland are best managed by distal resection, with control of the proximal duct and drainage. Extensive injuries to the head of the pancreas (type III) should be treated with distal resection if the remaining pancreas is clearly viable. When the head of the pancreas is severely contused or resection entails removal of more than 80 to 90 percent of the gland, a Roux-en-Y jejunal anastomosis to the distal pancreas should be considered.

Treatment of proximal pancreatic injury associated with injury to the second portion of the duodenum (type IV) depends on the integrity of the ampulla and distal common bile duct. If the ampulla and common bile duct are intact, the pancreatic injury is treated as described for type III injuries, the duodenum is repaired, and the pylorus is excluded. The rare injury with disruption of the ampulla requires a combined pancreatoduodenal resection. If the first portion of the duodenum is intact, the pylorus should be retained. Silastic stents through the pancreatic and common bile duct anastomosis are utilized. To ensure proximal decompression and eventual removal from the duct, the stents are brought out to the skin.

The Spleen

The spleen is the organ most commonly injured following blunt trauma and ranks second behind the liver as the source of life-threatening hemorrhage following injury. Prior to the past two decades, the lack of appreciation of the immunologic importance of this organ resulted in routine splenectomy for essentially all splenic injuries. Concern about postsplenectomy sepsis has prompted reappraisal of this approach. The options available to the surgeon caring for a patient with a rupture spleen include (1) splenectomy for all damaged spleens, (2) exploration and attempted salvage, and (3) nonoperative observation. The choice between these options requires weighing the risks and benefits of each. Although our current information is incomplete, there are some established facts that are useful in making such a decision.

The risk of developing sepsis following splenectomy in the otherwise healthy trauma victim is 1 to 3 percent. Vaccines against *Pneumococcus* and *H. influenzae* may reduce this incidence by half. Since the mortality from postsplenectomy sepsis is 30 to 50 percent, the risk of a septic death related to the splenectomy is 0.5 to 1 percent. Adding this figure to a 0.5 percent operative mortality from splenectomy for isolated injury results in a 1 to 1.5 percent overall long-term mortality rate. Less aggressive means of treating splenic injuries must equal or surpass this low mortality rate.

The benefits of nonoperative therapy must be weighed against the risk of missing an associated hollow viscus injury, the risk of blood transfusion, and the practicality of prolonged hospitalization and limitations on normal activity. Twenty percent of splenic injuries from high-velocity impact such as motor vehicle accidents and falls from heights greater than 20 feet are associated with hollow viscus injury. The morbidity of delayed recognition of these combined injuries strongly favors operative therapy unless hollow viscus perforation can be rapidly and reliably ruled out.

The incidence of associated injuries is undoubtedly lower in patients subjected to lesser forces. In such patients, this argument becomes less persuasive. Some reviews of nonoperative management of isolated splenic injuries report replacement of 30 percent or more of the estimated blood volume in "successfully" treated patients and two or more times the blood volume in patients who are eventually operated on. The risk of transfusion complications (e.g., viral hepatitis risk: 1% to 2% per unit transfusion with 20% progressing to the chronic state) may well outweigh the benefits of such an approach.

These issues are obviously not resolved. We believe that the nonoperative approach should be applied *very* selectively. The benefits of general application of such an approach are unproven. It is *not* applicable to patients who demonstrate hemodynamic instability, require significant blood transfusions, or are at risk for associated intra-abdominal injuries.

Splenic injuries are identified at our institution by positive peritoneal lavage or laparotomy for patients with obvious intra-abdominal hemorrhage. When *small* non-bleeding lacerations are identified, they should be left undisturbed. The potential of repairing more extensive wounds can only be assessed by mobilizing the spleen into the midline and removing the surrounding clot. Bleeding from superficial tears in the capsule can usually be controlled with direct pressure and application of topical hemostatic agents. Deeper lacerations or avulsions are best repaired with "pledgeted" mattress sutures placed 1 cm back from the wound edge. Partial splenectomy is employed for more extensive injuries if 50 percent of the splenic tissue can be preserved. Splenectomy is performed for diffuse parenchymal injuries and extensive injuries that do not permit preservation of 50 percent of the spleen. Patients who remain hemodynamically unstable and those with multiple associated injuries are not considered for splenic repair.

Since immunocompetence requires approximately 50 percent of viable splenic mass, omental implantation or salvaging of small fragments is not attempted. Drains are used only if there is a potential injury to the tail of the pancreas, and are removed the following day unless the fluid amylase is elevated.

Pneumovax is given following splenectomy, usually the day prior to discharge. Although antibiotic prophylaxis is controversial, low-dose penicillin is prescribed for children under the age of 6, and recommended for all splenectomized patients undergoing procedures likely to produce a bacteremia. Patient education and "medical alerts" are also important measures.

The Kidneys

Patients who require laparotomy and are suspected of having renal injury because of proximity or hematuria should generally undergo contrast pylography to establish renal perfusion and function prior to exploration. Rapid injection of 1 to 1.5 ml of water-soluble contrast medium per kilogram of body weight, followed by lower abdominal films at 5 minutes provides evidence of perfusion and usually excretion without delaying surgery. When hemodynamic instability necessitates immediate laparotomy, the pylogram can be done on the operating table.

Blunt injuries resulting in contusions or simple lacerations should be treated conservatively unless there is evidence of active perinephric bleeding. Nonexpanding perinephric hematomas following blunt trauma do not require exploration if contrast studies have documented adequate perfusion and function. Nonfunctioning kidneys, expanding perinephric hematomas, and wounds penetrating Gerota's fascia should be explored. Vascular control should be obtained prior to exploration.

The vast majority of renal injuries can be managed without nephrectomy. Isolation of the renal vessels prior to opening Gerota's fascia increases the frequency of renal salvage. Debridement of devitalized tissue or partial nephrectomy with adequate drainage provides excellent results.

INJURIES TO HOLLOW VISCERA

Specific surgical treatment of injuries to hollow viscera depends on the reliability of primary healing and the risk of leak, infection, or stricture. Organs such as the stomach, small bowel, and urinary bladder possess adequate circulation and sufficiently low resident flora to permit primary repair in nearly all cases. Rarely do injuries to these organs require a resection extensive enough to compromise their storage or absorptive functions. For the stomach and bladder, debridement of the wound margins, meticulous closure, and decompression provide excellent results. Limited resection with primary anastomosis is indicated for small bowel injuries when simple closure is not possible owing to a devitalized segment or compromised lumen. In contrast, repair of injuries to the extra-hepatic bile ducts, duodenum, colon, and rectum results in stricture or leak often enough to warrant a more detailed discussion (to follow).

Bile Ducts

Penetrating trauma accounts for the majority of injuries to the extrahepatic biliary tree. The rare isolated injury from blunt impact should be suspected when bile is recovered from the peritoneal lavage or when extravasated bile is present in the hepatoduodenal ligament. The presence and location of such injuries can be confirmed by an operative cholecystocholangiogram. This is accomplished by inserting a No. 16 or No. 18 angiocatheter into the fundus of the gallbladder. If no injury is seen, the puncture wound can be closed with a single absorbable suture.

Isolated injuries to the gallbladder are best managed by cholecystectomy. Cholecystostomy may be indicated in the unstable patient, although removal of a previously normal gallbladder rarely requires significantly more time than simple tube placement. The high incidence of stricture and bile leak following primary repair or end-to-end anastomosis of major injuries to the hepatic and common bile ducts favors the creation of an enteric anastomosis. Small clean lacerations can be closed primarily. With more extensive injuries, an anastomosis to the duodenum or jejunum is preferred. Stents brought out through the bowel are preferred to placement of a T-tube in a normal-sized duct. Closed-suction drains should be placed near the repair.

The Duodenum

Injuries to the duodenum are present in less than 5 percent of cases of blunt and penetrating abdominal trauma. Damage from anterior penetrating wounds is usually obvious. Duodenal injuries from bullets or knife wounds to the back or flank can be missed if the duodenum is not mobilized. Blunt injuries to the retroperitoneal portion of the duodenum may be subtle; in many cases the only early indication is an elevation in the serum amylase. Since the morbidity and mortality of duodenal injury is greatly increased by delays in diagnosis, early identification is critical. Contrast studies and computerized tomography are both useful in confirming a suspected injury.

The management of isolated injuries to the third and fourth portions of the duodenum is basically the same as that outlined for the small bowel. The second portion requires special consideration because of its limited collateral blood supply and integral relationship with the common bile duct and pancreas. As with other organs, the preferable approach depends on the degree of injury. Lacerations resulting in minimal tissue loss (grade I), where closure would not compromise the bowel lumen, should be closed primarily. If there is concern about the closure, decompression with a small catheter through a retrograde jejunostomy or lateral duodenostomy is advisable. When closure would result in significant narrowing (grade II), a Roux-en-Y jejunal anastomosis provides satisfactory repair. Pyloric exclusion with a gastrojejunostomy may be necessary with more extensive or combined injuries (grade III). As previously discussed, only when the duodenal injury has resulted in destruction of the ampulla (grade IV) is a pancreatoduodenal resection required.

Colon and Rectum

The morbidity of producing and closing intestinal stomas and the reported safety of primary closure or resection and primary anastomosis have resulted in the reappraisal of routine fecal diversion for all abdominal colon injuries.

The safety of leaving or returning the repaired colon into the abdominal cavity is clearly dependent on the degree of fecal contamination, associated injuries, delay between injury and surgery, and hemodynamic stability (Table 1). Leaving the bowel in continuity should be considered only in stable patients who are operated on im-

TABLE 1 Management of Abdominal Colon Injuries

Grade	Location	Treatment
Isolated injury, no delay, hemodynamically stable	Right Transverse Left	Closure Exteriorize Colostomy
Through-and-through perforation, lacerations, moderate contamination	Right Transverse Left	Right colectomy Exteriorize/colostomy Colostomy
Severe tissue loss, devascularized segment, heavy contamination	Right Transverse Left	Ileostomy Colostomy Colostomy

mediately following injury and have minimal fecal spillage. We primarily repair or resect and anastomose only grade I injuries of the right colon. Increased bacterial concentration and possibly collagenase activity favors complete diversion for left colon injuries. When technically possible, single perforations of the transverse and left colon can be satisfactorily managed by exteriorizing the injured segment as a loop colostomy. Our enthusiasm for early colostomy closure 2 to 3 weeks following injury has waned owing to the difficulty of dissection and increased blood loss from the ongoing inflammatory response.

Injuries to the rectum below the peritoneal reflection result from massive pelvic fractures, penetrating wounds to the pelvis and perineum, or foreign bodies passed through the anus. Sigmoidoscopy is the only reliable means of identifying mid- and lower rectal injuries. Perforations of the extraperitoneal rectum require complete fecal diversion with an end-colostomy and prevention of continued contamination by irrigation of the distal segment and closure of the wound if possible. Presacral drainage of the contaminated perirectal space is crucial and is far superior to anterior drainage with closed-suction drains.

Broad-spectrum antibiotics are administered to all patients suspected of having a bowel perforation, particularly colon injuries. The risk of bowel injury from penetrating wounds is great enough to justify routine administration preoperatively. Wound infection following colon injuries can be effectively prevented by leaving the skin and subcutaneous fat open. Delayed primary closure at 5 days provides excellent results.

NONPRODUCTIVE VERSUS UNNECESSARY LAPAROTOMY

Much of the decision making in patients with abdominal injuries involves weighing the risk of missing (or delaying treatment of) a significant injury against morbidity of a nonproductive laparotomy. The word nonproductive is used to describe operations at which no injury is found (negative) and those at which the injuries found do not require treatment (e.g., nonbleeding liver lacerations). Although we all wish to reduce nonproductive laparotomies to a *safe* minimum, we must avoid doing our patients harm by considering all such nonproductive procedures to be "unnecessary." For instance, in a young healthy patient with isolated (e.g., penetrating) abdominal trauma and equivocal findings, the short- and long-term risks of anesthesia and celiotomy are minimal and the surgery is justified by the potential for identifying and repairing an injury that might be life-threatening. In such circumstances, laparotomy is necessary even though it may be nonproductive. In contrast, in an elderly patient with multisystem disease, the risk of operative intervention rises. In such patients, especially following blunt injury, equivocal findings may well justify extensive efforts to specify the injuries by noninvasive means, accepting the slightly increased risk of missing a significant injury.

SHOCK

ARTHUR E. BAUE, M.D.

The treatment of shock is second nature to surgeons who must deal with problems of circulatory failure on a daily basis in treating patients after injuries and operations. The classification of shock into hypovolemic, septic, cardiogenic, and neurogenic categories is well known and serves as an initial framework for discussion and therapy. However, in an individual patient, therapy must be directed toward his particular circumstances and not to a classification. Thus, a patient with an acute myocardial infarction may be hypovolemic or an elderly patient with gastrointestinal bleeding may have cardiac failure or a septic patient may be hypovolemic or have myocardial depression or require a higher cardiac output than the cardiovascular system can develop. Thus, the initial evaluation of a patient with shock (hypotension, low urine output, inadequate organ perfusion) must be an assessment of vascular volume, cardiac function, and the presence of organ dysfunction or failure and complications such as infection. Shock, although common and well under-

stood by surgeons, remains a critical factor in survival after an injury or an operation. In the recent experiences of the Regional Trauma Center at Yale and in our reviews of multiple organ failure after injury, the most important factors predicting increased morbidity and mortality were the severity and duration of shock after injury. Thus, shock remains a problem, particularly if it persists or is not treated expeditiously or adequately.

INITIAL THERAPY

In all patients with circulatory inadequacy, initial assessment must include not only measurement of blood pressure and urine output, but also an estimate of vascular volume as determined by filling pressures of the ventricles. Initial observation of collapse or distention of neck or peripheral veins may suffice to initiate therapy or for an uncomplicated and easily treatable problem. Depending on the urgency and severity of the situation, large-bore intravenous cannulas should be inserted, and therapy should begin immediately with volume replacement or a challenge with a fluid load unless the patient has a high filling pressure, as indicated by venous distention, or high CVP or wedge pressure, which by definition indicates cardiogenic shock. If there is any doubt about the adequacy of vascular or extracellular fluid volume, a fluid challenge of 200 to 500 ml should be given over 10 to 15 minutes. Ringer's lactate is the best fluid for initial resuscitation and replacement or treatment of any patient; it is given as rapidly as needed and in as large a quantity as needed until blood pressure begins to increase, urine output begins again or increases, skin perfusion is improved, organ functin (particularly of the heart and brain) seems reasonable, and central venous or right atrial pressure increases. In the injured patient in the emergency room, 1 to 2 liters of balanced salt solution may be given in the first half-hour depending on the severity of injury and depth of hypotension. If the patient does not respond quickly to initial therapy, this should be followed by percutaneous insertion of a subclavian or internal jugular vein catheter for central venous (CVP) or right atrial pressure measurement and/or insertion of a Swan-Ganz catheter for pulmonary artery and capillary wedge pressure measurement. If, during the initial assessment or after initiation of a fluid challenge or volume replacement, there is evidence of increased venous pressure above 15 cm H_2O or venous distention to high normal or abnormal levels, then by definition there is a cardiogenic problem regardless of the original etiology of shock. This indicates that the myocardium (ventricles) cannot keep up with the circulatory demand either because of inherent problems within the myocardium itself, such as myocardial disease or myocardial depression, or because of external forces, such as tamponade or an abnormal heart rate. In such a circumstance, relief of compression, if present, or control of heart rate by correcting bradycardia or active control of tachycardia or a tachyarrhythmia by giving an inotropic agent is necessary. The best all around inotropic agent is dopamine, which not only has a potent positive effect on ventricular contractility (inotropic effect), but also improves blood flow to the kidneys. An initial infusion of 2 to 5 μg per kilogram per minute is given. A response should be apparent within a few minutes or the dose may be increased up to a maximum of 50 μg per kilogram per minute.

At this point in time, more sophisticated and invasive monitoring is necessary rather than just observation of the patient. This should include a right atrial catheter and/or a Swan-Ganz catheter (if not inserted earlier) with the capability of measuring pulmonary artery wedge pressure and also cardiac output by the thermodilution method, a Foley catheter in the bladder for continuous measurement of urine output, access to the arterial circulation for direct measurement of arterial pressure, and on-line continuous observation of arterial pressure and blood gas tension measurements. The pulmonary artery wedge pressure (PAWP) or pulmonary capillary pressure is measured with a Swan-Ganz catheter wedged into a distal pulmonary artery. This pressure is a reflection of left atrial pressure (left ventricular filling pressure). Electrolyte and fluid balance require monitoring. A continuous EKG monitor should be used and a 12-channel EKG obtained for assessment of myocardial ischemia and/or infarction.

During initial resuscitation of injured patients in the field and during transport, the MAST garment (military anti-shock trousers) has been used with some success to splint extremity injuries and decrease venous bleeding from extremity, pelvic, or lower abdominal injuries. Only a low pressure should be used. The abdomen should not be compressed with high pressures, and the garment should not be let down until the patient is in the operating room or blood volume is being restored.

Decision Regarding Operative Control of Losses

With internal and/or external hemorrhage and vascular volume loss, it is necessary to decide early whether continued resuscitation and treatment of shock is possible or reasonable or whether operative intervention to control fluid or blood loss is required. After initiation of therapy, this decision becomes a critical factor in the care of the patient. In the face of continuing losses, the patient's circulatory status cannot be stabilized.

Volume Replacement

The most common problem in surgical patients with shock is inadequate volume replacement. We frequently underestimate how much has been lost or the loss is hidden. A patient often requires more fluid replacement than predicted, estimated, or actually lost. Continuous monitoring is the best guide, not only to the volume of blood and fluids needed, but also to the rate of administration required. The goal is to achieve an effective circulating blood volume. This effective volume is a functional concept and is that volume which produces a reasonable arterial pressure, good urine output, good peripheral perfusion as judged by palpable full-peripheral pulses, warm dry skin, and good organ function (heart, lungs, brain, liver, kidneys) without excessive elevation of atrial pressures. The best initial solution is Ringer's lactate solution (balanced salt solution). Normal saline can be used and has as its only disadvantage the initial dilutional increase in metabolic acidosis that may occur. This is usually of little or no consequence. The primary ingredient in a crystalloid solution for volume replacement is the sodium ion. A salt solution given intravenously disperses into the entire extracellular fluid space including the vascular space. Thus if blood is being replaced, it is necessary to give the salt solution in an amount approximately 2.5 times the amount of blood that has been lost. Other solutions for initial volume replacement and resuscitation are primarily of historic interest and no longer have a firm place in therapy. These include plasma, albumin, purified protein fraction, and the like. They are expensive and in general are no longer necessary. It is well accepted now that during resuscitation from shock and volume replacement, fluids (other than whole blood) that provide colloid osmotic pressure are not necessary. Plasma was helpful in the past and can be given, but even in single donor units of plasma, hepatitis remains a small risk. Other solutions that provide colloid osmotic pressure include the dextrans and hydroxyethyl starch. Low-molecular-weight dextran, because of its size (40,000 daltons), does not stay in the circulation long and has no place in the initial treatment of shock. Clinical dextran (average molecular weight, 75,000 daltons) can be used for initial resuscitation. However, when given in a volume of more than 2 liters, it has been associated with increased bleeding from sites of injury due to hemodilution, increasing capillary blood flow, and dilution of clotting factors. Hydroxyethyl starch has been used in certain circumstances, but like dextran, it has no particular advantage in the initial therapy of hypovolemic shock.

Blood Transfusion

When more than one or two units of blood have been lost, replacement of red blood cells becomes necessary. Most patients with an injury or an operation can tolerate the loss of one unit of blood, and many tolerate loss of two units of blood as long as there is adequate replacement with a crystalloid solution. Hemodilution also can improve peripheral blood flow, particularly in the microcirculation, although exact clinical documentation of the value of this approach is difficult to obtain. However, if hemodilution by volume replacement with crystalloid solution decreases the hematocrit to 30 or below, reduced oxygen transport to peripheral tissues by the smaller number of red cells may be problem. With a hematocrit below 30, and particularly at 25, cardiac output may not be able to increase sufficiently to compensate and maintain oxygen delivery, and peripheral tissue hypoxia may occur.

Most blood banks now prefer to provide blood in its component parts. Packed red cells are satisfactory for elective replacement of blood loss in the operating room or on the surgical ward. However, the patient with massive blood loss may be in jeopardy because of the difficulty in infusing packed red cells rapidly. Whole blood is preferable when there has been massive blood loss. Fresh blood has some advantages, but is almost impossible to obtain. Blood from the blood bank is cold, hyperkalemic, acidotic, and hypocalcemic. In spite of this, blood should be given as rapidly as it is needed and can be given when massive transfusions are required. However, it should be warmed during infusion. If, with massive transfusion, the blood is not warmed, core body temperature may be reduced, and the result may be ventricular fibrillation. One ampule of sodium bicarbonate can be given empirically with each two units of bank blood. Usually the increase potassium in bank blood is of little moment if urine output is normal. The low calcium in blood from the ACD or CPD solution (acid citrate dextrose, citrate phosphate dextrose) is not a problem unless the patient has liver disease. Giving supplemental calcium infusions empirically is not wise. With massive transfusions, coagulation abnormalities are frequent problems. In such circumstances, coagulation and its components are measured, and administration of fresh frozen plasma and platelet transfusions may be necessary.

If blood replacement is needed in an emergency situation before proper rapid crossmatching can be carried out, type-specific uncrossmatched blood should be given. Universal donor, type O, Rh-negative, low-antibody-titer blood was previously kept on hand for this purpose, but it is no longer readily available and type-specific blood is better.

Blood stored in a blood bank accumulates particles or debris of platelet and white cell aggregates and red cell ghosts. These embolize to the pulmonary capillary bed during transfusion. If a patient receives ten or less transfusions, such particles seem to be of little consequence and are probably broken up in the lungs. With massive transfusions, these microaggregates could produce a problem. However, this has not been well documented in patients. Microfilters to remove these particles are available and are helpful during extracorporeal circulation for cardiac surgery. However, no differences in pulmonary function have been demonstrated in patients transfused through such microfilters during operations. If microfilters are used, they should not interfere with the need to give blood as rapidly as it is needed.

Autotransfusion using a device to suction and collect blood from the operating field can be lifesaving. This requires the use of filters in the system and is worthwhile only when a large amount of blood may be lost quickly. The use of stroma-free hemoglobin to replace red blood cells is not yet ready for clinical use.

Vasoactive Agents

Vasoconstrictor agents (drugs with strong alpha-adrenergic action) have little if any place in the initial therapy of shock. These drugs include norepinephrine (Levophed), phenylephrine (Neo-Synephrine), metaraminol (Aramine), and other agents. The only role for a vasoconstrictor agent is in a patient whose blood pressure is so low that cardiorespiratory arrest is imminent or has ocurred. Then an initial increase in central perfusion pressure to the heart and brain by the use of one of these agents for a short period of time, along with volume replacement, may be necessary. Otherwise, vasoactive agents should be used only if volume replacement does not correct the problem or if there is a problem with myocardial depression and cardiogenic shock. In such a circumstance, as indicated earlier, dopamine is the initial drug of choice. Isoproterenol (Isuprel) can also be useful in certain circumstances. It is a pure beta-stimulating agent with a positive inotropic and chronotropic effect and produces peripheral vasodilation in certain vascular beds. Isoproterenol can be given at a rate of 1 to 2 μg per minute, with several milligrams mixed in 500 ml of intravenous fluid. Since isoproterenol has a potent chronotropic effect, caution is advised so that heart rate is not increased beyond an effective level (130 to 140 per minute). Digitalis is not as helpful in an emergency situation. Even the rapidly acting digitalis preparations

(Digoxin, Oubain, Deslanoside) take a half-hour or so for the initial effect, and they cannot be controlled minute-to-minute as can an intravenously infused inotropic agent. If a patient responds to an intravenous inotrope infusion, digitalization can be done slowly to supplement or take the place of the other drug. Epinephrine and dobutamine (Dobutrex) may be helpful. Other inotropic agents such as amrinone (Inocor) have had insufficient use in the treatment of shock in surgical patients to recommend their use at the present time. However, such agents may be used if dopamine, isoproterenol, epinephrine, and digitalis are not effective. Pure vasodilator drugs such as alpha-adrenergic blocking agents (phenoxybenzamine) or ganglionic blocking agents (trimethaphan camsylate) are dangerous in the treatment of shock and should not be used.

Position

The patient in shock should be kept supine and horizontal. Elevation of the legs has the effect of a single-unit blood transfusion and can be done during initial resuscitaiton. However, the Trendelenburg position was developed for exposure of the pelvic organs during operation, not for the treatment of shock. The head-down position may compromise ventilation and provide a false gravitational stimulus to the baroreceptors.

Buffering Agents

Although it is recognized that shock produces metabolic (lactic) acidosis, the best way to correct this is to improve the circulation. In certain circumstnaces, correction of metabolic acidosis by sodium bicarbonate can be helpful, but by and large, metabolic acidosis is self-correcting by circulatory improvement provided by fluids and/or inotropic agents. Intravenous sodium bicarbonate can be given (1 to 2 ampules) as an adjunct during initial resuscitation and particularly with cardiac arrest. After that, it should be given only if blood pH measurements indicate significant acidosis. Even then such continuing metabolic acidosis indicates the need for greater improvement in the circulation and not just administration of a buffering agent. The lactate in Ringer's lactate does not contribute to the lactic acidosis since it is not an acid and is metabolized rapidly by the liver.

Oxygen

Since one of the problems with shock is decreased oxygen delivery to tissues, it may be thought that supplemental oxygen would be useful. However, if the patient's lungs are normal and the patient is breathing adequately, arterial blood oxygenation should be normal. Since there may be some small advantage in increasing the oxygen dissolved in arterial blood and in increasing alveolar PaO_2, oxygen by mask (with an FiO_2 of 50%) should be given to all patients in shock. If alveolar venti-lation is inadequate or there is arterial hypoxemia, assisted ventilation is needed. In any patient in shock who does not respond to initial therapy, it is best to measure blood gas tensions, including PaO_2, $PaCO_2$ and pH to determine whether the patient requires ventilatory assistance. This is particularly true with septic shock, in which ventilatory failure is a frequent occurrence.

Diuretics

Renal function should be restored in the shock patient by the administration of fluids, transfusions, and drugs that support the circulation. However, along with these methods of treatment, an ampule of mannitol, an osmotic diuretic, or a small dose (10 to 20 mg) of furosemide (Lasix) may be given to assist in beginning a diuresis and to decrease the risk of renal failure. Diuresis cannot be produced by a diuretic in a severely hypovolemic patient, and the hazard of producing or aggravating hypovolemia by diuresis must be kept in mind. With injury, myoglobin, hemoglobin, and other proteins from injured tissue may contribute to renal tubular injury so that flushing these substances through and out of the renal tubules may be helpful.

SEPTIC SHOCK

In addition to the general treatment of infection and support of the circulation in a septic patient, there are certain other important measures to be considered. First, the best treatment for septic shock is prevention. In any patient with sepsis, a high temperature, and the requirement for a higher than normal cardiac output, the circulation should be monitored so that vascular and ECF volume are maintained, urine output is maintained, and cardiac output is kept at whatever level is necessary to prevent circulatory failure. The prodrome, described by McLean, of anxiety and confusion, hyperventilation, and respiratory alkalosis in a febrile, septic patient should alert us to the possibility of circulatory failure and the need to improve the circulation. In a patient who is febrile or toxic, particularly if he has had a recent invasive procedure, instrumentation, or an indwelling catheter, the assumption must be made that circulatory inadequacy is due to a septic process. An abnormal circulation in a patient with sepsis requires (1) circulatory support, (2) antibiotics, (3) drainage of the infection or other surgical therapy as required, (4) consideraton of ventilatory support, and (5) a decision regarding steroids.

Shock due to sepsis is a complex and poorly understood phenomenon. Although endotoxin from infection with gram-negative organisms may be a critical factor, there is no practical way to treat this clinically as yet. Antitoxins may be helpful in the future. In addition, septic shock may be produced by any organism. Infection with an elevated temperature produces demands on the circulation with decresed peripheral resistance and the need for a higher than normal blood flow. Thus, cardiac output must increase to meet the demands of the infection and its metabolic stimulus. If this cannot be met by the individual, shock results. This is why patients who are otherwise normal and then develop septic shock often initially have a hyperdynamic circulation with warm skin, bounding pules, and high cardiac output with decreased peripheral vascular resistance (high output sepsis). However, if the septic patient's fluid volume (ECF) is low or the heart cannot keep up with the demand, a low-output state (hypodynamic circulation) may be present. Again, active support of the circulation in a patient with sepsis is the best treatment to prevent septic shock from occurring. This includes maintaining an adeqaute ECF and vascular volume, monitoring cardiac function to maintain it at an optimal level, and early and aggressive treatment of the infection. If shock occurs, a number of steps must be taken quickly.

1. Blood is drawn for culture and other specimens are obtained for culture as appropriate or available (e.g., sputum, urine, drainage, pus).
2. Crystalloid solution should be given rapidly to increase vascular volume and raise filling pressures. In many septic patients, this is sufficient to increase cardiac output and peripheral blood flow to an adequate level. Sequestration of fluid (third-space losses), high insensible loss with fever, and vasodilatation all contribute to the need for large amounts of fluid. This is particularly true in patients with peritonitis, intestinal obstruction, burns, and multi-system injury.
3. At the same time, broad-spectrum antibiotics must be given systemically before culture reports are available. The decision regarding antibiotics must be based on the most likely organism or organisms present, which in turn is based on the source of the infection, e.g., whether it be biliary tract (cholangitis), urinary tract with septicemia, peritonitis, pneumonia, or enteric infection. In general, treatment is best started with an aminoglycoside such as gentamicin or kanamycin. If the causative organisms are thought to be gram-positive cocci, a large dose of intravenous penicillin is required (20,000,000 units per day). If anaerobes are suspected, as with peritonitis or abdominal wall infections (a mixed infection), a combination of gentamicin, 3 to 5 mg per kilogram per day, clindamycin, 600 to 1,200 mg per day, and penicillin, 20 to 30 million units per day, is recommended. With certain infections such as nosocomial infections or enteric infections, penicillinase-resistant drugs should be used, such as Oxacillin or one of the cephalosporins (cefoxitin, cefamandole, or cefazolin), combined with an aminoglycoside such as gentamicin or tobramycin. Clindamycin has been used with an aminoglycoside for anaerobic infections. When pseudomonas infection is suspected or if the patient is neutropenic, carbenicillin or ticarcillin should be used with an aminoglycoside.

Chloromycetin is still effective in the treatment of peritonitis. When culture reports and antibiotic sensitivities are known, appropriate changes should be made in antibiotics.
4. Drainage of the septic process, resection of necrotic tissue, or exteriorization of a leaking anastomosis must be done as quickly as possible.
5. Sepsis and septic shock are often associated with, or produce, organ failure, particularly in the lungs. There may be a specific effect of a septic process on the pulmonary capillary circulation, producing endothelial damage, interstitial edema, and the respiratory distress syndrome. Early ventilatory assistance may be necessary.
6. The use of pharmacologic doses of steroids for septic shock has been an area of controversy because of the difficulty in establishing a clear-cut clinical benefit. The rationale for their use is that under adverse circumstances, cells and organs work better with high levels of steroids (membrane stabilization and other effects). When steroids have been given experimentally before septic or endotoxic shock develops, they are beneficial. When they have been given to patients early in the course and seem to have a beneficial effect, the argument is that the patient may have gotten better anyway. When steroids have been given late in septic shock, there may not be any effect because of the severity of the problem. There is sufficient evidence of potential benefit, however, to recommend that if a patient with septic shock does not respond to initial fluid and antibiotic therapy along with further treatment and drainage of the infection, a trial of a pharmacologic dose of steroids can be given. A drug such as methylprednisolone, 30 mg per kilogram IV, administered over a few minutes and repeated in 8 to 12 hours if necessary, may be given. Dexamethasone, or hydrocortisone in comparable doses can be used. After 12 to 24 hours, if the patient has improved, the drug is stopped. The hazards and complications of such large doses given over a short period are small. There is also the possibility of acute adrenal insufficiency developing in such septic, stressed patients.

CARDIOGENIC SHOCK

Certain specific measures must be considered where the heart is the limiting factor in providing adequate circulation. If measurement of right and/or left ventricular filling pressures (CVP-PAWP) indicate that there is no volume deficit and these pressures are high, a 12-lead ECG should help to determine the possibility of myocardial ischemia and infarction or right heart strain. A chest roentgenogram and ventilation perfusion lung scan may be necessary to determine the possibility of pulmonary embolism, and this may be followed by a pulmonary arteriogram or other diagnostic studies as necessary. Cardiogenic shock may result from myocardial (muscle) depression, bradycardia, excessive afterload on the left ventricle, excessive afterload on the right ventricle by pulmonary embolism, and pericardial tamponade. For myocardial depression, an inotropic agent is necessary, as described earlier. For severe bradycardia, isoproterenol and/or a pacemaker may be required. For tachyarrhythmias, digitalis, lidocaine, a beta-blocking agent (propranolol), cardioversion, or a calcium blocking agent (verapamil) may be necessary. For reduction of afterload on the left ventricle, nitroglycerin paste, sodium nitroprusside, or an intra-aortic balloon pump may be helpful. For reduction of afterload on the right ventricle, pulmonary embolectomy, intravenous heparin, streptokinase infusion, supplementary oxygen, and ventilatory assistance may be required. If tamponade is suspected, an ultrasound study of the heart and/or a diagnostic-therapeutic pericardiocentesis should be done.

REFRACTORY SHOCK

If a patient does not respond to initial resuscitative efforts and treatment by volume replacement, inotropic agents, and other measures, intensive monitoring, detailed evaluation, and a more aggressive approach to therapy are necessary. A search for occult bleeding, tamponade, hidden sepsis, necrotic tissue, metabolic problems, or other abnormalities must be sought. In such a circumstance, the patient must have, in addition to a Foley catheter and intravenous lines, an intra-arterial line to continuously monitor intra-arterial pressure and to obtain frequent arterial blood samples for blood gas tensions and pH. In addition, a Swan-Ganz catheter should have been inserted for measurement of pulmonary artery pressure, pulmonary capillary wedge pressure, reflecting left atrial pressure, and cardiac output by the thermodilution method. In some patients, because of differences in left and right ventricular function, both right atrial and left atrial (PAWP) measurements may be needed. Unless filling pressures are very low (2 to 4 cm water), indicating inadequate volume, or very high (20 to 25 cm water), in-

dicating ventricular failure, the important comparison is what happens to filling pressure with therapy (volume, inotropes). A simple programmed calculator then allows calcultion of peripheral and pulmonary vascular resistance, oxygen consumption, and left ventricular stroke volume and work. This can be plotted against left atrial pressure, constructing ventricular function curves. The effect on ventricular function of fluids and different inotropic agents and doses can then be evaluated. If the patient requires ventilator support, an optimal level of PEEP (positive end expiratory pressures) can be determined, and the effect of afterload reduction can be measured. PEEP at pressures above 5 cm of water may decrease cardiac output because of the high intrathoracic pressure. Careful balance of forces—preload, afterload, ventricular functional characteristics, PEEP, and heart rate—are necessary to successfully treat some patients. In certain patients, particularly cardiac surgical patients, combinations of drugs may be necessary, e.g., norepinephrine combined with a vasodilator such as phentolamine, sodium nitroprusside, or nitroglycerine; or dopamine combined with nitroprusside.

In most patients, the circulation can be supported so that shock per se seems to be treated adequately. However, if the underlying problems of organ injury after trauma or sepsis cannot be controlled, organ failure (pulmonary, renal, hepatic, metabolic, gastrointestinal, and cardiac failure) results in multiple organ failure (MOF) and death. Thus rapid and complete suport of the circulation (prevention or treatment of shock) is a key factor in preventing MOF.

NEUROGENIC SHOCK

Hypotension due to syncope, spinal anesthesia, or spinal cord injury is caused by reduction in vascular resistance. It may be self-limiting or responsive to an infusion of fluids and/or a mild vasoconstrictor agent such as vasoxyl or phenylephrine. Seldom should this form of hypotension be a problem and produce the effects of what we commonly think of as shock.

ADULT RESPIRATORY DISTRESS SYNDROME

CARL E. BREDENBERG, M.D.

Adult respiratory distress syndrome (ARDS) is not a diagnosis. The term serves as a convenient shorthand to be used in discussions of acute lung injury from diverse etiologies. In surgical patients, ARDS is seen in complex clinical settings that frequently include multiple trauma and/or sepsis and often follows episodes of hemodynamic

instability, resuscitation from which requires intravenous infusion of large volumes of fluid and/or blood. The sepsis is often nonpulmonary in origin and frequently includes necrotic wounds, peritonitis, intra-abdominal abscess, and visceral leaks. The source of hemodynamic instability may be sepsis or it may be hemorrhage resulting from the initial trauma, from a surgical misadventure, or as a postoperative complication. Hemorrhage is often prolonged, control of bleeding delayed, and transfusions multiple. The hemodynamic crisis may be complex, with varying degrees of hypovolemia and sepsis mixed with poor myocardial performance, as a consequence of either shock or coincident disease such as atherosclerosis. Other frequently associated complications include renal and hepatic failure as well as disseminated intravascular coagulation (DIC).

In short, ARDS rarely occurs as a single isolated event or even as a single isolated complication in an otherwise undisturbed clinical course. The current management of patients with ARDS is largely preventive and supportive. Prevention of ARDS begins with good surgical judgment and good operative execution. Expeditious assessment and operation, prompt control of hemorrhage, appropriate management of traumatic injuries, construction of secure anastomoses and visceral closures, adequate debridement, and timely drainage of abscesses are all aspects of traditional surgical skills that help prevent ARDS.

Physiologic abnormalities common to ARDS include lung edema, increased venous admixture or pulmonary "shunting," and a poorly compliant stiff lung. Lung water is increased secondary to varying degrees of interstitial edema and inflammation with vascular congestion. Left heart failure usually is not the primary cause of this edema. However, poor cardiac function, in which increased left heart filling pressure is required to maintain cardiac output, may be a major contributing factor. The increase in lung water with ARDS is often seen without markedly elevated microvascular hydrostatic pressure, and an increase in pulmonary microvascular membrane permeability is a frequent consequence of the lung injury. Pulmonary hypertension and increased pulmonary vascular resistance are present in many patients. The source of these pulmonary hemodynamic changes and their effect on microvascular pressure and membrane permeability are still unclear.

Increased pulmonary venous admixture and "shunting" result from continued perfusion of non-ventilated or underventilated alveoli. Alveoli may be nonventilated because of collapse and microatelectasis or because they are filled with edema or pus. If perfusion of nonventilated alveoli continues, venous blood is returned to the arterial system without additional oxygen. As a consequence, one of the hallmarks of ARDS is the persistence of arterial hypoxemia despite high concentrations of inspired oxygen.

The result of lung injury, alveolar collapse, vascular congestion, and parenchymal edema is a "stiff" poorly compliant lung that requires high peak pressure for ventilation. The volume in the lung at the end of expiration, that is, functional residual capacity (FRC), is reduced. At a low FRC, more alveoli become unstable and tend to collapse, further reducing FRC and increasing pulmonary shunt and hypoxemia.

ROLE OF HEMODYNAMICS

Aggressive fluid administration is often required in these patients to provide the filling volumes for adequate cardiac output. The increase in microvascular permeability frequently seen with ARDS increases the vulnerability of the lung to edema even with small increases in hydrostatic pressure. With a porous microvascular membrane, relatively small increases in cardiac filling pressures with secondary increases in pulmonary microvascular pressure can contribute to interstitial pulmonary edema. Lung edema and the frequent occurrence of hemodynamic instability make precise hemodynamic management and avoidance of increased microvascular hydrostatic pressure critical to prevention and treatment of ARDS.

The choice of fluid for resuscitation remains controversial, depending largely on how one interprets the roles of plasma oncotic pressure and the microvascular membrane in pulmonary edema. When hematocrit is low, administration of red cells is useful. This increases oxygen-carrying capacity of blood and also provides a volume expander which, all agree, remains within the intravascular space whatever changes occur in microvascular permeability. As long as one does not "overtransfuse" to hematocrits greater than 40, the rheologic limitations from the increased viscosity of high hematocrit are probably more theoretical than real. There are preliminary experimental data suggesting that increased hematocrit may protect against pulmonary edema. It is also agreed that isotonic salt solutions are necessary. Plasma volume usually needs to be expanded along with red cell mass, and frequently there are extra-cellular volumes that need to be repleted.

It is controversial whether protein or some other large molecule should be added to this agreed-upon mixture of isotonic salt solution and red cells. The lack of a definitive answer to this controversy in the face of abundant experimental and clinical work suggests that this particular question may not be as important as the loyalists on either side claim. The effectiveness of plasma oncotic pressure in preventing pulmonary edema depends on an intact microvascular membrane to maintain the oncotic gradient between the plasma and interstitial fluid. Since pulmonary microvascular membrane permeability is increased in many of the injuries leading to ARDS, the theoretical benefit from intravascular colloid may not apply, particularly in the case of sepsis and shock. On the other hand, evidence that colloid solutions are injurious to the lung is insecure. Intravenous fluid is like any drug; it must be given in sufficient volumes to be therapeutically effective, but one must avoid overdose. I favor a combination of red cells and isotonic salt solution (Ringer's lactate or normal saline, usualy in 5% dextrose) without the routine addition of colloid. Careful hemodynamic monitoring is far more important than whether or not protein is added to the resuscitation fluid. An intra-arterial catheter for pressure measurements and blood sampling and a Swan-Ganz catheter with thermister tip for measurement of cardiac output and pulmonary artery wedge pressure and for mixed venous blood sampling are necessary in complex situations.

In administering stored bank blood or packed cells, the contribution of particulate debris to the development of ARDS is probably not so great as it was once believed. Experimental evidence in subhuman primates as well as human clinical studies indicate that at least 10 unit transfusions are necessary before debris can be identified in the lungs and that, even then, the role of this debris in the development in ARDS is a secondary one. A place for microaggregate filters (pore size 20 to 40 μ) would appear to be only in patients who receive truly massive transfusion (more than 10 to 15 units). Because of obstruction by debris on the micropore filter, blood must be administered under pressure and the filters changed every 3 to 5 units. This may limit the usefulness of these filters in the very settings in which one might want them, i.e., emergent resuscitation of the patient suffering massive hemorrhage.

Using intravenous fluids to increase cardiac output solely by increasing left ventricular filling volume may be one way that increases in microvascular hydrostatic pressure are created that are large enough to be hazardous to the lung with an injured and therefore leaky microvascular membrane. If both cardiac output and filling volumes are low, initial efforts are directed at rapid volume infusion. This approach is usually effective. However, if filling pressures increase without an adequate increase in cardiac output, I add adrenergic support with either dopamine or dobutamine. In low and moderate doses, dopamine and dobutamine increase the force of ventricular contractility. They are not "vasopressors," and in low and moderate doses they may even decrease systemic vascular resistance. Dopamine includes a specific pharmacologic effect of increasing renal blood flow. These drugs usually are not necessary in previously healthy ptaients with pure hemorrhage. In complex hemodynamic situations in which elements of sepsis and pump failure are present, they may help to achieve hemodynamic resuscitation and urine output with less overexpansion of intravascular and extracellular volume and thus less potential for injury to the lung.

Aggressive fluid therapy includes the necessary rapid administration of large volumes of blood and isotonic salt solution during the acute resuscitative interval of trauma, hemorrhage, and sepsis. Aggressive fluid therapy also includes early and definitive turning off of the "faucet" when resuscitation has been accomplished. The early use of loop diuretics (Lasix or ethacrynic acid) in the post-resuscitative interval may help to prevent lung edema. It is particularly important to identify those patients in whom fluid overload and expanded extracellular volume are contributing to pulmonary failure. It is this subgroup of patients with ARDS which responds particularly well to diuretic therapy and in whom the full-blown picture of ARDS may be prevented by judicious fluid management.

PULMONARY COLLAPSE AND INFECTION

The assiduous applicaton of standard maneuvers in the nonintubated patient to prevent pulmonary collapse and clear bronchial secretions deserves emphasis in discussions of more exotic, but perhaps less controllable, factors. In getting the patient to cough and take a deep breath, verbal encouragement and incentive spirometers are standard and useful techniques. Position change is

important to prevent pooling of secretions and persisting hydrostatic pressure gradients, which lead to dependent lung edema. No position is ideal for all patients and no single position is good for any patient. Percussive therapy of the chest, when applied by skilled practitioners, is an effective adjunct. Endotracheal suctioning, using sterile technique to prevent airway contamination and caution to prevent hypoxemia, also helps to clear secretions and expand the lungs. Flexible bronchoscopy for airway aspiration can be more easily applied than its rigid counterpart.

The occult aspiration of oral and pharyngeal contents or of small-volume gastric contents may be a source of pulmonary infection. Adequate gastric decompression, pharyngeal suctioning, and proper inflation of cuffs on endotracheal and tracheostomy tubes are important preventive measures. Frequent sputum cultures help to monitor microbial growth in the lower airway. The indiscriminate use of broad-spectrum antibiotics may lead to the emergence of resistance organisms in the lungs, contributing to a terminal pneumonia superimposed on whatever other pulmonary and nonpulmonary crises already exist. Current use of prophylactic antibiotics generally limits them to within 24 hours or less of surgery or trauma. The decision whether to start therapeutic antibiotics should be approached with the same gravity as surgical decisions. Failure to treat infection has an obvious consequence. The development of drug-resistant super-infection when antibiotics are administered unnecessarily, or when too many are given, or when they are continued too long is a less frequently recognized but potentially devastating consequence of that decision.

The foregoing discussion is not meant to imply that ARDS is simply another name for pulmonary edema or bacterial pneumonia. Nevertheless, it reflects a conviction that pulmonary infection and fluid overload are frequent contributors to ARDS. They are contributions that often can be effectively prevented or treated.

MECHANICAL VENTILATION

Patients with ARDS receive mechanical ventilation. The goal of mechanical ventilation is to sustain the patient until the underlying pulmonary and nonpulmonary problems can be corrected and the lung heals sufficiently to allow effective gas exchange during spontaneous ventilation. In the unintubated patient, the goal is anticipation and early detection of respiratory failure so that intubation can be performed in controlled circumstances rather than as a hectic, emergent procedure. Serial arterial blood gases, careful clinical observation particularly for tachypnea or signs of increased respiratory effort, and a "prepared mind" are most important. The use of compliant high-volume tube cuffs has markedly reduced the frequency of tracheal injury. I usually leave endotracheal tubes in place for 10 to 14 days before considering tracheostomy unless I know sooner that long-term ventilation will be required. Sterile handling and suctioning are observed as well as regular changes of respirator tubing and humidifiers to reduce the chances of nosocomial superinfection. With today's sophisticated ventilators, use of controlled ventilation is unnecessary. The patient's own ventilatory pattern usually can be more readily adapted to the machine's, using either intermittent mandatory ventilation (IMV) or an assist/control ventilatory pattern.

With intubation and mechanical ventilation, positive end expiratory pressure (PEEP) may be added to the ventilatory cycle. PEEP does not drive water out of the edematous lung, but it can be a useful technique for maintaining gas transport until lung and patient are healed. The hysteresis of the lung during volume change means that it takes a higher pressure to achieve a given lung volume during inspiration than it does to maintain that same lung volume during expiration. Although the origins of this phenomenon are complex, the clinical implications are straightforward: it is easier and takes less pressure to maintain the volume of alveoli that are already open than it is to reopen collapsed alveoli. Thus the goals of ventilator therapy are to recruit (open) closed alveoli and then to maintain alveolar patency by ventilating the lung from an increased functional residual capacity (FRC).

Alveolar recruitment is largely a function of peak inspiratory pressure. Recruitment maneuvers include intermittent sighing, either by regularly spaced large ventilator breaths or by manual breaths with an Ambu bag. Normal exhalation is to zero (atmospheric) pressure. Increasing the pressure at end expiration (PEEP) increases the volume in the lung at the end of expiration (FRC). Since the lung begins inflation at a higher volume and pressure, peak inspiratory volume and pressure are also increased, thus aiding recruitment. More significantly, with higher lung volume at the end of expiration, alveoli are less likely to collapse and thus alveolar and airway patency are maintained for the next inspiration. The usual result is better matching of ventilation and perfusion and thus improved oxygenation of blood. There may be a critical lung volume that must be reached before alveoli are recruited and stabilized. Thus, occasionally sequential increases in PEEP may have relatively little effect on PaO_2 until a critical level is reached when a small additional increase in FRC and/or additional recruitment maneuvers markedly improves PaO_2.

The addition of PEEP to the ventilator requires the judicious balance of the benefits to the lung of increased FRC with the depressant effect on cardiac output of increased intrathoracic pressure. Five management variables include (1) the concentration of inspired oxygen (FiO_2), (2) the level of PEEP, (3) the arterial Po_2 [PaO_2] that is acceptable, (4) intravascular volume, and (5) adrenergic support of the left ventricle. The relative importance of these factors varies, depending on the priorities of heart and lung at a given moment.

Because of the dangers to the lung of oxygen toxicity, I try to maintain FiO_2 at 0.4 or below. My usual goal with the FiO_2 is to achieve a PaO_2 above 90 mm Hg. Although this is significantly less than the PaO_2 that would normally be achieved with an FiO_2 of 0.4, it is sufficient for full oxygenation of hemoglobin. If this PaO_2 is not achieved

and there is hemodynamic stability, I progressively increase PEEP to levels of 15 cm H_2O, if necessary, to achieve the desired PaO_2. If, on the other hand, the patient has a severely reduced cardiac output, I do not add PEEP or limit PEEP to 5 cm H_2O. In this situation, I try to achieve a satisfactory PaO_2 by temporarily increasing FiO_2 as high as 0.9 without challenging cardiac output with a further increase in PEEP. Ideally, these high levels of FiO_2 are maintained for less than 12 to 24 hours. Once hemodynamic stability has been restored, FiO_2 is lowered and PEEP increased. I am also willing to accept a lower FiO_2 in critical situations, if necessary, to avoid prolonged high FiO_2 or very high levels of PEEP. A PaO_2 of 65 mm Hg, for example, should provide adequate oxygenation in most patients.

There is a contrary opinion that seeks to "optimize" PEEP by increasing it until the minimum level of intrapulmonary shunt is achieved regardless of PaO_2. Using this technique, PEEP may be increased to levels above 20 to 25 cm H_2O (so called "super PEEP"). Maintenance of cardiac output at high levels of super PEEP often requires administration of large volumes of intravenous fluids and/or adrenergic support. The addition of moderate amounts of PEEP (5 to 15 cm H_2O) may unmask occult hypovolemia, requiring replacement of these intravenous deficits. On the other hand, I see no value in overexpanding intravascular volume or adding adrenergic support simply to allow levels of PEEP above 15 to 20 cm H_2O unless one is struggling to achieve a minimally adequate PaO_2 and all other measures have failed. The critical balance of cardiac output and lung function with PEEP further underlines the importance of thoughtful hemodynamic management and precise ventilator control in patients with ARDS.

ONGOING RESEARCH

It has been suggested that high-frequency jet ventilation may allow the addition of PEEP without large increases in mean intrathoracic pressure. To be clinically effective, high-frequency jet ventilation must be combined with the regular insertion of conventional tidal volumes to recruit alveoli. On the other hand, in my own experimental work, jet ventilators have been ineffective in very stiff lungs, and this technique of ventilatory management remains experimental.

Failure, despite abundant research, to demonstrate a conclusive benefit of steroids persuades this observer that they are unnecessary in the treatment of ARDS. Current research is exploring the interactions of cellular injury and bacteria with host defenses, including the byproducts of dead white cells and killed bacteria. The impact of these and fibrin breakdown products on the complement and immune systems of the patient is providing a complex but fertile ground for linking nonpulmonary sepsis and injury to lung failure. In this experimental work, enzymes that break down proteins (proteases) and free oxygen radicals appear to play an important role in lung injury. It is possible that protease enzyme blockers and/or free oxygen radical scavengers may someday be administered to prevent or treat ARDS. Installation into the airway of artificial surfactant has had limited application in infantile respiratory distress

syndromes and conceivably could make the alveoli of adult lungs more stable with consequent better matching of ventilation and perfusion. However, given the vagaries inherent in the shorthand term "ARDS," specific therapy remains a speculative glimmer on a distant horizon.

LIVER INJURY

CHARLES E. LUCAS, M.D.

The three main principles in the treatment of liver injury are (1) control of bleeding, (2) adequate debridement, and (3) appropriate drainage. The most important determinant of survival is control of bleeding. Consequently, preparation for laparotomy is done in conjunction with rapid volume restoration and with appropriate blood bank back-up and support.

LIVER EXPOSURE

A midline laparotomy extending from xiphoid to or below the umbilicus facilitates rapid exposure of the injured liver. The degree of liver mobilization varies according to the site and severity of injury. The falciform ligament is divided in most patients to facilitate exposure. Cholecystectomy may be required in patients with injuries to the gallbladder bed. Division of the right and left triangular ligaments permits excellent exposure to the superior liver margins, whereas taking down the liver off the "bare area" of the right hemidiaphragm facilitates exposure to the superior and medial portion of the right lobe and the right hepatic vein. Often this latter maneuver must be made by "Brail technique" in the actively bleeding patient. Once the right or left lobes have been completely mobilized in this manner they can be delivered to the midline incision, where definitive hemostasis can be obtained more easily.

Anatomic resection requires complete mobilization of either the left or the right lobe in order to permit dissection and ligation of the respective hepatic veins. A median sternotomy with bisection of the diaphragm in the median plane permits visualization of the right hepatic vein, which is about 1.5 cm long prior to its entrance into the inferior vena cava. The left hepatic vein may be visualized by mobilizing the left lobe anteriorly and medially away from the left hemidiaphragm. Control of the midhepatic vein is accomplished during resection since this vein bifurcates within the substance of the liver.

CONTROL OF BLEEDING

Often the liver injury has stopped bleeding or will stop bleeding with temporary pack compression; when this occurs in the stable, fully restored patient, no hemostatic technique is required. When bleeding persists, the simplest and most effective means of hemostasis is the liver suture, using 2–0 chromic suture swaged onto a 2-inch blunt-tip "liver needle." Deep liver sutures placed 2 cm from the injury margins permits gentle but effective approximation of the underlying tissue and thus hemostasis (Fig. 1). Deep buttress sutures placed parallel to the margin of injury may be used to anchor perpendicular sutures placed across the margin of injury. This technique provides hemostasis in most stab wounds, many gunshot wounds, and some blunt liver disruptions.

When the liver wound does not lend itself to liver suture hemostasis, the injury may be unroofed as a tractotomy or hepatotomy, thereby exposing partially severed arteries or veins within the substance of the liver. This technique permits these individual cross-linking vessels to be clamped, divided, and secured, after which the margins of the tractotomy are reapproximated by liver sutures. Tractotomy with intraparenchymal ligation of cross-linking vessels permits good hemostasis in many deep gunshot wounds and deep blunt injuries.

When the actively bleeding liver cannot be controlled by sutures or tractotomy, hepatic artery ligation (HAL), resectional debridement, or anatomic resection may be needed. Hepatic artery ligation, which is effective for controlling arterial bleeding but not portal venous or hepatic venous bleeding, should be performed as close to the site of injury as possible. It seldom causes hepatic necrosis. A cholecystectomy should be added when blood flow through the cystic artery is compromised by HAL.

Resectional debridement is a good technique in patients with ragged injuries sometimes seen after "blowout" deceleration trauma or close-range shotgun blasts involving the liver periphery. The area of ragged liver parenchyma is resected by performing a sharp debridement near the margins of injury, followed by approximation of the fresh margins by liver sutures, if possible, or by control of bleeding from the fresh cut by means of deeply placed liver sutures across the fresh margin.

Anatomic resection, which is best reserved for bleeding wounds that cannot be made hemostatic by some lesser technique, is also mandated when HAL leads to irreversible ischemia. When anatomic resection is needed, mobilization of the involved segment or lobe must be accomplished while temporary control of the bleeding segment is achieved by pack compression, temporary occlusion of the porta hepatis, or placement of a retrohepatic shunt to achieve inflow and outflow occlusion.

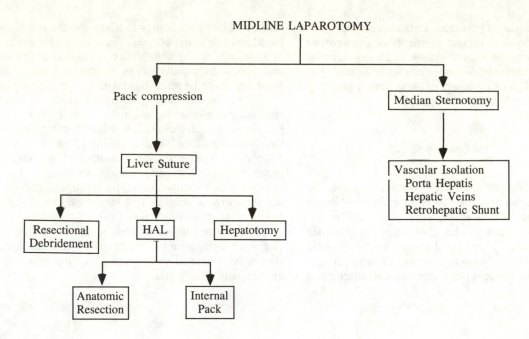

Figure 1 Approach to the bleeding liver

This latter technique, namely the insertion of a retrohepatic inferior vena cava shunt, has been widely discussed, but in practice seldom leads to patient survival. The technique used to obtain hemostasis during the placement of this shunt usually ends up being the definitive technique for hemostasis; continued bleeding during placement of the shunt is almost always lethal. This technique should be held in reserve, however, for the rare patient in whom it can be lifesaving.

When all other techniques fail, the liver injury may be made hemostatic by the placement of an internal pack. The use of a pack is reserved for patients who have an ongoing coagulation problem despite component therapy, for refractory bleeding despite multiple hemostatic attempts, and for injuries requiring anatomic resection when the surgeon is not prepared to do that operation. Internal packing and closure permits transfer to another facility for a second attempt at definitive hemostasis by means of anatomic resection by a more experienced surgeon. This definitive procedure may be deferred for 1 or 2 days when appropriate coagulation support has been instituted and the blood bank is fully stocked for back-up support.

INTRAHEPATIC HEMATOMA

Many intrahepatic hematomas may resolve spontaneously. Consequently, when this diagnosis is made prior to laparotomy in a patient without hemoperitoneum or other organ injury requiring laparotomy, the patient may be observed nonoperatively by serial liver scans. When the intrahepatic hematoma is associated with a capsular tear and hemoperitoneum, laparotomy is mandatory in order to evacuate and drain the intrahepatic hematoma and obtain hemostasis by the aforementioned

techniques. Prior to full evacuation, care must be taken to control hepatic artery and portal venous inflow, and one must be prepared to secure hepatic venous outflow.

HEMOBILIA

Hemobilia is a complication of hepatic trauma due to a fistula formation between the hepatic artery and one of the intrahepatic biliary radicles. Hemobilia is suspected by the triad of (1) a history of trauma, (2) right upper quadrant pain, and (3) hematemesis followed by relief of pain. Once suspected, hemobilia is confirmed by arteriography and may be treated by HAL, hepatotomy with intraparenchymal division of the fistula, anatomic resection of the involved area, or nonoperative embolization of the involved artery. The site and extent of the fistula determine the desired mode of therapy (Table 1).

DEBRIDEMENT

Debridement of liver tissue is seldom required since most patients with liver injury have no liver tissue that

TABLE 1 Approach to Hemobilia

Operative	*Nonoperative*
Peripheral fistula	Embolization
Tractotomy and ligation	
Central fistula	
HAL	
Central fistula refractory	
to inflow occlusion	
Anatomic resection	

is not being adequately perfused. Debridement therefore should be confined to ragged segments of liver parenchyma which are obviously nonviable and will otherwise lead to intra-abdominal infection. Portions of injured liver that are attached by a thin bridge of tissue to the remaining liver are resected between clamps.

DRAINAGE

A small nonbleeding liver wound requires no drainage. Larger wounds are treated by soft rubber drains placed in a dependent location. Sump drains are recommended by many, although I have noted a higher incidence of bleeding from adjacent solid viscera or fistulization from hollow viscera following the use of sump drains. Drains should be brought out a separate stab wound that readily admits two fingers to allow for the free flow of blood and bile to the outside. These drains should be left in place only as long as they continue to drain, after which they should be rapidly advanced over the next 2 days. Most drains can be removed at 5 days, although occasionally persistent drainage of a serosanguineous material requires that a drain be left in for several weeks. When bile flows through these drains, a biliary cutaneous fistula has been identified. These usually close in 3 weeks. Supportive therapy during this interval includes total parenteral nutrition and timely antibiotics. In rare instances, such fistulas persist for prolonged periods and require operative closure. This may occur in a patient who has an obstruction of the distal common bile duct owing to an associated unrecognized injury to the bile duct. Definitive drainage of the biliary tree by choledochostomy should be restricted to patients who have injury to the extrahepatic biliary tree.

PANCREATIC AND DUODENAL INJURY

GEORGE L. JORDAN, Jr., M.D., M.S.(Surg.)

Injuries to the duodenum and/or pancreas occur in approximately 8 percent of patients who sustain abdominal trauma. All types of injuries are encountered, including lacerations, through-and-through penetrations, and contusions. Blunt force may crush the neck or body of the pancreas and/or the third portion of the duodenum against the vertebral column and result in an isolated injury to either of these organs. In most patients, however, there are associated injuries of other organs. Elevation of the serum amylase concentration may be noted in injuries to either of these organs as amylase spilled from a ruptured duodenum is rapidly absorbed and causes abnormal serum values. This test is helpful only in patients in whom the diagnosis of intra-abdominal injury is in doubt.

The usual preoperative diagnosis is that of intra-abdominal injury based on the history and physical examination, leading to the diagnosis of peritonitis or intra-abdominal hemorrhage rather than delineation of the specific organs involved. When the diagnosis of intra-abdominal injury is in doubt, peritoneal lavage is a valuable test with a high degree of accuracy. It is utilized in patients with knife wounds and in patients with blunt trauma without clinical findings of organ injury. Gastrografin swallow has been advocated by some as a diagnostic tool in questionable cases of duodenal rupture, but this test is not recommended. CT scan has been recommended as a method to diagnose specific organ injury preoperatively. This modality may be helpful in the occasional patient in whom other modalities of diagnosis are negative or equivocal. It is used in only a small percentage of patients.

Occasionally a patient who on initial evaluation appears to have no intra-abdominal injury will develop signs of duodenal obstruction after a few days or a week, owing to an intramural hematoma. Similarly, an undiagnosed pancreatic injury may result in formation of a pseudocyst. Ultrasound and a CT scan are unequivocally the best diagnostic modalities for detecting the latter abnormality. Some have used endoscopic retrograde cholangiopancreatography (ERCP) for the diagnosis of pancreatic ductal disruption, but we have not because injuries of this severity can be suspected on clinical grounds and may be diagnosed on CT scan without the use of this invasive technique.

Exploration of patients with suspected upper abdominal trauma requires a careful examination of the duodenum and the pancreas for final diagnosis as well as delineation of the pathology must be made at the time of operation. The possibility of a duodenal injury should be immediately suspected if there is gaseous crepitation and/or bile staining of periduodenal tissue. Similarly, damage to these organs must be suspected when there is a retroperitoneal hematoma in the immediate proximity. When the possibility of injury exists, careful examination of the entire duodenum and the entire pancreas must be accomplished. The first, second, and proximal third portions of the duodenum as well as the head of the pancreas can be explored by a Kocher maneuver, incising the peritoneal attachment along the posterolateral border of the duodenum and dissecting bluntly in the plane just anterior to the vena cava. This allows inspection of both anterior and posterior surfaces of the duodenum as well as the posterior aspect of the head of the pancreas. The remainder of the duodenal examination requires division of the ligament of Treitz and reflection toward the right to expose the fourth and the entire third portion of the duodenum, after retracting the small intestine and the superior mesenteric vessels to prevent injury to these structures. The completion of the pancreatic examination requires division of the gastrocolic omentum to expose the entire anterior surface of the head, neck, body, and tail. When posterior pancreatic wounds are suspected, the peritoneum along the inferior border of the gland can be incised and the entire body and tail of the gland rotated upward to allow inspection of this area.

PANCREATIC WOUNDS

Management of wounds of the body and tail of the pancreas is determined by the type of injury. Simple contusions or superifical lacerations may be treated by drainage of the injured area. Deep lacerations are sutured. Pancreatic transections and wounds that may have traversed the main pancreatic duct may be managed in a variety of ways. The most common technique is distal pancreatectomy which also requires a splenectomy in most cases. Although the spleen may be preserved in some individuals by ligation of the splenic artery and vein near the splenic hilum, maintaining the blood supply to the spleen through retrograde flow via the gastroepiploic and short gastric vessels, in most instances the spleen is removed. The spleen should be removed when it has been injured in association with pancreatic injury. Closure of the splenic vein and artery is best done with vascular suture rather than a simple tie. The proximal transected end of the pancreas should be closed. The pancreatic duct should be specifically identified and individually ligated. The transected pancreas can then be closed either by staples or by suture. I continue to prefer sutures and place a row of interrupted Prolene sutures reinforced by a running suture of Prolene. This closure is further protected by placement of a tongue of omentum so sutured that it occludes and forms a seal over the closed end of the pancreas. This area should be well drained. The alternate method of treating pancreatic transection is anastomosis to a Roux-en-Y loop. The Roux-en-Y loop may be brought only to the distal end with closure of the proximal transected end, or anastomosis of the loop to both transected ends. This latter technique is more complicated and has been used in relatively few patients. Reconstruction in this manner should be accomplished in only good-risk patients in whom there are no, or few, associated injuries, and particularly when there has been no associated injury of the splenic vessels or the spleen itself.

Fortunately, bleeding directly from the pancreas is rarely severe. When severe bleeding occurs from the region of the pancreas it is almost invariably due to injury to an associated major vessel—the splenic, hepatic, or superior mesenteric vessels, or the gastroduodenal artery. Massive bleeding from the superior mesenteric vein may on occasion require division of pancreatic tissue for exposure, and one should not hesitate to do so if necessary to control life-endangering hemorrhage. Exposure of an injury of the superior mesenteric artery or aorta can be accomplished by reflecting the pancreas, spleen, and left colon to the right, thus allowing exposure of the origin of the superior mesenteric artery and aorta.

Wounds of the head of the pancreas, despite the increased possibility of fistula formation, can be primarily repaired in most instances. When the major duct is injured, drainage with a Roux-en-Y loop of jejunum should be considered before resection. On rare occasions, pancreatoduodenectomy is required because destruction of the head of the pancreas and the duodenum is so extensive that salvage is impossible. Total pancreatectomy should be considered only when there is total destruction of all pancreatic tissue. Salvage of even a relatively small remnant of pancreatic tissue, which will prevent diabetes, is highly desirable.

Injury to the common bile duct in its intrapancreatic portion associated with a wound of the head of the pancreas should be treated by placement of a T-tube that approximates the size of the common bile duct, passing it through the area of the injury. The injury itself can be repaired if it is easily exposed; however, division of the pancreas to expose the common bile duct injury is not justified. Some of these injuries heal satisfactorily without stricture formation. In other patients, however, stricture formation occurs and requires late operative repair. In my experience, this has been extremely uncommon.

DUODENAL WOUNDS

Duodenal perforation allows escape of active digestive juices into the retroperitoneal space or into the free peritoneal cavity. There is a potential for severe fluid and electrolyte loss, particularly if a major fistula develops. Lack of a serosal surface on the lateral and posterior portions of the duodenum makes repair or anastomsis less secure than gastric or small bowel anastomoses. In actuality, however, most duodenal wounds can be repaired successfully. We have reported primary repair of 100 minor and moderate wounds of the duodenum without fistula formation. All fistulas occurred from major wounds that devitalized large segments of the duodenal wall, necessitating special procedures in their management and defying closure or repair. I close duodenal wounds with three rows of sutures in the line of the damage of the duodenum, either transversally or longitudinally. The inner row is a running baseball stitch of 4–0 chromic catgut, taking full-thickness bites of the duodenal wall, sufficiently deep to provide adequate tensile strength, but small enough to avoid turning in a large cuff. The second row is a running horizontal mattress stitch of 4–0 chromic catgut, and the third row consists of interrupted sutures of silk or Prolene placed as horizontal mattress sutures. The entire repair is then protected by suturing omentum or adjacent mesenteric structures to seal this area. This latter coverage also prevents direct contact with drains, which should be placed into the general region of the wound but not against the actual repair. Most severe wounds require special procedures for treatment. Occasionally there is total division of the duodenum with sufficient tissue remaining so that debridement and a primary end-to-end anastomosis is accomplished. In other patients, the destruction is so great that the distal end must simply be closed and gastrointestinal continuity established by anastomosis between the proximal transected end and a loop of jejunum. Wounds that destroy so much of the lateral wall that a primary closure cannot be accomplished without fear of stricture formation or undue tension on the suture line, increasing the chances of fistula formation, may be repaired by a number of special techniques. A side-to-side duodenojejunostomy may be performed, an onlay serosal patch of jejunum may be utilized, or a patch of jejunum created specifically to fit this defect. The latter procedure is actually rarely used as it is unduly time-consuming and more complicated than the other techniques mentioned. Pancreatoduodenectomy has never been utilized in our institution for a patient who had injury to the duodenum alone. Even injuries directly to the papilla of Vater can be satisfactorily repaired. As noted in the section on the pancreas, pancreatoduodenectomy is justified only when there has been massive destruction of the head of the pancreas as well as injury to the duodenum.

Destructive wounds of the first portion of the duodenum are special in the sense that this portion of the duodenum can be easily resected and managed by limited gastrectomy, and injuries to the fourth portion can always be managed, if necessary, by anastomosis to the proximal jejunum.

When complicated wounds of the duodenum increase the probability of wound disruption or of stricture formation, some adjunctive procedure to prevent rises in pressure within the duodenum should be employed. Tubes for duodenal decompression can be placed directly into the duodenum by Witzel duodenostomy or a tube jejunostomy threaded back into the duodenum. When these techniques are used, a tube jejunostomy is also placed for feedings. In complicated cases, I prefer total diversion of all gastrointestinal contents from the duodenum by closure of the pylorus and performance of a gastrojejunostomy, which eliminates the need for a feeding jejunostomy and allows a patient to resume normal oral alimentation as soon as bowel function has returned.

Intramural Hematoma of the Duodenum

Blunt injury to the duodenum may result in the development of a hematoma in the submucosal plane. This may reach sufficient size to compress the bowel lumen and produce obstruction. The mucosa characteristically remains intact as does the serosal surface, and there is no intestinal perforation. The diagnosis is confirmed by a roentgenographic study with barium, which shows obstruction to the duodenum and a characteristic "coil spring" appearance of the area of obstruction. If obstruction is incomplete, the patient may be treated by nasogastric suction and parenteral nutrition for the lesion may resolve spontaneously. This can be confirmed by a repeat barium study. If improvement has not occurred in 7 to 10 days, operative intervention is indicated, which consists of longitudinal incision of the duodenal wall to the submucosal plane and evacuation of the hematoma, ligation

of the bleeding vessels, and partial closure of the seromuscular defect.

When a hematoma of the duodenum is identified at the time of an emergency operation, it should be evacuated if it is sufficiently large to encroach on the lumen of the bowel. Care must be taken to ensure that there has been no actual perforation.

DRAINAGE

The most common recommendation for drainage of pancreatic and severe duodenal injuries found in the literature is use of a sump drain. In the past, sump drains were made of hard plastic or rubber and there was danger of erosion of adjacent organs. Today, a number of softer plastic drains are available which have a lower probability of erosion. However, I continue to use simple Penrose drains as the initial technique of drainage because most pancreatic and duodenal wounds heal primarily. Our incidence of duodenal fistula is only 2 percent. The incidence of pancreatic fistula remains high, ranging from 25 to 30 percent, as will be discussed subsequently, but most are small fistulas, and Penrose drainage is all that is needed. The routine use of sump drains makes treatment of these wounds unduly complicated, restricts the activities of the patient, and requires an entirely different level of nursing care. On the other hand, sump drains are extremely valuable if a large pancreatic or duodenal fistula develops. Under these circumstances, either the sump drain can be inserted beside the Penrose drains to ensure adequate evacuation of fistulous drainage or the Penrose drains can be completely removed and the sump drain substituted. Sump drainage should be maintained as long as the fistulous drainage is excessive in order to protect the skin and to allow an accurate collection of drainage material for calculation of fluid and electrolyte requirements.

In the uncomplicated case, the Penrose drains are left in place for 12 days and are then shortened. They are then removed over the next 2 or 3 days, gradually, to allow healing of the deeper portions of the tract prior to the time that they are removed from the abdominal wall.

COMPLICATIONS OF PANCREATIC INJURY

Patients with pancreatic injuries may develop a multitude of complications as may patients with any intra-abdominal injury. With the exception of pancreatic fistula, the intra-abdominal complications are more commonly related to wounds of other organs than to the pancreas itself. Complications that may result specifically from the pancreatic injury are fistula formation, pancreatic abscess, pancreatitis, and pseudocyst.

The most common complication, as previously noted, is pancreatic fistula. The fistula may occur even when it appears that only small pancreatic ducts have been transected. Although pancreatic wounds should be repaired by suture when possible, the absence of serosa and the low tensile strength of pancreatic tissue are such that disruption may occur. In our experience with over 500 pancreatic wounds, fistulas developed in almost 30 percent. Most fistulas are small (less than 200 to 300 cc per day) and require no specific therapy. If adequate drainage is maintained and infection is prevented, these fistulas close spontaneously, most within a few weeks, though some take a longer time. Even large pancreatic fistulas draining in excess of 1,000 cc a day frequently close spontaneously with conservative management. Hyperalimentation has been advocated as an adjunct in treating pancreatic fistulas to reduce the stimulation of the flow of pancreatic juice by the presence of food in the gastrointestinal tract. There is also some evidence that hypertonic glucose solutions given intravenously specifically decrease the flow of pancreatic juice. Rarely is hyperalimentation necessary for treatment of pancreatic fistula, however. If the remainder of the gastrointestinal tract is intact and the patient is able to resume a normal diet, the value of oral alimentation far exceeds the theoretic advantages of putting the tubular gastrointestinal tract at rest.

Pancreatic abscess is fortunately a relatively uncommon complication of pancreatic injury, occurring in less than 2 percent of patients. Intra-abdominal abscesses are more likely to result from associated organ injuries than from the pancreatic injury itself. When pancreatic abscess is suspected, however, confirmation of the diagnosis by ultrasound or CT scan is indicated, and prompt drainage should be undertaken. There is current interest in the use of percutaneous catheters inserted under ultrasound or CT guidance to avoid open laparotomy, but pancreatic abscesses are not well drained by this technique. The ability to place a catheter into the abscess cavity without injuring other structures is more difficult than when treating a hepatic abscess or intra-abdominal abscesses in other locations. More importantly, the abscess may be multiloculated and the thick purulent material does not drain well through a small catheter. Consequently, open drainage with large drains and the use of appropriate antibiotics remains the treatment of choice.

Although some degree of inflammation occurs as a response to injury, true diffuse pancreatitis as a complication of pancreatic injury occurs in no more than 2 percent of patients. Fear of pancreatitis should not alter the treatment of the patient with a pancreatic wound. Oral alimentation should be resumed when there is good function of the gastrointestinal tract and food is tolerated without symptoms. When pancreatitis develops, the clinical picture is the same as that of spontaneously developing pancreatitis and treatment should be the same: nasogastric suction, proper fluid and electrolyte administration, and, in severe cases, parental hyperalimentation. The development of hypocalcemia or diabetes is managed as in other types of pancreatitis. In rare patients, recurring pancreatitis develops in the late postoperative period. This usually is due to a stricture of the major pancreatic duct. This diagnosis can now be made by ERCP, and surgical treatment is the same as that of pancreatic ductal destruction from other causes.

Pseudocyst formation most often occurs in patients sustaining blunt injury, in which the pancreatic injury was not appreciated and operative intervention with drainage was not accomplished. When operative intervention is undertaken with adequate drainage of the pancreatic wound, pseudocyst formation is uncommon. The diagnosis can be suspected on the basis of symptoms, a persistent elevation of the serum amylase concentration, and ultrasound or CT scan documentation of the presence of a fluid-filled lesion. Surgical treatment should be the same as that used for pseudocysts that develop as a complication of pancreatitis: cystgastrostomy, cystjejunostomy, cystduodenostomy, or, when the cyst wall is poorly developed or secondary infection has occurred, external drainage.

COMPLICATIONS OF DUODENAL INJURY

Suture line disruption with consequent generalized peritonitis or the development of duodenal fistula is the most serious complication of the duodenal wound. Because of the high fatality rate associated with generalized peritonitis due to rupture of the suture line, drainage of duodenal wounds should always be performed. Thus, if leakage occurs, a track has been established which allows egress of the duodenal contents and the formation of an enterocutaneous fistula without the development of infection. Such fistulas carried a high mortality rate only a few years ago, and duodenal fistulas still constitute one of the most serious forms of enterocutaneous fistulas. This is particularly true of a lateral duodenal fistula because all gastrointestinal contents pass the fistulous opening after leaving the stomach. Procedures that prevent the passage of gastrointestinal contents through the duodenum result in the development of an end-duodenal fistula rather than a lateral duodenal fistula should suture line disruption occur. End duodenal fistulas almost all close spontaneously. With the use of hyperalimentation there has been an increased frequency of spontaneous closure of lateral duodenal fistulas as well. However, many of these still require surgical intervention. I utilize sump suction and parenteral nutrition for the treatment of lateral duodenal fistulas, and with rare exceptions, such treatment is maintained for a period of 4 to 6 weeks before surgical intervention is considered. When tube jejunostomy has been employed at the time of the original operation, this may be used for alimentation. When diverticulization has been utilized, the fistula is an end fistula, and resumption of oral alimentation in the normal manner is possible.

When surgical closure of a duodenal fistula is necessary, simple closure of the chronically inflamed fistulous opening is doomed to failure. Either closure with a serosal patch or conversion to an end fistula with tube duodenostomy is a viable procedure.

When severe injuries to the duodenum occur, closure of the duodenal defect may result in compromise of the duodenal lumen, and the healing process may constrict the lumen more severely, resulting in duodenal obstruction. Should this complication occur, anastomosis of the proximal duodenum to the jejunum is the treatment of choice, though gastrojejunostomy is an alternate procedure. Anticipation of this possibility should lead one to perform a gastrojejunostomy at the time of the original operation.

Hemorrhage may complicate the development of either a duodenal or a pancreatic fistula. When transections of major arteries such as the splenic or gastroduodenal artery are necessary and fistulous drainage comes into contact with these transected vessels, erosion or secondary infection involving the ligatures of these vessels may lead to their destruction and massive hemorrhage. This requires prompt control of hemorrhage, which in some cases can be accomplished by simple tract occlusion, but in most instances requires re-operation and control of the bleeding vessel.

MORTALITY RATE

Better treatment of patients with complicated and multiple intra-abdominal injuries has reduced the mortality rate from both pancreatic and duodenal injuries. However, because of the multiplicity of organs commonly injured in association with pancreatic or duodenal injuries, the mortality rate remains high. In recent reports mortality rates of 19 to 25 percent are still reported for pancreatic injuries. However, in our own institution it has been possible to reduce the mortality rate to 12 to 15 percent in recent years. Only rarely is the pancreatic wound itself the specific cause of death. In a study of 175 duodenal wounds reported from our institution a few years ago, the mortality rate had been reduced to 14 percent, and in only one patient was death due to a duodenal fistula; this eroded into the repair of an associated aortic wound and caused fatal hemorrhage.

SMALL AND LARGE BOWEL INJURY

JAMES W. HOLCROFT, M.D.

INITIAL EVALUATION, RESUSCITATION, AND TREATMENT

Initial resuscitation and treatment proceed hand-in-hand in all trauma patients, including those with potential injuries to the small bowel, colon, or rectum. Inspection of the patient should begin as he is brought into the emergency room, with a conscious effort to inspect the patient's back as he is transferred from the ambulance stretcher to the emergency room guerney. The airway and ventilation should be established, external bleeding controlled, and intravascular volume replenished, as appropriate. A Foley catheter should be inserted if the patient is hypovolemic, assuming he does not show signs of a urethral tear, and a nasogastric tube should be placed if there is any suspected trauma to the neck, chest, abdomen, or pelvis or if the patient is likely to require an anesthetic. A portable anteroposterior chest roentgenogram, the only laboratory test that is mandatory in the injured patient, should be obtained. The physical examination should be completed, including inspection of the perineum and performance of a rectal examination, while initial resuscitation is proceeding. After initial resuscitation, the patient should be re-evaluated. If he remains or becomes unstable, the underlying abnormality causing the instability should be corrected promptly. Physical examination and the chest film may reveal pericardial tamponade, pneumothorax, or hemothorax. In the absence of chest abnormalities, and in the absence of blood loss from or into the extremities, persistent cardiovascular instability implies bleeding into the abdomen. That bleeding should be controlled at celiotomy. Injuries to the small bowel, colon, and proximal rectum are recognized at that time.

Patients who, after initial resuscitation, become and remain stable—stability being good skin perfusion, a normal blood pressure, and a brisk urine output—should be evaluated more thoroughly before deciding on, or against, celiotomy. The approach to the patient depends, in part, on whether the injury is caused by blunt or penetrating forces. The bowel is only rarely damaged after blunt trauma. Far more common is damage to the solid organs—spleen, liver, kidneys, or pancreas. Damage to these organs usually manifests itself by signs of continuing blood loss, signs of peritoneal irritation, a falling hematocrit, return of blood with peritoneal lavage, or findings of damage to parenchymal organs on a computed tomogram of the abdomen. Blunt trauma can rupture the bowel, however, typically in automobile accidents in which the bowel is compressed against the vertebral column by a poorly placed seat belt or by the lower rim of a steering wheel. Perhaps because these injuries are unusual (less than 5% of bowel injuries are caused by blunt trauma in most series), and perhaps because they are frequently associated with only minimal blood loss, they are all too often missed initially. The resulting peritonitis can cost a life from an injury that would have been easy to repair if recognized early enough. A normal blood pressure, physical examination, hematocrit, abdominal film, peritoneal lavage, and even computed tomography of the abdomen do not necessarily rule out rupture of the bowel. Only repeated physical examinations over 24 hours, with vigilance for tenderness, guarding, spasm, reluctance to shift position in bed, and other signs of irritation of the parietal peritoneum can rule out such an injury.

Blunt trauma that fractures and disrupts the pelvis can also tear the rectal wall. Perineal lacerations or bleeding into the rectal lumen, detected by rectal examination, in patients with major pelvic fractures must be assumed to be associated with a rectal laceration. Proctosigmoidoscopy should be performed in these patients, but a negative examination does not rule out a rectal injury. Blood and feces in the rectal vault can all too easily hide the damaged area.

Any stab wound to the torso, from the fifth intercostal space to the pelvis, can penetrate the abdomen and lacerate the small bowel or colon. The diaphragm, during forced expiration, a phase of ventilation frequently assumed by a frightened victim, can easily rise to the level of the fifth intercostal space, and a stab wound to the lower chest can readily penetrate the diaphragm and lacerate abdominal organs directly beneath it. Any stab wound to the lower chest, anterior or posterior, that produces pneumothorax or hemothorax can enter the abdomen. All patients with air or blood in the chest with such a wound should undergo celiotomy. Patients with stab wounds to the lower chest that produce neither pneumothorax nor hemothorax can be followed without celiotomy, remembering that occasionally a knife can slide into the peritoneal cavity from the chest without introducing air or blood into the pleural cavities.

All patients with stab wounds to the abdomen anterior to the posterior axillary line must either undergo celiotomy or thorough local exploration of the wound with good lighting, good instruments, and good assistance. If local exploration indicates penetration of either the anterior rectus sheath or the external oblique muscle, the abdomen should be explored. If local exploration clearly indicates, with no question, that the penetration is confined to the skin and fat, the patient can be observed without celiotomy.

Patients with stab wounds to the abdomen posterior to the posterior axillary line can be watched for 24 hours without celiotomy as long as they show no signs of damage to abdominal organs. Any signs of abdominal injury such as unexplained hypovolemia, abdominal tenderness or guarding, ileus, blood in the stomach or rectum, or abdominal air or retroperitoneal hematoma on the x-ray film of the abdomen should prompt celiotomy.

All patients with gunshot wounds to the lower chest that produce pneumothorax or hemothorax and all patients with gunshot wounds to any part of the abdomen should undergo exploratory operation, except for the rare patient with what seems to be an obvious superficial, glancing wound. Patients with these latter wounds can be explored locally. If the wound is found, with complete certainty, to be indeed superficial, celiotomy is unnecessary.

The overriding consideration in deciding whether to explore patients with penetrating injuries of the lower chest and abdomen is to miss no injury that, if undetected, could kill a patient. Of particular risk are missed injuries to the small bowel, colon, and rectum. In some patients bowel contents take hours to produce detectable irritation of the peritoneum. Continued peritoneal or retroperitoneal soilage can prove fatal, even in patients who are operated on promptly after signs of peritoneal irritation become evident.

The risk of a negative celiotomy is minimal. Many centers, including our own, have reported series of hundreds of negative explorations (collected over years) with no deaths. Results with a policy of early exploration for patients with penetrating torso injuries are superb; it would be hard to improve on them.

INITIAL OPERATIVE ASSESSMENT AND MANAGEMENT

Systemic antibiotics of the surgeon's choice should be started before any celiotomy is performed for trauma. An antibiotic with a limited spectrum should be adequate in patients with blunt trauma (unless a rectal injury is suspected) because, in all likelihood, the bowel will be intact. Antibiotics with a broad-spectrum should be used in patients with penetrating torso trauma. If the bowel is found to be intact at celiotomy, the antibiotics should be stopped at that time. If the bowel is violated, the antibiotics should be continued during the postoperative period.

The abdomen should be entered through a midline incision. Free blood should be evacuated by inserting and removing Mikulicz tapes. (Tapes are more effective than suctioning; suction devices are too easily clogged with clotted blood.) The most obvious site of bleeding may not be the major source; for example, bleeding from the small bowel rarely leads to exsanguination, even though hemorrhage from that site is usually evident on opening the abdomen. Clot frequently forms at the primary sites of hemorrhage; nonclotted blood settles wherever gravity dictates, without relation to origin of the bleeding.

Rapid continued bleeding should be controlled by packing and tamponade. Obvious holes in the bowel should be closed, either with a quickly placed suture or with an Allis or Babcock clamp. Complete hemostasis within the abdomen should then be obtained. The bowel should then be inspected again, this time thoroughly. The small bowel should be eviscerated to the right and inspected from the ligament of Treitz to the cecum. The right colon should be taken down and reflected on its mesentery if any hematoma surrounds it. The left colon should be similarly mobilized if there is any suspicion of injury. Hematomas next to the bowel wall should be dissected off the serosa, and the bowel wall inspected, even if it is necessary to divide and ligate some of the small vessels in the mesentery in immediate proximity to the bowel. The number of holes in the bowel should be even; an odd number dictates an even more compulsive inspection. The trajectory of missiles and weapons should be visualized so that the injury is understood and so that associated injuries are anticipated and sought.

Once all of the injuries to the bowel are identified and temporarily closed, definitive therapy should begin.

REPAIR OF SMALL BOWEL INJURIES

Repair of injured small bowel can be successful only if the vascular supply to the bowel is intact. The pulse in the superior mesenteric artery should be assessed by grasping the root of the small bowel mesentery with the right hand and compressing it between the thumb anteriorly and the fingers posteriorly. If no pulse is present, attention must be directed first to re-establishing blood flow into the gut with arterial reconstruction as necessary. Assuming that a pulse is present, and assuming that gross leakage from the bowel has already been controlled, the next priority is exposure and control of bleeding into the mesentery. Small stable hematomas should not be explored, but large expanding hematomas have to be. Bleeding from small branches of the superior mesenteric artery and superior mesenteric vein should be controlled by ligation. Bleeding vessels larger than 5 mm in diameter should be repaired with fine vascular sutures. Care should be taken in applying clamps to veins in the mesentery (or to veins anywhere); clamps can tear veins and worsen any damage that might already be present. It is better to compress the vein proximally and distally, manually or with sponge sticks. The damaged area can then be repaired.

The small bowel itself should be repaired next, either with primary closure of defects or with resection and primary anastomosis. Defects that involve less than one-half of the circumference of the bowel can be closed primarily. An effort should be made to close the defects transversely, but they can be closed longitudinally as long as the bowel lumen is not compromised. Badly damaged or devascularized bowel should be resected, maintaining as much length as possible. Open end-to-end anastomosis is preferable, using a running suture of absorbable material for the inner layer and interrupted sutures of a nonabsorbable material for the outer. Open anastomoses allow inspection of the mucosa, the most metabolically active layer of the gut wall and the layer that shows ischemia the most readily. Bleeding mucosa ensures healing of the anastomosis. Nonbleeding mucosa suggests possible failure of healing: if more bowel can be resected without compromising its resorptive capacity, the anastomosis should be re-done with clearly viable tissue; if the bowel is short and no more can be resected, the anastomosis should be completed, even though the margins are questionable, and the patient re-explored the next day.

The decision to re-explore should be made at the time of the first operation. If such a decision is made at that time, the patient should be re-explored, no matter how good he may look the next day. Injured patients can hide dead or dying gut with no manifestations on physical examination. The point of re-exploring selected patients who have had repair of extensive mesenteric or small bowel injuries is to detect correctable abnormalities before they progress to dead gut. To wait for signs of peritonitis is to wait too long.

REPAIR OF COLON INJURIES

The most lethal of all bowel injuries is the missed colonic (or rectal) laceration. The gut must be thoroughly examined. There should be no hesitation in taking down the hepatic or splenic flexure and no hesitation in dissecting pericolonic fat off of the bowel wall in order to completely inspect the colon. Once detected, defects in the colonic wall can be treated either by primary closure or by resection with ileostomy or colostomy. Primary closure in patients with penetrating injuries to the colon is safe as long as the wound is clean, fresh, and isolated, and as long as the patient's overall condition is good with no pre-existing systemic disease and no shock. An example of a clean wound would be one that is produced by a knife; gunshot wounds are rarely clean; colon disruption by blunt trauma is never clean. Any wound associated with fecal contamination is by definition unclean. Fresh wounds are those less than 6 hours old. Isolated wounds are those that involve only the colon with no damage to other organs. All substantial injuries to the colon—those with ragged edges or fecal contamination, those incurred more than 6 hours previously, or those associated with other injuries—and all colonic injuries in patients in shock or general poor health require resection and isolation by proximal diversion of the fecal stream.

Substantial injuries to the colon or colonic injuries in compromised patients should be treated with resection of the damaged gut and creation of a proximal end ostomy and mucous fistula. Such injuries to the right colon should be treated with resection from the distal ileum to the proximal transverse colon. There is little point in attempting to salvage right colonic length. The patient will require resection of the ascending colon when the ileostomy is taken down. Removal of the entire ascending colon at the time of the initial surgery leaves behind a neater operative field and perhaps decreases the risk of the patient's developing an intra-abdominal abscess. In the case of injuries to other parts of the colon, only enough need be resected to ensure healthy bowel for creation of the proximal colostomy and mucous fistula or, in the case of injuries to the distal sigmoid, a Hartmann pouch.

Creation of proximal diversion requires mobilization of enough bowel to permit the stoma to be brought out through the skin *under no tension*. Few observations in medicine are more distressful than watching a colostomy sink back into the abdomen when abdominal wall edema and distention reach their extreme in the postoperative period.

Thus, my usual treatment of colonic injuries is either primary closure or resection of the damaged area with proximal fecal diversion and creation of a mucous fistula or Hartmann pouch. I rarely use other operative strategies such as primary repair with proximal diversion, primary repair with exteriorization of the repaired segment, resection with primary anastomosis, or resection with primary anastomosis and proximal diversion. Primary repair with proximal diversion subjects the patient to an ostomy and subjects him to the risk of intraperitoneal breakdown of the repair. Primary repair with exteriorization has not worked well in my hands except in cases so favorable that a primary repair by itself would have been successful. Resection of a major injury with primary anastomosis is too risky with unprepared bowel. Resection with a primary anastomosis and proximal diversion subjects the patient to the risk of the primary anastomosis and the inconvenience of an ostomy.

Occasional exceptions to the policy of either primary closure or resection with complete proximal diversion of the fecal stream can be made. In selected cases in which time is critical, injured areas of the transverse or sigmoid colon can be brought out as loop colostomies and opened 24 hours later. Loop colostomies can also be used for proximal diversion if time is limited. They do not completely divert the fecal stream, however, and are hard to fit with appliances.

After treatment of the colonic injury, the abdomen is copiously irrigated, using Mikulicz tapes to remove the irrigating fluid and to remove fecal matter that may be imbedded in raw tissue surfaces. An antibiotic solution is instilled into the peritoneal cavity. The fascia is closed with monofilament suture, and the skin is either closed with a few staples or left open, depending on the degree of contamination and shock. (If the skin is closed with staples, these are removed 24 hours later and paper tapes applied to maintain skin approximation. Many of these wounds will heal by first intention; those that suppurate do so readily between the tapes, which can be removed at the time of suppuration with little disadvantage to the patient.)

REPAIR OF RECTAL INJURIES

All patients with compound pelvic fractures and all patients with penetrating injuries of the rectum or perineum should have a proximal diverting end colostomy and mucous fistula performed. The anal sphincter should be dilated and the rectal vault cleared of feces. In most instances, presacral drains should be placed, either through a surgically created perineal incision or through the perineal wound, if one is present and suitably close to the posterior aspect of the anal verge. I do not dissect out the presacral space from within the peritoneal cavity in order to place presacral drains. Neither do I perform abdominal perineal resections for trauma: the damaged rectum has remarkable capabilities for repairing itself. Neither do I suture rectal lacerations: large lacerations should be allowed to heal secondarily so as to allow free drainage; small lacerations heal quickly, no matter what the treatment, and repair is not necessary.

The ileostomy or colostomy, in cases of colonic or rectal trauma, is usually opened and matured, under local anesthesia, in 4 days unless peristalsis develops earlier, in which case the stoma is matured when abdominal cramps begin. The clamp on the mucous fistula, if one is created, is left on for 7 days.

Ileostomies and colostomies can sometimes be taken down as early as 3 weeks after the injury. In some cases, they should never be taken down. Relatively minor injuries in a good-risk patient who has recovered quickly from his injury lend themselves to early take-down. Patients with devastating injuries, especially those that damage anal sphincter function, are best left with a permanent stoma. The majority of patients tolerate take-down of their stomas 1 to 2 months after the initial injury.

Rectal examination to assess sphincter tone should be performed on all patients before re-anastomosis. A proctosigmoidoscopy should be performed and a barium enema should be obtained before take-down in any patient in whom there is any chance of obstruction distal to the mucous fistula or the Hartmann pouch.

SPLENIC INJURY

ROGER SHERMAN, M.D., F.A.C.S.

The incidence of overwhelming postsplenectomy sepsis following splenectomy for trauma is not yet accurately defined. It is estimated, from the available data, that between 1 and 2 percent of patients who undergo splenectomy following trauma will develop serious postoperative infections. The majority of these infections occur within 2 years after splenectomy, but some patients have developed overwhelming postsplenectomy infections more than 30 years following removal of the spleen. Despite difficulty in establishing the precise incidence of these overwhelming infections, there is no doubt that a small, but finite, number of patients are at risk indefinitely for a characteristic highly lethal septic syndrome following removal of the spleen for trauma. Unfortunately, at present, it is not possible to identify these patients.

However low the incidence of overwhelming sepsis following splenectomy for trauma, the consequences are so devastating that several measures to reduce or eliminate this complication have been developed and evaluated over the past 10 to 15 years by a number of surgeons. They include nonoperative management, splenorrhaphy, partial splenic resection, and, in patients in whom splenectomy cannot be avoided, deliberate autotransplantation of splenic tissue, antibiotic prophylaxis, administration of pneumococcal vaccine, and careful education of the patient regarding appropriate measures to be taken for a febrile illness.

NONOPERATIVE MANAGEMENT

Initial enthusiasm for conservative or nonoperative management of patients with trauma to the spleen has grown from the original reports of success in management of pediatric patients with splenic injuries to include adults as well. Consequently, a number of reports of successful nonoperative management of both children and adults following splenic injury have appeared in the literature. It has been adequately demonstrated that many patients with isolated splenic injury following blunt abdominal trauma who are hemodynamically stable and are in an appropriate hospital setting for close observation can be satisfactorily managed without laparotomy.

As more experience has been gained with the conservative management of splenic trauma, the nonoperative approach has been relegated, for the most part, to children with splenic injury, and it is generally thought that all adults, with few exceptions, should be managed by laparotomy.

In children who have experienced blunt abdominal trauma, conservative management requires accurate diagnostic studies consisting primarily of computerized tomography to delineate the presence and degree of splenic damage. The patient is admitted to the surgical intensive care unit where total blood replacement up to 25 or 30 cc per kilogram during the first few hours after injury may be required. If the child remains stable following transfusion or remains stable without it, he is observed in the intensive care unit for 48 hours during which time his activity is considerably restricted. After discharge from the intensive care area, children are usually kept in the hospital for a minimum of 10 days to 2 weeks, where restriction of their activity is perhaps somewhat easier than at home. After discharge the child is followed by serial computerized tomographic studies at monthly intervals until evidence of complete healing of the splenic injury is obtained. It is usually recommended that for an additional 3 months following evidence of healing, the child should be restricted from any vigorous physical activity.

For adults who have received blunt abdominal trauma, the prolonged period of reduced activity (in many instances requiring interruption of income-producing work) necessary for successful conservative management of splenic injury seems unwarranted. Following operative intervention with splenic repair or splenectomy where indicated, full activity can be resumed without risk at a maximum of 6 weeks following injury.

After stabilization and appropriate supporting measures, adult patients with blunt abdominal trauma who are suspected of splenic injury undergo peritoneal lavage which, when positive, is followed by laparotomy and abdominal exploration. In some instances computerized tomography is indicated, especially in patients with head injuries. However, the reliability of peritoneal lavage in our hands makes the expensive CT study unnecessary in all but a few instances. Prompt laparotomy for adult patients following stabilization permits careful abdominal exploration, identification of the splenic injury, and the absolute exclusion of associated intraperitoneal injuries. Abdominal exploration is usually approached through a long midline incision so that easy access to mobilization of the spleen is possible. Capsular avulsion injuries that are not bleeding and small nonexpanding subcapsular

hematomas can usually be left in place without further surgical management. However, continued oozing from capsular tears is easily managed by the application of microfibrillar collagen followed by the application of pressure. When more complex injuries of the splenic parenchyma are present, the posterior peritoneum should be incised parallel to the entire length of the spleen, and the splenocolic ligament should be divided. The spleen and tail of the pancreas should then be mobilized onto the anterior abdominal wall by gentle blunt dissection. Control of the splenic artery in the lesser sac through the gastrocolic or gastrohepatic ligament can be achieved when time permits and if bleeding is excessive. Identification of hilar divisions of the splenic artery, when indicated, must be carried out gently if partial splenectomy is to be successful. Special care to avoid injury to hilar branches of the splenic vein must be exercised as the vessel is quite thin and easily injured. Control of parenchymatous bleeding during partial splenic resection is afforded by temporary occlusion of the splenic artery. Individual ligation or clipping of parenchymatous vessels in intersegmental planes should be accomplished. Through-and-through 2–0 catgut mattress sutures are adequate for hemostasis. Bleeding from raw surfaces should be controlled by microfibrillar collagen. Splenic artery ligation for control of hemorrhage may be necessary and is compatible with viability of the spleen, as long as blood supply through the short gastrics is not compromised. Many techniques for suture repair, partial splenectomy, and even total wrapping of a fragmented spleen in absorbable mesh have been reported. Since apparently nearly every technique that has been utilized has been successful, it would seem that only the principles of careful hemostasis and gentleness in suturing are the essential ingredients of successful splenorrhaphy.

When these principles of management have been followed, reports of the necessity to reoperate for continued bleeding following suture repair or splenorrhaphy have been exceedingly rare.

Our policy using splenic salvage techniques, when possible, for adult patients with injury to the spleen is based on the argument that laparotomy eliminates even the remote possibility of a missed associated abdominal injury. In addition, the hospital stay can be shortened, and time missed from work decreased with minimal risk to the patient from laparotomy.

SPLENECTOMY

Despite the clear evidence that splenic preservation procedures are safe and probably effective in preserving splenic function, as well as the development of technical procedures for repair of even gross disruptions of splenic parenchyma, there will always be patients with massive splenic injury who require splenectomy.

Indications for splenectomy include total avulsion of the hilar vessels, extensive splenic fragmentation, avulsion of the splenic vein in the splenic hilus, and continued bleeding after attempted splenic repair. In patients with severe associated injuries requiring prompt attention or extensive peritoneal contamination from visceral perforations, it is good surgical judgment to weigh the benefits of splenic salvage against splenectomy.

Following splenectomy, three avenues for protection against severe postsplenectomy infections are currently available: deliberate autotransplantation of splenic tissue, long-term antibiotic prophylaxis, and immunization with polyvalent pneumococcal vaccine.

DELIBERATE AUTOTRANSPLANTATION

Considerable experimental evidence clearly demonstrates that autotransplanted splenic tissue placed in the peritoneal cavity will develop vascular ingrowth and become viable. Many of these implants have been shown to restore the ability of the animal to form antibody, raise leukophilic gamma globulin levels, remove red cell imperfections, and take up injected radiocolloid. Their ability to protect against pneumococcal challenge is less clear. There are extensive and conflicting experimental data concerning the ability of autotransplanted splenic tissue to protect against, or to ameliorate, overwhelming sepsis following bacterial challenge. In addition, clinical reports of severe infections in patients with accessory spleens or with splenosis discovered at autopsy raise questions about the ability of autotransplanted splenic tissue to protect humans against infection. It has been suggested that a minimum of 50 percent of functioning splenic tissue is necessary for adequate protection against severe infections.

Despite the controversy, a number of surgeons believe that deliberate autotransplantation provides a logical, simple, and safe alternative for possibly preserving some splenic function. Clear recommendation for or against autotransplantation of splenic tissue following splenectomy based on available data is not possible at this time. Techniques that have been described include placing two or three thin (3 mm) cross-sectional slices of splenic tissue from the central portion of the resected spleen into a pocket of omentum made by folding the omentum back upon itself, and careful search and removal of splenic fragments from the peritoneal cavity. Placement of the transplant into omental pouches permits venous drainage of the splenic tissue into the portal system, which is apparently important, and should prevent complications of splenosis.

ANTIBIOTIC PROPHYLAXIS

There are a number of disadvantages to antibiotic prophylaxis against overwhelming postsplenectomy infections. Compliance is a major disadvantage, in light of the fact that splenectomized patients are probably at risk for the rest of their lives. Patient compliance with long-term antibiotic prophylactic programs has been disappointing.

A recent death at our institution from overwhelming postsplenectomy infection in a child 2 years after splenectomy, in whose case compliance with an antibiotic prophylaxis regimen was questionable, is a case in point.

Selection of an appropriate antibiotic for prophylaxis as well as an effective dosage schedule is difficult. Although penicillin is the usually recommended antibiotic of choice, the efficacy of this agent is compromised by the fact that a number of penicillin-resistant organisms may produce the syndrome of postsplenectomy sepsis. Until controlled studies are available that indicate the usefulness of long-term antibiotic prophylaxis for prevention of postsplenectomy overwhelming infections, long-term prophylactic antibiotics are not recommended.

There are some exceptions to this recommendation, the most important being the use of penicillin prophylaxis following splenectomy in children under 2 years of age. This is an important consideration because there is a variable response to pneumococcal vaccine in children under the age of 2, and accordingly, antibiotic prophylaxis is indicated in addition to immunization. Oral penicillin is the antibiotic of choice, with a dosage schedule tailored to the individual patient.

VACCINE PROPHYLAXIS

All patients undergoing splenectomy for trauma should receive polyvalent pneumococcal vaccine. All patients who sustain major splenic injury, whether managed by nonoperative intervention or by surgical salvage, should also receive this vaccine as the long-term ability of salvaged spleens to protect against pneumococcal sepsis has not been established. Following administration of pneumococcal vaccine after splenectomy, adequate antibiotic titers take 2 to 3 weeks to develop. During this period, prophylactic penicillin, 250 mg orally every 12 hours, or erythromycin, 250 mg orally every 12 hours, to patients allergic to penicillin should be administered. The duration of protection induced by the vaccine is unknown. Available data show elevation of titers 3 to 5 years after immunization. Initial vaccination is well tolerated, but because of a marked increase in adverse reactions with reinjection of the vaccine, second or "booster" doses are not recommended at this time.

PATIENT EDUCATION

Patients undergoing splenectomy and parents of children who have undergone splenectomy must be fully informed of the possible occurrence of serious postoperative infection. The rapidity of development of these overwhelming infections and the need for early medical attention should be well understood. Documentation of the absence of the spleen should be carried by the patient at all times.

RETROPERITONEAL INJURY

ALFRED S. GERVIN, M.D., F.A.C.S.

Injuries to the retroperitoneal organs are extremely difficult to diagnose, and require a constant awareness and concern on the part of the trauma surgeon. This concern must be directed to the mechanism of injury as preoperative laboratory and x-ray studies may be entirely normal. At the time of surgery, retroperitoneal organs must be adequately mobilized and visualized so that no injury will be missed. Once injuries are identified, proper repair with adequate drainage must be undertaken. To miss or inadequately repair a retroperitoneal injury is to subject the patient to a risk of retroperitoneal sepsis that has mortality rates in excess of 40 percent.

The abdominal cavity has as its lining a complex tissue of mesothelial origin, the peritoneum. Classically, the peritoneum has been divided into two portions, the visceral and parietal peritoneum. The parietal peritoneum lines the walls of the abdominal cavity. It reflects over all intra-abdominal organs as the visceral peritoneum. Several intra-abdominal organs have a portion of their structure covered only by parietal peritoneum. These abdominal structures are therefore considered "retroperitoneal." The retroperitoneal organs are listed in Table 1.

In addition to the organs listed, the retroperitoneal area contains the pelvic bones, the vertebral column, and several sets of muscles—the PSOAS major and minor, the Iliacus, and the Quadratus Lumborum muscles.

Injury to the retroperitoneal structures may occur in both blunt and penetrating trauma. The most commonly injured retroperitoneal organs in order of frequency are presented in Table 2.

The early diagnosis of retroperitoneal injury is extremely difficult. In fact, the retroperitoneum has long been considered a "silent area" in its manifestations of response to trauma. Routine abdominal x-ray films are usually unrevealing. Diagnostic peritoneal lavage, well appreciated as insensitive to retroperitoneal injury, may be positive only if significant intra-abdominal injury is present. It is estimated that injury to retroperitoneal structures is associated with concomitant intra-abdominal injury in approximately 60 to 80 percent of patients. Major

TABLE 1   Retroperitoneal Organs

Gastrointestinal System
  Terminal esophagus
  Duodenum - 2nd, 3rd, 4th portions
  Common bile duct
  Pancreas
  Ascending and descending colon -
    posterior and lateral walls
Genitourinary System
  Kidneys
  Ureters
  Posterior bladder
  Vagina

TABLE 2   Most Commonly Injured Retroperitoneal Organs (Decreasing Frequency)

Kidney	Bladder
Pancreas	Ureter
Colon	Common bile duct
Duodenum	Rectum
Retroperitoneal muscle	

genitourinary tract injury may occur without blood in the urine. The use of body scanning techniques for the diagnosis of pancreatic and duodenal trauma has given controversial results. Specific diagnostic tests, as they relate to particular retroperitoneal organ injury, will be discussed in the following sections.

TERMINAL ESOPHAGUS

As the terminal esophagus exits through the crus of the diaphragm, it is covered by parietal peritoneum. The esophagus becomes intraperitoneal at the esophagogastric junction. Injury to the terminal esophagus is extremely rare. In my experience, the most common source of injury to the terminal esophagus is a penetrating injury to the upper abdomen. Almost always, concurrent intra-abdominal injury is present. I have now seen eight patients with gunshot wounds to the liver in whom the bullet crossed the posterior midline to the left side of the abdomen, penetrating the esophagus. On exploration, hematoma in the area of the cardia of the stomach is a telltale sign. The greater curvature of the stomach and the peritoneum over the esophagus must be mobilized and the esophagus circumferentially explored. A missed esophageal injury condemns the patient to retroperitoneal sepsis and ascending mediastinitis, resulting in death. Techniques for repair of esophageal perforations depend on the extent of the injury and the time lapse from injury to operation. For small perforations, I advocate direct suture repair with interrupted sutures of monofilament nylon. It is my protocol to reinforce such suture lines with a serosal patch of the stomach or with a wrap of the Nissen fundoplication type. For extensive lacerations of the esophagus, primary repair should be undertaken with fundoplication and diversion of the cervical esophagus. I believe that all repairs of the intra-abdominal esophagus should be drained with soft, closed drainage systems of the Jackson-Pratt type. Decompression of the stomach by tube gastrostomy may also be indicated.

THE DUODENUM

The diagnosis of duodenal injuries is extremely difficult. The mechanism of trauma must be taken into consideration when assessing this injury. Any blunt trauma to the upper abdomen should initiate (in the mind of the surgeon) concern for pancreaticoduodenal injury. On abdominal examination, some tenderness may be present.

On kidney, ureter, and bladder (KUB) x-ray study of the abdomen, retroperitoneal air may be present. However, in my opinion this is a rare finding. At laparotomy, hematoma in the mid-central abdomen may be a telltale sign of duodenal trauma. Bile staining and retroperitoneal air may also be present. Whenever there is concern for duodenal injury, wide mobilization of the duodenum using the Kocher maneuver must be performed. This mobilization must be carried to the superior mesenteric vessels so that all walls of the duodenal can be visually inspected. Additionally, the fourth portion of the duodenum to the left of the major vessels must also be explored. This may necessitate taking down the ligament of Treitz. As trauma to the pancreas frequently accompanies duodenal injury, I advocate the wide opening of the lesser sac whenever a duodenal exploration is undertaken so that the body of the pancreas may also be observed (to be discussed). Full mobilization of the duodenum is extremely important for gunshot wounds as penetration of the duodenum may produce little in the way of retroperitoneal hematoma or bile staining.

A simple and logical classification of duodenal injuries has been advocated by Lucas and Ledgerwood (Table 3). Class 1 injury consists of intramural hematoma without perforation of the duodenum. When an intramural hematoma is encountered in penetrating trauma, I believe that the serosa over the hematoma should be carefully opened and the clot evacuated to determine whether a perforation of the duodenum has occurred. If no perforation is encountered, the serosa should be carefully approximated with seromuscular Lembert sutures after successful hemostasis is obtained. If the intramural hematoma is related to blunt trauma, the decision must be made at operation whether or not to excise the serosa and drain the hematoma. I believe that intramural hematoma from blunt trauma can be safely observed without evacuation. Decompression of the stomach with a nasogastric tube or a tube gastrostomy is indicated. No bypass of the hematoma, such as by gastrojejunostomy, is indicated even if relative obstruction is present. If, after 2 weeks of gastric decompression, obstruction exists, then a bypass procedure should be considered. Drainage is not routinely utilized in the treatment of intramural hematoma of the duodenum.

Class 2 injuries, perforation without pancreatic injury, is treated by primary suture repair. I use a running 3–0 absorbable suture for an internal layer and interrupted 4–0 nonabsorbable sutures for a seromuscular layer. Most class 2 injuries occur along the latter wall of the duodenum in a transverse fashion. If an adequate suture line can be achieved and if the duodenal lumen is not compromised, the area should be drained. I advocate the use of soft, external closed drainage systems. An alternative might be internal drainage created by threading a soft catheter through the duodenum from a gastrostomy or jejunostomy site or from a nasogastric tube extended through the pylorus. Various combinations of double and triple internal catheter drainage have been described. Our experience with internal drainage has not been satisfactory. An older technique of closing the perforation around a catheter or "T" tube to create a "controlled" lateral fistula is to be condemned. Additionally, the use of omental patching, such as that used in the Graham closure for perforated duodenal ulcer, has not worked in my hands.

If the suture lines appear precarious, external reinforcement is indicated. This may be accomplished by mucosal or serosal patching. Drainage should be utilized in this situation. If the duodenal closure is precarious or if the duodenal lumen has been compromised, a diversionary procedure is indicated. Initially, Bern and his associates advocated antrectomy, tube duodenostomy, suture of the duodenal laceration, and external drainage for severe duodenal injury, particularly if pancreatic injury was present. For these injuries, I advocate the use of a pyloric exclusion technique. This consists of opening the greater curvature of the stomach as for creation of gastrojejunostomy, internally suturing shut the pylorus with a nonabsorbable suture, and creation of a gastrojejunostomy. The majority of these pyloric exclusions open with restoration of normal gastrointestinal continuity in 3 to 4 weeks. An alternative technique is external stapling of the pylorus and creation of a stapled gastrojejunostomy. If this is utilized, it is important to ensure that the staple line is slightly distal to the pylorus to avoid a "retained antrum" ulcerogenic situation. In my experience, the incidence of permanent occlusion of the pylorus is slightly higher with the stapled technique. However, the stapled exclusion can be created more rapidly if the patient's condition is unstable intraoperatively.

The techniques for the repair of class 3 injuries are essentially the same as those for class 2, with the inclusion of pancreatic drainage. The general principle is that the more extensive the pancreatic injury, the greater should be the tendency of the surgeon to consider multiple tube decompressions, diverticularization, or pyloric exclusion.

THE PANCREAS

Injuries to the pancreas may be subdivided as follows: class 1, superficial capsular tear; class 2, deep lacerations of the body or tail involving major ductal structures; class 3, lacerations of the head with suspected ductal injury; and class 4, severe injury of the head with associated duodenal injury.

When class 1 (laceration or capsular tear) of the pancreas is encountered, meticulous hemostasis should be achieved. Subcapsular hematomas should be unroofed and evacuated; no attempt should be made to repair the capsule. Drainage of the lesser sac should be undertaken with

TABLE 3 Duodenal Injuries

Class 1—intramural hematoma without perforation

Class 2—perforation without pancreatic injury

Class 3—perforation with minor pancreatic injury

Class 4—perforation with major pancreatic injury

soft rubber drains placed adjacent to the injury. I routinely use a closed drainage system of the Jackson-Pratt variety, although Penrose drains and sump drains have been enthusiastically advocated by many. With major injuries to the body of the pancreas, distal pancreatectomy may be required. It is often possible to achieve this without a concomitant splenectomy. Closure of the pancreatic stump can be achieved with interrupted silk sutures into the capsule or with a stapling device. An effort should be made to find and suture-ligate the main pancreatic duct. Following distal pancreatectomy, the area should be drained with soft rubber drains. An alternative technique is the drainage of the pancreatic stump into a Roux-en-Y loop. Whether this technique is utilized depends on the amount of pancreas injured and the general condition of the patient. A double Roux-en-Y technique with loops to the pancreatic stump and to the distal pancreas is not wise in my opinion. Likewise, a Roux-loop to cover a stellate laceration of the anterior body of the pancreas is fraught with failure. Severe injuries to the head of the pancreas may require either 90 percent pancreatic resection or pancreatic transection and drainage of the body and tail to a Roux-en-Y loop. If the patient's condition is extremely unstable, simple drainage of this area may prove lifesaving.

For severe injuries to the head of the pancreas with concomitant duodenal injury, I recommend achievement of hemostasis, drainage of the pancreatic injury, duodenal repair, and pyloric exclusion.

Radical pancreaticoduodenal resection (Whipple procedure) for trauma is rarely undertaken. When this procedure must be performed (rarely), it is usually debridement of a dissection done by nature's forces rather than a formal surgical procedure.

COLON AND RECTUM

The majority of injuries to the retroperitoneal colon involve penetrating trauma. Most of these are discovered during laparotomy for gunshot wounds penetrating the anterior abdominal fascia. If the colon is found intact at laparotomy for an anterior abdominal wall wound, there is no need to open the retroperitoneum. However, if the anterior wall of the ascending or descending colon is lacerated or an odd number of holes are found in the colon, the white line of Toldt must be excised and the colon mobilized so that both intra- and extraperitoneal aspects of the bowel wall are visualized. The retroperitoneal colon may sustain an isolated injury with tangential penetrating wounds to the flank. This has occurred most frequently in our series with obese patients who have large protuberant penetrating wounds. Diagnostic peritoneal lavage should be performed, and if any blood is present, laparotomy should be undertaken. If not, the patient should be admitted to the hospital for close observation and laparotomy undertaken at the first sign of abdominal symptoms. A CT scan with Gastrographin enema may prove to be a useful technique for the diagnosis of this injury.

Treatment of a penetrating injury to the retroperitoneal colon is essentially the treatment for any penetrating colon injury. For patients with through-and-through perforations produced by a low-velocity gunshot wound or by stab wound in whom there are (1) fewer than three associated injuries, (2) no hypovolemic shock, (3) minimal blood transfusion requirements, (4) minimal spillage, (5) clear margins of the wounds, and (6) less than 6 hours from injury, primary repair can be considered. This repair should be in two layers with an inner running layer of absorbable suture and an outer seromuscular layer of nonabsorbable suture, after debridement of the edges of the wound. Evidence now suggests that injuries to both the right and left colon can be primarily repaired under these criteria. For wounds that do not meet these stringent criteria for primary closure (and I believe that colon wounds *rarely* do), other forms of therapy may be indicated. These consist of (1) primary repair and exteriorization of the injury over a rubber catheter, through a transverse incision away from the midline or the area of injury; (2) resection of the injury with colostomy and mucous fistula or Hartmann procedure if the distance from the injury to the sigmoid colon is less than 24 inches; or (3) primary repair with proximal diversion.

In my experience, the exteriorized colon can be successfully interiorized in only about 50 percent of cases. Frequently, severe serositis develops necessitating resection or opening of the loop as a colostomy. The Hartmann procedure should not be performed if the distal closed loop is long, as cleansing preparation of this segment may be difficult for reanastomosis.

If the right colon has sustained a severe injury requiring resection, the operating surgeon must decide whether to attempt a primary ileocolonic anastomosis or to create an ileostomy and colon mucous fistula. In my experience, the main determinants are the degree of contamination and the condition of the patient. For massive injury to the ascending or descending colon, with marked contamination, I recommend resection, colostomy, or ileostomy and mucous fistula or long Hartmann procedure.

Injuries to the extraperitoneal rectum are uncommon in civilian practice. In my experience, the major injuries are penetrating wounds from spikes, stakes, or fence posts. For penetrating wounds of the perineum, rectal examination should be done initially. Blood in the stool is infrequent. Sigmoidoscopy and examination and exploration of the wound should be performed in the operating suite. If there is any suggestion of rectal injury, exploration should be undertaken through the abdomen. Peritoneal reflection should be open and dissection carried out as for an abdominal perineal resection. Wounds to the rectum must be identified, debrided, and sutured, and adequate presacral drainage established. A diverting sigmoid colostomy should then be performed.

A form of penetrating rectal injury that may be missed occurs with major pelvic fractures. For all patients with pelvic fracture, a rectal examination should be performed. If perforation by a spicule of bone is appreciated, then proper debridement, reduction of the pelvic fracture if possible, operative repair, and diverting colostomy should be performed. For women with pelvic fractures, a pelvic examination should be performed to rule out concomitant vaginal laceration.

THE KIDNEY

The kidney is the most frequently injured retroperitoneal organ. The classic hallmark of renal injury has been the presence of post-traumatic hematuria. Today, however, it is appreciated that major injuries both to the bladder and the kidneys can occur without significant hematuria. Statistically, when hematuria is present, gross hematuria correlates with either bladder or kidney injury, whereas microscopic hematuria is most frequently associated with renal parenchymal or renal pedicle injury.

All patients who have been involved in a major blunt or penetrating trauma should have a urinalysis performed. If the patient's condition is unstable, the first urine obtained should be tested by dipstick for hematuria and decisions regarding radiologic evaluation based on these results. If the patient is stable, decision making should be delayed until the results of the formal urinalysis return, if this time interval is less than one hour. This should be done because of the high incidence of false positive dipstick studies for hematuria. For patients with three to five red cells or more in their urine, or patients who have sustained a blunt or penetrating trauma to the flank or mid-lower abdomen or who have been involved in deacceleration injuries irrespective of the presence or absence of hematuria, radiographic assessment of the genitourinary tract should be performed. In the trauma room, an intravenous urogram should be performed after the patient has been resuscitated to a blood pressure greater than 80 mm Hg. Following injection of a bolus of dye, a single KUB film of the abdomen is then taken, in search of bilateral nephrograms or gross extravasation. The Foley catheter, which has been placed in the absence of urethral injury, can be clamped and the dye collected as an antegrade cystogram. If gross extravasation of the bladder is identified, surgery is undertaken. If no extravasation is identified, a formal retrograde cystogram is performed by distending the bladder with 400 cc of radiopaque material. Rarely are the ureters delineated with these techniques (to be discussed). If the screening intravenous urogram demonstrates the absence of nephrogram effect on one side and the patient's condition is stable, arteriography is indicated. If the patient's condition is unstable from other injuries, laparotomy should be undertaken with either an intraoperative arteriogram or exploration of the involved renal pedicle.

The most common injury to the kidney is a contusion. This is manifested by a normal roentgenographic study and hematuria that rapidly clears. If dye extravasation from the renal pelvis is present and there are no other indications for operation, this may be observed. If at the time of laparotomy a hematoma is discovered around the kidney and the preoperative intravenous urogram revealed normal renal vasculature and extravastion, this hematoma should not be explored. If the hematoma is ex-

panding or if there is evidence of active bleeding, the perirenal hematoma must be opened and the kidney inspected. Prior to this, control of the renal artery and vein should be secured. For most penetrating injuries of the kidney, repair can be achieved by interrupted mattress sutures of 2–0 chromic catgut. When the damaged portion of the kidney is too extensive for salvage, a partial nephrectomy should be performed along the lobar planes. The renal capsule overlying the resected segment of the kidney should be saved to fold over the salvage margin prior to suturing. If extensive renal injury is present with marked bleeding that cannot be easily controlled, a nephrectomy may be performed if the presence of a contralateral kidney has been established.

URETERAL INJURY

Injury to the ureter following blunt trauma is extremely rare. The majority of ureteral injuries occur following gunshot or stab wounds to the abdomen. These injuries are usually discovered when laparotomy is undertaken for these penetrating injuries.

Injuries to the ureter are rarely defined by the techniques for emergent intravenous urogram and cystogram. If the trauma patient's condition is stable after his initial work-up and time permits, a formal intravenous pylogram with oblique views and nephrotomograms should be undertaken. Ureteral transection is best treated by primary end-to-end repair by spatulated technique, using interrupted 5–0 chromic catgut sutures. If the integrity of the repair is in question, I splint the ureter from below with ureteral stints. If primary anastomosis cannot be performed, the ureter may be brought out as a temporary ureterostomy with plans for reconstruction at a later date.

RETROPERITONEAL HEMATOMA

Retroperitoneal hematoma, when discovered at laparotomy, may challenge the decision-making abilities of even the most skilled trauma surgeon. Retroperitoneal hematomas can be divided into those caused by blunt trauma and those caused by penetrating trauma. A general principle is that the retroperitoneal hematoma that is expanding rapidly at the time of surgery must be explored irrespective of etiology. If the hematomas are stable and not expanding, they should be explored selectively. It is my routine to explore all retroperitoneal hematomas caused by penetrating trauma. Even if the hematoma is in the perinephric area and preoperative urography demonstrates no significant injury, it is my routine to explore this area. Retroperitoneal hematoma in the deep pelvis caused by penetrating trauma must be explored to rule out major vascular injury. Hematomas in the mid-central portion of the abdomen must be explored to rule out pancreatic, duodenal, or common bile duct injuries.

Hematomas of the mid-central abdomen caused by

blunt trauma should always be explored. Perinephric hematomas from blunt trauma need not be explored if a preoperative intravenous urogram reveals a normal arterial supply and contained extravasation. Hematomas in the deep pelvis from blunt trauma should not be explored. On occasion, a massive retroperitoneal hematoma that seems to involve all areas of the retroperitoneal space may be encountered. The best judgment of the surgeon should then be employed to determine whether the hematoma started laterally and dissected medially, or medially with lateral extension. Retroperitoneal hematomas that seem to have their source in the mid-central area of the abdomen should be explored.

When pelvic retroperitoneal hematomas from penetrating trauma are explored, bleeding can usually be controlled by repair of major vascular structures. However, in rare instances the bleeding from the retroperitoneal musculature cannot be controlled. In this situation, I advocate the retroperitoneal packing of the abdomen and postoperative arteriography for embolization if the bleeding continues. Fortunately, in my experience, this occurrence is rare.

VASCULAR INJURY

DONALD. D. TRUNKEY, M.D.

The primary effects of acute vascular injury are hemorrhage and ischemia. Arterial injury may be obvious when there is pulsatile external hemorrhage, but bleeding may also occur into body cavities and in deeper tissues contained by fascial compartments. Until proved otherwise, ischemia of an extremity must be treated as though it were primarily due to vascular injury. Paralysis or anesthesia that develops rapidly indicates anoxia of peripheral nerves. Occlusion of the carotid artery results in brain damage within minutes of the injury in approximately 20 percent of patients, although extremity ischemia can be tolerated for 6 to 8 hours. Nevertheless, a delay in restoring perfusion may cause a vicious cycle to develop; subfascial edema, venous occlusion with resultant venous hypertension, propagation of thrombi within vessels, and disruption of arterioles and capillaries that will bleed and produce progressive swelling and necrosis when perfusion is re-established. Time is a critical factor in the management of all vascular injuries.

Late changes associated with major vascular injuries include false aneurysms and traumatic arteriovenous fistulas. False aneurysms are prone to rupture without warning. Fistulas can compress adjacent nerves or collateral circulation and ultimately may also rupture. They occur after simultaneous injury to adjacent arteries and veins, usually a result of stab wounds or muscle injury. Both entities can occur following catheterization and angiographic procedures. With time, the fistula enlarges and makes increasing demands on cardiac output, which results in an obvious thrill or a continuous bruit, or both, and dilated veins in the extremity.

PRINCIPLES OF DIAGNOSIS

Vascular injury must be assumed in any wound in proximity to major blood vessels. Unless they are hemodynamically unstable, all trauma patients should have a complete vascular examination, including palpation of carotid, subclavian, brachial, radial, femoral, popliteal, dorsalis pedis, and posterior tibial pulses. Neurologic function must be assessed. Any injured part should be examined by auscultation over the area of obvious or suspected injury. The Doppler flow probe may be useful in detecting diminished pulses and determining whether there is flow in a vein in which injury is suspected. The best single test for confirming a suspected vascular injury is arteriography. However, arteriography should not be performed in the patient who is unstable and needs emergency laparotomy, thoracotomy, or control of peripheral vascular bleeding. In these instances, arteriography should be postponed until resuscitation and treatment of the life-threatening emergency, in either the emergency room or the operating room, have been carried out. Specific indications for arteriography are shown in Table 1.

TREATMENT

General Measures

Most injuries involving large vessels, particularly those in the chest and abdomen, require only lateral repair.

TABLE 1 Indications for Arteriography Following Trauma

Neck injuries—zones I and III

Chest injuries
  Mediastinal widening
  First rib fracture
  Deviation of trachea to the right
  Obscuration of the aortic shadow

Abdominal injuries
  Nonvisualization of a kidney by pyelogram
  Selected pelvic fractures

All penetrating wounds of extremities in
    proximity to major vessels

Dislocation of the knee

All fractures associated with abnormal pulses

Larger wounds are usually incompatible with survival and the patient's reaching the emergency room. Exceptions include wounds that may be contained, such as those around the crus of the diaphragm and peripheral vascular injuries. When there is segmental loss of vascular tissue, it is generally a good rule to replace with autogenous tissue or to perform an extra-anatomic bypass if there is gross contamination. Substitution of vessels with synthetic material should be avoided if there is fecal contamination or contamination from another hollow viscus. I prefer to use a monofilament suture such as Prolene, 3–0 for large vessels and 4–0 or 5–0 for smaller vessels.

The same principles outlined for arterial injuries also apply to venous injuries except that many venous injuries can be ligated, particularly if there are other life-threatening problems. Exceptions to this would be the superior vena cava, inferior vena cava above the renals, and the portal vein; although the portal vein can be ligated, it is preferable to repair. Another vein that should be repaired is the popliteal since this will reduce venous hypertension and significantly increase the chance of repair to the popliteal artery to remain patent.

Treatment of Specific Injuries

Neck Injuries

Injuries to the neck can be anatomically divided into zone I, II, and III injuries. Zone I injuries include those rostral to the clavicles, and these are also called thoracic outlet injuries. Zone II injuries affect the area from the clavicles to the angle of the mandible (mid-cervical), and zone III injuries are high in the cervical area, cephalad from the angle of the mandible. All patients with zone I and zone III neck injuries should undergo arteriography as soon as vital signs are stable. Arteriography is helpful in the planning of a surgical approach in the patient with such an injury, particularly if there is a suspected injury to the left subclavian artery. If the patient is hemodynamically unstable, however, our general approach would be to do a midline sternotomy with extensions either up the sternocleidomastoid or out along the clavicle, and removing the medial head of the clavicle if necessary. If the patient turns out to have a left subclavian artery injury, exposure can be enhanced by converting the incision into a so-called trap-door incision by extending it out the third or fourth intercostal space on the left. Zone III injuries also require arteriography because of the anatomy of the vessels and nerves at the base of the skull. Some of these injuries can best be managed by either nonoperative techniques or maneuvers remote from the injury site, such as balloon tamponade or embolization of a vertebral artery injury in the intervertebral canal. Operative approach to zone III injuries may be enhanced by dislocating the jaw forward after succinylcholine has been administered or by performing an osteotomy of the ramus, sparing the lingual nerve.

Some surgeons recommend arteriography in zone II as well. This may be rational for posterior wounds, but for anterior zone II injuries I believe that exploration is warranted if the injury penetrates beneath the platysma muscle. Arteriography will not rule out significant injury to the venous system, trachea, or the esophagus. The selective versus mandatory approach is controversial, but a review of the literature shows that there are unacceptable deaths when selective management is used.

Blunt trauma to cervical vessels is relatively uncommon, but should be considered in any patient with hyperextension injury with neurologic deficits and/or physical findings of expanding hematoma. Unexplained focal neurologic findings would also lead one to suspect disruption of the intima with embolization.

Thoracic Injuries

Arteriography should be mandatory in any patient who has a widened mediastinum following blunt chest trauma. Associated findings include first or second rib fractures and deviation of the trachea to the right and an apical hematoma. Obscuration of the aortic shadow and depression of the left main stem bronchus are also common findings.

Controversy exists regarding the management of thoracic aortic rupture. Most of these occur at the isthmus, and although there are proponents of left heart bypass, of shunts, and of clamp and repair, a recent review shows that there is no difference in outcome or paraplegia rates among the three techniques. I personally prefer to clamp and repair. Injuries at the aortic valve usually require cardiac bypass. As a general rule, one should try to avoid heparinization in the multiply injured patient, particularly when there is associated head injury.

Abdominal Injuries

Major vessel injuries within the abdominal cavity present as hemorrhagic shock that does not respond to resuscitation; thus, immediate surgery becomes an important part of the resuscitative effort as well as treatment. Direct or proximal control of the vessel is mandatory for success. A pneumatic antishock garment may stabilize the situation long enough for the patient to be transferred to a center capable of definitive treatment. Arteriography is only rarely of benefit in the management of major abdominal vascular injuries. Exceptions include nonvisualization of a kidney by pyelogram and severe pelvic trauma with continuing bleeding. In this instance, demonstration of a bleeding site also allows the radiologist to embolize the vessel.

Injuries to the abdominal aorta are approached by taking down the left colon and mobilizing all viscera to the midline, including the pancreas and spleen. This allows direct access to the abdominal aorta from the crus of the diaphragm to the bifurcation and beyond. If the injury is at the crus of the diaphragm, a thoracoabdominal incision may be necessary. Injuries to the inferior vena cava or portal vein are approached by taking down the right colon and mobilizing all the viscera to the midline.

In some instances, it may be necessary to transect the neck of the pancreas to get access to portal vein injuries directly beneath the pancreas. Injuries to the hepatic veins are approached through a midline sternotomy incision. The surgeon must then consider use of an intracaval shunt to control bleeding or, alternatively, finger-fracturing the liver around the hepatic veins and getting direct access to them. Injuries to branches of the aorta and the inferior vena cava are usually treated by gaining proximal and distal control and then dissecting into the mesentery or lesser sac. Injuries to the pelvic vessels can be difficult to treat. As a general rule, I would only attempt repair on major arterial injuries. Venous injuries deep in the pelvis are best left to tamponade since the veins often shear off and retract into sacral foramina or otherwise are inaccessible for direct control.

Extremity Injuries

Vascular injuries are present in 25 to 35 percent of all penetrating trauma to extremities. A significant percentage of these patients have no physical findings suggesting vascular trauma; thus, routine use of arteriography is necessary. Significant vascular injury to the extremity also may be associated with blunt trauma, particularly posterior dislocation of the knee. This dislocation results in a 50 percent injury rate to the popliteal artery. Arteriography is mandatory in all dislocations of the knee if catastrophic consequences are to be avoided.

Fractures are often associated with decreased or absent pulses. Even if the distal pulses are restored after splinting and traction, an arteriogram is frequently indicated to rule out a significant intimal injury that may precipitate later arterial thrombosis.

There are several adjunctive measures that need to be considered when one is treating extremity vascular injuries. Although fasciotomy is controversial, recent advances in measurement of compartment pressures has now allowed a scientific approach to this problem. Fasciotomy is indicated if compartment pressures are above 40 centimeters of water. Another useful adjunctive measure concerns destructive soft tissue wounds, such as those that follow shotgun blasts, farm accidents, or industrial accidents. In these instances, it is desirable to immediately cover any reconstructed vessel or prosthesis with autogenous tissue. I prefer immediate muscle flaps with skin grafting or myocutaneous flaps if the area lends itself to that technique.

POSTOPERATIVE COMPLICATIONS

The most common postoperative complications are thrombosis and infection. Thrombosis can lead to ischemia or gangrene. Repeat physical examinations and arteriograms, as necessary, can detect early thrombosis and prevent irreversible loss. Infections are not uncommon following hollow viscus injury within the peritoneal cavity or devitalizing soft tissue injuries in the extremities. Antibiotics are indicated for 3 days following such injuries. Established infections are best treated by debridement, drainage, and covering with autogenous tissue as soon as possible. Synthetic grafts that become infected may require removal and extra-anatomic bypass.

BURN WOUND

ANDREW M. MUNSTER, M.D., F.R.C.S.(Eng.), F.A.C.S.

The overall goal of burn therapy is expeditious closure of the wound, with the best possible functional and cosmetic result. The prognosis of the injury depends on the extent and depth of the burn, the age of the patient, and the coexistence of complicating factors, particularly smoke inhalation and serious pre-existing medical disease. Management of the wound itself, particularly surgical intervention, has to be planned with a great deal of judgment in light of the general condition of the patient and the success of resuscitation. The timing of surgery in relationship to these factors will be discussed in this chapter, but the principles of resuscitation, the airway management, and the treatment of complications are dealt with elsewhere in this book. Of the prognostic factors influencing outcome, extent of burn and age of the patient are the most important. Because so many unpredictable factors can influence outcome, it is wise not to predict prognosis based on the early appearance of the patient or of the burn wound.

DETERMINATION OF THE EXTENT AND DEPTH OF BURNS

The rule of nines is the traditional field method, also suitable for emergency room use, for determining the extent of the burn in terms of total percentage of the body surface involved. The body of an adult is divided into nines or multiples thereof: the head and each upper limb are 9 percent, the anterior trunk 18 percent, the posterior trunk 18 percent, and each lower limb 18 percent, which adds up to 99 percent, the remaining 1 percent being the genital area. In children, the surface-to-weight ratio of the body is altered, so that in infants and small children a larger surface (up to 16% at age 1) is represented by the head and a comparatively smaller percentage by the trunk and limbs. Smaller burns may be assessed by comparing the burn size to the palm of the patient's hand;

each palm-sized area is approximately equivalent to 1 percent of the total body surface. In special burn care units, more accurate diagrams are available for the estimation of total burn size, and these are usually drawn up on admission.

The depth of a burn is defined by the extent of necrosis of the skin and underlying structures. A first-degree burn involves death of superficial epithelial cells; sunburn is characteristic of this type of injury. Second-degree or partial-thickness burns are conveniently divided into superficial and deep. A superficial partial-thickness injury causes necrosis of the superficial layers of the dermis, and these injuries usually heal spontaneously within 10 to 14 days, provided there is no infection and the patient's nutritional status is good. Deep partial-thickness burns involve most of the dermis, sparing only the deep dermal elements and the skin appendages. Such burns heal spontaneously, but may take up to 6 weeks to do so and, in the process, often cause a great deal of hypertrophic scarring with a poor cosmetic and functional outcome.

Full-thickness (third-degree) burns involve the destruction of all skin elements down to the hypodermis. Small injuries that are no more than 1 or 2 cm in size are capable of healing by contracture through myofibroblast action and some epithelial ingrowth from the edges, but larger areas of loss either do not heal or heal with extreme contracture and must be surgically covered.

Occasionally, the term fourth-degree is applied to very deep injuries involving muscle, bone, or tendon; these are characteristic of high-voltage electrical injuries or flame burns in patients with impaired consciousness or sensation.

Clinically, partial-thickness burns are characterized by moist appearance and a great deal of pain. The color is usually reddish or pink, and hair persists in hair-bearing areas. In superficial partial-thickness injuries, the necrosed skin or eschar is thin, and it is often possible to see deep dermal elements or "buds" through the eschar on examination. Full-thickness injuries are dry, insensate, and may vary in appearance from dark red to white; occasionally, there is a charred black appearance. The evaluation of the depth of burns is difficult, with error rates up to 30 percent being reported even in the hands of experienced observers. There are currently no reliable laboratory aids for the diagnosis of the depth of burns. As a general rule, burns tend to be deeper than they initially appear. The history may be helpful: flash burns, hot water burns, and chemical burns that have been immediately and copiously lavaged tend to be partial-thickness burns; flame burns, scalds by hot grease, gravy, or soup, chemical burns that have not been immediately lavaged, and high-voltage electrical injuries tend to be full-thickness burns.

NATURAL HISTORY OF THE BURN WOUND AND INITIAL CARE

It is essential to understand that the burn wound evolves in dynamic fashion. During the first 48 hours following the burn, there is a zone of stasis and capillary sludging underlying the area of immediate necrosis, and this zone can either return to normal or proceed to further necrosis. Thus, it becomes imperative to scrutinize the burn wound daily and note changes in the appearance of the wound. Within 5 to 7 days, the necrotic skin or eschar slowly begins to separate from the underlying granulation tissue by a process of autolysis and by bacterial action, slowly revealing the underlying burn bed. In the case of partial-thickness burns, particularly when superficial, as the eschar separates viable dermal elements become apparent. In the case of full-thickness burns, separation of the eschar reveals underlying hypodermic fat. This process of separation occurs more rapidly in the presence of heavy wound colonization by bacteria and in infants and small children, more slowly in the elderly. As the eschar continues to separate, the underlying bed is revealed to an increasing extent until by the end of 3 to 4 weeks the eschar has either separated completely or, in the case of a partial-thickness injury, the wound has healed. Inadequate nutritional support can completely arrest wound healing at any time, and the importance of providing adequate calories and protein cannot be overemphasized.

The initial care of the wound involves gentle cleansing with saline or a mild antiseptic agent, the opening of blisters, and the application of a topical chemotherapeutic agent to the wound, followed by appropriate dressings. This process is then repeated twice daily until the wound has either closed or a decision has been made for surgical intervention. Details of available chemotherapeutic agents and their indications will be discussed subsequently. Whether debridement and cleansing are carried out with the patient in bed or in a hydrotherapy tub, such as the Hubbard tank, is a matter of individual preference; hydrotherapy has as many enthusiastic supporters as adamant opponents. If daily hydrotherapy is chosen as the method of preference, it is wise to add a mild antiseptic agent to the water in order to prevent cross-contamination of the wound; we use sodium hypochlorite (Clorox), one part in 20,000. Early surgical intervention in terms of escharotomy or fasciotomy may be required within the first 3 hours of admission, and this will be discussed under surgical management.

TOPICAL AGENTS

Topical chemotherapeutic agents represent a major advance in the care of burns over the last 20 years. The most widely used agents are listed in Table 1, together with their advantages and drawbacks. Although it is probably fair to say that silver sulfadiazine is the most popular in use today and is the first choice of most specialty centers, definite indications exist for at least three or four other topical agents, and any hospital treating a substantial number of burn patients should keep all of them on the formulary. We use silver sulfadiazine as the primary agent, but are guided by bacteriologic cultures of the burn wound. Biopsy cultures of the wound are routinely obtained approximately twice

TABLE 1 Topical Chemotherapeutic Agents

Name	Advantage	Side Effects	Dressing Orders
Silver sulfadiazine (Silvadene)	Broad antibacterial action, painless, washable	Only fair penetration of eschar; incidence of sulfonamide sensitivity (rash); absorption into fetal circulation unknown and drug is contraindicated in pregnancy; occasional leukopenia (reversible upon discontinuation)	Apply b.i.d. and cover with a light layer of Kling or Kerlix bandage on extremities; leave face and chest open
Mafenide (Sulfamylon)	Excellent antibacterial action, particularly against gram-positive and gram-negative organisms and *Clostridia*; rapid eschar penetration	Pain; sulfonamide sensitivity (rash); carbonic anhydrase inhibition leading to an acid load that has to be compensated for by lungs and kidneys	Face, chest, and abdomen open; one light layer of gauze dressings elsewhere; apply b.i.d.
Aqueous silver nitrate solution	Universal antibacterial action	Poor penetration of eschar; leaking of chloride into the dressings with potential hypochloremic alkalosis; strong staining of tissues, equipment, linen, and floor	All areas to be dressed with thick layers of burn dressings and gauze bandage, wet down with silver nitrate solution q4h; change dressings daily
Iodophors (e.g., Efodine)	Universal antibacterial action	Poor penetration of eschar; strong staining of tissues; iodine absorption	Apply twice daily and dress with a light layer of gauze dressings
Topical bacitracin cream	Transparent, cosmetically acceptable, easy to apply	Limited antibacterial action; poor eschar penetration, rapid development of resistance; conjunctivitis if in touch with the conjunctiva	Should only be applied to small areas of cosmetic importance, e.g., second-degree burns of the face; leave open; apply b.i.d.

a week, beginning about the end of the first week. These biopsies are processed by the microbiology laboratory by grinding of the tissue and bacteriologic plating following serial dilution. In this manner, individual organisms, *in* rather than *on* the burn wound can be identified and cultured for sensitivity to systemic and topical antimicrobial drugs. It is not uncommon, using this technique, to discover that the organisms in the burn wound are resistant to the topical agent used; for example, there is a definite incidence of silver sulfadiazine resistance by *Staphylococcus aureus* and *Enterobacter cloacae*; in case of staphylococcal infection, topical therapy may be switched to mafenide (Sulfamylon) cream; in case of *Enterobacter cloacae* infection, therapy may be switched to nitrofurantoin (Furacin) cream. With the exception of 0.5% silver nitrate solution, which is applied to bulky dressings and changed daily, all other agents require twice daily dressing changes, and these, as previously described, may be carried out in the hydrotherapy tank or in bed. When the wound has healed either with surgery or spontaneously to the point where it may be left open to the air with only a few spots remaining unhealed, topical cream therapy may be discontinued, and antiseptic solutions may be dabbed on the open spots twice daily; Mebromine and Mercurochrome are suitable. At this point, most patients are ready for discharge from the hospital and may continue therapy at home.

SURGICAL MANAGEMENT

The terminology applied to the surgery of burns is sometimes confusing and has not been universally agreed upon. The terms used in this chapter are therefore defined in Table 2.

Regular debridement is an essential part of burn wound management throughout the patient's hospital course, the purpose being to remove devitalized tissue and allow topical agents to reach the burn bed. Blisters, separating nonviable eschar, necrotic fat, devitalized skin grafts that show nonadherence, and other necrotic debris should be removed from the wound at daily intervals. Wet-to-dry dressings may help in preparing a burn bed that is almost completely debrided for surgery.

Escharotomy is an operation that usually needs to be undertaken within a few hours of the injury and is necessitated by circulatory, neurologic, or respiratory embar-

TABLE 2 Definition of Surgical Terms

Term	Definition
Early excision	Excision within 5 days of injury
Late excision	Excision beyond 5 days of injury
Debridement	Gentle removal of separating necrotic tissue, usually without anaesthesia
Escharectomy/necrectomy	As above, but accomplished by sharp dissection under anesthesia
Tangential excision	Excision of burn eschar layer by layer until viable bleeding tissue is encountered
Sequential/staged excision	Excision not accompanied by immediate closure
Fascial excision	Excision of all tissue to the level of investing (deep) fascia

rassment caused by tissue swelling under a constricting full-thickness eschar. In the limbs, the clinical indications for escharotomy are pain in the extremity, immobility of the fingers or toes, a diminished or absent circulation as judged by Doppler auscultation, and diminishing sensation. When in doubt, elevation of the affected extremity combined with vigorous exercises may be undertaken for 30 to 60 minutes in an attempt to avoid the need for escharotomy. Pressure measurements of closed fascial spaces of the hand, arm, foot, or leg may be undertaken in cases of doubt, but there is no universal agreement on the exact pressure that indicates the need for intervention. In my experience, an intrafascial pressure of 50 mm H_2O or higher is an indication for escharotomy, and following escharotomy, these pressure measurements need to be repeated. If escharotomy fails to relieve the increased pressure, fasciotomy may need to be undertaken. Escharotomy may be performed with a scapel or a razor blade while the patient is in bed. Since a properly performed escharotomy leads through areas of third-degree burn, which are insensate, anesthesia is not necessary, and bleeding should be minimal and easily stopped with pressure, epinephrine-soaked dressings, or minimal local electrocautery to the wound. Escharotomy incisions should be placed in the affected limb along axial lines, i.e., the medial and lateral border of the arm or leg, with care being taken to avoid crossing flexion or extension creases of joints. The escharotomy should encompass the entire extent of full-thickness injury and should be carried in both directions for an inch or two beyond this area into zones of partial-thickness injury. Usually, the effect is immediate, and the edges of the incision separate for a distance of 1 or 2 cm with improvement in the peripheral circulation. The escharotomy wound is then treated the same way as the remainder of the burn wound, (i.e., with topical chemotherapeutic agents and dressings) and eventually requires coverage by skin grafting.

Fasciotomy needs to be performed more rarely, the indication being the failure of escharotomy to relieve the symptoms and signs of compression. Fasciotomy is commonly necessary in instances of high-voltage electrical injury, particularly in the area of the median nerve at the wrist, where extensive carpal tunnel decompression is usually necessary. Fasciotomy is a formal surgical procedure performed in the operating room under anesthesia, and should be extensive enough to allow for wide decompression of all involved areas. To salvage neurologic structures such as a median nerve, a fasciotomy, when indicated, must be performed within 6 hours of injury. Once a fasciotomy has been performed, it is impractical to close the skin incision surgically, and other forms of wound coverage must be utilized: I customarily allograft the fasciotomy site.

Elective Excision of Burn Wounds

The most important aspect of surgical excision and coverage of the burn wound is *timing*. Excision and closure of the wound has been shown to decrease length of hospital stay and improve function, although there is as yet no definite proof that it reduces mortality. Theoretically, all full-thickness and deep partial-thickness wounds are an indication for surgical excision and closure, but the decision to perform this procedure must be tempered with considerations of the clinical condition of the patient. Wounds smaller than 10 to 15 percent of the total body surface that are full-thickness or deep partial-thickness can be excised with confidence within a day or two of injury provided the patient's general condition is stable enough to permit anesthesia and there are not complicating factors such as severe smoke inhalation necessitating respirator support. In the presence of a serious systemic complication, it is wise to defer surgery until the patient's condition has been stabilized and either weaned off respirator support or at least close to the weaning point. Optimal "take" of skin grafts is so dependent on adequate capillary circulation and oxygenation that any cardiovascular or pulmonary impairment results in reduced graft take. If that should occur, the clinician has to contend with both a failed graft and the additional trauma of a new donor site, thereby enlarging the effective wound surface. It is our practice to defer surgery on unstable or respirator-dependent patients for several days. In the case of a major burn exceeding 30 or 40 percent of the total body surface and having a dominant full-thickness component, early surgery is advisable in order to avoid life-threatening complications; these patients should undergo initial excision and closure of the wound as soon as possible. For burns of this size, and for larger injuries, it is wise not to attempt to close the entire wound in one sitting; as a general rule, I restrict the operating time on such patients to 2 hours, during which period it is possible to excise and close approximately 15 percent of the body surface, reserving the remainder for a subsequent session. Very large burns, exceeding 60 to 70 percent of the total body surface, must be operated on expeditiously because septic complications are inevitable, and every attempt must be made to reduce the total body surface involvement as swiftly as possible.

In order to perform successful excision and closure of large burns, several requirements exist. The operators must be experienced in the techniques of burn excision, there should be at least two assistants available in the operating room, the operating room itself should be well equipped, spacious, and well lit, and the anesthesia team must be conversant with the specific problems and difficulties of burn patients.

Techniques of Wound Excision

Tangential excision is performed with a hand-held instrument such as the Goulian-Weck dermatome or Humby knife, or with a mechanical dermatome. Successive layers of eschar are resected in thin slices until a healthy, bleeding capillary bed is encountered. Following hemostasis, the wound is closed. Tangential excision is best suited to deep partial-thickness burns and is most commonly practiced on burns of the back of the hand, where this kind of surgery has been very successful in accomplishing excellent early closure and mobilization. Fascial excision is a technique employed when, in the opinion of the clinician, full-thickness injury exists down to and perhaps involving the hypodermic fat. Because the hypodermic fat is relatively avascular and takes grafts poorly, while the underlying investing fascia is more vascular and readily accepts grafts, fascial excision is aimed at electively removing all tissue down to the level of the investing fascia. This procedure may be performed with a scalpel, cutting cautery, or laser. Incisions are made circumferentially, emcompassing the area to be resected; a plane is dissected down to the investing fascia, and all tissues superficial to this layer are removed with careful hemostasis. This procedure usually involves less blood loss than tangential excision, but because of the loss of subcutaneous fat, it involves greater cosmetic deformity, and occasionally severe distal lymphedema may result.

On occasion, a procedure that begins as a tangential excision may have to be converted to a fascial excision when nonviable or poorly viable subcutaneous fat is reached. Escharectomy and necrectomy are examples of delayed excision and consist of the surgical removal of separating eschar and underlying necrotic tissue and the preparation of a burn bed adequate for grafting.

At this point, the surgeon is faced with a burn bed from which, by one technique or another, all dead and devitalized tissue has been removed, and the wound is now ready for operative closure.

Techniques of Wound Closure

Wound closure is best accomplished immediately after excision. Occasionally, however, even after excision, and removal of the eschar and debris, the wound is so contaminated and colonized that the surgeon may elect not to close the wound immediately, but apply dressings and return the patient for delayed wound coverage the next day or the day after. In our experience, this is a technique to be avoided whenever possible because the wound invariably desiccates in the ensuring 24 to 48 hours and is less suitable for closure than immediately after excision of an eschar.

The best method of coverage of the burn wound is autograft. Autograft is harvested with a hand dermatome or an electric or air-driven instrument, the thickness of the graft being tailored to the needs of the recipient area and the age of the patient. Generally, the thinner an autograft the better it will take, and we rarely take autografts thicker than eleven thousands of an inch. Even thinner autografts should be taken in the elderly and in children. In the vast majority of cases, for the coverage of burn wounds, the autograft should be meshed in a mesh dermatome with a carrier board setting of 1½ to 1, allowing for slight expansion. This technique allows for the escape of serum from the wound through the interstices of the graft, and allows for superior take. Fully expanded 1½ to 1 mesh, or the use of 3 to 1 mesh, will result in a visible reticular pattern on the grafted skin which will be cosmetically visible for the rest of the patient's life.

Therefore the mesh should be expanded just slightly enough to allow for the escape of fluid. In the case of very large burns, for which donor sites are scarce and coverage is imperative, the eventual cosmetic appearance must take second place to maximal utilization of skin, and in these instances I expand the mesh fully. Currently there is controversy about the use of mesh grafts on cosmetically exposed areas such as the hands and face, but meshed grafts, when unexpanded, give perfectly acceptable results on the back of the hand. On the face it is my custom not to use mesh grafts on the cheeks, but I do place them on the forehead, the direction of mesh being laid down in Langer's lines. This gives an extremely acceptable cosmetic result, but it is fair to say that this technique has not found widespread acceptance, and most surgeons prefer to place sheet grafts on the forehead as well. Grafts may simply be laid on the wound and dressed, or they may be secured with Steri-Strips, metal clips, or sutures. The placement of dressings on meshed skin graft is of utmost importance and must be aimed to prevent shearing stress on the graft. Next to the grafts, I usually place an impregnated dressing such as Adaptic gauze, which is then covered with a 16-ply gauze dressing ("burn dressing") moistened in polymyxin-bacitracin solution, then secured in place with Kerlix or Kling bandages and splinted as necessary. In restless children, or in areas that are difficult to bandage such as the shoulder, the dressing themselves may be sutured in place or held in place with clips. If meshed grafts have been used, dressings must be wetted down with saline or antibiotic solution every 4 to 6 hours until the first dressing change on the third postoperative day; otherwise the skin graft desiccates and is lost. Patients should be at bed rest until the first dressing change unless the donor site, usually on the thigh, is very small. I allow patients with grafts above the waist to walk after 3 days, patients with burns of the thigh to walk after 7 days, and patients with grafts below the knee to begin ambulation on the twelfth postoperative day. At all times, when the patient begins ambulation, elastic support in the form of an Ace or similar bandage should be provided.

If autograft is not available in sufficient quantities to cover the excised burn wound, other alternatives must be looked for, and the next best alternative is allograft. Allograft is harvested from cadaver donors, usually quick-frozen in liquid nitrogen, and stored at −70 °C. It is now available from commercial sources. Allograft does not need to be meshed and can be applied as a sheet to the wound. Sheet allograft can be left open in the same way as sheet autograft and "rolled" by the nursing staff to avoid the accumulation of underlying serum or pus. In addition to providing comfort and coverage, allograft diminishes colonization of the burn wound and renders the wound moist and suitable for later autografting. After approximately the fifth day, allograft becomes vascularized and needs to be surgically removed, a step that is not desirable. I therefore remove all allograft on the third or fourth day after application and replace it with fresh allograft, this procedure being repeated until the patient is ready for further autografting. In the case of very extensive burns (over 60%), it may be preferable

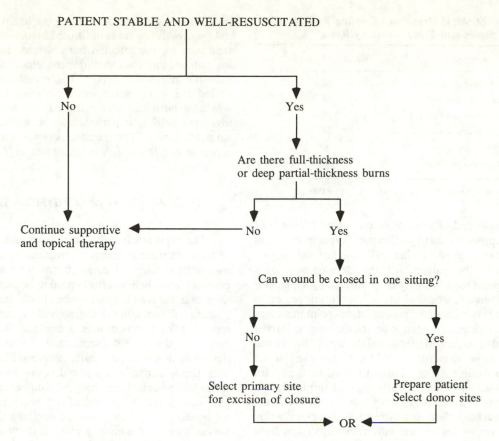

PATIENT STABLE AND WELL-RESUSCITATED

No / Yes

Are there full-thickness
or deep partial-thickness burns

No / Yes

Continue supportive
and topical therapy

Can wound be closed in one sitting?

No / Yes

Select primary site
for excision of closure

Prepare patient
Select donor sites

OR

Figure 1 An algorithm for surgical intervention (Close daily observation of the wound is necessary for decision making).

to consider the allograft as a method of prolonged wound closure and leave it until rejection occurs; because of the immunosuppressed state of the burn patient, this is usually delayed several weeks.

If allograft is unavailable, amniotic membrane may sometimes be used to achieve the same purpose, and several skin substitutes are available for this purpose. Although several of these artificial skin substitutes are reasonably satisfactory physiologically, none is as good as allograft in obtaining the desired quality of wound closure. Various types of cultured skin are currently under intensive investigation and will probably become available for clinical use within the next few years. An algorithm for decision making with regard to surgical intervention is shown in Figure 1.

Donor Site Management

There are many techniques for dressing donor sites, and all are satisfactory. Provided there is no infection, the donor skin is the correct thickness, and the patient's nutritional status is good, healing of the donor site occurs within 7 to 10 days, and the donor site is ready for recropping if necessary. Wound infection rate in donor sites should be under 2 percent. The simplest and cheapest method of management, and the one that I prefer to use, is the application of dry fine mesh gauze to the bleeding

donor site, which is kept dry in the postoperative period by the application of heat lamps to the exposed gauze. If the burn wound is heavily colonized and cross-contamination at the operating table is feared, the application of a donor site dressing impregnated with an anti-septic, such as scarlet red, is preferable. Synthetic skin substitutes (already discussed) may also be used to cover the donor site, and they usually achieve superior pain relief in contrast to fine mesh gauze; however, they are a great deal more expensive.

Severe infection in a donor site must be vigorously treated the same way as the burn wound, i.e., by application of topical chemotherapeutic agents. Infection may led to the conversion of the donor site to full-thickness injury, and rarely, the donor site itself may need to be grafted.

The Septic Wound

There is probably no more difficult problem in burn wound management than the surgical management of the infected wound. Burn wound sepsis may be diagnosed by the unhealthy appearance of the wound that becomes discolored, develops a foul-smelling discharge or a dark appearance, or areas of punctate hemorrhage and surrounding cellulitis. Previously partial-thickness burns, when infected, take on the appearance of full-thickness injury and indeed are full-thickness. The infected appear-

TABLE 3 Etiologic Organisms Causing Burn Wound Sepsis and Their Mortality Rates*

Organism	Mortality Rate (%)
Pseudomonas aeruginosa	30
Enterobacter cloacae	43
Streptococcus fecalis	50
Staphylococcus aureus	33
Staphylococcus epidermidis	0
Klebsiella pneumoniae	50

* Statistics from Baltimore Regional Burn Center, 1983–1984.

ance of the wound is usually accompanied by signs of systemic sepsis such as hyperthermia, hypothermia, and an elevated or depressed white cell count as well as disorientation in the patient and the development of a paralytic ileus. Diagnosis may be confirmed by a quantitative wound biopsy, which yields 10^5 organisms per gram or more, and commonly the patient, at this point, develops septicemia. Adequate systemic antibiotic treatment must be instituted at once, and the topical therapy of the wound may have to be changed to reflect sensitivities of the dominant organism in the wound. Limited areas of burn wound sepsis can be successfully excised surgically and closed, but with areas larger than 5 or 10 percent of the total body surface, there is serious risk of contaminating the freshly excised burn bed with microorganisms from the invaded wound, thereby perpetuating the infection. Attempts at excising large septic burns usually fail with a dismal outcome. Subeschar antibiotic infusion has been practiced in some burn centers, but again, it is usually only successful in areas of limited involvement. The best treatment for the infected burn wound, in my opinion, is continued vigorous topical management combined with systemic antibiotic support. If the patient survives this period, the septic eschar will rapidly separate, following which the burn bed can be cleaned with wet-to-dry dressings over a 48-hour period, and the wound can then be surgically closed. The recent experience with burn wound sepsis at our institution is illustrated in Table 3.

OCCUPATIONAL AND PHYSICAL THERAPY

The importance of the entire team in the management of the burn patient cannot be overemphasized. With the national mortality of major burns now around 6 to 7 percent, rehabilitative efforts need to be emphasized more than ever before. Injured limbs should be splinted in a position of function. If the patient is capable of some movement of fingers or toes, splints may be worn at night only, and the patient encouraged to undertake activity during waking hours at regular intervals. Physical therapy, with gentle active and assisted active movement of all joints of the burned extremity, should begin on admission and, except for the period of necessary immobilization following skin grafting, should continue throughout the patient's hospital course. I place particular emphasis on maximal mobilization prior to surgery to mitigate the unavoidable effects of the immobilization that follows surgical intervention.

FLUID AND NUTRITIONAL MANAGEMENT OF THE BURN PATIENT

RONALD G. TOMPKINS, M.D., Sc.D.
JOHN F. BURKE, M.D.

FLUID MANAGEMENT

The early fluid management of the serious burn injury consists of two phases during the first 24 hours. The initial empiric delivery of sodium-containing fluid, designed to prevent the development of serious "burn shock," is begun as soon as the patient is available for treatment and continued until a thorough evaluation of the patient's injury can be made and an individual fluid treatment plan for the patient is developed. The initial rough estimate of fluid administration carried out in this first 1 to 2 hours allows fluid resuscitation to begin immediately and is delivered according to the "Rule of Fourths." The Rule of Fourths roughly estimates the patient's needs for the first hour or so after injury according to the number of fourths of his body that are burned. The body surface area (BSA) can be quickly divided into fourths when the patient is first seen. For example, face and anterior chest and abdomen to the umbilicus total approximately one fourth. The remaining abdomen and anterior legs also constitute another one-fourth. The number of fourths is then multiplied by the flow rate of 1 liter per hour. Thus, if the face and anterior chest including the abdomen to the umbilicus are burned (approximately one-fourth of the total body surface area), the initial fluid is delivered as Ringer's lactate at a rate of 1 liter per hour. This infusion rate can be continued during the first 1 to 2 hours until a more detailed physical examination and accurate calculation of fluid requirements can be made. This rough estimate is intended as an initial guide only. The proper fluid replacement is determined by the careful monitoring of the patient, and the initial rough estimate as well as the more definitive calculated plan should be modified to optimize blood pressure, pulse, and urinary output. If hypovolemic shock is not aggressively treated during the early phase following a large thermal injury, renal failure or, worse, irreversible shock results. This initial guide, using the Rule of Fourths, is intended to give a rough calculation that allows one to immediately begin reasonable fluid resuscitation. One major error in early resuscitation is in not giving enough crystalloid to the severely burned patient during the first few hours after the injury.

After initial fluid therapy is begun, a more detailed evaluation by means of history and physical examination can be used to determine a more accurate estimate of fluid requirements. If intravascular fluid loss is extensive enough to cause hypovolemia, re-establishment of plasma volume requires sodium-containing water. This is the case if injury is deep and involves more than 10 to 15 percent BSA. The need for fluid replacement is related to both the extent of the burn (% BSA) and depth of injury. The predicted volume of replacement is therefore based on the percentage of the body surface area involved. This is taken as the sum of the areas of second- and third-degree burn as determined by comparisons with the Rule of Nines in adults or the Lund Browder chart in children.

The indications for use of central venous catheters, pulmonary artery catheters, and arterial lines in burn patients are identical to those for any trauma victim. The burn injury does not contraindicate their use if needed. Nonburned areas are preferred for all peripheral and central venous insertion sites owing to problems with infection as well as difficulties in securing a catheter to eschar. However, entrance through a burned site is indicated if the catheter is needed and no suitable unburned site is available. Central lines, when needed, are placed early if central venous access will be required for total parenteral nutrition, high-dose potassium replacement, or pulmonary artery pressure monitoring. We believe that placement of central lines may be difficult and dangerous in the hypovolemic patient. We reserve the placement of central lines for the specific indications already mentioned. In patients whose burns are not severe and whose needs for venous access will be brief, peripheral lines are used for fluid delivery. Femoral vein lines may be used for 24 hours if the patient is hypovolemic and the placement of a central line is difficult or if peripheral vasoconstriction makes the placement of more peripheral lines impossible. Cutdowns are avoided because of the prohibitively high associated infection rate.

The requirement of sodium-containing fluid in the resuscitation of burns is generally accepted for all burned patients requiring fluid resuscitation. However, the inclusion of colloid, such as fresh frozen plasma, as part of the fluid resuscitation is a matter of judgment. We use colloid based on the size of the burn, the age of the patient, and the patient's associated medical diseases. Small burns do not require colloid, whereas large burns benefit from colloid. Our treatment plan is based on prompt excision and immediate wound closure with grafting for all portions of the burn injury that will not heal spontaneously within 3 weeks. In this treatment plan, a normal colloid osmotic pressure with normal coagulation parameters is essential for the patient to tolerate the excision and grafting opera-

tions. Young children, the elderly, and patients with cardiac disease benefit most from the inclusion of colloid and the resulting decreased volume of the resuscitation fluid required. As with all the formulas, the exact volume of crystalloid and the amount and rate of colloid administration depends on the response to the fluids already administered.

Most formulas suggest 2 to 4 ml per kilogram per percent BSA for the first 24 hours. At the Massachusetts General Hospital, the patient's resuscitation is begun with Ringer's lactate. On careful clinical evaluation, if it is determined that the patient will benefit from colloid, the colloid is added as fresh frozen plasma. This is usually begun 4 to 6 hours after the beginning of resuscitation. The formula used as a guide is 0.5 ml per kilogram per percent BSA of colloid, 1.5 ml per kilogram per percent BSA of Ringer's lactate, and 100 ml per hour of maintenance Ringer's lactate is given. One-half is given in the first 8 hours, and one-quarter is given each of the next 8 hours. A sample calculation and sample orders for a 70-kg man with a 40 percent BSA burn are given in Figure 1. The calculated figures seldom are correct for the total period of resuscitation. The formula is intended only as a guide. For the next 24 hours, usually half the calculated volumes are used, depending on the patient's condition and urine output. From 48 to 72 hours, the requirements become maintenance plus considerations for increased insensible water losses and electrolyte balances. Again, adjustments are made, based on the patient's clinical state as determined by blood pressure, heart rate, urine output, mental status, and ventilatory function. The optimal urinary flow rate chosen is 50 to 100 ml per hour in the adult and 1 ml per kilogram per hour in the child. Catheters for monitoring pulmonary artery pressure are reserved for patients with signficant left ventricular congestive heart failure and are not used routinely, even in patients with large burns.

The two major errors in resuscitating the burn patient are delay in resuscitation and failure to vary from the calculated requirements when signs of adequate resuscitation are not achieved. All formulas are only guidelines for planning fluid therapy and must be adjusted on the basis of the patient's clinical response.

NUTRITIONAL MANAGEMENT

An important part of early management of a burn injury is the method chosen to solve the two critical problems for nutritional management of an injured patient: (1) What level of caloric intake will be required to allow the patient to meet the caloric needs in response to his injury? (2) What should the mixture of substrates (proteins, carbohydrates, and fats) contain that will optimally meet the patient's metabolic needs without incurring a negative nitrogen balance?

To answer the first question, oxygen consumption studies have shown that the metabolic rate of burn patients does not exceed twice the normal basal metabolic rate (BMR), as predicted by the Harris–Benedict table of cor-

0.5 × 70 × 40 = 1,400 ml colloid

1.5 × 70 × 40 = 4,200 ml replacement Ringer's lactate

100 × 24 = 2,400 ml maintenance Ringer's lactate

SAMPLE CALCULATION	SAMPLE ORDERS
FIRST 4 HOURS	
1,050 ml replacement Ringer's lactate	Ringer's lactate at 360 ml/h
400 ml maintenance Ringer's lactate	
SECOND 4 HOURS	
700 ml Fresh frozen plasma	Fresh frozen plasma at 180 ml/h
1,050 ml replacement Ringer's lactate	Ringer's lactate at 360 ml/h
400 ml maintenance Ringer's lactate	
SECOND 8 HOURS	
350 ml Fresh frozen plasma	Fresh frozen plasma at 45 ml/h
1,050 ml replacement Ringer's lactate	Ringer's lactate at 220 ml/h
800 ml maintenance Ringer's lactate	
THIRD 8 HOURS	
350 ml Fresh frozen plasma	Fresh frozen plasma at 45 ml/h
1,050 ml replacement Ringer's lactate	Ringer's lactate at 220 ml/h
800 ml maintenance Ringer's lactate	

Figure 1 Total fluid requirements for the first 24 hours for a 70-kg patient with a 40 percent BSA burn. According to the Massachusetts General Hospital formula for the first 24 hours, 0.5 ml per kilogram per percent BSA of colloid is used. Fresh frozen plasma is usually the colloid chosen. Half of this is given in the second 4 hours, and one-fourth of this is given in each of the remaining 8-hour periods; 1.5 ml per kilogram per percent BSA of replacement Ringer's lactate is given. One-fourth of this is given in the first 4 hours, in the second 4 hours, and in each of the remaining 8-hour periods. An additional 100 ml per hour of maintenance Ringer's lactate is given continuously over the 24-hour period.

relations. Prompt excision and immediate wound closure with grafting may contribute to this lower metabolic rate than the metabolic rate reported by other investigators. The Harris–Benedict correlation is as follows:

Male (Equation 1)

$$BMR = 66 + (13.7 \times W) + (5 \times H) - (6.8 \times A)$$

Female (Equation 2)

$$BMR = 665 + (9.6 \times W) + (1.7 \times H) - (4.7 \times A)$$

where BMR is normal basal metabolic rate in kcal, W is ideal body weight in kg, H is height in cm, and A is age in years. Equations 1 and 2 consider age, sex, height, and weight as factors determining basal caloric requirements. These variables normally control individual metabolic rates. In actual clinical practice, tables that list the results of Equations 1 and 2 for various heights, weights, and ages—rather than the equations—are used in the calculation of BMR.

Studies have demonstrated that although the size of the open burn wound and body temperature contribute to the hypermetabolism, their contribution is small and, for clinical purposes in the treatment of burn patients, may be disregarded in determining daily caloric requirements. Since twice the BMR has been shown to slightly over-estimate even the largest burn, we have chosen to ignore burn size and body temperature to simplify the clinical calculation of caloric need. That is, the daily caloric need for a seriously burned patient who is doing no muscular exercise may be calculated using the simple formula:

Total Daily Caloric Requirement = BMR × 2

with BMR as defined with the Harris–Benedict correlation for the individual patient in question.

The answer to the second question is more complex. The total caloric requirement is met with carbohydrate, protein, and fat. Carbohydrate at 5 mg per kilogram per minute has been shown to provide enough calories to prevent amino acid breakdown as an energy source and to suppress endogenous glucose production via hepatic gluconeogenesis, which requires mobilization of amino acids as gluconeogenic precursors. This glucose infusion rate approximates the maximum rate of glucose oxidation for an injured patient at strict bed rest. Additional glucose in a patient at rest is not used from ATP production, but is converted to fat. At this infusion rate, the respiratory quotient is just below unity, indicating that the glucose is oxidized to CO_2, H_2O, and energy and is not being stored as fat.

Protein is infused at 1.5 to 2.5 g per kilogram per day. For moderate injuries, the lower rate is used, and for severe injuries, the higher rate is used. Using nitrogen

TOTAL DAILY CALORIC REQUIREMENTS: (BMR × 2)
Male, 70 kg, 180 cm, and 20 years old

BMR = 66 + (13.7 × 70) + (5 × 180) − (6.8 × 20)
BMR = 1,800 kcal/day
BMR × 2 = 1,800 × 2 = 3,600 kcal/day

PROTEIN REQUIREMENT: 2.5 g/kg/day

70 × 2.5 = 175 g/day
175 g × 4 kcal/g = 700 kcal/day

CARBOHYDRATE REQUIREMENT: 5 mg/kg min

5 mg/kg/min × 1,440 min/day × 70 kg × 10^{-3} g/mg = 500 g/day
500 g/day × 4 kcal/g = 2,000 kcal/day

FAT REQUIREMENT: Remainder of total calories

3,600 = 700 + 2,000 + FAT
FAT = 900 kcal/day
900 kcal/day ÷ 9 kcal/g = 100 g/day

Figure 2 Total daily caloric requirements for a male, 70 kg, 180 cm, and 20 years old. The caloric need is estimated as BMR (normal basal metabolic rate) × 2. His BMR is estimated with the Harris–Benedict correlation as 1,800 kcal per day. His total daily caloric need is 3,600 kcal per day. Of this, 700 kcal per day (175 g of protein per day) should be protein to deliver 2.5 g per kilogram per day. He should have 2,000 kcal per day (500 g glucose per day) in order to receive 5 g glucose per kilogram per minute. The remaining calories are 900 kcal per day of fat or 100 g fat per day. In actual clinical practice, tables of the results of the Harris–Benedict correlation are easier to use than the equations.

balance analysis and kinetic amino acid turnover studies, this rate of administration was shown to maintain a positive nitrogen balance in adults and in children. Until we are able to measure muscle protein, collagen, and other protein synthesis rates in vivo, these will remain estimates and are as accurate as any other estimates. The exact protein and amino acid requirements for seriously injured patients are not known. While burn wounds are open and healing, the nitrogen requirement is known to be higher than normal. Unfortunately, these nitrogen balance studies do not translate into exact information about the quantity and composition of the proteins required.

Calculating the caloric equivalent given to a seriously burned patient when glucose is given at 5 mg glucose per kilogram per minute and protein at 2.5 g per kilogram per day shows that the patient's caloric requirement calculated as BMR × 2 is not achieved. Fats are therefore given to meet the remaining caloric requirement in either an enteral or a parenterally delivered diet. Fats are

included for two reasons: (1) to supply calories and minimize the need for mobilization of endogenous proteins for energy and gluconeogenesis, and (2) to provide essential fatty acids. For burn patients, usage of parenteral lipids as intravenous fat emulsions has been associated with significant thrombocytopenia, particularly in infants and children, and therefore must be given with care.

Early, aggressive metabolic support is given to (1) patients with burns of more than 20 percent BSA, (2) patients with preinjury malnutrition, (3) patients with complications such as sepsis or associated injuries, and (4) patients admitted late in their burn course who have a weight loss in excess of 10 percent of premorbid weight. This is begun as soon as possible after the injury and not later than postburn day 1 or 2 on completion of the immediate resuscitation phase. This support is accomplished by oral feeding, tube feeding, or total parenteral nutrition (TPN), depending on the patient's ability to receive nutritional support. The enteral route is preferred because of fewer complications and lower cost associated with enteral feedings as compared to parenteral feeding. However, anorexia, facial burns, or dysphagia may make oral feeding difficult or impossible. If these are present, but gastric motility and absorption is normal, tube feedings are given. These tube feedings are given as a constant infusion rate as either a supplement to oral feedings or as a replacement of the oral feedings as the total caloric source. Total parenteral nutrition is used if intestinal motility or absorption is abnormal, or if multiple excision and grafting procedures are anticipated over the first week of the admission so that the gastrointestinal tract is not allowed to recover between operations.

A sample calculation is given in Figure 2 for a 20-year-old male, 5 feet 11 inches tall (180 cm), weighing 155 pounds (70 kg) with a 20 percent BSA burn (combined second- and third-degree burns). His preburn weight is his ideal body weight according to tables such as the Metropolitan Life Insurance Company Standard Tables of Ideal Body Weight. The sample calculation shows the recommended daily enteral diet to be 175 g protein, 500 g carbohydrate (primarily glucose), and 100 g fat. This provides 3,600 kcal of which 700 kcal is from protein, 2,000 kcal from glucose, and 900 kcal from fat. The same nutrients would be used in a parenteral diet. The enteral diet could be constructed by the burn unit dietitian. If these goals were not met after careful determinations of daily caloric intake, commerically available tube feedings could be used to supplement the caloric intake or entirely replace oral feedings.

PENETRATING INJURY TO THE NECK

CHARLES R. SACHATELLO, M.D.

My approach to the patient with penetrating trauma to the neck is based on the framing and answering of a series of straightforward questions:

1. Is this injury immediately life-threatening?
2. What structures are most likely to have been injured?
3. Will I need to operate on the patient?
4. What other diagnostic procedures, if any, are necessary to evaluate this patient more completely?

Implicit in these questions and the resulting evaluation and treatment of the patient with penetrating neck trauma are several assumptions:

1. It is not necessary to explore every patient with penetrating neck trauma.
2. There are basically only three structures in the neck that warrant exploration when injured—the airway (larynx and trachea primarily), major arterial structures, and the esophagus. Excluding major external venous bleeding, injuries to veins rarely require operative treatment.
3. It is generally easier and more accurate to reconstruct the depth, path, and trajectory of gunshot wounds than stab wounds.
4. The site of injury (low neck, midneck, or high neck) determines the probability of a given injury.
5. There are substantial differences between the potential and magnitude of injury produced by stab wounds and those produced by gunshot wounds.
6. Intelligent planned observation with repetitive re-examination of the patient with penetrating neck trauma cannot be construed as neglect or negligence.

Some surgeons, perhaps even a majority, believe that all neck injuries require exploration and, without much cognitive thought, immediately schedule the patient for operation. This practice, which has generally prevailed since the mid-forties, evolved from a combination of wartime experience and earlier surgical practice that failed to appreciate that some neck injuries can be lethal if neglected. The neck is simply not another extremity.

Mandatory exploration of neck injuries should be considered in the same historical context as the wartime dictum that every colon injury required a proximal diverting colostomy or the more recent civilian practice whereby every abdominal stab wound required an exploratory laparotomy. These rules were both appropriate and necessary for their time. They were certainly well intentioned. However, all outlived their usefulness.

The decision to explore or observe a patient with penetrating neck trauma should be based on a number of factors, including the nature of the injury, the trajectory and depth of penetration, physical signs, and ancillary diagnostic tests such as endoscopy or arteriograms as necessary.

IMMEDIATE LIFE-THREATENING INJURY

Immediate life-threatening penetrating injuries to the neck are characterized by one or more of the following physical signs: (1) massive exsanguination, (2) destruction or obstruction of the airway, (3) unexplained hypotension or respiratory embarrassment, generally due to a tension pneumothorax (hemothorax?) or major intrapleural bleeding, and (4) respiratory paralysis due to cervical cord injury.

In the absence of one or more of these dramatic injuries, sudden death from penetrating neck trauma is not likely to occur. Evaluation and treatment should be both expedient and deliberate.

The two injuries that demand immediate emergency attention are major bleeding and/or airway obstruction or destruction. Neck injuries are unique in their potential to produce severe and even fatal external bleeding with seemingly innocuous soft tissue injury. External bleeding can almost always be controlled temporarily by direct manual pressure. The observation that fatal external bleeding can occur with only venous injury emphasizes the importance of direct digital pressure. Blind clamping is unlikely to be successful and is more apt to be associated with substantial additional blood loss.

Intraoral bleeding can cause death either by direct blood loss or, more likely, by drowning due to the aspiration of blood. Severe intraoral bleeding may require bimanual intraoral and external tamponade. The technical maneuvers are easier to discuss than to perform owing to the associated anxiety and combativeness of the hypoxic struggling patient.

Airway control with major intraoral bleeding presents one of the most difficult and challenging problems encountered in an emergency situation. The patient is invariably combative, anxious, struggling, and coughing to clear his airway. An immediate crycothyroidotomy is necessary. Under these circumstances a number of strong hands are necessary to restrain the patient while suctioning his mouth and airway simultaneously.

These hypoxic restless patients are usually struggling to sit up and spit out the blood coughed up. It may be necessary to perform the crycothyroidotomy while the patient is sitting. The procedure is facilitated by a strong assistant standing behind the patient both supporting and restraining him simultaneously. As soon as the airway is controlled, a large nasogastric tube should be placed to evacuate the large quantities of air, blood, and gastric contents that are invariably present.

Repetitive suctioning of the airway is mandatory to remove residual aspirated blood. A short-acting muscle relaxant to paralyze the patient is frequently necessary so that the pharynx can be packed to stem the tide of intraoral bleeding.

Both the surgeon and the anesthesiologist must be alert to the potential for residual intratracheal blood to clot and act as a ball valve causing progressive airway obstruction. The clue to this phenomenon is increasing airway pressure due to the initially insidious nature of the air trapping. Inspiration appears to be normal and suctioning the patient does not solve the problem. The intratracheal clot moves to and fro with respiration. Expiration is partially blocked by the ball-valving blood clot, the lungs become more distended, and greater airway pressure is required for inspiration. Venous pressure rises, and hypotension develops as a result of impaired venous return. The only solution is to remove the tube and immediately replace it with another larger tube. Tension pneumothorax becomes a distinct possibility and can occur almost instantaneously owing to the increased airway pressure.

Gunshot wounds in particular can lead to destruction of the airway. The nearly severed trachea tends to retract toward the mediastinum. Bleeding from the injured soft tissue, thyroid gland, and strap muscles enters the trachea to cause paroxysms of coughing and straining. These soft tissues tend to flop over the injured trachea, interfering with inspiration. Emergency first aid requires manual retraction of the injured soft tissue to facilitate inspiration. The injured trachea needs to be intubated immediately with a medium-sized endotracheal tube. In this and other similar acute airway problems, an endotracheal tube is easier to insert than standard tracheostomy tubes. The beveled edge and extra length permit more rapid insertion and better airway control. Even a tube as small as a No. 5 or No. 6 can provide an adequate temporary airway. It is not advisable to struggle to insert a No. 8 cuffed tracheostomy tube under these circumstances. The downward pressure necessary to insert a larger tracheostomy tube may disrupt the trachea even further. The surgeon should not be reluctant to use short-acting muscle relaxants to calm the struggling patient once the airway is controlled.

Crycothyroidotomy

A crycothyroidotomy is performed by first identifying the inferior border of the large prominent thyroid cartilage. The taut membrane separating this cartilage from the inferior cricoid cartilage is relatively superficial. The membrane should be punctured with a scalpel and spread open with a hemostat or Kelly clamp. A small endotracheal tube (No. 5 or No. 6) should be rapidly inserted and the balloon inflated. The tube should be held in place firmly until it is secured by tape or suture. This type of airway should be considered only as a temporary procedure until a more formal adequate-sized tracheostomy tube can be inserted under controlled circumstances.

EVALUATION OF PENETRATING NECK TRAUMA

Once the surgeon has ruled out the likelihood of an imminently fatal neck injury, he should proceed with a more detailed evaluation of the area of injury, based on the following questions:

1. What structures are most likely to have been injured?
2. Will I need to operate on the patient?
3. What other diagnostic tests are indicated?

In attempting to answer these questions, it is helpful to recognize the distinct anatomic areas in the neck. The high neck is that part of the neck above the angle of the mandible. The mid-neck, or free neck, extends from the mandible inferiorly to the insertion of the trapezius. The low neck extends from the trapezius to the suprasternal notch. When viewed in this context, it is apparent that penetrating trauma may involve or extend from one area of the neck to another. Similarly, the trajectory of penetration can be sagittal (anterior-posterior—front to back), or transverse (left to right), or coronal. An approximation of the depth and trajectory of penetration gives a relatively accurate first impression of the potential severity of injury.

It is surprisingly easy to obtain a working approximation of the depth and trajectory of gunshot wounds by means of a simple roentgenographic examination. A standard paper clip should be taped vertically over the entrance wound and horizontally over the exit wound. The patient can then be examined fluoroscopically to superimpose one paper clip over the other to produce a cross sight of the two wounds. Plain films taken in this projection give an approximation of the trajectory of the injury. The same technique is equally valuable when the bullet is still lodged in the neck. The vertically placed paper clip marking the extrance wound is aligned over the bullet in situ and plain films are taken. Detailed inspection of the neck films should be made in search of any sign of bony injury or fragmentation that would suggest ricochet.

This simple roentgenographic technique demonstrates that low-caliber missiles frequently "bend," especially as they travel around the mandible. It is not unusual to align an entrance and exit wound fluoroscopically and sight a path that is presumed to be through the mandible, only to find that detailed views of the mandible do not show any osseous injury. It appears that the missile travels along the contour of the mandible, "bending" as it travels. This type of approximation of trajectory is valuable in determining the necessity for arteriograms, endoscopic examination, or esophagrams.

It is much more difficult, if not impossible, to make any type of preoperative accurate assessment of the trajectory or depth of penetration of stab wounds. A number of experienced surgeons have explored a neck for a supposedly deep stab wound only to find virtually no evidence of penetration and virtually no clue as to the trajectory.

Such recurrent experiences force the experienced surgeon to ask himself, ''What was I looking for? How can I be sure I didn't miss it? Could I have done other tests to prevent this unnecessary exploration?'' Ancillary x-ray studies surely could have helped.

A stab wound of the low neck is extremely difficult to evaluate clinically. With a downward thrust, the central mediastinal vascular structures, the trachea, and the esophagus are at risk. Tension pneumothorax or hemothorax may result. Neck exploration might serve to delineate the depth and trajectory. Unfortunately, the exposure is totally inadequate for effective management of injuries in the upper mediastinum. More than any other injury, stab wounds of the low neck demand a thorough nonoperative evaluation initially. Arteriograms and esophagrams should be obtained in many of these patients. Follow-up chest films in search of small apical pneumothoraces are indicated. Although stab wounds of the low neck may prove to be totally innocuous, they can be associated with injuries that are serious and difficult to diagnose. Neck exploration offers little help for patients with central mediastinal injuries and is of no value for patients with only superficial stab wounds.

Unexplained hypotension or respiratory insufficiency with penetrating neck trauma generally indicates that a tension pneumothorax or hemothorax is present. Stab wounds of the low neck are particularly likely to produce mediastinal or intrapleural injury since stab wounds generally have a downward trajectory. Immediate insertion of a chest tube to re-expand the lung can improve respiratory dynamics. The re-expanded lung generally provides tamponade for major central venous bleeding. The combination of major intrapleural bleeding and a stab wound of the low neck mandate thoracotomy. A variety of alternative approaches to central mediastinal vessel injuries have been advocated, including sternal splitting and flap-type incisions. A high third or fourth intercostal thoracotomy is generally easier to perform in emergency situations and affords the opportunity for manual control of the injured vessels.

Major bleeding or an expanding hematoma is usually present with major arterial disruption in the neck. The tight vesting fascial compartments of the neck are efficient in providing tamponade for major arterial injury. Expanding hematomas in the neck warrant arteriography at a minimum. Many patients with a normal arteriogram may be observed carefully and be spared an unnecessary exploration. It should be recognized that only two decades ago, large numbers of carotid arteriograms were done with direct carotid artery sticks. It was not at all unusual to stick the carotid two or three times before the needle could be advanced enough to allow injection of medium contrast. These patients frequently developed impressive cervical hematomas, but hardly ever needed any treatment other than bed rest. Airway obstruction, even with fist-sized hematomas, was rare.

Arterial thrombosis without bleeding can occur from gunshot wounds. Arterial thrombosis due to gunshot wounds is more common in the vertebral artery than in the carotid artery. There is minimal or no hematoma present, and the injury is frequently an unanticipated arteriographic finding. Thrombosis without bleeding is virtually an impossibility with penetrating stab wounds.

Injury to the airway is usually immediately obvious by virtue of simple physical examination, airway embarrassment, or the presence of blood-tinged sputum and paroxysms of coughing. Crepitus or extensive subcutaneous emphysema may be present with airway injury or with esophageal penetration.

Esophageal penetration is difficult to diagnose on physical examination. Even large esophageal perforations are rarely diagnosed by saliva exiting the wound. Subcutaneous emphysema is not a totally reliable finding. It is surprising how much subcutaneous emphysema can be present without detection of esophageal or tracheal injury. The possibility of esophageal perforation must be considered with every stab wound and mid-neck gunshot wounds. Since the esophagus is normally compressed in an anterior plane, lateral penetrating injuries are more likely to lead to esophageal injury than are direct anterior injuries.

Endoscopic examination or esophagrams are indicated and worthwhile in patients with subcutaneous emphysema or pain on swallowing.

SPECIFIC INJURIES

Cervical Spine

As with any injured patient, preliminary evaluation of cervical spine instability is important. Penetrating trauma is much less apt to produce instability than blunt trauma to the head and neck. Stab wounds in particular are extraordinarily unlikely, if ever, to lead to cervical spine instability. There are anecdotal cases of quadriplegia due to stab wounds with direct cord injury, but without cervical spine instability.

Severe gunshot wounds of the neck may cause enough osseous and ligamentous destruction to lead to cervical spine instability. Associated immediate quadriplegia is almost invariably present. The fear of producing quadriplegia by inserting an airway or applying pressure to control external bleeding is not warranted in patients with penetrating neck trauma. However, a rigid neck collar has no place in the triage or treatment of a patient with major external bleeeding from a neck wound.

The Esophagus

There is little disagreement regarding the management of esophageal injuries, which consists of closure with absorbable sutures and drainage. The problem in closing esophageal perforation is related to esophageal anatomy. The esophagus is normally compressed in an anterior-posterior plane and perforations may be missed or misjudged. Although a nasograstric tube aids in identifying the esophagus, it is not particularly helpful in defining the extent of perforation. A Foley catheter or endotracheal tube with the balloon inflated is far more useful in demonstrating the size, location, and extent of the perforation. Injecting a white antacid or contrast agent with 1 or 2 cc of hydrogen peroxide sometimes facilitates identification of a puncture-type perforation.

Traction sutures should be placed on each end of the perforation. Closure with a single layer of interrupted or running synthetic absorbable sutures is adequate. It is advisable to place a soft drain from the esophageal injury to the incision.

The Trachea

Simple perforations of the trachea can be closed with synthetic absorbable sutures. Intratracheal bleeding is rarely a problem, and tracheostomy is generally not necessary. More extensive tracheal wounds, especially those of blowout proportion, may require resection of one or more tracheal rings. Formal tracheostomy is almost always a necessity. The possibility of injury to one or both recurrent laryngeal nerves, owing either to the initial injury or to the exposure necessary for repair, should be evaluated as soon as it is practical.

Treatment of combined tracheal and esophageal wounds must be individualized. Ideally, viable tissue interposed between the trachea and esophagus may prevent development of a tracheoesophageal fistula.

Thoracic Duct

It is distinctly unusual for the thoracic duct to be the only structure injured as a result of penetrating neck trauma. This injury is generally associated with central vessel trauma or unusually zealous neck exploration. The duct is much easier to find in the emergency situation than in elective operation because of the presence of chyle drainage associated with recent ingestion of food. In my experience, silver clips are more effective in controlling lymph drainage than are sutures or ligatures. The latter have a tendency to sever the delicate vessels. Drainage of thoracic duct injury is mandatory, and soft suction drainage is preferred.

Spinal Accessory Nerve

The spinal accessory nerve can be severed by surprisingly superficial neck lacerations, and presence of this injury should be documented specifically prior to any incision in the lateral and posterior neck. The spinal accessory nerve innervates the trapezius muscle. The specific defect is the inability of the abducted arm to be raised over the head.

If there is a specific indication to explore the neck, the divided ends of the nerve should be repaired or marked to facilitate later nerve graft. Injury to this nerve results in a major disability. Injury to the nerve is not in itself a specific indication to explore the neck.

The Tongue

Penetrating injuries to the tongue, especially gunshot wounds, warrant special comment. This injury may appear so innocuous initially that it receives only passing notice as care is directed toward the more obvious buccal or mandibular injury. The injured tongue rarely requires operative control of bleeding, but it frequently swells progressively for 12 to 48 hours to such an extent as to totally occlude the airway.

Elective nasotracheal intubation is warranted for patients with gunshot wounds of the tongue who do not require neck exploration. Those who are explored for associated neck injuries should have the nasotracheal tube left in place for at least 24 hours.

The frequently associated buccal or mandibular injury may require little operative treatment. It is reasonable to delay any extensive mandibular or dental procedures until the swelling subsides. Intravenous antibiotics such as penicillin or a cephalosporin are worthwhile.

Blood Vessels

Venous injuries should be treated by ligation. Only rarely is venous repair of the internal jugular vein possible or worthwhile.

The common carotid artery and internal carotid artery should be repaired if possible. The controversy regarding delayed repair of the carotid artery in patients with a neurologic defect preoperatively is both real and unsettled. The possibility of converting an ischemic injury to a hemorrhagic infarct simply cannot be settled by any type of controlled study in this group of patients. The most useful and pertinent observations are made in patients who develop an immediate neurologic defect after a carotid endarterectomy. Many experienced surgeons have seen complete rapid neurologic improvement following prompt reoperation whereby an occlusive or thrombotic process could be satisfactorily corrected.

There is little justification for repair of the external carotid artery. Ligation is preferable.

The specific technique to approach the injured carotid artery through the invariably present hematoma varies somewhat from that used to do an elective carotid endarterectomy. A generous vertical incison is made at the anterior edge of the sternocleidomastoid. Every attempt is made to approach the carotid as low in the neck as possible before approaching the actual perforation. The carotid is encircled with a vessel loop, which is converted to a Rummel type tourniquet to ensure proximal control. For carotid injuries in the low neck, the patient should be so draped as to permit sternal splitting to gain proximal control if necessary. The partially severed carotid artery should not be further divided until adequate proximal control is obtained. An inexperienced surgeon will be astounded at the extent to which a divided common carotid can retract behind the sternum. Once this happens, it is difficult to rapidly regain proximal control.

Stab wounds of the carotid can usually be repaired with several interrupted nonabsorbable monofilament sutures.

Gunshot wounds usually require resection and end-to-end anastomosis. Only rarely is a saphenous vein graft necessary. The saphenous vein from the ankle area is adequate for an interposition graft. An indwelling shunt is useful to maintain cerebral flow while the vein is being harvested.

Vertebral Artery

Ideally, an experienced surgeon will not discover major vertebral bleeding spurting between two cervical vertebra without having suspected the injury preoperatively and performed arteriography. An arterial spurter pulsating from between osseous fragments of the cervical vertebra presents a humbling and unforgettable problem. Standard suture technique simply does not work. Jamming large silver clips toward the bleeding is more frustrating than successful. Bone wax used to help secure previously placed Gelfoam pledgets may or may not be successful.

Proximal ligation of the vertebral artery requires extensive dissection of its subclavian origin. In some patients, even proximal ligation does not totally arrest the bleeding as there can be extensive back bleeding. When back bleeding persists and is refractory to both proximal ligation and bone wax at the site of vertebral bleeding, there are only two choices. Once is to expose the vertebral artery as it enters the skull. Many surgeons, including the author, have had little experience with this approach. The other choice is to measured distance toward the skull. Inflating the balloon may well control retrograde bleeding. Detachable balloons have worked surprisingly well in this application. In the absence of detachable balloons, the catheter can be left in place and brought out through the incision. The balloon can be deflated several days later to determine whether there is any further bleeding.

COLD INJURY

ALAN R. DIMICK, M.D.

Localized cold injuries are due to either freezing or nonfreezing temperatures. Cold but not freezing temperatures produce trench foot, immersion foot, and chilblains. Frostbite is caused by freezing temperatures. There are significant differences between localized cold injury and generalized cold injury (hypothermia).

Localized cold injury is due to exposure to cold temperatures and usually is present in areas of reduced circulation, i.e., cheeks, nose, ears, fingers, and toes. Cold injuries of the face tend to be superficial because of the excellent blood supply to the face. Cold injury to the extremities is usually more serious because of poor circulation in the extremities.

TRENCH FOOT

Trench foot is commonly seen in the military and may occur with exposure to cold but not freezing temperatures. This exposure is usually prolonged, and the presence of moisture seems to be important. Sequelae after recovery from the acute phase usually consist of pain in the area, hypersensitivity to cold, and abnormal sensations.

IMMERSION FOOT AND HAND

Immersion foot and hand are usually seen after prolonged exposure to cold but not freezing water. Sequelae of this condition consist of paralyses of major nerves as well as chronic hypersensitivity to cold and paresthesias.

CHILBLAINS

Chilblains, the mildest form of cold injury, usually occurs after prolonged exposure to cold nonfreezing temperatures and requires the presence of moisture. Burning and itching usually occur, and vesicles may be seen in the acute phase. The chronic condition is characterized by cold hypersensitivity, paresthesias, itching, and sometimes skin breakdown. Treatment consists of protection from cold and heat. Chilblains usually does not result in tissue loss. Sympathectomy has an unproven role in the treatment of this condition.

FROSTBITE

Exposure to freezing temperatures causes frostbite. The damage due to frostbite is similar to that seen in burn injury and is classified similarly.

First-degree frostbite is a superficial injury to the skin similar to that of a first-degree burn. It is associated with erythema and edema, but unlike a first-degree burn, it is also associated with numbness. First-degree frostbite usually heals spontaneously in 7 to 10 days. Second-degree frostbite is also characterized by numbness, erythema, edema, and blister formation. These blisters may be either clear or bloody. Healing usually occurs in 14 to 21 days. Healing of second-degree frostbite is similar to that of second-degree burn injury, occurring with a thin epidermis that is easily traumatized and must be protected from further injury.

In third-degree frostbite, as with third-degree burns, there is full-thickness skin loss. Shortly after injury, the skin may appear bluish or black. With conservative therapy, the black eschar may take one or two months to separate.

Some clinicians consider fourth-degree frostbite as involvement of muscles, tendons, and bone. This condition is similar to the third-degree burn that involves these underlying structures, and therefore probably does not deserve a separate classification.

Pathophysiology of Frostbite

Mechanisms for the production of frostbite include vasoconstriction with damage to the microcirculation, and also direct damage to cells due to the cold injury. Experts disagree as to how much each of these mechanisms is responsible for the injury.

Cold injury may directly injure the capillary circulation, causing ischemia of the distal extremities. Tissue injury may occur from both direct damage to the cells and ischemia due to the loss of circulation in the area.

Tissue repair in frostbite is similar to that seen in burn injuries. Epithelium migrates to cover the wound from the surviving remnants of sweat glands, hair follicles, and the margins of the wound. Autoamputation may occur as a result of ischemic necrosis and gangrene, and this process may take several months without surgical intervention.

Environmental Influences

The most significant environmental influence is the ambient temperature, which can be modified by wearing protective clothing. This clothing must provide insulation in layers to protect against the loss of body heat through the clothing. The presence of wind and wet conditions will further accelerate the loss of heat. The wind chill index reflects the magnitude of the contribution of wind in heat loss. Even in a moderate temperature, the excessive wind chill can lower the temperature severely.

Clothing should be light, dry, and in layers (to trap air within the multiple layers) to be effective. Wet clothing reduces the insulation and therefore is detrimental to the conservation of heat. Proper protective clothing is important. In numerous studies, the majority of those suffering frostbite had inadequate protective clothing.

Prevention of Cold Injury

Obviously, there are two ways to prevent cold injury. The first is by increasing heat production and the second is by decreasing heat loss. The avoidance of wet clothing and contact with metal as well as wearing proper protective clothing helps one to avoid excessive heat loss and prevents cold injury. The extremities represent prime sites for heat loss and therefore should be protected. There are several factors that increase susceptibility to frostbite injuries. These include the use of tobacco and alcohol, anemia, and hemorrhage. The importance of working and keeping active so as to increase heat production has been documented in the literature, as has the need to avoid sweating so as to avoid wetness and further heat loss.

Frostbite in the areas of good capillary circulation is usually superficial, such as in the areas of the head and neck. In areas where circulation is poor, such as the fingers and toes, deeper frostbite usually occurs.

Therapy of Frostbite

Vigorous rubbing of frostbitten tissue should not be done because this further damages the skin. Slow thawing or rubbing the area with snow increases tissue damage. Furthermore, a frozen part should not be thawed if refreezing is likely to occur.

Therapy for frostbite should include restoration of core body temperature. Hypothermia, with a core body temperature of less than 35 °C, must be corrected prior to the specific treatment of frostbite. Death may occur at a body temperature of 28 °C. The patient should be wrapped in dry, warm blankets or other insulating material to maintain the body temperature and prevent the further loss of heat from the body. As in burn injury, the use of prophylactic antibiotics is not indicated. Patients with serious frostbite, primarily involving the extremities, should be admitted to the hospital. Once the generalized hypothermia has been corrected, the frozen area should be rewarmed in an agitated water bath at 104 ° to 108 °F (40 ° to 44 °C) for 15 to 30 minutes. The rewarming may be stopped when the involved part becomes hyperemic. Excessive rewarming results in further damage. Rewarming may be painful, and narcotic analgesia may be needed.

As in burn injury, it is now recommended that all wounds be dressed with some type of topical antibacterial to prevent the proliferation of bacteria. Hands and feet should be properly splinted.

The management of blisters in frostbite as well as in burn injury usually provokes controversy. Robson has definitively shown that blisters contain thromboxane derivatives, which can accelerate the progressive vascular thrombosis and ischemia in frostbite and burn injuries. Therefore, there is a therapeutic advantage to removal of the blisters. Robson also recommends the application of topical Aloe vera (Dermaide Aloe), and aspirin. Robson has reported no tissue loss with the use of this regimen.

It is important that affected parts be elevated and splinted as for burn injury. Exercise and range of motion should be applied accordingly.

Early surgical intervention usually is not necessary in frostbite. With the development of ischemia and gangrene, surgical intervention may be required. Escharotomy may be necessary in cases of circumferential constriction similar to that found in burns involving extremities.

Treatment aimed at the microcirculation has included anticoagulants and hyperbaric oxygen. Heparin has been shown to increase tissue survival in experimental frostbite injury, but clinical experience has not confirmed this. The same is true for low-molecular-weight dextran.

Regional sympathetic blockade also remains controversial. It has both its opponents and proponents. Some patients have benefited from the use of sympathectomy; others have had no improvement. Therefore it is difficult to determine whether regional sympathetic blockade would be beneficial in general. However, it may be of benefit in patients with sympathetic hyperactivity and cold sensitivity. This can only be determined on an individual basis.

Degenerative joint disease as well as stiff and painful joints with fibrosis may be sequelae of severe frostbite. Intrinsic muscle atrophy and fibrosis also may occur. Injury due to frostbite may involve the epiphyseal growth centers, and in children this may result in severe deformity. Parents should be advised that these sequelae are possible despite appropriate therapy of frostbite during the acute interval.

PELVIC FRACTURE

RENNER M. JOHNSTON, M.D.

Since the majority of pelvic fractures involve multisystem trauma, it is natural to expect a multispecialty approach to the management of these patients. Particularly at risk are those individuals who also sustain serious head, chest, or abdominal injury, as the mortality can reach over 10 percent for all accident patients in these categories. With the exception of the elderly and persons with osteopenia, it takes significant direct or indirect trauma to fracture the large, rugged flat bones of the pelvic ring. Twenty-five percent of these patients have associated major long bone fractures. Thus, prompt aggressive diagnosis and treatment are essential to diminish the mortality and morbidity.

IMMEDIATE CONCERNS

Head, neck, and chest trauma are primary in resuscitative measures. Fractures of the pelvis and long bone can cause steady, significant, but often insidious, blood loss. Intra-abdominal and major peripheral arterial bleeding may be the source of hemorrhage, but most commonly, the large vascular fracture surfaces and associated soft tissue venous rupture cause the continuous blood loss. It is crucial to emphasize that movement of these fracture surfaces is directly related to increased pain and apprehension as well as significant increased bleeding. Thus, if these patients are transported for various diagnostic studies (every time they are moved or rolled to another table or bed) bleeding may be accentuated.

Peritoneal lavage, IVP cystogram, and AP roentgenograms can all be done without moving the patient. If the film of the pelvis is combined with 40-degree-angled inlet and outlet views, sufficient information can frequently be obtained to assess the degree of instability of the pelvic ring, again without moving the patient. If a CT scan is to be done for the head or spine, remarkably accurate information can be ascertained by including several "cuts" through the sacroiliac area.

MANAGEMENT OF PELVIC RING INSTABILITY

Any suspected pelvic ring injury should be considered unstable until proved otherwise. Thus, if movement, crepitus, or pelvic pain is detected in the field or emergency room, a MAST compression garment should be used, and orders to restrict movements from the supine position should be given, especially if the patient is hypotensive. Close inspection of the various x-ray films may detect patterns of anterior fractures or symphysis diastasis which can combine with posterior sacral or iliac fractures or dislocations to make the unstable pelvic ring injury. A major clue to ring instability is upward (cephalad) displacement of one side of the pelvic ring, especially through the posterior fracture or SI separation. This would indicate an unstable vertical shear (Malgaigne) pattern.

The orthopaedist should plan the treatment of the pelvic fracture in conjunction with the specialists who are managing the patient's other injuries. The orthopaedic decision is based on the expected severity of the pelvic fracture in terms of blood loss, pain, limited mobility, and functional outcome (in that order of importance).

If the general surgeon performs a laparotomy, the orthopaedist should take the opportunity to feel the hemipelvic instability and to re-evaluate pelvic blood loss. Either before or after the laparotomy is an excellent time to quickly apply an external fixator to the pelvic ring. By stabilizing the fractures, this further facilitates control of venous bleeding and dramatically relieves fracture pain. If there is continued heavy blood loss after external fixator application and laparotomy, it should then be investigated by arteriography and possible selective embolization of a ruptured artery in the pelvic distribution. It should be pointed out that major arterial branch rupture is uncommon with pelvic fractures.

If no laparotomy or other surgery is to be done emergently on the patient with a pelvic fracture, the MAST suit and/or bed rest in a pelvic sling is acceptable while the blood loss and pelvic pain are assessed. Skeletal traction can reduce any upward displacement of the hemipelvic fracture as well. If long bone fractures are to be internaly fixed over the next few days, internal or external fixation of the unstable pelvic fracture should again be strongly considered because the patient may then be mobilized from bed with less pain. Sometimes this shortens the hospitalization significantly.

INTERNAL FIXATION OF THE UNSTABLE HEMIPELVIC FRACTURE

This decade has brought increased awareness of the functional problems with malunion and non-union of pelvic ring injuries, especially with the increased number of severe pelvic fractures and polytrauma patients that now survive the initial shock and tissue damage to their systems. Chronic pain, leg-length inequality, and pelvic dysfunction have been used as reasons to justify the trauma orthopaedist's renewed surgical efforts to improve pelvic fracture reductions. Many of these surgical procedures are difficult and unfamiliar to the orthopaedist and have sometimes resulted in disastrous consequences from renewed blood loss, further tissue damage and sepsis, especially if performed within the first 3 to 4 days after injury. The reader is cautioned that I greatly prefer to approach these pelvic ring disruptions only after thorough analysis of the x-ray studies (usually including a CT scan) and after blood loss and other injuries are stabilized for 5 to 7 days. During this time, the external fixator is of great help in stabilizing the pelvic ring. Not uncommonly, the fixator maintains a satisfactory enough reduction to allow the orthopaedist to use it in place of an open surgical fixation of the pelvic ring disruption.

Other than the application of the external fixation to the pelvic ring, the least traumatic and simplest surgery is to reduce and internally fix the symphysis diastasis or adjacent pubic ring fracture with plate and screws. This technique then stabilizes the anterior ring and allows the external fixator to compress the posterior injury, if necessary. Unfortunately, in my experience, this relatively simple anterior diastasis is well managed by a fixator alone (an open-book injury), or all four pubic rami are fractured and difficult to fix internally. Studies have also shown that non-unions or mild (less than 2 cm) anterior diastases are usually asymptomatic because only tension forces are applied to the anterior ring in daily activities.

Posterior pelvic ring disruptions are another matter entirely. No specific guidelines exist to determine when and where the sacroiliac fracture or dislocations should be surgically approached. However, it appears that patients with posterior or superior displacement of the iliac wing through the SI joint are especially prone to problems with malunion and non-union. Some of this dysfunction and pain may be irreparable damage owing to the severe trauma, but for the most part, the disorder apparently can be reversed by satisfactory open reduction and stable fixation of fractures and dislocations of the SI joint. I am being hesitant because there are only limited data, at this time, to confirm our impressions that this rather risky surgery is justified by the expected positive, long-term results. The anatomy of the sacroiliac joint and its surrounding structures, such as the sciatic plexus, ureter, and iliac and gluteal vessels, make exposures demanding and fixation exacting, often with poor visualization of the fracture reduction and the position of the screw fixation. The posterior iliac crest overhangs the SI joint, making direct vision of the fracture reduction difficult, and requires screw placement by indirect means. Successful reduction and fracture stability is indeed rewarding to the surgeon and the patient. The ability to be mobile and relatively pain-free is satisfying and justifies the risks taken in the properly selected patient. There is a 5 to 10 percent incidence of such complications as increased blood loss, nerve palsy, and sepsis. Damage to the ureter, large vessels, nerve roots, and bowel is always possible if the screw is not placed with extreme caution.

With either internal or external fixation, the unstable pelvic fracture should be united and able to take added stresses after 2 to 3 months. At that time, the external fixator pins can be removed and more vigorous physical therapy pursued.

ACETABULAR FRACTURES

The pelvic ring can also be injured by fractures of the acetabulum. These are indirect injuries by forces directed through the femur to the femoral head and acetabulum. Associated injuries to the patient are much less frequent, and blood loss is usually only mild, not requiring resuscitative measures. However, the fractures and their displacement can cause serious and permanent damage to the hip joint and adjacent sciatic nerve. While associated injuries are being treated, the acetabular fracture is managed in traction after AP and angled views of the acetabulum have been obtained. Associated dislocation or subluxation of the hip joint should be promptly reduced, under anesthesia if necessary. A few days after traction is applied, the decision should be made regarding internal fixation of the acetabular fracture.

A detailed classification of acetabular fractures has been developed to assist the surgeon in determining the proper surgical approach and the prognosis for the patient with or without surgical fixation. Basically, the acetabulum is divided into two major columns (anterior and posterior). Fracture lines and displacement can occur in either column or in both. If the fracture fragments are large and are displaced more than 2 to 3 mm, the hip joint reduction is probably incongruent between the femoral head and acetabulum. In the relatively young individual (physiologically under age 60), internal fixation of a displaced, incongruent acetabulum is strongly indicated. I rely on CT scanning and skeletal models showing the fracture lines to assist me in deciding when to attempt internal fixation and what approach to use. These are usually comminuted fractures and extremely difficult to reduce surgically without considerable experience and expertise. Transfer of these patients in skeletal traction to a major trauma center is safe once the patient's condition is stable.

The incidence of acceptable results with nonoperative traction treatment of displaced, incongruent acetabular fractures is about 55 percent. The remaining patients have stiffness and pain and may require a prosthetic arthroplasty or arthrodesis within a few years. When surgical fixation is performed by an experienced surgeon, satisfactory results are the rule in 75 percent of cases. Complications include infections, nerve palsies, failure of fixation, and heterotopic bone formation with stiffness. The complication rate is under 3 percent for infections and nerve palsy, but around 20 percent for significant heterotopic bone formation.

SKIN AND SOFT TISSUE

SKIN TUMOR

HAROLD V. GASKILL III, M.D.
J. BRADLEY AUST, M.D., PH.D.

Lesions of the skin, both benign and malignant, are common. Although most surgical texts review a wide variety of pathologic entities, the clinical approach to skin lesions is straightforward. The surgeon has three primary objectives: (1) establish a diagnosis, (2) eradicate the lesion, and (3) preserve function and cosmesis.

ESTABLISHING THE DIAGNOSIS

With experience, one can diagnose many skin tumors with reasonable certainty based on their clinical presentation and gross appearance. This does not in any way lessen the importance of objective histologic examination of the tissue by a pathologist. In almost all instances, then, evaluation of skin tumors begins with a biopsy.

Excisional Biopsy

Lesions confined to the dermis and having a diameter of less than 1 cm are ideally managed by excisional biopsy. This should be performed on an outpatient basis under local anesthesia. Prior to commencement of the procedure, an appropriate container for the specimen, properly labeled and filled with fixative, should be prepared. The area is then scrubbed and draped. Xylocaine, 1% or 2%, should be infiltrated into the surrounding tissue with a 26-gauge or smaller needle. Epinephrine, 1%, may be included for hemostasis if desired (except on the fingers!). Direct infiltration of the lesion proper disrupts the histologic architecture and should be avoided. An elliptical incision is then created with the long axis parallel to natural skin creases in the area. Dissection should be limited to the subdermal plane. Although traction on the tissue with fine-toothed forceps aids dissection, care must be taken not to crush or fragment the specimen. Extension of the dissection to or through fascial boundaries is contraindicated. On removal, the specimen is immediately dropped into fixative before it can be lost or damaged. Closure of the wound is accomplished with two to four

inverted dermal sutures of 3–0 or 4–0 synthetic absorbable material. Final approximation of the wound edges is achieved with sterile wound strips or a running subcuticular suture of 4–0 or 5–0 synthetic absorbable material. Alternatively, in areas where cosmesis is not a primary concern, the wound may be closed with simple sutures of monofilament material.

Incisional Biopsy

For larger lesions, especially those that may be malignant, histologic diagnosis is best established by incisional biopsy. The basic principles of incisional biopsy are similar to those of excisional biopsy (already discussed). Several important differences should be noted. First, the incision should be designed as an ellipse encompassing both normal and abnormal tissue. Second, effort should be made to include any unusual areas of the lesion such as ulcerations or pigmentations. However, tissue from frankly necrotic areas is not likely to be helpful. Again, although a full-thickness section of the lesion is desirable, no attempt should be made to extend the dissection to or through fascial planes. Wound closure is accomplished with simple sutures of monofilament material. It is usually sufficient to close only the uninvolved skin as attempts to suture tumor tissue frequently result in fragmentation and bleeding.

Punch Biopsy

Punch biopsy is well suited for diffuse, superficial lesions as well as for very small lesions. Disposable, presharpened punch biopsy instruments are readily available and extremely convenient. Anesthesia is provided by injection with a small amount of Xylocaine, and a full-thickness punch biopsy, usually 3 to 6 mm in diameter, is obtained. By applying gentle traction, the punched tissue can be snipped off below the dermis with fine scissors. Closure is effected with a single simple suture of monofilament material. For smaller punch biopsies, no closure at all is necessary.

Tissue submitted to the pathologist should be accompanied by a brief history including the patient's age and sex as well as a description of how long the lesion has been present and its exact location on the body.

Information about systemic diseases, occupational exposure, and previous biopsies may also prove helpful.

CYSTS

Sebaceous Cysts

These lesions are common on the face, back, and other areas where sebaceous glands are found. They occur when the duct becomes obstructed and the production of sebum continues without drainage. Small lesions can be recognized by identifying the obstructed duct near the apex of the mass. Although excision is curative, care must be taken to ensure removal of the entire cyst wall and duct without rupture of the cyst. If the lesion is excised without rupture, the skin may be closed primarily. If rupture of the cyst has occurred, the wound should be left open or drained with a knotted rubber-band drain. Recurrence requiring re-excision may result. Large cysts should be reduced in size prior to excision. This may be accomplished in some cases by injection of steroids into the lesion every week for several weeks. Alternatively, the cyst may be opened with a circular incision and allowed to drain and involute. Often, patients present with a large cyst that has beome secondarily infected. In such cases, the lesion must be opened and drained and the infection allowed to resolve. Given sufficient time, most large lesions can be reduced in size substantially. They may then be excised and the skin closed primarily.

Epidermal Inclusion Cysts

These cysts result when squamous epithelium becomes lodged beneath the dermis, usually as a result of trauma. As the tissue attempts to mature and desquamate, it creates a cyst filled with cornified epithelium. Unlike the sebaceous cyst, these lesions do not necessarily connect with the surface. Simple excision is curative. Again, care must be taken not to rupture the cyst during dissection if recurrence is to be avoided.

Dermoid Cysts

The dermoid cyst (branchial cleft cyst, congenital keratinous cyst) is a congenital variant of the epidermal inclusion cyst already described. It may also contain epidermal appendages such as sebaceous glands and hair follicles. Any cyst appearing near the head, neck, or dorsal midline in a child or young adult should be assumed to be a dermoid cyst until proved otherwise. Since these lesions may communicate with the aerodigestive tract or the central nervous system, appropriate preoperative studies should be obtained. The surgeon should be prepared to totally excise the cyst, including any associated tracts or sinuses. Failure to recognize and appropriately treat a dermoid cyst results uniformly in recurrence.

PIGMENTED LESIONS (NEVI)

Intradermal Nevus

The intradermal nevus is the most common pigmented lesion of adults. It has no malignant potential. Excisional biopsy is indicated only to rule out malignancy. No further treatment is required.

Junctional Nevus

Compared to the intradermal nevus, the junctional nevus is more irregular in shape, color, and texture. Unlike the intradermal nevus it may occur on the palms, soles, and genitalia. Since this lesion may undergo malignant degeneration, excisional biopsy is indicated. Further treatment is not required. The *compound nevus* contains both intradermal and junctional elements. It is treated as a junctional nevus.

Giant Pigmented Nevus

The giant pigmented nevus (giant hairy nevus, bathing trunk nevus) is so called because of its characteristic clinical appearance. Although this lesion resembles the intradermal nevus histologically, it has a strong tendency to undergo malignant degeneration. Since they are usually too large to excise primarily, frequent follow-up and biopsy of any unusual areas is indicated.

Juvenile Melanoma

The juvenile melanoma is a pigmented lesion that appears prior to puberty and is histologically identical to the malignant melanoma. It is essential that the juvenile melanoma be recognized as a benign lesion. Excisional biopsy is curative. More aggressive treatment is not indicated.

KERATOSES

Seborrheic Keratosis

The seborrheic keratosis (basal cell papilloma, verruca senilis) is a raised, waxy-appearing lesion found commonly on the face and trunk of older adults. Although these lesions have no malignant potential, they may mimic basal cell carcinoma or even melanoma. Excisional biopsy is clearly indicated in such cases. Other lesions may be cosmetically objectionable or become irritated by undergarments, jewelry, or eyeglasses. These may be treated initially by curettage with histologic examination of the tissue. Once the diagnosis has been established, seborrheic keratosis responds well to cryotherapy with liquid nitrogen. Multiple lesions are ideally managed by this method.

Actinic Keratosis

The actinic keratosis (solar keratosis, senile keratosis, farmer's or sailor's disease) is associated with chronic exposure to the sun. It is usually seen on the forehead, ears, nose, and hands. Involvement of large areas is common. The diagnosis is easily established by punch biopsy. Treatment is essential since these lesions may degenerate to squamous cell carcinoma. Topical therapy with 5% 5-fluorouracil cream twice each day for 2 to 3 weeks is usually effective. With adequate treatment, a severe inflammatory reaction with moist desquamation is produced. Subclinical lesions may also become evident. The skin is extremely sensitive during this period, and additional sun exposure is prohibited. After the reaction has resolved the patient should be advised to avoid the sun as much as possible or to use a therapeutic sunscreen lotion. These patients should be followed closely for recurrent lesions.

Keratoacanthoma

The keratoacanthoma (molluscum sebaceum, molluscum pseudocarcinomatosum) is a benign tumor of the hair follicle. The classic lesion is volcano-shaped with a keratotic plug at the apex. It is often confused clinically *and histologically* with squamous cell carcinoma. The diagnosis is most often confirmed by histologic examination of an entire excisional biopsy specimen in cross section. Although some lesions undergo spontaneous regression, excision is curative.

KELOIDS

Keloids are masses of dense fibrous tissue that form at sites of injury. They are distinctly more common in young black patients and tend to occur on the head, neck, and upper body. Unfortunately, simple excision frequently results in recurrence. Small lesions are best treated by steroid injection. For larger lesions, excision may be the only alternative. Both low-dose radiation (less than 500 rads) and coverage with skin grafts have been advocated after excision of recurrent lesions. Since the tendency to form keloids diminishes with age, repeated excisions should be delayed as long as possible.

BASAL CELL CARCINOMA

Basal cell carcinoma is the most common malignant tumor of the skin and accounts for half of all skin cancers. It occurs most often on sebaceous areas exposed to sunlight, trauma, or chemicals. Accordingly, almost 90 percent appear at the hair margin, on the forehead, or near the nose. Small lesions are treated by excisional biopsy and plastic closure. Treatment of larger lesions is more difficult. Because they are frequently located on the face, surgical excision must be carefully planned. Once the specimen has been removed, it should be carefully marked and its exact orientation in the wound recorded. Although rotation flaps provide a superior cosmetic result, they may obscure local recurrence. Accordingly, many surgeons prefer coverage with a thin split-thickness skin graft and delayed reconstruction. If the pathologist cannot confirm that the margins are free of tumor, the area in question should be re-exised and submitted for further study. An alternative to conventional excision is microscopically controlled surgery (Moh's surgery, chemosurgery). In practice, the tissue is fixed in situ and a dish-shaped specimen is excised and its orientation in the wound carefully marked. The entire convex surface of the specimen is immediately examined, and all areas where tumor is present are identified. Each positive margin is then fixed in situ, re-excised, and immediately examined. This sequence is continued until the tumor has been eradicated. The wound may then be left to heal by second intention with delayed reconstruction if necessary. Since this technique was first reported, many physicians have learned how to use it efficiently and effectively. Cure rates approach 95 percent. Although most basal cell carcinomas can be cured by simple excision, recurrent lesions, lesions near the orbit or facial nerve, and morphea-type lesions are ideally treated by microscopically controlled surgery. Basal cell carcinoma also responds to radiotherapy. In each particular case the decision to use excisional treatment versus radiotherapy may be debated depending on the location, the number of lesions, the character of the surrounding skin, and the patient's preference.

SQUAMOUS CELL CARCINOMA

Squamous cell carcinoma comprises approximately 25 percent of all skin cancers. It is strongly associated with solar exposure, ionizing radiation, and chronic irritation. Like the basal cell carcinoma, it is commonly found on the head, neck, and upper extremities. The squamous cell carcinoma differs in that it tends to grow more rapidly with involvement of deeper layers and eventual metastasis to regional lymph nodes. Clinically, the lesion is more likely to demonstrate ulceration, satellitosis, and inflammation. The diagnosis is readily confirmed by biopsy, as already described. For both small and large lesions, the preferred treatment is surgical excision with adequate margins. Again, microscopically controlled surgery may be recommended for selected lesions. Squamous cell carcinoma also responds to radiation therapy. This modality is most often employed as an adjunct to surgical excision or for lesions that are not amenable to excision. Both intravenous and intra-arterial combination chemotherapy have been recommended for treatment of unresectable or recurrent tumors. Again, chemotherapy also may be used in combination with radiation and surgical excision. Although both topical chemotherapy with 5-fluorouracil and cryotherapy with liquid nitrogen have been advocated, they are still considered experimental. At best, they are effective only for superficial lesions. Most squamous cell carcinomas require surgical excision with histologic confirmation of clear margins.

DERMATOFIBROSARCOMA PROTUBERANS

Dermatofibrosarcoma protuberans is uncommon, comprising about 1 percent of skin cancers. It most often appears after the age of 40 as a slow-growing, protuberant lesion appearing anywhere on the body except the palms and soles. Because it is usually asymptomatic, patients may present with lesions that have ulcerated or become quite large. Satellitosis is common. Incisional biopsy reveals fibroblasts or spindle cells in a characteristic cartwheel appearance. Treatment consists of complete excision of the lesion, including an adequate margin of surrounding tissue. A more limited excision frequently results in recurrence.

PRESACRAL TUMOR AND CYSTS

CHARLES O. FINNE III, M.D.

Lesions of the presacral space are rare and have a small but significant malignant potential. Involvement of the sacrum and the peripheral and central nervous systems is frequent enough to require considerable caution in the surgical approach to the lesions. A simple three-category clinical classification is presented in this chapter to help the surgeon avoid serious mistakes in the management of these lesions. Such a classification does not replace a thorough understanding of the pathology of these lesions; rather, it encourages a systematic evaluation that can often predict the correct pathology and avoid encountering unsuspected associated disease. Proper assessment, not biopsy, should be the first step in the treatment of these lesions.

INCIDENCE

Presacral lesions are so unusual that accurate incidence figures are unavailable. An average of one or two sacrococcygeal teratomas per year are seen in children's hospitals such as at Harvard and the University

KAPOSI'S SARCOMA

Kaposi's sarcoma has recently gained notoriety as a common manifestation of the acquired immune deficiency syndrome (AIDS). Although this lesion is still rare, its incidence is 100 times greater in AIDS patients than in the general population. It appears most often as multiple reddish-blue nodules involving the arms and legs. The diagnosis is established by excisional biopsy. Since AIDS is probably caused by a transmissable agent, special precautions are indicated during any surgical procedure. Anesthesia and operating room personnel should be informed in advance when the diagnosis of AIDS is being considered. Double gloving is advised for all members of the operative team. Knives, needles, and all other sharp instruments should be handled with particular care. The specimen container should be clearly marked so that other operating room and pathology personnel can take similar precautions. After the diagnosis has been established, combination chemotherapy is the treatment of choice. Radiation therapy may also be effective.

of Pittsburgh. Ulig and Johnson (1975) were able to find only 60 such adult cases over a 30-year period in the Portland metropolitan area. The Mayo clinic has estimated that a presacral lesion occurs once in 40,000 admissions to its facility and is seen once in every 7,000 proctoscopic examinations. Gardiner (1968) estimated four retrorectal tumors in 2,500 barium enemas.

A rare inherited form of presacral cyst has been reported: 26 teratomas were found in 106 members of six families.

DEFINITIONS

The presacral (or retrorectal) space is really a potential space that normally contains mesenchymal tissue. It is bounded superiorly by the peritoneal reflection of the rectrum, inferiorly by the levator ani muscle group, and laterally by the iliac vessels and ureters. The rectal wall and sacrum mark the anterior and posterior boundaries.

PATHOLOGY

Although congenital lesions predominate as the most common lesions, the presacral space is a virtual Pandora's box of pathologic findings. Over 40 distinct lesions have been described in this region, reflecting its complicated embryonic development. The presacral space, which in the adult contains mostly nerves and blood vessels, develops from the primitive streak in the embryo, a region containing so-called "totipotential cells," intimately related to the formation of the three germ cell layers, thus accounting for the wide variety of germ-cell-derived pathology seen in this area (Fig. 1).

The differential diagnosis of presacral lesions is presented in Table 1. In general, age at diagnosis and solid or cystic character are important prognostic factors. Although this chapter is concerned mainly with the non-pediatric age group, it is worthwhile noting that presacral lesions diagnosed in the neonatal period carry approximately a 4 percent malignancy rate, whereas those diagnosed in the postnatal and pediatric period are 95 percent malignant with a grave prognosis. In the adult, cystic lesions carry a 10 percent malignancy rate, whereas the malignancy rate for solid lesions approaches 60 percent.

TYPES OF LESION

Congenital Lesions

The congenital lesions account for slightly more than half of all presacral tumors, and two-thirds of these are developmental cysts. A postanal dimple occurs in association with some of the congenital cysts and may be a clue to the diagnosis. The congenital cysts are important because they occasionally become infected, they can be confused with supralevator abscess and fistula in ano, and they occasionally become malignant. Their presentation is sometimes bizarre, as when hair protrudes from the rectum after the cyst has ruptured into the rectum, giving the appearance of a rectal wall sinus with protruding hair. In other cases, the cyst wall may have everted, becoming a pseudo-rectal wall with a patch of different epithelium that has hair growing out of it.

The cysts and teratomas are attached to the coccyx and derive their blood supply from the middle sacral vessels. One pediatric series reported a 37 percent recurrence rate when the coccyx was not removed at the time of cystectomy. The incidence of malignant degeneration in adult teratomas is significant, about 30 percent. Teratomas have a definite female predilection, occurring in a female:male ratio of 3:1.

Duplications of the rectum are rare, even among large series at children's hospitals. They present as cystic lesions and must be differentiated from teratomas.

Congenital bony abnormalities of the sacrum and coccyx are frequently associated with the congenital lesions, and teratomas may occur in association with anterior sacral meningocele. Familial inherited forms of presacral cysts are especially likely to have a sacral deformity.

Chordomas are serious lesions arising from fetal notochordal remnants in the sacrum. Their benign physical characteristics (smooth, soft, cystic lobulation) belie their aggressive local behavior with invasion of soft tissue and bone. Though some pathologists classify benign and malignant varieties on the basis of metastasis occurring in 10 percent of cases, this distinction is artificial and does not connote the seriousness of nonmetastasizing lesions. A review of the world's literature reveals only a 4 percent cure rate out of almost 300 reported patients, with 9 percent surviving longer than 10 years. The average

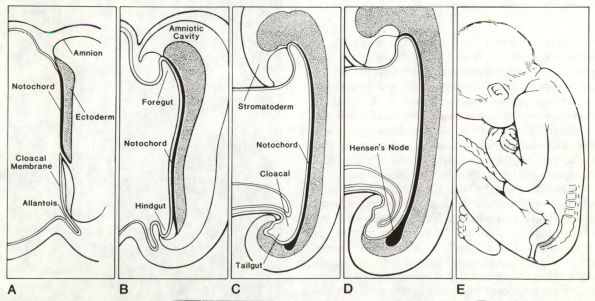

Figure 1 Embryologic development of the presacral space. The area surrounding the primitive pit and Hensen's node comes to lie in the presacral and coccygeal area in the fully developed human (stippled area). In the early embryo, this important area contains the so-called totipotential cells, which dedifferentiate into the three germ cell layers. Germ cell lesions are relatively common in this area and probably result from stimulation of rests of these embryonic cells. It is easy to understand how cysts or duplications might form by pinching off a fragment of the hindgut.

TABLE 1   Differential Diagnosis of Presacral Lesions

Congenital lesions
    Developmental cysts (epidermoid, dermoid,
      enteric, teratoma)
    Chordoma
    Teratocarcinoma
    Adrenal rest tumor
    Anterior sacral meningocele
    Duplication of rectum
Inflammatory lesions
    Foreign body granuloma
    Perineal abscess
    Internal fistula
    Pelvirectal abscess
    Chronic infectious granuloma
Neurogenic lesions
    Neurofibroma and sarcoma
    Neurilemoma
    Ependymoma
    Ganglioneuroma
Osseous lesions
    Osteoma
    Osteogenic sarcoma
    Simple bone cyst of sacrum
    Ewing's tumor
    Chondromyxosarcoma
    Aneurysmal bone cyst
    Giant cell tumor of bone
Miscellaneous lesions
    Metastatic carcinoma
    Lipoma and liposarcoma
    Endothelioma and hemangioendotheliosarcoma
    Lymphangioma
    Extra-abdominal desmoid
    Plasma cell myeloma
    Fibroma and fibrosarcoma
    Leiomyoma and leiomyosarcoma
    Pericytoma
    Hemangioma
    Malignant tumor, indeterminate type

Data from Ulig, Johnston.

patient survives 5 years from the time of diagnosis, but even the long-term survivors usually die as the result of recurrent chordoma. Chordoma is one of the few tumors known to implant from operative spillage and along biopsy tracts, and preoperative biopsy, if done at all, should be done in such a way as to allow resection of the biopsy site with definitive operation. Because these lesions arise in bone, they require sacral resection as part of their treatment and may be diagnosed with the aid of plain films, tomography, and computed tomography. Most series report significant benefit from palliative and debulking resection in symptomatic patients. Radiation therapy, when pushed to toxic limits with special techniques (6,000 rads for palliation; 8,000 to 12,000 rads for control) can be of significant benefit, and can occasionally ''cure'' patients. In four small recently reported series of patients, radical en bloc resection was performed, and an approximate 50 percent ''cure'' rate can be expected. En bloc resection is the only technique that has resulted in permanent cure.

Anterior sacral meningocele is extremely rare, with fewer than 150 cases reported in the world's literature. Untreated, there is a significant fatality rate from rupture or infection complicating delivery or surgical misadventure with the unsuspected lesion. Approximately 10 to 20 percent of these patients have associated teratomas and cysts that may distract the unwary from the correct diagnosis and lead to disaster when transrectal biopsy or surgery is performed. Characteristic sacral bone deformity (scimitar sacrum) is the rule and usually is diagnostic of this lesion (Fig. 2). Ligation of the dural sac at operation is imperative to avoid recurrence and to prevent meningitis. These meningoceles rarely have neural elements within them, patients usually do not have neurologic deficits, and hydrocephalus is rare.

Inflammatory Lesions

The inflammatory lesions, as grouped in Table 1, ignore the infected congenital lesion. Most inflammatory lesions are secondary to other disease such as diverticulitis or Crohn's disease. The barium granuloma is uncommon and may well be clinically silent, but should be obvious on the plain film. The old granuloma usually presents as a submucosal lesion, and this may ulcerate and bleed and be confused with carcinoma. Biopsy, therefore, is always indicated for lesions accessible to the proctoscope.

Foreign body granuloma, fungal infections, intestinal

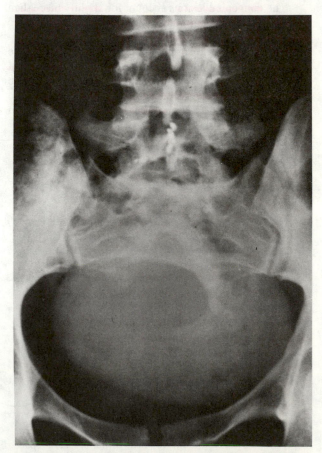

Figure 2   The ''scimitar sacrum'' deformity. This finding on plain film is virtually diagnostic of anterior sacral meningocele. The apparent soft tissue mass is the meningocele sac filled with dilute metrizamide at myelography.

tuberculosis, and Crohn's disease should be readily diagnosed if the evaluation and history are complete and thorough.

Neurogenic Tumors

The neurogenic tumors are standard peripheral nerve tumors that require standard treatment. They are not associated with von Recklinghausen's disease. Since ganglioneuromas tend to occur in children and young adults, a solid lesion in this age group is highly suggestive of ganglioneuroma. As a group, the neurogenic tumors have a particularly favorable prognosis.

Bony Lesions

Primary osseous tumors span the spectrum of bone tumors. The prognosis of these lesions is the same as that associated with bone tumors elsewhere: osteogenic sarcomas tend to be rapidly lethal, being discovered at an unresectable stage, and the prognosis of benign bone tumors depends on the location and amount of neurologic damage required for their removal.

Miscellaneous Group

The most common lesion in this group is metastatic tumor. All of the others are found scattered throughout most series in small numbers and except for leiomyoma, do not have any remarkable characteristics.

Leiomyoma of the rectum is somewhat different from the garden variety of leiomyoma because there is a 30 percent recurrence rate, and because histologically benign lesions have produced metastasis. To make matters more confusing, many benign-appearing lesions, when they recur, do so as obvious sarcomas. The only distinguishing characteristic of malignancy is size: a diameter of less than 5 cm is not associated with recurrence. After resection of a suspected benign lesion, recurrence tends to be late, the majority occurring between 4 and 8 years after the original resection. Careful follow-up is necessary for long periods after resection of the large leiomyoma.

SYMPTOMS

The presentation of these tumors may be varied and is often unremarkable. One frequent symptom is pain, which is poorly localized to the base of the spine and may radiate to the buttocks or legs. It may be exaggerated by sitting and relieved by changing position. The pain is often thought to be low back strain because many patients date the onset of symptoms to an episode of minor trauma such as slipping on ice or falling on stairs.

Headache with straining, defecation, or intercourse may be a clue to anterior sacral meningocele. Refractory meningitis or the presence of enteric pathogens in the spinal fluid after delivery or pelvic or rectal surgery is an all too frequent presentation of sacral meningocele.

All of the cystic lesions may be complicated by infection presenting as an abscess or recurring fistula and may easily be confused with primary rectal or pelvic disease. Failure to cure fistula in ano may lead to the diagnosis of a presacral cyst at fistulography.

Pelvic outlet obstruction causing difficult delivery or requiring cesarean section is not uncommon.

Rectal obstruction or a feeling of unsatisfied defecation may result from tumor impingement on the rectum and levators. Mechanical or neurologic interference with sphincter function may produce incontinence in rare instances.

Urinary symptoms may range from frequency due to mechanical interference with bladder filling to overflow incontinence from neurologic damage.

CLINICAL CLASSIFICATION

Although many of these lesions are straightforward, it is useful to classify them according to the following scheme: (1) both bony and central nervous system involvement, (2) bony without CNS involvement, and (3) pure soft tissue lesion. Clinical judgment determines how extensive a work-up should be, but if a lesion cannot be classified, the work-up is likely to be incomplete. With bony or CNS involvement, neurosurgical participation to identify and preserve the sacral nerves is imperative, and operative planning should be a collaborative effort between specialties.

PREOPERATIVE WORK-UP

The clinical investigation of these lesions should proceed in an orderly manner from the simple to the complex, either omitting biopsy or undertaking it as the last procedure. An adequate work-up, in the majority of cases, makes biopsy unnecessary, except as a prelude or guide to palliative therapy. Examination under anesthesia may sometimes be necessary. Infected cysts need little work-up other than physical examination (Fig. 3), but judgment and caution are necessary to avoid pitfalls in this complex set of lesions. *The guiding principle of work-up should be that too much information might be enough.*

Plain roentgenograms can reveal characteristic or diagnostic congenital bony deformity; bony destruction that may be characteristic of chordoma, primary bone tumor, or metastasis; calcified markers such as bones or teeth typical of teratomas; or foreign body.

Because the presacral space is surrounded by hollow organs (blood vessels, ureters, rectum, spinal canal) and bone, it is an ideal region for contrast studies. Such studies can show the extent of disease, secondary involvement (hydronephrosis, neurogenic bladder), and the presence of primary or secondary bowel disease (diverticulitis, Crohn's disease, fistulas, obstruction). Fistulagrams may be the first clue to an unsuspected presacral cyst. Myelog-

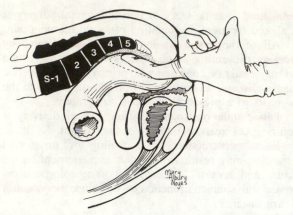

Figure 3 Digital examination of the presacral space. Digital examination is the most useful maneuver to detect abnormalities in the presacral area. The ability to palpate most of a mass from below suggests that a mass can successfully be resected via a posterior approach, since this corresponds roughly to the S4 sacral segment.

raphy has great utility in confirming or denying CNS involvement, although meningoceles with necks too small to permit the passage of dye have been described. Myelography also can be useful in determining operability of sacral lesions, those involving disc spaces about L5-S1 being inoperable by any technique. Computed tomography should always be done; it permits precise determination of cystic or solid nature, loculated cystic structure, and involvement of ureter, bone, and the spinal canal. It does not replace the use of plain films and the contrast enema, however, and should be used in addition to the other modalities. Ultrasound, because of the depth of the pelvis and proximity of bone, has limited application in this region, and computed tomography is far preferable. Arteriography may show diagnostic vascular patterns and delineate the blood supply of a given tumor.

There are times when biopsy may be appropriate as part of the work-up. When deemed necessary for chordoma, because of implantation, a technique allowing resection of the biopsy site should be chosen. Transrectal needle biopsy is remarkably safe for solid lesions and is particularly applicable for suspected metastatic lesions. Because of the risk of infection in cystic lesions, biopsy other than total excision is probably not indicated. Transperineal needle biopsy is another option and should be used if appropriate.

SURGICAL APPROACHES

All surgery in the presacral space should be accompanied by complete mechanical and antibiotic bowel preparation and systemic antibiotic prophylaxis as with any colon surgery. The risk of bowel injury is real, bone is sometimes exposed, and on occasion the dural sac is opened. Palpation of the tumor mass through the rectum can be a practical aid at surgery and, when coupled with the use of topical antibiotics or antiseptics in the irrigating solutions, should not result in significant contamination.

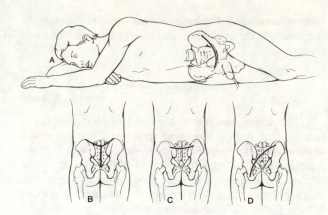

Figure 4 Incisions for operation in the presacral space. When simultaneous anterior and posterior access is desired, the right lateral position allows the mobilized sigmoid and rectum to fall away from the operative field. Alternatively, the posterior portion may be done first with the patient in the prone position, and the abdominal portion completed at a later time with the patient supine; in other cases the sequence might be reversed.

In general, the location, size, and classification of the tumor dictate the surgical approach to individual lesions (Fig. 4). The four basic approaches are pure abdominal, combined abdominosacral (either synchronous or sequential), pure posterior or sacral, and transrectal. Sphincter-dividing procedures (Schuchardt and York-Mason) have been advocated by some, but may be hazardous to function and are unnecessary. Delineation of neuroanatomy requires a posterior approach and laminectomy (Fig. 5), whereas the abdominal approach offers control of the blood supply and a better assessment of tumor for lesions extending about the S4 level. In general, lesions that can be encircled with the examining finger by rectal examination at surgery can be safely approached from below, although larger lesions with significant sacral deformity may permit more extensive surgery from the pure posterior approach. If one can palpate one-half of the tumor or less on rectal examination, an abdominal approach is required for adequate control of the blood supply, but this may have to be combined with the posterior approach for removal of coccyx or bone.

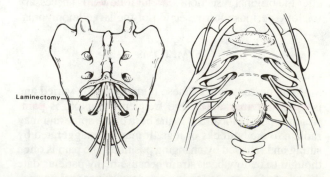

Figure 5 Posterior sacral laminectomy. Laminectomy is required to properly identify the anterior sacral nerve roots which penetrate through the sacrum and are not accessible anteriorly. The S3 roots are so important to sphincter function that unwitting bilateral sacrifice renders the patient incontinent.

Lesions with CNS and Bony Involvement

Lesions involving CNS and bone require laminectomy via a posterior approach to identify nerve roots since it is impossible to properly identify them from an anterior approach. A discourse on sacral resection is beyond the scope of this chapter, but some general observations are in order. Bilateral resection of S2 and distal nerve roots can be tolerated with intermittent bladder catheterization and bowel training programs, but this leaves a significant functional deficit. Preservation of one S3 nerve results in considerably better function, and when both are preserved, essentially normal sensation and function result. Unilateral sacrifice of S1 through S5 results in hemisensory loss and occasionally some leg dysfunction, but crossover motor innervation results in normal bowel and bladder sphincter function. Spinal stability is maintained with preservation of S1 vertebral body and its lumbosacral attachments. Integrity of the dural sac to spinal fluid must be assiduously preserved. Such extensive resections are best done through a combined approach with the patient in a right lateral position. The anterior operator controls blood supply, protects the iliac vessels, and delimits the extent of sacral resection to the posterior operator, who has the nerves identified and preserved and cuts through the sacrum. Smaller lesions from S4 and below do not have identifiable neurologic dysfunction and, because the sacral hiatus is a reliable landmark, may be resected by a pure posterior approach.

Occasionally certain meningoceles with a small high sac may be approached from the abdomen, if care is taken to ligate the dural connection at the sacral defect.

Closed suction drains are highly advisable in this situation to protect against lymphatic and unsuspected spinal fluid leaks. Occasionally, prolonged drainage may ensue (200 to 500 cc per 24 hours), and the suction drain should be left in place until the flow decreases to 30 to 40 cc per 24 hours.

Lesions with Bony but No CNS Involvement

Lesions involving bone may be of two types: (1) congenital lesions with deformity, and (2) those with bone destruction due to invasion or compression. For the most part, deformity implies only the need for coccygeal resection as part of the definitive procedure. The size and upper extent of the lesion determines whether supplemental abdominal access will be required (already discussed).

The requirements for sacral resection are the same as for the resection already discussed, but significant sacral resection (above the sacral hiatus or S4 level) will require laminectomy and precise attention to dural control and nerve sacrifice.

Lesions of Soft Tissue Only

This group constitutes the vast majority of the tumors encountered. A rule of thumb can be applied: these tumors can be safely approached from below if at least half of the lesion can be palpated with the index finger on rectal examination. The sacral hiatus is a reliable, palpable landmark at surgery, allowing safe sacral resection below this level for accessibility to the presacral space. For smaller tumors and cysts, coccygeal resection allows access and is a required part of the procedure. Lesions less than 4 cm in diameter are easily approached through a straight transverse incision centered over the coccyx. If a larger incision is required, this may be enlarged cephalad or caudad with a second incision at right angles to the first (final shape of a T). The anococcygeal ligament is divided as the first step in access to the presacral space. Once the space is entered, the levator and anal sphincter musculature are pushed inferiorly, allowing one to stay away from the neurovascular bundles to the sphincter. The lateral soft tissue attachments to the coccyx are then divided, and the coccyx separated from the sacrum. Often this dissection is aided by a finger in the rectum after division of the coccyx, which allows elevation of the cyst or tumor out of the presacral space up into the operative field. The anterior and superior attachments of the tumor are then divided and the tumor removed en bloc with the bony specimen. Depending on the degree of hemostasis or contamination, a suction drain such as a Jackson-Pratt may be used and subsequently irrigated with an antibiotic solution.

MELANOMA

CHARLES M. BALCH, M.D., F.A.C.S.

The incidence of melanoma is increasing at a faster rate than almost any other cancer in man, but fortunately, most melanomas treated today are curable with appropriate surgical management. Surgery is the primary treatment for cutaneous melanomas, for regional node metastases, and, in selected patients, for palliation of isolated distant metastases. There is no single treatment approach, only surgical options to be selected for the individual patient, depending on the anatomic location of the melanoma, its growth pattern, and prognostic features of the tumor (especially tumor thickness and ulceration) that predict the risk of microscopic metastatic disease.

THE PRIMARY MELANOMA

Appropriate surgical excision consists of a wide excision of the primary melanoma or the biopsy site with a margin of normal-appearing skin. Until recently, cutaneous melanomas were removed with radical excisions employing a 5-cm margin of skin and a split-thickness skin graft. This recommendation originated from a single autopsy study of a recurrent melanoma reported by Sampson Handley in 1907. During the past decade, it has become evident that such radical excisions are unnecessary and that more conservative excisions can be safely employed. In my practice, the surgical margins are adjusted according to the measured tumor thickness since this factor correlates best with the risk for local recurrences (Table 1).

The earliest lesion is a melanoma in situ. Although the natural history of these noninvasive lesions is not completely understood, there is a risk of local recurrence (either as an in situ melanoma or an invasive melanoma) if they are not re-excised after biopsy. It is therefore recommended that the biopsy site of an in situ melanoma be excised, usually with a 0.5- to 1-cm margin of skin.

For thin melanomas (measuring less than 0.76 mm in thickness), there is only a minimal risk of local recurrence in all reported patient series. A wide excision consisting of a 2-cm minimal margin of skin is recommended. This can be performed as a generous elliptical incision and a primary skin closure (Fig. 1). In one study of 936 patients with melanomas less than 1.0 mm thick, there was not a single local recurrence, despite the fact that 61 percent of patients had conservative margins of excision (2 cm or less).

For intermediate and thick melanomas (i.e., those greater than 0.76 mm in thickness), a 3-cm margin is usually employed because of an increased risk of local

TABLE 1 Recommended Surgical Margins for Excising Cutaneous Melanomas*

Type	Margin (cm)
In situ lesions	1
Lentigo maligna melanomas	1
<0.76 mm thickness	2
>0.76 mm thickness	3

* Where anatomically feasible

recurrence and satellitosis. This risk may exceed 10 percent for melanomas over 4 mm in thickness, especially if they are ulcerated.

Lentigo meligna melanomas do not require a wide excision since they have a low risk for recurrence. They generally occur on the face and neck and can be safely excised with a 1-cm margin of excision. Other types of melanomas located on the hands, face, and feet generally do not lend themselves to a wide surgical excision because of their anatomic location. In these circumstances, the surgeon must use his best judgment to excise the lesion as widely as possible within the anatomic constraints of surrounding structures.

The underlying fascia is generally incorporated into the surgical resection, especially for thicker melanomas (i.e., greater than 1.0 mm). The rationale for incorporating the fascia is to interpose a barrier between the surgical boundary and the melanoma. However, a recent retrospective study showed no difference in results between patients who had a subfascial excision and those who did not.

The overall risk for local recurrence is extremely low, being around 3 percent of all patients. Patients at highest risk for local recurrence have tumors with one or more

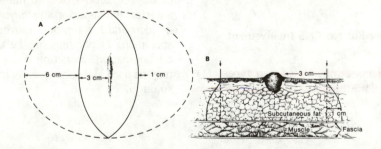

Figure 1 Technique of excising a primary melanoma with an elliptical excision and primary skin closure. *A*, The surgical margin consists of a 3-cm radius of normal-appearing skin surrounding the biopsy site or the lateral margin of the intact melanoma. The long axis of the incision should be three to four times the width of the incision. After the melanoma is excised, skin flaps are raised in a plane above the deep fascia for a sufficient distance to close the skin edges without undue tension. The most extensive area of mobilization is near the center of the flaps, and it often is necessary to mobilize the skin flaps for a distance twice that of the excised skin margin. Skin flaps can be closed primarily in two layers by approximating the subcutaneous tissues and deep dermis in one layer while the outer layer is approximated with either a standard suture material or subcuticular skin closure. It is often necessary to place a suction drain in the surgical wound. *B*, Cross-section of the excision site. A skin margin of 3 cm from the tumor is shown. Flaps of gradually increasing thickness are raised for an additional 1 cm to 2 cm to remove any surrounding subdermal lymphatics. Excising the fascia is optional. (From Urist MM et al. Surgical management of the primary melanoma. In: Balch CM, Milton GW, eds. Cutaneous Melanoma. Clinical Management and Treatment Results Worldwide. Philadelphia: J.B. Lippincott, 1985; 71–90. Used with permission.)

of the following features: (1) thickness of 4 mm or more (13% incidence), (2) ulceration (11%), or (3) location on the foot, hand, scalp, or face (5% to 12%).

Technique of Surgical Excision

A standard elliptical incision is most commonly employed to excise melanomas. With generous skin flaps, even large defects can be moblized for primary skin closure. To achieve adequate skin for closure, the long axis or length of the incision should be three to four times the width of the incision. After excision of the specimen and mobilization of the flaps, the incision is closed with interrupted subcutaneous sutures, and the skin approximated with either nylon sutures or a subcuticular closure with a suitable absorbable suture.

Another means of avoiding a skin graft for covering a defect is to use skin flaps. A rotational advancement flap is especially well suited for melanomas involving the face and neck, where the cosmetic result is more important than at other sites. I commonly use this approach for closing surgical defects that are not otherwise amenable to primary closure with an elliptical excision. An advancement flap also provides better padding over bony prominences (e.g., scapula) and a superior cosmetic effect compared to a skin graft.

For larger defects, a split-thickness skin graft may be required, except on the face, where small defects may be covered with a full-thickness graft using skin from behind the ear or the supraclavicular fossa. Donor skin is taken with a dermatome with a skin thickness usually at 0.014 inches (0.36 mm). The skin graft is usually taken from skin over the anterolateral thigh or the lateral shoulder (Fig. 2). It is important not to take donor skin from a site of potential intransit metastases, such as the ipsilateral thigh for a melanoma of the foot. In some cases, it may be necessary to mesh the graft to increase the amount of tissue it can cover. However, this results in a less suitable cosmetic appearance. A meshed graft may be preferable for covering a large defect on the back, especially over the scapula, since it is difficult to stabilize the graft in this area.

Special Sites

Fingers and Toes

A melanoma located on the skin of a distal digit or beneath the fingernail must be removed by a digital amputation. When such a biopsy-confirmed lesion is located on the fingers (especially the thumb), it is important to save as much of the digit as possible to maximize function. This depends on the extensiveness of the lesion (e.g., some have significant nailbed or paronychial involvement) and the location of its proximal border. In general, an amputation of a digit is performed proximal to the distal interphalangeal joint of the thumb

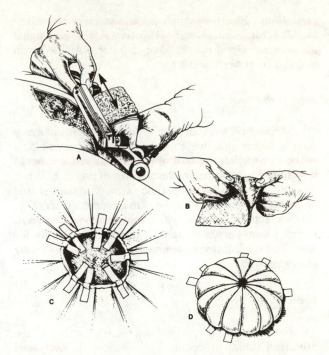

Figure 2 The Reese technique for skin grafting. *A*, The dermatome is applied to the skin and the blade moved sideways to split the skin (usually with a 0.14-inch thickness). It is sometimes helpful for the first assistant to apply two straight hemostats alongside the dermatome as the graft is being taken to enable a smoother edge. *B*, The tape is split to separate the two rubber backings. *C*, The skin graft and the flexible rubber backing is fashioned to the defect and then placed in the defect (skin side down). The edges of the rubber backing are then attached to the skin edges with Steri-strip. In some cases, it is necessary to partially close the defect with horizontal stent sutures of 3–0 silk. *D*, A standard stent bolus dressing is then applied to maximize donor skin apposition to the recipient site. For extremity lesions, a posterior mold splint is used to further immobilize the graft site. The Reese technique gives a better texture, color, and cosmetic appearance of the skin graft compared to a freehand-sewn technique. (From Urist MM et al. Surgical management of the primary melanoma. In: Balch CM, Milton GW, eds. Cutaneous Melanoma. Clinical Management and Treatment Results Worldwide. Philadelphia: J.B. Lippincott, 1985; 71–90. Used with permission.)

and at the middle interphalangeal joint for the fingers, as long as the lesions are small and confined to the nailbed. The excision should include a border of normal-appearing skin of at least 1 cm from the border of the tumor. This approach of partial amputation retains the maximal function of the digit and is especially important for the thumb. An amputation of the entire finger or thumb (as a ray amputation) is recommended for more extensive lesions, especially those with satellites.

For melanomas located on a toe, an amputation of the entire digit at the metatarsophalangeal joint is indicated, and this generally does not cause any significant morbidity. Subungual melanomas, especially those involving the toes, are more frequently associated with local recurrences, intransit metastases, and nodal metastases. Elective lymph node dissection is recommended for clinical stage I patients with subungual melanomas. Good results have also been obtained with isolated limb perfusion as well.

Sole of the Foot

Melanomas on the plantar surface often involve a sizable defect in a weight-bearing area. If possible, a portion of the heel or ball of the plantar surface should be retained to bear the greatest burden of pressure. When possible, the deep fascia over the extensor tendons should be preserved as a base for the skin coverage. Generally, these defects are covered with a split-thickness skin graft. Isolated limb perfusion may be of value, especially for large and thick lesions. Amputation of the foot is rarely indicated.

The Ear

For a small suspicious lesion of the helix, the preferred initial procedure for diagnosis is excisional biopsy followed by a wedge re-excision if the diagnosis of melanoma is confirmed. A partial amputation may be necessary for larger lesions. A total amputation of the ear is restricted to patients with widespread local disease or those with recurrence after partial amputation.

Female Breast

There is some controversy whether melanomas overlying the breast should be treated by a wide excision of the skin and subcutaneous tissue or by a total mastectomy. In our experience, such lesions could safely be treated as any other cutaneous melanoma, with skin margins determined by the tumor thickness and other criteria as described earlier.

REGIONAL NODE METASTASES

Regional lymph nodes are the most frequent site of metastasis. They may occur clinically as enlarged, firm lymph nodes or as microscopic metastases in lymph nodes that are clinically occult. These two settings require different types of clinical assessment and surgical judgment regarding lymph node management.

Clinically Enlarged Nodal Metastases

In patients with clinically evident lymph node metastases, the treatment approach consists of a radical lymphadenectomy involving the regional lymph node basin. A partial lymph node dissection or simple excision of nodal metastases is insufficient treatment for patients with metastatic melanoma. In two-thirds or more of these patients, metastatic disease is present in other lymph nodes. Since the surgeon's ability to detect nodal metastases by clinical criteria is not optimal, a philosophy of limited excision for only clinically detectable nodes often compromises both the palliative and the curative goals of surgical treatment.

In-continuity resection of the primary melanoma and radical lymph node dissection are performed together whenever feasible, rather than as two separate procedures. This approach incorporates the lymphatics between the primary melanoma site and the regional lymph nodes into the specimen to remove any in-transit disease trapped in major lymphatics or in regional lymph nodes at the periphery of the primary nodal basin. This is particularly important for trunk melanomas, but not exclusively so.

For patients with demonstrable inguinal node metastases, a combined dissection of the iliac and femoral lymph nodes is recommended. This is because 25 to 50 percent of patients with femoral node metastases have iliac nodal involvement as well. Excision of the obturator lymph nodes is important because they can also be involved with metastases. Suction catheters, antibiotics, and prophylactic measures (elastic stockings, diuretics, and leg raising) are recommended for 6 months postoperatively to minimize edema of the leg.

For patients with axillary node metastases, a complete axillary lymphadenectomy is important, including the level III lymph nodes medial to the pectoralis minor muscle. It is important to incorporate metastatic nodes that may be present at the perimeter of a traditional axillary node dissection. Lymph nodes that might be missed include those along the posterior axillary line, the lower chest wall, and the long thoracic nerve. Suction catheter drainage and antibiotics are recommended. Mobilization of the arm is not encouraged during the first 7 to 10 days after surgery. Gradually over the ensuing 4 weeks, mobilization of the arm is increased with active exercises. The complication rate for axillary lymph node dissection is low, the most frequent complication being a wound seroma.

Metastases to cervical lymph nodes require a radical neck dissection. A superficial parotidectomy may also be necessary, depending on the anatomic site of the primary melanoma. Melanomas that occur anterior to the pinna of the ear generally produce nodal metastases to the parotid, submandibular, submental, upper jugular, and posterior triangle (spinal accessory, transverse cervical) lymph nodes. Lesions that occur inferior to the lateral commissure of the lip usually spread to cervical lymph nodes rather than to parotid nodes. Melanomas that occur on the scalp posterior to the pinna of the ear usually spread to occipital, postauricular, posterior triangle, or jugular chain nodes. Parotid lymph node metastases may be extraglandular or intraglandular. The most common extraglandular metastases are located in the preauricular nodes and the nodes located about the tail of the parotid. Intraglandular nodes are within the substance of the parotid gland and are usually located superficial to the seventh cranial nerve. The parotid chain of nodes is contiguous with the cervical nodes, and for this reason, it is generally advisable to combine neck dissection with parotid lymph node dissection when parotid nodes are involved with metastatic melanoma.

The postoperative management of the patient who has undergone cervical or parotid lymphadenectomy consists of suction drainage and elevation of the head to minimize edema. Complications are infrequent, but may include seroma, skin slough, nerve dysfunction, or chylous leak from a thoracic duct fistula.

Clinically Normal Regional Lymph Nodes

Decisions regarding management of suspected microscopic (or occult) metastases in regional lymph nodes are more difficult. The central question in this decision revolves around the timing of the operation to excise regional lymph nodes. The surgeon has two options. First, he can perform an elective (immediate) lymph node dissection (ELND) to remove suspected microscopic or clinically occult metastatic tumor. The second option would be to defer this procedure until any nodal metastases have grown sufficiently large for clinical detection by palpation. A therapeutic (delayed) regional node dissection is then performed.

The efficacy of elective lymph node dissection for melanoma is still controversial. Since it is clear that all melanoma patients do not benefit from this procedure, the debate centers around whether a subgroup of patients can be identified with improved survival rates after elective lymphadenectomy compared to those whose initial management of the lymph nodes is observation only.

Elective lymphadenectomy thus has the major theoretic advantage of definitive treatment given at a relatively early stage in the natural history of nodal metastases, when the tumor burden is generally less than several million cells. It has the disadvantage that some patients may be subjected to an operation when they do not have metastases in the lymph nodes. Conversely, the advantage of delayed lymphadenectomy is that only patients with demonstrable metastases undergo a major operation. It has a disadvantage in that treatment is delayed until the metastases are clinically palpable, when the tumor burden is much greater (i.e., many billions of metastatic cells). As a consequence, the chances for cure are diminished. Thus, by the time regional nodal metastases can be detected clinically, 70 to 85 percent of patients have distant micrometastases from which they will eventually die.

Since the cure rate for delayed lymph node dissection is so poor (i.e., 25% survival at 10 years), I advocate immediate excision of the regional lymph nodes in *selected* patients to remove nodal micrometastases before they can disseminate. In this setting, the surgical decisions depend on knowing which prognostic factors can reliably identify those patients at risk for occult metastatic disease.

The measured tumor thickness of the melanoma provides a quantitative estimate of the risk for occult metastatic melanoma at regional and distant sites (Table 2). In fact, melanoma thickness is the most important guide, but not the sole guide, for selecting patients who

TABLE 2 Estimated Risks of Regional and Distant Micrometastases in Clinical Stage I Melanoma Patients

Location of the Primary Melanoma	Risk of Occult Regional Metastases Only*	Risk of Occult Distant Metastases* (± Regional Metastases)
Female extremity		
<0.76 mm	2%	1%
0.76 mm–1.49 mm	5%–7%	7%–10%
1.50 mm–3.99 mm	7%–19%	10%–24%
≥4.00 mm	0%	48%
Male extremity		
<0.76 mm	2%	2%
0.76 mm–1.49 mm	22%–24%	22%–24%
1.50 mm–3.99 mm	24%–29%	24%–34%
≥4.00 mm	0%	70%
Female axial		
<0.76 mm	8%	10%
0.76 mm–1.49 mm	14%–17%	21%–29%
1.50 mm–3.99 mm	17%–21%	29%–41%
≥4.00 mm	0%	60%
Male axial		
<0.76 mm	9%	14%
0.76 mm–1.49 mm	27%–28%	29%–32%
1.50 mm–3.99 mm	28%–30%	32%–45%
≥4.00 mm	0%	79%

* Estimated risk for microscopic metastases at the time of initial diagnosis in patients with clinically localized cutaneous melanoma based on a mathematical model that did include ulceration as a factor.

might benefit from ELND. The major advantage of using tumor thickness for these surgical decisions is that they can provide a quantitative estimate of the risk for occult metastatic melanoma in both regional and distant sites. Thus, *thin melanomas* (less than 0.76 mm) are associated with localized disease and with a 95 percent or greater 10-year survival rate. An ELND would provide no therapeutic benefit in such patients. *Intermediate thickness melanomas* (0.76 mm to 4.0 mm) have an increasing risk (up to 60%) of harboring occult regional metastases, but a relatively low risk (less than 20%) of distant metastases. Patients with these lesions might therefore benefit from an ELND. *Thick melanomas* (greater than 4.0 mm) not only have a high risk of regional node micrometastases (greater than 60%), but they also are associated with a high risk (greater than 70%) of occult distant metastases at the time of initial presentation. These patients often fare poorly, since the distant metastases in most instances would negate the curative potential of surgically excising micrometastases in the regional lymph nodes.

The anatomic site of the melanoma is also an important criterion in predicting the risk for regional node micrometastases. Patients with extremity melanomas have a more favorable outlook, whereas those with melanomas on the trunk or head and neck area have a higher risk of microscopic metastatic disease, even with equivalent tumor thicknesses. Extremity melanomas in women have the lowest biological potential for metastatic melanoma compared to lesions of equivalent thickness on the extremities of men (Table 2), whereas patients with melanomas located on the trunk or head and neck areas fare worse, regardless of sex. Finally, ulcerative melanomas are at higher risk for microscopic metastases than their nonulcerated counterparts, even when matched for other prognostic indicators such as tumor thickness. The growth pattern is also an important consideration in this decison-making process. Since lentigo maligna melanomas have a low biological risk for metastases, an ELND is not recommended in these patients.

Tumor thickness thus should not be the sole criterion for making surgical treatment decisions. Other factors, such as the presence or absence of tumor ulceration, the growth pattern, the patient's sex and age, the anatomic location of the melanoma, and the operative risk should all be considered when making the decision to perform ELND in an individual patient.

Melanomas located on the trunk can have ambiguous lymphatic drainage, making it difficult for the surgeon to accurately assess which nodal basins are at risk for harboring microscopic metastases. The sites of multidirectional lymphatic drainage on the trunk are much greater than previously appreciated. In these circumstances, a radionuclide cutaneous scan is an accurate and reproducible test for determining the lymphatic drainage of trunk melanomas.

With proper surgical judgment and technique, ELND can be performed in selected patients with minimal morbidity and virtually no mortality (Table 3). Older patients and obese patients have an increased risk of developing wound complications. Some modifications of the lymphadenectomy can be considered to minimize the operative morbidity. Thus, when an ELND of the cervical nodes is planned, a modified neck dissection is usually performed. This modified procedure spares the spinal accessory nerve and decreases the morbidity of shoulder function. The sternomastoid muscle, but not the jugular vein, is also spared in most cases. Partial cervical dissections generally are not performed, since it is difficult to

TABLE 3 Surgical Morbidity After Lymphadenectomy

Site	Number	Short-Term*	Long-Term†
Cervical	48	19%	6%
Axillary	98	27%	9%
Inguinal	58	23%	26%

* Nerve dysfunctions, seroma
† Edema, functional deficit, pain

precisely define the pathways of nodal drainage to various parts of the neck. When ELND is planned for melanomas located on the arm or upper trunk, a standard radical axillary lymphadenectomy is performed. The postoperative morbidity is extremely low (less than 5%). In patients undergoing ELND for leg or lower trunk melanomas, generally only the femoral nodes are excised (i.e., a superficial inguinal dissection). The iliac nodes are spared to minimize the risk of significant leg edema. However, an iliac node dissection is recommended if there are demonstrable metastases to the femoral nodes at the time of ELND. Using this approach, the long-term operative morbidity is low and is certainly at an acceptable level in patients with a life-threatening illness.

FOLLOW-UP

At present, there is no proven benefit of adjuvant therapy, including immunotherapy, chemotherapy, or radiation therapy. There is a limited but definite role of isolated limb perfusion for administering regional chemotherapy and hyperthermia, especially for patients with documented in-transit metastases, satellitosis, or local recurrences involving an extremity.

SOFT TISSUE SARCOMA OF THE EXTREMITY

ARMANDO E. GIULIANO, M.D.
FREDERICK R. EILBER, M.D.

Soft tissue sarcomas are unusual tumors. Only 4,500 malignant soft tissue tumors occur annually in the United States. They occur with equal frequency in men and women and may occur at any age. Most soft tissue sarcomas occur in young children 3 to 5 years old and in adults 40 to 50 years old. These malignant tumors comprise less than 1 percent of all malignant tumors treated annually in the United States.

There are no obvious etiologic factors for the development of soft tissue sarcoma. Trauma often is implicated. Patients recall a minor injury that ultimately leads to the diagnosis of the tumor. However, there is no evidence to support the suggestion that trauma is etiologically related to sarcomas. Approximately 10 percent of patients with von Recklinghausen's disease develop neurofibrosarcoma, and occasionally, sarcomas arise in scars, irradiated tissue, or chronic lymphedematous extremities. Such involvement is rare, and most tumors arise with no predisposing factors.

The overwhelming majority of patients with soft tissue sarcoma of the extremity present with a painless, slowly growing mass. In rare instances, the mass may cause symptoms. Symptoms are usually the result of pressure on adjacent nerves or blood vessels, causing paresthesias, weakness, or swelling of the extremity. Most patients give a history of having had the mass for approximately one year. There is often a long time from the appearance of the mass to the diagnosis because of the patient's delay in seeking treatment and the physician's delay in recognizing the disease. Most physicians rarely treat patients with primary soft tissue sarcomas, and these tumors are frequently mistaken for muscle pulls or chronic hematomas. Muscle pulls and chronic hematomas are extremely unusual in the patient who is not an athlete. The natural history of both these benign abnormalities is rapid resolution. Any mass that persists longer than 3 to 4 weeks should be suspected of being a tumor, and the diagnosis of chronic hematoma or muscle pull should no longer be entertained.

DIAGNOSIS, PREOPERATIVE EVALUATION, AND STAGING

Few diagnostic tests are helpful in the preoperative diagnosis of soft tissue sarcomas. Complete history and physical examination are the first steps in evaluating a patient with a suspected extremity sarcoma. X-ray studies of the soft tissue or bone may be helpful to show whether there is cortical bone destruction or whether an extremity mass is a soft tissue tumor or a primary bone tumor. Soft tissue tumors occurring in the thigh or arm of a young adult could, on physical examination, be confused with osteosarcoma. In general, angiography is not helpful in diagnosis because these tumors are often avascular and do not reveal a tumor blush. Sometimes the angiogram is helpful in defining vascular displacement or in planning the operation. Most recently, computed tomographic (CT) scanning of the extremities has proved to be the most reliable method of determining the anatomic extent of tumor. The CT scan should be used after a diagnosis is made prior to determining definitive therapy.

After a complete history and physical examination, the only necessary and definitive diagnostic test for the evaluation of a soft tissue mass is biopsy. The benign counterparts to malignant tumors of the extremity are far more common than soft tissue sarcomas. Such benign tumors as lipoma, fibroma, neurofibroma, and nodular fasciitis are the most common soft tissue tumors of the extremity. The overwhelming majority of benign soft tissue tumors are located in the subcutaneous tissue and are less than 2 to 3 cm in diameter. For this reason, a small subcutaneous mass should be totally excised, since local excision is the appropriate treatment for these benign tumors. Recurrence of benign tumors is possible if excision margins are narrow; however, this is not a significant clinical problem.

On the other hand, most malignant soft tissue tumors are deep to the subcutaneous space and tend to be larger than 5 cm. Several methods of biopsy are available for such tumors. We prefer a needle biopsy with a Vim-Silverman or Tru-cut needle, which is used to remove a core of tissue for histologic examination. A pathologist who is familiar with soft tissue sarcomas is able to diagnose such a tumor accurately from an adequate needle biopsy specimen. The advantages of needle biopsy are that the large mass is not disturbed, and the boundaries between tumor and normal tissue are not obscured.

Similarly, fine-needle aspiration cytology can be used for the diagnosis of soft tissue sarcomas. With this technique, individual tumor cells are aspirated from the mass, and many areas of the tumor can be sampled at one time. The diagnosis can be made quickly, with little disturbance of fascial planes or hematoma formation. However, since any type of needle biopsy removes a limited amount of tissue, interpretation of the specimen by the pathologist is difficult, and open biopsy is often necessary to determine the malignant nature of the soft tissue mass.

For large, deep-seated tumors, we recommend incisional rather than excisional biopsy. Frozen section should be obtained at the time of incisional biopsy to be certain that malignant tissue is obtained rather than fibrous reaction to the tumor. The surgeon performing the incisional biopsy should plan the incision to facilitate definitive operation. In general, vertical incisions are preferable, since subsequent removal of a transverse scar would lead to a large skin defect on the extremity. In addition, blood vessels, nerves, and muscle groups are ultimately exposed most easily through a longitudinal incision.

Once the histologic diagnosis of sarcoma is made, further studies should include whole lung tomography or CT scanning of the chest (to determine whether the tumor has spread to the lungs), complete blood count, liver function tests, and calcium and alkaline phosphatase determinations. Both CT scans of the affected extremity and angiography are helpful in the planning of definitive therapy. Soft tissue sarcomas in previously untreated patients rarely spread to the liver, brain, or bone. If the patient has no symptoms suggestive of the involvement of these organs and if there are no abnormalities on physical examination or routine blood testing, then bone, liver, or brain scans are not indicated for preoperative evaluation.

Clinical staging, terminology, and histologic diagnosis of soft tissue sarcomas of the extremity are confusing and difficult. Currently, approximately 60 different histologic types of soft tissue sarcoma have been identified. These tumors are all derived from mesenchymal or neural crest cells and are pluripotential, exhibiting the ability to dedifferentiate into any of the soft tissue elements. In addition, large tumors may exhibit histologic features suggestive of a number of different soft tissue cell types, making histologic labels extremely difficult to apply. The most common histologic subtypes of soft tissue sarcoma are liposarcoma, malignant fibrous histiocytoma, synovial cell sarcoma, rhabdomyosarcoma, and fibrosarcoma in descending order of frequency.

Because of the multiple histologic types and diagnostic difficulties, a uniform staging system is essential for the study and treatment of these diseases. The American Joint Committee on Staging and End Results developed a system that has a major advantage in that it bypasses the problem of histologic identification of the tumor. In this system, malignant soft tissue tumors are graded according to the number of mitoses per high-power field; the tumor size and the presence or absence of regional lymphatic metastases and distant metastases also are considered. There is no consideration for anatomic location of the tumor or histologic subtype. This staging system correlates well with prognosis. Although, in general, some histologic subtypes of sarcoma may tend to be of a lower grade than others, the deviations of grade among the different histologic subtypes make this classification a more accurate predictor of clinical course than reliance on histology alone, as has been done in the past.

TREATMENT

Once the soft tissue mass is determined to be a sarcoma, and there is no evidence of distant spread, definitive therapy should be instituted. In the adult, soft tissue sarcomas of the extremity have been treated primarily by surgery. Although surgical resection still plays an essential role, the addition of chemotherapy and radiation therapy may afford superior local control with less morbidity. Various therapeutic modalities include local excision, compartmental excision, amputation, and multimodality therapy.

Local Excision

Early attempts to treat soft tissue sarcomas surgically by local excision or enucleation of the tumor through the capsule were unsuccessful. It readily became apparent that local recurrences were inevitable, and the reported local recurrence rate was as high as 90 percent after this type of operative treatment. This is because soft tissue sarcomas are not encapsulated. However, they form a pseudocapsule of compressed normal tissue that is infiltrated microscopically by tumor cells. Enucleation or excision through this capsule is, by definition, incomplete, and local recurrence is nearly certain. This technique should not be used.

Compartmental Excision

Soft tissue sarcomas arising within a particular muscle group can be treated successfully by resection of the entire muscle group from origin to insertion. Several studies indicate that local recurrence could be reduced to approximately 30 to 40 percent with muscle group excision alone. In practice, however, sarcomas rarely are confined to one muscle group. Indeed, with large tumors of the proximal thigh, the sarcoma crosses multiple fascial planes and the site of tumor origin remains uncertain. Most operative procedures must therefore involve multiple muscle groups and fascial planes, rendering this technique extremely difficult in practice.

Amputation

Amputation has been a mainstay of therapy for soft tissue sarcomas of the extremity. In theory, an amputation should be done one joint above the anatomic region involved by the sarcoma. In practice, above-the-knee amputations are done for lesions of both the calf and the foot. Hemipelvectomy or hip disarticulation is performed for large proximal sarcomas of the thigh, and intrascapular thoracic amputations for large proximal arm lesions. Despite these radical operations, the local recurrence rate can be as high as 10 to 15 percent with amputation alone. This seemingly high recurrence rate is probably because most sarcomas treated by amputation are large, bulky proximal lesions. Although a hemipelvectomy may be performed for a proximal thigh lesion, there still could be a close proximal margin.

Multimodality Therapy

As the field of radiation therapy developed, radiation oncologists attempted to treat soft tissue sarcomas with radiotherapy. It rapidly became apparent that the overall response rate was too low to continue the use of radiation therapy alone for patients with unresected disease. Later work showed that while radiation therapy alone was relatively ineffective in controlling primary tumors, the combination of surgical resection followed by radiation therapy for microscopic residual disease was extremely effective. Complete excision of extremity sarcoma followed by approximately 5,000 rads of radiation therapy can achieve local control in 80 to 85 percent of patients.

Certain treatment principles have evolved on the basis of early experience with combination surgery and radiation therapy. First, by not treating the entire extremity, the severe complications of subcutaneous fibrosis and subsequent vascular and neurologic problems can be avoided. Usually a strip of skin is spared opposite the primary tumor, and only the compartment involving the tumor is treated with radiation therapy. Second, radiation therapy should be used only in combination with complete surgical excision of gross tumor since local control, when irradiating for macroscopic disease, falls to approximately 50 percent. In general, the control rate with the combination of surgery and radiation therapy is better for tumors located distal to the elbow or distal to the knee than for tumors located more proximally in the extremity. Third, radiation therapy has been used successfully by some oncologists prior to surgical resection of the tumor. However, preoperative administration has an associated higher incidence of wound complications.

In 1974, Haskell and associates at UCLA infused doxorubicin intra-arterially into limbs of patients with soft tissue sarcoma. Evaluation of resected specimens revealed marked tumor cell necrosis, a finding that led to the subsequent use of chemotherapy as part of the multimodality approach. The rationale for using chemotherapy was to treat the tumor prior to excision in an attempt to kill cells at the periphery, cells that might lead to subsequent local recurrence. Doxorubicin was selected because it is a known radiation sensitizer and was effective against metastatic sarcomas. Patients then received 3,500 rads of radiation therapy over a 2-week period (10 days). This preoperative treatment was followed by wide local excision of the tumor.

The aim of this operation is to remove the tumor and a rim of 3 to 4 cm of surrounding normal tissue. Wherever tumor abuts bone, blood vessels, or nerves, the respective periosteum, adventitia, or perineurium is removed with the operative specimen. Numerous intraoperative biopsy specimens and frozen sections are taken to ensure tumor-free margins.

The use of this technique, in an initial series of 86 patients with extremity sarcomas, showed only two local recurrences for an overall local control rate of 97 percent. However, five patients developed a subsequent fracture of adjacent bone. These patients had large proximal thigh lesions where the periosteum was stripped during the wide excision. The cause of these fractures could have been either the surgical procedure or the relatively high radiation fractionation and chemotherapy.

To reduce the incidence of this serious complication and of the fibrosis that was seen in some patients, a second series of patients was treated with the same intra-arterial chemotherapy, but with only 1,750 rads of radiation therapy over 5 consecutive days. Since 1981, 105 patients have been treated in this manner. There have been only two local recurrences in this group and only one pathologic fracture. The lower dose of radiation therapy appears to reduce postoperative complications while achieving local control rates similar to those of the higher dose of radiation or even amputation.

Clearly, multimodality therapy affords excellent local control and has the major advantage of limb salvage with a viable functional extremity. The overall survival appears similar to that achieved with amputation.

Adjuvant Chemotherapy

The study by the American Joint Committee on Staging and End Results showed that patients with high-grade soft tissue sarcomas (clinicopathologic stage III or IV) have at least a 70 percent chance of disease recurrence with a survival of less than 20 percent. For this reason, several investigators had used doxorubicin as a single agent or with other various drug combinations in an adjuvant setting. The overall survival rate appeared to be much better than that of the historical controls, approximating 60 to 70 percent. It seemed reasonable that adjuvant chemotherapy was the reason for the enhancement of survival. However, it also was noted that, in most studies, the local recurrence rate had decreased markedly. Thus, several investigators began to question whether improved survival was, in fact, due to the adjuvant chemotherapy or perhaps to better local control or improved earlier treatment of the primary tumor. Conflicting reports led to a questioning of the value of adjuvant chemotherapy in improving survival.

Recently, Rosenberg and colleagues at the National Cancer Institute described their experience with adjuvant doxorubicin, cyclophosphamide, and high-dose methotrexate in a randomized trial. Sixty-five patients have been entered into this study, and early results suggest that adjuvant chemotherapy reduces the incidence of metastases. However, the occurrence of significant toxicity, such as cardiomyopathy and subsequent heart failure, may preclude an improved survival in this group, and complications may outweigh benefits. A subsequent investigation with a different drug regimen is currently being investigated.

At present, we are conducting a trial at UCLA that compares adjuvant intravenous, postoperative doxorubicin with no further chemotherapy in patients who are treated with multimodality limb salvage therapy. Sixty-five patients have been entered into this study, and conclusions cannot yet be entertained. Clearly, the use of adjuvant chemotherapy appears promising, but its exact role remains to be determined. In general, there is an improved survival for patients with soft tissue sarcoma of the extremity.

SOLITARY NECK MASS

MARSHALL M. URIST, M.D., F.A.C.S.

When a patient presents with a mass in the neck or when a physician discovers a neck mass on routine examination, there is a tendency to proceed immediately to open (excisional) biopsy for diagnosis. Surgeons should resist this temptation and develop the philosophy that evaluation of a neck mass is an orderly progression of examinations and tests which are aimed at obtaining an appropriate amount of information prior to biopsy. When open biopsy is performed, the surgeon must be prepared to render definitive treatment. For possible causes of a mass in the neck, see Table 1 and Figure 1.

DIAGNOSTIC EVALUATION

The diagnostic evaluation of a neck mass begins with a thorough medical history. Important considerations are age, sex, history of irradiation to the head and neck area, family history of cancer, occupation, and personal habits

TABLE 1 Masses in the Neck Region

Congenital masses
  Branchial cysts and sinus tracts
  Thyroglossal duct cysts and tumors
  Cystic hygroma or lymphangioma

Acquired neck masses
  Benign
    Salivary gland tumors
    Thyroid nodules and tumors
    Lymph nodes
  Malignant tumors
    Salivary gland
      Mucoepidermoid carcinoma
      Adenoid cystic carcinoma
      Acinic cell carcinoma
      Adenocarcinoma
      Epidermoid carcinoma
    Thyroid gland
      Papillary carcinoma
      Follicular carcinoma
      Medullary carcinoma
      Anaplastic carcinoma
    Lymph nodes
      Primary tumors
        Hodgkin's disease
        Non-Hodgkin's lymphoma
      Secondary (metastatic) tumors
        Leukemic infiltrate
        Sarcoma
        Carcinoma
        Melanoma

Sources of tumors metastatic to the neck
  Skin
    Melanoma
    Squamous cell carcinoma
    Basal cell carcinoma
  Salivary gland
    Parotid
    Submandibular
    Minor glands in lining of mucosa
    Sublingual
  Thyroid gland
  Upper aerodigestive tract
    Squamous cell carcinoma arising from mucosal lining
      of oral cavity, pharynx, larynx, and esophagus
  Lung
  Gastrointestinal and genitourinary tracts
    Adenocarcinoma

such as smoking and alcohol intake. Particular attention should be paid to a history of previous benign and malignant tumors. A review of reports, slides, and blocks of

previously excised specimens may be helpful, especially in the case of skin lesions.

The physical examination should also be comprehensive, particularly as regards the precise location and character of the neck mass. A solitary neck mass is defined as a mass located between the clavicle inferiorly and the margin of the mandible superiorly. On the posterior surface of the neck, the area included is between the spinous process of C7 and the occiput. The location of the mass should be described in reference to the major muscular and bony laryngeal landmarks. A particularly important location is the area at the angle of the jaw. A mass in the tail of the parotid may be difficult to differentiate from enlarged lymph nodes in the jugulodigastric area or upper jugular chain. These parotid-associated structures lie external to the sternocleidomastoid muscle, whereas nodes of the upper portion of the jugular chain lie medial to the sternocleidomastoid muscle. Jugulodigastric lymph nodes lie slightly anterior between these two locations. The submandibular gland must also be identified. This is best accomplished by means of bimanual palpation with an examining finger in the floor of the mouth. Careful attention to anatomic details aids in the diagnosis. Nodes of the lower jugular chain may be difficult to differentiate from masses in the thyroid gland. If the mass moves upward on deglutition, it is under the strap muscles and most likely of thyroid origin. Supraclavicular lymph nodes should be located posterior or lateral to the lower aspect of the sternocleidomastoid muscle, whereas lower jugular chain lymph nodes are medial to the muscle. By precisely describing the location of the mass, the examiner's attention should be drawn to the most likely origins for a tumor metastasizing to the solitary node. Table 2 lists sites of origin for lymph nodes appearing in various anatomic regions.

Biopsy

A biopsy of a solitary neck mass can be obtained by either a closed or open technique. The closed technique involves the use of an aspiration needle (21- to 26-gauge) to obtain cytologic material. This method is not preferred by all surgeons because it does not always provide as much information as an open biopsy. On the other hand, aspiration needle biopsy is often expeditious and cost-effective, and has not been shown to increase the risk of tumor dis-

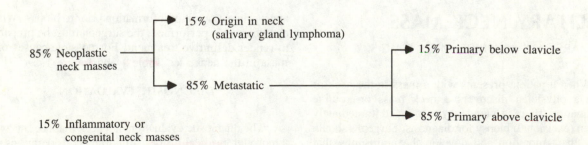

Figure 1 Etiology of neck masses (exclusive of thyroid).

TABLE 2 Sites of Origin for Lymph Node Metastasis

Lymph Node Area	Primary Site
Occipital	Scalp
Spinal accessory chain	Nasopharynx
Submandibular	Lip, oral cavity, salivary gland
Upper jugular	Oral cavity, oropharynx, nasopharynx, salivary gland
Mid-jugular	Larynx, pharynx, oral cavity, thyroid
Lower jugular and supraclavicular	Thyroid, breast, lung, gastrointestinal tract

semination or local recurrence if the proper precautions are observed. In order to perform an aspiration needle biopsy, the physician must be absolutely certain that the tip of the aspirating needle can be guided into the tumor mass. Several passes with the needle may be required for thyroid masses. The puncture site of the aspiration should be marked to identify the portion of skin to be excised with the specimen in the event that a cancer is diagnosed. When surgeons begin to use this technique, there should be a clear line of communication with the pathologist, and all results should be discussed between these two individuals. During the learning period with this technique, several authors have recommended that aspiration needle biopsy be performed immediately prior to open biopsy in order to confirm findings. Slides can be read within hours of the needle biopsy procedure and therefore a great deal of time can be saved. In addition, it is possible for the physician to discuss recommendations and options for therapy with the patient when a precise diagnosis is known. False-positive findings are extremely uncommon when strict cytologic criteria are observed. Aspiration needle biopsy is not recommended for masses in the parotid area because of the danger of implanting cells in the adjacent nerves or salivary gland tissue. A negative needle biopsy (nonmalignant cytology) should be considered as an incomplete answer, and the next step would be open biopsy.

Open biopsy should be planned with future treatment in mind. A small incision is made over the mass, and as little dissection as possible is carried out. If the mass is small, it can be excised in its entirety. For masses larger than approximately 1 cm, an incisional biopsy can be performed if the mass is obviously a malignant tumor. This decreases the amount of dissection and facilitates subsequent resection. If the diagnosis of cancer is confirmed, the surgeon can proceed with definitive management of the mass. Masses near the angle of the mandible may be within the tail of the parotid gland and require partial or total parotidectomy for safe management of the facial nerve. The surgeon should approach masses in this area with a plan of limited exploration, using an incision that can be enlarged to resect the mass with an appropriate operation. Local recurrence of a mixed tumor of the tail of the parotid gland would be much more likely to occur if an excisional biopsy were performed instead of a super-

ficial parotidectomy. As with many facets of the evaluation of neck masses, the plan must be individualized.

Further Evaluations

When the physical examination and a biopsy have revealed the presence of metastasis, further evaluations in search of a primary site may be indicated prior to definitive management of the neck. These tests include chest roentgenogram, liver function tests, chest and abdominal CT scans, intravenous urogram, and upper and lower gastrointestinal series. When squamous cell carcinoma is found in cervical metastases without a site of origin after physical examination (including indirect laryngoscopy), then direct laryngoscopy, esophagoscopy, and bronchoscopy should be performed. Biopsy should be obtained from any areas that appear abnormal. Adenocarcinoma in the lower neck is usually of gastrointestinal, breast, or pulmonary origin. In the upper neck, a primary in a salivary gland should be suspected. Metastases from thyroid carcinoma may appear in any of these areas, although the middle and lower jugular chain or posterior triangle positions are most common.

MANAGEMENT OF UNKNOWN PRIMARY CARCINOMA IN THE NECK

When unknown primary squamous cell carcinomas are manifested by enlargement of a single cervical node, careful attention should be paid to the most likely sites of origin and biopsies obtained if there is any evidence of an abnormality. Metastatic lymph nodes are removed with an appropriate neck dissection based on their location. If they are adjacent to the course of the spinal accessory nerve, a standard radical neck dissection is performed. When the isolated mass is not approaching the course of the spinal accessory nerve, either a modified or a standard radical neck dissection may be performed. Irradiation of the neck up to the base of the skull is designed to treat suspected (but unproven) primary tumors in the nasopharynx. This results in high morbidity (complete drying of the mucous membranes) and appears to be unjustified when only 2 percent of patients subsequently develop primary tumors in the nasopharynx after neck dissection alone. Although fewer patients eventually develop a demonstrable primary tumor after elective irradiation, the overall survival is similar to that of patients treated by neck dissection as the only initial therapy. The delayed appearance of primary cancers can be treated by surgical resection or irradiation as appropriate. The controversy over neck dissection alone versus neck dissection plus irradiation will remain unsettled until randomized studies are available. All patients should have monthly follow-up visits for the first year, every 2 months for the second, and every 3 months for the third year, regardless of the type of initial treatment. If patients are not available for close follow-up, postoperative irradiation is essential. When multiple nodes or nodes with extracapsular invasion are present, postoperative irradiation is also recommended.

INFECTION OF THE HAND

GAYLORD L. CLARK, M.D.

Our hands, because of their constant exposure to the environment, are highly susceptible to infection. The use of them in our day-to-day activities in our homes, at recreation, at our avocations, and at our work places make them vulnerable. The potential seriousness of hand infections cannot be minimized in spite of the availability of antibiotics. Damage to the critical anatomy that allows for the function of precision can occur quickly if an infection is allowed to progress uncontrolled. In the era before antibiotics, irretrievable loss of normally functioning parts as well as the threat of death were more common. The latter is rare today, yet the seriousness of infection cannot be diminished.

BACTERIOLOGY

Bacteria penetrate the protective skin barrier through puncture wounds, hair follicles, lacerations, or open fractures. Bacteria are also blood-borne and set up a focus of activity in regions of tissue compromise or injury such as a hematoma, a foreign body, or a scar. The most common organisms found in infections of the hand are *Staphylococcus aureus*, streptococci, and coliform bacilli. These organisms are usually sensitive to penicillin or its derivatives. They are also sensitive to many of the broad-spectrum antibiotics such as cephalosporins, erythromycin, or tetracyclines. I prefer, when possible, to obtain a culture and sensitivity of the organisms from an infected area and to perform a Gram stain to aid in the immediate choice of the correct antibiotic. The treating physician is also responsible to determine whether the patient has an allergy to the antibiotic.

ANATOMY

As with all medical or surgical problems, an accurate history is required. The physical examination that follows should bring to light the location and degree of involvement. The treating physician must know his hand anatomy well and be able to recognize the deep structures and

PROGNOSIS

Specific prognoses of cancers that present as a solitary neck mass are based on the location, histologic type, and degree of differentiation of the primary tumor.

spaces beneath the skin that may contain the infection. This is often manifested by a specific pattern of swelling and erythema (Fig. 1).

NONSURGICAL MANAGEMENT

Many cases of infection can be treated nonoperatively if recognized early. I treat such cases with therapeutic doses of antibiotics in conjunction with splinting and

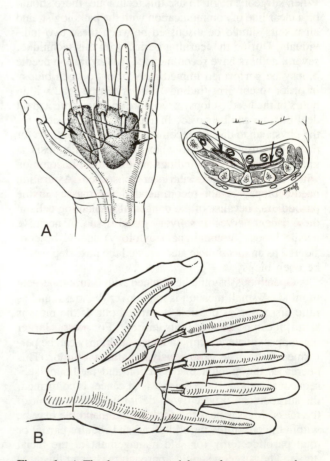

Figure 1 *A*, The thenar space and deep palmar space are shown in the frontal and cross-sectional drawings. The arrows point to their locations. The digital synovial sheaths are, as outlined, covering the flexor tendons in their fibro-osseous tunnels. *B*, This drawing shows the connection of the radial and ulnar bursae at the carpal tunnel level.

elevation. One effective method of supplementing this treatment is the use of a "continuous compress," whereby the involved digit or hand is wrapped with warm, moist, absorbent cotton and then covered with a plastic wrap to retain the moisture and heat. This application should be renewed every 12 hours. Although the skin appears white and shriveled when this compress is removed, this treatment may bring the problem to a head or allow for its resolution. If there is no improvement after 24 to 48 hours, a more aggressive approach to treatment must be considered. The use of appropriate intravenous antibiotics in conjunction with carefully considered surgery may be necessary. Signs of improvement are a decrease in pain, reduction of swelling, a decrease in localized erythema and heat, and correction of systemic fever.

SURGICAL MANAGEMENT

Surgery is frequently necessary in well-established infections or in those that are unresponsive to the initial treatment. The surgeon must have a thorough knowledge of the appropriate incisions to use for a particular diagnosis (Fig. 2). It is essential that an abscess be adequately flushed out and drained. This drainage must be maintained in order that the body's healing processes can take over and that systemic antibiotics reach the involved area. The surgery must not damage any critical structures such as arteries, nerves, and tendons and must be so designed as to prevent scar contractures across joints during the healing phase. In the fingers and thumb, mid-axial incisions along the borders of the digits are preferred. At the tip of the finger, an incision close to the fingernail is required with the longitudinal limb of that incision in the mid-axial plane. If possible, these incisions should be placed on the side away from thumb-finger pinch in case a tender scar develops. In the palm area, the incisions should be slightly curved or transverse and parellel to the folds and creases of the distal palm or thenar eminence. At the wrist, a zigzag pattern is used. Incisions should not cross flexor creases at a right angle because of the potential of a

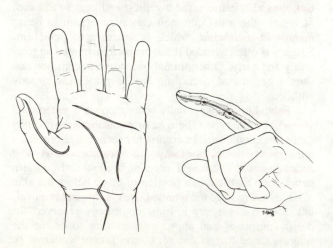

Figure 2 The appropriate skin incisions are shown and are to be used for the purpose of draining infected areas.

crippling scar contracture. Wounds should be left open or adequately drained. Often a polyethelene catheter is placed in the wound for irrigation with physiologic saline or antibiotic solutions.

Paronychia

Infection about the fingernail is termed paronychia. This can be treated in the early stages as outlined above and by surgically decompressing any pocket of pus. With a more established infection, removal of a portion of the nail overlying the abscess is necessary. When incising the pocket of pus, I prefer to direct the scapel away from the nail matrix at its edges to avoid creating a scar that might ultimately deform the nail itself.

Felon

Infection of the finger pulp, a felon, requires surgery under adequate anesthesia to open the skin with a J-shaped incision close to the fingernail itself and with the longitudinal limb of the incision on the side away from the thumb. It is necessary to divide the small fibrous septa of the pulp to appropriately drain the abscess. The wound is packed open for 24 to 48 hours, then soaked and redressed on a daily basis until healed. During the operation, one should avoid entering the digital flexor sheath unless it is suspected of having infection within it.

Tenosynovitis

Infection within the tendon sheaths, termed purulent tenosynovitis, is an emergency because of the danger of irretrievable flexor tendon damage. I prefer to make a transverse palmar incision combined with a mid-axial incision in the finger in its distal portion, then opening the sheath at both ends. The sheath is thus decompressed, and thorough catheter irrigation is carried out. If the catheter is left in place, periodic irrigation may be performed and the finger allowed to move within its dressing to minimize tendon adhesions.

Major Hand Spaces

There are two major spaces within the palm and one on the dorsum of the hand (see Fig. 1). There is the mid-palmar space located beneath the finger flexors and superficial to the interosseous muscles. The second is the thenar space lying superficial to the adductor pollicis and deep to the thenar musculature. On the dorsum of the hand, deep to the extensor tendons, is the subaponeurotic space. The importance of the palmar space as related to the subaponeurotic space is the type of infection that can occur here which penetrates around the metacarpals and is contained dorsally by this fascial barrier, creating a collar-button configuration—thus the term "collar button abscess.'' These infections should be drained on both the volar and dorsal aspects of the hand. If left uncontrolled, an infection can spread beyond the confines of a single space and occupy contiguous areas, thus putting many critical structures in jeopardy.

The so-called radial and ulnar bursae are in reality synovial coverings of the flexor tendons in the region of the carpal tunnel. The ulnar bursa is continuous with the flexor sheath of the little finger, and the radial bursa continuous with the digital sheath of the thumb (see Fig. 1). If one or the other becomes infected, there is risk of a horseshoe-shaped abscess, which has the potential of involving the thumb, little finger, and the carpal tunnel. Appropriate drainage is necessary, following the pattern of treatment already outlined.

Clostridial Infections

Clostridial infections do occur in the hand and arm. They are associated with wounds that cause considerable soft tissue damage such as gunshot wounds, agricultural injuries, and tissue damage caused by crushing. The treatment must be aggressive with excision of all devitalized parts; the wound must be left wide open, and heavy antibiotic coverage has to be administered. The use of anti-gas-bacillus serum is controversial, and I have not used it. The employment of a hyperbaric chamber, if available, may be a useful adjunct to the treatment. Patients with this type of infection must be monitored carefully and blood transfusions administered as required. Uncontrolled spread of the process can lead to the loss of a limb or life. The morality rate for gas bacillus infections remains high. Less virulent infections may be encountered in narcotic addicts. It is probable that these individuals may develop some resistance to such infections because of their life style.

Joint and Bone

Infections within joints or involving bone require immediate attention. The surgeon must not wait for roentgenographic changes, and suspicion of infection can sometimes be proved by needle aspiration and culture of the aspirate. It must be remembered that bacterial action on articular cartilage or bone, once advanced, can create permanent damage that may impair function permanently.

Fractures

Fractures in conjunction with infection must be treated with proper and appropriate immobilization. Frequently, internal bone fixation in the form of Kirschner wires, screws, and even bone plates are required for strong stabilization. Occasionally an external fixation device is indicated. These devices are now sophisticated and designed for the hand. The main effort is toward skeletal alignment and prevention of motion at a fracture site. Motion of bone fragments may retard resolution of an infection. The wounds underlying the infected area must be left open to allow for appropriate drainage, and with good bone fixation this can be achieved with minimal risk of complications.

POSTOPERATIVE CARE

Postoperative care allows for wound healing and maintaining function. In many cases, I refer the patient to a hand therapist for whirlpool baths with sterile solutions, range of motion exercises, dressing changes, and appropriate splinting. Debridement of devitalized tissues is facilitated during or after whirlpool baths. Concern about hand swelling from an infection can be monitored and well controlled by a knowledgeable therapist. By using well-designed physical therapy modalities, post-infection complications are greatly reduced.

UNCOMMON INFECTIONS

The treating surgeon must be aware of uncommon infections. These include such organisms as atypical *Mycobacterium* including *M. marinum, M. Kansaii, M. avium,* and *M. intracellularis.* These are chronic problems and may mimic other diseases such as rheumatoid arthritis or sarcoidosis. If such an infection is suspected, special culture and histologic studies are indicated. I frequently invite a pathologist to be present in the operating room so that the chances of a clear-cut diagnosis are maximal.

Tuberculosis, although uncommon today in our society, still occurs. Also infrequently seen is *Mycobacterium lepraemurium,* which produces leprosy or Hansen's disease.

Human and animal bites can introduce infection to the hand. Human bites are particularly dangerous because of the variety of organisms that may be introduced into a tooth penetration wound such as *Eikinella corrodens, Staphylococcus aureus,* and beta-hemolytic *Streptococcus.* Cat bites also cause rapid swelling and pain in the area of injury, the most common causative organism being *Pasturella multocida,* which is sensitive to penicillin. Surgery is often avoided if the problem is treated aggressively and early. Other animal bites are less common and should be treated according to the principles already outlined.

Fungal infections usually occur through a penetration wound of some type. The rose or pyracantha thorns may cause this condition. The commonly seen fungal problems are sporotrichosis, blastomycosis, cryptococcosis, and actinomycosis. The fungal infection brought on by a thorn penetration that leaves a portion of thorn below the skin surface may require the retained thorn's surgical removal, but otherwise surgery is most commonly reserved for biopsy purposes and appropriate culture to define the fungus. Once this is complete, the proper systemic or topical drugs are administered.

Herpes simplex infections must also be mentioned.

These can easily mimic a felon or paronychia. They frequently occur on the fingers of individuals such as dentists, anesthesiologists, respiratory therapists, and certain specialty personnel who must place their hands in the mouths of the humans for whom they are caring.

CLOSTRIDIAL GAS GANGRENE OF THE EXTREMITY

FRANK B. CERRA, M.D.

Clostridial gas gangrene of the extremities is an uncommon surgical infection; a given surgeon may see only a few cases in a lifetime of practice. In most cases, a pure clostridial infection is not present; the signs and symptoms of the pure and mixed forms are not easily distinguished; and the mainstay of therapy continues to be appropriate surgical control of the wound.

CLINICAL PERSPECTIVE

Clostridial organisms are ubiquitous; wound contamination is common in surgical practice and is usually of little clinical significance. With the right combination of factors, however, a virulent clinical infection ensues that continues to carry a high morality risk. Although the precise details of the "right combination" of local factors is not well understood, a number of predisposing factors and conditions have been identified (Table 1).

TABLE 1 Predisposing Factors of Clostridial Gas Gangrene

Deficits of oxygen delivery
  Vascular compromise
  Low cardiac output
  Low oxygen content

Underlying metabolic abnormality
  Diabetes mellitus
  Closed space
  Acidosis
  Malnutrition
  Chronic renal failure
  Alcohol

Immunocompromise
  Chemotherapy
  Transplanted organ
  Underlying carcinoma or sarcoma

Source
  Dead or injured tissue
  Open bowel or biliary tree
  Gross contamination: dirt, debris, stool

Surgery to treat this problem is not indicated because secondary bacterial infection may occur. Local care with protection of the affected area is all that is necessary. The problem is self-limited.

A source of infection is usually necessary. As the organisms are ubiquitous, this criterion is not difficult to fulfill. Gross contamination by such agents as dirt, debris, or stool in the presence of dead or injured tissue is a common history in cases of trauma. The opened bowel or biliary tree in elective surgery may be incriminated. A problem of oxygen delivery is usually present. This may take the form of direct vascular compromise, or it may be the result of such physiologic abnormalities as an acute low flow state or low oxygen content. Underlying metabolic abnormalities or disease, especially diabetes mellitus, potentiate the infection. Other predisposing factors are a closed space, acidosis, malnutrition, alcohol, and chronic renal failure. Immune compromise constitutes another potent predisposing condition. The immune compromise may result from an underlying condition such as carcinoma or sarcoma or from chemotherapy, radiation therapy, or immunosuppression after organ transplantation.

The organisms involved can be pure clostridial or a mixture of obligate and facultative anaerobes. In either case, an anaerobic environment is a necessary condition. Gas in the tissue occurs with both groups of pathogenic organisms and results from the metabolic processes of denitrification, fermentation and deamination. The gas produced in aerobic infections is carbon dioxide, which is water-soluble and does not accumulate in tissue.

Pure clostridia are gram-positive bacilli that are obligate anaerobes and form spores. They are ubiquitous; they are part of the normal flora of stool. More than 90 forms of the organism are known to exist. Infection commonly involves only six: *C. perfringens, C. septicum, C. fallax, C. histolyticum, C. bifermentans*, and *C. noyvi* or *edematiens*.

Most infections are mixed. The other bacteria are usually coliforms such as *E. coli*; anaerobic gram-negative bacilli such as *Bacteroides fragilis* or *melaninogenicus*; and anaerobic streptococci. Sometimes anaerobic organisms interact to create a synergistic infection that is tissue-necrosing and gas-forming.

The pathogenesis of the infection proceeds on two levels. The first is the wound itself. It is the primary site of infection and consists of a direct, spreading, tissue-necrosing infection. This focus is surrounded by an intense local inflammatory response. The primary infecton may originate in either muscle or subcutaneous tissue. The inflammatory response involves surrounding tissue and eventually skin. The necrosing process can eventually spread to include all tissues from skin to muscle.

The second level in the pathogenesis is the systemic (inflammatory) response, more properly called sepsis. The dead and injured tissue and the toxins of bacterial growth activate the mediators of the systemic response: the classic neuroendocrine system and the microendocrine or cell-to-cell mediating system. Such mediators as interleukin 1, prostanoids, cortisol, catecholamine, and the autonomic nervous system are involved. These mediators act to modulate and control the end-organ responses seen in the systemic response. The classic "toxic" picture results with its hyperdynamic cardiovascular picture (tachycardia, high cardiac output, low systemic vascular resistance) and with all the characteristics of hypermetabolism (high oxygen consumption, hypercatabolism, glucose intolerance, and insulin resistance).

CLINICAL SYNDROMES

Given the previous discussion, four clinical syndromes of systemic toxicity, tissue necrosis, gas formation, and infection occur in surgical practice (Table 2). Typical or classic clinical presentations can and do occur. However, the usual case is mixed in its clinical manifestations. A coagulopathy is also usually present, most commonly as disseminated intravascular coagulopathy. Because of the hemolysins that can be produced by the *Clostridium* or the anaerobic *Streptococcus*, frank, fulminant hemolysis can also occur. This latter complication is difficult to treat except with control of the infection, whereas the former usually responds well to blood product support.

The major factors associated wth mortality have been (1) the time interval from onset of disease to definitive surgical therapy and (2) the type of surgical therapy performed. The longer the time interval, frequently occupied by "expectant or hopeful watching," the higher the mortality rate. Incision rather than excision of dead tissue likewise potentiates the mortality. In reality, the former seems to be another form of expectant therapy.

DIAGNOSIS

The clinical setting usually signals that the patient is sick with a surgically remediable disease. Since the clinical findings overlap significantly, this function is probably all that should be required of the clinical setting and the clinician. The clinical setting, then, provides the *high index of clinical suspicion* that such an infection is present (Fig. 1).

Once this suspicion has occurred, the involved area should be explored. At least two processes should occur during this exploration: a Gram stain of fluid and tissue and a determination of the presence of dead tissue. The Gram stain is useful in attempting to differentiate pure clostridial infection from the mixed variety. Cultures take more time than is usually available for initial definitive therapy, but are helpful in adjusting antibiotic therapy in the subsequent clinical course. The presence of pure clostridial infection is important, as there may be some benefit to hyperbaric oxygen in that setting.

The determination of the presence of necrotic tissue is critical. If it is present, surgical intervention is necessary for the removal of all necrotic tissue. Fasciotomy and inspection of the underlying muscle is frequently necessary. The pathologist may be of considerable assistance in evaluating biopsies in this setting.

TREATMENT

Definitive therapy must proceed rapidly and efficiently. The first order is to resuscitate the patient and begin antibiotics. Resuscitation requires the restoration and maintenance of oxygen transport. Usually invasive flow monitoring is required to adequately assess blood volume, cardiac function, and oxygen consumption. A PaO_2 over 100 mm Hg may be useful. Preparations also need to be made with the blood bank for the large numbers of blood products and platelets that are necessary during and after the surgical intervention. Antibiotic therapy should be broad-spectrum, covering clostridial species and the usual other anaerobes, facultative anaerobes, and

TABLE 2 Clinical Syndromes

Characteristic	Clostridial Cellulitis	Clostridial Myonecrosis	Synergistic Necrotizing Cellulitis	Necrotizing Fasciitis
Onset	3–5 days	Hours–days	Days	Hours–days
Tempo	Moderate	Rapid	Rapid	Rapid
Temperature (F)	101–102	101–105	100–102	102–105
Systemic toxicity	Low	High; hemolysis	High; hemolysis	High; hemolysis
Skin-wound appearance	± Crepitus blebs, necrosis, red-brown fluid, edema, extreme wound pain	Crepitus, necrosis, tan color, "bronze erysipelas," sickly sweet odor	Crepitus, blebs, necrosis, dishwater fluid edema	Red-purple color, blebs, edema, hypoesthesia
Bacteriology	Clostridia, mixed Gm + and Gm −	Clostridia, mixed Gm + and Gm −	*Streptococcus, Bacteroides,* coliforms, (aerobe-anaerobe)	*Bacteroides, Peptococcus,* coliforms (aerobe-anaerobe)
Depth involved	Subcutaneous tissue	Muscle to skin	Skin through muscle	Skin through muscle

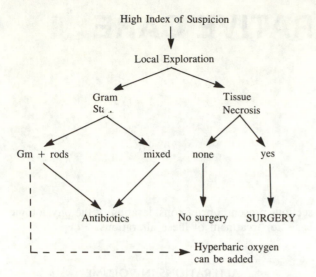

Figure 1 High index of clinical suspicion.

TABLE 3	Treatment Summary for Clostridial Gas Gangrene

High index of suspicion

Local exploration

Resuscitation

Antibiotics; tetanus prophylaxis

Surgery

Adjunctive therapy
  Nutrition
  Hyperbaric oxygen
  Wound coverage

aerobes that may be present. Penicillin, clindamycin, and an aminoglycoside constitute an effective combination. The antibiotics can be readjusted when definitive fluid and tissue cultures are available. Tetanus prophylaxis should be given.

Surgical therapy must then occur. Appropriate tissue for aerobic and anaerobic cultures should be taken. Dead tissue must be removed. This latter mandate is sometimes difficult, as it is not always possible to determine which tissue is dead or the extent of the necrosis. In this setting, the commitment to redebride as necessary is important; the tissue will demarcate over time. During the debridement, a search for a source must also be made. A perineal or perirectal abscess, a retroperitoneal perforation of a colonic diverticulum, and carcinoma are examples of disease that can present with a "clostridial syndrome" of the extremity.

Once this point has been reached, adjuvant therapy should be instituted. Hyperbaric oxygen is one such therapy and is the subject of continued controversy. There are currently no prospective or randomized prospective trials to establish the efficacy of this resource-dependent therapy. The anecdotal literature and experience suggest a possible role for hyperbaric oxygen in the management of pure clostridial infections. It may have a potential tissue-saving function, particularly following debridement, or when there are questionable areas of viability. The use of this technique with the mixed type of infection is less well established. The risk/benefit ratio of transfer to a hyperbaric center needs to be considered.

Aggressive nutritional support then needs to be started. The metabolic demands are probably similar to those of a burn of comparable size. Thus, malnutrition can develop rapidly and contribute to the mortality risk.

Local wound care is also an important component of therapy. Poor wound care can reactivate infection, result in continued infection, lead to more tissue loss and resultant disability, or produce superinfection. To manage the wound, frequent dressing changes with saturated saline packs, debridement as necessary, and tissue cultures are the rule. Topical antibiotics do not seem to be of the same use as in burns and can make it difficult to determine whether more dead tissue needs to be debrided. Artificial skin coverings such as porcine skin in the presence of active infection seem to be of little use and can produce superinfection and septicemia. Once the infection is over, the rapid achievement of wound covering is essential. Treatment is summarized in Table 3.

PRE- AND POSTOPERATIVE CARE

FLUID AND ELECTROLYTE THERAPY

WILLIAM R. DRUCKER, M.D., F.A.C.S., F.R.C.S.(C)

The mechanisms protecting the homeostasis of body fluids are organized in an hierarchical manner. Numerous physiologic studies since the pioneering work of Adolf, Peters, Darrow and Yannet, and McCance have demonstrated clearly that circulatory volume has the top priority for defense. The solute content and composition of body fluids are relegated to secondary and tertiary positions in this biological ordering of homeostatic priorities. Thus, when the intrinsic defense mechanisms are forced to make a choice among these three basic priorities by the vicissitudes of a disease process or, more likely, because of inappropriate therapeutic intervention, the defense of circulatory volume always wins. Once this essential fact is understood, many of the apparent enigmas of electrolyte and fluid balance become comprehensible. Although it is unusual to find the problems of individual patients neatly packaged within this framework, it does provide a conceptual basis for planning therapy. In real life one must, of course, assess and reconcile the challenges to homeostasis from alterations in each category—volume, solute content, and composition—for any given patient.

The surgeon must possess sufficient understanding of the mechanisms that maintain fluid homeostasis to provide rational therapy in support of these mechanisms. Rules and formulas are not only inadequate for this purpose, but their use compromises the intellectual satisfaction engendered by the application of an understanding of body fluid physiology to the care of patients. Realistically, the fluid regimen instituted by the surgeon rarely maintains normality or corrects an abnormality. Rather, this goal is achieved by the homeostatic processes of the body when supplied with fluids and substrates of appropriate volume, content, and composition. Careful attention to the daily balance between the volume and solute content of fluid intake and all losses provides the rationale for judging the quantity and type of fluids to be administered in the perioperative period. Nevertheless, there are many alterations in body fluids and their electrolyte content (Table 1), which the surgeon must manage. The following sections present a brief consideration of the physiologic basis for treatment of these alterations.

ALTERATIONS IN VOLUME

Hypervolemia

Most surgeons are aware of the dangers incurred by the administration of an excessively rapid or an excessively large volume of isotonic fluid. Admittedly, the usual causes of an increase in total body water reflect profound alterations in the function of specific organs, such as the heart, liver, and kidneys, which ordinarily do not fall within the province of surgeons for therapy. However, surgeons must be aware of these alterations in their management of fluids and electrolytes pre- and postoperatively. It is the subtlety of fluid composition that may cause problems. The excessive administration of water or hypotonic fluids in the early postoperative period can be dangerous to the patient who is unable to excrete a water load. Unfortunately, the complication of an acute excess of body water continues to be produced in surgical patients, in spite of the clear-cut warning from the studies of Zimmerman and Wangensteen. This is particularly apt to occur as a result of overly enthusiastic infusion (more

TABLE 1 Alterations in Body Fluids and Electrolytes

Volume
  Hypervolemia
    Chronic organ failure (heart, liver, kidney)
    Iatrogenic (Isotonic fluid overload, water intoxication)
  Hypovolemia
    Total body dehydration ("pure" water loss)
    Extracellular dehydration (salt and water loss)

Solute content
  Hyponatremia
  Hypernatremia

Composition
  Potassium
    Hypokalemia
    Hyperkalemia
  Acid-Base
    Metabolic acidosis
    Metabolic alkalosis
    Respiratory acidosis and alkalosis

than 2 liters) of water or hypotonic fluid to normovolemic patients in the immediate postoperative period, when there is an increased secretion of the antidiuretic hormone (ADH) and aldosterone. These two hormones are primarily responsible for maintenance of fluid and electrolyte homeostasis. Despite correction of the loss of fluid volume that occurs with surgical procedures (blood loss, wound edema), other stresses associated with an operation combine to induce an apparent ''inappropriate'' antidiuresis and retention of sodium (Na). When this occurs, the daily urine volume is less than one liter with a negative free water clearance and an increased specific gravity due to the increased concentration of solute and urea. This type of metabolic response to stress may not occur at all, and it rarely persists more than 2 or 3 days following an uncomplicated injury. Careful attention to reducing the pain, anxiety, and prolonged bed rest, coupled with avoidance of drugs known to stimulate an output of these hormones (narcotics, psychoactive agents, chemotherapeutic compounds, oral hypoglycemic agents, thiazide diuretics), minimizes the proclivity of postoperative patients to retain fluid beyond their need to restore an adequate circulatory volume. The acute ''water intoxication'' that can be produced in the normovolemic postoperative patient by the administration of excess hypotonic fluids differs significantly from the hyponatremia produced when solute-free fluids are used to treat hypovolemia resulting from isotonic losses (discussed in section on *Hyponatremia*). The postoperative patient with water intoxication has an increased circulatory volume that defies correction by the normal homeostatic mechanisms because of the stress-induced transient increase in ADH.

Curtailment of water intake, possibly coupled with the administration of furosemide, which enhances ''free'' water excretion, is adequate therapy. This allows the urinary output plus the insensible losses of fluid to reduce the overloaded circulatory volume and raise, thereby, the total body solute concentration to the normal range. However, if the neurologic signs of acute hypo-osmolality develop (lassitude, headache, seizures, coma), one must cautiously administer hypertonic saline to correct the hypo-osmolality without exaggerating the fluid overload. Ultrafiltration can be effective therapy of this problem. Only rarely is it necessary to use an infusion of hypertonic saline (3% to 5%) to treat these patients. Osmotic diuretics are potentially dangerous because they may expand too rapidly an already overexpanded extracellular fluid (ECF) and circulatory volume.

Hypovolemia

There are two different types of dehydration. These will be considered in the following section, but hypovolemia due to blood loss is omitted as a subject sufficient unto itself.

Total Body Dehydration (primarily water loss). This type of dehydration is uncommonly seen in surgical patients because most of their fluid disorders involve the loss of salt as well as water. When total body dehydration does occur, it usually happens in an unconscious patient who cannot express the severe sensation of thirst, a cardinal symptom of intracellular dehydration. This is most apt to occur in patients with head injuries, or following a neurosurgical procedure that has produced diabetes insipidus, or as a consequence of an osmotic diuresis. Clinical signs of circulatory volume depletion are lacking even with volume deficits equivalent to 10 percent of total body water because *in total body (''pure'') dehydration, the water loss is shared by all body fluid compartments*. This is in marked contrast to the hypovolemia produced by the loss of salt and water (extracellular dehydration), which rapidly induces clinical signs of increased sympathetic activity. Blood pressure is well maintained with total body dehydration, but owing to the loss of water in excess of salt, the concentration of all bodily solutes begins to increase. In time, the circulatory volume becomes sufficiently reduced to induce renal conservation of sodium, despite the increased plasma concentration of this solute (hyperosmolality),* which ordinarily induces naturesis. This ''dehydration reaction,'' described so clearly by John Peters, is applied to reabsorption of Na by the kidneys to conserve water (volume). It is an excellent example of the ordering of homeostatic priorities. Circulatory volume is defended at the expense of osmolality. The concentration of plasma proteins and hematocrit (Hct) also are increased by depletion of total body water, and there is a rise in blood urea nitrogen (BUN) reflecting prerenal azotemia.

Obviously, the therapy of patients with ''pure'' dehydration is administration of water and, not so obviously, these patients also benefit from adding some salt to the water (to be discussed). Since many of these patients are obtunded or otherwise incapable of taking oral fluids, therapy is usually given by the intravenous route. However, one must be careful not to reduce too rapidly hyperosmolality produced by the relative lack of body water (see section on *Hypernatremia*).

Extracellular Dehyration (Desalting Dehydration or Volume Depletion). For the surgical patient, the three primary causes of large losses of fluid volume are (1) hemorrhage, (2) gastrointestinal disorders, and (3) sequestration of fluid in various areas of the body (third space) owing to such disorders as intestinal obstruction, trauma, infection, and burns. From a therapeutic standpoint, the common denominator of the several disorders causing extracellular volume depletion in surgical patients is a loss of isotonic fluid.

In assessing the nature and extent of volume depletion, the clinical history and examination of the patient are the most important sources of reliable information. A distinction between dehydration and depletion of salt and volume is initially evident from historical information regarding mental status, head injury, previous medical

---

* In health, the concentration of sodium in our hospital varies between 135 and 145 mEq per liter of serum. A more precise expression of concentration, osmolality, is based on a liter or kilogram of serum water. Since serum ordinarily has a water content of 93 percent, this expression is about 7 percent higher than the usual values obtained from the hospital laboratory.

disorders, and acute losses of fluid such as vomiting and diarrhea. In marked contrast to total body dehydration, patients with salt and water depletion begin to demonstrate, relatively early in the course of their fluid loss, the signs, symptoms, and laboratory changes characteristic of a reduced circulatory volume. The 10 percent reduction of total body water tolerated by a total body dehydrated patient (about 6% of body weight) is equivalent to a 20 to 30 percent reduction of plasma volume in patients with salt and water dehydration because these losses are confined largely to the ECF. An acute depletion of circulatory volume greater than 15 to 20 percent can be expected to produce orthostatic hypotension (a drop to 70 mm Hg or below within 1 to 2 minutes on rising to a standing position) in all but well-conditioned individuals. The conventional signs of decreased skin turgor, sunken eyeballs, diaphoresis, tachycardia, reduced pulse pressure and, in more advanced states, a fall in systolic pressure generally are dependable clinical indices of circulatory insufficiency. In children, dry mucous membranes and lack of tears when crying are the best signs. Skin turgor is hard to evaluate in children.

To a great extent, these clinical signs are manifestations of the increased activity of the sympathetic nervous system, induced to defend homeostasis of circulatory volume. In an oliguric patient, the laboratory data usually reveal an elevated urine specific gravity with rise in BUN, plasma creatinine, and Hct. Conversely, the Hct falls rapidly within 1 to 2 hours following any significant hemorrhage in a well-hydrated patient. The distinction between an extrarenal cause for fluid loss, "prerenal azotemia," and renal losses of Na from intrinsic kidney disease can be facilitated by measurement of the concentration of Na in the urine. The homeostatic mechanisms protecting circulatory volume restrict renal Na excretion to less than 5 mEq per liter (upper limit is 20 mEq per liter with prerenal azotemia) when extrarenal fluid losses are present, whereas the loss of Na in the urine rises above 20 mEq per liter when renal (or adrenal) problems are responsible for the loss of salt and water. A more precise assessment is the fractional excretion of sodium:

$$(FeNa) = \frac{urine\ Na}{plasma\ Na} \div \frac{urine\ creatinine}{plasma\ creatinine}$$

(Values < 1 = prerenal causes; > 1 = intrinsic renal disease. This calculation is applicable only if the patient is oliguric.)

The degree to which intracellular fluid (ICF) volume participates in defense of circulatory volume depends on (1) the duration and extent of depletion, and (2) whether or not there is a rise in plasma osmolality that would serve to pull fluid out of the cells. Through mechanisms as yet poorly understood, it is probable that ICF volume, in time, does help to defend against acute isotonic losses of ECF greater than 10 to 15 percent. The concentration of serum sodium is totally worthless as a test for determining volume loss because it may be reduced, normal, or elevated in dehydrated patients. The serum concentration

reflects only a ratio, the number of milliequivalents of sodium per liter of serum. At issue is the deficiency in the number of liters. Thus, with isotonic losses, one should not expect to find a change in serum Na. In these patients a change in serum Na results from either iatrogenic causes or movement of water from the cells to protect the circulation when there has been a large loss of volume. Administration of potassium can cause a rise in serum Na. The problems associated with hypo- and hypernatremia are to be discussed subsequently.

Treatment of hypovolemia is based largely on clinical judgment. Although the rise in Hct is a good indicator of the extent of a volume deficit due to combined water and salt losses, the fall in Hct is an imprecise guide, at best, for the treatment of blood loss. The change in Hct is also useful for estimating the volume loss in "pure" dehydration if one takes into account that, in this circumstance, the change in hematocrit reflects loss of total body water rather than loss confined to the ECF. Usually, serial measurements of Hct combined with observations of urine output, blood pressure, and the clinical response to infusion of fluids is sufficient to provide dependable guides for the rate and volume of fluid therapy. Naturally, patients must be observed with care to preclude an excessive administration of fluid. When the extent of fluid loss necessitates the rapid infusion of fluid or when the patient has precarious cardiovascular compensation, the use of a catheter to monitor the central venous pressure or insertion of a Swan-Ganz catheter to monitor the pulmonary capillary wedge pressure as an index of left atrial pressure will provide more precise quantitation of the cardiovascular response to restoration of fluids. It is often forgotten that crystalloid fluids can be infused, even to a patient with borderline cardiac decompensation, at the rate of 250 ml per hour without precipitating acute pulmonary edema provided there is a need for additional fluid to be administered. Measurement of the concentration of electrolytes in plasma is not a substitute for clinical judgment supported by hemodynamic monitoring during the restoration of fluid volume. However, these laboratory values are critically important to assess the appropriate solute content and composition of the fluids used in this therapy (to be discussed).

The four basic principles of therapy for acute volume depletion are soundly based on the physiologic mechanisms that support body fluid homeostasis:

1. All losses incurred by hemorrhage, gastrointestinal disorders, and sequestered fluid are detrimental—none are "sensible" in terms of body needs. Therefore, all of these losses must be replaced.
2. Since these losses almost invariably are isotonic, they produce acute depletion of ECF (most importantly intravascular volume) with scant mobilization of intracellular water to replace the defect. Consequently, replacement fluids, other than allowing for insensible losses of approximately 800 ml per day, should reflect the *solute content* + composition of the fluid that is lost.

Coexisting alterations in *plasma solute content* + composition will be "fine-tuned" by mechanisms supporting homeostasis after an adequate circulatory volume has been restored. Colloids other than blood are rarely needed during the initial 24 hours of therapy for an acute depletion of ECF or blood volume. A possible exception is the use of fresh frozen plasma to treat disseminated intravascular coagulation.

3. The fluid losses frequently involve loss of fixed acid or base. Although the body cannot replace these losses, it can compensate partially for them. It cannot be overemphasized how well the kidney can correct acid-base imbalances if only it is given the fluid volume and electrolytes (including potassium) with which to work. Therapy must be oriented initially toward volume replacement even in the face of acid-base (composition) alterations.

4. An important adjunct to restoration of an adequate fluid volume is provision of sufficient calories to prevent or minimize the undesirable sequelae of starvation-acidosis, loss of potassium (K), and loss of nitrogen (N). The classic studies of Gamble demonstrated that a minimum of 100 g carbohydrate per day will approach these objectives as well as foster renal conservation of sodium.

ALTERATIONS IN SOLUTE CONTENT OF BODY FLUIDS (OSMOLALITY)

Hyponatremia

Since Na salts constitute more than 95 percent of the total body solutes in extracellular fluid and since water generally moves freely and rapidly across all compartments of body fluids, the measured concentration of Na in the serum provides a reasonable precise and useful guide to the osmolality of total body water. Consequently, a rise or fall in serum sodium concentration indicates a corresponding shrinking or swelling of cellular size in response to an osmotic gradient induced by sodium which, in the absence of K depletion, remains confined largely to the ECF space. When hypo-osmolality occurs, one can be confident that the body fluids have become diluted by an excess of water relative to total solute. The use of serum concentration of Na as a guide to total body osmolality is valid with two exceptions: (1) hyperlipidemia or extreme hyperproteinemia cause a spurious hypo-osmolality because the lipid or protein occupies a disproportionate space in the sample of serum analyzed for its electrolyte content, and (2) hyperglycemia acting as an osmotic agent draws cellular fluid into extracellular spaces, thereby diluting the serum concentration of sodium. There is a decrease of 1.6 mEq per liter for each rise of 100 mg per 100 ml of glucose. Calculation of total body fluid osmolality on the basis of the serum concentration of sodium with correction for the contribution of glucose and urea in the serum can be made by the formula:

$$2 \times ([Na^+ + [K^+]) + \frac{Glucose \ mg/100 \ ml}{18} + \frac{BUN \ mg/100 \ ml}{2.8}$$

Although hyponatremia otherwise reflects hypo-osmolality, hyponatremia is not equivalent to total body sodium depletion, nor does it inform us about the volume of plasma or total body water.

Hyponatremia can occur with expanded, normal, or depleted body fluids. Ordinarily a fall in osmolality induces prompt diuresis by inhibition of ADH. Thus, when plasma sodium falls, it reflects one or more of the following: (1) secretion of ADH in defense of plasma volume which has superseded the role of ADH in defense of plasma volume which has supersceded the role of ADH in protecting osmolality, (2) advanced disease of the liver, kidney, or heart with retention of water in excess of sodium, (3) the syndrome of inappropriate secretion of ADH (SIADH), or (4) there may be rare clinical situations in which the osmoreceptors become "reset" to control serum sodium at a lower level. This may occur after prolonged or marked hypovolemic shock, or it may be a part of the mechanism responsible for the edema associated with cardiac, renal, or hepatic dysfunction.

For the surgical patient, however, acute hyponatremia usually reflects one of two iatrogenic errors:

1. Infusion or ingestion of a large volume of free water at a time when a compensatory diuresis is inhibited by high levels of ADH. This is most likely to occur, as noted in the section on hypervolemia, in the early postoperative period when there may be a high level of circulating ADH released in response to pain, anxiety, and many drugs.

2. Use of hypotonic fluid to replace isotonic losses. In the well-hydrated patient, hypotonic fluids are excreted to protect total body fluid osmolality. In the presence of significant hypovolemia, however, the compensatory renal and hormonal mechanisms defend volume by retention of the administered water, leading to a dilution of serum sodium, instead of protecting osmolality by diuresis. A 7 to 10 percent depletion of circulatory volume initiates this defense of volume over osmolality. One can be virtually certain that any volume deficiency that requires more than two liters of fluid for treatment will induce hyponatremia if the fluid administered is not iso-osmotic.

Although the level of serum sodium establishes the diagnosis of hypo-osmolality of total body fluids, it does not reflect the existing volume of the circulation. The mechanisms responsible for hyponatremia can be determined with fair confidence from the patient's history, fluid intake and output record, and the composition of the fluid administered. Circulatory volume must be evaluated on the basis of hemodynamic functions, as already noted. Specific therapy depends on the physician's judgment whether the decrease in osmolality reflects an iatrogenic problem, an inappropriate secretion of ADH, or a pre-existing medical disorder; multiple factors may be responsible for the hyponatremia in some cases.

The need for therapy and the urgency with which it should be provided is determined by (1) the severity of clinical symptoms produced by hypo-osmolality and (2) whether or not there is an associated excess or deficit in circulatory volume. Although correction of volume deficit or excess must receive the first priority, one must remember that hypo-osmolality can lead to neurologic manifestations such as increasing confusion leading to coma and hyperexcitability progressing to twitches, tremors, convulsions, and ultimately death. One becomes concerned when the serum sodium concentration falls rapidly (within a day or two) from its normal level by more than 10 to 15 mEq per liter. The rate of fall has a significant influence on the proclivity for symptoms to develop. This probably explains why patients with chronic hyponatremia may be free of adverse symptoms even at low levels of sodium in the serum. A reset of the osmostat or a compensatory increase in the solute content within the cells may be mechanisms that help to prevent dangerous neurologic consequences in the patient with chronic hyponatremia.

Often no therapy is needed. In the postoperative patient given excess water, the necessary diuresis will ensue as the stimulus for ADH declines.

If hypervolemia is present and the kidneys are still under control of an increased secretion of ADH, it may be necessary to resort to ultrafiltration to reduce the fluid overload and raise the serum osmolality. The main danger with this approach is the rapid change in osmolality that may occur. If hypovolemia is responsible for an apparent inappropriate retention of water, the therapeutic priority clearly is to restore an adequate circulatory volume with isotonic fluid. This provides some of the required intake of solute in excess of water and, as the hypovolemic stimulus for ADH is turned off, the remaining relative excess water is excreted. Thus, one can depend on the homeostatic mechanisms of the body for the fine tuning of osmotic adjustments.

Only rarely is a hypertonic solution required for therapy. When neurologic symptoms dictate the need for urgent therapy, hypertonic solutions of NaCl (3% to 5%) are infused. The amount to be given can be calculated easily by multiplying the deficit in plasma sodium concentration by the estimated normal volume of total body water (60% body weight in kilograms). The planned correction of the deficit must take into account that fluids will shift from the intracellular to extracellular fluid to maintain iso-osmolality as the hypertonic sodium is infused. Thus *the correction fluid must be given slowly* to prevent rapid expansion of plasma volume with the attendant danger of inducing pulmonary edema. Generally, administration of one-half the calculated deficit of sodium over a 24-hour period raises the osmolality above the level that induced

symptoms. Additional hypertonic fluid can be administered cautiously over the next day or two, but usually further adjustments can be left to the intrinsic mechanisms supporting body fluid homeostasis.

Therapy also must be constrained by knowledge that overly rapid correction of osmotic alterations induces potentially lethal neurologic changes. Apparently the brain cells compensate to a variable extent for osmotic changes in their environment by an increase or decrease in the number of intracellular solute particles. Vigorous correction of a changed ECF osmolality (hyper- or hypona-tremia) may adversely affect cellular size if this internal adjustment has occurred before therapy is provided.

Attempts to correct longstanding hyponatremia are contraindicated because the cells have become adjusted to the altered osmolality. When SIADH is responsible for the low level of serum sodium, a restriction in water intake usually is sufficient to help restore osmolality to a more nearly normal level.

Hypernatremia

Hypernatremia reflects a deficiency in total body water relative to solute content. For the surgeon, the situations most commonly encountered with hypertonic body fluids result from (1) the acute onset of diabetes insipidus in a postoperative neurosurgical patient or following a head injury; fever, especially the hypothalmic fever from head trauma, increases insensible water loss, thereby causing even a greater deficit of total body water; (2) the excessive administration of solutes without sufficient water; and (3) the "dehydration reaction" in which there is a marked deficiency in circulatory volume in association with a defect in total body water. It is important to remember that hypernatremia can be produced by intrinsic renal disease and by an excess of salt-retaining hormones (Table 2). Common to all of these disorders is the failure of the patient to manifest or to be capable of responding to the strong stimulus of thirst that develops from hyper-tonicity. Many of these patients are either comatose or restrained in a manner that prevents easy access to water.

A rise in plasma sodium establishes the diagnosis of hypertonicity of all body fluids, but it does not provide

TABLE 2   Causes of Hypernatremia

Failure of renal conversion of water
   Diabetes insipidus
      Chronic neurohypophyseal deficiencies
      Acute response to injury
   Loss of renal tubule response to ADH
      Intrinsic renal disease
      K, Ca, Li, and pH

Osmotic Diuresis
   High-solute tube feeding in comatose patients
   Diuretics
   Glycosuria

Excess of Na-retaining hormones
   (Cushing's syndrome, hyperaldosteronism)

Dehydration reaction

information as to whether the relative deficit of water represents inability of the kidney to retain water or a disorder that overwhelmed the renal mechanisms to conserve water. Finding a urine hypotonic to serum in the presence of hypernatremia in a patient who responds to the administration of ADH establishes the diagnosis of diabetes insipidus and helps to determine the therapy. Failure of renal tubule response to ADH can be produced by alterations in serum electrolytes and, more rarely, it occurs in patients with nephrogenic diabetes insipidus. The contribution of osmotic diuresis to hyperosmolality is usually easily determined from a history of a large solute loss in a patient who did not receive sufficient water. Renal retention of Na due to adrenal hyperfunction can be detected by a measured increase in the plasma level of the responsible hormones.

By the time the hypernatremia becomes clinically evident, there has been loss of fluid from the intracellular to the extracellular compartment to compensate for the rise in tonicity of ECF. Thus, the presenting clinical signs reflect intracellular dehydration primarily manifested in the central nervous system by confusion followed by stupor, convulsions, and death. Since the defect in water is shared across all body compartments, these patients usually do not show signs of an acute deficiency in circulatory volume, and they often have a loss of Na in the urine. The one major exception, however, is the "dehydration reaction," as noted previously, in which sodium is retained and potassium is excreted in excess despite a normal blood potassium level. The naturesis ordinarily associated with a rise in serum osmolality is replaced by renal retention of Na subservient to the homeostatic hierarchy of protecting circulatory volume before osmolality. This effect on Na retention is mediated by increased aldosterone output.

The treatment of hypernatremia is directed toward restoring normal osmolality of body fluids. But caution must be observed; an overly vigorous rate of reduction in serum Na is not tolerated well by the central nervous system. Since the water deficit is shared by all fluid compartments, calculation of replacement fluid should be based on total body water (60% body weight in young men; 50% in young women).

$$\text{Total Body Water} \times \frac{\text{Existing Serum Na}}{\text{Desired Serum Na}} - \text{Total Body Water}$$

$$= \text{Vol. Water Needed}$$

The calculated volume of water ordinarily is given over a 2- to 3-day period. Often the composition of the fluid should include some salt (0.25 normal saline) to correct a deficit of Na and Cl because total body solutes usually are decreased by conditions that produce hypernatremia. Additional salt (0.5 normal or isotonic saline) is required for therapy of the "dehydration reaction" that develops in the hypovolemic patient with hypernatremia. Antidiuretic hormone is administered when diabetes insipidus is present. An osmotic diuresis is brought under control by attention to the causative factors. Overall, until the patient is capable of expressing thirst and drinks water, it remains the responsibility of the attending physician to provide sufficient water on a continuing basis to prevent a recurrence of hyperosmolality.

ALTERATIONS IN COMPOSITION OF BODY FLUIDS

Potassium

Potassium (K), the major determinant of intracellular solute concentration, is involved in many metabolic processes. The transcellular movement of this important ion is influenced greatly by the acid-base balance of body fluids. Acidosis promotes the loss of K from its high intracellular concentration (150 mEq per liter) into a low extracellular concentration (3.5 to 5.0 mEq per liter). Alkalosis causes K^+ to move in the opposite direction, into cells, against a concentration gradient.

Hypokalemia. Renal retention of K in response to a low intake or an increased loss of K from the body requires several days to reach its maximum effectiveness. Nevertheless, it is usually operational by the time clinical symptoms of K deficiency become apparent. The usual causes for K depletion in surgical patients are disorders of the gastrointestinal tract and renal losses under the influence of diuretics, mineral corticoids, or intrinsic renal disease. The diagnosis of hypokalemia is confirmed by neuromuscular abnormalities, particularly weakness, by EKG changes of flattening and inversion of the T wave, and by a low level of K in the serum. The urine loss is less than 20 to 25 mEq per liter when gastrointestinal disorders are responsible for hypokalemia, but the loss exceeds these values when renal abnormalities are responsible. Diarrhea may also lead to large potassium deficits because the concentration of potassium may be 40 to 60 mEq per liter in liquid stool. Acting through incompletely understood mechanisms, hypokalemia impairs renal concentrating abilities. Potassium depletion is rarely, if ever, found without an associated deficit of water and sodium which should also be replaced.

Therapy depends largely on the cause for the loss of K and the extent of clinical signs of its deficiency. Oral supplementation with KCl is preferred, particularly in alkalotic patients. The gastrointestinal disorders usually require administration of K by intravenous infusion. If the concentration of KCl exceeds 40 mEq per liter, it is likely to cause burning at the site of infusion. Unless the rate of infusion is monitored carefully, it may induce cardiac arrhythmias. There is a slow exchange of administered K with the cellular K of many organs. If rapid administration of fluids containing K is required, electrocardiographic monitoring is essential. Also, it is probably wise to reduce the concentration of K in these fluids. A change in the clinical symptoms of weakness and serial determinations of the level of K in the serum assist in monitoring the response to K therapy. A word of caution relates to the not-uncommon association of hypokalemia with hypocalcemia. Correction of one disorder without attention to the other may precipitate the signs and symptoms of a deficiency of the neglected electrolyte.

Hyperkalemia. This condition is probably the most feared early complication for surgical patients who develop acute oliguria or anuria. In these patients the concentration of K in plasma increases about 0.5 mEq per liter per day even in the absence of abnormal loads. Situations most likely to cause this complication are episodes of hypotension and hypovolemia associated with cellular damage. A rapid desalting dehydration secondary to peritonitis, intestinal obstruction, vomiting, or diarrhea causes an increased loss of K into plasma, owing to the associated acidosis and/or cellular injury. However, it is the combination of renal shutdown with acidosis and tissue damage that usually leads to dangerous hyperkalemia rather than any one cause acting alone. The plasma K rises rapidly (2 to 4 mEq per liter per day) under these circumstances. The cardinal signs of danger relate to cardiac arrhythmias manifested by high peaked T waves in the EKG and atrial asystole leading to terminal ventricular tachycardia with fibrillation. Cardiac arrest occurs in systole. Therapy becomes urgent when the serum potassium exceeds 7 or 8 mEq per liter, although certain patients may tolerate considerably higher levels before signs of toxicity develop. In the presence of severe hyperkalemia, the EKG record also has absent P waves with of the QRS complex. Ventricular arrhythmias indicate that therapy is urgently required. An infusion of as much as 30 ml of a 10% solution of calcium gluconate over a 5-minute period with EKG monitoring should ameliorate the immediate dangerous cardiac and neuromuscular responses to the high level of potassium. This "buys time" for the effect of an infusion of 10 to 20% glucose containing 10 to 20 units of regular (crystalline) insulin. Potassium is carried into the cells with glucose. To become effective, this infusion is usually safely given at the rate of 200 ml within the initial 30 minutes, followed by additional quantities depending on changes in symptoms, the EKG, and serum levels of K. Since acidosis is present in renal failure with hyperkalemia, the effect of this infusion is enhanced by the addition of 100 mEq of sodium bicarbonate (NaHCO₃ to a liter of the infusion media. This alkalinization also drives K into the cells. The hypertonic media made by combining 100 to 200 g glucose and 100 mEq NaHCO₃ in a liter of water may have additional therapeutic value owing to the osmotically induced dilution of plasma potassium. A hypertonic solution has an indirect inhibitory effect on the neuromuscular toxicity induced by hyperkalemia. If calcium, glucose, and bicarbonate are needed, either dialysis or a cationic exchange resin (Kayexalate) is needed as definitive treatment. Patients with persistent renal insufficiency may require repeated dialysis to maintain a normal level of serum potassium.

Acid-Base Balance

From a practical standpoint, the acid-base status of total body fluids can be characterized with reasonable, clinically useful, precision by knowledge of the hydrogen ion concentration (H^+) and the partial pressure of carbon dioxide (Pco_2[6]). For the purist, the total dissociated bicarbonate is related to H^+ as expressed in the Henderson-Hasselbalch equation:

$$pH = pK \text{ bicarb} + \log \frac{HCO_3}{0.03 \times Pco_2}$$

where 0.03 represents the solubility coefficient of CO_2 in plasma. The concentration of dissolved CO_2 determines the carbonic acid (H_2CO_3) for this equation. As long as a ratio of 20:1 of HCO_3 to dissolved CO_2 is maintained, the pH is protected within the optimal range for cellular functions. Alterations in ventilation regulate the loss of H_2CO_3 (Pco_2) while renal excretion controls the rate of HCO_3 loss. These organs function to maintain the 20:1 ratio of base to acid (HCO_3 to H_2CO_3) rather than to maintain the absolute quantity of either. Metabolic disorders disturb the concentration of HCO_3, whereas respiratory disorders alter the concentration of CO_2. Acidosis, which may have a metabolic or a respiratory cause, occurs when acid (H^+) is added or alkali (HCO_3) is removed from the body fluids. On the other hand, physiologic disturbances that either remove acid or add base to body fluids cause alkalosis. Homeostasis of pH is protected when a primary change in HCO_3 induces a respiratory response that alters the plasma carbonic acid in the same direction to protect the 20:1 ratio. Conversely, a primary change in CO_2 induces a compensatory increase or decrease in renal excretion of HCO_3, although this response requires one or more days to become effective in contrast to the immediate influence of respiratory alterations.

Metabolic Acidosis. The leading causes of metabolic acidosis in surgical patients are (1) accumulation of nonvolatile acids and the end products from anaerobic metabolism from (a) hypoperfusion of tissues, (b) reduced arterial oxygen saturation, or (c) ketoacids produced by starvation or diabetes mellitus; (2) excessive loss of alkaline gastrointestinal (GI) fluids, and (3) decreased acid excretion by the kidney owing either to an associated reduction of circulatory volume or to intrinsic renal failure. When the H^+ rises in body fluids, HCO_3 falls through immediate action of the HCO_3/H_2CO_3 buffer system; quickly thereafter respiration is stimulated to produce a compensatory reduction of the carbonic acid content of plasma in order to maintain the 20:1 ratio of the buffer system that is required for protection of the pH of body fluids.

Treatment directed exclusively to correct an abnormality in acid-base balance without attention to the underlying cause of the abnormality fails to recognize the hierarchical ordering of homeostatic priorities. As a result, single-minded devotion to correcting pH may be unnecessary, ineffectual, or actually detrimental. When the metabolic acidosis is due to low flow, diarrhea, or loss of alkaline gastrointestinal secretions, restoration of an inadequate circulatory volume is mandatory. Return of renal perfusion usually allows the kidney to correct the acid-base abnormality. It is rarely necessary to use intravenous sodium bicarbonate to supplement volume therapy of acute metabolic acidosis. However, if it is used, the amount required can be calculated from a change in the "anion gap." Subtraction of the sum of serum Cl and HCO_3 concentration from the serum Na concentration is a simple, convenient expression of the "anion gap." Normally, this is in the range of 4 to 12 mEq per liter (or, since these are monovalent ions, the gap can be expressed as milliosmoles). Some laboratories add the serum concentration of K to serum Na in calculating the "anion gap"; the range of normal values is 10 to 16 mEq per liter with this calculation. Probably the most valuable result of calculating the "anion gap" is the clue this provides to the etiology of the acid-base imbalance. When the metabolic acidosis is due to a loss of HCO_3 by diarrhea or upper intestinal fluid loss, the anion gap is not increased because there is an equivalent loss of sodium. However, it increases when there is an accumulation of lactic or ketoacids with low perfusion states, starvation, or diabetes. In these conditions, the HCO_3 is removed to "make room" for the acids. An increased respiratory loss of CO_2 compensates in turn to maintain the 20:1 ratio of the bicarbonate buffer system that protects pH. By multiplying the increase in the anion gap (mEq per liter) by the volume of ECF (20% of body weight), one can derive a reasonable estimate of the safe quantity of bicarbonate that can be given intravenously to supplement therapy of the depleted circulatory volume. At best, this is an underestimate of the deficit because at least one-half of the administered bicarbonate is taken up by intracellular buffers. However, it is unwise to seek total correction of the deficit in bicarbonate because of the potential toxic effects of raising the pH too rapidly or of overshooting the mark and producing alkalosis. Alkalosis may induce hypokalemic cardiac toxicity, or tetany from hypocalcemia. Furthermore, as the circulatory volume is restored, the accumulated lactic acid and ketone bodies are metabolized to bicarbonate, thereby adding endogenous assistance to correction of the acid-base imbalance. The one circumstance in which urgent $NaHCO_3$ may be valuable is in the treatment of cardiac arrest.

Metabolic Alkalosis. In the surgical patient, metabolic alkalosis usually results from loss of acid from the stomach owing to prolonged vomiting or gastric aspiration. Today it rarely occurs as a result of prolonged intake of alkali. It is also a secondary phenomenon associated with syndromes involving hyperadrenocorticism (Cushing, Conn, Bartter). Extreme depletion of K, which can occur if there is a deficit of water and sodium, causes metabolic alkalosis. If the plasma concentration of K^+ falls below 2 mEq per liter, it intensifies the problem induced by other causes. Since the kidney possesses such a tremendous capacity to excrete HCO_3, development of a metabolic alkalosis almost invariably means that renal defense has been altered, either by reduced circulatory volume or in response to hyperadrenocorticism or potassium deficiency.

Once again, treatment directed solely to the acid-base imbalance can be dangerous. Administration of HCl or NH_4Cl temporarily corrects the alkalosis, but it ignores the possibility of a fundamental defect in the circulatory volume. Administration of NaCl is essential for correction of the depleted ECF volume. If K depletion also exists, this must be corrected. In fact, if it does not exist, it will develop as a result of NaCl therapy. After the circulatory volume, solute content, and K loss have been restored, the kidneys excrete Na with HCO_3 to correct the alkalosis. Many additional days may be required to fully correct the K depletion. A misleading term "chloride depletion alkalosis" refers, in fact, to a deficit of both Na and Cl. But the term does signify the necessity to restore Cl, as well as Na, in the therapy of this disorder. The excessive loss of H^+ and Cl^- in conditions such as the Zollinger-Ellison (ZE) syndrome can be controlled by use of the H_2 antagonist, cimetidine, or its newer derivative, ranitidine, rather than by resorting to administration of dilute HCl or NH_4Cl. Unless sufficient NaCl is provided to correct a volume deficit, a "paradoxical aciduria" can develop. This is usually found in children who have prolonged vomiting caused by pyloric stenosis or in adults with "subtraction alkalosis." In this situation, the kidneys excrete K and H in order to conserve Na after circulatory volume has become threatened. Later, as the K deficiency becomes pronounced, the production of NH_4 is augmented, leading to a greater renal loss of hydrogen ion. The urine pH is usually near 7.0 in these patients despite the substantial metabolic alkalosis in their body fluids. Although the mechanisms are not fully understood, it seems likely that the K deficiency causes a shift of H^+ into cells. In the renal epithelial cells, the change in ratio of these two ions promotes the secretion of H^+, while HCO_3 reabsorption is maintained at a high threshold. Thus, therapy must be directed to the correction of the three dominant defects, volume, sodium, and potassium.

In view of the frequent use of diuretics in surgical patients, it behooves the surgeon to be aware of the proclivity of these potent agents to induce metabolic alkalosis. This complication of diuretic therapy is produced by direct inhibition of Cl transport in the kidney and loss of Cl combined with secretion of hydronium, ammonium, and K. The consequential hypokalemic metabolic alkalosis may require therapy with KCl as well as adjustment of the diuretic medication.

Respiratory compensation for metabolic alkalosis is rapid, but it is limited by hypoxia. Thus, ventilation decreases sufficiently to raise the P_{CO_2}, but it rarely causes a rise of P_{CO_2} above 50 to 55 mm Hg.

Respiratory Acidosis and Alkalosis. The pulmonary control of CO_2 excretion constitutes the first line of defense of the pH of body fluids. By the same token, acute pulmonary disorders promptly induce a serious threat to homeostasis of pH; any compensation the body can make beyond the limited modulation afforded by tissue buffers is dependent on renal alteration in the excretion of HCO_3 and acid. This compensation requires time. For instance, the respiratory acidosis that develops as a result of acute respiratory insufficiency is due to an inability to excrete the rapidly produced CO_2 from daily metabolic activity. The renal adjustment to protect the 20:1 ratio of HCO_3 to Pco_2 requires several days. If the disorder is sustained, the kidneys do respond by excretion of acid and reabsorption of HCO_3 to minimize the degree of acidemia.

Respiratory alkalosis due to a decrease in arterial Pco_2 may be caused by a large number of disorders that produce hyperventilation. All of us are familiar with the characteristic clinical picture of numbness, tingling, light-headedness, and even tetany that can be induced by voluntary hyperventilation. The body buffers and renal compensatory mechanisms are not sufficiently prompt to prevent these changes induced by a sudden respiratory loss of carbonic acid. In time, the kidney reduces reabsorption of bicarbonate to bring the plasma level of bicarbonate closer to the required ratio with Pco_2.

In both respiratory acidosis and alkalosis, the only appropriate therapy is directed to correct the underlying respiratory disorder. Rapid infusion of alkali may be justified in the treatment of cardiopulmonary arrest, but it is dangerous to give bicarbonate to a patient with respiratory acidosis because the respiratory drive from an elevated H^+ concentration may be reduced. These disorders are properly treated by discovery of the underlying respiratory problem and dealing directly with this alteration.

NIH Grant GM30095 provides support for ongoing studies relevant to the concepts presented in this chapter.

INTRAVENOUS HYPERALIMENTATION IN THE SURGICAL PATIENT

JAMES V. SITZMANN, M.D., F.A.C.S.

In 1904, William Stewart Halsted declared that "pain, hemorrhage, infection, the three great evils which had always embittered the practice of surgery" would eventually be controlled. Today, we would also add a fourth evil, malnutrition. There is no longer doubt that operative morbidity and mortality are greatly affected by a patient's nutritional status. However, although malnutrition has embittered the practice of surgery, this evil can be better overcome today than at any time before.

Just as a surgeon needs to understand control of hemorrhage and infection, so he must also know how to reverse or prevent malnutrition. From a practical standpoint, this involves (1) knowledge of the pathophysiology of starvation as it interacts with each disease state, (2) knowledge of biochemical adaptation and response of the body to disease andd starvation, and (3) knowledge of the pharmacology of nutrients required by the body and, in the case of hyperalimentation, surgical techniques needed for vascular access.

INDICATIONS

Indications for nutritional support (whether enteral or parenteral) are discovered in the same fashion as are the indications for any other therapy of any other disease. Thus the physician must first diagnose the condition and then determine treatment. Nutritional support is a treatment for the disease of malnutrition.

The diagnosis of malnutrition is occasionally problematic, and if it is straightforward, it has been delayed. As with any illness, the diagnosis is arrived at by history, physical examination, and laboratory examination. A careful history brings to light most of the general indications for hyperalimentation. The actual need for support is confirmed by laboratory and physical examinations.

In general, any patient who has lost 10 percent of his or her body weight and is unable to absorb enough calories from his gut is a candidate for hyperalimentation. This becomes more critical if a "catabolic load" such as an operation or chemotherapy is to be placed on the patient.

Thus any patient who already has lost weight or is expected to be unable to maintain oral intake, or is expected to become "hypermetabolic," will need support. In general these states include:

1. Pediatric patients of low birth weight or those who have congenital or developmental gut defects such as gastroschisis, malrotation, tracheoesophageal fistulas, Hirschsprung's disease, omphaloceles, short gut syndrome, or metabolic abnormality precluding normal gut function (e.g., VIP syndrome, cystic fibrosis).
2. Adult short gut syndromes following massive bowel resection for vascular catastrophe or volvulus, or multiple resection for Crohn's disease or small bowel obstruction.
3. Malabsorptive syndromes of which inflammatory bowel disease (Crohn's, ulcerative colitis), Whipple's disease, celiac sprue, angiodysplasia, and abetaliproteinemia are the most common causes. Other major causes of malabsorption are radiation enteritis and, less frequently, idiopathic malabsorption, adult Hirschsprung's disease, or aganglionosis.
4. Secondary gut failure, due to major organ system failure such as pancreatitis, intestinal fistulas, biliary fistulas, hepatic failure, chronic partial bowel obstruction, or high bowel obstruction.

5. Gut insufficiency in the face of overwhelming catabolic demand. In these instances the patient is stressed to such a degree that the gut could not conceivably absorb the amount of calories needed for recovery. These include multiple trauma, major (greater than 30%) body burns, major sepsis with concomitant organ failure (e.g., respiratory failure, anuric renal failure).

6. Preoperative preparation. The patient scheduled for a major operative procedure can be fed preoperatively with oral supplements and postoperatively with jejunal feeding catheters. Nonetheless, many patients with high intestinal malignant disease are not able to absorb a nutrient load, and the large postoperative catabolic demand cannot be met via gut alimentation. Thus patients with gastric, pancreatic, biliary, or esophageal carcinomas frequently require hyperalimentation.

7. Chemotherapy or radiotherapy. Patients undergoing combined chemotherapy, radiotherapy, or surgical therapy of malignant tumors have long periods of sustained stress without adequate gut function. Although hyperalimentation does not improve the efficacy of chemotherapy or radiotherapy, it certainly improves the patient's overall status and well-being.

In theory, most patients who are considered for hyperalimentation should manifest some abnormality on anthropometric examination (a measure of somatic protein and fat stores) or laboratory examination (a measure of visceral protein stores). However, anthropometric examination has been amply criticized in the last several years, mainly on the grounds that it is subject to interpretive errors, lacks sensitivity, and does not reflect early changes in nutritional status. All these criticisms merely reflect the fact that somatic protein and fat stores change slowly in response to catabolic stress. Nonetheless, in the newly hospitalized patient, anthropometric examination can document certain starvation states that laboratory examination cannot. This is especially true in the chronic starvation state, in which a patient "adapts" to starvation. Its usefulness is limited, but when viewed as one of several ways to assess nutritional status, its value is clear.

The laboratory determination of nutritional status is also subject to error, depending on the disease state of the host. The most commonly used laboratory value of nutritional status is serum albumin. This, like the anthropometric examination, is of some worth, especially in the newly hospitalized patient, but has little value as a long-term measure of response to nutritional support. It loses its value during long hospitalizations when patients receive exogenous albumin or undergo major fluid shifts, or in the event of liver dysfunction due to parenchymal disease, cor pulmonale, or sepsis. Owing to the long half-life of serum albumin this value is slow to react to positive changes in nitrogen balance. More useful is the serum transferrin level, which should manifest an increase after 10 to 14 days of adequate nutrition. Rarely used are pre-albumin and retinal binding protein, two proteins that have even shorter half-life than transferrin, but are more costly to measure.

In addition to liver proteins, immune competence is a readily available measure of nutritional status. Two measures of immune competence are used: skin test to antigen stimulation and lymphocyte count. Skin testing is cumbersome, time-consuming, and painful to the patient and thus is not commonly used. Absolute lymphocyte count is simpler and cheaper. Generally an absolute lymphocyte count of less than 1,500 indicates depressed immune competence. Unless the patient has received radiotherapy, chemotherapy, or steroids, this is a straightforward indication of malnutrition.

In summary, when assessing a patient's initial nutritional status, a good rule of thumb to determine malnutrition is to look for three abnormalities: (1) weight loss of 10 percent or greater in the previous 2 months, (2) a serum albumin less than 3.4 g per deciliter, and (3) an absolute lymphocyte count less than 1,500. Patients who manifest one abnormality are malnourished; those who manifest three are severely malnourished. For the patient with an ongoing disease state who is unable or will be unable to maintain oral intake, intravenous hyperalimentation should be employed. Finally, if a patient manifests malnutrition to the extent that intravenous support is indicated, the common trace elements—magnesium, copper, and zinc—should be measured as unexpected deficiencies are frequently discovered.

PHARMACOLOGY OF INTRAVENOUS ALIMENTATION

Once the decision is made to support a patient intravenously, the physician must choose the correct nutrient solution. No longer is it acceptable for the physician to view intravenous feeding as a "one size fits all" proposition. The simple fact is that major complications can occur from inappropriate feeding regimens or from excessive or inadequate feeding of patients.

The first determination the physician must make is the caloric needs of his patient. To derive this, the basal energy expenditure (BEE) of the patient is determined by means of the Harris-Benedict equation:

$$BEE = (males) \quad 664 + 13.7W + 5H - 6.7A$$

$$BEE = (females) \quad 655 + 9.6W + 1.8H - 4.6A$$

where A is age in years, H is height in centimeters, and W is weight in kilograms.

Few patients achieve positive nitrogen balance if they receive only basal caloric intake. The number of calories must be increased by a certain factor, depending on the disease or activity level of the patient. Thus daily activities of living increase caloric needs by 20 percent above the BEE (i.e., BEE × 0.2). Operation increases the BEE by 10 to 20 percent, major trauma by 20 to 30 percent, and major concurrent infection by 50 percent. Only in simple starvation do caloric needs fall below the BEE by approximately 10 percent. It is important to realize that this is just an estimate, which needs to by confirmed by performing a 24-hour urinary nitrogen excretion and calculating nitrogen balance. Typically, a positive nitrogen balance of 3 to 5 g is a reasonable target.

Once the total number of calories to be given is known, the physician must tailor the composition of the caloric intake. Typically, the bulk of calories are given as hypertonic glucose, and only 10 percent of calories are given as fat to avoid essential fatty acid deficiency. Some researchers have recently used fat as a substantial calorie source without any major problems and recommend using increased fat calories as a more "balanced diet." However, I do not recommend fat unless there is specific indication. However, these indications occur fairly frequently in dealing with a sick patient population. Thus a number of patients have significant glucose intolerance (e.g., owing to diabetes, pancreatitis, or steroid therapy). They benefit if the amount of glucose calories is decreased and replaced by fat. Other patients are in respiratory failure and ventilator-dependent. By changing to lipid as a major calorie source and decreasing glucose, the respiratory quotient and net carbon dioxide production are diminished, thus facilitating the ventilator weaning process. Still other patients have problems accepting the high volumes of fluid sometimes necessary to achieve positive nitrogen balance. Fat, being more calorie-dense than glucose, can be substituted as a calorie source while reducing the total volume given. I recommend 25 to 50 percent of the total caloric intake as fat in these situations. Once calorie composition is determined, the physician must also determine the amount of protein to be given. Too high a protein intake results in toxicity and too low an intake results in a negative nitrogen balance. Protein is delivered as amino acids, the amount being expressed as a ratio of nonprotein calories to grams of nitrogen. The typical calorie-nitrogen ratio is 150:1. In hypermetabolic states such as severe sepsis or trauma, this ratio should be lowered, thus raising the amount of protein given to 100:1.

While most crystalline amino acid solutions manufactured by commercial companies have basically the same amino acid compositions, several solutions have been introduced which dramatically alter the amino acid composition. One of these is a solution containing only essential L-amino acids, which is a solution designed for patients in severe renal failure. In theory, this solution spares protein and leads to less urea production than the standard crystalline amino acid solutions. The other new formula has high concentrations of branched-chain amino acids and is designed to reduce or ameliorate hepatic encephalopathy in liver failure patients. Normally, patients in liver failure are unable to tolerate a protein load and branch-chain amino acid enriched formula is thought to allow peripheral, as opposed to hepatic, metabolism of nitrogen, thus avoiding encephalopathy.

In summary, when designing the formula for a particular patient the physician must (1) estimate caloric needs and later confirm positive nitrogen balance, (2) decide the composition of calories (either primarily glucose or glucose plus fat), and (3) decide the amount of protein to be given. These decisions can be simplified by having the hospital pharmacy manufacture several base solutions with fixed glucose-protein ratios. The physician only needs to vary the fat concentration and the electrolyte additives. Table 1 lists the base solutions used at The Johns Hopkins Hospital. The physician can thus easily choose a high, low, or intermediate glucose-protein ratio. In addition, if fat is used as a calorie source, the calorie-nitrogen ratio can be lowered even further if needed. Since most solutions have negligible electrolyte content, the physician is at liberty to manipulate this as indicated.

TABLE 1 Solutions Used for Intravenous Hyperalimentation

	Unit Volume (ml)	Amino Acids (g)	Nitrogen (g)	Dextrose (g)	Total kcal	Na (mEq)	K (mEq)	Mg (mEq)	Ca (mEq)	Phos* (mM)	Cl (mEq)	Acetate (mEq)	mOsm/L
Standard THAS	1,000	41 (4.25%)	6.5	250 (25%)	1,020	30	20	5	5	5	30	67	1,850
Peripheral HAS	1,000	29 (3%)	4.6	70 (7%)	360	35	24.5	5	4	3.5	40	44	800
Low-nitrogen THAS	750	14 (2%)	2.3	350 (47%)	1,250	1.8	--	--	--	1.8	--	13	2,550
Concentrated THAS	1,000	58 (6%)	9.2	280 (28%)	1,190	6	--	--	--	6	--	53	2,050
Hi-cal THAS	1,000	41	6.5	350 (35%)	1,360	5	--	--	--	5	--	37	2,200
Renal THAS (essential amino acids only)	750	14 (1.8%)	1.6	350 (47%)	1,250	1.5	--	--	--	--	--	11	2,500
Fat emulsion 10%	500	--	--	--	550	--	--	--	--	7.5	--	--	280
Fat emulsion 20%	500	--	--	--	1,000	--	--	--	--	7.5	--	--	330

* 1 mm phosphate = 2 mEq phosphate.

NUTRIENT SOLUTION: MONITORING

While hospitalized, patients receiving TPN solution should be infused continuously. However, for patients who receive TPN at home, every effort is made to confine the infusion to 12- to 16-hour periods. The reason for continuous infusion is to allow for maximum safety; that is, to give the needed nutrients without exceeding the host capability to metabolize glucose, fat, protein, or water and electrolyte loads.

Thus, it is when parenteral nutrition is initiated that most metabolic complications are seen. This is the time when the body must adapt to the nutrient loads. Once the maintenance level of TPN is established, metabolic abnormalities are less frequently encountered. To minimize the risk of complications a low volume of infusion is begun, usually 40 to 42 ml per hour (1 liter per day). The infusion rate is increased by 24 cc to 42 cc per hour each day, not to exceed an increment of one liter per day. This is to prevent the most common metabolic complications of TPN: fluid overload, glucose intolerance, protein intolerance, hypokalemia, or hypophosphatemia.

Accurate daily input and output measurements and weights are mandatory as are urine sugar and ketone determinations every 6 hours and daily serum electrolytes, blood sugar, and blood urea nitrogen determinations (Table 2). Complete blood count and total serum protein, albumin, calcium, and phosphorus determinations should be obtained twice a week initially. Hepatic and renal function tests should be evaluated initially and every 2 weeks thereafter. Periodic determinations of arterial blood gases are also needed in the critically ill patient. The trace elements—magnesium, zinc, and copper—should be determined at the onset of therapy. I have noted a high incidence of trace element deficiency in my critically ill patients. I repeat the measurement of serum magnesium and zinc during therapy at 2-week intervals as these sometimes need to be replenished. As TPN patients stabilize, the frequency and number of laboratory determinations can be greatly decreased.

At times, the needed amount of protein or calories cannot be delivered owing to a pre-existing disease state. When this occurs, the solution must be modified or treatment of the rate-limiting condition must be established. Thus if the patient cannot tolerate the volume of standard solution, a more concentrated solution may be given. Lipid is often used as a calorie source because of its high caloric density (20% intralipid has 2 calories per cubic centimeter). Judicious use of diuretics is also employed, but diuretics alone are rarely the answer to fluid overload in the TPN patient.

If a patient cannot tolerate high glucose loads, insulin may be added to the TPN bottle in amounts of 5 to 50 units per 1,000 calories. Although convenient, this practice can also be dangerous, especially if the glucose intolerance is aggravated by sepsis or steroids. For example, if the infection causing sepsis responds to treatment, the insulin needs of the patient may fall precipitously, and then profound hypoglycemia can ensue if the patient is receiving high-dose insulin in the TPN

TABLE 2 Monitoring of the Parenterally Supported Patient

Daily measurements
  Weight
  Intake and output
  Temperature
  Blood pressure
  Pulse
  Urine
    Sugar and acetone
    Specific gravity
  Blood
    Electrolytes (Na, Cl, K, HCO_3)
Biweekly measurements
  Blood, serum
    Creatinine, glucose, urea, total protein, albumin, magnesium, calcium, phosphorus, alkaline phosphatase, SGOT, SGPT, bilirubin
  Hematology
    Hemoglobin, hematocrit, WBC with differential, PT, PTT, platelets
As indicated
  Anthropometrics
  Urine
    Nitrogen, creatinine, urea
  Blood
    Retinal binding protein, transferrin, pre-albumin, triglycerides, ammonia, zinc, copper

bottle. For this reason, I recommend that only 50 to 75 percent of the daily insulin need be given by bottle and the rest subcutaneosly by sliding scale. Thus the blood glucose is "titrated" to a level below 250 mg per deciliter but above 150 mg per deciliter with insulin in the TPN bottle, and further control is obtained with subcutaneously administered crystal and zinc insulin (CZI). If 50 units of regular insulin per 1,000 cc is given and hyperglycemia is still a problem, I frequently change to a 25 to 50 percent fat calorie solution, thus enabling the physician to reach the caloric goals without hyperglycemia.

If the patient is uremic (BUN greater than 40 or a BUN/creatinine ratio over 35), I recommend a solution with less than 4 percent amino acids. This protein-calorie ratio can be lowered further if necessary by adding fat (either 500 calories per day or 1,000 calories a day). If the patient is profoundly oliguric or anuric, I prefer to treat the patient with dialysis and concurrently administer a high-calorie, moderate-protein solution. However, this practice remains controversial, and most other centers would recommend a high-glucose, very-low-protein solution in order to reduce the level of blood urea nitrogen, ammonia, potassium, and phosphorus. The drawback to this "minimal" nutrition approach is that the patient's caloric needs are not met. Thus, I prefer a more aggressive regimen that attempts to meet the expected catabolic demands and then, as necessary, to treat with dialysis.

If the patient has liver failure, the physician must reduce the protein load drastically or use a branched-chain enriched formula. Frequently, a parenterally administered protein load cannot be given at all. Thus if the serum ammonia is 90 or greater and the patient manifests signs of encephalopathy, I recommend that TPN be discontinued until adequate liver function is present.

Virtually any conceivable electrolyte abnormality can occur in a patient who is receiving TPN, but there are a few that occur frequently and can be attributed directly to the hyperalimentation. These abnormalities can be avoided by early intervention. Perhaps the most common is hypokalemia. This can occur at any time with diuretic use, but even in the "average" patient, it occurs on the fourth to sixth day of TPN, when net positive nitrogen balance is achieved and potassium is drawn into the cell. Thus it is not unusual to see a stable patient suddenly experience a fall in the serum potassium. Hypophosphatemia also is a problem, for essentially the same reasons, at this time. Profound hypophosphatemia (levels below 1.5) are sometimes seen and can lead to such extreme muscle fatigue that respiratory arrest occurs.

The other common abnormality is acidosis. This is caused in part by a high load of crystalline amino acids. Since the amino acids are given as chloride and acetate salts, a hyperchloremic acidosis ensues. In many cases the physician does not note the steady gradual rise of serum chloride levels and concurrent fall in serum bicarbonate level until the patient's respiratory rate is 40 per minute and the blood pH actually drops. Thus the acidosis is particularly insidious and sometimes masked by a diuretic-induced alkalosis or concurrent lactic or keto acidosis. All amino acid solutions have acetate added by the manufacturer to buffer the titratable acidity of the protein solution. In some patients this is not sufficient, and the physician must then add sodium or potassium as the acetate rather than the chloride salt in order to correct the metabolic acidosis.

If severe metabolic derangements occur while the patient is receiving TPN, it is generally a good rule to reduce or temporarily discontinue hyperalimentation and establish biochemical stability. Then hyperalimentation can be restarted at a low rate and slowly increased to meet caloric needs. This is far safer than trying to manage a patient with severe abnormalities and concurrently delivering large volumes of protein, glucose, and fluids. Many physicians also prefer to withhold TPN during operative procedures, anticipating large fluid and electrolyte shifts. Actually, I have not found this to be a major problem and rarely withhold TPN during operations, although I recommend that lipid not be infused during the operation (owing to the risk of decreased platelet function and subsequent bleeding, or risk of pulmonary sequelae); I routinely recommend reducing the total volume of infusion to 2 liters per day or less to avoid perioperative fluid overload.

HOME TPN

While important TPN is certainly well accepted and widespread, home TPN remains in its infancy as a therapeutic modality. Many physicians are reluctant to consider home TPN because of inconvenience and anxiety over its effectiveness or risk. Yet home TPN offers a physician greater therapeutic flexibility rather than less, and is probably as safe as in-hospital TPN. The general indi-

cation for home TPN is gut failure of any cause in any otherwise medically stable patient (Table 3). The majority of patients suffer from various inflammatory bowel diseases or short gut syndrome. Owing to the cost pressures of prolonged hospitalization, home TPN is now being offered to patients for short periods of time (3 to 4 months). This allows dramatic savings to all involved and frees the patient from the hospital. Consequently, patients with terminal cancer can be nourished and sent home for weeks or months instead of languishing in the hospital. Patients with Crohn's disease or chronic pancreatitis who need a prolonged period of gut rest can also be treated at home.

The major difference between in-hospital and home TPN is the duration of delivery of the hyperalimentation solution. Instead of a continuous infusion, the formula is delivered over a 12- to 16-hour period, thus giving the patient more freedom to pursue work or interests. Patients who have problems with glucose tolerance have more difficulty adjusting to this regimen as the peak glucose infusion rate is higher on home than on in-hospital TPN. Since the patient must also be trained in the use of the delivery pump and catheter care, a certain amount of motivation, responsibility, and intelligence are required, but this requirement is frequently overestimated. My patients are trained within a 4- to 6-day period without problems. Various home care companies provide intensive home nursing and the pharmaceutical supplies and equipment needed to safely proceed with home TPN.

CENTRAL VENOUS CATHETERIZATION METHODS

Owing to the hyperosmolality of most parenteral solutions, it is necessary to deliver the solution into a high-flow vessel, thus immediately "diluting" the solution to serum osmolality. The superior vena cava is the only vessel that meets this criterion adequately. Thus the tip of

TABLE 3 Indications for Home Parenteral Nutritional Support

Enterocutaneous and entero-enteral fistulas
Biliocutaneous fistulas
Shortgut syndrome
Inflammatory bowel disease
Crohn's disease
Ulcerative colitis
Sprue
Whipple's disease
Chemotherapy of malignant disease
Colonic pseudo-obstruction
Anorexia nervosa
Stroke
Coma
Chronic relapsing pancreatitis
Prolonged ileus
Radiation enteritis
Intractable diarrheal disease

TABLE 4 Metabolic Complications of Parenteral Nutrition

Glucose metabolism
Hyperglycemia
Osmotic diuresis
Hyperosmolar nonketotic dehydration
Ketoacidosis
Hypercarbia, increased ventilatory work
Post-infusion rebound hypoglycemia

Amino acid metabolism
Hyperchloremic acidosis
Amino acid imbalance
Hyperammonemia
Prerenal azotemia

Fat metabolism
Essential fatty acid deficiency
Hyperlipemia
Increased pulmonary vascular resistance
Decreased platelet adhesiveness

Electrolyte metabolism
Hypernatremia
Hyponatremia
Hypokalemia
Hyperkalemia
Hypomagnesemia
Hypermagnesemia

Calcium and phosphorus metabolism
Hypophosphatemia
Hypocalcemia
Hypercalcemia

Hepatic function
Cholestasis, possible gallstones
Fatty liver syndrome

any catheter must be positioned in the superior vena cava prior to commencement of TPN. This is accomplished by placing a catheter either percutaneously in the subclavian vein and threading it centrally or by cutd vn.

Percutaneous placement is the standard technique used for in-hospital TPN. In most hospitals, the catheter used is made of Teflon, polyvinyl, silicone, polyethylene, or polyurethane. Not all catheter materials are equally suited for long-term hyperalimentation. Teflon, polyvinyl, and polyethylene catheters are all rigid and are more thrombogenic than either silicone or polyurethane. Therefore the former materials cause a higher incidence of vessel erosion or vessel thrombosis than either silicone or polyurethane catheters.

Another point that is often overlooked is the design of the catheter. Many centers utilize a technique of passing the catheter through a large-bore needle used to locate the subclavian vein. This is to be condemned as unsafe owing to the risk of shearing the catheter in half with the locator needle. The Seldinger technique of locating the vein with a small-gauge needle and passing a guidewire into the central circulation, removing the locator needle, and then passing a catheter over the guidewire is a far safer technique, resulting in a lower incidence of technical complications at the time of catheter insertion.

In additon to factors of catheter design, the major source of complications during catheter placement is physician error. Most of these errors result from failure to observe a few simple guidelines: (1) absolute sterility must be maintained throughout the procedure, (2) all patients should be in Trendelenburg position with a roll towel under the scapulae, (3) the patient's coagulation and hydration should be normal or optimized prior to catheterization, and (4) there should not be urgency or hurry associated with the procedure. It is purely elective, and there is no need to increase risks by rushing the operator or the patient or the support staff.

For patients who are to receive prolonged TPN or home TPN, a tunneled catheter is needed. The catheter used is a 90-cm barium-impregnated silicone rubber catheter with a Dacron velour cuff 30 cm from the catheter hub. Placement is done in the operating room under local anesthesia. The catheter is tunneled subcutaneously from a stab wound over the lower sternum to a second larger incision placed in the infraclavicular fossa lateral to the sternum. A 2-inch 18-gauge needle attached to a syringe is directed through the infraclavicular incision into the subclavian vein. A J-wire is introduced through the needle to the superior vena cava. A large introducer, consisting of an internal obturator and an external cannula which can be split apart, is then threaded over the guidewire into the SVC. The catheter, having been passed through the subcutaneous tunnel, is then cut to the appropriate length, flushed with heparin solution, and passed through the cannula after the guidewire and obturator have been removed. Care must be taken at this point to avoid inadvertent introduction of an air embolus. The cannula is then gently "peeled apart" and removed, leaving the catheter in the superior vena cava.

This technique is the simplest available and can be used for children and adults. However if the patient's coagulation status prohibits the risk of a percutaneous approach, the catheter can be passed into the central circulation by simple cutdown to an accessible vein, such as the pectoral, cephalic, thyroid, facial, or internal or external jugular vein.

Complications

The complications of central venous catheterization by percutaneous insertion are listed in Table 4. Most are avoidable if catheter design is appropriate and the operator placing the line is experienced. However, the most frequent complication of the central line is not a technical one, but rather sepsis. Early on, TPN central line sepsis was a significant and frequent complication. With the institution of rigorous sterile techniques during line insertion and of special nursing staffs to routinely change the central line dressings and vigorous aseptic standards adopted by hospital pharmacies in the mix of TPN solutions, the infection rate in most hospitals is well below 7 percent.

However, in many hospitals central line sepsis is still a problem of diagnosis, with over 25 percent of lines suspected of sepsis and thus removed immediately. Recently, some centers have advocated guidewire catheter exchange for suspected line sepsis and subsequent catheter culture. It is important to stress that the intracutaneous portion of catheters, not the tip, should be cultured quantitatively, as a colony count over 15 is considered evidence of catheter infection. Tip cultures have a low correlation with actual catheter sepsis. Thus a catheter can be exchanged over a guidewire and cultured without stopping therapy. If the culture is positive, the exchanged line should be removed. Currently, there is no evidence that weekly or twice weekly "prophylactic" guidewire exchange alters the risk of sepsis.

POSTOPERATIVE WOUND INFECTION

CARLOS A. PELLEGRINI, M.D.

Postoperative wound infection is a major cause of morbidity in surgical patients; it also increases hospital stay and health care costs. The risk of developing postoperative wound sepsis is related to the extent of bacterial contamination during surgery, and therefore, the incidence varies from less than 1 percent in clean, primarily closed wounds to more than 20 percent in heavily contaminated wounds. Table 1 presents the classification of operative wounds according to the National Research Council. This classification makes comparisons possible and emphasizes the usefulness of prophylactic antibiotics in certain types of operations. Although there is no hard rule about it, infection rates should not surpass 1.5 percent for clean cases, 5 percent for clean-contaminated cases, and 15 percent for contaminated cases. Illnesses such as cirrhosis, cancer, and renal failure; certain drugs such as steroids and anticancer medications; and severe malnutrition increase the risk of wound infection because they compromise the intrinsic defense mechanisms.

Most wound infections become apparent between the fifth and tenth postoperative day, and over 80 percent are clinically evident before discharge from the hospital. However, in immunodeficient patients and in patients with prosthetic devices, wound sepsis may not become apparent for several months. In these patients the infection is caused by organisms introduced into the wound at the time of surgery which become active at a later time.

CLINICAL FINDINGS AND MANAGEMENT

The first sign of wound infection is either fever (wound sepsis is the most common cause of postoperative fever between the third and seventh postoperative day) or wound pain. From a therapeutic point of view it is useful to divide wound infections into those in which the infection involves only tissues above the fascia (superficial wound infections) and those in which the main infection occurs below the fascia (deep wound infections).

If a subcutaneous catheter should become infected, it must be removed immediately and appropriate antibiotics given for a 7- to 10-day course. Frequently these catheters become clotted and can be opened with a flush of heparin solution, 1,000 u per cubic centimeter, or if that fails, with instillation of 2 cc of urokinase, 5,000 u per cubic centimeter. If that fails, a new catheter must be placed.

Superficial Wound Infections

This is the most common type of wound infection. Examination of these wounds discloses the presence of local edema and firm or fluctuant areas, and palpation elicits tenderness. Superficial wound infections should be treated by opening the wound and allowing it to drain. This can be done safely at the bedside. Certain rules, however, ought to be observed to make the procedure as smooth as possible and to avoid contamination within and outside the patient's room. For example, it is important to prepare, before opening the wound, a small sterile setting that includes all elements necessary to open, clean, and pack the wound as well as those needed to obtain adequate specimens for culture of aerobic and anaerobic bacteria. The surgeon must wear gloves and a protective apron, and an assistant ought to be present.

Local anesthetic infiltration of the surrounding skin is not necessary in most cases and may be deleterious. However, it is advisable to provide an adequate level of analgesia before opening the wound (75 to 125 mg Demerol or 10 to 12 mg morphine sulfate IM 30 minutes prior to the procedure). This increases the patient's cooperation, so that the surgeon may explore all areas of the open wound.

Wound opening should start at the area of maximal fluctuation, induration, or pain. I prefer to remove one or two stitches (or tapes) and then gently introduce a "Q" stick. In most cases one can break into the abscess easily, and the tip of the "Q" stick can be used as a specimen for culture and sensitivity. The wound should then be opened as needed to fully unroof the area of fluid collection. Gentle digital palpation should then be done to break fibrin adhesions and to explore for tracts. Dead tissue (usually fat) should be removed by sharp dissection. Extensive dissection is not needed in most superficial wound infections, and it may increase the risk of developing a ventral hernia. Once the wound has been cleaned, the integrity of the fascia should be examined. Pus draining between stitches may indicate the presence of a deep infection. The wound should then be lavaged gently, packed with wet-to-dry dressings (using saline or Dakin's solution), and sealed with a water-impermeable tape to prevent external contamination.

The frequency of dressing change is determined by

TABLE 1 National Research Council Classification of Surgical Wounds

| | | | Anticipated Infection Rate (%) | |
Classification	Definition	Example	Without Antibiotic	With Antibiotic
Clean	Intact technique; respiratory, gastrointestinal, and genitourinary tract not entered; no inflammation	Herniorrhaphy, thyroidectomy	1–2	(Antibiotics Not Recommended)
Clean-contaminated or potentially contaminated	Intact technique; GI, respiratory, or genitourinary tract entered; no inflammation	Gastrectomy, cholecystectomy	10–20	7
Contaminated	Major breakdown in technique; gross spillage from GI tract; inflamed biliary system	Choledochotomy for cholangitis	20–35	10–15
Dirty	Old traumatic wounds; per-forated viscus; presence of pus	Perforated diverticulum with peritonitis	25–50	15–35

the amount of drainage. The primary goal of a dressing program is to continue surgical debridement, to allow drainage, and to decrease bacterial colonization. When this is achieved, clean granulation tissue rapidly fills the wound. In most cases, three to four dressing changes a day are required initially. Generally, dressing changes can be done by the nurse, but the surgeon must inspect the wound at least once daily to determine the need for debridement of new necrotic tissue and the effectiveness of packing, which must include all recesses of the wound. One or two days after opening the wound, the patient should start showering. This contributes to wound debridement, increases the patient's comfort, and places him in charge of the wound. Once the wound is clean and granulating, there is no need to carry out dressing changes with sterile technique, and thus most patients can manage it well at home, without need of a visiting nurse.

Occasionally, superficial wound infections adopt a nonsuppurative form (cellulitis), in which case the inflammation is limited to the surrounding connective tissue. Cellulitis appears around the wound as a red area of edematous skin. Exploration of the wound reveals no pus. Most cases of cellulitis are caused by streptococci, but other bacteria may be involved. Since there is no suppuration, bacteria are often difficult to obtain for culture. However, one must be aware that cellulitis is a rare form of wound infection, and redness around the skin of an operative wound usually means that there is a collection of pus superficial or deep within it. Patients with bona fide cellulitis are best treated with penicillin, 600,000 units every 6 hours intramuscularly. If a clear response has not occurred in 12 to 24 hours, one should suspect an abscess,

or consider the possibility that the causative agent is *Staphylococcus* or another organism resistant to penicillin.

Deep Wound Infections

Infections deep to the fascia may be more difficult to diagnose, as in these patients the wound may appear normal. However, fever is almost always present, and spiking temperatures after the fourth or fifth postoperative day should always raise the suspicion of a wound infection. The diagnosis of deep laparotomy wound infections is particularly important, as they are frequently associated with more serious intra-abdominal infection (e.g., intra-abdominal abscess, leaking anastomosis). Patients who have spiking fever and a normal-looking wound should have a CT scan (or ultrasonography) of the abdomen. Ultrasonography is useful to detect fluid collections deep to the fascia, but may miss other intra-abdominal abscesses.

Once the diagnosis is clear, the treatment is adequate drainage. Patients in whom the fluid collection has been localized by a CT scan, and those who have other associated intra-abdominal abscesses, may benefit from percutaneous CT-guided catheter drainage. However, the majority of deep wound infections can be drained directly through the operative wound. In addition to the analgesics recommended for superficial wound infection, intravenous diazepam should be given. If an adequate exploration and debridement cannot be carried out with intravenous or intramuscular sedation, the patient should be taken to the operating room where, under general anesthesia, the wound can be explored and adequate debridement can be performed. However, this is rarely required.

The superficial portions of the wound should be opened according to the guidelines set forth for superficial wound infections. When the fascia is exposed, pus is usually seen leaking between fascial stitches. The stitches overlying the abscess cavity should then be removed, and the adjacent devitalized tissues (including portions of the fascia) should be debrided. Although the goal is to remove all dead tissue, care must be taken not to remove an excessive amount, as many areas of the fascia that are covered by fibrinous exudate may still be viable. When large portions of the fascia have to be removed, and bowel is exposed, it may be better to take the patient to the operating room, perform a complete debridement, and close the abdominal wall using full-thickness, heavy (e.g., No. 22) wire stitches. This should be done when the wound is relatively fresh, when the risk of evisceration is greater. As the time from operation increases, the risk of evisceration following extensive wound debridement decreases.

During the debridement it is important to be careful with the underlying bowel, as it is easy to penetrate its wall. When the collection is large, or when pus or other body fluids continue to pour from within the abdominal cavity after cleaning the wound, it is preferable not to pack the wound as this may interfere with drainage. Instead, I prefer to use colostomy bags, mounted over large colostomy rings. This protects the adjacent skin and allows the surgeon to measure the amount of fluid draining from the wound. Samples of wound discharge may also be taken and analyzed as needed (i.e., amylase determination). Drains are not as effective when the wound has been widely opened. On the other hand, drains of the red rubber type may be reinserted through previous drain tracts (only if they are passed easily; they are not to be pushed) when there is a discharge from these tracts. Although softer drains (Silastic) are preferred at the time of operation, it is almost impossible to thread old tracts with them.

Continuous irrigation of deep cavities helps debridement. However, this is only possible when there is an inflow tract into the cavity (usually a drain) and an outflow tract. The outflow tract may be another drain connected to suction or, if the lavage fluid emerges from the wound, a bag connected to a drainage system. A closed system should be used whenever possible to prevent contamination of adjacent areas of the wound.

When continuous lavage is not possible, intermittent lavage of all deep recesses of the wound, tracts, and cavities should be done at every dressing change to prevent accumulation of debris.

Deep wound infections always have several tracts that must be identified, drained, and packed. In deep wound infections, or in those that drain considerably after the first day or two, I perform fistulograms, as it is not unusual to find an even deeper undrained area or a fistula to the bowel or biliary tract. Subsequent care of these deep wounds varies, depending on the clinical response to drainage and the presence of associated fistulas or intra-abdominal abscesses. The patient and the wound should be inspected frequently by the surgeon. CT should be repeated if the patient does not respond to the initial treatment or if there are other reasons to suspect an intra-abdominal collection.

Gram Stain and Culture in Superficial and Deep Wound Infections

A specimen from the wound should always be sent to the laboratory for culture and sensitivity. Evaluation of a stained smear is important in wound infections that develop within the first 48 to 72 hours following the operation since *Clostridia perfringens* or other *Clostridia* species may be the causative agent. It is also important in the occasional patient that requires immediate antibiotic therapy, as it may help the surgeon in the choice of antibiotic. Identification of the offending organism is useful for two reasons. From the standpoint of *infection control*, it provides bacteriologic data and it may help to locate the source and prevent further infection in other patients. From the standpoint of the *patient's treatment*, it helps in the selection of an appropriate antibiotic if infections develop in other areas (e.g., intra-abdominal abscess), the wound must be re-entered (preoperative antibiotic), or the wound infection becomes invasive. Bacterial identification is particularly important in patients who have prosthetic devices and in immunocompromised patients.

Antibiotics

The key to the treatment of all wound infections is adequate surgical unroofing and debridement. Most wound infections, even those that are deep and complex, can be treated successfully with local measures only. Antibiotics are needed when (1) there is marked surrounding cellulitis, (2) the patient is immunodeficient or at high risk for systemic complications, (3) the patient has a prosthetic device (e.g., graft, valve, pump, artificial joint), or (4) the infection is invasive (i.e., there are signs of systemic infection). When an infected wound is complicated by signs of sepsis (fever, tachycardia, and hypotension), blood cultures should be obtained and intravenous antibiotics immediately started. If the patient does not improve rapidly after the wound is opened, the surgeon must search for undrained infection deeper in the wound or elsewhere in the body. These patients often have other sources of infection that require additional drainage.

Selection of an antibiotic initially is based on the Gram stain and the surgeon's guess as to the most likely organism involved. For example, wound infections following intra-abdominal procedures are usually secondary to gram-negative organisms, often anaerobic bacteria, and a broad-spectrum antibiotic is called for. Multiple antibiotics usually are not necessary in the treatment of wound infections. Within 24 to 48 hours, culture and sensitivity reports provide information necessary to select the specific antibiotic.

Clostridial Infections

Clostridia causes a broad spectrum of disease, ranging from negligible surface contamination to invasive infection of muscle with massive tissue necrosis and profound toxemia. This type of infection is discussed separately as it is much more serious and potentially life-threatening. Three factors are important in the development of clostridial infections: (1) the contamination of the wound, (2) the presence of devitalized tissue, and (3) an anaerobic environment. Thus, these infections are more frequently seen following massive tissue injury and less frequently following colonic and biliary operations.

In its lesser form, clostridial infection produces *crepitant cellulitis*, an invasive infection of subcutaneous tissue. This type of cellulitis is occasionally seen after appendectomy. Invasion is superficial to the deep fascia, but may spread very fast, often producing discoloration of the skin and edema as well as crepitus. Systemic symptoms and signs are remarkably absent, and this is one of the features that distinguishes cellulitis from myositis. *Clostridial myositis* (gas gangrene) is a rapidly progressive, life-threatening toxemic infection caused by *Clostridium perfringens*. The incubation period is much shorter than that of other pyogenic infections. Severe wound pain is the first sign and may appear as early as 24 hours after the operation. Toxemia, delirium, and hypotension may follow. The wound itself usually appears swollen and pale, but may exhibit a yellowish-brown discoloration. However, the superficial changes are always less extensive than the underlying muscle necrosis.

The major emphasis in the treatment of clostridial infection is *prompt* and *ample* wound debridement. The patient should be taken to the operating room as soon as the diagnosis is made. Under general anesthesia, wide debridement of necrotic areas back to healthy, bleeding tissue should be performed. Patients with clostridial cellulitis should be treated by a wide excision of skin and infected subcutaneous tissue, leaving the wound widely opened. In patients with clostridial myositis, all involved areas of the muscle must be excised. Amputation may be necessary when there is diffuse myositis with complete loss of blood supply or when adequate debridement is so extensive that it leaves the limb useless. Many of these patients require serial debridement at 24-hour intervals under general anesthesia for the first 3 to 4 days.

The second major component of treatment of gas gangrene is antibiotic therapy. Two to three million units of penicillin G every 2 hours (24 to 30 million units per day) are required. Clindamycin or metronidazole is an alternative for patients with penicillin allergy.

Hyperbaric oxygenation is useful in treating clostridial infections as it inhibits bacterial invasion and toxin production, *but it cannot replace (and should not delay) surgical therapy*. Treatment for 1 or 2 hours at three atmospheres repeated every 6 to 12 hours is recommended for a total of three to five exposures. Unless hyperbaric therapy and debridement can be done simultaneously (large hyperbaric chambers), surgery should always precede hyperbaric oxygenation.

PREVENTION OF WOUND INFECTION

Although a detailed discussion of this subject is not within the scope of this chapter, there are certain aspects that must be emphasized as they have been shown to decrease markedly the risk of wound infection.

Delayed closure of heavily contaminated operative wounds markedly decreases the chances of wound infection. In these patients the wound should be packed loosely with fine-mesh gauze at the end of the operation, leaving the skin open. The dressing should be left undisturbed for 4 to 5 days. If, when the packing is removed, the wound contains only serous fluid or a small amount of exudate, the skin edges can be approximated with tapes. If drainage is considerable or infection is present, the wound should be allowed to close by second intention, treating it as one would a superficial wound infection.

Early Correction of Wound Hematomas. Hematomas represent an excellent culture medium and frequently lead to wound infection. Hematomas that are detected shortly after surgery are best treated by opening the wound under sterile conditions, evacuation of the blood clots, gentle lavage, control of the bleeding vessel (rarely found), and reclosure of the wound. A hematoma discovered days after surgery may be evacuated by gentle compression of the wound edges without formally opening the wound.

Adequate Treatment of Wound Seromas. Seromas are fluid collections in the wound that usually follow operations involving elevation of skin flaps or transection of numerous lymphatic vessels. Seromas should always be evacuated because they delay healing and provide an excellent medium for bacterial growth. They should be evacuated by needle aspiration. A compression dressing should be used to seal lymphatic leaks and prevent reaccumulation. If the seroma recurs, I prefer to place a drain through a stab wound incision. The drain should be connected to suction in a closed system, and a compression dressing should be used.

Prophylactic antibiotics are only useful in certain clean-contaminated and contaminated wounds (see Table 1). Prophylactic antibiotics should (1) be given before the operation starts, (2) be specific against the most likely organism to contaminate the wound, (3) be stopped 24 hours later.

Good surgical technique, avoiding spillage and contamination of the operative wound, careful handling of tissues, and leaving no devitalized tissue on the wound edges, is one of the most important ways to prevent infection of the operative wound.

PREOPERATIVE NUTRITIONAL ASSESSMENT

JOHN M. DALY, M.D., F.A.C.S.

The aim of all treatment during the preoperative period is to prepare the patient to withstand the stress of operation and to minimize the risk of any surgical procedure. The appropriate duration of the preoperative preparatory period depends on the relative urgency of the procedure, the surgical risk, and the natural history of the disease without operative intervention. Major preoperative risk factors include the patient's age and presence of obesity, chronic illness, cardiopulmonary dysfunction, and malnutrition. Thus, evaluation of nutritional deficits is critical to the calculation of operative risk since it often influences the timing and type of operative intervention.

Protein-calorie malnutrition is a common problem in hospitalized medical and surgical patients. Several studies have shown that 20 to 50 percent of hospitalized patients suffer from moderate-to-severe malnutrition as a result of their primary disease or as a result of the diagnostic and therapeutic regimens employed in the management of their disease. Protein-calorie malnutrition is generally the result of decreased oral intake, increased enteral losses secondary to malabsorption or intestinal fistula, or increased nutritional requirements secondary to hypermetabolism caused by major burns, sepsis, or multiple trauma. The degree and type of malnutrition are determined by the nutrient intake and amount of stress. Semi-starvation alone leads to a marasmic condition, with loss of body weight and skeletal muscle mass but normal serum protein levels. Addition of severe stress can produce hypoalbuminemia and depressed immune function, similar to a kwashiorkor syndrome. Often a vicious cycle occurs in which the patient's primary disease leads to malnutrition which results in impaired wound healing, reduced immunocompetence, anemia, decreased resistance to infection, generalized sepsis, and further malnutrition. The end result may be multiple organ system failure and death. Successful interruption of this cycle requires a comprehensive knowledge of body composition, energy requirements, quantitative nutritional assessment techniques, and current methods of enteral and parenteral nutritional support.

BODY COMPOSITION, FUEL STORES, AND ENERGY REQUIREMENTS

Body composition studies show that the normal 70-kg man has approximately 17 kg of fat, 11 kg of protein, and 0.22 kg of glycogen in liver and muscle (Fig. 1). Carbohydrates, stored as glycogen, can provide only 800 to 1,200 kcal and ordinarily are consumed within the first 16 to 18 hours of fasting. Body protein, skeletal muscle and visceral protein mass, theoretically could provide 24,000 kcal, but protein is not truly an energy storehouse.

Each molecule of protein serves a specific structural and functional purpose as in the contractile elements of cardiac, smooth, and skeletal muscle; hormones; enzymes; carrier circulating proteins; or antibodies. Loss of body protein decreases structural reserve (motion, strength) and functional reserve (hormonal response to stress, immunocompetence). Body fat is an efficient storehouse of energy (approximately 141,000 kcal), but is utilized differentially compared with glucose, depending on the hormonal mileau associated with starvation or stressed states. Nutritional assessment techniques attempt to calculate these compartments of body composition using direct and indirect methods.

Balanced against these energy reserves are the daily energy requirements determined from the basal metabolic rate (BMR), which can be calculated using age, sex, body habitus (height), and body weight plus the estimated energy expenditure of activity plus 10 percent for the specific dynamic action of food. In normal individuals, basal metabolic rate correlates directly with measurements of lean body mass. However, in hospitalized patients, chronic undernutrition usually results in decreased energy requirements whereas stress, sepsis, or trauma increases metabolic requirements from 5 to 100 percent above predicted normal values. Actual measurements of energy requirements may be made by indirect calorimetry (measurement of oxygen consumption and carbon dioxide production). Using the modified Weir formula, energy requirements can be determined with reasonable accuracy. These measurements have correlated well with direct measurements of body heat production using direct calorimetry. Actual measurement of energy expenditure may become important in certain clinical conditions that alter basal metabolic rate from standard values, such as

Body Weight (kg)

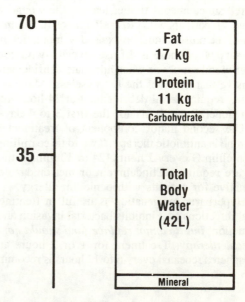

Figure 1 Components of body composition.

TABLE 1 Indications for Nutritional Assessment

Patient Unable to Eat	Patient Unwilling to Eat	Patient Unable to Eat Enough	Patient With Specific Nutritional Requirements
Cancer of mouth, pharynx, larynx, or esophagus	Anorexia secondary to malignancy, depression, chronic illness, psychiatric disorder	Increased nutritional requirements: severe catabolism secondary to burns, sepsis, multiple trauma	Cardiac failure
Trauma to mouth or throat		Impaired digestion and absorption, short-gut syndrome	Liver failure
Radiation stomatitis, enteritis	Radiation effects: stomatitis, xerostomia, enteritis, intestinal		Renal failure
Stupor, coma, stroke or paralysis	Chemotherapy effects: stomatitis, mucositis, enteritis		
Oropharyngeal or esophageal stricture	Acute or chronic inflammatory bowel disease		
Esophageal achalasia			
Upper gastrointestinal tract fistulas or obstruction			

stress (sepsis or multiple trauma), inflammatory bowel disease, malignant disease, chronic obstructive pulmonary disease, pregnancy, and cardiopulmonary failure.

NUTRITIONAL ASSESSMENT

General indications of the need for nutritional assessment and therapeutic intervention with enteral or parenteral nutritional support include the patient's inability to eat, unwillingness to eat, inability or unwillingness to eat enough, and specific nutritional requirements due to cardiac, hepatic, and/or renal dysfunction (Table 1). Using data obtained from the patient's history, physical examination, and laboratory tests, together with knowledge of the anticipated method of treatment, the degree and duration of nutritional disability can be estimated.

The ability to ingest adequate quantities of nutrients orally is evaluated by dietary history and the extent of recent weight loss. A history of a recent (within 3 months) loss of 10 percent of more body weight signifies substantial protein-calorie malnutrition. In our society, this determination is more important than measurement of the percent ideal body weight since obesity is more the norm than the exception, and the rapidity of weight loss indicates the severity of illness. This information provides an approximate assessment of the patient's nutritional status and also indicates to some extent the method and magnitude of nutrient therapy required during the perioperative period. Patient history includes questions regarding usual body weight; recent weight changes; special diets; problems with taste, chewing, or swallowing; food allergies and medications; alcohol ingestion; and bowel habits

related to dietary intake. Physical examination may reveal evidence of undernutrition such as dry, scaly, and atrophic skin, muscle wasting, pitting, presacral or pretibial edema, and loss of muscle strength. A thorough history and physical examination by an experienced physician is the simplest and perhaps the best method of nutritional assessment.

An excellent correlation has been demonstrated between the clinical diagnosis of malnutrition and nutritional status as determined by a battery of anthropometric and laboratory tests as well as analyses of total body potassium and total body nitrogen. Thus, although laboratory tests and research tools such as total body potassium and nitrogen measurements allow quantification of nutritional status for comparative purposes, the diagnosis of malnutrition can be made by an experienced physician.

A variety of sophisticated tests have been devised to detect milder forms of malnutrition and to evaluate quantitatively the patient's response to nutritional therapy. Anthropometric measurements quantify body habitus and body compartments can relate them to measurements of an age- and sex-matched normal population. Measurement of skin-fold thickness (mm) at the triceps, iliac crest, and thigh areas provides an estimate of the subcutaneous fat layer and total body fat compartment since approximately 50 percent of the body fat is located in the subcutaneous tissue. Arm muscle circumference is calculated as the arm circumference minus $0.314 \times$ triceps skin-fold thickness (mm). This determination allows a rough estimate of lean muscle mass, which is the largest portion of the body's protein compartment. The creatinine-height index, defined as the 24-hour creatinine excretion by a patient divided by the expected 24-hour excretion of creatinine by a normal adult of the same height, provides another estimate of skeletal muscle mass in a patient with normal renal function. Substantial protein-calorie malnutrition would be defined by a level approximately 75 percent of standard. A method for estimating body cell mass has also been developed by determining the ratio of exchangeable sodium to exchangeable potassium using isotope dilution techniques. This ratio increases with chronic malnutrition to a value greater than 1.22. Use of a whole body counter allows determination of 40_K present in small amounts, primarily intracellularly, within the skeletal muscle mass. From this measurement, one can calculate total body potassium, which allows an estimate of lean body mass. Measurement of total body nitrogen by gamma neutron activation is the "gold standard" for the determination of total body protein. However, these last three tests are not available for routine use in hospital centers, but have been useful research tools in the assessment of body compositional changes.

The degree of visceral protein depletion can be estimated by determining concentrations of serum proteins such as retinal-binding protein, prealbumin, transferrin, and albumin. Depression of serum protein levels owing to protein-calorie malnutrition is directly related to the metabolic half-life of the individual serum proteins and the patient's hydrational state. Prealbumin and retinal-binding protein have the shortest half-lives and are depressed first, followed by serum transferrin and serum albumin levels. The half-lives of these compounds are $\frac{1}{2}$, 2, 8, and 20 days respectively. A decrease in the serum concentration of these proteins may also be related to changes in the patient's salt and water balance. For example, serum albumin concentrations are commonly decreased when a malnourished patient is started on total parenteral nutrition. This depression in albumin concentration results from hydrational effects and is not a reflection of a worsening malnourished state.

The degree of visceral protein depletion has also been evaluated by determining the status of cell-mediated immunity as manifested by recall antigen skin testing and by the total blood lymphocyte count. Loss of immunocompetence is not a sensitive indicator of visceral protein depletion because weight loss usually exceeds 10 percent of the body weight before anergy develops secondary to malnutrition. Therefore, anergy associated with malnutrition signifies a significant deficiency of visceral protein and portends increased morbidity and mortality in hospitalized patients. Similarly, total lymphocyte counts are often reduced below 1,500 cells per cubic millimeter in the malnourished patient and may correlate with depressed delayed skin-test reactivity. A number of factors result in anergy to recall skin testing. Age, presence of malignant disease, immunosuppression due to exogenous medications, such as steroids, radiation therapy, stress, or sepsis, and a variety of other factors result in anergy to recall skin tests. In the absence of these factors, nutritional repletion of the malnourished patient can result in reversal of skin-test anergy, and this reversal is associated with improvement in the outcome of treatment. Usually,

however, improvement in other measurements of nutritional status such as body weight occur much in advance of improvement in delayed cutaneous hypersensitivity.

T-cell immunity rather then humoral immunity is depressed by malnutrition and can be measured in vivo by determining delayed cutaneous hypersensitivity responses to a battery of recall antigens. One-tenth milliliter each of Dermatophytin, Dermatophytin-0, Varidase (10 units streptokinase and 2.5 units streptodornase), mumps antigen and intermediate-strength purified protein derivative of tuberculin is injected separately intradermally into the volar aspect of the forearm. Skin reactions are measured 24 and 48 hours after injection. A positive reaction is defined as an area of induration at least 5 mm by 5 mm to one or more antigens at 48 hours.

Complete nutritional assessment provides an estimate of body composition—fat, skeletal muscle protein, and visceral protein—to help identify and quantify the magnitude of clinical or subclinical malnutrition. A nutritional status scale can be devised from which patients may be placed into nutritional categories of normal status, mild malnutrition, or severe malnutrition. The nutritional assessment also may help to determine whether maintenance or anabolic nutritional therapy should be used. Recent body weight change, anthropometric measurements, serum albumin and transferrin values, the creatinine-height index, and delayed cutaneous hypersensitivity skin-test responses help to quantify nutritional status during the initial assessment of the patient. All of these measurements have proved accurate in population surveys, but they have varying sensitivity and lack specificity. Thus, their major value lies in supporting the clinical diagnosis of malnutrition made by an experienced observer. Finally, blood analysis documents specific deficiencies that require correction.

Objective data can thus define the rather nebulous term "nutritional status" and allow both initial assessment of the patient and repeated evaluation of the efficacy of nutritional therapy. A prognostic nutritional index (PNI) has been developed by Mullen and colleagues in which the PNI (calculated as a percentage) equals 158 minus 16.6 × serum albumin (per deciliter) minus 0.78 × the triceps skin-fold thickness (mm) minus 0.20 × serum transferrin (per deciliter) minus 5.8 × delayed cutaneous hypersensitivity. The delayed cutaneous hypersensitivity score is graded as 0 = negative, 1 = less than 5 mm reactivity, and 2 = greater than or equal to 5 mm reactivity. In a large retrospective series of surgical patients, a PNI less than 30 (low risk) was associated with an 11.7 percent complication rate and a 2 percent mortality. A PNI greater than or equal to 60 (high risk) was associated with an 81 percent complication rate and a 59 percent mortality. Studies such as these have helped to establish the relative importance of nutritional indices as predictive factors for postoperative morbidity and mortality in surgical patients. Almost all nutritional support teams have devised nutritional status scoring systems that allow repeated estimates of nutritional status during diagnostic and therapeutic management of the patient (Fig. 2). A simple, practical definition of malnutrition that can be readily applied

NUTRITIONAL PROFILE

PATIENT NAME_____

ASSESSMENT DATE_____

SEX____ AGE ____(yrs) HEIGHT_____(cm) WRIST_____(cm) BODY FRAME ____

DIAGNOSIS_____

COMMENTS_____

_____

_____

TYPE TREATMENT AND DATE_____

_____

_____

MEASUREMENTS

Present weight_____ kg

Usual weight_____ kg

% Usual weight_____

Ideal weight_____ kg

% Ideal weight_____

Triceps skin-fold_____ mm

% Standard (TSF)_____

Midarm muscle circumference_____ cm

% Standard (MAMC)_____

Other (specify)_____

LAB RESULTS

Serum albumin_____ g/100 ml

Serum transferrin_____ mg/100 ml

Creatinine-height
   index (CHI)_____ %

Figure 2 Nutritional status scoring system.

clinically includes an unintentional or unexplained loss of 10 percent or more of body weight, a serum transferrin level less than 150 mg per deciliter, and a serum albumin level less than 3.4 per deciliter. Any combination of two of these three criteria is an indication for nutritional support or therapy.

After the need for preoperative nutritional support has been established, the most appropriate feeding regimen and the duration of nutritional support are determined. The optimal duration of preoperative nutritional support is ill-defined, however, and varies with each patient. Generally, patients with moderate-to-severe malnutrition should receive a minimum of 10 days of preoperative nutritional therapy before a major elective procedure and should continue to receive postoperative intravenous nutritional support until oral intake is adequate. Obviously, the urgency of the operation determines the length of time available to correct existing nutritional deficiencies. Retrospective and prospective studies substantiate that preoperative nutritional support of the malnourished patient improves postoperative outcome.

PREOPERATIVE ASSESSMENT OF THE ELDERLY PATIENT

JACQUELINE McCLARAN, B.S., M.D., C.C.F.P.

By convention, the term "elderly" refers to individuals who have reached the age of 65 or more. Most elderly are healthy, feel well most of the time, and function independently. Most elderly want to work, and work as efficiently as younger workers. Most elderly retain sexual desire and capacity. Only a very few elderly acquire dementia or confusion, or must live in protected housing or institutions. Yet both young and old are captured by negative aging perceptions or myths. In 1974, in an extensive survey, the U.S. National Council on

Aging determined that in regard to health status, access to care, having enough money, shelter, social interactions, and job opportunities, the subjective experience of the elderly is less serious than expected per condition, and is similar to the experience of the young.

If illness or disability does occur in the elderly, the surgeon must look for hidden problems, anticipate unusual presentations, and expect multiple complex ongoing problems that require special therapies and management techniques. For example, continence maintenance training and aggressive mobilization throughout the perioperative period may ensure the patient's return to his milieu, even where surgery is not specifically related to these areas of function. In elective hernia repair, preoperative physiotherapy for longer length of stride and narrower posture oscillation may subsequently promote early mobilization.

Regardless of pathology, illness and disability are likely to present in one of seven potential problem areas (Table 1): trouble with balance and falls, impaired mobility, compromised activities of daily living (ADL) or functional level, altered homeostasis, incontinence, confusion, and iatrogenesis. The surgeon should memorize these seven signals of disease. A fall and the resulting fractured hip may herald a urinary tract infection. Failed appetite may point to myocardial infarction or acute cholecystitis. Hypothermia and dehydration may mimic an acute abdomen, or occur as its result. The frail elderly individual arriving in an emergency room, deprived of sensory input because of removal of his hearing aid, glasses, clothes, and family, and/or left in unfamiliar surroundings, appears confused to clinicians. In addition, the patient without appropriate shoes and his usual walking aid makes the staff fearful of his even more impaired mobility; hence, protective restraints are provided. Now the patient is unable to get to the toilet, is labeled incontinent of urine and stool, confused and/or disoriented, delirious, immobile, and a placement problem. It is not hard to see how he may become totally demoralized. This sequence of events, entirely too common, is also seen postoperatively and/or following injury.

For example, a 78-year-old deaf gentleman of extremely spare lean body mass, speaking only Ukrainian and recovering from stroke incurred in the recovery room after resection of a colon carcinoma, awaits his transurethral prostatectomy. This last is meant to ensure that he is continent of urine and can therefore return to his home environment to be cared for by his wife and daughter. However, he also has stool incontinence, thought not to be due to surgery, nor to the cancer itself, nor to his stroke, but rather attributable to poor communication, occasional use of restraints, and impaired but improving mobility. Surgery alone cannot repair this patient's functional level; supportive therapies and nursing techniques must be simultaneously introduced. Total care must be coordinated.

Most at risk to become ill are the frail elderly, characterized as unable to recognize their own health problems. They are likely to live alone, be recently bereaved, have locomotor difficulty, show signs of mental impairment, be recently discharged, display self neglect, and tend to isolate themselves.

There is also evidence to suggest that another population of elderly, usually octogenarians, exhibit a survivorship effect and are less at risk for disease and disability.

BIOLOGY AND PHYSIOLOGY OF AGING

The elderly population are a biologically distinct entity because they are in a particular stage of human development, and also because of the particular diseases associated with this age group. Aging is not something that happens only to the aged. Each organ system ages at is own rate, and these rates are not altered in old age; however, the result is diminished functional reserve (Fig. 1).

TABLE 1   Seven Signals of Health Problems in the Aged

Trouble with balance and falling

Impaired mobility

Compromised activities of daily living
    or functional level

Altered homeostasis

Incontinence

Confusion

Iatrogenesis

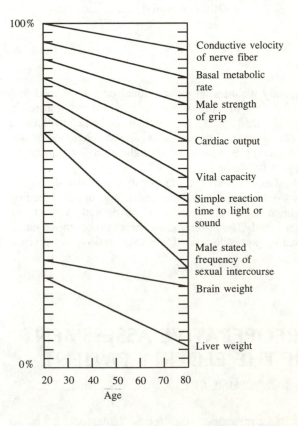

Figure 1   Relative physiologic rates and decrement of age.

Decreased pulmonary reserve, elasticity, and compliance are part of normal aging. Gas exchange surface per unit of mechanical surface is decreased. Consequently, the arterial/alveolar oxygen difference increases with age; however, this difference becomes significant only under the stress of injury (or disease) when muscular and cardiac as well as respiratory reserve are all called into play. Acid-base balance may be affected. These system responses may be adequate initially, but perhaps cannot be sustained in the aged.

Renal mass, number of glomeruli, and filtration rate decrease with aging. Response to fluid loading and dehydration is less dramatic and takes longer to correct. Since lean body mass is diminished and protein intake is decreased in most elderly, serum creatinine is no measure of renal function; creatinine clearance measures are necessary.

Cardiac ejection fraction diminishes with aging as does cardiac rate and output. Again, it may not be possible to sustain an adequate initial response.

Immune response, measured by number of circulating white blood cells, fever, phagocytosis, wheal and erythema, and response to antigens diminishes with age. The response may be variable; for example, high fever (40 °C) and low white count (3,800) may coexist in documented septicemia. Central temperature is more difficult to maintain. Response to external environment is delayed or may become impaired even in self-limited illness. Response to dehydration, electrolyte shifts, and fluid balance is also impaired.

Metabolic rate decreases with age; consequently, a diet rich in nutrients must be packed into fewer and fewer calories to ensure physiologic function. Controversy exists regarding normal protein intake in elderly. Although low protein intake keeps serum creatinine low, minimal protein intake recommendations for adults are thought to be inadequate in the elderly, in whom gastrointestinal absorption is likely to be decreased and nitrogen product synthesis is diminished.

Medication doses required are smaller, and a narrower therapeutic range is present before toxicity results. Response is less dramatic and side effects are frequent.

Some neurologic functions change. For example, the static mechanoreceptors in the neck decrease in number and function; therefore, more postural sway is required before dynamic mechanoreceptors and optic and auditory feedback loops can allow correction to upright posture. A 300 percent light requirement is normal in the very elderly to achieve the same degree of clarity and interpretation at a particular refraction. Hearing deficit may be an adaptive screen of sensory overload. Some functions are enhanced with aging; for example, crystallized intelligence or ability to integrate culturally associated knowledge improves throughout the life span.

Changes of normal aging must be recognized as separate from any systemic deterioration due to disease and must be taken into account during illness and the stress of surgery.

CLINICAL APPROACH TO THE PATIENT

Physical Examination

Physical examination is altered in the elderly. The skin becomes a less reliable indicator of degree of hydration in the aged. Turgor and elasticity are reduced. These changes contribute to an inadequate response to cold stress, centrally monitored. Muscle mass is known to decrease with normal aging; however, further small decrements associated with short-term illness may be interpreted as normal, and therefore signs of poor nutrition are missed. In fact, chronically poor nutrition has a high incidence even in community-dwelling elderly. Degenerative changes of the cervical spine and temporomandibular joint and poor dental hygiene influence anesthesia management. In the cardiovascular system, the left jugular venous system may be dilated during deep inspiration owing to compression of the left innominate vein during systole. The cardiac apex may be displaced by kyphosis, and kyphosis may also compromise pulmonary capacity. Slight hyperinflation and depressed diaphragms make pulmonary examination less reliable in the aged. Abdominal landmarks may be altered. The epigastrium is compressed, and the rib cage may sit on the iliac crests. In regard to the nervous system, pupillary reflex is not reliable, and other reflexes may be decreased. Primitive reflexes may reappear. Vibration sense is diminished. A degree of increased postural sway is part of the normal aging picture; however, sway beyond the standard deviation for age denotes disease and increases the risk of falls. Function is not predictable from physical examination alone in the elderly. For example, a high risk of falls may exist in the face of intact musculoskeletal and neurologic findings. Conversely, a steady gait may be observed in severe osteoporosis, poor muscle mass, and multiple motor and sensory deficits. The clinician should pay special attention to examination of the mouth, dentition, feet, gait, hearing, and the cardiovascular system.

Factors Associated with Morbidity

Although the surgical gerontology literature is substantial, the predicted benefit of each type of operation and the relative risks of particular ongoing conditions, functions, and habits for each age group remain to be established. Surgical studies describing the elderly patient exhibit the same problems as the rest of the age and aging literature. For example, trends by age are assumed to apply in the extreme to the very old. Authors use too many and too-wide age groups and publish studies that include too few elderly. Not surprisingly, studies are not comparable; nevertheless, some interesting observations have been made.

Half of the population reaching the age of 65 undergo operation. Twenty-five percent of laparotomies are currently performed on aged patients. Since in the elderly surgical candidate remaining life span is diminished, recovery time will be longer, and other conditions may compromise expected outcome, preoperative assessment has more implications. Expected deterioration of other conditions with and without surgery must be considered. Quality of life considerations also play a larger role for these frail individuals.

For the elderly, most perioperative morbidity is secondary to cardiovascular and pulmonary complications, as is true in the overall population. In noncardiac surgery, an age greater than 70 years is an independent risk factor for life-threatening cardiac complications (0.4% versus 5.0%). Previous infarct is more important than age. In moderate-to-severe pulmonary disease, age does not add to risk. This is one of many examples that specific disease is a more important indicator of risk than age alone. On the other hand, diminished immunologic reserve of the aged is associated with increased morbidity, even when no infection is identified.

Operative Benefits. Can surgeons make clinical decisions based on more refined judgement than age parameters alone permit? Will it make any difference to the functional level, placement milieu, and quality of life of the older patient? Trends indicate that surgeons already make clinical decisions based on more refined judgment than age alone. For example, over the past twenty years, surgical mortality in octogenarians has decreased from 20 percent in the 1960s to approximately 10 percent in the 1980s. This trend is not explained by a diminished rate of elective procedures in the elderly or by improved health among octogenarians, but is rather a true improvement of outcome. In fact, the numbers of elective procedures available to the frail elderly have increased. In my opinion, and insofar as it is safe to generalize, not enough elective procedures are offered to the frail elderly. Geriatricians beg for surgical intervention for such procedures as transurethral prostatectomy, cataractectomy, lens implantation, cholecystectomy, hip prosthesis, debriding and draining of undermined bed sores, and skin grafts.

Case Example. A 65-year-old woman, functioning independently in a church residence, was admitted for a 14- to 20-day geriatric assessment for withdrawal of psychotropic drugs and investigation of urinary frequency. On day 1, a urinary tract infection (UTI) was identified and treated. On day 2, carpal pedal spasm occurred and was thought to be due to withdrawal of medication. On day 3, the patient fell and fractured her hip and was put on bed rest. The fall was thought to be due to the UTI, and to a combination of factors including her gait, altered by the carpal pedal spasm, and perhaps by either interstitial pneumonia, or congestive heart failure appearing as a new finding on chest film. While receiving intravenous fluids, this very skinny dry old lady began to retain fluid and had a very poor urinary output. On day 5, the anesthesia service refused to permit the patient to be operated on because she was in congestive heart failure. The cardiologist insisted that the patient was not in congestive heart failure. On days 6, 7, and 8, the patient continued to be booked for the operating room and starved until 3:00 PM every afternoon, whereupon she was bumped by the anesthesia department. On day 9, the cardiologist identified a cardiomyopathy on ultrasonography and stated that she should be kept on the "wet" side during surgery rather than reducing fluid volume as had been planned. On day 10, the patient sloughed full-thickness skin over both heels and the sacral region because of incontinence and immobility since day 3. On day 32, the patient had improved enough to be able to sit in her wheelchair and pedal down the hall with her feet. On day 137, the plastic surgeon could not be persuaded to open the draining sinus over her sacrum and break up loculations because she had no fever, and because if the geriatric ward had packed the wound properly in the first place, this would never have happened. And so the patient was punished for our stupidity. Finally, the wound did close on its own, and the patient returned to the protected residence. Two months later, it was noted that she had not made an adequate social readjustment and was no longer welcome. Perhaps immediate hip repair would have prevented bed sores and incontinence. Skin grafts may have led to discharge soon enough to permit adequate social reintegration.

In spite of many such examples, access to surgery is improving for the elderly, and better surgical decision making is leading to lower rates of morbidity and mortality. For example, the rate of cognitive impairment in acute hospital beds is lower for surgical admissions than for medical admissions (32% vs 40%). Half of this 32 percent is explained by reversible conditions, such as urinary tract infection or environmental change. In fact, these odds can be further ameliorated. In elderly patients who are urgent surgical admissions, an 8 percent mortality rate occurs if the emergency room diagnosis is correct. A 20 percent mortality rate occurs if the emergency room diagnosis is wrong, even if the surgeon is in the appropriate cavity and the patient proves to have a surgical disease. Proper diagnosis improves the odds in emergency surgery in the elderly.

How can the surgeon improve his diagnostic skill and reduce complications in the elderly in the face of a poverty of clinical signs and history, and when existing signs do not correlate with surgical pathology as encountered in younger patients? It would appear that even altered presentations can be specific in the elderly. Only one-third of elderly patients with acute appendicitis have classic pain, starting centrally and moving to the right lower quadrant. Ileus may present as steady pain in the elderly. Only 47 percent of perforated gastroduodenal ulcers present with pain. Only 39 percent of perforated ulcers present with roentgenographic evidence of air under the diaphragm. For this biologically distinct entity, the elderly patient, these distinct clinical signs and symptoms must be identified and shared in the literature. That illness and impaired function are more predictive of well-being than age alone will become evident, and surgical risk will be

TABLE 2 Saskatchewan Short Mental Status Questionnaire*

1. What is your full name?
2. What is your address?
3. What year is this?
4. What month is this?
5. What day of the week is this?
6. How old are you?
7. What is the name of the president?
8. When did the first World War start?
9. Remember these three items, I will ask you to recall them in a few minutes.... bed, chair, window.
10. Count backward from 20 to 1.

* 7–10 correct = probably intact; 3–6 correct = moderately impaired; 0–2 correct = intellectual impairment.

individualized based on the pathophysiology of the patient's condition.

ASSESSMENT: A GERIATRICIAN'S VIEWPOINT

Unlike pediatrics, geriatrics highlights a high degree of individual variability and function, from patient to patient, for the same age, sex, and disease. To select elderly candidates for surgery, the following elements of assessment are appropriate: a mental status assessment (Table 2), the Selected Symptom Review for the elderly (Table 3), assessment of sensory deficit, a medication review, a reliable report of home environment and social supports, and basic laboratory screen (Table 4). The Saskatchewan Short Mental Status Questionnaire is favored because it can be memorized and administered in the office and at bedside. Major mental impairment, coupled with other measures of quality of life, may be a relative contraindication in elective procedures. In the acutely ill patient, the initial assessment is a baseline from which to measure progress of delirium. Severe sensory deficit may be a relative contraindication; for example, the elderly person who is afraid to leave his home environment because of impaired vision does not improve ambulation and socialization after joint replacement or hernia repair. A baseline assessment of sensory deficit permits the surgeon to anticipate management problems. For example, elderly patients who cannot see or hear may pull out tubes, may subsequently become incontinent, and may not regain function as rapidly as younger patients postoperatively. These patients are at risk for a long hospital stay.

The medication review may influence selection of patients, but is particularly important in predicting the management of the frail elderly person, once admitted. The elderly take multiple medications; interactions are common, and consistency of dosage is difficult to maintain. Consequently, the clinician can be fooled. For example, 0.25 mg per day of digoxin was once considered the appropriate dose for the elderly as well as for younger adults. Today we know that 0.125 mg per day or every

other day is a more suitable dose for most elderly patients. It has been demonstrated that noncompliance among those in community dwellings has in the past kept the dosage below that instructed, and consequently digoxin toxicity has been avoided. When hospitalized, however, the patient receives the "correct" dose, and homeostasis is altered. To complicate matters, digoxin toxicity is difficult to recognize in the elderly, and serum levels are not reliable within the individual, nor consistent among patients in the same narrow age group.

A set of laboratory screens in selecting surgical candidates is suggested (see Table 4). These tests identify potential problems during surgery and anesthesia which can be managed effectively when anticipated. Beware of laboratory normals in the elderly. Most laboratories give a range by age. Although it is unreasonable to delay urgent surgery to obtain these laboratory tests, they are an integral part of any baseline geriatric assessment and therefore so much more important when invasive procedures are considered.

Verify the home environment. The surgeon must assure himself that the requested cataract operation is not the family strategy to get mother out of the too large, too dark apartment with too many stairs. If the environment is already unsuitable, the surgeon cannot expect to send his patient back there after surgery. Knowledge of the support system allows the surgeon to prepare for convalescent hospital or respite admission as an appropriate interim measure.

TABLE 3 Selected Symptom Review

Anorexia
Fatigue
Weak all over
Weight loss
Headache
Insomnia
Visual impairment
Transient visual disturbance
Hearing impairment
Dental/denture discomfort
Exertional chest discomfort
Orthopnea
Edema
Claudication
Abdominal pain
Usual bowel habit (meds?)
Urinary frequency/urgency
Nocturia
Incontinence
Dizziness/unsteadiness
Falls
Focal weakness or sensory loss
Forgetfulness
Disruptive behavior/wandering
Verbally/physically aggressive
Suffers verbal/physical abuse
Weakness
Syncope

TABLE 4 Suggested Laboratory Screen

CBC
Cell differential
Cell sedimentation rate
Serum B_{12} level
Serum and cell folate levels
Iron studies
VDRL
Serum calcium
BUN
Creatinine
Serum protein
Alkaline phosphatase
Electrolytes
Serum glucose
Urinalysis
Urine culture
Electrocardiogram
Chest film
Mammogram
Blood gases

The traditional complete history and physical examination are cumbersome in the elderly, yet a complete assessment is necessary. By using a selected symptom review suited to the elderly, the surgeon can take a global view of his patients and yet complete assessment in the office in a reasonable period of time (see Table 3). The preoperative clinical evaluation always has a view to the postoperative course.

For ongoing monitoring of progress of the elderly, the preoperative baseline should include a simple measure of functional level. In conjunction with the Saskatchewan Mental Status, the Katz Scale of Independence measures activities of daily living, and provides a reliable clinical picture (Fig. 2). The Katz ADL assessment is simple and easy to memorize. It provides a biological hierarchy that predicts the order of loss and return to function. The basic elements are: independence in feeding, continence, transferring, toileting, dressing, and bathing. Dressing and bathing are the highest functional levels, akin to ritual behavior in animals. Hundreds of functional level schemata have been developed; however, the Katz is a simple practical score reflecting a universal progression. The order of return to function reflects human development; for example, feeding (or sucking) is the first skill learned in the newborn. The other skills are learned in the order of the Katz' hierarchy. Independence in continence, then in transferring, and finally in toileting (meaning the child is able to get to and from the toilet alone, accompanied by the appropriate degree of dressing and undressing) follows. This same sequence reflects phylogeny. All organisms feed, but other functions are acquired in evolution, in the order of the Katz hierarchy. The higher the class or level of organism, the more functions it can carry out. In illness, regardless of age group, these functions are lost in reverse order. For example a young healthy person with a viral illness may stay home and not dress or bathe. If he is very ill, he may not be able to get to the toilet nor to walk unaccompanied. If he is incontinent, he is likely to be in an intensive care unit. These functions are regained in reverse order as he mends. Any variation in the order of loss or acquisition of function should be a signal that there is an unidentified illness, or must be explained by a particular ongoing disability. For example, an individual with an above-the-knee amputation may not be able to ambulate independently and yet might be able to dress or bathe. An individual dependent only for continence may have a urinary tract infection or a chronic condition such as prolapsed uterus. One point is given for each area of dependence; the lower the score, the more independent the individual. The score ranges from "0" for total independence to "6" for total dependence. The score can be assigned by any member of the health care team. The Katz serves as a monitor of health status and as a signal for illness; it helps the surgeon to select the appropriate special therapies and to predict outcome for his patients.

With the clinical profile provided by these simple tools, the surgeon prevents chronic disability and serves more effectively his elderly patients, regardless of their biological age. Consultation from family physicians, psychogeriatricians, the geriatric assessment team, and/or the internists, can help the surgeon complete the preoperative assessment. But expect more than clearance for surgery. Consultation should mean that your patient arrives in the operating room sooner and in better condi-

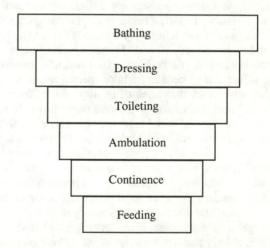

- Independent in feeding, continence, ambulating, going to the toilet, dressing, and bathing
- Independent in all but one of these functions
- Independent in all but bathing and one additional function
- Independent in all but bathing, dressing, and one additional function
- Independent in all but bathing, dressing, going to the toilet, ambulating, and one additional function
  (fully independent = 0; any impairment regardless of reason = 1; maximum score = 6)

Figure 2 The Katz hierarchy of activities of daily living.

TABLE 5 Preoperative Regimen
Exercise 3 times per week for 20 minutes
Hydration
Supplement calcium
Vitamin C
Folate
Vitamin B$_{12}$
Vitamin D
Stop smoking
Taper selected medications
Institute breathing exercises

TABLE 6 Geriatric Survival Kit
Calendar
Glasses
Hearing aid
Walking aid
Familiar objects
Radio
Night light
Clock

tion, that he is among the 70 to 80 percent of the elderly discharged home postoperatvely, and that he is not readmitted.

MANAGEMENT PRINCIPLES

Management of elderly patients rests on these principles: special therapies, maintenance of function, and reality orientation. The elderly are likely to exhibit delirium in the face of environmental change (admission to hospital) and sensory deprivation (aggravated by poor vision and hearing, and later by lack of clues as to the time of day in recovery). Elderly patients who are accustomed to glasses and hearing aids should wear these aids throughout the hospital stay. Glasses may be removed for the operation, but should be replaced in the recovery room. Sensory deficits are known to cause delirium, confusion, and disorientation, sometimes difficult to-reverse in the elderly.

Unexplained mental deterioration and incontinence are not normal aging changes and must be investigated. Such patterns may develop during admission and may be reversible only with great difficulty, if at all. To compensate, insist that the patient's glasses and hearing aid be in place every day all day, that a calendar and familiar photo are in view, and that a small night light signals time of day. Do not stand in the doorway to greet your patient; come to the bed-side, touch him, say your name and the patient's name. Assure yourself, on each visit to the bed-side, that he remembers the circumstance of admission. Otherwise suspicion, confusion, and even combativeness may occur.

The elderly also exhibit different responses to additional stresses; for example: medications, the surgery itself, anesthesia, a cold operating room, and bed rest. The chronically starved, then acutely starved (preoperatively), then cold stressed (OR), anesthetized, and traumatized (surgery) frail elderly individual exhibits rapid loss of function not unlike that seen in concentration camps. This loss is difficult to reverse in the frail elderly and results in disorientation, contractures, and bed sores. High caloric intake, warmed intravenous solutions and thermal blankets in the operating room, emergency room, and recovery room are recommended. Monitor the elderly aggressively. Once you have decided to operate, use high-tech support to help you. Consider Swan-Ganz catheterization and continued cardiac monitoring. It is strongly recommended that the frail elderly be booked first thing in the morning when possible, and that they take priority. The frail elderly individual with a hip fracture is not infrequently alternately starved from 6 in the evening till 12 noon, and then encouraged to eat and drink as much as possible and then starved again, because more acute trauma cases arriving in the emergency room "bump" the eldery off the operating schedule. Thus, the behavior of professionals leads to further loss of function, further disease, and institutionalization among the aged.

In elective cases, advise the patient to institute a presurgery regimen for 2 to 4 weeks before surgery (Table 5). Then advise the patient to arrive in the hospital the evening before surgery with the geriatric survival kit (Table 6): a calendar that can be displayed at all times in view of the patient, eyeglasses, hearing aid, walking aid, sturdy safe shoes, a few familiar objects, a radio, a night light, and a clock. Assure yourself that your patient is oriented and hydrated, then book him at 8:00 AM and do not postpone. For urgent surgery, do as much preparation as is possible in the time available, and recruit the family to assist.

POSTOPERATIVE INTRA-ABDOMINAL INFECTION

RICHARD D. GOODENOUGH, M.D.

Intra-abdominal infection after surgical intervention continues to be a complication of major importance. Despite newer techniques of diagnosis and drainage, the continuing development of broad-spectrum antibiotics, and increasing sophistication in the care of the critically ill patient, the mortality rate for clinically evident intra-abdominal infections approximates 30 percent.

A discussion of postoperative intra-abdominal infections requires consideration of the anatomy of the infection and its subsequent presentation. There exists a continuum from abscess to generalized peritonitis based on the body's ability to localize the infection and eradicate it via local defense mechanisms. However, all abscesses exhibit some degree of a surrounding cellulitis (peritonitis). Furthermore, the systemic effects of an abscess also depend upon the body's ability to locally contain it. For this reason, intra-abdominal abscesses present with a much broader clinical spectrum of illness than does generalized peritonitis.

GENERALIZED PERITONITIS

Peritonitis is a cellulitis that spreads radially from the site of contamination along tissue planes within the abdomen. Patients frequently present with a generalized intra-abdominal infection some hours to days after the initial contamination has occurred and are at risk for the catastrophic sequellae of systemic sepsis, including death. Generalized peritonitis develops as a result of the number and virulence of the bacterial innoculum and from the inability of host defenses to eliminate this innoculum.

Patients with generalized peritonitis require intensive perioperative and operative care. The objectives of care are (1) to return the metabolic and hemodynamic responses of severe sepsis toward normal physiology, (2) to surgically control the source of contamination, and (3) to remove necrotic and heavily contaminated tissue by debridement and lavage. The timing of operative intervention hinges only on the length of time required for intensive resuscitation and operative preparation. Generalized peritonitis requires urgent operation. Furthermore unless the patient is nonsalvageable at the time of presentation or refuses operation, surgical intervention is mandatory.

Preoperative preparation includes fluid resuscitation, hemodynamic and metabolic monitoring and support, and broad-spectrum antibiotic coverage. Adequate intravenous access is obtained, and with pulmonary artery catheter monitoring, rapid fluid resuscitation is performed with lactated Ringer's solution. These patients may present in septic shock, necessitating pressor support if rapid volume infusion does not maintain blood pressure and cardiac index. The drug of choice is dopamine. These patients require an additional pressor only if maximal pharmacologic doses of dopamine are inadequate. Direct pressure monitoring via arterial catheter is usually required. In addition, urinary output should be followed by catheter. Nasogastric decompression is necessary. If adult respiratory distress syndrome (ARDS) has intervened, oxygenation may become difficult, necessitating the use of positive end-expiratory pressure (PEEP) and oxygen concentrations above 40 percent.

Antibiotic coverage must include drugs active against the normal colonic species, including anaerobes. In practice, this usually requires a two- or three-drug regimen, e.g., ampicillin, tobramycin, and clindamycin. These choices cover the gram-negative rods, *Enterococcus* species, and anaerobes until finer selection can be made on the basis of peritoneal culture data. The use of an aminoglycoside mandates dose adjustment based on blood levels.

Operative intervention follows satisfactory fluid and pharmacologic resuscitation. The incision used in generalized peritonitis should be midline and is extended as necessary after the source of the intra-abdominal disease is clear. The purpose of the operation is to identify and repair the initiating process, to debride necrotic tissue, and to reduce the bacterial load by means of debridement of exudate and lavage.

Once the abdomen is open, cultures should be taken and a Gram stain performed. A systemic search is then performed and the initiating process corrected. In the case of bowel perforation or anastomotic leak, a diversion of the enteric contents is required. Frequently, resection of a segment of bowel also is necessary. Anastomosis should not be performed in the setting of generalized peritonitis as dehiscence and leak can result.

Debridement of all necrotic tissue and exudate is then gently performed. Gentle debridement is defined as that which does not incite significant bleeding from denuded surfaces. These operative efforts reduce the existing bacterial load and culture material for future bacterial growth. Copious lavage with isothermic normal saline is then performed in order to dilute the remaining bacterial load. Irrigation in the presence of already generalized peritonitis does not spread bacterial contamination. Abdominal drains are not used, however, as they are ineffective.

Further methods toward control of generalized peritonitis have also been advocated, but are less widely accepted. The first is the continuous irrigation of all four abdominal quadrants postoperatively with saline, antibiotic, or povidone-iodine solutions. Radical debridement of the abdomen has also been advocated, but may lead to significant blood loss and provision of a blood culture medium for further bacterial growth. Intraoperative antibiotic lavage is also employed by many surgeons, but may not add further tissue resistance to the broad-spectrum intravenous antibiotics already used.

The midline fascia is closed preferentially with a monofilament running suture. Retention sutures may provide added wound support. Generally, the skin and subcutaneous tissues are left open and 5 days later undergo delayed primary closure. Quantitative wound cultures are lowest at that time.

Postoperatively, these patients require prolonged intensive care and may develop any of the complications to which critically ill patients are subject. Particular postoperative concerns are respiratory complications, including ARDS and prolonged ventilatory support, renal failure, coagulopathy, and sepsis-related catabolism leading to malnutrition. A therapeutic course of antibiotics must be used.

The overall risk of mortality in generalized peritonitis is 30 to 40 percent, depending on its source. Further operative intervention is indicated if abscess formation occurs or if continued peritoneal soilage is present.

ABDOMINAL ABSCESS

Postoperative abdominal abscesses are discrete collections of purulent and necrotic tissue that are bounded by surrounding anatomic structures. They are best defined anatomically and can be grouped as intraperitoneal, visceral, and retroperitoneal. Intraperitoneal abscesses most frequently follow abdominal operation, whereas visceral abscesses are more commonly due to bacteremic seeding or primary organ disease, such as pancreatitis or ascending biliary infections. Retroperitoneal abscesses may arise from any of these mechanisms. The most common sites for intraperitoneal abscesses, in order of frequency, are (1) right paracolonic, (2) left paracolonic, (3) pelvic, (4) subphrenic (right or left), (5) retroperitoneal, (6) subhepatic, and (7) hepatic. Hepatic abscesses are by far the most common visceral abscesses. Altemeier has divided retroperitoneal abscesses into anterior, posterior, and retrofascial. The anterior retroperitoneal space is limited by the peritoneum, anterior renal fascia, quadratus lumborum, diaphragm, and pelvic rim. The posterior space extends to the transversalis fascia and communicates inferiorly as the renal fascia is not fused. The retrofascial space is posterior to the transversalis fascia. These spaces may become obliterated by chronic or widespread infections.

The diagnosis of postoperative abdominal abscess must be suspected in any patient with fever, leukocytosis, and abdominal tenderness. However, because these abscesses may not irritate the abdominal wall, the abdominal findings may be absent. Furthermore, the clinical spectrum ranges from indolent, chronic infection to abscesses presenting with septic shock.

Computed tomography (CT) provides the best imaging technique in the diagnosis of abdominal abscesses and has revolutionized their evaluation. Ultrasound, gallium or indium scanning, and plain abdominal films can each be helpful in diagnosis. However, the CT scan is clearly the most sensitive and specific test.

The bacteria responsible for abdominal abscesses are similar to those responsible for peritonitis. The gram-negative rods, enteric streptococci and anaerobes predominate. Pathogens that cause abdominal abscess, in order of frequency, are (1) *E. coli*, (2) *B. fragilis*, (3) *Streptococcus*, (4) anaerobic cocci, (5) *Clostridia*, (6) *Proteus*, (7) fusobacteria. These are polymicrobial infections and must be treated with broad-spectrum antibiotics capable of interrupting the symbiosis between the multiple organisms present. Of course, the choice of antibiotics is tailored after appropriate culture and sensitivity data are available. Antibiotics are continued until the systemic signs of sepsis are eliminated for a reasonable period of time. However, antibiotic therapy does not need to continue until the drains are completely removed. In practice, 7 to 14 days of intravenous antibiotic coverage is usually required.

The choice of an aminoglycoside with clindamycin or metronidazole is still the most secure one in the treatment of abdominal abscess. If the patient is in extremis or does not respond completely with surgical therapy, possible enterococcal infection should be treated with ampicillin or penicillin, in addition. The second- and third-generation cephalosporins and the uredopenicillin derivatives may be shown adequate as single-drug therapy of intra-abdominal infection in the future. However, consensus does not currently support this position.

Treatment

Treatment of intra-abdominal abscesses consists of adequate drainage of the abscess in conjunction with appropriate antibiotic coverage to augment local host defense. Drainage of the abscess cavity must address all purulent foci and must continue until the abscess cavity collapses and eliminates the infected space. In addition, any communication with the gastrointestinal tract as the source of continuing contamination must be corrected. This usually requires a diversionary procedure in addition to abscess drainage, with definitive repair staged at a later time.

Drainage may be performed percutaneously via ultrasound or CT-guided catheter placement, or surgically in the operating room. Percutaneous drainage of abscesses has been shown to be efficacious and well tolerated when the following basic criteria are met. There must be a "window" for clear access to the abscess without traversing bowel or contaminating previously sterile spaces. Multiple abscesses or loculated abscesses are not well drained percutaneously. Continued contamination from anastomotic leak or nonviable bowel is not treated percutaneously. This form of therapy is not appropriate for thick pus or necrotic tissue requiring debridement, as in pancreatic abscesses. However, percutaneous drainage is clearly a valuable therapeutic tool and may be much safer than open drainage. It should always be considered.

Operative drainage of abscesses must be predicated on adequate dependent drainage, debridement of necrotic tissue, diversion of the enteric stream if appropriate, cavity lavage, and, above all, avoidance of contamination of surrounding sterile spaces. The classic "extraserous" drainage approaches the abscess from an extraperitoneal route and dependently drains it without

TABLE 1 Operative Approach to Abdominal Abscess

Site	Primary	Secondary
Right subphrenic	Subcostal	Posterior
Left subphrenic	Subcostal	Posterior
Subhepatic	Subcostal	Posterior
Paracolonic	Lower quadrant transverse	
Pelvic	Transrectal or vaginal	Abdominal midline
Interloop	Midline transabdominal	
Retroperitoneal	Flank or posterior	

transgressing the peritoneal cavity. This approach may not be practicable if multiple abscesses exist, or if the abscess is loculated in the central abdomen, or if enteric communication exists. In general, the purulent material is carefully drained, all loculations are manually explored so that a single cavity then exists, judicious debridement is performed, the cavity is irrigated with saline, and multiple soft rubber and/or soft sump drains are placed in a position that favors dependent drainage. These drains are left in position until all signs of systemic sepsis are gone, drainage is scant, and the cavity has collapsed. They are then serially advanced.

The timing of drainage depends on the individual patients' illness. Treatment of profound systemic sepsis precedes operative drainage, as discussed in the therapy of peritonitis, but should not delay therapy unduly.

The mortality rate in patients with postoperative abdominal abscesses is 20 to 30 percent and depends on the underlying disease and the patient's general health, as well as the execution of adequate therapy. Complications include profound sepsis, fistulas, recurrent abscess formation, hemorrhage, bowel obstruction, wound complications, renal failure, pulmonary failure, and malnutrition. A significant complication occurs in approximately 40 percent of patients.

Surgical Approach to Specific Abscesses

The right subphrenic space is bounded by the liver, diaphragm, and their ligamentous attachments. Abscesses arise here after gastric, duodenal, or biliary operations and also as a result of distant, septic, peritoneal contamination. The accumulation of infected material in this potential space is favored by the lower relative pressure in this region and the circulation of intra-abdominal fluid. Drainage is best performed via an extraperitoneal approach using a standard right subcostal or lateral subcostal incision, with dissection superficial to the transversalis fascia until the abscess is localized (Table 1). Purulence is verified by needle aspiration and drainage is then performed, as already described. An alternative approach is through the bed of the twelfth rib posteriorly. However, some authors state that this posterior approach requires transgression and contamination of the posterior recess of the peritoneal cavity.

Frequently, the left subphrenic abscess occurs after distant contamination due to peritonitis or leakage and after operations on the spleen or stomach. They are posterior and may be approached through a standard left subcostal, a lateral left subcostal, or a posterior incision. Care is necessary to avoid splenic injury if the spleen is to remain.

The subhepatic abscess lies caudad to the right lobe of the liver and usually involves its deep recess, Morrison's pouch. These abscesses occur frequently after gastric, biliary, colonic, and appendiceal surgery. Furthermore, they may occur in conjunction with subphrenic collections. These abscesses are best drained through a lateral right subcostal incision and extraperitoneal approach. A posterior approach may also be employed.

Paracolonic abscesses occur on either side and commonly follow appendectomy or colonic surgery. The possibility of a fecal communication must always be considered. An extraperitoneal approach over the most direct avenue of entry is performed. A counterincision with enteric diversion may be necessary with or without resection of a segment of bowel.

Pelvic abscesses are usually palpable through the anterior rectal wall and occur after colonic and appendiceal surgery, or after drainage of primary intra-abdominal abscesses or generalized peritonitis. Drainage is best performed transrectally or through the vagina, with manual exploration to break down loculated areas of purulence. Digital exploration should be repeated daily until the cavity collapses, to ensure adequate drainage, as surgical drains frequently do not stay in place. Transabdominal drainage is carried out, if necessary, if drainage cannot be performed from below.

Interloop abscesses occur between adjacent loops of bowel and may involve the abdominal wall and omentum. These are frequently multiple and follow widespread contamination of the abdominal cavity after colonic surgery or peritonitis. They require transperitoneal drainage via a midline incision, with careful debridement and cavity irrigation. Drains should not be brought through previously clean areas of the abdominal cavity. Interloop abscesses frequently recur, requiring close attention on the part of the clinician.

Hepatic abscess may follow operation on the colon or appendix, usually in conjunction with established intraperitoneal infections. They may be polymicrobial, but also can be due to a single organism, usually E. coli or a staphylococcal species. Small abscesses respond to antibiotic therapy alone. Larger abscesses require drainage, but can usually be drained percutaneously.

Retroperitoneal abscesses may follow appendicitis, posterior colonic perforations, or anastomotic leaks. They can grow to a large size and may be indolent. Occasionally, they present as groin sepsis. Drainage is done through the posterior or flank approach and requires multiple drains in all of the involved areas. As already noted, diversion of the enteric stream is necessary if a communication exists.

ACUTE RENAL FAILURE

ARLIE R. MANSBERGER, Jr., M.D.
JOSEPH T. WATLINGTON, M.D.

Renal failure in the patient with diseases unique to the discipline of surgery continues to be accompanied by a distressingly high mortality rate. The clinical course of acute renal failure in surgical patients is complicated by problems in volume, electrolyte and catabolic disturbances, metabolic acidosis as a result of and complicating the above, wound healing deficiencies, and immunosuppression with resultant infection and sepsis.

Significant groups of the population for whom the surgeon must provide therapy are literally "patients with renal failure waiting to happen." These include those with advancing age, diabetics, patients with pre-existing chronic compensated renal disease from a variety of etiologies, those with major vessel arterial disease, and patients with major cardiovascular (particularly left ventricular) dysfunction.

Trauma, the third leading killer in our population, adds to the incidence (especially in the young) via transfusion reactions, myoglobinuria from crush injuries, shock, hypoxia, and multiple organ failure from multisystem injury and sepsis.

The incidence of renal failure in surgical patients has not decreased over the past two decades. However, the incidence of oliguric renal failure (ARF) has decreased and that of nonoliguric or high-output renal failure (HORF) has replaced ARF as the most common presentation of renal damage. Reasons for the continuing magnitude of the problem are many, some of which are overlooked by the individual surgeon who may be lulled into a sense of false security by (1) a relatively low incidence of ARF and HORF in his or her individual practice, (2) a lack of recognition of the more subtle forms of renal failure in their early stages, (3) the availability of modern methods of vascular access, ultrafiltration, peritoneal dialysis, hemodialysis, and transplantation, and (4) incomplete comprehension of polypharmacy as that, in turn, relates to nephrotoxicity.

Drug-induced acute renal failure has become more common. We physicians subject our patients to multiple medications, some of them well-known nephrotoxins, others less well understood. Each surgeon undoubtedly knows that aminoglycosides and radiocontrast materials are potentially nephrotoxic *but* does he or she recognize that the toxicity is related to the number of free amino groups in the compound, that the various aminoglycosides have different numbers of free amino groups, and that the half-life of the antibiotic in the renal tubular cell exceeds that of the serum by 218 times? In fact, each surgeon must answer the question: Have I adequately evaluated this patient's renal function and volume status prior to writing my orders for an aminoglycoside or for study with radiocontrast materials?

Furthermore, he or she must respond to such queries as: Am I aware that aspirin and indomethacin may predispose this geriatric arthritic patient to severe ischemia since those drugs are prostaglandin inhibitors and since postglandins (particularly PGE) act as renal vasodilators and work toward balancing the vasoconstrictor effects of renin and angiotensin (particularly angiotensin II)?

An awareness of the aforementioned possible hazards allows the surgeon to institute *preventive* measures. Surgeons must take this course if the overall incidence and mortality rates for this entity are to be reduced significantly in surgical patients.

DIAGNOSIS OF RENAL FAILURE

Azotemia in the surgical patient is properly classified by the anatomic site in which the initiating disturbance occurs, that is, prerenal, postrenal, or renal. The classes and broad causal relationships are as follows:

1. Prerenal azotemia results from events leading to a decrease in renal perfusion pressure, increased vascular resistance, or both; glomerular filtration is diminished to such a degree that endogenous nitrogenous waste cannot be eliminated.
2. Postrenal azotemia is due to obstruction in the lower or, more rarely, the upper urinary tract.
3. Renal azotemia results from intrarenal causes of renal failure, oliguric or nonoliguric, secondary to a wide variety of causes.

Prerenal Azotemia

In patients with prerenal azotemia, the concomitant rise in serum creatinine usually is not of the same magnitude as the rise in blood urea nitrogen (BUN). The urinary osmolality is greater than 500 m0sm, the urine-to-plasma (U/P) urea ratio greater than 30, and U/P creatinine ratio greater than 40, and examination of the urinary sediment shows nothing remarkable (Fig. 1).

In some patients, differentiation of prerenal from other causes may be difficult because of an overlap in laboratory values. In these circumstances, calculation of the "renal failure index" (RFI) = (urine sodium (Una) divided by U/P Cr) and of the fractional excretion of sodium (FeNa) = (U/P Na divided by U/P Cr $\times$ 100) is helpful. A value of less than 1 is characteristic of prerenal azotemia, whereas values of 2 or greater are associated with acute renal failure or urinary obstruction. One should not rely on RFI or FeNa in patients who have received diuretics or in patients in hepatic decompensation or congestive heart failure.

Postrenal Azotemia

Evaluation of laboratory parameters is of less aid in the differentiation of postrenal and renal azotemia than in separating the latter from prerenal azotemia. The urine

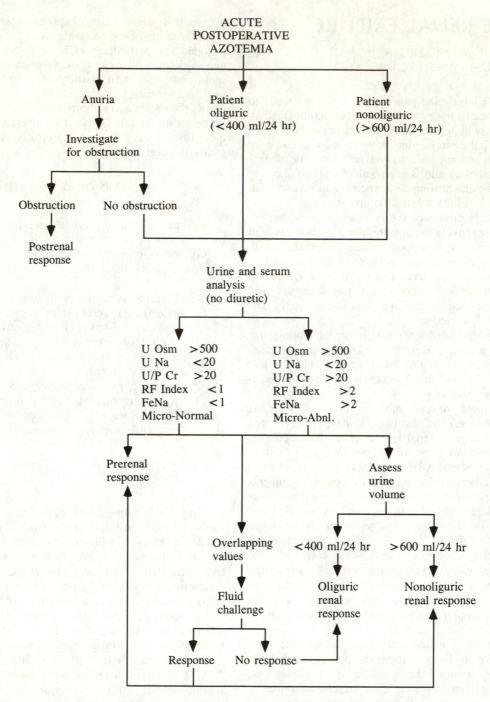

Figure 1 Algorithm for differential diagnosis of acute postoperative azotemia.

in patients with acute obstruction of the urinary tract may show a composition similar to that of prerenal azotemia for a short interval. By contrast, chronic obstructive uropathy causes varying degrees of tubular dysfunction, and when acute obstruction is superimposed, the urinary composition is similar to that in renal azotemia.

The differential diagnosis is made by virtue of a sudden onset of complete anuria, a prior history of frequency, nocturia, difficulty in initiating or terminating the act of voiding leading to a high index of suspicion,

anatomic knowledge of the operative procedure (in proximity to the ureters) or appropriate indicated studies (catheterization, sonography, computerized tomography, and pyelography).

Renal Azotemia

The diagnosis of renal azotemia is based on rapid and sequential elimination of prerenal and postrenal azotemia through history, physical examination, and laboratory tests, including a qualitative examination of the urine. The urinary osmolality is less than 400 mOsm, urine sodium values are usually in excess of 40 mEq per liter, U/P creatinine ratio less than 20, U/P urea less than 10, FEna and RFI greater than 2, and a microscopic examination that is abnormal and includes brown granular casts, tubular cells, red cells and/or protein or cellular casts (see Fig. 1).

The analysis of urine (both the quantitative measurement of osmolality, sodium, and creatinine, and the microscopic examination) is essential in the diagnosis of renal azotemia. Some use the RFI and FeNa value, but Baxter believes the U/P area to be the most reliable test; in renal azotemia it is usually less than 10 and, not uncommonly, less than 5.

There are two forms of renal azotemia: oliguric (less than 400 ml urine in 24 hours) and nonoliguric (greater than 600 ml urine in 24 hours). A high index of suspicion and awareness are keys to the diagnosis of nonoliguric renal azotemia. The diagnosis is usually first suspected postoperatively by virtue of a rising BUN in the face of "adequate" urinary output.

PREVENTION OF RENAL FAILURE

Preoperative Prevention

In the patient with an elective surgical problem and with known and recognized chronic compensated renal failure, a safe course through anesthesia and operation may be ensured by determining the urinary volume required for compensatory mechanisms and ensuring maintenance of that volume before, during, and after the operation. The clearance of any substance may be determined by the formula $C1 = UV/P$ (urine concentration × volume ÷ plasma concentration). When the concentration of urea (the main contributor to urinary osmolality) is consistently less than 400 mOsm and the blood urea is maintained at 60 mg per decilter, for example, the only mechanism by which the BUN can remain at 60 mg per deciliter occurs via an increase in daily urinary volume excretion. Therefore, preoperative determination of the 24-hour urine volume necessary to maintain a constant BUN, divided by 24, will give the surgeon the hourly quantitative urinary output necessary to maintain compensation. The patient can ill afford to be permitted *any* degree of volume contraction preoperatively, since that state causes decreased hydrostatic pressure in the juxtaglomerular apparatus and results in an increase in the level of renin, angiotensin, and aldosterone. It is imperative that intravenous fluid loading be instituted when that type of patient is undergoing an operative procedure so that the usual order, NPO after midnight, will not result in volume depletion. Preoperative loading with solute solution (i.e., Ringers lactate) not only prevents the elaboration of aldosterone, but also acts as a solute diuretic since the sodium is not resorbed in the proximal tubules and, on reaching the distal convoluted tubules, by virtue of the sodium gradient, "bypasses" the antidiuretic hormone effect of anesthesia and operation. The resultant solute diuresis, if stimulated in sufficient quantity, provides for maintenance of renal compensation and results in a normal postoperative course.

If, for example, a patient with a BUN of 60 mg per deciliter and a urinary osmolality of 340 has a daily urinary output of approximately 2,400 ml, then an hourly urinary output of 100 ml prior to, during, and after operation, stimulated by solute diuresis, as already outlined, will result in abortion of renal decompensation, provided there is no significant episode of hypovolemia or hypoxia during the conduct of the operation.

As a matter of fact, preloading should be the standard not only for patients who have renal disease, but also for all patients who are in the "high risk for renal failure" category and for those who are undergoing operative procedures with high hypotensive potential (i.e., for abdominal aortic aneurysm) or operations with potential large third-space losses (i.e., pelvic exenteration).

In patients sustaining trauma and/or those with hemorrhagic shock, volume depletion must be treated vigorously, and hypoxia must be avoided if renal insult is to be negated. Initial resuscitation of patients in hemorrhagic shock or those sustaining severe trauma typically consists of 2,000 ml of balanced salt solution, which not only permits time for crossmatching of type-specific blood, but also abets the avoidance of hemolytic transfusion reactions. Because of the sequestration of large volumes of fluid into the extracellular space, or into the intestinal lumen in patients who sustain trauma, volume losses are often difficult to estimate with any degree of accuracy. A sine qua non of accurate volume replacement in the severely traumatized patient, therefore, is the careful and accurate monitoring of urinary output, cardiac output, and central venous and pulmonary wedge pressures in response to resuscitative efforts before operation, during operation, and in the postoperative period until hemodynamic stabilization is realized.

Should the patient develop a hemolytic response to mismatched blood, the presence of an established diuresis greatly diminishes the chances of renal failure secondary to heme pigment and protein cast deposits in the renal tubules. Precipitation potential is further reduced by alkalizing the urine.

Similarly, renal failure prevention in patients with myoglobinuria is enhanced by maintaining volume, alkalinizing the urine with sodium bicarbonate, and stimulating diuresis with mannitol, 12.5 g per hour, until the urine is myoglobulin-free.

When alkalinizing the patient to raise urinary pH, serum calcium levels must be followed to avoid hypocalcemia, with its life-threatening complications.

Intraoperative Prevention

Intraoperative measures to prevent renal failure in patients who are in severe shock and/or ischemic or hypoxic states (to include temporary renal or suprarenal aortic cross-clamping) includes regional renal hypothermia carried out by bathing the kidneys with chilled isotonic solution (4 °C) for 5 minutes prior to removal of the sluice by suction. The process should be repeated every 1 to 1½ hours for the duration of the procedure.

Maintenance of adequate tissue oxygenation during operation is mandatory. The fact that alkalosis, hypothermia, and deficiencies of 2,3-diphosphoglycerate (DPG) all detract from the ability of the red cell to give up its oxygen via a left shift of the oxyhemoglobin dissociation curve mandates that careful attention be paid to prevention of hypothermia by warming fluids and blood, and that fresh blood be given preferentially because of the presence of 2,3-DPG. It should be remembered that blood preserved in dextrose-citrate-phosphorus solution maintains adequate levels of 2,3-DPG for up to 7 days of storage.

Postoperative Prevention

Acute renal failure may happen as a result of sepsis and in conjunction with the failure of other organs. The alert observer notes that the early renal response to septic insult is polyuria and hyponatremia, the latter associated with an intracellular migration of the sodium ion. At this stage of insult, antibiotics, especially aminoglycosides, may be given overenthusiastically and in inappropriately large doses. All surgeons are familiar with the fact that dosages may be adjusted on the basis of serum creatinine levels, but many do not recognize that creatinine values often do not rise until significant numbers of nephron units (approximately 50%) have been compromised. In this group of patients, daily creatinine clearance, rather than serum creatinine levels, should be the basis of dose calculation. If available, accurate peak and trough levels should be continuously determined.

It is possible to ascertain aminoglycoside renal toxicity in advance of rising creatinine levels. Rises in urinary alkaline phosphatase and beta-2 microglobulin often precede elevations in serum creatinine by 5 to 7 days.

In the postoperative and/or the post-trauma period, increased intra-abdominal pressure (above 30 mm Hg) may potentiate the onset of ARF. One factor in this saga resides in resultant inferior vena caval compression with consequent decreased cardiac filling pressure and reduced cardiac output.

Recent information suggests that ARF can be initiated by this phenomenon (intra-abdominal pressure greater than 30 mm Hg) early in the postoperative period without a decrease in blood pressure or cardiac output. Kron et al reported their observations in 11 patients who had acute elevations of intra-abdominal pressure greater than 30 mm Hg. Four of their patients who were observed developed renal failure and died. The other seven were reoperated on and decompressed and responded with immediate diuresis.

The technique for measuring intra-abdominal pressure is as follows:

1. Sterile saline (50 to 100 cc) is injected in the empty bladder through the indwelling Foley catheter.
2. The sterile tubing of the urinary drainage bag is cross-clamped just distal to the culture aspiration point.
3. The end of the urinary drainage is connected to the indwelling Foley catheter.
4. The clamp is released just enough to allow the tubing proximal to the clamp to flow with fluid from the bladder, then reapplied.
5. A 16-gauge needle is then used to Y-connect a cup manometer or pressure transducer through the culture aspiration port of the tubing to the drainage bag.
6. The top of the symphysis pubic bone is used as the zero point with the patient supine.

Recently, we substantiated Kron's observation in four of five patients in our trauma unit (Fig. 2) in whom adequate urinary output decreased to oliguria over 1 or 2 hours and who had elevated intra-abdominal pressures with adequate hemodynamics.

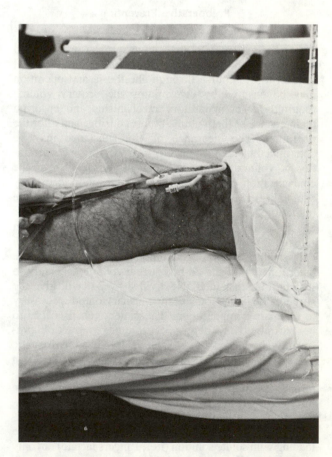

Figure 2 Equipment in place to monitor intraperitoneal pressure.

TREATMENT

In patients with ARF, maintenance of fluid balance is essential. Fluid intake must be restricted and is best adjusted by obtaining the daily weight of the patient on an accurate scale. In the absence of fistulas or other significant extrarenal fluid loss, daily fluid intake should rarely exceed 500 to 700 ml plus urine output in the previous 24 hours; in some instances, as little as 300 to 400 ml per day is required for maintenance. Amounts must be added to the daily requirement to compensate for extrarenal losses through drain tracts, fistulas, nasogastric tubes, and diarrhea stools. The body weight should be permitted to decrease by 0.2 to 0.3 kg per 24 hours.

The most common fluid and electrolyte abnormalities are hyponatremia and hyperkalemia. The former is not uncommonly an iatrogenic dilutional phenomenon, but may also be secondary to a primary sodium deficit or to a primary potassium deficit.

Even mild fluid overload may lead to congestive heart failure or subtle forms of water intoxication, which may be managed by fluid restriction. More severe fluid overload with pulmonary edema and/or symptomatic water intoxication are indications for dialysis or ultrafiltration.

When there is clear evidence that hyponatremia and hypochloremia are not dilutional and that potassium deficits are not responsible for the hyponatremia, small amounts of hypertonic (3%) sodium chloride may be used for replacement on the basis of calculated deficiencies. Similarly, small amounts of sodium bicarbonate, added to the infusate as necessary, are beneficial in combating acidosis and hence hyperkalemia. (Care must be taken to ensure that the serum lactate level is not excessive when bicarbonate is used.)

A significant and immediately life-threatening problem associated with renal azotemia is hyperkalemia. In fact, it is the leading biochemical cause of death in patients with ARF and occurs in both the oliguric and nonoliguric varieties, although its incidence is less in the latter form of failure.

In less severe conditions, the body tolerates moderate elevations of potassium by compensation through potassium fluxes across cellular membranes. Rapidly developing increases in serum potassium (from decreased renal potassium excretion and extracellular shifting from catabolism and metabolic acidosis) are not accompanied by the similar elevation of intracellular potassium and may alter the membrane potential severely, leading to neuromuscular dysfunction and cardiac arrhythmias.

Acute increases in serum potassium in the vicinity of 5.5 mEq per liter generally are not associated with symptoms. As the level of potassium rises, the patient may experience fatigue, lassitude, and parethesias. Decreased tendon reflexes follow. When serum levels approach 7.5 to 8 mEq per liter, complete neuromuscular paralysis, vascular collapse, ventricular fibrillation, and cardiac arrest are imminent.

Although there is no distinct or absolutely accurate correlation between serum potassium levels and electrocardiographic changes, definite trends may be noted. The earliest sign is peaking T waves (usually not seen until K levels exceed 5.5). The QRS complex widens when the serum potassium level reaches 6.5 mEq per liter. As the serum potassium level rises, P-wave amplitudes decrease and the PR interval is prolonged. When the level of 7.5 mEq per liter is approached, the P wave may disappear and the QRS complex may resemble a sine wave. A distinct bradycardia may be noted; ventricular fibrillation or ventricular standstill follows.

The treatment of acute hyperkalemia should be considered in two parts as follows: (1) the treatment of hyperkalemic cardiac toxicity and (2) the immediate and long-term therapy of acute elevations of serum potassium levels through (a) first, intracellular flux and (b) later, potassium removal.

The cardiac toxicity of acute elevations in potassium levels is best managed by the intravenous administration of a 10% calcium solution (one ampule of calcium chloride) given over a 5- or 10-minute period. Calcium gluconate in 2- to 4-g doses given intravenously is also effective therapy. The infusion of calcium causes rapid reversion of the QRS complex to normal. Because the result is directly dependent on the calcium ion, the cardiac effects of calcium infusion last only as long as the calcium levels are effectively maintained. Continuous electrocardiographic monitoring is essential, and calcium infusions are repeated as indicated.

Hyperkalemia is treated by causing potassium flux from the extracellular space and by effectively lowering the total body potassium. The former is accomplished by raising the arterial pH and by stimulating the formation of glycogen. One ampule (44 mM) of sodium bicarbonate should be given directly intravenously over a 5- to 10-minute time span. An additional two or three ampules should be added to 500 ml of 10% glucose. Ten to 15 units of regular insulin should be given subcutaneously at the start of the infusion or added to the infusate, which should be given over a 2- to 4-hour period. Neither of these methods of therapy reduces total body potassium. Generally speaking, the serum potassium level is reduced by 1 mEq per liter for every 0.1 unit rise in arterial pH.

Total body potassium can be lowered by the administration of the cation exchange resin, polystyrene sodium sulfonate (Kayexalate), which effectively exchanges sodium for potassium. Thirty grams mixed with 200 to 300 ml of solution are given as a high retention enema. Approximately 1 mEq of potassium is removed for every gram of polystyrene used. The process can be repeated two or three times in 24 hours. If mixed with Sorbitol, the cation exchange resin can be given effectively by mouth, provided the patient can tolerate oral intake. Sodium levels must be monitored as a precaution against hypernatremia when large quantities of cation exchange resin are used to lower the total body potassium content.

When conservative measures are unable to stem the clinical problem associated with ARF, more aggressive and invasive techniques are indicated. Dialysis is indicated when severe metabolic acidosis and severe hyperkalemia are present. Ultrafiltration, a recent clinical development, can be used in oliguric ARF when volume removal is required because of congestive heart failure or to allow increased fluid therapy (parenteral hyperalimentation).

Dialysis

In surgical patients who develop ARF, many nephrologists recommend dialysis when the BUN or serum creatinine reaches an arbitrary level (i.e., 90 mg per deciliter or 8 mg per deciliter respectively). The goal of "prophylactic" dialysis is to prevent uremic signs and symptoms (frost, pericarditis, neurologic symptoms) and to allow increased nutrient intake in an attempt to lower the high mortality rate accompanying ARF.

The recommended frequency of dialysis varies. However, in the postoperative period or the post-trauma period, frequent or even daily dialysis is indicated because of the increased catabolic rate associated with trauma and/or operation.

Peritoneal Dialysis

Peritoneal dialysis is a relatively safe and effective form of therapy in which the peritoneum acts as a simple semipermeable membrane. This method of dialysis is approximately 25 percent as effective as hemodialysis per unit time. Individual solute transfer is inversely proportional to the molecular weight of the solute. For example, creatinine with its larger molecular weight is removed less rapidly than urea.

The composition of commercially available dialysates is roughly that of extracellular fluid, with sodium values of 137 to 140 mEq per liter; chloride, 97 to 103 mEq per liter; magnesium, 2 mEq per liter; calcium, 3 to 5 mEq per liter; and glucose, 1,500 mg per deciliter. Acetate or lactate is used as an alkalizing agent in place of bicarbonate since sodium bicarbonate causes precipitation of calcium and magnesium salts in the dialysate and since acetate or lactate is ultimately converted to bicarbonate when absorbed. Glucose in higher concentration (4.25 g per deciliter) is utilized when significant water removal is indicated. The lack of potassium in the dialysate enhances a decrease in the serum potassium level, which is further aided by glucose absorption and alkalinization (intracellular shift of potassium). When high glucose concentrations are utilized, acute volume depletion must be avoided by maintenance of strictly monitored weight and fluid balance records.

Among the advantages of peritoneal dialysis are the following: (1) it can be carried out in the patient's room because the mechanics are uncomplicated and commercially available materials are employed; (2) hemodynamic and biochemical changes are moderate per unit time; (3) anticoagulation and blood transfusion are unnecessary and the complications attendant to both or either are thus avoided; and (4) it is less costly than hemodialysis.

The choice of peritoneal dialysis versus hemodialysis depends in large measure on the capacity of the method to prevent uremic symptoms. In general, those disorders associated with severe catabolic states requiring optimal clearances require hemodialysis because even continuous peritoneal dialysis is inadequate under those circumstances. The latter is to be discouraged since there is a definite relationship between the length of peritoneal dialysis and the incidence of complications (notably peritonitis).

Patients who have dense adhesions or the probability of same are not candidates for peritoneal dialysis. However, recent abdominal operations are no longer considered contraindications for dialysis by this route as long as one is prepared to cope with increased leakage and increased albumin loss through fresh incisions and drainage sites.

Hemodialysis

In hemodialysis, blood is passed through tubing composed of a series of semipermeable membranes that allow low-molecular-weight molecules to be passed from the blood to the dialysate and dialyzable material from the dialysate to the blood stream. Thus, low-molecular-weight toxins can be removed, and acid base balance and electrolyte homeostasis can be achieved. Standard commercial dialysate is available as a concentrate and must be diluted with deionized water. Again, dialysate concentrations of electrolytes mirror ideal extracellular fluid and are similar in concentration to that described previously for peritoneal dialysis except that hemodialysate contains potassium (2.0 to 4.0 mEq per liter) and lesser concentrations of glucose (0.0 to 0.200 g per deciliter).

Vascular access for hemodialysis can usually be secured through double-lumen venous catheters placed in either the subclavian or the femoral vein. These catheters allow a blood flow of 200 to 250 ml per minute to the dialyzer and can be inserted at the patient's bedside. Long-term venous access is usually obtained through shunts, although venous catheters have been used for as long as 6 to 8 weeks at times.

In the usual situation, the patient's blood is anticoagulated prior to and during dialysis. However, in patients in whom bleeding would be enhanced by systemic heparin therapy (as those requiring dialysis in juxtaposition to operative procedures), regional heparinization can be accomplished by heparinizing the blood as it leaves the patient and enters the dialyzer and by infusing the returning blood with protamine after it leaves the dialyzer and before it enters the patient.

Ultrafiltration

Some critically ill patients do not tolerate volume removal on dialysis and require ultrafiltration. This can be accomplished either with dialysis equipment over 3 to 4 hours or with a slow continuous ultrafiltration (SCUF) device.

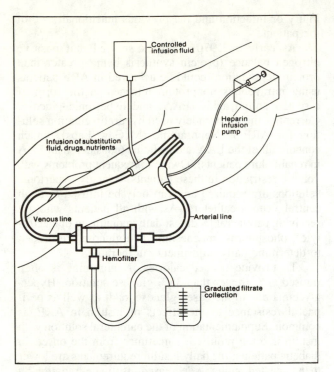

Figure 3 Continuous arteriovenous hemofiltration with femoral cannulation. (Courtesy AMICON Corporation)

Slow continuous ultrafiltration is performed by connecting arterial and venous catheters through a hemofiltration cartridge and allowing the patients own blood pressure to provide the needed gradient for fluid removal. The primary function of the cartridge is to remove plasma fluid. The ultrafiltration can be regulated by adjusting a clamp on the ultrafiltration line (not the arterial line). Heparin is infused into the arterial line at approximately 10 to 15 units per kilogram per hour (usually 700 to 1,000 U per hour) (Fig. 3).

Ultrafiltration can be applied by the surgeon, and even at systolic pressures of 60 to 80 mm Hg, filtration rates of 300 cc per hour can be obtained. The removal of fluid in oliguric patients allows the surgeon to institute appropriate hyperalimentation and drugs and, in some cases, may facilitate control of uremia and hyperkalemia. Constant monitoring of intravascular volume is recommended to determine safe UF rates.

Adjuvant Drug Therapy

The pharmacokinetics of drugs is relatively complex. Under physiologic conditions, first-order kinetics is characterized in terms of three variables (1) the serum half-life, (2) the elimination constant, and (3) the volume of distribution.

Some drugs are eliminated by the renal route, others by way of the liver, and others by varied combinations of the two. Elimination by the renal route is obviously altered in renal failure. Further, renal elimination may, under normal circumstances, be through glomerular fil-

tration or by tubular secretion. Certain drugs compete for secretory transport sites within the tubular cells. Tubular luminal pH has a definite role in the efficient elimination of drugs. These facts are but a few of the variables of drug kinetics cited only to suggest the complexity of same.

Impedance of renal execretion then is the most obvious pharmokinetic consequence of renal failure. The obvious, however, is potentially compounded by changes in the uremic patient's ability to handle drugs and includes alteration in absorption, protein binding, metabolism, and drug sensitivity.

Absorption in the patient with ARF is altered not only by vomiting and diarrhea, as well as by edema of the gastrointestinal tract, but also by a reduction in the biotransformation capacity of the damaged kidney (i.e., vitamin D_3 metabolism).

Patients in renal failure are often hypoproteinemic. Drugs are bound to protein in variable concentrations. Since the unbound drug is active at tissue binding sites, slight decreases in serum protein can lead to significant alteration in drug activity, especially those with a high affinity for protein binding.

The metabolism of drugs dependent on renal function for reduction is obviously altered in ARF. Thus, for example, the insulin requirements in diabetic patients in renal failure is reduced.

Finally, alterations in tissue receptor sites and increased permeability of the blood-brain barrier may in part account for the increased drug sensitivity seen in patients with renal failure.

Although the initial recommended loading dose of drugs is appropriate to obtain therapeutic levels, maintenance delivery doses must be altered to compensate for the changes in kinetics. This can be accomplished in one of two ways: (1) by increasing the interval between dosages, or (2) by maintaining the normal interval and decreasing the dosage. Most of the formulas available as guides for drug therapy are based either on the serum creatinine or on creatinine clearances and relate to the relatively steady state of chronic renal failure. In ARF, the "steady state" does not exist, and it is appropriate to assume a GFR of less than 10.

The safest method, when available, is that of serum assays for achieving therapeutic but nontoxic levels of drugs.

Some drugs can be removed by either peritoneal dialysis or hemodialysis, some by just one of these methods, and some are unaffected by either method of dialysis.

Comprehensive dosing guidelines for drug therapy in renal failure are available in the literature. In general, there are three therapeutic classes of drugs in renal failure: (1) those that require no dosage modification, (2) those that do, and (3) those that should be avoided in patients with ARF (Table 1).

NUTRITION

Surgical patients in ARF are usually catabolic and often malnourished. The importance of reversing

TABLE 1   Dose Modification of Some Drugs Commonly Used in ARF Patients*

Drugs requiring no dosage modification
  Antibiotics
    Erythromycin
    Chloramphenicol
    Clindamycin
    Oxacillin-dicloxacillin
    Nafcillin
    Cefoperazone
  Others
    Propranolol-Metoprolol
    Diazoxide
    Quinidine
    Codeine-morphine
    Meperidine**
    Nifedipine
    Theophylline
    Steroids

Drugs requiring dosage modification
  Antibiotics
    Gentamicin-Tobramycin
    Penicillin G
    Ampicillin
    Carbenicillin
    Cephalothin
    Cefomandole
    Cefoxitin
    Cefotaxime
    TMP/SMZ
    Doxycycline
    Metronidazole
    Vancomycin
  Others
    Digoxin
    Methyldopa
    Nadolol
    Procainamide
    Allopurinol
    Cimetidine

Drugs to avoid in renal failure
  Antibiotics
    Tetracyclines (except doxycycline)
    Methenamine mandelate
    Nitrofurantoin
  Others
    Chloral Hydrate
    Spironolactone
    Triameterene
    Probenecid
    Chlorpropamide
    Terbutaline

* Data from Bennett WM, et al. Drug prescribing in renal failure: dosing guidelines for adults. Am J Kid Dis 1983; 3:155.
** A metabolite of meperidine accumulates in ARF and can cause seizures.

catabolism and providing calories and nutrients for tissue repair should not be overlooked.

In most patients, nutrition through enteral routes is not possible, although this route is preferred when available. Hyperalimentation through central intravenous lines can be used successfully to provide all of the daily requirements or as a supplement to enteral feedings.

Specific requirements in ARF are determined not by the degree of renal insufficiency, but by the extent of injury or infection and the previous nutritional state of the patient.

As early as 1970, Dudrick showed that positive nitrogen balance (protein synthesis being greater than protein degradation) could be achieved in ARF patients using intravenous nonprotein nitrogen in the form of essential amino acids (EAA) and hypertonic glucose. Currently, the most widely used hyperalimentation solution for ARF is Nephramine (McGaw Labs), which contains all of the EAA and histidine (considered an EAA in renal failure patients). Owing to frequent problems with volume restriction in these patients, strongly hypertonic solutions are required and can only be infused through central venous catheters. As with all patients who are receiving parenteral feedings, daily monitoring of electrolytes, phosphorus, magnesium, and glucose are needed to determine daily adjustments in therapy.

To provide needed calories, Nephramine is often infused as a greater than 35% glucose solution. Hyperglycemia due to increased glucose load, as well as peripheral resistance to the effects of insulin in ARF, is common. Supplementation of the parenteral solution with insulin is often required, sometimes from the onset. In diabetic patients, the daily insulin requirements are lower than expected owing to decreased insulin degradation by the damaged kidneys.

High carbohydrate loads may increase the ventilatory load of carbon dioxide in acutely ill patients enough to cause respiratory acidosis and difficulty with respiratory failure.

For patients who can utilize the enteral route, nitrogen requirements should be provided either as high biologic value protein (containing high ratio of EAA to total AA, i.e., egg whites, lean meat) or as commercially available enteral feedings with only EAA (Amin-aid; McGaw) or EAA plus non-EAA including histidine (Travasorb Renal; Travenol), both essentially electrolyte-free. The caloric intake needs to be supplemented with monosaccharides. In many cases, duodenal feeding tubes and continuous infusion pumps are needed to secure adequate intake.

Daily requirements for ARF patients should be determined in each patient by means of urea nitrogen balance studies, but some guidelines exist. Most catabolic ARF patients require 40 to 55 cal per kilogram per day. This should be provided as less than 80 percent carbohydrates and greater than 20 percent fat, either enterally or parenterally. Daily nitrogen requirements vary from 80 mg per kilogram (0.5 g per kilogram protein) in noncatabolic patients to 240 mg per kilogram (1.5 g per kilogram protein) in highly catabolic ARF patients. Use of nonprotein nitrogen sources (EAA) decreases the urea nitrogen appearance and reduces the need for dialysis.

Ketoanalogs of branched-chain EAA have been shown experimentally to further decrease protein breakdown in renal insufficiency. At present, no clinical studies have been done in ARF.

Dialysis (both hemo and peritoneal) removes amino acids, proteins, and vitamins from patients. When ARF patients undergo dialysis, additional nitrogen intake is required, along with therapeutic doses of water-soluble vitamin supplements.

When, despite preventive measures, ARF occurs in surgical patients, proper attention to nutrition, volume, and electrolytes (plus timely dialysis, or ultrafiltration, when needed) can greatly improve the chances of a successful outcome.

ABNORMAL BLEEDING

CHI V. DANG, M.D., PH.D.
WILLIAM R. BELL, M.D.

An open surgical wound in a patient whose blood will not coagulate or cannot be made to coagulate may result in catastrophe. Hence, preoperative screening for potential abnormal bleeding in surgical candidates is of utmost importance. Abnormal bleeding may result from vascular abnormalities, quantitative or qualitative platelet abnormalities, factor deficiencies, circulating anticoagulants, consumptive coagulopathy, or massive transfusion therapy (Table 1). These abnormalities may be detected preperatively or may be causes of intraoperative and postoperative bleeding.

Effective management of abnormal bleeding disorders relies on their early preoperative identification. Preoperative screening consists of obtaining a thorough history and physical examination (Table 2). The extent of laboratory evaluation (Table 3) depends on the clinical suspicion of a bleeding disorder based on the history and physical examination.

VASCULAR DISORDERS

With vascular defects (see Table 1), purpuric lesions may be apparent. Telangiectases may reflect the Osler-Weber-Rendu syndrome. Body habitus and skin texture may be characteristic of hyperadrenalism or certain heritable diseases of connective tissues. Most of the vascular disorders with hemorrhagic complications are not treatable, but recognition of such disorders allows for optimal management of surgical candidates.

PLATELET DISORDERS

Essential to normal hemostasis are platelets, which must be present in adequate numbers (normally 150,000 to 350,000 per cubic millimeter) and normal in function (maintain vessel wall integrity, support clot retraction). When the platelet count falls below 50,000 per cubic millimeter, derangement of the hemostatic mechanism may occur. Spontaneous hemorrhage may be expected when the count falls below 20,000 per cubic millimeter. Whenever thrombocytopenia (automated platelet count less than 100,000 per cubic millimeter) is identified, this count must be verified by direct examination of the peripheral blood prepared from a finger puncture. In some patients, platelets enumerated by automated devices may be spuriously low for a variety of reasons.

TABLE 1 Causes of Abnormal Bleeding

Vascular disorders
 Scurvy
 Adrenocortical hyperfunction
 Amyloidosis
 Heritable disorders of connective tissues: Marfan
  syndrome, Ehler-Danlos syndrome, pseudoxanthoma
  elasticum, and osteogenesis imperfecta
 Osler-Weber-Rendu syndrome
 Vascular tumors
Platelet disorders
 Quantitative
  Thrombocytopenia
   Decreased production: congenital, aplastic anemia,
    marrow infiltration, radiation, drugs, nutritional
    deficiency, viral infections, renal failure,
    paroxysmal nocturnal hemoglobinuria
   Increased destruction: infection, drug, chronic and
    acute idiopathic thrombocytopenic purpura, post-
    transfusion purpura, disseminated intravascular
    coagulopathy, thrombotic thrombocytopenic
    purpura, and hemolytic uremic syndrome
   Sequestration: hypersplenism
   Dilutional: massive transfusion
 Qualitative
  Enzyme defects (cyclo-oxygenase): acetylsalicylate
   ingestion
  Uremia
  Liver disease
  Bernard-Soulier syndrome (giant platelet, adhesion
   defect)
  Glanzmann's thrombasthenia (aggregation defect)
  Gray platelet syndrome (agranular large platelet)
  Pseudo-von Willebrand's disease
Disorders of blood coagulation
 Congenital factor deficiencies
  Relatively common:
   Hemophilia A (factor VIII deficiency)
   Hemophilia B (factor IX deficiency)
   von Willebrand's disease
   Factor XI deficiency
   Factor VII deficiency
  Uncommon: deficiency of factors II, V, X, XII, XIII
 Acquired
  Liver disease
  Vitamin K deficiency
  Amyloidosis (decreased factor X)
  Circulating anticoagulants
  Disseminated intravascular coagulation

TABLE 2 Preoperative Screening

History
    Prolonged minor bleeding
    Easy bruisability
    Bleeding complications with previous
        surgical or dental procedures
    Medical illnesses: liver disease, neoplasia,
        connective tissue disorders, malabsorption
    Medications: especially acetylsalicylate
    Family history of bleeding disorders

Physical examination
    Petechiae
    Ecchymoses
    Mucosal bleeding (gingiva, gastrointestinal)
    Signs of liver failure
    Hepatomegaly
    Splenomegaly

Laboratory studies*
    Negative history and minor surgery:†
        no screening
    Negative history and major surgery:
        platelet count, prothrombin time, partial
        thromboplastin time, thrombin time
    Positive history and minor surgery:
        platelet count, prothrombin time, partial
        thromboplastin time, thrombin time,
        bleeding time, and fibrin clot solubility
    Positive history and major surgery:
        platelet count, prothrombin time, partial
        thromboplastin time, thrombin time,
        bleeding time, fibrin clot solubility,
        platelet function studies, factor VIII
        level, factor IX level, and alpha$_2$-
        antiplasmin level

* Laboratory studies suggested are for patients without previously identified coagulopathy based on history and physical examination.
† Minor surgery consists of simple excisional biopsy and dental procedures.

Reduced platelet numbers may result from a defect in production or from premature removal from the peripheral blood via destruction or hyperactivity of the reticuloendothelial system (hypersplenism). Destruction may result from a variety of mechanisms including infectious agents of all varieties, direct action of drugs, drug-induced immune mechanisms, autoimmune mechanisms, or disseminated intravascular coagulopathy. Among the common offending drugs are quinine, quinidine, procainamide, thiazides, sulfonamides, gold salts, and heparin. In general, the onset of drug-induced thrombocytopenia occurs within 1 to 3 weeks after exposure, and recovery of the platelet count occurs in about 10 to 14 days (or longer if renal or hepatic dysfunction is present) following discontinuance of the offending agent. Thrombocytopenia secondary to dilutional mechanisms can occur with massive transfusion (20 to 30 units of red cells over 1 to 2 hours), but it is extremely rare.

When thrombocytopenia is identified at the time of preoperative screening, during surgery, or in the immediate perioperative or postoperative period, the following must be urgently carried out:

1. Verify that the platelet count is low.
2. Begin attempts to identify the etiology.
3. Remove all potentially offending agents.
4. Unless absolutely essential, abort further surgery and avoid all invasive procedures.
5. Institute studies to identify whether the thrombocytopenia is resulting from peripheral destruction or removal or from production failure.
6. Obtain hematology consultation to aid in administration of appropriate therapy.

If abnormal bleeding is present and the platelets are normal in number, platelet function must be studied. The agent most commonly involved in causing platelet dysfunction is acetylsalicylic acid (ASA, aspirin). Identification of dysfunctional platelets is most reliably determined by performing (1) bleeding time (this should be performed preoperatively anytime a history of ASA ingestion within 10 days is elicited), (2) clot retraction test, (3) tourniquet test, and (4) specialized studies in the coagulation laboratory such as prothrombin consumption and platelet aggregation.

The management of bleeding problems due to abnormal platelets (too few in number or dysfunctional) is most successfully accomplished by removal of the cause. Transfusion of platelets is not commonly indicated. However, some situations are promptly remedied by the judicious use of platelet concentrates. Such situations include thrombocytopenia due to bone marrow production failure, dysfunctional platelets resulting from ASA ingestion, dysfunctional traumatized platelets as seen in blood that is circulated through extracorporeal machinery or damaged by such intravascular devices as the intra-aortic pulsatile balloon. Currently, the physician must be cognizant that conditions exist where, in the presence of thrombocytopenia, platelet transfusions are not only without benefit but may induce a catastrophic disaster.

TABLE 3 Laboratory Findings and Therapeutic Goals in Factor Deficiencies*

Deficient Factor	PT	PTT	TT	Bleeding Time	Therapeutic Goal (Percent Normal)	Half-Life (Hours)
I	+	+	+	±	> 100 mg/dl	96–144
II	+	+	−	−	> 20	50–80
III†	·	·	·	·	·	·
IV†	·	·	·	·	·	·
V	+	+	−	−	> 25	24
VII	+	−	−	−	> 10	5
VIII	−	+	−	−	> 50	12
VIII:vWF‡	−	+	−	+	> 25	24
IX	−	+	−	−	> 50	20–30
X	+	+	−	−	> 20	25–60
XI	−	+	−	−	> 20	40–84
XII	−	+	−	−	< 10	−
XIII	−	−	−	−	> 5	150

Abbreviations: PT = prothrombin time; PTT = partial thromboplastin time; TT = thrombin time; + = prolongation; − = normal.
* Therapeutic goals are for major surgery.
† Deficiency affecting coagulation is unknown. Factor III is thromboplastin and factor IV is calcium.
‡ von Willebrand's disease.

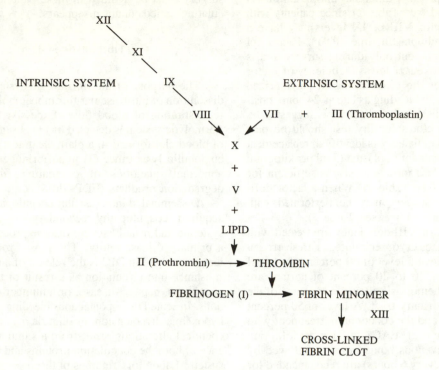

Figure 1 The coagulation cascade.

In the case of abnormal bleeding in the surgical patient with a normal platelet system, one must immediately proceed to evaluation of the glycoproteins, serine proteases, and cofactors that constitute the coagulation cascade scheme.

DISORDERS OF BLOOD COAGULATION

The classic coagulation cascade is depicted in Figure 1. The functional status of this aspect of the coagulation process is best asssessed by the (1) whole blood coagulation time, (2) prothrombin time (PT), and (3) nonactivated partial thromboplastin time (PTT) or activated partial thromboplastin time (APTT). The whole blood coagulation time provides an overall view of the interaction of all the components of the coagulation cascade. This test must be performed in clean glass tubes (nonsiliconized and without anticoagulants). Normal blood coagulates in less than 10 minutes. By observation of the clot that forms, considerable information can be gained. If the size of the clot that forms approximates the volume of blood placed in the tube, the plasma fibrinogen concentration is greater than 100 mg per 100 ml and more than adequate for normal hemostasis. Within 1 hour the formed clot normally begins to undergo retraction, signifying that 75,000 or more platelets per cubic millimeter are present and functional. The color of the serum extruded from the clot may provide information about the presence of red cell hemolysis if it is pink in contrast to the normal clear yellow color. If a clot forms and, a few minutes later, undergoes dissolution, this suggests excessive activity of the fibrinolytic system and DIC may be the problem. The prothrombin time assays for factors II, V, VII, and X. When time is prolonged, a disturbance of one or more of the components of the extrinsic system is suggested. The PTT and APTT systems assay primarily for factors VIII, IX, XI, and XII, but also provide a general view of the function of all coagulation proteins with the exception of factor VII. Since clot formation is the end point of these assay systems, both the PT and PTT-APTT indirectly provide information on the amount of factor I (fibrinogen) present. When an abnormality of either the PT or PTT-APTT occurs, further definition of the problem requires individual specific assays. Both of these assay systems may be abnormal because of a deficiency of a given component(s), or there may be an additional component in the circulating blood (designated circulating inhibitor) that interferes with normal coagulation factor activity.

Assay techniques that monitor the function of the coagulation factors should be performed whenever abnormal bleeding is encountered (before transfusion of any blood components) or preoperatively in patients who have blood relatives with known factor deficiency states (e.g., hemophilia A, Christmas disease, and von Willebrand's disease) or patients with a past history of significant bleeding (especially those requiring transfusion). Patients with factor deficiencies (see Table 1) usually have associated laboratory abnormalities (see Table 3). If the clinical suspicion is high for a bleeding disorder, specific assays for factors VIII and IX, the thrombin time, and possibly an alpha$_2$-antiplasmin level should be determined (see Table 2) since patients with 20 to 40 percent factor VIII or IX levels may have a normal partial thromboplastin time (PTT). Factor XI deficiency may be apparent only during surgery and is more common in Ashkenazi Jews. Deficiency of factor XIII, which catalyzes the crosslinking of polymerized fibrin, may present with bleeding as late as 24 hours postoperatively. When this peculiar disorder is suggested by the history, a fibrin clot solubility test should be performed. If factor XIII deficiency is identified, replacement therapy with a small amount of plasma (5 ml per kilogram body weight in one dose intravenously) is sufficient for effective hemostasis (see Table 3). When a factor deficiency is identified, surgery may be performed with adequate replacement therapy (see Table 3).

Patients with factor VIII deficiency are treated with factor VIII concentrate, cryoprecipitate, or fresh frozen plasma (FFP) to achieve a level of 20 percent of normal or greater. Levels of 10 to 20 percent of normal are usually adequate for hemostasis after minor trauma of the oral cavity or genitourinary tract. A level of 50 percent of normal or greater and the concomitant treatment with epsilon aminocaproic acid (EACA) (0.1 g per kilogram body weight in intravenous bolus infusion followed by the same dose orally every 6 hours) are recommended for patients undergoing major surgery. Factor IX deficiency requires similar replacement therapy with factor IX before surgery. For the purpose of calculating replacement therapy, one unit of factor is defined as that amount present in one milliliter of normal plasma. In order to achieve 50 percent of normal activity in a patient with 0 percent activity, 50 percent of the patient's plasma volume must be replaced by fresh plasma (or an equivalent number of VIII units that is present in cryoprecipitate or factor VIII concentrate). Plasma volume is estimated to be 40 ml per kilogram of body weight. For a 60-kg patient, the plasma volume is about 2,400 ml. To achieve 50 percent normal activity, 1,200 units of factor must be administered. For factor VIII deficiency, the dose is administered every 8 hours to maintain the desired level.

Circulating Anticoagulants

Circulating anticoagulants are endogenous, spontaneously appearing immunoglobulins directed against one or more components of the coagulation system. These anticoagulants may be incidently found in patients with systemic lupus erythematosus (SLE), patients treated with certain drugs such as penicillin, procainamide, or phenytoin, or even in apparently normal patients. Most of these patients bleed abnormally with the slightest trauma; the exception is a patient with SLE who has a circulating anticoagulant. An isolated elevation of the PTT is characteristic of this disorder, but this may also be associated with heparin-like anticoagulants seen in patients with neoplasms. In either case, treatment consists of therapy for the underlying disease. If at all possible,

surgery must be avoided in these patients until the circulating anticoagulant disappears.

Fibrinolytic System

The purpose of the fibrinolytic system is to induce dissolution of intravascular thromboemboli and to permit reconstitution of blood flow. Excessive activity of the fibrinolytic system is detected by (1) observing rapid lysis of blood clot formed in a plain clean test tube, (2) rapid euglobulin lysis time, (3) hypofibrinogenemia, and (4) abnormal quantities of circulating fibrinogen-fibrin degradation products (FDP-fdp).

Disseminated intravascular coagulopathy (DIC) is an acquired coagulopathy secondary to an underlying systemic and usually severe disease process. DIC is not a primary disease entity. The most probable etiologic factor involved in DIC is the release of a thromboplastic substance into circulation as a result of trauma, sepsis, neoplasms, hepatic disease, or a number of other conditions. In acute DIC, spontaneous bleeding, acral cyanosis, hypoxemia, hypotension, or oliguria may occur. The biochemical alterations result from a simultaneous disturbance of both the coagulation proteins and the fibrinolytic system. Laboratory findings of thrombocytopenia, hypofibrinogenemia, prolonged PT and PTT, and elevated fibrin(ogen) degradation products (FDP-fdp), and a microangiopathic blood smear are diagnostic of DIC in the appropriate clinical setting. Effective treatment of DIC is dependent on the identification and control or eradication of the underlying disease process. If hemorrhage is excessive, replacement with packed red blood cells is indicated. Although transfused platelets are usually immediately consumed, platelet transfusion may be appropriate if thrombocytopenia is severe and the bone marrow is suppressed. The use of heparin and antifibrinolytic agents (EACA or tranexamic acid) in DIC is controversial and in fact may sometimes worsen bleeding or enhance thrombotic complications. Before employing these agents in this situation, guidance from a hematologist is suggested.

Major consumptive coagulopathy may occur with the onset of laparotomy. Significant mortality has been associated with continuation and completion of the operation despite vigorous replacement therapy with plasma and platelets. Upon recognition of the coagulopathy, surgery is terminated immediately, all nonvital severed vessels are ligated, and laparotomy pads are packed tightly into the peritoneal cavity. The abdomen should be closed under high tension. Surgery may be resumed when hemostasis returns to normal.

Vitamin K Deficiency

Vitamin K deficiency may be seen in severely malnourished patients, in patients with malabsorption, or in those receiving antibiotics. The vitamin K-dependent clotting factors are factors II, VII, IX, X, protein C, protein S, and protein Z. Characteristically, the prothrombin time is prolonged, and often the partial thromboplastin time is also abnormally long. The diagnosis of vitamin K deficiency is established when laboratory abnormalities are corrected with vitamin K therapy. Vitamin K may be administered intravenously (10 mg over 10 minutes) or subcutaneously for reversal of the deficiency state. If rapid correction is essential, FFP (20 ml per kilogram of body weight) may be administered. The use of cephalosporins, such as cefamandole or moxalactam, probably should be avoided since the use of these antibiotics has been associated with bleeding due to hypoprothrombinemia and platelet dysfunction.

INDEX

Page numbers followed by (f) indicate figures; those followed by (t) indicate tables.

A

Abdominal infections, postoperative, 532–534
  antibiotics in, 532
  surgical approach to, 534
  treatment of, 533–534
Abdominal injuries of, 427–433
  blunt, 428
  hemorrhage in, 429
  to hollow viscera, 432–433
  identification of visceral injuries, 427–429
  penetrating, 427–428
  to solid organs, 429–432
  vascular, 459–460
Abscess
  abdominal
    in appendicitis, 131
    postoperative, 533–534
    small bowel obstruction due to, 62
  anorectal, 137–138
    cryptoglandular, 138
  in Crohn's disease of small bowel, 67
  diverticular, of colon, 91
  drainage of, in Raynaud's syndrome, 394
  of liver, 153–157
  pancreatic, in trauma, 447
  perirectal, in Crohn's disease, 95
  pilonidal, 150–151
  plantar, in diabetic foot, 407–408
  splenic, 266
Acetabulum, fracture of, 477–478
Achalasia, esophageal, 3–5
Acid-base balance, 510–512
Acid burns, of esophagus, 1
Acid secretion
  in gastric ulcers, 27
  in short bowel syndrome, 85
  in Zollinger-Ellison syndrome, 47
Acidosis
  hyperchloremic, 516
  in mesenteric ischemia, 75–76
  metabolic, 510–511
  respiratory, 511–512
Acquired immune deficiency syndrome
  (AIDS), Kaposi's sarcoma and, 482
ACTH production, by tumors, 284–285
Actinic keratosis, 481
Addison's disease, 287–288
Adenocarcinoma, *See also* Carcinoma
  Barrett's esophagus and, 14–15
  of gallbladder, 223
  of stomach, 34–38
Adenoma
  aldosterone-producing, 283
  cortisol-producing, 285
  of liver, 161

Adenopathy, multiple endocrine (MEN I),
  family history of, 47
Adenosis, sclerosing, 315
Adhesions, small bowel obstruction due to, 61
Adrenal gland
  cortex of, 281–288
    in Addison's disease, 287–288
    in adrenocortical neoplasms, 285
    in aldosteronism, 282–283
    anatomy of, 281–282
    carcinoma of, 286–287
    in Cushing's syndrome, 283–285,
      285–286
    insufficiency of, in Crohn's disease, 65
    myelolipoma of, 287
    in Nelson's syndrome, 286
    tumors of, 287
  hyperplasia of, 282
  insufficiency of, 287–288
Adrenalectomy
  in aldosteronism, 283
  in metastatic breast cancer, 329
  preoperative and postoperative
    management of, 288
Adult respiratory distress syndrome
  (ARDS), 438–442
  endotracheal intubation in, 440–441
  fluid administration in, 439–440
  mechanical ventilation in, 440–441
  and PEEP, 441
  physiologic abnormalities common to, 439
  pulmonary collapse and infection in, 440
  role of hemodynamics in, 439–440
  and sepsis, 438
Aging, biology and physiology of, 526–527
Airway management, in penetrating neck
  trauma, 470–471
Alcoholism
  in chronic pancreatitis, 246–247
  and Mallory-Weiss syndrome, 31
Aldosteronism, 282–283
  diagnosis of, 282–283
  differential diagnosis and localization
    of, 283
  treatment of, 283
Alkali burns, of esophagus, 1, 19
Alkalosis
  metabolic, 511
  respiratory, 511–512
Allografts, in burn management, 464–465
Altemeier method, 104
Amebic abscess, of liver, 153–154, 156–157
Amebicidal agents, for amebic liver
  abscess, 156
Amino acid
  deficiency of, in short bowel syndrome, 85

in hepatic encephalopathy, 189
Aminoglutethimide, in breast cancer, 330
Ampicillin, in caustic burns of esophagus, 21
Amputation
  in arterial embolism, 383–384
  in Buerger's disease, 387–388
  in diabetic foot, 408
  in digital melanoma, 489–490
  in gangrene foot
    above-knee, 380
    below-knee, 380
    postoperative pain in, 380
    toe, 379
    transmetatarsal, 379–380
  in Raynaud's syndrome, 394
  in soft tissue sarcoma, 494
Anal canal, carcinoma of, 124–125
Anal incontinence, 144–150
Anal verge, carcinoma of, 125–126
Anastomosis, lymphatic, in lymphedema of
  extremity, 425
Anemia
  hemolytic
    hereditary, splenectomy in, 263
    immune, 263–264
  sickle cell, splenectomy in, 263
Anesthesia
  in carotid endarterectomy, 362
  in pheochromocytoma, 290
Aneurysm
  abdominal aortic, 349–354
    postoperative complications of, 351
    presentation and evaluation of, 349–350
    ruptured, 352–354
      pain symptoms in, 352
      postoperative complications of, 354
      postoperative results of, 354
      preoperative evaluation in, 353
      presentation of, 352
      surgical procedure in, 353–354
    surgical problems in, 351
    surgical procedure in, 350–351
  false, 357–360
    diagnosis of, 357
    nonsurgical management of, 357–359
    shunts in, 359
    surgical management of, 359–360
    vascular repair in, 359–360
  femoral, 355–356
  popliteal, 355–356
    blue toe syndrome in, 355
    diagnosis of, 355
    management of, 355
    symptoms of, 355
Angelchik prosthesis, in gastroesophageal
  reflux, 13

Angiography
  in asymptomatic bruits, 361
  in cerebrovascular occlusive disease, 363
  in false aneurysms, 358
  in Mallory-Weiss syndrome, 32–33
  in pancreatic carcinoma, 251
  in portal hypertension, 178
  in tibioperoneal occlusive disease, 370
Angioplasty, percutaneous transluminal, in
    femoropopliteal occlusive disease, 368
  in renovascular hypertension, 391
Anoplasty, for anal strictures, 140, 142
Anoscopy, in hemorrhoids, 132
Antacid therapy
  in gastric ulcer, 28
  in Mallory-Weiss syndrome, 33
  in short bowel syndrome, 86
Antibiotics
  in biliary tract surgery, 226–231
  in Buerger's disease, 386
  in burns, 461–462
    in caustic burns of esophagus, 21
  in cholangitis, 209, 210
  in cholecystectomy, 197–198
  in clostridial gas gangrene, 502–503, 521
  in diabetic foot, 406
  in enterocutaneous fistula, 83
  in hand infections, 499
  in liver abscess, pyogenic, 154
  in pancreatic abscess, 237
  in postoperative infections
    abdominal, 532
    of wounds, 520
  against postsplenectomy infections, 453
  in preoperative bowel preparation, 126–128
    in appendicitis, 129–130, 131
    in Crohn's disease of small bowel, 65
    duration of, 127
    kanamycin in, 127
    prophylactic, 128
  in Raynaud's syndrome, 393
  in septic shock, 437
Anticoagulants
  circulating, 546
  in venous thrombosis, 414
Antidiuretic hormone (ADH), inappropriate
    secretion of, 507–508
Anti-inflammatory agents, in venous
    thrombosis, 414
Antireflux surgery, indications for, 9–10
Antithyroid drugs, in hyperthyroidism, 299
Antrectomy and vagotomy, gastroduoden-
    ostomy with, in duodenal ulcer, 44
Anus
  carcinoma of, 124–126
    squamous cell, 124–126
  fissure in ano, 137
  fistula-in-ano, 138–139
  hemorrhoids of, 132–136
  melanoma of, 126
  strictures of, 139–143
    etiology of, 139–140
    nonoperative treatment of, 140
    signs and symptoms of, 140
    surgical management of, 140–143
Aorta, abdominal, aneurysms of, 349–354.
    See also Aneurysm
Aortoiliac occlusive disease, 364–366
  aortic reconstruction in, 365
  aorto-bifemoral bypass in, 365
  aortofemoral and femoropopliteal bypass
    in, 366
  diagnosis of, 364
  femorofemoral bypass in, 364

  therapy for, 364–366
    evolution of, 366
Aortorenal bypass, in renovascular
    hypertension, 391
Appendectomy, in Crohn's disease of small
    bowel, 67
Appendicitis
  acute, 129–131
    complications of, 131
    diagnosis of, 129
    operative approach in, 130
    postoperative management of, 131
    preoperative management of, 129–130
    perforated, alternative management of, 131
APUD cells, 258
Apudoma, 258
Arterial embolus(i), peripheral, 381–384
Arterial occlusion, in mesenteric
    ischemia, 78–79
Arterial reconstruction, in upper extremity
    ischemia, 375–376
Arteriosclerosis, Buerger's disease vs., 385
Arteriovenous fistula, 357–360
Ascites, 183–187
  cardiogenic, 184
  chylous, 177–178, 184
  infected, 184
  malignant, 183–184
  pancreatic, 184, 241–243
    clinical features of, 241–242
    diagnosis of, 242
    irradiation in, 243
    nonoperative management of, 242–243
    operative management of, 243
    results of treatment of, 244–245
  in patients on hemodialysis, 184
  peritoneovenous shunt in
    indications for, 183
    operative technique in, 185
    postoperative care in, 185–187
    risk factors for, 184–185
  postoperative, 184
  recurrent, 186
  secondary to cirrhosis, 183
Aspiration
  of amebic liver abscess, 156
  needle, of pneumothorax, 340
  of pyogenic liver abscess, 154–155
  recurrent, in gastroesophageal reflux, 10
  of stomach, in caustic burns of
    esophagus, 21
Aspirin, and platelet dysfunction, 544
Autografts, in burn management, 464
Autotransplantation
  parathyroid, 314
  splenic, 452
Axillary vein valve transplant, 411–412
Azotemia
  postrenal, 535–536
  prerenal, 535
  renal, 536–537

B

Bacterium(a), in positive bile
    cultures, 226–227
Bacteroides, in short bowel syndrome, 86
Bacteroides fragilis
  in acute cholangitis, 209
  in positive bile cultures, 227
Bactibilia
  antibiotic therapy in, 227
  incidence of, 226
  types of bacteria in, 226–227

Balloon catheter embolectomy, 383
Balloon dilatation
  in anal incontinence, 144
  in aortoiliac occlusive disease, 364
  of biliary tract strictures, 211–212
  Sengstaken-Blakemore, in Mallory-Weiss
    syndrome, 34
Banding, rubber, in hemorrhoids, 133
Barium studies, in Mallory-Weiss
    syndrome, 33
Barium swallow, in caustic burns of
    esophagus, 21
Barrett's esophagus, 10, 14–16
  and adenocarcinoma, 14–15
  clinical presentation and prevalence of, 14
  diagnosis of, 14
  management of
    controversies in, 15
    suggestions in, 15–16
  pathogenesis of, 14
Basal cell carcinoma, of skin, 481
Basal energy expenditure (BEE), calculation
    of, 513
Basal metabolic rate (BMR), calculation
    of, 468
Bathing trunk nevus, 480
Belsey Mark IV fundoplication, for
    gastroesophageal reflux, 4–5, 10–11
Bile acids, in short bowel syndrome, 85–86
Biliary cysts, 216–219
  anatomic classification of, 216
  surgical options in, 217–219
  surgical treatment of, rationale for, 216–217
Biliary tract
  antibiotics for, 226–231
    in acute cholangitis, 230
    in acute cholecystitis, 230
    in cholangiograms, 230–231
    cost of, 228–229
    distribution of, 227–228
    in elective cases, 229–230
    half-life of, 228
    pharmacokinetic properties of, 227–228
    spectrum of, 227
    toxicity of, 228
  bacteriology of, 226–227
  cholangitis, acute, 208–210
  cholecystitis, acute and chronic, 195–198
  common duct conditions. See Common
    bile duct
  disease of, treatment of, 214–215
  extrahepatic cysts of, 217
  fistulas in, and gallstone ileus, 219
  gallstones in. See Gallstones
  intrahepatic cysts of, 218–219
  nonbiliary diseases of, treatment of, 215
  strictures in, 211–212
  trauma of, 432
  tumors of, 223–226
Biopsy
  excisional, of colorectal polyps, 115
  of neck mass, 496–497
  of nevi, 480
  of soft tissue lesions, 479
Bleb resection, in pneumothorax, 342
Bleeding. See Hemorrhage
"Blind loop" syndrome, 86
Blisters, in frostbite, 475
Blood cells, altered surface properties of,
    splenectomy in, 263–264
Blood transfusion. See Transfusions
Blood urea nitrogen (BUN), in acute renal
    failure, 537
Blood vessels. See Vascular system

Blue toe syndrome, in popliteal aneurysm, 355
Body composition, components of, 522
Body warmth, maintenance of, Raynaud's
   syndrome in, 393
Boerhaave's syndrome, 2–3, 31
Bone, infection involving, 500
Bowel conditions. *See* Intestines
Bowel management program, in anal
   incontinence, 144–145
Breast, 315–332
  carcinoma of, 317–332
    adrenalectomy in, 329
    aminoglutethimide in, 330
    axillary lymph node staging and, 319–320
    bilateral, 325–326
    bilateral oophorectomy in, 329
    chemotherapy in, 321
      hormonal therapy with, 330–331
    clinical variants of, 324–326
    cystosarcoma phylloides in, 326
    disseminated, 329–332
      chemotherapy in, 330
      combined hormonal and chemotherapy
        in, 330–331
      endocrine therapy in, 329–330
      local treatment and supportive care
        in, 331–332
      radiation therapy in, 331–332
      systemic therapies in, 329–331
    early detection of, 318–319
    histologic type and multicentricity of, 319
    hormonal therapy in, 321, 329–330
      ablative, 329
      additive, 329–330
      chemotherapy with, 330–331
    hypophysectomy in, 329
    inflammatory, 325
    lobular, in situ, 326–328
      clinical data in, 327
      multicentricity vs. bilaterality, 327
      optimal therapy for, 327–328
      pathologic data in, 326–327
      and subsequent invasive
        carcinoma, 327–328
    local control of, 321–322
    in males, 326
    mastectomy of
      modified radical, 320
      partial, 320–321
      reconstruction after, 321
    megestrol acetate in, 330
    nonpalpable mass in, 318–319
    Paget's disease in, 324–325
    palpable mass in, 318
    pathologic variants of, 324
    postoperative radiation in, 320, 321–324,
      331–332
    in pregnancy, 325
    psychologic impact of, 323–324
    risk factors in, 317–318
    stage I and II, 317–321
    surgical options for primary
      operable, 320–321
    surgical staging of, 321–324
    tamoxifen in, 329
    unusual forms of, 324–326
  fibrocystic disease of, 315–317
    clinical evaluation of, 316
    clinical spectrum of, 315
    management of, 316–317
    microscopic appearance of, 315
    relationship to cancer, 315–316, 317–318
    surgical considerations in, 317
  melanoma of, 490

Bromocriptine, in hepatic encephalopathy, 189
Brooke ileostomy, in ulcerative colitis, 94
Bruit, asymptomatic, carotid endarterectomy
   in, 361
Budd-Chiari syndrome, 189–192
  diagnosis of, 189–190
  Johns Hopkions experience, 191–192
  medical management of, 190
  mesoatrial shunt in, 191
  mesocaval "C" shunt in, 190
  surgical management of, 190
  with thrombosis of inferior vena
    cava, 190–191
Buerger's disease, 385–388
  aggressive diagnostic evaluation in, 385
  amputation in, 387–388
  vs. arteriosclerosis, 385
  bypass grafts in, 387
  immunologic considerations in, 388
  medical management of, 385
  pharmacologic management of, 385–386
  surgical management of, 386–388
  sympathectomy in, 387
  wound care in, 386–387
Buffering agents, in shock, 436
Bupivacaine, in rib fractures, 335
Burns, 460–469
  acid, of esophagus, 1
  alkali, of esophagus, 1, 19
  allografts in, 464–465
  antibiotics in, 21, 461–462
  autografts in, 464
  caustic, of esophagus, 19–22
  debridement of, 462
  donor site management in, 465
  elective excision of, 463
    technique of, 463–464
  escharotomy in, 462–463
  excision of, 463–464
  extent and depth of, 460–461
  fasciotomy in, 462–463
  fluid management in, 464–465, 466–467
  hydrotherapy in, 461
  initial care of, 461
  natural history of, 461
  nutritional management in, 467–469
  occupational therapy for, 466
  septic wound in, 465–466, 466t
  shock, 467
  surgical management of, 462–466
  technique of wound closure for, 464–465
  topical chemotherapeutic agents
    for, 461–462
Bypass procedures, vascular. *See*
    Revascularization

C

Calcium
  as therapy in hypocalcemia, 310
  ulcerating subcutaneous, in Raynaud's
    syndrome, 394–395
Calculus(i)
  bile duct, treatment of, 214–215
  common duct, 201–204
    exploration for, 198–201, 202
    primary, 204–208
      diagnosis of, 205
      operative management of, 205–206
      pathogenesis of, 204–205
      surgical procedures in, 206–208
      vs. secondary, 204
    retained
      dissolution of, 203
      endoscopic papillotomy in, 204

    extraction of, 203–204
  gallstones. *See* Gallstones
  retained, treatment of, 202–204
Calories, daily requirements of, 513–514
Carbohydrates, absorption of, in short bowel
    syndrome, 85
Carcinoid tumor, gastric, 39
Carcinoma. *See also specific anatomic sites
    of carcinoma*
  adrenal cortical, 286–287
  of anus, 124–126
  of bile ducts, 223–225
  of breast, 317–332
  of colon, 120–121
    polypoid, 115
    and ulcerative colitis, 93
  colorectal, metastatic to liver
    infusion chemotherapy in, 169–175
    resection in, 164–168
  of esophagus, 22–25
  of gallbladder, 223
  of liver, 162
  of pancreas, 249–255
  of rectum, 120–123
  of skin, 481–482
  of stomach, 34–38
  of thyroid gland, 295–297
Cardia, lesions of, surgical treatment of, 23
Caroli's disease, 216–219
  with intrahepatic cysts, transhepatic tube
    insertion in, 218–219
Carotid artery, endarterectomy of, 360–363
  anesthesia for, 362
  complications of, 363
  diagnostic studies in, 361
  emergency, 361–362
  indications for, 360–361
  selective shunting in, 362
  technique of, 362–363
Catecholamine levels, in pheochromo-
    cytoma, 289
Catheter, intercostal, insertion of, 334
Catheterization, for parenteral
    nutrition, 516–517
Caustic burns, of esophagus, 19–22
Caustics
  liquid, 20–22
  solid, 20
Cefazolin, in biliary tract surgery, 229
Cefoxitin (Mefoxin), 207
Celiac axis compression syndrome, 404–405
Celiotomy
  in esophageal perforation, 21
  for trauma, 451
Cellulitis
  crepitant, 521
  in diabetic foot, 407
  penicillin in, 519
Cerebrovascular occlusive disease, 360–364
  asymptomatic bruits in, 361
  carotid endarterectomy in
    completion angiography after, 363
    coronary bypass grafting and, 363
    emergency, 361–362
    indications for, 360–361
    morbidity and mortality following, 363
    technique of, 362–363
  obesity and, 39
  subclavian steal syndrome in, 363–364
Cervical esophagus, lesions of, surgical
    treatment of, 24
Cervical spine, trauma of, 472
"Chemopreventors," of colon carcinoma,
    118

Chemotherapy
  in anal cancer, 125
  in breast cancer, 320–321, 330
  in gastric cancer, 37
  in gastric lymphoma, 38
  infusion, in metastases to liver, 164,
    169–175
  in large bowel cancer, 123
  in soft tissue sarcoma, 495
Chenodeoxycholic acid (CDCA), in gallstone
    dissolution, 194
Chest wall, 333–344
  flail chest, 335–336
  hemothorax, 343–344
  penetrating wounds of, 333
  pneumothorax, 339–343
  rib fractures, 334–335
  sternal fractures, 336
  trauma of, 333–336
    blunt, 333–334
  tube insertion in, 334
  tumors of, 336–339
    benign, 337
    malignant, 337–338
Chilblains, 474
Child(ren)
  fibropolycystic disease in, 159
  frostbite in, 476
  polyps in, 117
  splenic trauma in, nonoperative
    management of, 452
Chloroquine, in amebic liver abscess, 156
Cholangiography
  endoscopic retrograde, in chronic
    pancreatitis, 246
  intraoperative, 201–202
  operative, 199
  percutaneous transhepatic, in pancreatic
    carcinoma, 251–252
  prophylactic antibiotics during, 230–231
  in sclerosing cholangitis, 220–221
  T-tube insertion after, 200
Cholangiopancreatography, endoscopic retro-
    grade, in pancreatic carcinoma, 251–252
Cholangitis
  acute, 208–210
    antibiotics in, 230
    bacteriology of, 209
    clinical course of, 210
    clinical presentation of, 208–209
    initial management of, 209–210
    toxic, 210
  sclerosing, 220–222
    clinical manifestations of, 220
    liver transplant in, 222
    medical management of, 221
    prognosis of, 222
    surgical procedures in, 221–222
  toxic, 210
Cholecystectomy
  in acute cholecystitis, 196–197
  in chronic cholecystitis, 197–198
  early, in asymptomatic gallstones, 193–194,
    196
  postcholecystectomy syndrome, 212–215
    assessment and investigation of, 213–214
    treatment of, 214–215
Cholecystitis, 195–198
  acute, 196–197
    antibiotics in, 230
  chronic, 197
  surgery for, 197–198
Cholecystojejunostomy, in carcinoma of
    pancreas, 254

Cholecystostomy, in bile duct trauma, 432
Choledochal cysts, 216–217
  Lilly's technique of excision of, 217
Choledochoduodenostomy, in common duct
    stones, 206–207
Choledocholithotomy, endoscopic
    papillotomy with, 208
Choledochoscopy, 200
Choledochotomy, 199
  incisions for, 199
  indications for, 198
  T-tube insertion after, 200
Cholelithiasis. See Gallstones
Cholera, pancreatic, 260–261
"Cholera solution," 85
Cholestyramine (Questran), in short bowel
    syndrome, 86
Chondroma, 337
Chondrosarcoma, 337–338
Chordoma, of presacral space, 483–484
Cimetidine
  for gastrinoma, 48
  for lesser curvature ulcers, 28
  in Mallory-Weiss syndrome, 33
Cirrhosis, ascites secondary to, 183
Clindamycin
  in caustic burns of esophagus, 21
  in pancreatic abscess, 237
  in septic shock, 437
Clostridial gas gangrene, 521
  antibiotics in, 521
  of extremities, 501–503
    antibiotics in, 502–503
    clinical perspective of, 501–502
    clinical syndromes of, 502
    diagnosis of, 502
    hyperbaric oxygen in, 503
    treatment of, 502–503
Clostridial infection
  of hand and arm, 500
  postoperative, 521
Clostridium difficile, pseudomembraneous
    colitis caused by, 96
Clostridium perfringens, in positive bile
    cultures, 227
Coagulation
  blood, disorders of, 545–547
  after peritoneovenous shunts, 184
Coagulopathy, postshunt, 186
Cold injuries, 474–476
Colic, biliary, 193
Colitis
  Crohn's, 95–97
  granulomatous, 95–97
    differential diagnosis of, 95–96
    medical management of, 96
    surgical management of, 96–97
  ischemic, 110–114
    gangrenous, 114
    in mesenteric ischemia, 80
    shock-associated, 113–114
    spontaneous, 111––113
  pseudomembranous, caused by Clostridium
    difficile, 96
  ulcerative, 92–95
    Brooke ileostomy in, 94
    and cancer, 93
    continent ileostomy in, 94
    endorectal pull-through procedure
      in, 93–94
    hemorrhoids in, 136
    indications for surgery in, 92–93
    postoperative complications in, 94–95
    proctocolectomy in, 93

Colitis cystica profunda, 108
Collagen vascular disorders, of esophagus, 6
"Collar button abscess," 499–500
Collis-Nissen operation
  clinical experience with, 11–12
  technique of, 11–12
Colon
  acute diverticulitis in, 90
  carcinoma of, 118–121
    adjuvants to surgery in, 123
    diagnosis of, 119
    etiology of, 118
    follow-up in, 123
    metastasis to liver, 162
    obstruction in, 97–99
    and polyps, 115, 119–120
    resection of, 120
    screening of, 118
  Crohn's disease of, 95–97
    diverticular disease of, 90–92
      abscess in, 91
      complications of, 90–92
      elective operations in, 92
      fistulas in, 91
      hemorrhage in, 91–92
      obstructions in, 91
      perforation and peritonitis in, 91
  obstruction of, 97–99
    carcinoma in, 97–99
    in diverticulitis, 91
    neoplastic disease and, 97–99
    palliative surgery in, 98
    treatment of, 98
      "curative," 98–99
  polyps of, 114–117
    diminutive, 115–116
    multiple, 117
    nonmucosal, 117
    pedunculated, 116
    sessile, 116
  trauma of, 432–433, 448–449, 450–451,
    456–457
    operative assessment and management
      of, 451
    repair of, 450–451
  tumors of, 118–123
  volvulus of, 100–102
    acute, 101–102
    ileosigmoid knot, 102
    intermittent, 102
    sigmoid colon, 100–101
    transverse colon, 102
Colonoscopy
  in ischemic colitis, 112
  of polyps, 115
Colonostomy, in trauma of rectum, 451
Colorectal injury, 109–110
Colostomy, in diverticular abscess, 91
Coma, hepatic, 184
Common bile duct
  calculi of. See Calculus(i), common duct
  carcinoma of, 223–225
    diagnosis and clinical findings in, 224
    treatment of, 224–225
      operative ultrasound in, 225
      results of, 225–226
  exploration of, 198–201, 202
    incision in, 199
    indications for, 198–199
    irrigation of, 199
    tumors of, 223–226
Compress, in hand infections, 499
Compression syndrome, thoracic
    outlet, 395–398

Computerized tomography
  in diagnosis of pancreatic abscess, 236
  in pancreatic carcinoma, 250–251
  preoperative, in Crohn's disease of small
      bowel, 65
Constipation, and hepatic encephalopathy, 188
Coronary artery bypass, and carotid
      endarterectomy, 363
Corrosive agent, and esophageal perfora-
      tion, 1
Corticosteroid therapy
  in caustic burns of esophagus, 21
  in idiopathic thrombocytopenic
      purpura, 264
  postadrenalectomy, 288
Cricopharyngeal myotomy, in diverticula, 5
Crohn's disease
  of colon, 95–97
    aphthous ulcers in, 95
    differentail diagnosis of, 95–96
    loop ileostomy in, 96–97
    medical management of, 96
    perianal disease and, 95
    surgical management of, 96–97
    vs. ulcerative colitis, 95
  hemorrhoids in, 136
  of small bowel, 63–69
    abscess in, 67
    appendectomy in, 67
    complications after surgery for, 67–68
    fistulas in, 66–67
    gastroduodenitis in, 67
    indications for surgery in, 63–64
    obstructive uropathy in, 67
    operative strategy, 65–67
    perforation in, 67
    perianal suppurative lesions in, 67
    postoperative management of, 67
    postoperative recurrence of, 68
    preoperative management of, 64–65
    prognosis and follow-up after
        surgery, 67–69
    recurrent, 66
    survival and quality of life, 68–69
    timing of surgery in, 64
  small bowel obstruction due to, 62
Cricothyroidotomy, in penetrating neck
      trauma, 471
Cryotherapy, in hemorrhoids, 133
Cushing's syndrome, 283–286
  adrenocortical neoplasms in, 285
  diagnosis of, 284
    differential, 284–285
  ectopic ACTH production in, 284–285
  management of, 286
Cyst(s)
  biliary, 216–219
  choledochal, 216–219
  dermoid, 480
  epidermal inclusion, 480
  of liver, 157–160, 161
  pancreatic, in chronic pancreatitis, 245
  pilonidal, 150–152
  sebaceous, 480
  of spleen, 265–266
Cystadenoma, of liver, 161
Cystduodenostomy, in pancreatic pseudo-
      cysts, 240
Cystgastrostomy, in pancreatic pseudo-
      cysts, 240
Cystjejunostomy, in pancreatic
      pseudocysts, 240
Cystosarcoma phylloides, of breast, 326

D

Dale procedure, 412
Debridement
  in burn management, 462
  in clostridial infections, 521
  in liver trauma, 443–444
  in wound infections, 520
Decompression
  biliary, in carcinoma of pancreas, 254
  percutaneous transhepatic, in acute toxic
      cholangitis, 210
  of small bowel, in obstruction, 60
Dehydration
  extracellular, 505–507
  in mesenteric ischemia, 75
  total body, 505
de Quervain's thyroiditis, 304
Dermatofibrosarcoma protuberans, 482
Dermoid cysts, 480
Desmoid tumors, 337
Devascularization procedure, in portal
      hypertension, 178–179
Dexamethasone, in variceal de-
      compression, 177
Dexamethasone suppression test, in hyper-
      cortisolism, 284
Dextran infusions, in Buerger's disease, 386
Diabetes, insulin-dependent, and chronic
      pancreatitis, 246
Diabetes mellitus
  early cholecystectomy in, 194
  foot in, 405–408
  obesity and, 39–40
Dialysis, peritoneal, in acute renal failure, 540
Diarrhea
  postoperative, in ulcerative colitis, 94
  postvagotomy, 56
  in short bowel syndrome, 85–86
    treatment of, 87
  in Zollinger-Ellison syndrome, 47
Diet
  and hepatic encephalopathy, 188
  high fiber, for fissure in ano, 137
  in variceal decompression, 177–178
Digitalis, in shock, 435–436
Digits, melanoma of, 489–490
Dilatation
  of anal stricture, 140
  of anus, in hemorrhoids, 133
  balloon
    in aortoiliac occlusive disease, 364
    of biliary tract strictures, 211–212
  manual, in fissure in ano, 137
Dissolution of stones, in common duct, 203
Diuresis, and hepatic encephalopathy, 188
Diuretics, in shock, 436
Diverticulectomy, esophageal, 5
Diverticulitis, acute, of colon, 90
Diverticuloplexy, esophageal, 5
Diverticulum(a)
  of colon, 90–92
  duodenal, 72
  esophageal, 6–8
  jejunoileal, 72–73
  Meckel's, 73
  of small bowel, 72–73
  of thoracic esophagus, 5–6
Doxorubicin, in soft tissue sarcoma, 494–495
Dragstedt ulcer, 30
Drainage
  of abscess, in Raynaud's syndrome, 394
  of amebic abscess, 156–157

  of common bile duct, 206–207
  in duodenal injury, 446
  fistula, control of, 82
  after hepatic resection, 164
  in liver trauma, 444
  of pancreatic abscess, 237–238
  in pancreatic injury, 446
  of pancreatic pseudocysts
    external, 240
    internal, 239–240
  of pyogenic abscess, 155–156
  of sacrococcygeal pilonidal cyst, 150–151
  of thyroidectomy wounds, 294
Drug abuse, intra-arterial, 389–390
Drug therapy, adjuvant, in acute renal
      failure, 541
Dumping syndrome, 36
  postgastrectomy, 55
Duodenum
  diverticula of, 72
  hematoma of, intramural, 446
  obstruction of, in chronic pancreatitis, 245
  trauma of, 432, 444–448, 454–455
    classification of, 455, 455t
    complications of, 447–448
    drainage in, 446
    mortality rate in, 448
  ulcers of. See Ulcer, duodenal
Dysphagia, 3
Dysplagia, fibrous, 337

E

Eagle Barrett syndrome, herniation in, 277
Ear, melanoma of, 490
Echinococcus granulosis, hydatid disease
      caused by, 160
Edema
  and lymphedema of extremity, 423–426
  pulmonary, reexpansion, 342–343
Elderly patient
  gastric ulcer in, 30
  preoperative assessment of, 525–531
    factors associated with morbidity
        in, 527–529
    management principles and, 531
    physical examination in, 527
Electrolyte therapy, 504–512
  management of, in enterocutaneous
      fistula, 81–82
Embolectomy, 383–384
  postoperative treatment following, 384
  pulmonary, in venous thrombosis, 415
  in pulmonary embolism, 422–423
  reperfusion injuries following, 383
  results of, 384
Embolism, arterial, 381–384
  in abdominal aortic aneurysm, 350
  acute mesenteric ischemia in, 400
  amputation in, 383–384
  embolectomy in, 383–384
  heparinization in, 381
  initial patient management in, 381–383
  limb evaluation in, 381
  in popliteal aneurysm, 355
  pulmonary
    anticoagulants in, 421–422
    caval interruption in, 422
    clinical presentation of, 421
    diagnosis of, 421–422
    embolectomy in, 422–423
    Greenfield filter insertion in, 422
    surgical management of, 422–423

in venous thrombosis, 419–420
superior mesenteric artery, 400
thrombolytic therapy in, 382–383
Embolization
arteriographic, 357–359
transhepatic, in bleeding esophageal
varices, 176
Emetine, in amebic liver abscess, 156
Encephalopathy, hepatic, 184, 187–189
amino acids in, 189
bromocriptine in, 189
intestinal sterilization in, 189
L-dopa in, 189
lactulose in, 189
pathogenesis of, 187–188
therapy for, 188–189
Endarterectomy, carotid, 360–363
Endocrine glands, 281–314. *See also specific glands*
Endocrine neoplasia, multiple, 262
pheochromocytoma in, 291
thyroid medullary cancer in, 297
Endocrine tumor, of small bowel, 69–70
Endorectal pull-through procedure, in
ulcerative colitis, 93–94
Endoscopy
of large bowel, 118
in Mallory-Weiss syndrome, 32
Enema, preoperative, in Crohn's disease of
small bowel, 65
Energy requirements, disease
affecting, 522–523
Enolase, neuron-specific (NSE), 258
Enteritis, radiation, 109–110
operative management of, 109–110
preoperative evaluation of, 109
small bowel obstruction due to, 62
Enterobacter, in positive bile cultures, 226
Enterococcus, in positive bile
cultures, 226–227
Enterocutaneous fistula. *See* Fistula,
enterocutaneous
Epidermal inclusion cysts, 480
Epigastric hernia, 274–275
clinical findings and differential diagnosis
of, 275
treatment of, 275
Epiphrenic diverticulum, 8
Epithelial cell neoplasm, papillary-cystic, 257
Epithelial tumor, of small bowel, benign, 69
malignant, 70
Erythromycin
preoperative, in ulcerative colitis, 93
after splenectomy, 453
Escharotomy
in burn management, 462–463
in frostbite, 475–476
Escherichia coli
in acute cholangitis, 209
in positive bile cultures, 226
Esophagectomy
for carcinoma, 23–24
radical vs. standard, 24
Esophagitis
endoscopic grades of, 9
ulcerative, 9
Esophagogram, radiocontrast, in caustic burns
of esophagus, 21
Esophagoscopy, in caustic burns of
esophagus, 20
Esophagus, 1–26
achalsia of, 3–5
Barrett's. *See* Barrett's esophagus
carcinoma of, 22–25

in Barrett's esophagus, 14–15
esophagotomy for, radical vs.
standard, 24
postoperative care, 25
special problems, 25
surgical treatment of, 22–25
survival rates, 25
treatment modalities for, 22t
caustic burns of, 19–22
antibiotics in, 21
corticosteroid therapy in, 21
liquid, 20–22
solid, 20
treatment protocol for, 22
cervical, lesions of, 24
collagen vascular disorders of, 6
diverticulum of, 6–8
epiphrenic, 8
midesophageal, 7–8
Zenker's (pharyngoesophageal), 5, 6–7
hernia of, paraesophageal, 10, 16–19
motility disorders of, 3–6
myotomy of
in achalasia, 4–5
in diffuse spasm, 6
in epiphrenic diverticulum, 8
gastroesophageal reflux from, 4
perforations of, 1–3
clinical presentation of, 1–2
corrosive agents in, 1
etiology of, 1
foreign bodies in, 1
instrumentation causing, 1
spontaneous, 2–3
traumatic, 1
treatment of, 2
reflux in. *See* Reflux, gastroesophageal
spasm of, diffuse, 6
strictures of
in gastroesophageal reflux, 9–10
undilatable, management of, 13
thoracic, diverticulum of, 5–6
trauma of, 1, 454, 472–473
tumors of, 22–26
benign, 26
Ewing's sarcoma, 338
Excision
in burn management, 463–464
of skin lesions, 479
Extraction of stones, in common
duct, 203–204
Extremity(ies)
clostridial gas gangrene of, 501–503
lower, varicosities of, 409–412
lymphedema of, 423–426
soft tissue sarcomas of, 492–495
upper, ischemia of, 373–376
diagnosis of, 374–375
therapy for, 375–376
vascular injuries of, 460

F

Fasciotomy, in burn management, 463
Fats, absorption of, in short bowel
syndrome, 85–86
Felon, 499
Femoral aneurysm, 355–356
Femoral hernia, 270–271
inguinal hernia recurrence as, 273
Femoral vein valvuloplasty, technique
of, 410–411
Femoropopliteal bypass, in popliteal
aneurysm, 356

Femoropopliteal occlusive disease, 366–369
causes of, 366
lumbar sympathectomy in, 368
percutaneous transluminal angioplasty
in, 368
postoperative care in, 368–369
profundaplasty in, 368
prosthetic bypass in, 367–368
Femorotibial bypass, in tibioperoneal
occlusive disease, 371
using prosthetic material, 372
Fever, in wound infections, 519
Fibrinolysis, in venous thrombosis, 414
Fibrinolytic system, 546
Fibrocystic disease, of breast, 315–317
Fibropolycystic disease, 158–159
in children, 159
Fibrosis, hepatic, congenital, 159
Fibrous dysplagia, 337
Fingers, melanoma of, 489
Fissure, and cracks, in diabetic foot, 405
Fissure in ano, 137
Fistula
arteriovenous, 357–360
diagnosis of, 357
nonsurgical management of, 357–359
surgical management of, 359–360
biliary, and gallstone ileus, 219
colonic, in diverticular disease, 91
in Crohn's disease of small bowel, 66–67
duodenal, in trauma, 445, 447–448
enterocutaneous, 81–84
cause of death in, 81
definitive therapy for, 83–84
etiology of, 81
healing phase in, 84
investigation of, 83
late complications in, 84
management of, 81–84
recognition/stabilization in, 81–83
treatment goals in, 81
hemorrhoidal disease and, 136
in ano, 138–139
pancreatic, in trauma, 446–447
from radiation
rectovaginal, 110
rectovesical, 110
in vascular injury, 458
Fistulography, preoperative, in Crohn's
disease of small bowel, 65
Flail chest, 335–336
Floxacillin, in Raynaud's syndrome, 393
Fluid management, in variceal decompression, 177
Fluids of body
absorption and secretion of, in short bowel
syndrome, 85
acid-base status of, 510–512
alterations in composition of, 509–512
alterations in solute content, 507–509
alterations in volume, 504–507
potassium in, 509–510
replacement therapy, 504–512
in burns, 466–467
9∝-Fluorohydrocortisone (Florinef), in
adrenalectomy, 288
5-Fluorouracil
in anal cancer, 125
in gastric carcinoma, 37
Fogarty embolectomy catheter, 383
Foot
in diabetes, 405–408
abscess in, 407–408
amputations in, 408

cellulitis in, 407
fissures and dry skin in, 405
gangrene in, 408
hyperkeratosis in, 405–406
ingrown toenails in, 406
inpatient management of, 406–408
outpatient management of, 405–406
ulcerations in, 406–407
gangrene, 376–380
above-knee amputation in, 380
acute, 378–379
amputation vs. revascularization plus
amputation in, 376–378
below-knee amputation in, 380
in diabetes, 408
infected, 378
ray amputation in, 379
toe amputation in, 379
transmetatarsal amputation in, 379–380
immersion, 474
melanoma of, 490
trench, 474
Foreign body, and esophageal perforation, 1
Fractures
acetabular, 477–478
in conjunction with infection, 500
pelvic, open treatment of, 476–478
rib, 334–335
sternal, 336
Frostbite, 474–476
blisters in, 475
in children, 476
dressings in, 475
environmental influences in, 475
hypothermia in, 475
pathophysiology of, 475
prevention of, 475
rewarming in, 475
surgery in, 475–476
sympathetic blockade in, 476
therapy in, 475–476
Fuel stores, 522
Fungal infections, 500
Furosemide (Lasix), in shock, 436

G

Gallbladder
adenocarcinoma of, 223
cholecystectomy. See Cholecystectomy
cholecystitis, 195–198
cholelithiasis. See Gallstones
Gallstones
asymptomatic, 193–195, 196
management options in, 193
recommendations for, 195
risk factors in, 194–195
therapeutic alternatives in, 193–194
cholecystitis in, 195–198
early cholecystectomy in, 193–194
ileus from, 219–220
obesity and, 40
in pancreatitis, 196
in short bowel syndrome, 87
Ganglioneuroma, of presacral space, 485
Gangrene
in foot, 376–380
in diabetes, 408
gas, clostridial, 501–503, 521
in ischemic colitis, 114
in volvulus of colon, 100
Gardner's syndrome, 117
Gas gangrene, clostridial, 501–503, 521
Gastrectomy

in carcinoma, 35
complications of, 36–37
palliative, 36
reconstruction after, 36
hemigastrectomy, in lesser curve ulcers, 29
total, in Zollinger-Ellison syndrome, 49
Gastric, hypersecretion, in short bowel
syndrome, 86
Gastric mucosal barrier, damage to, 27
Gastric partitioning, technique of, 41–42
Gastric ulcer. See Ulcer, gastric
Gastrin levels, in Zollinger-Ellison
syndrome, 47–48
Gastrinoma, 47
treatment of, 48–49
Gastritis
preoperative prevention of, in Crohn's
disease of small bowel, 65
reflux, remedial reoperation for, 50–51
technique, 51–52
Gastroduodenitis, in Crohn's disease of small
bowel, 67
Gastroduodenostomy and vagotomy, in
duodenal ulcer, 44
Gastroenterostomy, in carcinoma of
pancreas, 254
Gastroesophageal reflux. See Reflux,
gastroesophageal
Gastrografin swallow examination, 3
Gastrojejunostomy, closing, 56
Gastroscopy, fiberoptic, in carcinoma, 34
"Gay bowel" syndrome, 96
Genetic predisposition, to breast cancer, 317
Gentamicin, in septic shock, 437
Giant pigmented nevus, 480
Glucagon, in ischemic colitis, 112
Glucagonoma syndrome, 261
Glucose, and electrolyte solutions, in short
bowel syndrome, 85
Goiter
intrathoracic, 293–294
mediastinal, posterior, 294
nontoxic, 291–294
pathophysiology of, 291–292
treatment of, 292–293
recurrent, 294
substernal, 293–294
thyroidectomy in, 293
drainage following, 294
toxic adenomatous, 298
Grafts
skin, in burn management, 464–465
vascular. See Revascularization
Granulomatous colitis, 95–97
Graves' disease, 298–303
thyroidectomy in, 301–303
Greenfield filter
in pulmonary embolism, 422
in venous thrombosis, 414–415
Groin hernia, 268–271
etiology and pathogenesis of, 268
incidence of, 268
surgical management of, 269–271
treatment of, 268–269

H

Hand
immersion, 474
infections of, 498–501
bacteria and, 498
nonsurgical management of, 498–499
postoperative care in, 500
surgical management of, 499–500
uncommon, 500–501

Hashimoto's thyroiditis, 305
Healing process
of enterocutaneous fistula, 84
of solitary rectal ulcer syndrome, 108
Hemangioma
cavernous, of liver, 160–161
of spleen, 265
Hemangiosarcoma, of spleen, 265
Hematoma
intramural, of duodenum, 446
in penetrating neck trauma, 472
retroperitoneal, 457–458
wound, early correction of, 521
Hemobilia, in liver trauma, 443
Hemodilysis, in acute renal failure, 540
Hemodynamics
role of, in adult respiratory distress
syndrome, 439–440
venous, 409–410
Hemolytic anemia
hereditary, splenectomy in, 263
immune, 263–264
Hemorrhage
in abdominal injuries, 429
abnormal, 543–547
blood coagulation disorders in, 545–547
platelet disorders in, 543–545
vascular disorders in, 543
and acute pancreatitis, 234
in diverticular disease of colon, 91–92
in duodenal ulcer, 45
in gastric ulcers, 29–30
gastrointestinal, 186–187
and hepatic encephalopathy, 188
in hemorrhoids, 135–136
in liver trauma, 442–443
in Mallory-Weiss syndrome, 31–32
in pancreatic pseudocysts, 240
in penetrating neck trauma, 470
in pneumothorax, 342
in portal hypertension, 176–180
pharmacologic control of, 180
in reflux esophagitis, 10
in ulcerative colitis, 92
Hemorrhoids, 132–136
diagnosis and classification of, 132
dilatation of anus in, 133
external, thrombosed, 133–134, 134f
office management of, 132–134
operative hemorrhoidectomy in, 134–135
complications following, 135–136
operative management of, 134–136
special cases of, 136
Hemothorax, 343–344
in penetrating neck trauma, 472
spontaneous, 343–344
traumatic, 344
treatment of, 344
Heparin therapy
in abdominal aortic aneurysm, 350
in arterial embolism, 381
in Buerger's disease, 386
in deep venous thrombosis, 415
in diabetic foot, 406
in embolism, arterial, pulmonary, 421–422
in venous thrombosis, 414, 421–422
Hepatic artery, ligation of, in liver
trauma, 442
in metastases to liver, 164
Hepatic duct, carcinoma of, 223–224
Hepatoma, 162

intrahepatic, 443
Hepatorenal syndrome, 184
Hepatotomy, in liver trauma, 442
Hereditary spherocytosis, splenectomy
  in, 263
Hernia, 268–280
  abdominal wall, 187
  epigastric, 274–275
  femoral, 270–271
  groin, 268–271
  inguinal, 269–274
    direct, 269–270
    indirect, 269
    recurrent, 271–274
    sliding, 270
  lumbar, 278–279
  obturator, 279–280
  ''pantaloon,'' 270
  paraesophageal, 10, 16–19
  paraesophageal hiatal, 10
  small bowel obstruction due to, 61–62
  spigelian, 280
  umbilical, 275–276
  ventral, 276–278
Herpes simplex infections, 500–501
Hill posterior gastropexy, in gastroesophageal
  reflux, 10–11
Histamine antagonist, in gastric ulcer, 28
Hormonal therapy, in breast cancer, 321,
  329–330
Hydatid disease, 160
Hydrocortisone, in adrenalectomy, 288
Hydrotherapy, for burn wounds, 461
Hydrothorax, high-pressure, 184
Hyperalimentation, intavenous, in surgical
  patient, 512–518
Hypercalcemia, in hyperparathyroidism,
  306–307
Hyperchloremic acidosis, 516
Hypercortisolism, and Cushing's
  syndrome, 284
Hypergastremia, in short bowel syndrome, 86
Hyperkalemia, 510, 539
Hyperkeratosis, in diabetic foot, 405–406
Hypernatremia, 508–509
Hyperoxaluria, in short bowel syndrome, 87
Hyperparathyroidism, 306–310
  diagnosis of, 306–307
  election for parathyroidectomy in, 307
  localization procedures in, 307–308
  pathology of, 309
  recurrent and persistent, 309, 310–314
  surgical treatment of, 308–309
Hyperplasia, focal nodular, of liver, 161
Hypersplenism, secondary, splenectomy
  in, 264
Hypertension
  in pheochromocytoma, 288–289
  portal, 176–180
    Budd-Chiari syndrome and, 189–192
    devascularization procedure in, 178–179
    distal splenorenal shunt in, 177–178
    in hemorrhoidal disease, 136
    total shunt in, 178
  renovascular, 390–392
    drug therapy in, 391
    operative therapy in, 391
      results of, 391–392
    percutaneous transluminal angioplasty
      in, 391
Hyperthyroidism, 298–303
  preparation for surgery in, 299–301
Hypervolemia, 504–505
Hypoglycemia, periodic, 259–260

Hypokalemia, 509–510
Hyponatremia, 507–508, 539
Hypophosphatemia, 516
Hypophysectomy, in metastatic breast
  cancer, 329
Hypotension, in ruptured abdominal aortic
  aneurysm, 352
Hypothermia, in frostbite, 475
Hypovolemia, 505–507
  in mesenteric ischemia, 75

I

^{125}I-labeled fibrinogen, in venous
  thrombosis, 413
Iatrogenic injury, of esophagus, 1
Idiopathic thrombocytopenic purpura (ITP),
  splenectomy in, 264
Ileitis, Crohn's, 66
Ileocolitis, Crohn's, 66
Ileocolostomy, in ischemic colitis, 114
Ileosigmoid knot, 102
Ileostomy
  loop, in Crohn's colitis, 96–97
  in trauma of rectum, 451
  in ulcerative colitis
    Brooke, 94
    continent, 94
Ileum
  Crohn's disease of, 63–69
  jejunoileal diverticula of, 72–73
  Meckel's diverticulum of, 73
Ileus, gallstone, 219–220
  diagnosis and treatment of, 220
  etiology of, 219
  symptoms of, 219–220
Immersion foot and hand, 474
Immunocompromised patient, early
  cholecystectomy in, 195
Incision and drainage. See Drainage
Incisional biopsy, of skin lesions, 479
Incontinence, anal, 144–150
  causes of, 144, 144t
  medical treatment of, 144–145
  postoperative care in, 145
  results of treatment of, 150
  supplementing sphincter mechanism
    in, 145, 149–150
  technique of, 149–150
  surgical treatment of, 145
Infants, umbilical hernia in, 275–276
Infection. See also Sepsis
  of burn wounds, 465–466
  catheter, in parenteral nutrition, 517–518
  and clostridial gas gangrene, 501
  fungal, 500
  of hand, 498–501
  and hepatic encephalopathy, 188
  herpes simplex, 500–501
  intra-abdominal, postoperative, 532–534
  postoperative, of wounds, 518–521
    antibiotics in, 520
    clinical findings and management
      in, 518–521
    clostridial, 521
    deep, 519–520
      gram stain and culture in, 520
    prevention of, 521
    superficial, 518–519
      gram stain and culture in, 520
  in ulcerative colitis, 92
  wound, as complication of appendicitis, 131
Inguinal hernia, 269–274
  direct, 269–270
  indirect, 269

  recurrent, 271–274
    anterior approach to, 272
    complications of repair of, 274, 274t
    diagnosis of, 271–272
    etiology of, 271
    as femoral hernia, 273
    through inguinal floor, 273
    at internal inguinal ring, 272–273
    nonsurgical management of, 272
    peritoneal approach to, 273–274
    prosthetic repair of, 271, 273
    at pubic tubercle, 273
    sites of, 272
    surgical management of, 272–274
Inguinal metastasis, in anal cancer, 125
Innominate artery, compression of trachea
  by, 346
Insulinoma, 259–260
  complications of, 260
  diagnosis of, 259
  operative management of, 259–260
  preoperative localization of, 259
Intercostal catheter, insertion of, 334
Intestines
  enterocutaneous fistulas in, 81–84
  ischemia in
    chronic, 403–404
    focal, 404
    revascularization in, 404
  large bowel, 90–152. See also Anus; Colon;
    Rectum
  obstruction of. See Ileus
  preoperative preparation of, 126–129. See
    also Preoperative state
    antibiotics in, 126–128
    in elective operations, 127–128
    in emergency operations, 128–129
    mechanical cleansing, 127–128
  radiation enteritis and proctitis of, 109–110
  small bowel, 57–89. See also Small bowel
  trauma of, 432–433, 448–451, 454–457
Intra-abdominal infections, postoperative, 532–534
Intra-arterial injections and infusions, 388–390
Intradermal nevus, 480
Intraoperative injury, to esophagus, 1
Intrasplenic cell destruction, conditions
  associated with, splenectomy in, 264
Intubation
  in enterocutaneous fistula, 82–83
  in penetrating neck wounds, 471
Intussusception, internal, 107
Iodine, radioactive, in hyperthyroidism, 298–299
Ischemia
  Buerger's disease in, 385–388
  cerebrovascular, transient carotid
    endarterectomy in, 360
  changes in, in solitary rectal ulcer
    syndrome, 107–108
  in diabetic foot, 406–407
  in embolic arterial occlusion, 381–384
  femoropopliteal occlusive, 366–369
    severity of, 366–367
  intestinal
    chronic, 403–404
    focal, 403
  mesenteric, 74–80, 399–405
    acute, 399
      diagnosis of, 400–401
      etiology of, 400
      incidence of, 399–400
      management plan for, 401–402
      prognosis of, 402–403
    anatomy and physiology of, 399

nonocclusive, 400
  Raynaud's syndrome in, 392–395
  renovascular, and hypertension, 390–392
  tibioperoneal occlusion, 369–373
  of upper extremity, 373–376
Isoproterenol (Isuprel), in shock, 435

J

J-tube insertion, in Caroli's disease, 218–219
Jaundice
  in chronic pancreatitis, 245
  in fibropolycystic disease, 159
  in periampullary cancer, 250
  in solitary liver cysts, 158
"Jeep drivers disease," 150
Jejunoileal diverticula, 72–73
Jod-Basedow phenomenon, 292
Joint, infection within, 500
Junctional nevus, 480

K

Kanamycin, in preoperative bowel
    preparation, 127
Kaposi's sarcoma, 482
Kayexalate, in hyperkalemia, 539
Keflex, in diabetic foot, 406
Keloids, 481
Keratoacanthoma, 481
Keratosis
  actinic, 481
  seborrheic, 480–481
"Key-hole-deformity," 137
Kidney
  failure of, acute. *See* Renal failure, acute
  fibropolycystic disease of, 159
  trauma of, 431–432, 457
"Kissing" ulcer, 45, 356, 405
Klebsiella, in acute cholangitis, 209
Klebsiella pneumoniae, in positive bile
    cultures, 226
Kock pouch, in ulcerative colitis, 93

L

L-dopa, in hepatic encephalopathy, 189
L-thyroxine therapy, in goiter, 292
Lactose intolerance, in short bowel
    syndrome, 85
Lactulose, in hepatic encephalopathy, 189
Large bowel, 90–152. *See also* Anus; Colon;
    Rectum
Laser resection, in mucosal tracheal
    stenosis, 347
Laser therapy, in hemorrhoids, 133
Lavage
  peritoneal
    in acute pancreatitis, 233
    in blunt trauma, 428
    in stab wounds, 428
  preoperative, in bowel preparation, 127–128
Leiomyoma
  of rectum, 485
  of stomach, 38–39
Leiomyosarcoma, of stomach, 38
Lesions
  of presacral space, 483–485
  skin, pigmented, 480
Leukemia, hemorrhoidal disease and, 136
Lidocaine, in rib fractures, 335
Lilly's technique, of choledochal cyst
    excision, 217
Liver, 153–175

abscess of, 153–157
  amebic, 156–157
    aspiration of, 156
    drainage of, 156–157
    drugs in, 156
    results of treatment of, 157
    vs. pyogenic, 153–154
  pyogenic, 154–156, 157
    antibiotics in, 154
    aspiration of, 154–155
    drainage of, 155–156
    vs. amebic, 153–154
adenoma of, 161
in ascites, 183–187
cysts of, 157–160, 161
  congenital hepatic fibrosis, 159
  echinococcal (hydatid), 160
  fibropolycystic disease, 158–159
  neoplastic, 159
  parasitic, 160
  posttraumatic, 159–160
  solitary congenital nonparasitic, 157–158
    diagnosis of, 158
    pathology of, 157–158
    recurrent, 158
encephalopathy, hepatic, 187–189
hemangioma of, cavernous, 160–161
hepatoma of, 162
hyperplasia of, focal nodular, 161
metastases to, 162
  colorectal cancer and
    infusion chemotherapy in, 169–175
    resection in, 164–168
  infusion chemotherapy in, 164
in portal hypertension, 176–180
resection of, technical refinements
    in, 162–164
transplant of, in sclerosing cholangitis, 222
trauma of, 429, 442–444
  debridement in, 443–444
  drainage in, 444
  exposure in, 442
  hemobilia in, 443
  hemorrhage control in, 442–443
tumors of, 160–164
  benign, 160–162
  hepatic artery ligation and chemotherapy
    for, 164
  malignant, 162
  technical refinements in resection
    of, 162–164
Lobular carcinoma, of breast, in situ, 326–328
Loop ileostomy, in Crohn's colitis, 96–97
Lumbar hernia, 278–279
Lumbar sympathectomy
  in Buerger's disease, 387
  in femoropopliteal occlusive disease, 368
Lungs. *See also* pulmonary entries
  collapse of, and infection, in adult
    respiratory distress syndrome, 440
  in flail chest, 336
Lye, ingestion of, 19
Lymph nodes
  dissection of
    in breast cancer, 320
    in melanomas, 491–492
  staging of, in breast cancer, 319–320
Lymphadenectomy, in metastatic
    melanomas, 490–491
Lymphedema, of extremities, 423–426
  classification of, 423–424
  medical management of, 424
  preoperative management of, 424
  surgical management of, 424–426

  indications for, 424
Lymphoid tumor, malignant, of small
    bowel, 70
Lymphoma
  hemorrhoidal disease and, 136
  non-Hodgkin's, of stomach, 38
  of spleen, 265
  of stomach, 38

M

Mafenide (Sulfamylon), in burns, 462
Magaldrate (Riopan), in short bowel
    syndrome, 86
Malabsorption, in short bowel
    syndrome, 85–86
Males, breast cancer in, 326
Mallory-Weiss syndrome, 31–34
  angiography in, 32–33
  barium studies in, 33
  endoscopy in, 32
  initial management of, 31–32
  nonoperative management of, 33–34
  operative management of, 34
  vasopressin infusions in, 32–33
Malnutrition
  diagnosis of, 512–513
  protein-calorie, 522
Mammography, of nonpalpable breast
    cancer, 318–319
Manometry, anorectal, 144
Marlex mesh, in recurrent hernia repair, 271,
    273
Mastectomy
  modified radical, 320
  partial, 320–321
  reconstruction after, 321
Meckel's diverticulum, 73
Megestrol acetate, in breast cancer, 330
Melanoma, 487–492
  anorectal, 126
  of breast, 490
  of digits, 489–490
  of ear, 490
  of foot, 490
  juvenile, 480
  lymph node metastases in, 490–492
  and nevi, 480
  primary, 488–490
    excision of, 488–489
Meningocele, of presacral space, 484
Meperidine hydrochloride (Demerol)
  in acute cholecystitis, 197–198
  in wound infections, 518
Mesenteric vascular occlusive disease, 74–80,
    399–405
  acidosis in, 75–76
  acute arterial occlusion in, 78–79
  dehydration and hypovolemia in, 75
  diagnosis of, 74–75, 76t
  intraoperative determination of viability
    in, 77–78
  ischemic colitis in, 80
  management of
    general principles in, 74–78
    specific entities in, 78–80
  multisystem failure syndrome in, 76–77
  nonocclusive mesenteric ischemia in, 80
  sepsis in, 75
  strangulation obstruction in, 79–80
  surgical intervention in, 77
  venous thrombosis in, 79
Mesoatrial shunt, for Budd-Chiari
    syndrome, 191

Mesocaval "C" shunt, for Budd-Chiari
    syndrome, 190
Metabolic acidosis, 510–511
Metabolic alkalosis, 511
Metabolism
    complications of, in parenteral nutrition, 517
    in Crohn's disease of small bowel, 64–65
Metastasis
    of colorectal cancer, 120
    inguinal, in anal cancer, 125
    to liver, 162
        colorectal cancer and
            infusion chemotherapy in, 169–175
            resection in, 164–168
        of melanomas, 490–492
Methylprednisolone, in septic shock, 437
Metronidazole (Flagyl)
    in amebic liver abscess, 156
    in preoperative bowel preparation, 127
Midesophageal diverticulum, 7–8
Mitomycin-C, for anal cancer, 125
Monooctanoin (Capmul), in dissolution of
    common duct stones, 203
Morbidity
    in carotid endarterectomy, 363
    postoperative, in Crohn's disease of small
        bowel, 67–68
Morphine sulfate, in wound infections, 518
Mortality rate
    in carotid endarterectomy, 363
    in duodenal trauma, 448
    in pancreatic trauma, 448
    postoperative, in Crohn's disease of small
        bowel, 67–68
Motility disorders
    of esophagus, 3–6
    in short bowel syndrome, 86–87
Multisystem failure syndrome, in mesenteric
    ischemia, 76–77
Muscle spasms, pelvic, 105–106
Myelofibrosis, splenectomy in, 264
Myelolipoma, 287
Myeloma, in chest wall, 338
Myositis, clostridial See Clostridial gas
    gangrene
Myotomy
    cricopharyngeal, in diverticula, 5
    esophageal
        in achalasia, 4–5
        in diffuse spasm, 6

N

Nasogastric tube, in enterocutaneous
    fistula, 82–83
Neck
    mass in, solitary, 495–498
        biopsy in, 496–497
        diagnostic evaluation of, 495–497
        management of, 497–498
        prognosis of, 498
    penetrating wounds of, 470–474
        crycothyroidotomy in, 471
        evaluation of, 471–472
        life-threatening injury in, 470–471
        specific injuries in, 472–474
        vascular injuries of, 459
Necrosis, in acute pancreatitis, 234
Needle aspiration, of pneumothorax, 340
Nelson's syndrome, 286
Neomycin
    preoperative, in ulcerative colitis, 93
Neoplastic cyst, of liver, 159
Nerve, intercostal block in rib fractures, 335

Neuroendocrine neoplasm, 257
Nevus(i), 480
Nipple, Paget's disease of, 324–325
Nissen fundoplication
    for gastroesophageal reflux, 4, 10–11
    in paraesophageal hernia, 19
Nitrofuratoin (Furacin), in burns, 462
Non-Hodgkin's lymphoma, of stomach, 38
Nonepithelial tumor, of small bowel, 69
Nonocclusive mesenteric ischemia (NOMI),
    in mesenteric ischemia, 80
Nutrition
    in acute renal failure, 541–543
    in burns, 467–469
    in Crohn's disease of small bowel, 64–65
    in enterocutaneous fistula, 82
    parenteral, 512–518
        complications of, 517–518
        at home, 516
        incidence of cholelithiasis in, 194
        indications for, 512–513
        monitoring of, 514–516
        in pancreatic ascites, 242–243
        solutions used in, 513–514
        venous catheterization methods
            in, 516–518
    preoperative, assessment of, 522–525
    in short bowel syndrome, 87

O

Obesity
    gallstones and, 40
    gastric restriction procedure, 39–43
    and venous thrombosis, 40
Obstruction, intestinal. See also Ileus
    of large intestine, 97–99
    of small intestine, 57–63
    in radiation enteritis, 109
Obturator hernia, 279–280
Occlusive disease, vascular. See Ischemia
Omental flaps, Goldsmith's, in lymphedema
    of extremity, 424–425
Oophorectomy, bilateral, in metastatic breast
    cancer, 329
Organ dysfunction, surgery for, in acute
    pancreatitis, 233
Osmolality of fluids, 507–509
Osmotically effective agents, preoperative, in
    bowel preparation, 127
Osteochondroma, 337
Osteogenic sarcoma, 338
Oxygen therapy
    hyperbaric, in clostridial gas gangrene, 503
    in shock, 436

P

Paget's disease, of breast, 324–325
Pain
    in abdominal aortic aneurysm, 352
    in Buerger's disease, 385, 386
    in chronic pancreatitis, 245
    in periampullary cancer, 250
    postamputation, 380
    in presacral tumors, 485
Palliation
    in colon obstruction with carcinoma, 98
    in gastric cancer, 36
Pancreas, 232–262
    abscess of, 235–238
        antibiotics in, 237
        clinical presentation of, 236
        diagnosis of, 236–237

drainage of, 237–238
        pathogenesis of, 235
        pathology of, 235–236
        prevention of, 237
        treatment of, 237–238
    and ascites, 241–243
    carcinoma of, 249–255
        incidence of, 249
        lapartomy and intraoperative decisions
            in, 252–254
        preoperative diagnosis and staging
            of, 250–252
        prognosis of, 254–255
    insulinomas of, 259–260
    islet cell tumors of, 258–262
        glucagonoma syndrome in, 261
        insulinoma in, 259–260
        management of, 258–262
        mixed, 262
        multiple endocrine neoplasia in, 262
        somatostatinomas in, 261
        Verner-Morrison syndrome in, 260–261
    and pleural effusion, 241–242, 243–245
    polypepidomas of, 261–262
    pseudocysts of, 238–241
        acute, 238–239
        and ascites, 241–242
        chronic, 239
        complications of, 240–241
        cystduodenostomy in, 240
        cystgastrostomy in, 240
        cystjejunostomy in, 240
        external drainage of, 240
        hemorrhage in, 240
        internal drainage of, 239–240
        obstruction from, 240–241
        operative therapy in, 239–240
        resection in, 240
        rupture of, 240
        size of, 239
    somatostatinomas of, 261
    trauma of, 430–431, 444–448, 455–456
        at body and tail, 445
        complications of, 446–447
        drainage in, 446
        at head, 445
        mortality rate in, 448
    unusual tumors of, 256–258
        diagnosis of, 256–257
        gross appearance of, 257
        technical considerations in
            approaching, 257–258
Pancreatectomy
    in carcinoma of pancreas, 253
    in tumors of pancreas, 257
Pancreaticoduodenectomy, See Whipple
    procedure
Pancreatitis
    acute, 232–235
        early phase of, 232–234
        late phase of, 235
        middle phase of, 234
        peritoneal lavage in, 233
        persisting, 235
        surgery in, 232–234
    alcoholic, 241
    chronic, 245–249
        complications of surgery in, 248
        indications for surgery in, 245
        nonoperation management of, 246–247
        operative management of, 247–248
        operation selection for, 246
        operative nerve blocks in, 248
        pancreaticojejunostomy in, 247

resection in, 247–248
results of surgical therapy in, 248–249
selection of patients for surgery in, 245–246
gallstone, 233
in pancreatic trauma, 447
Pancreatography, endoscopic retrograde, in chronic pancreatitis, 246
in pancreatic ascites, 243
Pancreatectomy, in chronic pancreatitis, 247
Pancreaticojejunostomy, in chronic pancreatitis, 247
"Pantaloon" hernia, 270
Papaverine, in ischemic colitis, 112
Papillary-cystic epithelial cell neoplasm, 257
Papilloma, basal cell, 480–481
Papillomatosis, 315
Papillotomy, endoscopic, with choledocholithotomy, 208
in retained common duct stones, 204
Paraesophageal hernia, 10, 16–19
definition of, 16
diagnosis of, 17
presentation of, 17
treatment of, 17–19
Parasitic cysts, 160
Parathyroid glands
anatomy of, 311
autotransplantation of, 314
hyperparathyroidism, 306–310
initial parathyroid exploration in, 311–312
mediastinal exploration in, 313
pathology of, 309
primary, 306
recurrent and persistent, 309, 310–314
evaluation of patient with, 312
reoperation in, 312–313
surgical treatment of, 308–309
Parathyroidectomy
complications of, 309–310
follow-up and results of, 310
preparation for, 308
selection for, 307
Paronychia, 499
Pauchet's operation, 29
Pelvic fractures, open treatment of, 476–478
Pelvic muscle spasm, 105–106
Pelvic ring instability, management of, 476–477
Pemberton's sign, 292
Penicillin
in cellulitis, 519
in septic shock, 437
after splenectomy, 453
Peptic ulcer, 43–46
Percutaneous transluminal angioplasty
in femoropopliteal occlusive disease, 368
in renovascular hypertension, 391
Perforation
in appendicitis, 129, 131
of colon, in diverticulitis, 91
in Crohn's disease of small bowel, 67
of duodenal ulcer, 44–45
of esophagus, 1–3
of gastric ulcers, 29–30
in radiation enteritis, 109
Periampullary cancer, 249–255
Perianal region. See Anal verge
Perianal suppurative lesions, in Crohn's disease of small bowel, 67
Perineum, strengthening exercises of, for anal incontinence, 145
Peristalsis, esophageal, 3

Peritoneovenous shunt, in pancreatic ascites, 243
Peritonitis
in appendicitis, 129
in diverticular perforation of colon, 91
generalized, 532–533
pH status, in acid-base disorders, 510–511
Phalanx, disruption of dorsal tissues of, in Raynaud's syndrome, 394
Pharyngoesophageal diverticulum, 5, 6–7
Phenoxybenzamine, in pheochromocytoma, 289
Pheochromocytoma, 288–291
anesthesia for, 290
localization of, 289–290
malignant, 291
in multiple endocrine neoplasia, 291
postoperative care in, 290–291
preoperative management of, 289–290
surgery in, 290
Phlebography
contrast, in venous thrombosis, 414
radionuclide, 413–414
in varicosities, 410
Phlegmon, and acute pancreatitis, 234
Photocoagulation, infrared, in hemorrhoids, 133
Pilonidal sinus and cyst, sacro-coccygeal, 150–152
incision and drainage of, 150–151
operative managment of, 151–152
postoperative care of, 152
Pitressin infusions. See Vasopressin infusions
Plasmacytoma, in chest wall, 338
Platelets, disorders of, 543–545
Plethysmography, in venous thrombosis, 413
Pleural abrasion, in pneumothorax, 342
Pleural effusions, pancreatic, 241–242, 243–245
clinical features of, 242
diagnosis of, 242
nonoperative management of, 243–244
operative management of, 244
results of treatment of, 244–245
Pleurodesis, chemical, in pneumothorax, 342
Pneumococcal vaccine, after splenectomy, 453
Pneumothorax, 339–343
clinical presentation of, 339
complications of, 342–343
incidence and etiology of, 339
in penetrating neck trauma, 472
in pilots and air travelers, 343
spontaneous, 339
chest tube insertion in, 340–341
diagnosis of, 339
tension, 342
traumatic, 339
treatment of, 339–342
Polycystic disease, of liver, 158–159
Polyp(s), colorectal, 114–118
and cancer, 115, 119–120
gastric, 38
juvenile, 117
mucosal, 115–117
multiple, 117
nonmucosal, 117
polyposis syndromes in, 117–118
therapeutic principles in, 115
Polypectomy, of polyps, 116
Polypeptidoma, pancreatic, 261–262
Polyposis syndromes, 117–118
Polytetrafluoroethylene (PTFE) graft, in femoral aneurysm, 356
Popliteal aneurysm, 355–356

Portal hypertension, 176–180. See also Hypertension
Portal systemic shunt, in portal hypertension, 178
Positive end expiratory pressure (PEEP), adult respiratory distress syndrome and, 441
Postcholecystectomy syndrome, 212–215
Postgastrectomy and postvagotomy syndromes, 49–56
diarrhea after vagotomy, 56
dumping syndrome, 55
multifacets of, 49
reflux gastritis, 50–51
remedial operations for
investigations prior to, 50
operative technique, 51–52
ulcer recurrence, 50
Postthrombotic syndrome, 416, 418f, 419
Potassium
hyperkalemia, 510
hypokalemia, 509–510
"Pouchitis," postoperative, in ulcerative colitis, 94
Pregnancy
breast cancer and, 325
hemorrhoids in, 136
Preoperative state
assessment of, in elderly patient, 525–531
bowel preparation in, 126–129
nutritional assessment in, 522–525
Presacral space
bony lesions of, 485
congenital lesions of, 483–484
definition of, 482
inflammatory lesions of, 484–485
neurogenic tumors of, 485
tumors and cysts of, 482–487
clinical classification of, 485
incidence of, 482
pathology of, 482–483
preoperative work-up in, 485–486
surgical approach to, 486–487
symptoms of, 485
Processus vaginalis, and inguinal hernias, 268–269
Proctalgia fugax syndrome, 132
Proctitis, radiation, 109–110
operative management of, 109–110
preoperative evaluation of, 109
Proctocolectomy, in ulcerative colitis, 93
Profundaplasty, femoral, in femoropopliteal occlusive disease, 368
Prolapse
mucosal, 107
rectal, 103–105, 107
Propranolol, in pheochromocytoma, 289
Propylthiouracil (PTU), in hyperthyroidism, 299
Prostaglandins
in Buerger's disease, 386
intra-arterial, in Raynaud's syndrome, 393–394
intravenous, 393
Prosthesis, in recurrent hernia repair, 271, 273
Prosthetic bypass, in femoropopliteal occlusive disease, 367–368
Protein deficiency, in short bowel syndrome, 85
Proteins, absorption of, in short bowel syndrome, 85
Proteus, in positive bile cultures, 226
Pseudocyst(s)
and acute pancreatitis, 234
hepatic, 159–160

pancreatic, 238–241
 vs. pancreatic abscess, 235–236
 in trauma, 447
Pseudolymphoma, of stomach, 39
Pseudomembranous colitis, caused by
 Clostridium difficile, 96
Pseudomonas, in positive bile cultures, 226
Psyllium (Metamucil), in short bowel
 syndrome, 86
Psyllium seeds, in anal fissures, 137
''Puffyhand'' syndrome, 390
Pulmonary edema, reexpansion, 342–343
Pulmonary embolism, in venous
thrombosis, 419–420
Punch biopsy, of skin lesions, 479–480
Purpura, thrombocytopenic, idiopathic, 264
 thrombotic, 264
Pyloroplasty, reconstruction of, 56
Pyogenic abscess, of liver, 153–156, 157

R

Radiation therapy
 in anal cancer, 124–125
 in breast cancer, 320, 321–324, 331–332
 complications of, 323
 controversies in, 323
 technical aspects of, 322–323
 in chordomas, 484
 enteritis and proctitis from 109–110
 in gastric cancer, 37
 in pancreatic ascites, 243
 in pancreatic cancer, 255
 in rectal cancer, 121–122, 123
 in soft tissue sarcoma, 494–495
Ranitidine
 for gastrinoma, 48
 for lesser curvature ulcers, 28
Raynaud's syndrome, 392–395
 digital amputation in, 394
 local surgery under prostaglandin cover
 in, 394–395
 maintenance of body and extremity warmth
 in, 393
 oral drug therapy in, 393–394
 reassurance in, 392–393
 sympathectomy in, 394
 treatment of, 392–395
 results of, 395
 wound management in, 395
Rectal ulcer syndrome, solitary, 105–108
 ischemic changes in, 107–108
 loss of support in, 107
 pelvic muscle spasm in, 105–106
 straining at stool in, 106
Rectopexy, posterior, 103–104
Rectosigmoidectomy, perineal, 104
Rectum
 carcinoma of, 120–123
 polyps of
 diminutive, 115–116
 pedunculated, 116
 sessile, 116–117
 prolapse of, 103–105
 preoperative preparation in, 103
 therapeutic options in, 103
 trauma of, 432–433, 448–449, 451,
 456–457
 operative assessment and management
 of, 451
 repair of, 451
 tumors of, 118–123
Recurrent inguinal hernia, 271–274
Red cell deformability, conditions with,

splenectomy in, 263
Reefing procedure, in anal incontinence, 145
Reflux
 gastritis, remedial reoperation for, 50–51
 technique of, 51–52
 gastroesophageal, 9–13
 Angelchik prosthesis in, 13
 Barrett's esophagus and, 10
 Belsey Mark IV fundoplication for, 4–5,
 10–11
 Collis-Nissen operation for
 clinical experience with, 12–13
 technique of, 11–12
 failure of medical management of, 9
 Hill posterior gastropexy for, 10–11
 indications for surgery in, 9–10
 as myotomy complication, 4
 Nissen fundoplication for, 4, 10–11
 recurrence risk factors in, 11
 stricture from, 9–10
Renal failure, acute, 535–543
 adjuvant drug therapy in, 541
 diagnosis of, 535–537
 drug-induced, 535
 hemodialysis in, 540
 intraoperative prevention of, 537–538
 nutrition in, 541–543
 peritoneal dialysis in, 540
 postoperative prevention of, 538
 preoperative prevention of, 537
 prevention of, 537–538
 treatment of, 539–541
 ultrafiltration in, 540–541
Renovascular hypertension, 390–392. *See also*
 Hypertension
Resection
 abdominoperineal, for anal cancer, 124
 vs. low anterior, of rectum, 123
 of anal strictures, 143
 of colorectal cancer, 120
 metastatic to liver, 164–168
 hepatic, technical refinements in, 162–164
Respiratory acidosis, 511–512
Respiratory alkalosis, 511–512
Resuscitation, in clostridial gas gangrene, 502
Retrohepatic shunt, in liver trauma, 442–443
Retroperitoneal injury, 453–458
 hematoma in, 457–458
Revascularization
 in abdominal aortic aneurysm, 350–351
 amputation and, 376–378
 aortofemoral, in aortoiliac occlusive
 disease, 366
 in aortoiliac reconstruction, 364–366
 aortorenal bypass in, 391
 in arteriovenous fistula, 359–360
 in Buerger's disease, 387
 in false aneurysm, 359–360
 in femoral aneurysm, 356
 femorofemoral bypass in, 364
 femoropopliteal bypass in, 356
 in intestinal ischemia, 404
 polytetrafluoroethylene graft in, 356
 in popliteal aneurysm, 355–356
 in tibioperoneal occlusive disease, 371–373
 in upper extremity ischemia, 375–376
Ribs, fractures of, 334–335
 intercostal nerve block in, 335
 transaxillary resection in thoracic outlet
 syndrome, 398
Riedel's struma, 305–306
Ringer's lactate
 in appendicitis, 129
 in shock, 434

Rocaltrol, in hypocalcemia, 310
Roux-en-Y choledochocystojejunostomy, in
 extrahepatic cysts, 217
Roux-en-Y loop
 in pancreatic ascites, 243
 in sclerosing cholangitis, 222
Rubber band ligation, in hemorrhoids, 133
Rupture
 of abdominal aortic aneurysms, 352–354
 of esophagus, 2–3
 of pancreatic pseudocysts, 240

S

S-plasty, for anal strictures, 142–143
Sacral meningocele, of presacral space, 484
Saphenous vein bypass, in tibioperoneal
 occlusive disease, 371–372
Saphenous vein stripping of, 410
Sarcoma
 Ewing's, 338
 Kaposi's, 482
 osteogenic, 338
 soft tissue
 chemotherapy in, 495
 diagnosis of, 493
 of extremity, 492–495
 multimodality therapy in, 494–495
 preoperative evaluation of, 493
 radiation therapy in, 494–495
 staging of, 493–494
 surgery in, 494
Scalenectomy, in upper extremity
 ischemia, 375
Scalenotomy, in thoracic outlet syndrome, 398
Scleropathy, endoscopic, in portal
 hypertension, 179–180
Sclerosing cholangitis, 220–222
Sclerosis, endoscopic, in bleeding esophageal
 varices, 176
Sclerotherapy
 endoscopic
 for esophageal varices, 180–183
 in portal hypertension, 179–180
 in hemorrhoids, 133
Sebaceous cysts, 480
Seborrheic keratosis, 480–481
Secretin challenge test, in Zollinger-Ellison
 syndrome, 47–48
Secretory studies, in pancreatic
 carcinoma, 250
Sepsis. *See also* Infection
 adult respiratory distress syndrome and, 438
 in burn management, 465–466
 in mesenteric ischemia, 75
 nail-related, surgery for, in Raynaud's
 syndrome, 394
 postsplenectomy, 431, 451
 shock due to, 436–437
Seroma, wound, treatment of, 521
Shock, 433–438
 burn, 467
 cardiogenic, 437–438
 initial treatment for, 433–436
 neurogenic, 438
 refractory, 438
 septic, 436–437
Short bowel syndrome, 84–89
 adaption and, 87
 bacteriology and, 86
 carbohydrate absorption in, 85
 cholelithiasis in, 87
 complications of, 87

diarrhea in, 85–86
treatment of, 87
endocrine effects on, 86
fats and bile acid absorption in, 85–86
fluid absorption and secretion in, 85
hyperoxaluria in, 87
lactose intolerance in, 85
malabsorption in, 85–86
motility and, 86–87
nutrition in, 87
protein absorption in, 85
steatorrhea in, 86
surgical therapy for, 87–89
team approach to, 89
treatment of, 85–87
Shunt procedures
in false aneurysm, 359
peritoneovenous, in cirrhotic
ascites, 187–187
in portal hypertension
distal splenorenal, 177–178
total portal systemic, 178
selective, in carotid endarterectomy, 362
Sickle cell anemia, splenectomy in, 263
Sigmoid volvulus, acute, 100–101
Silver nitrate, in burns, 462
Silver sulfadiazine, in burns, 461, 462t
Sinus, pilonidal, 150–152
Sipple's syndrome, 262
Skin
actinic changes in, 481
carcinoma of
basal cell, 481
squamous cell, 481–482
dermatofibrosarcoma protuberans of, 482
healing of, in enterocutaneous fistula, 82
Kaposi's sarcoma of, 482
tumors of, 479–482
diagnosing, 479–480
malignant, 481–482
Skin flaps, pedicle, in lymphedema of
extremity, 425
Skin grafts, in burn management, 464–465
Sliding hernia, 270
Small bowel, 57–89
Crohn's disease of, 63–69. See also Crohn's
disease, of small bowel
diverticular disease of, 72–73
duodenal, 72
jejunal and ileal, 72–73
Meckel's, 73
obstruction of, 57–63
acute postoperative, 63
diagnosis of, 57–59
gallstone ileus in, 219–220
identifying cause of, 59
mechanical, 57
partial, 62–63
vs. complete, 57–59
simple vs. strangulation, 59
treatment of, 59–63
decompression in, 60
operative vs. nonoperative, 60–61
systemic considerations in, 59–60
trauma of, 448–450
operative assessment and management
of, 451
repair of, 449–450
tumors of, 69–71
diagnosis of, 70
surgical considerations for, 70–71
Small bowel bypass, for obesity, 40
Smoking, and Buerger's disease, 385
Sodium bicarbonate, in shock, 436

Soft tissue, lesions of, 487
Soft tissue sarcoma, of extremities, 492–495
Solitary rectal ulcer syndrome, 105–108
Somatostatinoma, 261
Spasms
esophageal, diffuse, 6
pelvic muscle, 105–106
sphincter, in fissure in ano, 137
Spherocytosis, hereditary, splenectomy
in, 263
Sphincter mechanism, supplementing, in anal
incontinence, 145, 149–150
Sphincteroplasty, in common duct
stones, 206–207
Sphincterotomy
in hemorrhoids, 133
lateral internal, for anal strictures, 140
midline, 140, 142
Spigelian hernia, 280
Spinal accessory nerve, trauma of, 473
Spironolactone, in aldosteronism, 283
Spleen, 263–267
abscess of, 266
cysts of, 265–266
trauma of, 431, 451–453
antibiotic prophylaxis in, 453
autotransplantation of splenic tissues
in, 453
nonoperative management of, 451–452
patient education in, 453
spenectomy in, 452–453
vaccine prophylaxis in, 453
tumors of, 265
Splenectomy
in hematologic disorders, 263–265
technical aspects of, 266–267
in trauma of spleen, 452–453
Splenic flexure, volvulus of transverse colon
and, 102
Splenorenal shunt, in portal hypertension, 177–178
"Spring-water cysts," 161
Squamous cell carcinoma
of anus, 124
of skin, 481–482
Staging, of breast cancer, 321–324
Staphylococcus, in positive bile cultures, 227
Steatorrhea, in short bowel syndrome, 86
Stenosis
anal, 139–143
rectal, radiation-induced, 109–110
tracheal, 345–348
Stenting
in biliary tract strictures, 212
endoscopic, in chronic pancreatitis, 246
Sternum, fractures of, 336
Stomach, 27–56
carcinoid of, 39
carcinoma of, 34–38
choice of operation for, 35–36
clinical presentation of, 34
operative management of, 35
palliation in, 36
pathology of, 35
prognosis of, 37–38
radiation and chemotherapy in, 37
staging of, 35
leiomyomas of, 38–39
leiomyosarcoma of, 38
lymphoma of, 38
in Mallory-Weiss syndrome, 31–34
polyps of, 38
pseudolymphoma of, 39
restrictive procedure for obesity, 39–43

indications for, 40–41
patient selection for, 40–41
postoperative care in, 42–43
technique of, 41–42
tumors of, 34–39
benign, 38–39
malignant, 34–38
mesodermal, 39
ulcer of. See Ulcer, gastric
Stone formation. See Calculus(i)
Stool, straining at, 106
Strangulated conditions
in mesenteric ischemia, 79–80
in small bowel obstruction, 61
Streptococcus aureus, hand infections caused
by, 498
Streptococcus faecalis, in acute
cholangitis, 209
Streptococcus viridans, in positive bile
cultures, 227
Streptokinase therapy
for Budd-Chiari syndrome, 190
intra-arterial, 388–389
Stricture
anal, 139–143
bile duct, treatment of, 215
of biliary tract, 211–212
esophageal, undilatable, management of, 13
in gastroesophageal reflux, 9–10
Stripping, saphenous vein, 410
Stroke, in progress, carotid endarterectomy
in, 361–362
Subclavian steal syndrome, 363–364
Sucralfate, in gastric ulcer, 28
Surgery, emergency, in bleeding esophageal
varices, 176–177
Sympathectomy
in Buerger's disease, 387
cervical, in upper extremity ischemia, 375
in frostbite, 476
in Raynaud's syndrome, 394

T

T-tube insertion
after choledochotomy, 200
and postoperative cholangiography, 200
in structural tracheal stenosis, 348
Tamoxifen, in metastatic breast cancer, 329
Tamponade, balloon, in bleeding esophageal
varices, 176
Tenosynovitis, 499
Teratoma, of presacral space, 483
Thalassemia, splenectomy in, 263
Thoracic duct, trauma of, 473
Thoracic esophagus, diverticulum of, 5–6
Thoracic injuries, vascular, 459
Thoracic outlet syndrome, 395–398
conservative treatment of, 397–398
diagnosis of, 396–397
surgical treatment of, 398
Thoracic wall. See Chest wall
Thoracostomy
closed tube, in pneumothorax, 340–341
in hemothorax, 344
Thoracotomy
in hemothorax, 344
in pneumothorax, 341–342
Thrombectomy, in venous thrombosis, 414
Thromboangiitis obliterans, 385–388
Thrombocytopenia, 544
Thrombocytopenic purpura
idiopathic, 264
thrombotic, 264

Thromboembolism
  postoperative prevention of, in Crohn's
    disease of small bowel, 65
  pulmonary. *See* Embolism, arterial,
    pulmonary
Thromboendarterectomy, in renovascular
  hypertension, 391
Thrombolysis, of arterial emboli, 382
Thrombolytic therapy, 388–389
  in arterial embolism, 381–382
  complications of, 389
Thrombophlebitis, 412–420
Thrombosis
  and acute pancreatitis, 234
  acute superior mesenteric artery, 400
  arterial, in penetrating neck trauma, 472
  of inferior vena cava, Budd-Chiari
    syndrome with, 190–191
  venous, 412–420
    acute mesenteric, 400
    clinical syndromes of, 412
    deep
      acute, 415
      diagnosis of, 421
      recurrent, 415–416
    diagnosis of, 413–414
    in mesenteric ischemia, 79
    obesity and, 40
    pathophysiology of, 412–413
    and postthrombotic syndrome, 416, 419
    and pulmonary embolism, 419–420
    superficial, 416
    therapeutic options in, 414–415, 415–420
Thyroid gland
  anaplastic carcinoma of, 297
  follicular carcinoma of, 296–297
  goiter of. *See* Goiter
  malignant tumors of, 295–297
    operative approach to, 296
    pathology of, 295
  medullary carcinoma of, 297
    in multiple endocrine neoplasia, 297
  nodule of, solitary, 295
  papillary carcinoma of, 296
  surgery of, pathophysiologic principles
    of, 301
Thyroid hormone therapy, in goiter, 294
Thyroidectomy
  complications of, 294
  drainage with, 294
  in goiter, 292–294
  in Graves' disease, 301–303
  in hyperthyroidism, 299
  indications for, 292–293
  postoperative management of, 294
  technique of, 293
Thyroiditis, 303–306
  acute, 303–304
  chronic lymphoid, 305
  Hashimoto's, 305
  Riedel's, 305–306
  subacute (de Quervain's), 304
Tibioperoneal occlusive disease, 369–373
  angiographic evaluation in, 370
  femorotibial bypass in, 371
  femorotibial bypass using prosthetic
    material, 372
  physical evaluation in, 369–370
  postoperative care in, 373
  preoperative preparation in, 370–371
  sequential arterial bypass in, 372
  short-segment bypass graft in, 372–373
TNM classification, of gastric cancer, 35
Tobramycin, in pancreatic abscess, 237

Toes, melanoma of, 489–490
Tongue, trauma of, 473
Trachea, 345–348
  stenosis of, 345–348
    functional, 345–347
      diagnostic investigation of, 346
      innominate artery compression in, 346
      surgical management of, 346–347
    mucosal, 347
      laser resection of, 347
    structural, 347–348
      T-tube insertion in, 348
  trauma of, 473
Transfusions
  in Mallory-Weiss syndrome, 33
  in ruptured abdominal aortic aneurysm, 353
  in shock, 435
Transplant
  liver, in sclerosing cholangitis, 222
  valve, axillary vein, 411–412
Trauma, 427–478
  abdominal, 427–433
  of bile ducts, 432
  of blood vessels, 473–474
  burns, 460–469
  of cervical spine, 472
  cold, 474–476
  of colon, 432–433, 448–449, 450–451,
    456–457
  colorectal, 109–110
  of duodenum, 432, 444–448, 454–455, 455t
  of esophagus, 1, 454, 472–473
  frostbite, 474–476
  of kidney, 431–432, 457
  of liver, 429, 442–444
  of neck, penetrating, 470–474
  of pancreas, 430–431, 444–448, 455–456
  pelvic, 476–478
  of rectum, 432–433, 448–449, 451,
    456–457
  retroperitoneal, 453–458
  shock in. *See* Shock
  of small bowel, 448–450
  of spinal accessory nerve, 473
  of spleen, 431, 451–453
  of thoracic duct, 473
  of thoracic wall, 333–336
  of tongue, 473
  of trachea, 473
  of ureters, 457
  vascular, 458–460
    drug-induced, 389–390
Trench foot, 474
Truss management, of hernia, 272
Tumor markers, in pancreatic carcinoma, 251
Tumors. *See also specific anatomic sites of
    tumors*
  ACTH producing, 284–285
  of adrenal cortex, 286–287
    feminizing, 287
    virilizing, 287
  bile duct, treatment of, 215
  of biliary tract, 223–226
  of breast, 317–332
  of chest wall, 336–339
  colorectal, 118–123
  of esophagus, 22–26
  of liver, 160–164
  malignant, small bowel obstruction due
    to, 62
  neck mass, solitary, 495–498
  of pancreas, 249–262
  of presacral space, 482–487
  of skin, 479–482

of small bowel, 69–71
of soft tissue, 487
of spleen, 265
of stomach, 34–39
Turcot's syndrome, 117

U

U-tube insertion, in Caroli's disease, 218–219
Ulcer
  aphthous, in Crohn's disease, 95
  in Buerger's disease, 386
  in diabetic foot
    ischemic, 406–407
    neuropathic, 407
  Dragstedt, 30
  duodenal, 44–46
    bleeding, 45
    intractability of, 44
    obstruction due to, 45–46
    parietal cell vagotomy in, 44
    perforated, 44–45
    selective vagotomy in, 44
    vagotomy and drainage in, 44
    vagotomy, antrectomy and gastroduoden-
      ostomy in, 44
    in Zollinger-Ellison syndrome, 47–49
  gastric, 46
    benign, 27–30
    bleeding, 29–30
    in elderly patient, 30
    medical treatment of, 28
    pathophysiology and rationale of
      therapy, 27–28
    perforated, 29–30
    prepyloric, 30
    surgical treatment of, 28–30
    type I (lesser-curvature), 27–30
    type II and III, 30
    in Zollinger-Ellison syndrome, 46–49
  "kissing," 45, 386, 405
  peptic, 43–46
  rectal, solitary, 105–108
  recurrent, 46
    remedial reoperation for, 50
    technique, 51–52
  surgery for, in Raynaud's syndrome, 394
Ulcerative colitis, chronic, 92–95
Ulcerative esophagitis, 9
Ultrafiltration, in acute renal failure, 540–541
Ultrasonography
  in pancreatic carcinoma, 250
  preoperative, in Crohn's disease of small
    bowel, 65
  in treatment of biliary tumors, 225
  in venous thrombosis, 413
Umbilical hernia
  in adults, 276
  in infants, 275–276
Ureters, trauma of, 457
Urokinase, in thrombolysis of clot, 382
Uropathy, obstructive, in Crohn's disease of
  small bowel, 67
Ursodeoxycholic acid, in gallstone dissolution,
194

V

Vaccine, pneumococcal, after splenectomy,
  453
Vagotomy
  and antrectomy, gastroduodenostomy
    within duodenal ulcers, 44

diarrhea after, 56
and drainage
  in bleeding gastric ulcer, 30
  in perforated gastric ulcer, 30
parietal cell, in duodenal ulcer, 44
selective, 44
  in gastric ulcer, 29
Valvuloplasty, femoral vein, technique
  of, 410–411
Varices
  esophageal
    bleeding, portal hypertension in, 176–180
    diagnosis of, 180
    endoscopic sclerotherapy for, 180–183
      complications of, 182
      procedure in, 180–181
      prophylaxis for, 183
      results of, 182
      technique of, 181–182
  in lower extremity, 409–412
    auxillary vein valve transplant in, 411–412
    classification of, 409
    Dale procedure in, 412
    femoral vein valvuloplasty in, 410–411
    patient selection for surgery in, 410
    saphenous vein stripping in, 410
    venous hemodynamics in, 409–410
Vascular system, 349–426
  aneurysms. See Aneurysm
  disorders of, 543
  drug-induced injury to, 389–390
  occlusive disease of. See Ischemia
  trauma of, 458–460, 473–474
    abdominal injuries in, 459–460
    diagnosis of, 458
    extremity injuries in, 460
    neck injuries in, 459
    postoperative complications of, 460
    sutures in, 459
    thoracic injuries in, 459
    treatment of, 458–460
  varicosities of. See Varices
  venous, hemodynamics of, 409–410
Vasoactive agents, in shock, 435–436
Vasopressin infusions
  in bleeding esophageal varices, 176
  in Mallory-Weiss syndrome, 32–33
Veins, varicose. See Varices
Vena cava, thrombosis of, Budd-Chiari syndrome
  with, 190–191
Venography, in venous thrombosis, 413–414
Ventilation, mechanical, in adult respiratory
  distress syndrome, 440–441
Ventral hernia, 276–278
Verner-Morrison syndrome, 260–261
  clinical features of, 260
  operative management of, 260–261
  preoperative localization of, 260
Verruca senilis, 480–481
Vertebral artery, trauma of, 474
Vipoma, 260–261
Vitamin B_{12}, and gastrectomy, 37
Vitamin K deficiency, 546–547
Volume replacement, in shock patients, 434–435
Volvulus, of colon, 100–102
Vomiting
  and Boerhaave's syndrome, 2
  and Mallory-Weiss syndrome, 31
von Meyenburg complexes, 158

W

Warfarin (Coumadin)
  in deep venous thrombosis, 415

in femoral vein valvuloplasty, 411
WDHA syndrome, 260–261
Weight loss, in periampullary cancer, 250
Wermer's syndrome, 262
Whipple procedure (Pancreaticoduodenecotomy)
  in chronic pancreatitis, 246
  in pancreatic tumors, 257
  in Zollinger-Ellison syndrome, 48
Wounds
  burn. See Burns
  care of, in Buerger's disease, 386
  duodenal, 445–446
  management of, in Raynaud's syndrome, 395
  pancreatic, 445
  penetrating, of thoracic wall, 333–334

Y

Y-V advancement flap, for anal stricture, 142

Z

Z-plasty, for pilonidal sinus and cyst, 151–152
Zenker's diverticulum(a), 5, 6–7
  treatment of, 7
Zollinger-Ellison syndrome, 46–49
  acid secretion in, 47
  clinical characteristics of, 47
  diagnosis of, 47–48
  diarrhea in, 47
  gastrin levels in, 47
  provocative tests in, 47–48
  recurrent ulcer in, 47
  serum gastrin in, 47
  treatment of, 48–49
  tumor localization in, 48